Fourth Edition

Outdoor Emergency Care

Comprehensive Prehospital Care for Nonurban Settings

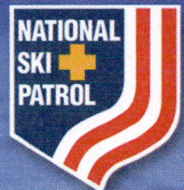

National Ski Patrol

Warren D. Bowman, MD, FACP

David H. Johe, MD

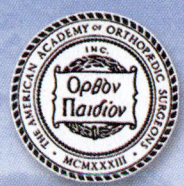

American Academy of Orthopaedic Surgeons

Bruce D. Browner, MD, FAAOS

Andrew N. Pollak, MD, EMT-P, FAAOS

Carol L. Gupton, BSEMS, NREMT-P

JONES AND BARTLETT PUBLISHERS

Sudbury, Massachusetts

BOSTON   TORONTO   LONDON   SINGAPORE

National Ski Patrol System, Inc.

Board of Directors
Bill Sachs, *Chairman*
Chris Ross, *Alaska Division*
Ronald Plumer, *Central Division*
Claude Kahn, *Central Division*
Trudy Olsson, *Central Division*
Linda Murphy Jacobs, *Central Division*
Jerry Sherman, *Eastern Division*
Gerit Lewisch, *Eastern Division*
Edmund Berry, *Eastern Division*
Bob McLaughlin, *Eastern Division*
Terry Petze, *European Division*
Ray Bryan, *Far West Division*
Bob Ashcraft, *Far West Division*
Kim Mills, *Intermountain Division*
Richard Everett, *Northern Division*
Mike Gooderham, *Pacific Northwest Division*
Robert Schroeder, *Pacific Northwest Division*
Barbara Dixon, *Pacific Northwest Division*
Bruce Malone, *Professional Division*
Bob Black, *Professional Division*
Chuck Tolton, *Professional Division*
Hap Burnham, *Rocky Mountain Division*
Frank Davis, *Rocky Mountain Division*
Eunice Singletary, *Southern Division*
Marilyn Burnside, *National Treasurer*
Michael Baker, *Assistant National Chairman*
Charles Martschinke, *Assistant National Chairman*
Bruce Ries, *National Legal Counsel*

Past NSP Board Members
John Clair, *National Chairman*
Douglas McCormick, *National Treasurer*
Jeff Olsen, *Assistant National Chairman*
Davis Olson, *National Legal Counsel*
Mary Davis, *Eastern Division*
Daryl Whitcher, *Far West Division*
Keith Underwood, *Pacific Northwest Division*
Brian Merryman, *Pacific Northwest Division*
Al Auten, *Rocky Mountain Division*
John Dobson, *Southern Division*

Editorial Credits
Judy Over, *National Education Director*
Leif Borgeson, *Assistant National Education Director*
Elizabeth Mason, *Education Assistant*
Rebecca W. Ayers, *Communications Director*
Mark Dorsey, *Marketing Director*
Brian Robb, *Photographer*
London Schertzer, *Photographer*
Ingrid Tistaert, *Photographer*
Reata Bitter, Bitter-Sweet Studio, *Illustrator*

First edition, 1988
Second printing, 1990
Second edition, 1993
Third edition, 1998

American Academy of Orthopaedic Surgeons

Vice President, Education Programs: Mark W. Wieting
Director, Department of Publications: Marilyn L. Fox, PhD
Managing Editor: Lynne Roby Shindoll
Senior Editor: Barbara A. Scotese
Associate Senior Editor: Susan Morritz Baim

Board of Directors 2002
Vernon T. Tolo, MD, *President*
James H. Herndon, MD
Robert W. Bucholz, MD
E. Anthony Rankin, MD
Andrew J. Weiland, MD
Edward A. Toriello, MD
Richard H. Gelberman, MD
S. Terry Canale, MD
Stephen A. Albanese, MD
Stephen P. England, MD
James N. Weinstein, DO
Gerald R. Williams, Jr, MD
Peter C. Amadio, MD
David G. Lewallen, MD
Glenn B. Pfeffer, MD
Lowry Jones, Jr, MD
Maureen Finnegan, MD
Peter J. Mandell, MD
William W. Tipton, Jr, MD *(ex officio)*

Jones and Bartlett Publishers

40 Tall Pine Drive
Sudbury, MA 01776
978-443-5000
info@jbpub.com
www.jbpub.com

Jones and Bartlett Publishers Canada
2406 Nikanna Road
Mississauga, ON L5C 2W6
CANADA

Jones and Bartlett Publishers International
Barb House, Barb Mews
London W6 7PA
UK

Production Credits
Chief Executive Officer: Clayton Jones
Chief Operating Officer: Donald W. Jones, Jr
Executive V.P. and Publisher: Robert W. Holland, Jr
V.P., Design and Production: Anne Spencer
V.P., Sales and Marketing: William Kane
V.P., Manufacturing and Inventory Control: Therese Bräuer
Publisher-Emergency Care: Kimberly Brophy
Associate Editor: Carol E. Brewer
Senior Production Editor: Linda S. DeBruyn
Senior Marketing Manager: Alisha Weisman
Director, Interactive Technology: Adam Alboyadjian
Design and Composition: Studio Montage
Cover Design: Studio Montage
Printing and Binding: The Courier Company
Cover Printing: Lehigh Press

The procedures and protocols in this book are based on the most current recommendations of responsible medical sources. The National Ski Patrol, the American Academy of Orthopaedic Surgeons, and the publisher, however, make no guarantee as to, and assume no responsibility for the correctness, sufficiency or completeness of such information or recommendations. Other or additional safety measures may be required under particular circumstances.

This textbook is intended solely as a standard of training for the appropriate procedures to be employed when rendering outdoor emergency care. It is not intended as a statement of the standards of care required in any particular situation, because circumstances and the patient's physical condition can vary widely from one emergency to another. Nor is it intended that this textbook shall in any way advise outdoor rescuers concerning legal authority to perform the activities or procedures discussed. Such local determinations should be made only with the aid of medical and legal counsel.

Notice: The patients described in "You are the rescuer" and "Assessment in Action" throughout this text and Appendix A are fictitious.

Copyright © 2003 by the National Ski Patrol System, Inc. and the American Academy of Orthopaedic Surgeons

Library of Congress Cataloging-in-Publication Data

Bowman, Warren D.
    Outdoor emergency care/Warren D. Bowman, David H. Johe. — 4th ed.
      p. cm.
    "National Ski Patrol"
    "AAOS"
    Includes bibliographical references and index.
    ISBN 0-7637-1715-0 (pbk.)
    I. Outdoor medical emergencies. I. Johe, David H., 1952- II. American Academy of Orthopaedic Surgeons.
    III. National Ski Patrol (U.S.) IV. Title
    RC88.9.O95 B68 2003
    616.02'5—dc21

                            2002069399

Additional credits appear on page 937 which constitutes a continuation of the copyright page.

Printed in the United States of America
06 05 04 03 02   10 9 8 7 6 5 4 3 2 1

Brief Contents

Contents

Section 1 Preparing to Be a Rescuer

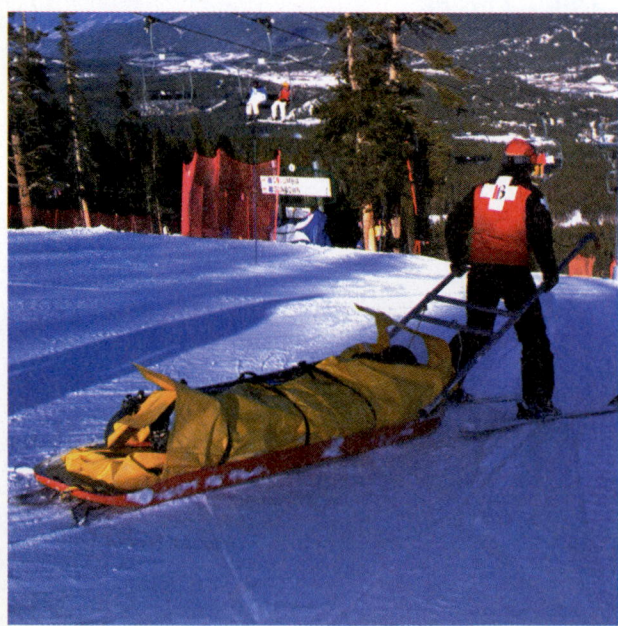

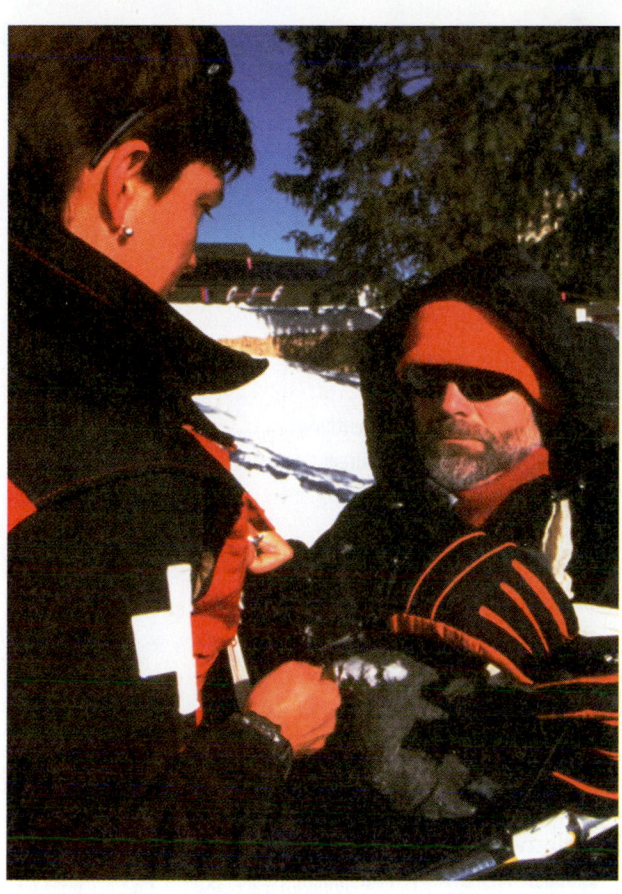

Section 2 Airway

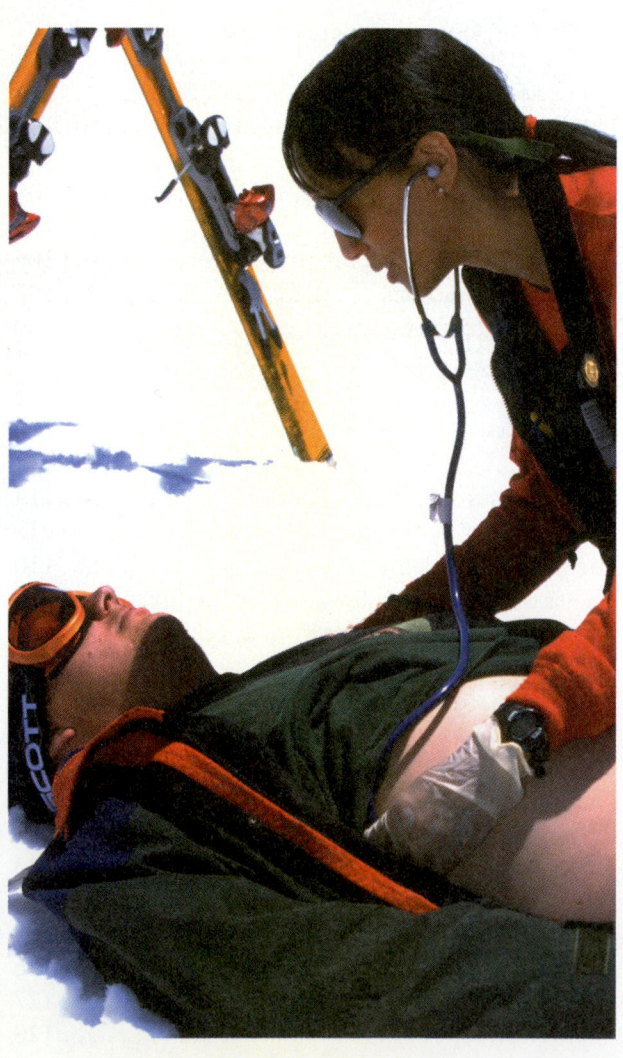

contents

Section 3 Patient Assessment

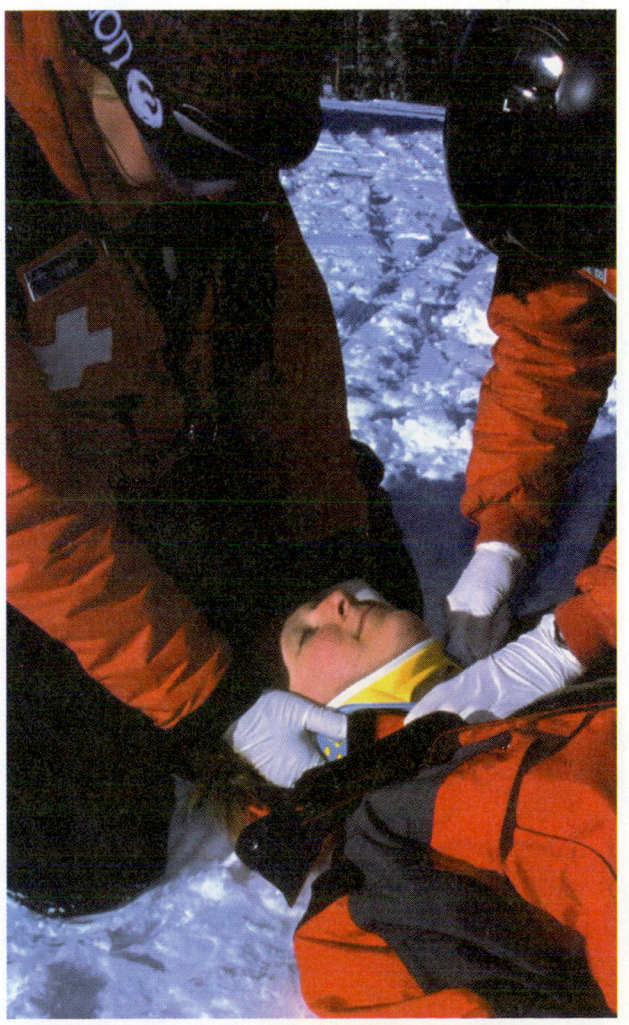

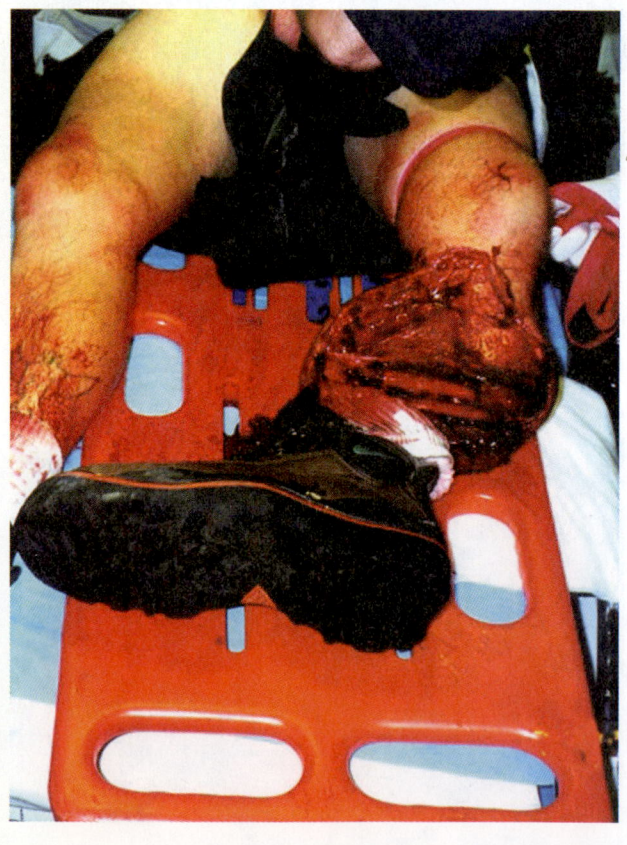

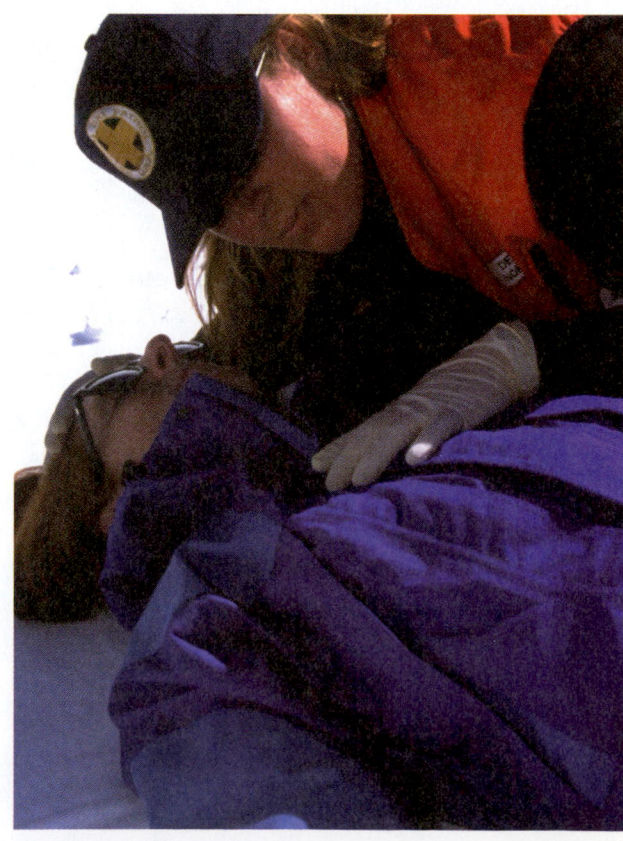

contents

Section 4 Medical Emergencies

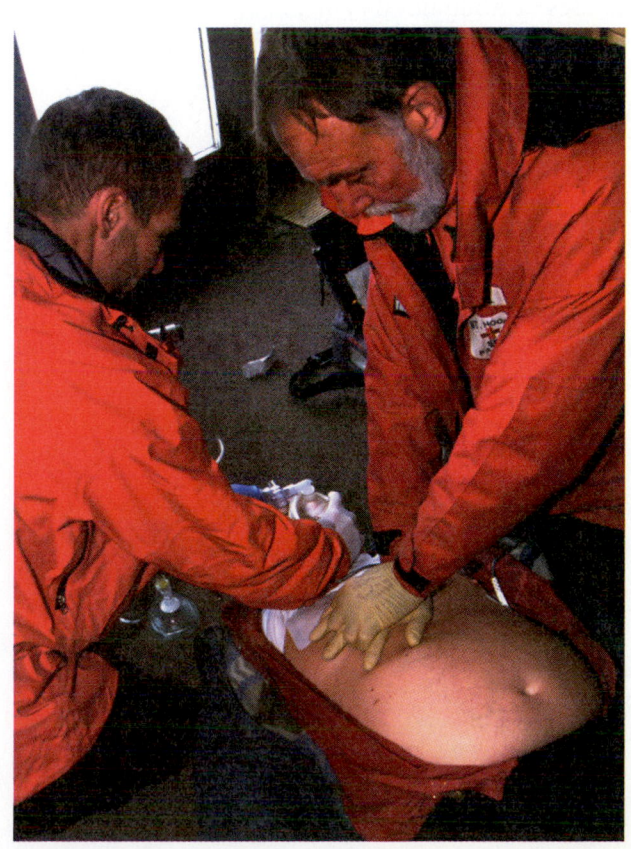

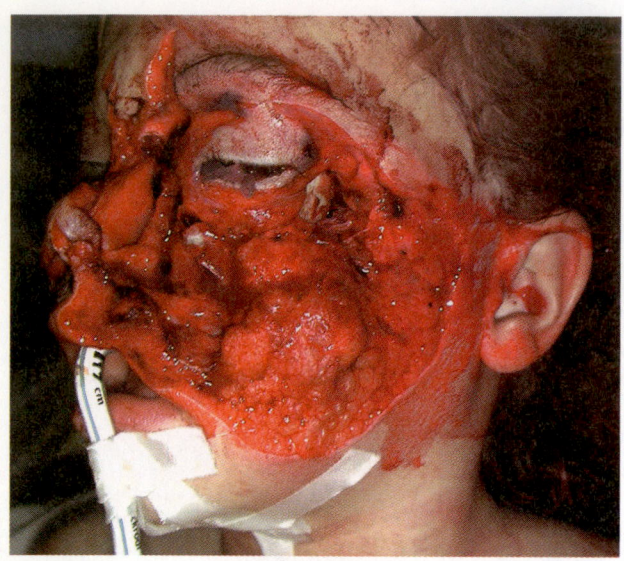

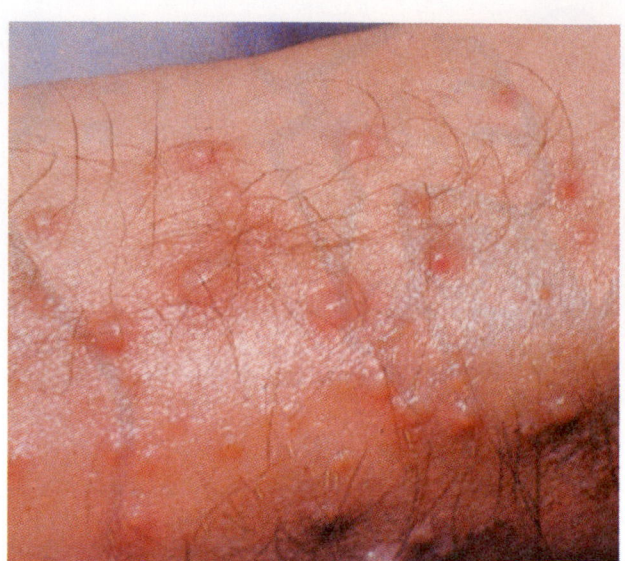

14 Snowsports and Mountain Biking Emergencies 396

15 Environmental Emergencies 412

Section 5 Trauma

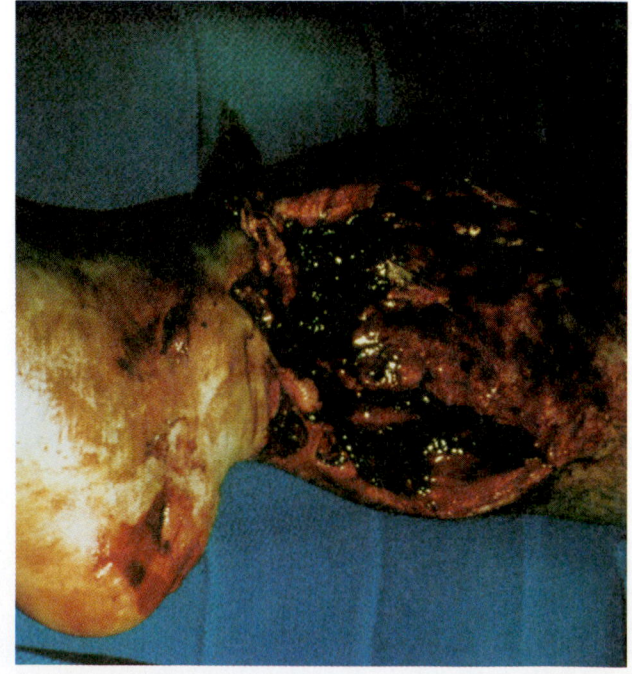

20 Eye Injuries 522

21 Face and Throat Injuries 536

22 Chest Injuries 548

23 Abdomen and Genitalia Injuries 560

contents

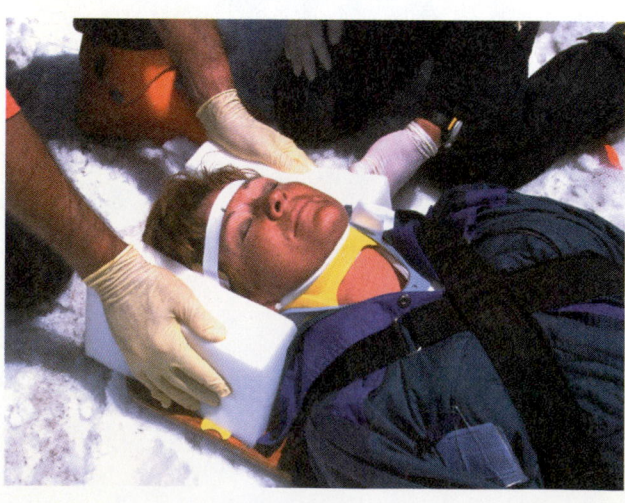

Section 6 Scene Techniques

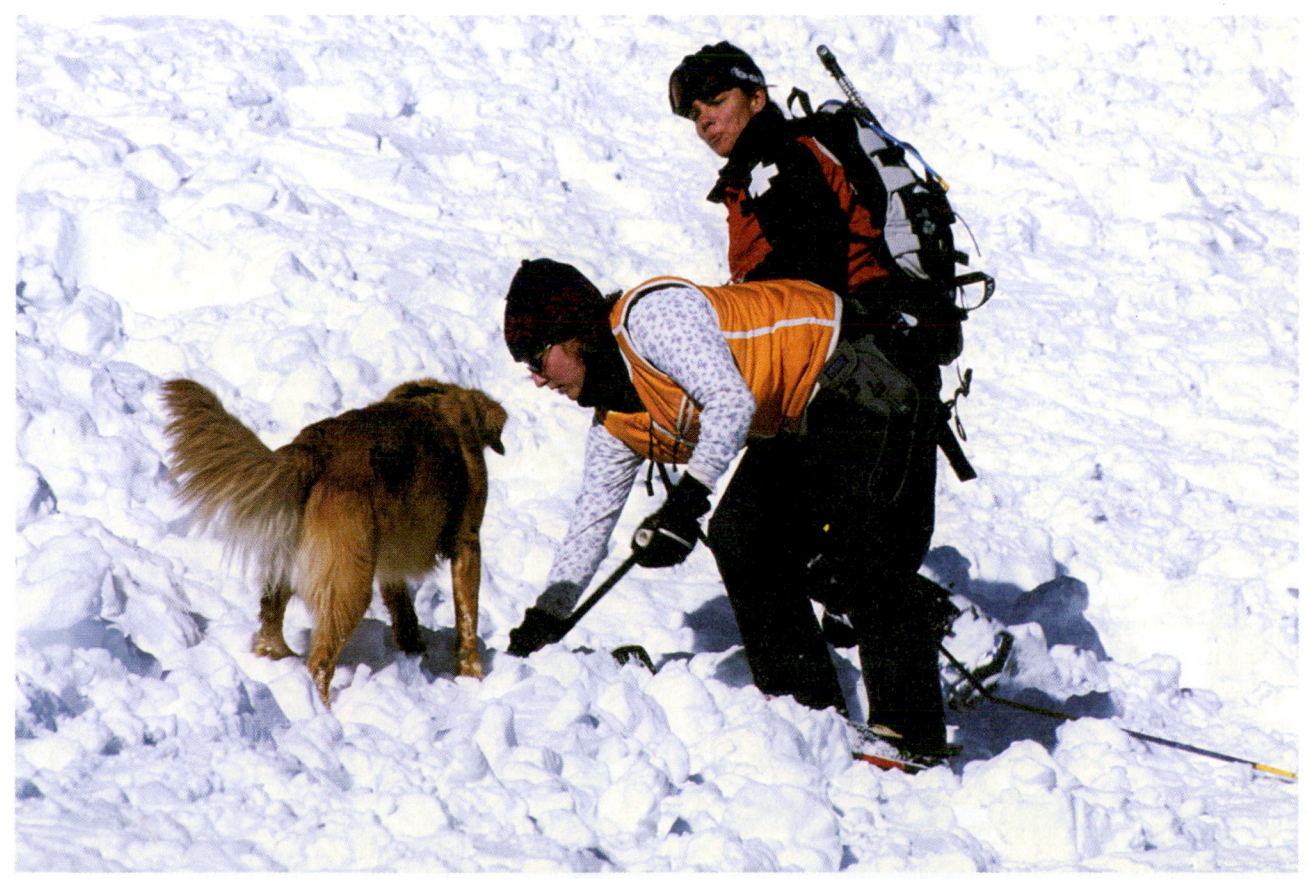

contents

Section 7 Special Populations

Rescuer Skill Drills

rescuer skill drills

Technology Resources

A key component in our program, www.OECzone.com, includes interactivities and simulations to help students become great outdoor rescuers.

www.OECzone.com

Anatomy Review—interactive anatomic figure labeling.

Web Links—present current information including trends in health care, the outdoor rescue community, and new equipment.

Online Outlook—activities further reinforce and expand on topics covered in each chapter.

Online Chapter Pretests—prepare students for training with instant results and feedback on incorrect answers.

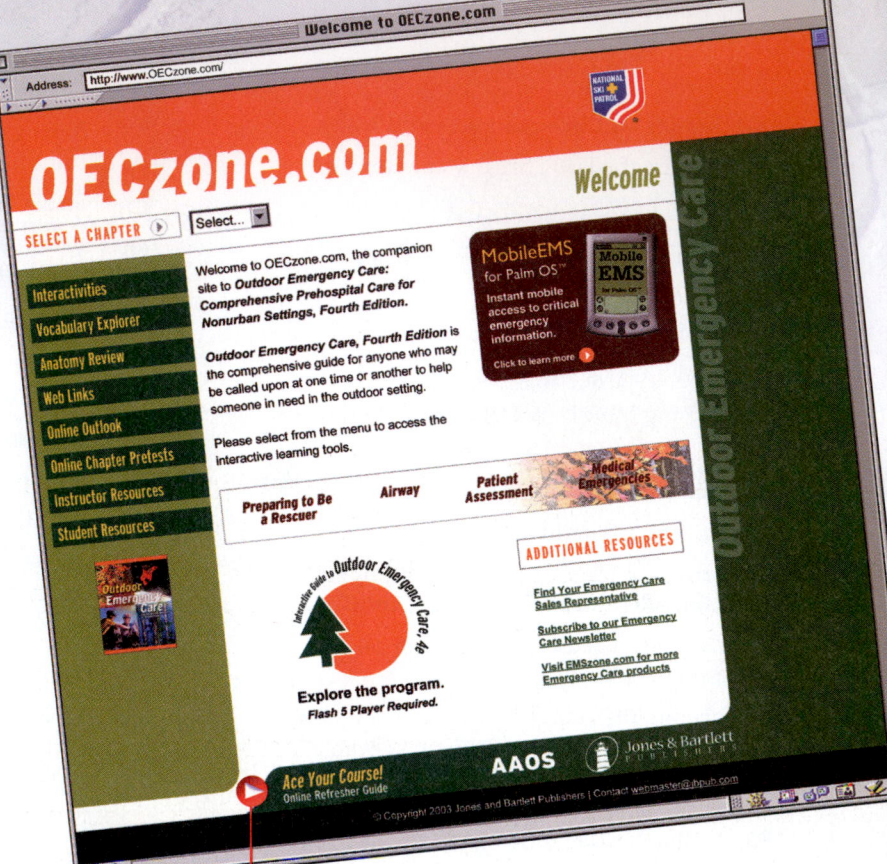

Online Refresher Guide—prepare for annual refreshers and continuing education sessions with this handy guide providing instant results, feedback, and page references.

Interactivities

Videos: Skills in Action— watch an experienced provider perform critical skills.

Interactive Simulations— experiment with rescuer skills in the safety of a virtual environment.

Assessment in Action— challenge students' problem-solving abilities using scenarios and get feedback.

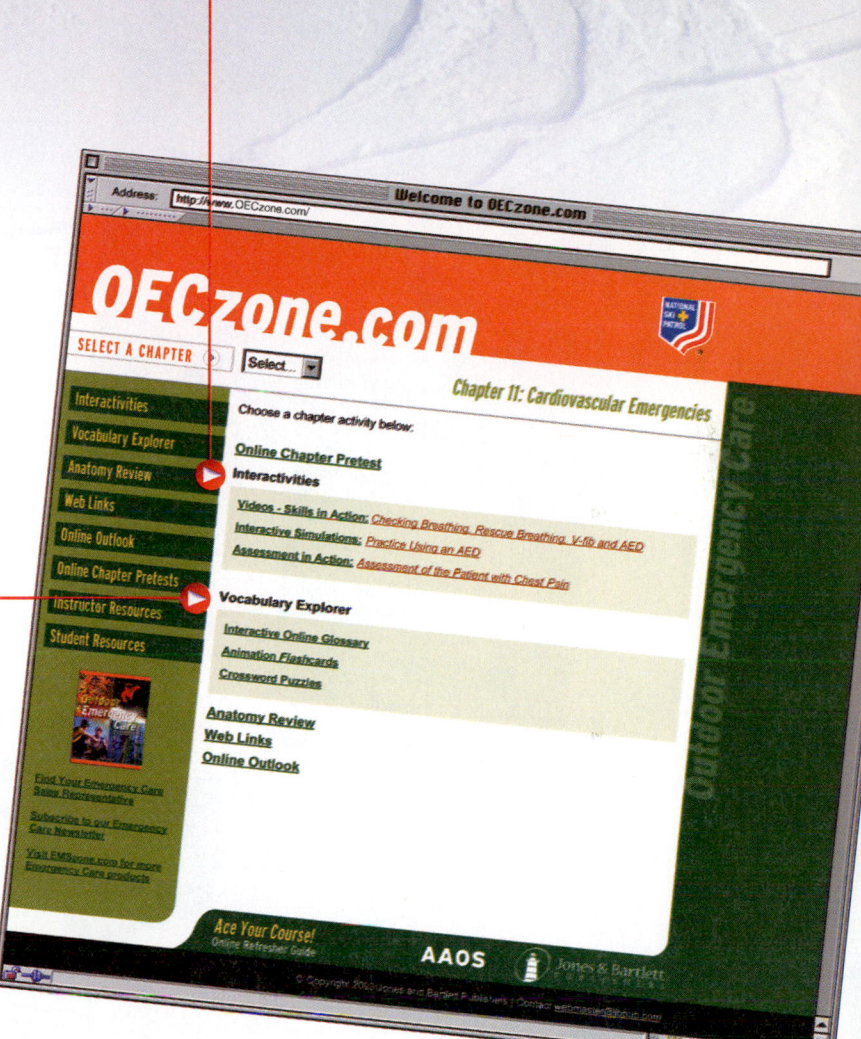

Vocabulary Explorer

Interactive Online Glossary— expand students' medical vocabulary, complete with sound and images.

Animated FlashCards— review vital vocabulary and key concepts.

Chapter Resources

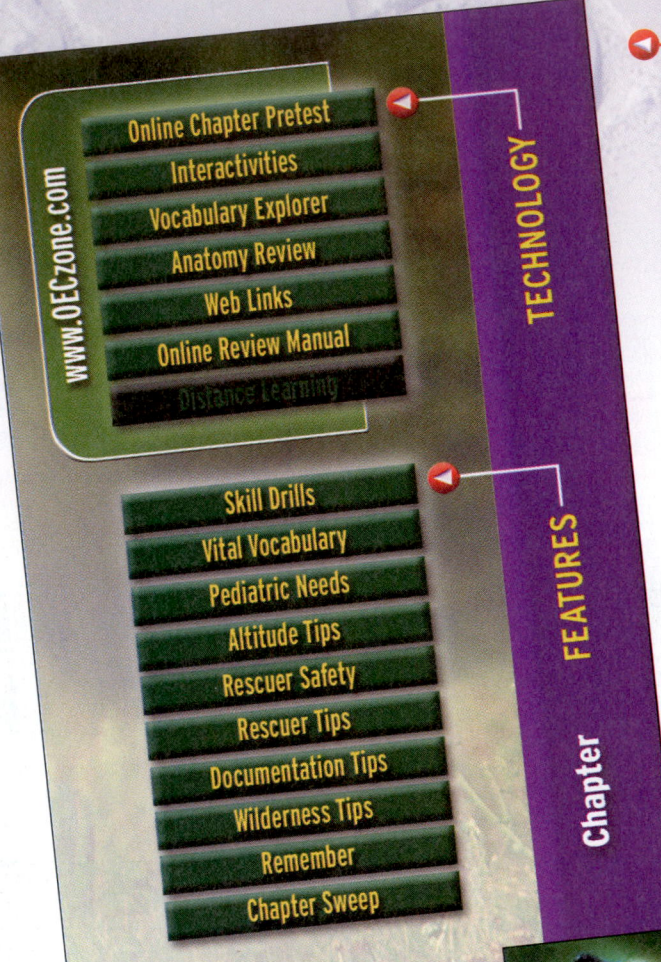

TECHNOLOGY

www.OECzone.com

- Online Chapter Pretest
- Interactivities
- Vocabulary Explorer
- Anatomy Review
- Web Links
- Online Review Manual
- Distance Learning

Chapter FEATURES

- Skill Drills
- Vital Vocabulary
- Pediatric Needs
- Altitude Tips
- Rescuer Safety
- Rescuer Tips
- Documentation Tips
- Wilderness Tips
- Remember
- Chapter Sweep

Navigation Toolbar

Found at the beginning of each chapter, the navigation toolbar will guide you through the technology resources and text features available for that chapter.

You are the rescuer

Each chapter opens with a case study that will stimulate classroom discussion, capture students' attention, and provide an overview of the chapter. Additional case studies and challenging questions are included in the end-of-chapter *Chapter Sweep*.

preview

You are the rescuer

While skiing a mogul run, you and your partner come upon a guest who has fallen against a large rock. The skier's lower arm and wrist are already showing signs of swelling and a hematoma, as well as some surface bleeding.

Blunt trauma can produce injuries ranging from minor soft-tissue wounds to fatalities, either of which can present with little visible outward signs indicating the severity of the injury. This chapter will provide information on the methods recommended to control bleeding along with helping you answer the following questions:

1. Why does internal bleeding often go unnoticed until the patient "crashes"?
2. Under what circumstances might the rarely used tourniquet be the best choice for bleeding control?

Bleeding

After managing the airway, recognizing bleeding and understanding how it affects the body are perhaps the most important skills you will learn as a rescuer. Bleeding can be external and obvious or internal and hidden. Either way, it is potentially dangerous, causing first weakness and, if left uncontrolled, eventually shock and death. The most common cause of shock after trauma is bleeding.

The purpose of this chapter is to help you understand how the cardiovascular system reacts to blood loss. The chapter begins with a brief review of the anatomy and function of the cardiovascular system. It then describes the signs, symptoms, and emergency medical care of both external and internal bleeding. The chapter concludes with a discussion on the relationship between bleeding and hypovolemic shock.

Anatomy and Physiology of the Cardiovascular System

The cardiovascular system circulates blood to all of the body's cells and tissues, delivering oxygen and nutrients and carrying away metabolic waste products ▶ Figure 8-1 . Certain parts of the body, such as the brain, spinal cord, and heart, require a constant flow of blood to live. The cells in these organs cannot tolerate a lack of blood for more than a few minutes. Other organs, such as the lungs and kidneys, can survive for short periods of time without adequate blood flow. After that, their cells begin to die. This can lead to a permanent loss of function or, if enough cells die, death.

- The pump (the heart)
- A container (the blood vessels that reach every cell in the body)
- The fluid (blood and body fluids)

The Heart

The heart is a hollow muscular organ about the size of a clenched fist. It is an involuntary muscle that is under the control of the autonomic nervous system, but it has its own regulatory system. Thus, it can function even if the nervous system shuts down.

The heart is always working; all other organs depend on it to provide a rich blood supply. For this reason, it has a number of special features that other muscles do not. First, because the heart can tolerate a serious interruption of its blood supply for only a few seconds, its blood supply is as rich and well distributed as possible. Second, the heart works as two paired pumps ▶ Figure 8-2 . Each side of the heart has an upper chamber (atrium) and a lower chamber (ventricle), both of which pump blood. Blood leaves each chamber of a normal heart through a one-way valve, which keeps the blood moving in the proper direction by preventing a backflow.

The right side of the heart receives oxygen-poor (deoxygenated) blood from the veins of the body. Blood enters into the right atrium from the vena cava, then fills the right ventricle. After the right ventricle contracts, blood flows into the pulmonary artery and the pulmonary circulation. The now oxygen-rich (oxygenated) blood returns to the left side of the heart from the lungs through the pulmonary veins. Blood enters the left

Figure 13-18 A snake bite wound from a poisonous snake has characteristic markings: two small puncture wounds about ½" apart, discoloration, and swelling.

Nostril —
Pit —
Vertical pupil
Fang —
Venom sac —
Teeth —
Tongue —

Wilderness Tips

Of all animals, venomous snakes are the most dangerous to humans. If you are in a remote area where transport to definitive medical care cannot be reached for hours, suggestions for emergency care include:

- Some experts recommend using a single constricting band to slow absorption of the venom in extremity bites. Tie a snug cloth or cravat around the extremity, directly over the bite, so there is pressure on the wound. This reduces blood flow to the area, decreasing systemic release of the venom. The pressure should not be so tight that peripheral pulses are absent.
- Use a commercial negative pressure device, which should be part of the emergency care kit carried in snake country. Use it immediately after the bite occurs.
- Send a member of the party for help.
- Clean the bite with soap and water and cover it with a sterile compress.
- Splint a bitten extremity.
- Give the patient electrolyte-containing fluids to replace fluid lost from the blood into the bitten area.

Set up camp and have the patient rest until help arrives. If the group is large enough and a litter can be improvised, carry the patient out. During tick season (spring and early

---

Wilderness Tips
Wilderness Tips provide advice on how to provide emergency care in remote areas.

When the blood pressure becomes elevated, the body's defenses act to reduce it. Some individuals have chronically high blood pressure from progressive narrowing of the arteries that occurs with age, and during an acute episode, their blood pressure may increase to even higher levels. Head injury or a number of other conditions may also cause blood pressure to rise to very high levels. Abnormally high blood pressure may result in a rupture or other critical damage in the arterial system.

You should measure blood pressure in all patients older than 3 years who have had a serious injury.

Blood pressure contains two key separate components: systolic pressure and diastolic pressure. Systolic pressure is the increased pressure that is caused along the artery with each contraction (systole) of the ventricle and the pulse wave that it produces. Diastolic pressure is the residual pressure that remains in the arteries during the relaxing phase of the heart's cycle (diastole), when the left ventricle is at rest. Systolic pressure represents the maximum pressure to which the arteries are subjected, and the diastolic pressure represents the minimum amount of pressure that is always present in the arteries.

Early blood pressure gauges contained a column of mercury and a linear scale that was graduated in millimeters. Even though different gauges are used today,

Altitude Tips

Recent ascent to altitude will affect baseline vital signs. Patients will normally show an increase in respiratory rate and depth, a mild increase in blood pressure, and a moderate increase in pulse rate. As acclimatization occurs, these signs will revert to more normal levels.

There are at least three sizes of blood pressure cuffs: adult, thigh, and pediatric (▼ Figure 5-11). The normal size cuff is designed to wrap around the arm one to one and a half times and take up two thirds the length from the armpit to the crease in the elbow of most adults. Use a thigh cuff with patients who are obese or have exceptionally well-developed arm muscles or to take the blood pressure of the thigh in patients who have injuries in both arms. Use a small pediatric cuff with children and exceptionally small adults.

You must be sure to select the appropriately sized cuff. A cuff that is too small may result in falsely high readings; a cuff that is too large may result in falsely low readings.

AUSCULTATION. Auscultation is the method of listening

Altitude Tips
Altitude Tips provide information on the effects of altitude and how it affects patient care.

TABLE 12-1 Common Causes of Seizures

Type	Cause
Epileptic	Congenital in origin
Structural	Tumor (benign or cancerous)
	Infection (brain abscess)
	Scar from injury
Metabolic	Abnormal blood chemistry
	Hypoglycemia
	Poisoning
	Drug overdose
	Sudden withdrawal from alcohol, medications
Febrile	Sudden high fever

Rescuer Safety

Patients may behave violently during the postictal phase. Though most seizure patients pose no threat to responders, signs of alcohol or drug abuse should heighten your awareness of the potential for dangerous behavior.

Documentation Tips

Physician evaluation of a patient who has had a seizure depends heavily on reports of the seizure pattern and changes in that pattern. Record all pertinent information about the seizure in terms of duration, areas of body movement, and possible triggering factors. This requires effective interviewing of available witnesses, family members, or caregivers.

routine and heavy alcohol or sedative drug usage or even from prescribed medications. Dilantin, a drug that is used to control seizures, can cause seizures itself if the person takes too much.

Seizures can also result from sudden high fevers, particularly in children. Such convulsions, known as febrile seizures, are usually very unnerving for parents to observe but are generally well tolerated by the child. Nevertheless, you should arrange for transport of a child who has had a febrile seizure, as this condition needs to be evaluated by a physician. The fact that a second seizure may occur is worrisome, and if it occurs, the patient requires hospital evaluation to identify possible causes, such as serious infection within the brain or tissues covering the brain.

THE IMPORTANCE OF RECOGNIZING SEIZURES. Regardless of the type of seizure, it is extremely important for you to recognize when a seizure is occurring or whether one has already occurred. You must also determine whether this episode differs from any previous ones. For example, if the previous seizure occurred on only one side of the body and this seizure occurs over the entire body, some additional or new problem may be involved. In addition to recognizing that seizure activity has occurred and/or that something different may now be occurring, you must also recognize the postictal state as well as the complications of seizures. Because most seizures involve a vigorous twitching of the muscles, they use a lot of oxygen.

the circulation to the vital functions of the body. It is similar to a situation in which you exercise vigorously without giving your body a chance to rest. As a result, there is a buildup of acids in the bloodstream. With lack of adequate oxygenation, the patient may turn cyanotic (bluish lips, tongue, and skin). Often, the seizures prevent the patient from breathing normally, making the problem worse.

Recognizing seizure activity also means looking at other problems associated with the seizure. For example, the patient may have fallen during the seizure episode and injured some part of the body; brain injury is the most serious possibility. Patients having a generalized seizure may become incontinent, meaning that they may lose bowel and bladder control. Therefore, one clue that unresponsive or disoriented patients may have had a seizure is to find that they urinated into their clothing. Although incontinence is possible with other medical conditions, sudden incontinence is very likely a sign that a seizure has occurred.

THE POSTICTAL STATE. Once a seizure has stopped, the patient's muscles relax, becoming almost flaccid, or floppy, and the breathing becomes labored (fast and deep) in an attempt to compensate for the buildup of acids in the bloodstream. By breathing faster and more deeply, the body can balance the acidity in the blood-stream. With a normal circulation

---

Rescuer Safety
Safety tips are included to reinforce safety concerns for both the rescuer and the patient.

Documentation Tips
Documentation Tips provide advice on how to document patient care and highlight situations where documentation is especially critical.

preview

Chapter Resources

approach can defuse frightening situations, but keep your safety and that of your team uppermost in mind. Expect the unexpected and remember: The drug user, not the drug, can pose the greatest threat.

Alcohol

The most commonly abused drug in the United States is alcohol (▼ Figure 13-31). It affects people from all walks of life and kills more than 200,000 of them each year. More than 50% of all traffic fatalities or injuries, 67% of murders, and 33% of suicides are related to alcohol, which impairs the capacity to think and function rationally. Alcoholism is one of the greatest national health problems, along with heart disease, cancer, and stroke.

Alcohol is a powerful central nervous system (CNS) depressant. It is both a sedative, a substance that decreases activity and excitement, and a hypnotic, meaning that it induces sleep. In general, alcohol dulls the sense of awareness, slows reflexes, and reduces reaction time. It may also cause aggressive and inappropriate behavior and lack of coordination. However, a person who appears intoxicated may have other medical problems as well. Look for signs of head trauma, toxic reactions, or uncontrolled diabetes. Severe acute alcohol ingestion may cause hypoglycemia, which may contribute to the symptoms. At the very least, you should assume that all intoxicated patients are experiencing a drug overdose and may require thorough examination by a physician. In most states, such patients cannot legally refuse treatment.

If a patient exhibits signs of serious CNS depression, you must provide respiratory support. This may be difficult, however, because depression of the respiratory system can also cause emesis, or vomiting. The vomiting may be very forceful or even bloody (hematemesis), since large amounts of alcohol irritate the stomach. Internal bleeding should also be considered if the patient appears to be in shock (hypoperfusion), as blood might not clot effectively in a patient who has a prolonged history of alcohol abuse.

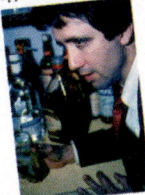

Figure 13-31   Alcohol intoxication causes altered mental status, slowed reflexes, and impaired reaction time.

Rescuer Tips

The human body has a limited number of ways to respond to the wide variety of illnesses, infections, and diseases. Being aware of the signs and symptoms that are common to many diseases—and their causes—will help you determine the nature of illness (NOI) during the initial assessment. Although it is important to be familiar with causes, the emergency care of a complaint may frequently be the same regardless of the underlying disease.

Remember

In all cases of substance abuse or poisoning, immediately arrange to have the patient rapidly transported to medical care.

A patient in alcohol withdrawal may experience frightening hallucinations or delirium tremens (DTs), a syndrome characterized by restlessness, fever, sweating, disorientation, agitation, and even convulsions. These conditions may develop if patients no longer have their daily source of alcohol. Alcoholic hallucinations come and go. A patient with an otherwise fairly clear mental state may see fantastic shapes or figures or hear odd voices. Such auditory and visual hallucinations often precede DTs, which are a much more severe complication.

DTs may develop 1 to 7 days after a person stops drinking or when consumption levels are decreased suddenly. Again, patients may experience one or more of the following signs and symptoms:

- Agitation and restlessness
- Fever
- Sweating
- Confusion and/or disorientation
- Delusions and/or hallucinations
- Seizures

Provide prompt transport for these patients after you have completed your assess... care. A person who is experi... DTs is extremely ill. Should... as you would any other seiz... be restrained, although you...

Rescuer Tips
Rescuer Tips provide advice from masters of the trade.

Remember
Remember boxes contain key points from the chapter to help students retain important information.

Pediatric Needs
Pediatric Needs highlight specific concerns and procedures for infants and children.

Pediatric Needs

Growth plate injuries in children are common, especially around the wrist, elbow, knee, and ankle. Injuries tend to occur through these cartilaginous growth centers because they are inherently weaker than the surrounding bone. Since longitudinal growth of the limb is dependent upon the function of the growth plate, it is extremely important to recognize the possibility of growth plate injuries, stabilize the injured limb, and transport the patient in timely fashion to an appropriate center with pediatric orthopaedic and surgical coverage. Proper functioning of the injured growth plate throughout the remainder of skeletal growth is dependent upon urgent anatomic reduction of the fracture and close follow-up by an orthopaedist.

Any deformity in close proximity to a joint in children younger than 16 years should be assumed to be a growth plate injury and transported and treated appropriately.

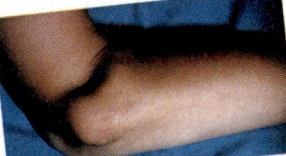

Figure 25-15   Posterior dislocation of the elbow makes the olecranon process of the ulna much more prominent.

the radius, the bone on the thumb side of the forearm, both join the distal humerus. The posterior displacement makes the olecranon process of the ulna much more prominent (▶ Figure 25-15). The joint is usually locked, with the elbow in partial flexion; this position makes any attempt at motion extremely painful. As with a fracture of the distal humerus, there is swelling and significant potential for vessel or nerve injury.

ELBOW JOINT SPRAIN. This injury is rare and is usually diagnosed by X-ray. Often, the real problem is a hard-to-detect fracture.

FRACTURE OF THE OLECRANON PROCESS OF THE ULNA. This fracture is usually the result of a direct blow, such as a fall onto the point of the elbow, and therefore is often accompanied by overlying lacerations or abrasions. The patient will be unable to extend the elbow. Almost always, the fracture requires surgical internal fixation for treatment (▶ Figure 25-16).

FRACTURE OF THE RADIAL HEAD. Occasionally missed even in the emergency department, this fracture generally occurs as a result of a fall on an outstretched arm or a direct blow to the lateral aspect of the forearm. Attempts to rotate the forearm or wrist are very uncomfortable. Again, surgery is usually required if the fracture is displaced (▶ Figure 25-17).

Care of Elbow Injuries

All elbow injuries are serious and require careful management. Always assess distal neurovascular functions periodically in patients with elbow injuries. If you find strong distal pulses and normal sensation in the hand,

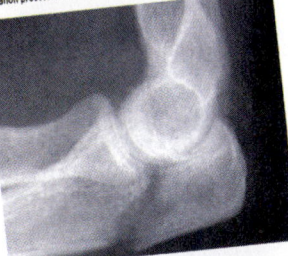

Figure 25-16   X-ray of a displaced olecranon fracture.

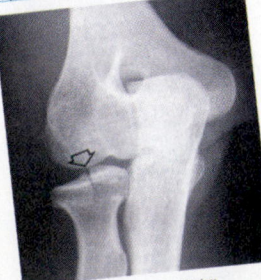

Figure 25-17   Displaced radial head fracture.

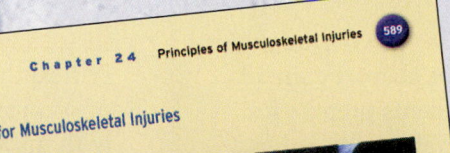

Skill Drills

Skill Drills provide written step-by-step explanations and visual summaries of important skills and procedures.

Skill Drill 24-2 — Caring for Musculoskeletal Injuries

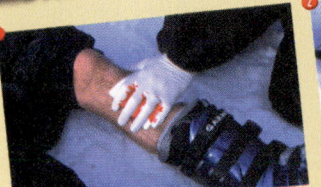

Cover open wounds with a dry, sterile dressing, and apply pressure to control bleeding. Assess distal CMS functions.

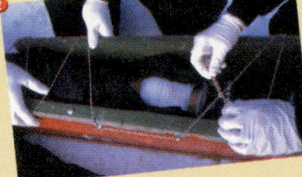

Apply a quick splint.

Elevate the extremity and position the patient for transport.

Assess distal CMS functions and position the patient for transport.

3. **Cover all wounds with a dry, sterile dressing** before splinting. Be sure to follow BSI precautions. Do not intentionally push protruding bones back inside the wound. Notify the accepting rescue squad of all open wounds.

4. **Do not move the patient before splinting** an extremity unless there is an immediate hazard to the patient or yourself or the patient's general condition requires immediate transport.

5. In a suspected fracture of the shaft of any bone, be sure to **immobilize the joints** above and below the fracture site.

6. With injuries in and around the joint, be sure to **immobilize the bones** above and below the injured joint.

7. **Pad all rigid splints** to prevent local pressure and discomfort to the patient.

8. While another patroller is applying the splint, **maintain manual immobilization** to minimize movement of the limb and to support and stabilize the injury site.

9. If fracture of a long bone shaft has resulted in severe deformity, **use constant, gentle longitudinal traction** to align the limb so that it can be splinted. This is especially important if the distal part of [the limb is cold] or pulseless.

10. **Expect to en[counter some pain when the] patient resist[s]** ... fractured limb ... splint the limb ...

Vital Vocabulary

Vital Vocabulary is easily identified and defines key terms students must know in the field. A comprehensive list follows each chapter, and Vocabulary Explorer on www.OECzone.com provides interactivities.

---

xiphoid process. The junction of the manubrium and the body forms a very prominent ridge on the sternum, called the angle of Louis. The angle of Louis lies at the level where the second rib is attached to the sternum; it provides a constant and reliable bony landmark on the anterior chest wall.

In the midline of the upper back, the spines of the 12 thoracic vertebrae can be palpated. Twelve ribs on each side form small joints with their respective thoracic vertebrae and extend around to the front to create the walls of the thoracic cage. The upper five ribs connect to the sternum through a short bridge of cartilage. The sixth through tenth ribs insert into the costal arch. The costal arch is a bridge of cartilage that connects the ends of the sixth through tenth ribs with the lower portion of the sternum. The eleventh and twelfth ribs are called floating ribs, because they do not attach to the sternum through the costal arch. The costal arch is easily palpable and represents the boundary between the lower border of the thorax and the upper border of the abdomen.

POSTERIOR ASPECTS. On the posterior chest wall, the scapulae overlie the thoracic wall and are surrounded by large muscles ▶ Figure 4-10B . When the patient is standing or sitting erect, the two scapulae should lie at approximately the same level, with their inferior tips at about the level of the seventh thoracic vertebra. In the lower part of the thorax on each side, an angle called the costovertebral angle is formed by the junction of the spine and the tenth rib. The kidneys lie deep in (beneath) the back muscles under the costovertebral angle.

DIAPHRAGM. The diaphragm is a muscular dome that forms the inferior boundary of the thorax, separating the chest from the abdominal cavity ▶ Figure 4-11 . Its contraction, along with that of the chest wall muscles, assists with allowing air to be drawn into the lungs. Anteriorly, it attaches to the costal arch; posteriorly, it attaches to the lumbar vertebrae. The diaphragm cannot be seen or palpated.

ORGANS AND VASCULAR STRUCTURES. Within the thoracic cage, the largest structures are the heart and lungs ▶ Figure 4-12 . The heart lies immediately under the sternum. It extends from the second to the sixth ribs anteriorly and from the fifth to the eighth thoracic vertebrae posteriorly. The inferior border of the heart extends into the left side of the chest. Diseased hearts may be larger or smaller. The major blood vessels that travel to and from the heart also lie in the chest cavity. On the right side of the spinal column, the superior and inferior venae cavae carry blood to the heart.

Just beneath the manubrium of the sternum, the arch of the aorta and the pulmonary artery exit the heart. The arch of the aorta passes to the left and

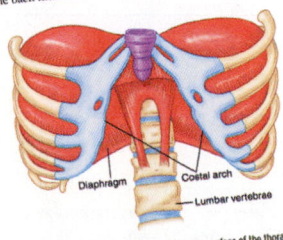

Figure 4-11 The diaphragm forms the undersurface of the thorax, separating the chest from the abdominal cavity.

Labels: Diaphragm, Costal arch, Lumbar vertebrae

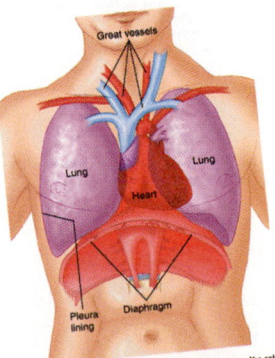

Figure 4-12 The anterior aspect of the thorax shows the relative positions of the principal organs beneath the surface.

Labels: Great vessels, Lung, Lung, Heart, Pleura lining, Diaphragm

Chapter Resources

Chapter Sweep
End-of-chapter activities reinforce important concepts and improve students' comprehension. Additional instructor support and answers to all activities are contained in the **Instructor's Manual** and **Instructor's ToolKit**.

Ready for Review thoroughly summarizes chapter content to help students prepare for practical evaluations.

Assessment in Action promotes critical thinking through the use of scenarios and provides you with discussion points for your course studies.

---

546 **SECTION 5** Trauma

Chapter *Sweep*

Ready for Review

Soft-tissue injuries and fractures to the bones of the face and neck are common and vary in severity. Proper emergency care can improve the patient's chances of making a complete recovery in health and appearance. Your priorities are to prevent further injury, especially to the cervical spine, and to manage any acute airway problems. These problems can result from heavy bleeding, swelling, and injuries to the brain or cervical spine that interfere with normal respiration.

To control the often heavy bleeding from soft-tissue injuries to the face and scalp, use direct manual pressure with a dry, sterile dressing, unless you suspect a skull fracture. Use a moist, sterile dressing for exposed parts of the brain or eye. Always check for bleeding inside the mouth. Open and clear the airway in all patients with facial injuries. Save any pieces of avulsed skin for possible attachment later; hold any avulsed flaps in place with a dry, sterile dressing. If the patient is bleeding heavily from an injury to the nose, apply a sterile dressing.

Injuries to the ear usually do not bleed very much. If local pressure does not control the bleeding, you can apply a roller dressing. Remember to place padding between the ear and the scalp, as bandaging the ear against the tender underlying scalp is extremely painful. Often, avulsed tissue from the ear can be reattached, so save any avulsed tissue. Always leave foreign bodies in the ear for a physician to remove. Watch for clear fluid coming from the ear or nose; this may indicate a basal skull fracture.

Assume that any patient who has sustained a direct blow to the nose or mouth has a facial fracture. Signs of fracture include irregularity of bite, inability to swallow or talk, and bleeding in the mouth. Check for airway obstruction if you notice swelling or if there is serious bleeding.

Both blunt and penetrating injuries to the neck can be life-threatening. With blunt injuries, you should palpate the neck and feel for the characteristic crackling associated with subcutaneous emphysema; patients with this sign may be in danger of complete airway obstruction within minutes. Direct pressure over the bleeding site will control most neck bleeding. However, bleeding may still occur within the tissues of the neck and compress the upper airway. If a vein has been lacerated, be alert for the possibility of air embolism. You may have to apply pressure both above and below the penetrating wound to control life-threatening bleeding from the carotid artery and jugular vein. Patients with a neck injury require spinal immobilization and prompt transport.

Vital Vocabulary

Adam's apple The firm prominence in the upper part of the larynx formed by the thyroid cartilage.

air embolism The presence of air in the veins, which can lead to cardiac arrest if it enters the heart.

avulse To pull or tear away.

cranium The skull.

eustachian tube The internal auditory canal that connects the middle ear to the nasal cavity.

external auditory canal The ear canal; leads to the tympanic membrane.

foramen magnum The large opening at the base of the skull through which the brain connects to the spinal cord.

hematoma The collection of blood in a space, tissue, or organ due to a break in the wall of a blood vessel.

mandible The bone of the lower jaw.

mastoid process The prominent bony mass at the base of the skull about 1" posterior to the external opening of the ear.

maxilla The bone that forms the upper jaw on either side of the face and contains the upper teeth, the orbit of the eye, the nasal cavity, and the palate.

occiput The most posterior portion of the skull.

pinna The external, visible part of the ear.

sternocleidomastoid muscles Muscles on either side of the neck that allow movement of the head.

subcutaneous emphysema The presence of air in soft tissue; palpation produces a characteristic crackling sensation.

temporomandibular joint (TMJ) The joint formed where the mandible and cranium meet, just in front of the ear.

tragus The small, rounded, fleshy bulge that lies immediately anterior to the ear canal.

turbinates Layers of bone within the nasal cavity.

tympanic membrane The eardrum, which lies between the external and middle ear.

www.OECzone.com

C h a p t e r 21 Face and Throat Injuries 547

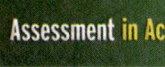

Assessment in Action

You respond to a call from a restaurant at your mountain where a diner, carrying a tray of food, tripped and hit his head on a glass decorative panel. He is reported to have head and neck lacerations with a lot of associated bleeding. The patient is 31 years old, in good health, and not taking any medication.

When his wife saw him bleeding on the floor, she applied pressure over her husband's wound with a large cloth napkin. She states that he did not lose consciousness. Your assessment reveals that the man is alert and oriented. He is talking in complete sentences, but is spitting blood. He has multiple lacerations to the face and neck. He has a 2" long laceration to the right cheek and a 4" long laceration to the right side of his neck, just below the ear, and down the shoulder. The bleeding from the neck appears to be controlled, but there is a large quantity of blood on the napkin that the wife used to apply pressure to the wound. Vital signs include a pulse of 110 beats/min, respirations of 22 breaths/min, and a blood pressure of 132/82 mm Hg.

1. What is the highest priority in caring for this patient?
   A. Administering low concentrations of oxygen.
   B. Treating potential or actual airway obstruction.
   C. Applying sterile dressings and bandaging the wound.
   D. Providing complete stabilization to a long backboard.

2. Which of the following interventions is acceptable for controlling bleeding of his neck injury?
   A. A wide band as a tourniquet
   B. A circumferential pressure dressing
   C. Direct pressure with a sterile dressing
   D. A pressure point

3. In most cases, a patient who sustains trauma to the face or throat should be placed in which of the following positions?
   A. Prone   B. Supine
   C. Sitting up   D. Turned to the side

4. Which of the following tools is considered an essential treatment adjunct for this patient, who has sustained face and neck trauma and is spontaneously breathing?

   A. AED   B. BVM device
   C. Portable suction   D. Hemostats

5. Which of the following statements about airway obstruction related to blunt trauma to the neck is true in this patient situation?
   A. Immediate transport is necessary because of the danger of possible obstruction.
   B. Airway obstruction is not likely to develop for at least 2 to 3 hours after the injury.
   C. Complete airway obstruction secondary to trauma is easily managed in the field by EMT-Bs.
   D. Airway obstruction rarely occurs as a complication of blunt trauma to the neck.

6. Additional injuries that you should suspect in this patient include:
   A. internal abdominal injuries.
   B. head and spinal injuries.
   C. injury to the respiratory system.
   D. disturbance with hearing and sight.

7. Assessment of this patient's neck should involve which of the following?
   A. Palpation for subcutaneous emphysema
   B. Palpation of the anterior cervical vertebra
   C. Listening over the carotid artery for abnormal sounds
   D. Listening over the wound site for subcutaneous emphysema

Challenging Questions

8. Every effort should be taken to prevent this patient from swallowing blood. Why is this important?

9. This patient is at risk for an air embolism if a major vein has been lacerated. How would you know if an air embolism occurred?

10. How would you appropriately bandage this patient's neck wound?

Points to Ponder

You respond to a call to find a skier who has been hit in the throat with a ski pole. The patient's throat is quite swollen, he is cyanotic, and he appears unable to breathe. You apply a cold pack to his throat and prepare to transport. Before you are able to get him loaded into the ambulance, he loses consciousness. You are not trained to perform a cricothyrostomy (create an artificial opening in his throat), but you have seen it done in the hospital twice. Would you ask medical control for permission to perform a cricothyrostomy? Why or why not? If medical control authorized the procedure, who would be liable for any damages that might occur? What other treatments might you try?

Issues Advanced Airway Management, EMT/Paramedic Relationships, Reporting Procedures, Impact of Reporting Treatment Issues.

Online Outlook

Soft-tissue injuries and fractures to the bones of the face and neck are common and vary in severity. Your priorities are to prevent further injury, especially to the cervical spine, and to manage any acute airway problems. Review your knowledge of these priorities by completing Exercise 21 at www.OECzone.com.

www.OECzone.com

Vital Vocabulary provides key terms and definitions from the chapter.

Points to Ponder tackles cultural, social, ethical, and legal issues through scenarios.

Online Outlook guides exploration of topics online, where additional activities reinforce and expand on important information from the chapter.

preview

Patient Assessment Flowchart

The Patient Assessment Flowchart provides a quick visual reference for the entire patient assessment process.

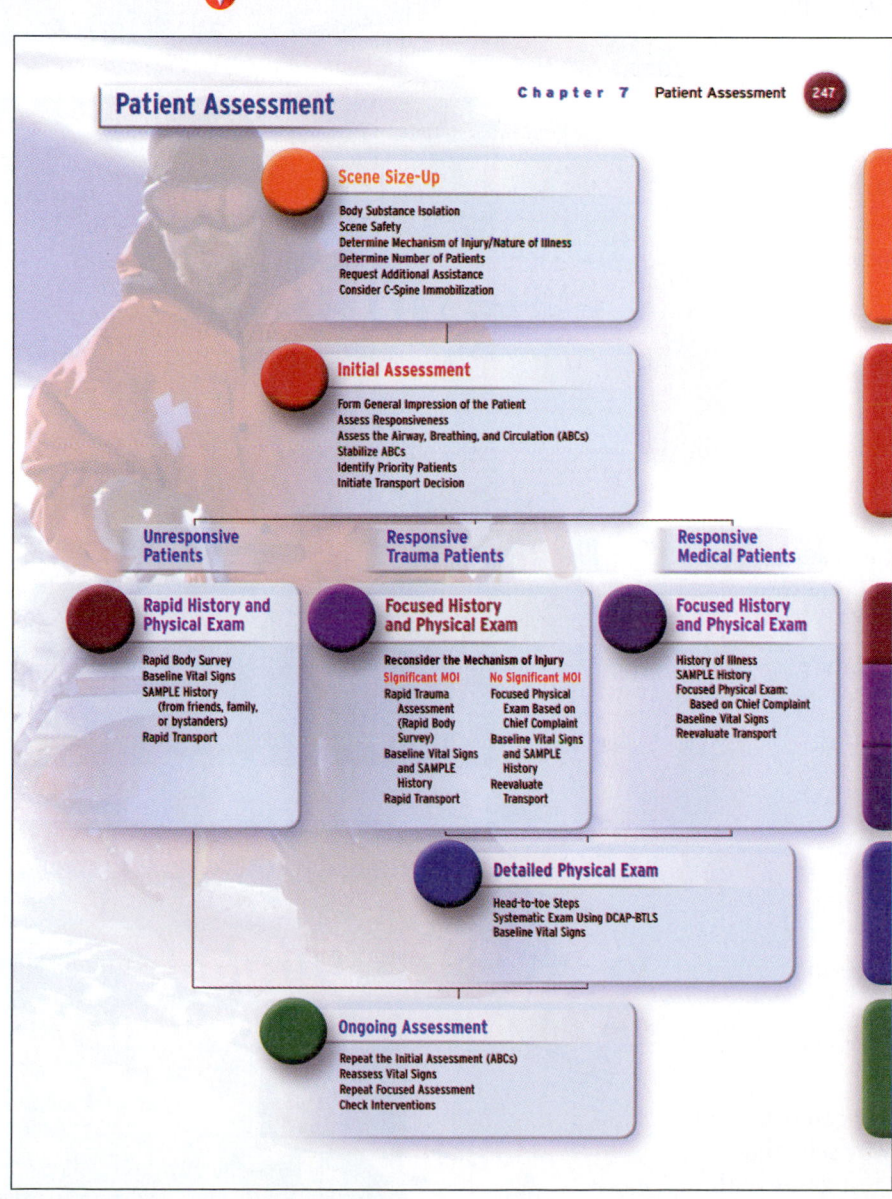

Patient Assessment

Chapter 7   Patient Assessment   247

Scene Size-Up

Body Substance Isolation
Scene Safety
Determine Mechanism of Injury/Nature of Illness
Determine Number of Patients
Request Additional Assistance
Consider C-Spine Immobilization

Initial Assessment

Form General Impression of the Patient
Assess Responsiveness
Assess the Airway, Breathing, and Circulation (ABCs)
Stabilize ABCs
Identify Priority Patients
Initiate Transport Decision

Unresponsive Patients

Responsive Trauma Patients

Responsive Medical Patients

Rapid History and Physical Exam

Rapid Body Survey
Baseline Vital Signs
SAMPLE History
   (from friends, family, or bystanders)
Rapid Transport

Focused History and Physical Exam

Reconsider the Mechanism of Injury

Significant MOI | No Significant MOI
Rapid Trauma Assessment (Rapid Body Survey) | Focused Physical Exam Based on Chief Complaint
Baseline Vital Signs and SAMPLE History | Baseline Vital Signs and SAMPLE History
Rapid Transport | Reevaluate Transport

Focused History and Physical Exam

History of Illness
SAMPLE History
Focused Physical Exam:
   Based on Chief Complaint
Baseline Vital Signs
Reevaluate Transport

Detailed Physical Exam

Head-to-toe Steps
Systematic Exam Using DCAP-BTLS
Baseline Vital Signs

Ongoing Assessment

Repeat the Initial Assessment (ABCs)
Reassess Vital Signs
Repeat Focused Assessment
Check Interventions

Divided into seven sections, the patient assessment flowchart is color-coded to the chapter content for easy reference. The flowchart is repeated at the beginning of each section to show students "at a glance" where they are in the patient assessment process.

preview

Instructor Resources

Instructor's ToolKit CD-ROM

ISBN: 0-7637-1195-0

Preparing for class is easy with the resources found on this CD-ROM, including:

PowerPoint Presentations, providing you with a powerful way to make presentations that are educational and engaging to your students. The slides can be edited and modified to meet your needs.

Sample Lesson Teaching Outlines, providing you with outlines that are keyed to the PowerPoint presentations and teaching strategies.

Image Bank, providing you with a selection of the most important images found in the textbook. You can use them to incorporate more images into the PowerPoint presentations, make handouts, or enlarge a specific image for further discussion.

Answers to all Chapter Sweep questions.

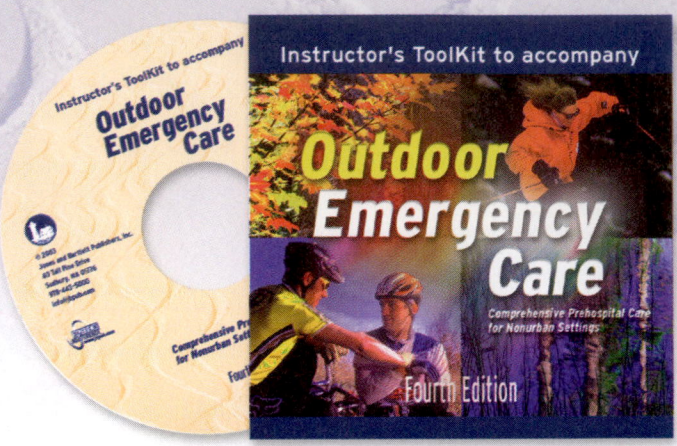

Instructor's Manual

ISBN: 0-929752-13-9

The Instructor's Manual is your guide to the entire teaching and learning system. This indispensable instructor material contains:

Detailed Lesson Guides provide the essential content and serve as reference for training strategies and resources.

Teaching Activities and Ideas to enhance presentations.

Answers to all Chapter Sweep questions.

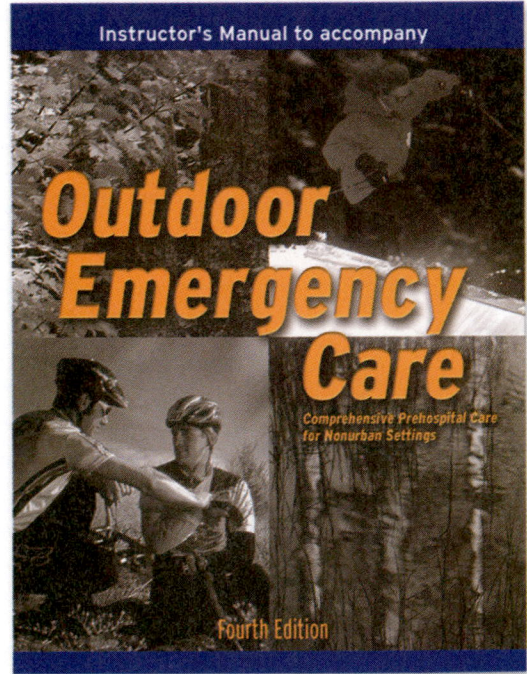

Instructor's TestBank

ISBN: 0-7637-1196-9 CD-ROM

This TestBank provides you with:

- more than 1,500 multiple-choice and scenario-based questions
- page references to *Outdoor Emergency Care, Fourth Edition*

With the TestBank on CD-ROM, you can originate tailor-made tests quickly and easily by selecting, editing, organizing, and printing a test along with an answer key.

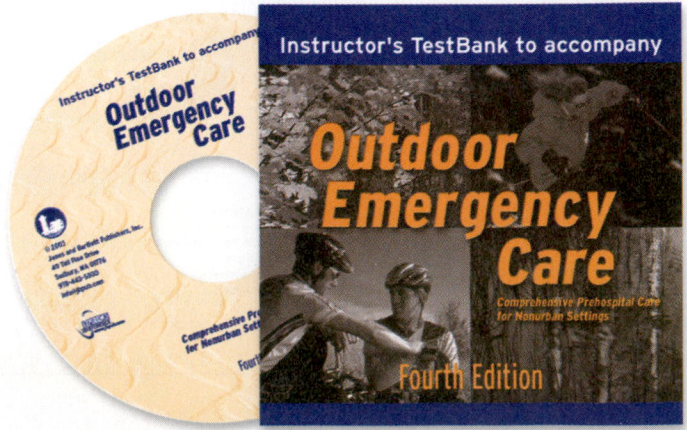

Student Resources

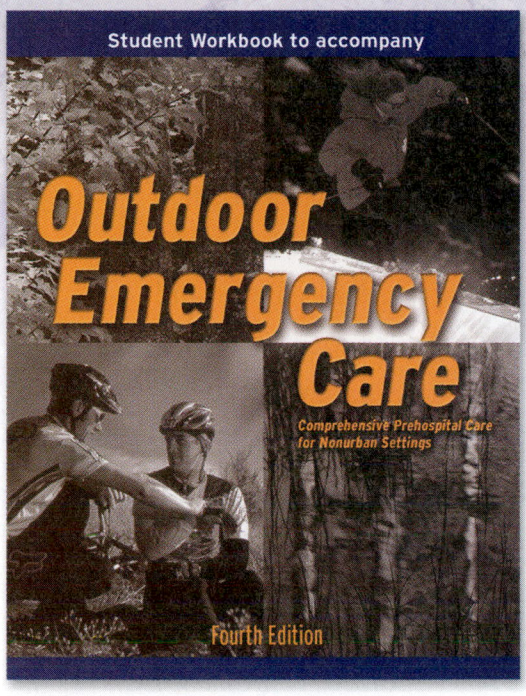

Student Workbook
ISBN: 0-7637-1194-2

This resource is designed to encourage critical thinking and aid comprehension of course material through:

- scenarios and corresponding questions
- figure labeling
- crossword puzzles
- matching, fill-in-the-blank, short answer, and multiple-choice questions
- skill drill activities

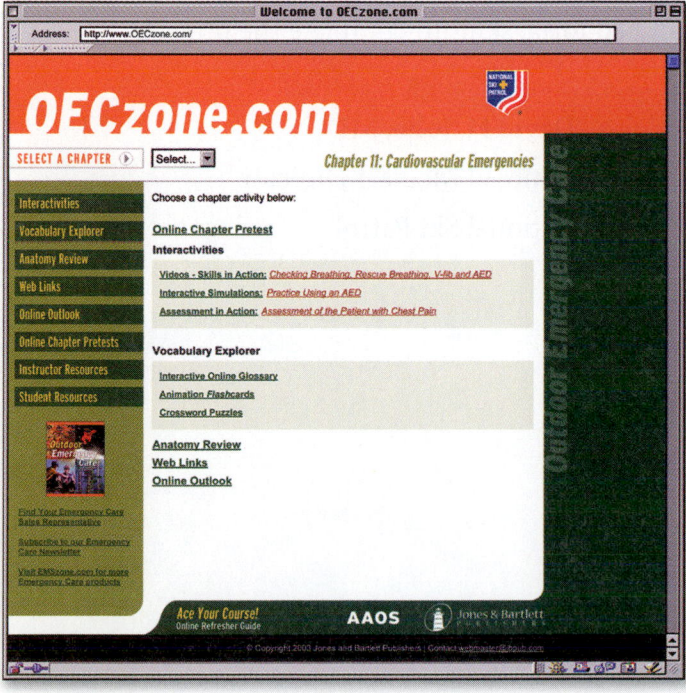

Online Refresher Guide
ISBN: 0-7637-1197-7
Online at www.OECzone.com

This online guide has been designed to prepare OEC technicians to complete the same type of scenario-based and multiple-choice questions that they are likely to see in the annual Refresher Study Guide. It provides answers to all questions with brief explanations and page references.

Acknowledgments

Producing a textbook of this magnitude and complexity would have been impossible without many useful suggestions and contributions from members of the National Ski Patrol (NSP) and others interested in Outdoor Emergency Care (OEC). The NSP Board of Directors had the insight to change this text's format, moving its presentation to a new level. The many authors, editors, and reviewers have spent countless hours putting the text together. Members of the National Ski Patrol's National Medical Advisory Committee, nationally known experts in nonurban and wilderness prehospital emergency care, NSP members, and other selected persons have carefully reviewed the entire manuscript.

The National Medical Director is particularly indebted to the NSP's National Chairman, Bill Sachs, and previous chairman, John Clair, for the opportunity to lead NSP's National Medical Advisory Committee. Mary Murrett, National OEC Program Director, and John Dobson, MD, Chair of the OEC Refresher Committee, have contributed to the educational aspect of the OEC program. Leif Borgeson tirelessly showed his dedication reviewing chapters and coordinating the photography. There was no one more dedicated than Judy Over, Education Director, who used her superb organizational and editorial skills to complete the project.

David H. Johe, MD
National Medical Director
National Ski Patrol

Editors

Warren D. Bowman, MD, FACP

Warren D. Bowman, MD, is a specialist in internal medicine and hematology with special interests in wilderness and mountain medicine. While semi-retired from the Department of Internal Medicine at the Billings Clinic in Montana, he continues to work part-time at Mammoth and Old Faithful Clinics and Lake Hospital in Yellowstone National Park and spends his leisure time hiking, cross-country skiing, and backcountry telemarking.

Dr. Bowman is a clinical associate professor of medicine emeritus at the University of Washington School of Medicine and is National Medical Director Emeritus of the National Ski Patrol. He is a fellow of the American College of Physicians (ACP) and a former governor of the Montana chapter of the ACP, which recognized him with the chapter's laureate award in 1995. He also belongs to the International Society for Ski Safety, the International Society for Mountain Medicine, and has been a US Commissioner of the medical committee, Union Internationale de Associations d'Alpinisme (UIAA).

Dr. Bowman has been a member of the medical committee of the American Alpine Club and is a founding member, board member, and past president of the Wilderness Medical Society. He is a former medical committee chairman for the National Association for Search and Rescue (NASAR) and a former board chairman of the Midland Empire chapter of the American Red Cross.

As a ski patroller, Dr. Bowman has served as a nationally registered avalanche and mountain travel and rescue instructor. He holds National Appointment #3537 and has twice received the NSP's national award as outstanding administrative patroller. In 1990, he was honored with the prestigious Minot "Minnie" Dole award, bestowed on rare occasions to those who personify the attributes of the NSP's founder.

Dr. Bowman is a member of the editorial board of the *Journal of Wilderness and Environmental Medicine*, and has written many journal articles on medical topics; textbook chapters on wilderness emergency care, cold injury, and wilderness survival; and first aid manuals, including the National Ski Patrol's *Winter First Aid Manual* and the first three editions of *Outdoor Emergency Care*.

National Medical Advisory Committee
National Medical Director Emeritus
Billings Clinic
Departments of Hematology/Oncology,
  Same Day Care
Billings, MT

David H. Johe, MD

David H. Johe, MD, is an orthopaedic surgeon who has a private practice and is part of the medical staff with the Elk Regional Health Center in Saint Marys, Pennsylvania.

Dr. Johe is a graduate of West Virginia University Medical School and completed his internship at Hartford Hospital, Hartford, Connecticut, and his orthopaedic residency at the University Hospitals of Cleveland. He is a member of the Pennsylvania Orthopedic Society and the American Board of Independent Medical Examiners.

Dr. Johe has been an active member of the Holiday Valley Resort Ski Patrol in upstate New York since 1995. He serves as the National Ski Patrol's National Medical Director and chair of the National Medical Committee. This committee serves as a resource on current issues and concerns such as trauma, emergency care, OSHA, pediatrics, ALS, new medical and rescue techniques, and equipment, etc. for NSP members and its outdoor affiliates. He participates in NSP education programs and continuing education as well as staying involved as an Outdoor Emergency Care instructor trainer. He holds National Appointment #8690.

Dr. Johe has been a contributor of numerous articles for *Ski Patrol Magazine* and NSP's *Refresher Study Guide*.

National Medical Advisory Committee
National Medical Director
Orthopaedic Surgeon
Elk Regional Health Center/
  Private Practice
Saint Marys, PA

Editors (continued)

Bruce D. Browner, MD, FAAOS

Dr. Browner is a senior member of the orthopaedic trauma community in the United States. He has been active at both the national and international levels in clinical program and technology development, education, research, and health policy. Prior to his orthopaedic residency, he completed a fellowship at the Shock Trauma Research Unit at Albany Medical College. Upon completion of his training, he spent 4 years on the faculty of the Maryland Shock Trauma Center. He subsequently spent 10 years at the University of Texas Medical School in Houston and Hermann Hospital where he served as Director of the Division of Orthopaedic Surgery and Chief of the Orthopaedic Service. Eight and one half years ago, he assumed his current position in Connecticut. Dr. Browner has served on the Board of Directors, and the Committees on Injuries, Health Care Finance, and International Affairs of the American Academy of Orthopaedic Surgeons. He is currently Chairman of the Advisory Council for Orthopaedic Surgery, member of the Health Policy Steering and International Committees, and a senior member of the Committee on Trauma of the American College of Surgeons. He has also been appointed the Founding Chairman of the Trauma Committee by Societe Internationale de Chirurgie Orthopedique et de Traumatologie (SICOT). Dr. Browner was a founding member and past President of the Orthopaedic Trauma Association. He is the senior editor of *Skeletal Trauma*, the leading textbook on fractures and dislocations in the world. He was the Chairman of the Editorial Panel for the Seventh Edition of *Emergency Care and Transportation of the Sick and Injured*. He is a member of the International Steering Committee for the Bone and Joint Decade: 2000–2010, and is currently involved in an international effort to control the global road traffic injury epidemic.

Gray-Gossling Professor and Chairman
Department of Orthopaedic Surgery
University of Connecticut Health Center
Farmington, CT

Director of Orthopaedic Department
Hartford Hospital
Hartford, CT

Andrew N. Pollak, MD, EMT-P, FAAOS

Dr. Pollak has been active in EMS activities since 1980 when he started as a volunteer firefighter and first responder. During his career, he has served as an EMT-A, an EMT-Paramedic, and as a flight physician with a hospital-based aeromedical ambulance service. He is currently an Attending Orthopaedic Trauma Surgeon at the R Adams Cowley Shock Trauma Center in Baltimore, Maryland. He remains active in EMS as Fire Surgeon for the Baltimore County Fire Department and as an educator and administrator. He is the director of the hospital-based rapid response field unit known as the Shock Trauma Go Team.

Associate Professor and Acting Chairman
Department of Orthopaedic Surgery
University of Maryland School of Medicine

Attending Orthopaedic Traumatologist
R Adams Cowley Shock Trauma Center
Baltimore, MD

Carol L. Gupton, NREMT-P

Carol Gupton has been involved in EMS since 1985 and has been a paramedic for 10 years. She is currently an EMS Instructor for the Omaha Fire Department. Her experience includes a faculty appointment with Creighton University's paramedic program and 5 years of service as a paramedic and EMS advisor for the La Vista Volunteer Fire Department. She is the Nebraska PHTLS state coordinator and co-chair of the Midlands EMS Protocol Committee and has authored several chapters in EMS textbooks. She received her Bachelor's of Science degree in EMS from Creighton University in 1994 and has been certified as a nationally registered paramedic since 1991. Carol has been actively teaching all levels of EMS including First Responders, EMT-B, Paramedic, AMLS, and PEPP, for 15 years.

Bachelor of Science, EMS
EMS Instructor
Omaha Fire Department
Prehospital Provider Education, Inc.
Omaha, NE

National Medical Advisory Committee

Ian D. Archibald, MD
Southern Division
Orthopaedic Surgeon
Clifton Forge, VA

Paul S. Auerbach, MD
Member at Large
Professor and Chief, Division
   of Emergency Medicine
Department of Surgery, Stanford
   University Medical Center
Stanford, CA

Jessica H. Bayless, MD
Northern Division
Urgent Care and Emergency Medicine
Missoula, MT

Warren D. Bowman, MD, FACP
National Medical Director Emeritus
Billings Clinic, Departments of
   Hematology/Oncology, Same Day Care
Billings, MT

Nancy Brooke, MD
Central Division
Assistant Clinical Professor of Pediatrics,
   Michigan State University
Grand Rapids, MI

John L. Dobson, MD
Member at Large
Retired Orthopaedic Hand Surgeon
Wintergreen, VA

Colin K. Grissom, MD
Intermountain Division
Assistant Professor, Pulmonary
   and Critical Care
Department of Internal Medicine,
   LDS Hospital, University of Utah
Salt Lake City, UT

Peter H. Hackett, MD, FACEP
Member at Large
President, International Society
   for Mountain Medicine
Division of Emergency Medicine,
   University of Colorado Health Sciences
Ridgway, CO

David J. Herfindahl, MD
Pacific Northwest Division
Diplomate, American Board
   of Family Practice
Director of Disaster Medical Services
County of Siskegan, Yrebia, CA

David H. Johe, MD
National Medical Director
Orthopaedic Surgeon
Elk Regional Health Center/
   Private Practice
Saint Marys, PA

Eric William Lamberts, MD, FAAFP, ASAM
Far West Division
Far West Division Medical Advisor
Clinical Professor, Departments of
   Family and Community Medicine
   and Psychiatry, University of Nevada
School of Medicine
Reno, NV

Michael Levy, MD, FACEP, FACP
Alaska Division
Medical Director Anchorage Fire
   Department, Aeromed International
   Medevac Services
Danali Emergency Medicine Associates
Anchorage, AK

Jeffrey Lozman, MD
Eastern Division
Clinical Professor of Orthopaedic Surgery,
   Albany Medical College
Capital Region Orthopaedic Group
Albany, NY

John S. Nichols, MD, PhD
Rocky Mountain Division
Neurological Surgeon
St. Anthony Central Hospital
Denver, CO

Steven G. Sutton, MD, FACS
European Division
LtCol, USAF, MC, FS
Chief, Department of Urologic Surgery
Landstuhl Regional Medical
   Center, Germany

John (Chip) Woodland, MD, FACEP
Professional Division
Emergency Medicine Physician
Vail Valley Emergency Physicians
Vail, CO

Other Contributors

R. Morgan Armstrong, JD
National Ski Patrol Member and Patroller
Collinsville, VA

Larry Bost, EMT-D, Paramedic
Assistant National OEC Program
   Director, Wilderness Medicine
   Instructor
Gastonia, NC

Les Chatelain
Health Promotion and Education
   Department
University of Utah
Salt Lake City, UT

Alice (Twink) Dalton, RN, MS
EMS Education Coordinator
Omaha Fire Department
Omaha, NE

Cressy Goodwin, MPH
EMS Coordinator
Hartford Hospital
Hartford, CT

Kermit Lowry, Jr., MD, FACS
Retired General Surgeon, Bristol Surgical
Associates, PC, Bristol, TN
Professor Emeritus of Surgery,
   East Tennessee State University,
   College of Medicine
Johnson City, TN

Captain Diane C. Lundy, MD
Staff Ophthalmologist,
   United States Navy
San Diego, CA

Gregg Margolis, NREMT-P
Director EMS Education
George Washington University
Washington, DC

Michael D. Panté, NREMT-P
EMS Educator
Robert Wood Johnson
   University Hospital
New Brunswick, NJ

Jeff Pollakoff, EMT-P
EMS Educator
UCLA Center for Prehospital Care
Los Angeles, CA

Harvey A. Ries, MD
Summit At Snoqualmie Ski Patrol
   Medical Advisor
Snoqualmie Pass, WA

Jose V. Salazar, MPH, NREMT-P
Training Officer
Loudoun County Fire & Rescue
Leesburg, VA

Marcus Sciadini, MD
Assistant Professor of
   Orthopaedic Surgery
Vanderbilt University
Nashville, TN

Other Contributors (continued)

Eunice M. Singletary, MD, FACEP
Clinical Associate Professor,
 Emergency Medicine
University of Virginia
Charlottesville, VA

Mike Smith, MICP
Vice President
Emergency Medical Training
 Associates, Inc.
Olympia, WA

Ed Travers, RN, CEN, EMT-P
Associate Professor and Department
 Chair EMS
Massachusetts Bay Community College
Burlington, MA

J. Douglas Yeakel, MD, FACEP
Director, Primary Care Sports Medicine
Spectrum Orthopaedics, Inc.
Canton, OH

Photographic Contributors

A special thank you to each of
the photography models who contributed time and expertise to help
the National Ski Patrol complete
this photographic project.

Photographers

Brian Robb

London Schertzer

Ingrid Tistaert

Other photographers are identified
on page 932, Additional Credits.

Participating Resorts and Organizations

Timberline Lodge
Pacific Northwest Division Members
Mt. Hood Ski Patrol
Timberline Ski Patrol
Mt. Hood National Forest, OR

Breckenridge Ski Resort
Breckenridge Ski Patrol
Breckenridge Outdoor Education Center
Breckenridge, CO

Keystone Resort
Keystone Ski Patrol
Keystone, CO

Copper Mountain Resort
Copper Mountain Ski Patrol
Copper Mountain, CO

Summit County Ambulance Service
Summit County, CO

**International Mountain
 Bicycling Association**
National Mountain Bike Patrol
Boulder, CO

The American Alpine Club
Golden, CO

Colorado Mountain College
Breckenridge, CO

**Cascade Toboggan
 Rescue Equipment Co, Inc.**
Hailey, ID

**St. Anthony's Central Hospital
 Trauma Services**
Denver, CO

**West Virginia Professional
 River Outfitters**
Class VI River Runners
Lansing, WV

**National Sports Center
 for the Disabled**
Winter Park, CO

Special Olympics Colorado

Salomon North America

Reviewers

A special thank you to each individual who contributed to the review
process for the Fourth Edition of the
Outdoor Emergency Care project.
*(Omission of any reviewer is
unintentional.)*

Wendy Adams, RN, MN
Philips Medical Systems
Andover, MA

Barbara Aehlert, RN, BSPA
Southwest EMS Education
Glendale, AZ

Kathy Alexander, EMT-I
Pacific Northwest OEC Supervisor
Mt. Bachelor Ski Patrol
Bend, OR

Janet Alfred
Timber Ridge Ski Patrol
Gobles, MI

Karen Anderson-Hadden, RN
Timber Ridge Ski Patrol
Gobles, MI

Ronald H. Baker
Windham Mountain Ski Patrol
Windham, NY

Greg Bala, MS
Kelly Canyon Ski Patrol
Ririe, ID

Eileen P. Barlage
Brighton Ski Patrol
Brighton, UT

Barbara L. Baxter, RN, JD, NRP
Big Bear Valley Ski Resort
Bear Valley, CA

Penny Beams, PT
Ausblick Ski Patrol
Sussex, WI

Rhonda Beck, NREMT-P
Macon Technical Institute
Macon, GA

Sandra Beecher, MS, CIH
Homewood Ski Patrol
Homewood, CA

James K. Benton
Snoqualmie Ski Patrol
Snoqualmie Pass, WA

Gloria Bizjak, EMT-A
Maryland Fire and Rescue
Berwin Heights, MD

Tom Blake, BA, MSE
Southern Maine Technical College
South Portland, ME

Ken Block
Timber Ridge Ski Patrol
Gobles, MI

Marc D. Bond, JD
Attorney at Law
Anchorage, AK

Larry Bost, Paramedic
Assistant National OEC
  Program Director
Hawksnest Ski Patrol
Seven Devils, NC

Carol Boughton
Reno Ski Patrol
Reno, NV

Kenneth O. Bradford, EMT-P
Santa Rosa Junior College
Petaluma, CA

Sandra Jo Bradley, EMT-P
Far West OEC Supervisor
Homewood Ski Patrol
Homewood, CA

Paul Brooks, MICP
Alaska OEC Supervisor
Alyeska Ski Patrol
Girdwood, AK

Anthony N. Brown
Grand Targhee Ski Patrol
Alta, WY

Cindy Budge, EMT
Jackson Hole Ski Patrol
Teton Village, WY

Vicki L. Callahan
Hyland Ski Patrol
Bloomington, MN

Elizabeth Cascio, EMT-D
Fire Department – New York City
Bayside, NY

Les Chatelain
University of Utah
Salt Lake City, UT

Michael J. Costa
Boyne Mountain Ski Patrol
Boyne, MI

Sharon Crockett
Nubs Nob Ski Patrol
Harbor Springs, MI

Andrew David, NA #7390, EMT-P
Ski World Ski Patrol
Nashville, IN

Corey Davis
Timber Ridge Ski Resort
Gobles, MI

Debra Delforge
Devils Head Ski Patrol
Merrimac, WI

Donald A. Dragon Jr., EMT-C, EMS-IC
Administrative Officer, National
  Disaster Medical System, RI-1 DMAT
School Emergency Medical Response
  Training Programs
Narragansett, RI

Elizabeth Dodge
Pacific Northwest OEC Supervisor
Ski Acres Ski Patrol
Snoqualmie Pass, WA

Steve Donelan
ASHI Wilderness Emergency Care,
  Chairman
Pinecrest Nordic Ski Patrol
Pinecrest, CA

Robert B. Doyle, EMT-B
Northeastern University
Burlington, MA

Ralph Elam, EMT-P, EMS-IC
Superior Medical Education
Madison Heights, MI

Gwendolin Ellis, EMT-CC
Broome County Emergency Services
Binghamton, NY

Lisa Ellis, RDH
Northern OEC Supervisor
Casper Mountain Ski Patrol
Casper, WY

Marcia Ellis, PA-C
Timber Ridge Ski Patrol
Gobles, MI

Richard Ellis, NREMT-P, AAS
US Air Force EMS Program
Sheppard Air Force Base, TX

Deb Endly
Central OEC Supervisor
Hyland Ski Patrol
Bloomington, MN

Adrian Fernandez
White Pass Ski Patrol
White Pass, WA

Jim Fillmore, EMT-A
Intermountain OEC Supervisor
Grand Targhee Ski Patrol
Alta, WY

Carol Fountain, RN, MN, ONC
Bogus Basin Ski Patrol
Boise, ID

Frederick E. Fowler
Adirondack Regional Emergency
  Services, Inc.
Glens Falls, NY

Donn E. Fox
Keystone Ski Patrol
Keystone, CO

Roberta Marie Fox
Maple Ski Ridge Ski Patrol
Schenectady, NY

Steve Francisco
OEC Refresher Committee
June Mountain Ski Patrol
June Lake, CA

Ann Gassman
Rocky Mountain OEC Supervisor
Keystone Ski Patrol
Keystone, CO

Janet T. Glaeser, MEd, NBCT
Central OEC Supervisor
Boston Mills/Brandywine Ski Patrol
Peninsula, OH

Kathy Glynn
Hyland Ski Patrol
Bloomington, MN

Daniel Goldberger, MD
Bittersweet Ski Patrol
Ostego, MI

Susan Gormley, EMT-B
Hyland Ski Patrol
Bloomington, MN

Mary Griffin
Central OEC Supervisor
Sugar Loaf Mountain Ski Patrol
Cedar, MI

Dayle Hadden
Timber Ridge Ski Patrol
Gobles, MI

Jonathan Hale, MAPS
Hawksnest Ski Patrol
Seven Devils, NC

Bryant F. Hall, BS (MT), MBA
West Virginia University,
  Pain Treatment Center
Canaan Valley Ski Patrol
Davis, WV

William F. Halsey
Eastern OEC Supervisor
Song Mountain Ski Patrol
Tully, NY

Drannan Hamby, PhD
Mt. Bachelor Ski Patrol
Bend, OR

Donnell Harvin, CIC, EMT-P
The City University of New York
New York, NY

Mike Helbock, MICP, NREMT-P
Emergency Medical Trainers
  and Consultants, Inc.
Woodinville, WA

Charles A. Herbert, PE
Squaw Valley Ski Patrol
Olympic Valley, CA

Victor Robert Hernandez, BA, EMT-P
Emergency Training & Consultations
Truckee, CA

acknowledgments

Reviewers (continued)

Barbara Hickman, MA
Prospector Ski Patrol
Pinecrest, CA

Douglas Hill
Far West OEC Supervisor
Big Bear Valley Ski Patrol
Bear Valley, CA

Edwin H. Humphrey, EMT-P, MBA (9206)
Perfect North Slopes
Lawrenceburg, IN

Michael E. Ingraham, AAS, Lic Paramedic
Medical Education Specialists Team
Temple, TX

Hugh W. Jernigan, Jr.
Hawksnest Ski Patrol
Seven Devils, NC

David Johnson, MD
Wilderness Medical Associates
Emergency Department Physician
Lewiston, ME

Rockey Johnson
Kentucky State Fire and Rescue/STAT Care
Louisville, KY

Jennifer Jones
Crystal Mountain Ski Patrol
Thompsonville, MI

Judith Kay-Monaghan, MA
Southern OEC Supervisor
Wintergreen Ski Patrol
Wintergreen, VA

Garrett P. Keane
Bromley Ski Patrol
Bromley, VT

John Keith, PhD
Beaver Mountain Ski Patrol
Logan, UT

Suzanne Kenney
Blackcomb Mountain Ski Patrol
British Columbia, Canada

Kevin P. Kesick, RN, EMT-P
Bearsville, NY

Brian Klebba
Crystal Mountain Ski Patrol
Thompsonville, MI

Nancy Knowles
Herman Mountain Ski Patrol
Stockton Springs, ME

James R. Kopp, MD, PC
Orthopaedic Surgeon
Anthony Lakes Ski Patrol
North Powder, OR

Erica Krol, PA-C
Timber Ridge Ski Patrol
Gobles, MI

Paula N. Larson
Nubs Nob Ski Patrol
Harbor Springs, MI

Shelia C. Leeds, RN, BSN
Brighton Ski Patrol
Brighton, UT

Charles L. Lentz, MA
Appalachian Ski Patrol
Blowing Rock, NC

Thomas Lipa
Greek Peak Ski Patrol
Ithaca, NY

David Long
Crystal Mountain Ski Patrol
Thompsonville, MI

Bob Lovelace, BF, EMT-P, I/C
Huron Valley Ambulance
Plymouth, MI

Don Lundy, BS, NREMT-P
Charleston County EMS
Charleston, SC

Edward Lynch, MEd
Wuerzburg Ski Patrol
Germany

David M. Magnino
California Highway Patrol Academy
West Sacramento, CA

Robert T. Mayberry, RN, CFRN, EMT-P
Flight Nurse, West Michigan Air Care
Timber Ridge Ski Patrol
Gobles, MI

Bonnie Maynard
Nashville Fire Department
Nashville, TN

Alan P. McCartney, CSP, CHCM, CHSP, EMT-P
Brigham and Women's Hospital
Boston, MA

Jeff McDonald, EMT-P
Tarrant County College – Northeast
Hurst, TX

Edward C. McNamara
Eastern OEC Supervisor
Wachusett Mountain Ski Patrol
Princeton, MA

Pamela Mead
Highland Forest Nordic Ski Patrol
Fabius, NY

Gwen Milley
Blackcomb Mountain Ski Patrol
British Columbia, Canada

Brian Murphy
Beartooth Ski Patrol
Red Lodge, MT

Michael E. Murphy, RN, CEN, EMT-P
Rockland Paramedic Services
Nanuet, NY

Mary Murrett, MS, MEd
National OEC Program Director
Kissing Bridge Ski Patrol
Glenwood, NY

Tim O'Brien
San Francisco Ski Patrol
San Francisco, CA

Robert Offerle
Southern Arizona Rescue Association
Tucson, AZ

Jeffrey J. Olsen, JD
Claims Specialist
Wild Mountain Ski Patrol
Taylors Falls, MN

Kathy Olsen, RN
Pebble Creek Ski Patrol
Inkom, ID

Michael Panté, NREMT-P
Robert Wood Johnson
   University Hospital
New Brunswick, NJ

Don Paul
Great Divide Ski Patrol
Helena, MT

Myllissa Pena-Wyatt
Pebble Creek Ski Patrol
Inkom, ID

Robert Persons
Keystone Ski Patrol
Keystone, CO

Kimberly Pollack, MS
Donner Ski Ranch Ski Patrol
Norden, CA

Jeff Pollakoff, EMT-P
UCLA Center for Prehospital Care
Los Angeles, CA

Mary Ann Porter
Keystone Ski Patrol
Keystone, CO

Monte Posner, MSW, EMT-B, CIC
TIMER
Staten Island, NY

Richard Prentiss
Miami-Dade Community College
Miami, FL

Dagmar Prout
Marquette Mountain Ski Patrol
Marquette, MI

Tom Raithby, EMT-2
Fairfield, New Brunswick
Canada

Paul G. Rauschke
Associate Professor, Ski Area Operations
Colorado Mountain College
Leadville, CO

Cathy Read
Beartooth Ski Patrol
Red Lodge, MT

Robb Rehberg, MS, ATC, NREMT
Montclair State University
Upper Montclair, NJ

Michael Reilly
Community Medical Center
Toms River, NJ

Gina Riggs, NREMT-P
Kiamichi Technology Center
Poteau, OK

Joe Riley
Cascade Ski Patrol
Portage, WI

Noel J. Rios, PhD
Labrador Mountain
Truxton, NY

Richard C. Roth
Big Bear Valley
Bear Valley, CA

Bill Sachs
Liberty Mountain Ski Patrol
Carroll Valley, PA

Jose Salazar, MPH, NREMT-P
Loudoun County Fire & Rescue
Leesburg, VA

Robert J. Schappert III
Maryland Fire and Rescue Institute
University of Maryland
Louege Park, MD

Paul Schifando
LA County Fire Department
Los Angeles, CA

Brigitte B. Schran, MEd, MA, EMT
OEC Refresher Committee
Ski Acres Ski Patrol
Snoqualmie Pass, WA

William H. Seifarth, MS, NREMT-P
Maryland Institute for Emergency
    Medical Services Systems
Baltimore, MD

Cathy Setzer, MEd
Boyce Park Ski Patrol
Pittsburgh, PA

Vince Shaffer
Medix School
Kennesaw, GA

Gary L. Shirley
Mississippi Gulf Coast
    Community College
Gulfport, MS

Kenneth L. Sicke, Jr.
Gore Mountain Ski Patrol
North Creek, NY

William Smith
Homestead Ski Patrol
Hot Springs, VA

Jan Stanford, RN
Bogus Basin Ski Patrol
Boise, ID

James Stefka
East Texas Medical Center
Brownsboro, TX

Jim Stevens
St. Louis Community College
Dayton, OH

Gail Stewart
Florida Association of Professional
    EMTs and Paramedics
Tallahassee, FL

Teresa Stewart, MHS, EMT
Hawksnest Ski Patrol
Seven Devils, NC

Keith Tatsukawa, MD, PhD
Neurosurgery
Mt. Waterman Ski Patrol
La Canada, CA

Denise Tiedeman, EMT-B
Tidewater Community College
Virginia Beach, VA

John Todaro, REMT-P, RN
Florida College of Emergency Physicians
Orlando, FL

Paul Tracy, MS
Eastern OEC Supervisor
Hidden Valley Ski Patrol
Ellicottville, NY

Ed Travers, RN, CEN, EMT-P
Massachusetts Bay Community College
Burlington, MA

Sherwin VanKlompenberg, MA, EMT-B
Crystal Mountain Ski Patrol
Thompsonville, MI

Sue F. VanOrden
Hidden Valley Ski Patrol
Ellicottville, NY

Ariel Villarreal
Broward Community College
Pembroke Pines, FL

Colleen A. Volmut
Bromley Ski Patrol
Manchester Center, VT

James E. Walker, Jr., EMT-B
Northeastern University
Burlington, MA

Lynore Ward
European OEC Supervisor
Stuttgart Ski Patrol
Germany

Susanne Wise
Hawksnest Ski Patrol
Seven Devils, NC

Donald D. Wolcott, EdS, LPC
Casper Mountain Ski Patrol
Casper, WY

David Worfel
Caberfae Ski Patrol
Cadillac, MI

Ann T. Wood, EMT
Hawksnest Ski Patrol
Seven Devils, NC

Don Wood, MD
Director, Bureau of EMS
Salt Lake City, UT

Willy Wright, EMT-P
Staten Island EMS
Staten Island, NY

Kathleen A. Young
Timber Ridge Ski Patrol
Gobles, MI

Dennis A. Zercher
Ski Roundtop Ski Patrol
Lewisberry, PA

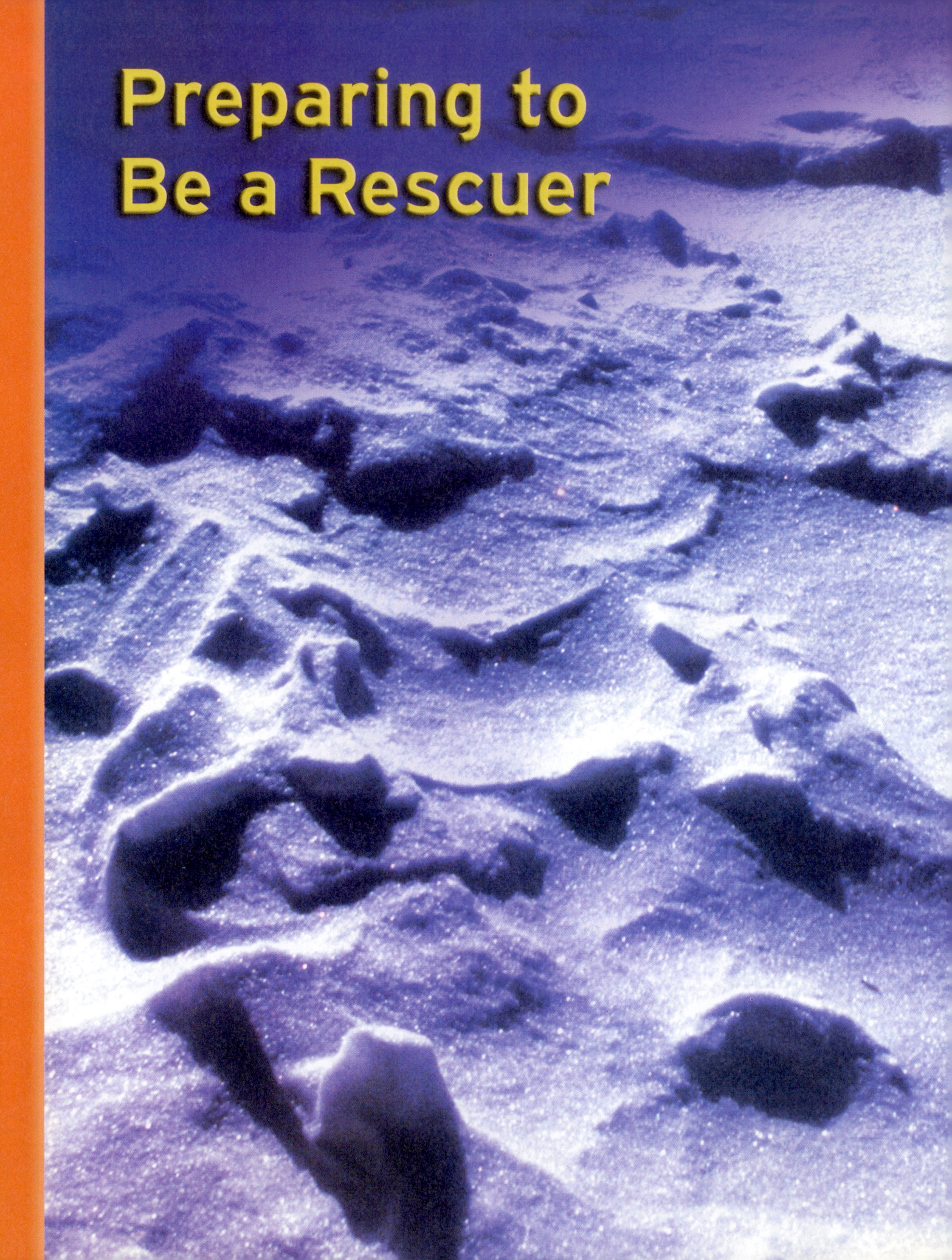

Preparing to
Be a Rescuer

Section 1

Introduction to Outdoor Emergency Care

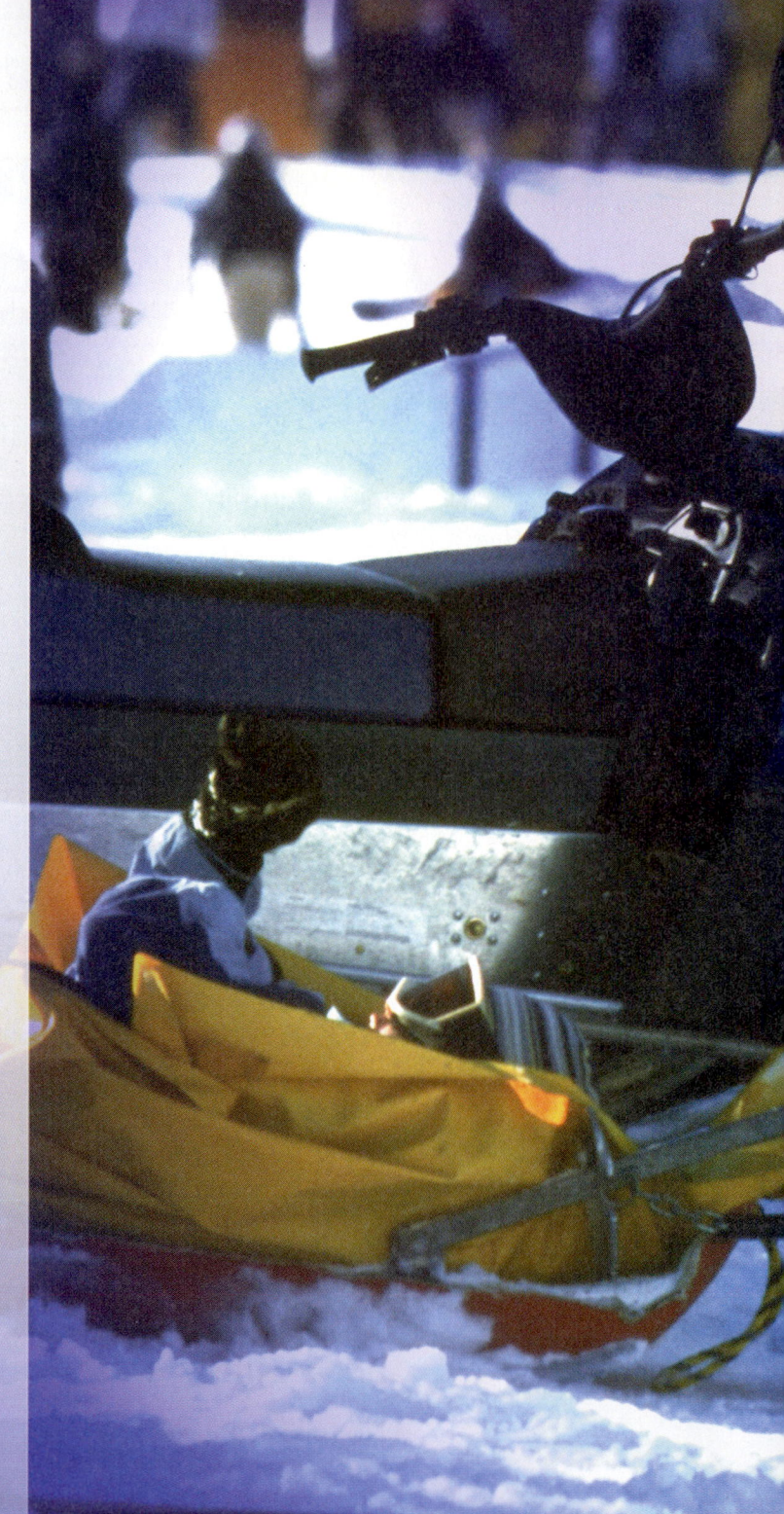

Objectives

Cognitive

1. Define the components of an OEC technician's education (p 4).
2. Differentiate the roles and responsibilities of the OEC technician from those of other prehospital care providers (p 5).
3. Discuss the roles and responsibilities of the OEC technician toward provider, patient, and bystander safety (p 12).
4. Define quality improvement and discuss the OEC technician's role in the process (p 10).
5. Define medical direction and the OEC technician's role in the process (p 10).

Affective

6. Define the medical, legal, and ethical issues you face as a rescuer (p 13).
7. Assess areas of personal attitude and conduct of the OEC technician (p 11).
8. Characterize the various methods used to support patrol operations and to access the EMS system in your community (p 9).

Psychomotor

None

🌲 These are core concepts in initial patrol training.

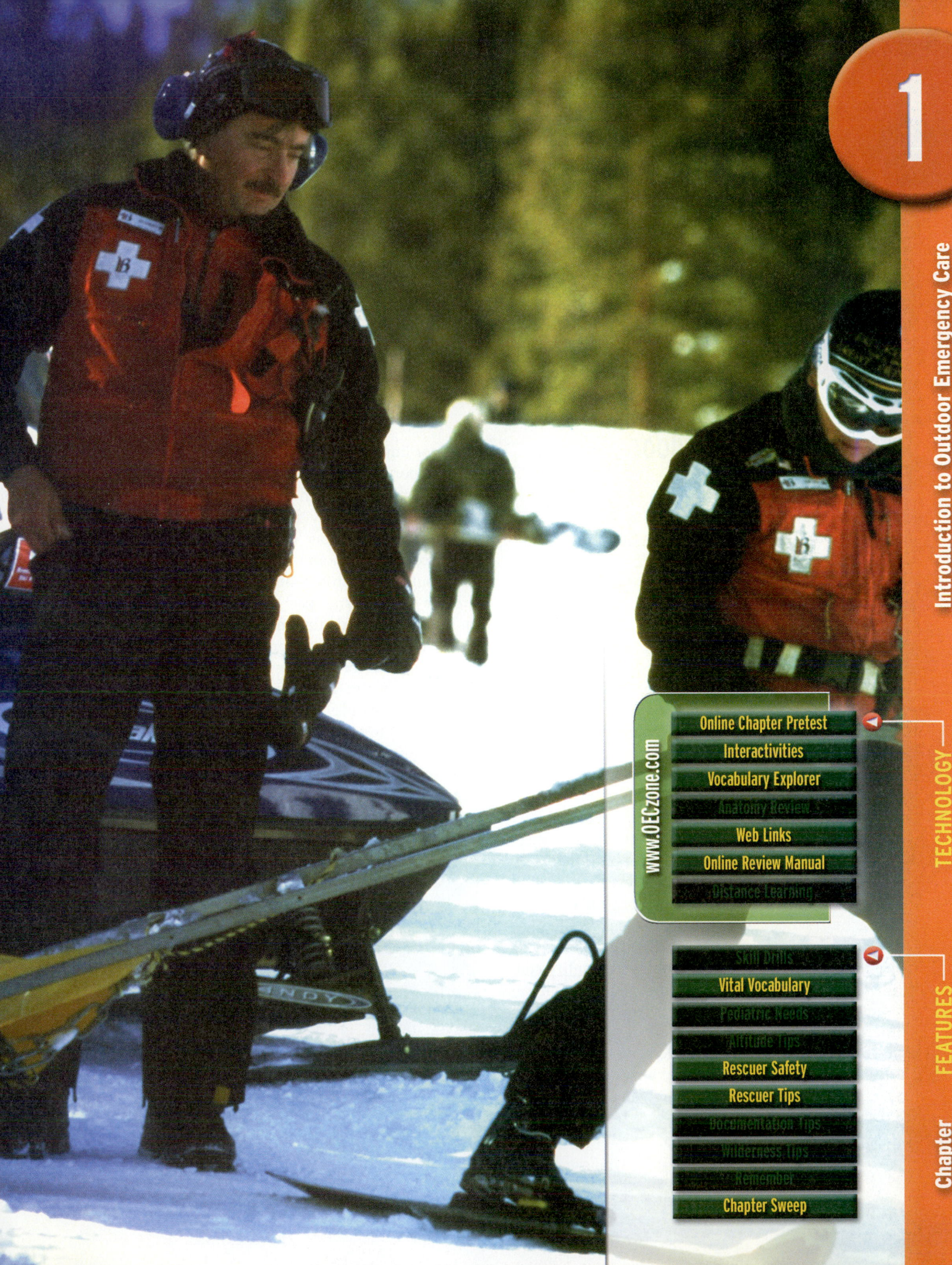

TECHNOLOGY

www.OECzone.com

- Online Chapter Pretest
- Interactivities
- Vocabulary Explorer
- Anatomy Review
- Web Links
- Online Review Manual
- Distance Learning

FEATURES

- Skill Drills
- Vital Vocabulary
- Pediatric Needs
- Altitude Tips
- Rescuer Safety
- Rescuer Tips
- Documentation Tips
- Wilderness Tips
- Remember
- Chapter Sweep

Chapter

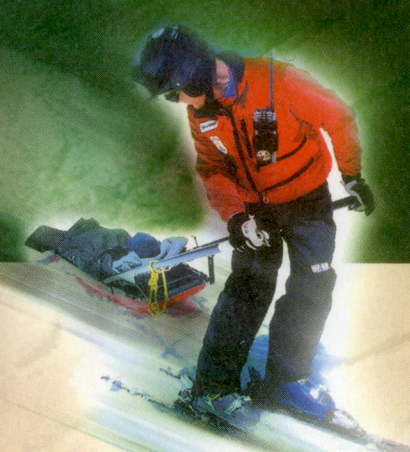

You have probably seen an injured skier being transported by a toboggan down a ski slope. The rescuer has gone through specialized outdoor emergency care (OEC) training. In this text, you will learn about this specialized training and how it has been developed.

This chapter will introduce you to the emergency care responsibilities of an OEC-trained prehospital emergency caregiver, hereafter called an "OEC technician." It will help you answer the following questions:

1. What are the components of an OEC technician's education?
2. Once trained, what are the responsibilities of an OEC technician?

Introduction to Outdoor Emergency Care

This text has been developed to serve as the primary resource for the **Outdoor Emergency Care (OEC)** course for the **National Ski Patrol (NSP)** member. It also can be used as an important source of information for other outdoor prehospital emergency care providers, such as wilderness medical technicians, river rafters, cavers, mountaineering guides, and search and rescue personnel, among others. This chapter describes the objectives and content of the OEC course. It also discusses what will be expected of you during this course and what you will need to learn to complete an OEC course successfully.

One of the functions of the NSP is to provide quality educational programs for the more than 28,000 members in its system. The key components of the emergency medical care part of this education and how they influence and affect the ski patroller and his or her delivery of emergency care will be addressed.

This chapter will discuss a brief history and evolution of OEC. Emergency care is dynamic, so changes in previous procedures and new information will be outlined. The administration, medical direction with **quality control**, and continuing education of the OEC program is presented. This chapter ends with a detailed discussion of the general roles and responsibility of patrollers as emergency prehospital care providers.

As an OEC technician, you will be part of the respected NSP system education programs, which have been active for more than 65 years.

Course Description

The emergency care of people in the outdoor environment can be exciting and challenging (▶ **Figure 1-1**).

Outdoor Emergency Care (OEC) has evolved into the most important current education program for individuals who provide care in the nonurban environment. **OEC technicians** provide prehospital care for the sick and injured at ski areas, wilderness settings, whitewater excursions, mountain bike events, and many other outdoor environments (▶ **Figure 1-2**). They also provide care at many special events such as local races and the Winter and Summer Olympic Games.

The NSP is the primary provider of medical educational programs for the patrollers who care for the snowsports public. The NSP encourages any other individuals who provide emergency care in the outdoor environment to be trained through its OEC course. All individuals completing this course are given a 3-year certification that notes course completion of all knowledge and skill objectives. Management personnel at nearly all mountain resorts in the United States recog-

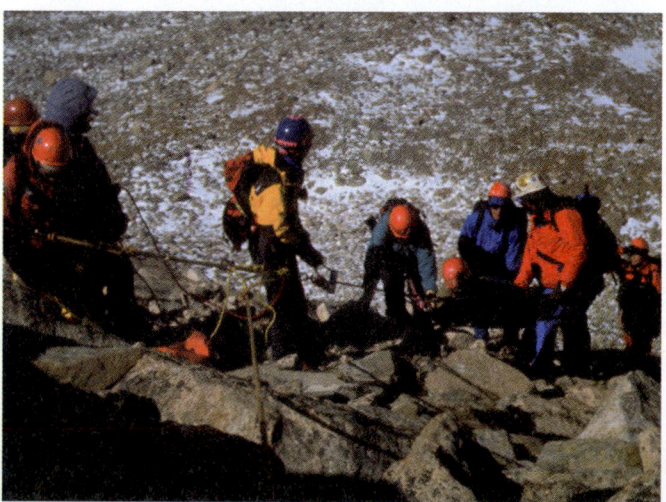

Figure 1-1 Outdoor emergency care is a comprehensive prehospital care training program for the nonurban environment.

nize the value of this OEC education program and use the completion of the course as a prerequisite for becoming a patroller. Other organizations, including white-water rafting companies, outdoor wilderness guide employers, and heli-ski companies, also use OEC as the basis for prehospital emergency care training.

This text occupies a unique niche in emergency care. Its principles, knowledge, and skills fall somewhere between urban care—in which response time is several minutes and includes an equipment-laden ambulance—and wilderness care, with long transport times and makeshift equipment. The sometimes harsh outdoor environment can make care difficult and present hazardous situations for the rescuer.

OEC technicians are trained in basic emergency skills:

- Using airway adjuncts
- Assisting patients with medications
- Splinting and bandaging
- Providing emergency care for environmental illnesses and injuries, spinal injuries, and ski/snowboard and other outdoor injuries
- Using special equipment and techniques particular to nonurban rescuers
- Managing prolonged transport
- In some cases, performing **automated external defibrillation (AED)** (▼ Figure 1-3)

The OEC curriculum contains the baseline knowledge and skills identified in the US Department of Transportation (DOT) 1994 *EMT-Basic National*

Standard Curriculum, but is tailored to the nonurban environment. For like topics, the OEC course content adheres to the same standard of training as the **EMT-Basic** course. Although the knowledge and skills presented in this course frequently go far beyond those included in **first responder** courses, all the components of the existing first responder curricula developed by DOT and the American Society for Testing and Materials (ASTM) have been included. The OEC course provides a national standard of training that is also compatible with local operational standards of care and protocols. This level of OEC care—the knowledge, understanding, and skills you acquire—also will serve as solid building blocks for any higher levels of training you might wish to pursue within the **emergency medical services (EMS)** system.

This textbook covers the knowledge and skills that are recommended by the NSP's National Medical Advisory Committee together with additional expert medical reviewers. Nearly all medical subspecialties are represented on the committee, which meets biannually and at other times as needed. The committee, chaired by the national medical director, consists of the division medical advisors plus members-at-large and includes well-known experts on wilderness medicine, altitude illness, and cold weather emergency care.

A knowledge of basic science provides the necessary background on which the more practical concepts and skills of emergency care can be built. An understanding of anatomy, physiology, and especially medical vocabulary are foundations for understanding emergency care principles.

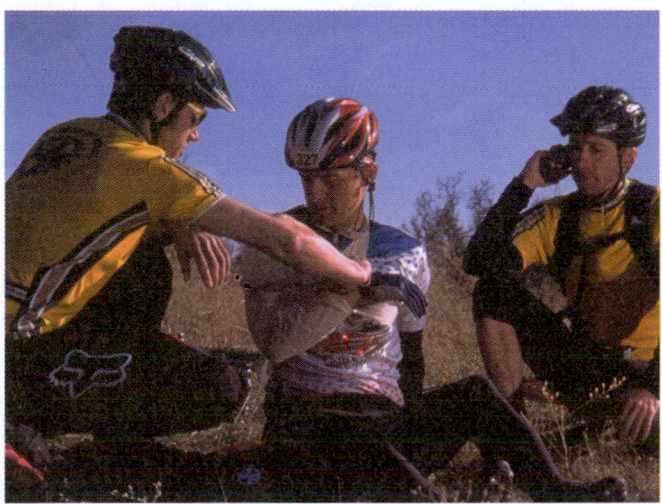

Figure 1-2 As an OEC technician, you will be part of a larger team that responds to a variety of calls and provides a wide range of prehospital emergency care.

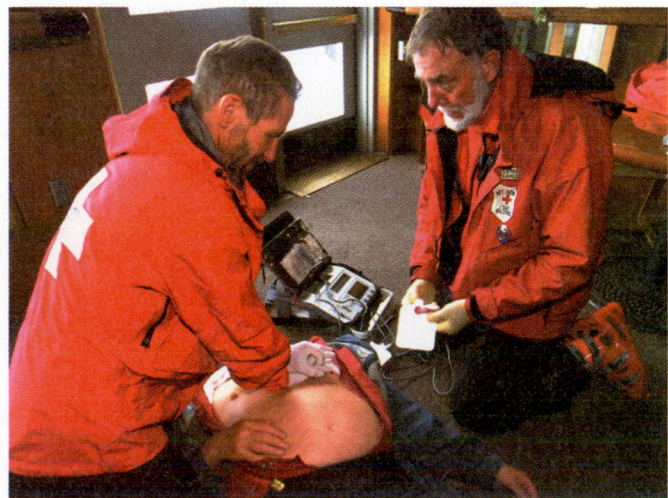

Figure 1-3 Many patrollers are trained to perform automated external defibrillation.

Certain additional emergency care skills may be required of individuals as defined by their management. This could include emergency care in summer months at ski resorts, water sport sites, or mountain bicycle events. The ability to use cardiac defibrillation equipment may also be required. This textbook not only provides the knowledge for the core curriculum, but also other important information that may be taught in an OEC course. The core curriculum is the base content covered in initial ski patrol training. Throughout this text, these topics are identified in the chapter objectives by a 🌲.

OEC Training Focus

OEC practical training is divided into four main categories. This text will take the reader through several components that build on each other. The first and most important category focuses on the care of life-threatening or potentially life-threatening conditions. To deal with these, you will learn how to do the following:

- Size up the scene and ensure scene safety
- Assess the patient's breathing and level of responsiveness
- Establish and maintain an airway
- Provide adequate ventilation
- Provide supplemental oxygen as necessary
- Assess circulation, performing CPR and defibrillation (using an AED) when needed
- Control bleeding
- Identify life-threatening injuries or conditions
- Obtain the patient's pertinent past medical history
- Recognize and provide emergency care for shock
- Recognize and provide emergency care for serious injuries
- Recognize and care for medical emergencies
- Assist patients to take their own medications as needed
- Care for individuals who have water emergencies, including near drowning
- Care for hypothermia and related conditions
- Care for altitude-related medical illness

The second category of training covers conditions that, although not life-threatening, are key components of emergency care or are necessary to prevent further harm before the patient is moved. You will how learn to do the following:

- Dress and bandage wounds
- Care for lacerations
- Care for different types of burns
- Care for frostbite
- Identify and care for vertebral or spinal injuries

The third category covers important additional skills that are related to your ability to provide outdoor emergency care. You will develop the following related skills:

- Techniques for safe extrication, positioning, packaging, and securing patients in a toboggan for rapid transport
- Learn triage and mass-casualty protocols and how to use them
- Understand unique illnesses and injuries of pediatric patients and how they differ from adult illnesses and injuries
- Understand the principles of immobilization and splinting
- Learn principles of spinal immobilization and how to immobilize a patient on a backboard
- Understand special populations such as disabled patients and the elderly and their unique needs when providing care

The last category deals with local protocols and other important issues. These include:

- Follow management's direction for local needs
- Follow local protocols developed by local medical directives
- Understand medicolegal and ethical problems
- Learn to proficiently apply rescue equipment
- Learn how to properly equip your rescue pack
- Develop proper communication skills with patients and bystanders at the incident scene and in the first aid room
- Learn how to prepare documents and written reports

The OEC course is performance driven. Completing the assigned reading and study exercises before each class is imperative for a better understanding of content. In class, the instructor will review the key parts of the reading assignment and will clarify any questions you have. Some presentations may be outdoors with a classroom in harsh weather, on steep slopes, and involve difficult extrications. Unless you have carefully read the assigned material, taken notes, and listed questions, you may not fully understand or benefit from classroom presentations, discussions, or outdoor sessions ▶ Table 1-1 .

Table 1-1   Study Tips for Using this Textbook

- Do each assignment diligently and carefully.
- Read the textbook like a resource, not like a newspaper, magazine, or novel; reread important sections. Take notes.
- Study objectives, tables, diagrams, and illustrations.
- Practice all the skill drills.
- Ask your instructor to clarify any questions you note in your reading or in class.
- Take additional notes when the assigned material is expanded upon in class.
- Go back and review the material taught, after class.

The OEC course will include four types of learning activities:

- **Reading assignments** from the textbook, in addition to the classroom presentations and discussions, will provide the necessary knowledge base.
- **Step-by-step demonstrations** will develop hands-on skills that you then need to practice repeatedly in supervised small group workshops.
- **Summary skills sheets** will help you to internalize the sequence of steps in complex skills, thus avoiding errors or omissions.
- **Case presentations and scenarios** will provide a practical environment to apply the acquired knowledge and hands-on skills learned in the classroom.

Certification Requirements

To be recognized and perform as an OEC technician, you must meet certain training and other requirements. The specific techniques, equipment, and local protocols may vary by location and area. You should ask your instructor or contact the area or agency to find out about the specific requirements for the position you seek. Because the OEC program is a prehospital emergency care program, the ability to ski or snowboard is not necessary. However, to become a patroller, you must be proficient as a skier or snowboarder.

To receive the 3-year certification, each OEC trainee must demonstrate the following:

- Successful completion of the NSP national written certification examination
- Successful completion of the NSP practical certification examination

Additionally, you may need to demonstrate additional skills and requirements deemed necessary by local management.

The **Americans with Disabilities Act (ADA)** of 1990 protects individuals who have a disability from being denied access to programs and services that are provided by state or local governments. NSP education programs are not subject to laws regulating **public accommodations**. Nevertheless, wherever possible, NSP desires to enroll any persons who can meet the requirements of the program. Within the significant time and budget constraints of a nonprofit organization, NSP instructors will strive to provide reasonable accommodations to students with disabilities before starting the course. It is incumbent upon prospective students to bring relevant disabilities to the attention of the instructor and to propose and work out a plan with the instructor for reasonable accommodations that will meet the requirements of the program and the needs of the student.

The instructor has discretion to restrict the participation of a student in all or any part of the program. The instructor also may restrict participation where, in the instructor's judgment, the student cannot complete the program objectives even with available reasonable accommodations, or the student's participation will be significantly detrimental to the completion of the program objectives for the other students.

Continuing Education

OEC technicians, in order to maintain their certification, must attend annual OEC **refreshers**. The NSP and its affiliates offer a structured learning environment to accomplish this goal. Each year, one third of the original course curriculum is covered. The OEC technician is able to refresh his or her skills predominately through hands-on participation. Each person must successfully complete three consecutive annual refreshers to maintain an OEC technician card. Also, working closely with other experienced rescuers (shadowing) after you obtain your OEC training will enhance your education.

Whether you take advantage of these continuing education opportunities depends on you. Whether you decide to remain an OEC technician or achieve a higher level of training and certification with the EMS or wilderness programs, the key to being a good prehospital care provider is your commitment to continual learning and increasing your knowledge and skills.

History of OEC

From its inception, the NSP's First Aid Program was the premier snow sport emergency care directive in North America. The principle of "immediate first aid treatment and speedy removal of the injured person in such a way as to keep secondary injury to a minimum" is essential in the outdoor environment.

The NSP began a long and fruitful association with the American Red Cross (ARC) when L.M. Thompson, MD, of the ARC wrote the first edition of *Ski Safety and First Aid* specifically for the NSP. Dr. Thompson, who was the first NSP national medical advisor, wrote the original 1938 edition of the *Winter First Aid* manual, which became the ski patroller's "standard of care." The national medical director, Warren D. Bowman, Jr, MD, wrote the next three editions of the *Winter First Aid* manual starting in 1976.

From the beginning, NSP rescue work was not confined to ski slopes—patrollers helped out whenever and wherever emergencies occurred. Because of the unique outdoor environment, including harsh weather, altitude problems, and steep, sometimes icy terrain, a need was demonstrated for a more specialized education process. The process recognized that the emergency care provided by patrollers occupied a unique position between urban and wilderness emergency care.

As first response care continued to evolve, the public looked to patrollers for better care "on the slope," and thus came the need for a more comprehensive program. By clarifying roles of ski patrols at ski areas, a legal basis was established for the Winter Emergency Care (now Outdoor Emergency Care) program, which prompted the NSP Board to adopt **Winter Emergency Care (WEC)** as the association's emergency care standard of training in 1987. In 1988, National Medical Director Warren D. Bowman, Jr, MD, wrote the first edition of *Outdoor Emergency Care* as a textbook for devising emergency care for people who become ill or injured at ski areas or in other nonurban locations. The original textbook for the WEC program has now evolved into this, the fourth edition of *Outdoor Emergency Care*. Other groups, such as search and rescue personnel, wilderness medical experts, and other outdoor emergency care providers use this text in their courses.

Most of the text in the three earlier editions of this book is credited to Dr. Bowman, now the Medical Director Emeritus of the NSP ▶ **Figure 1-4** . His deter-

mination, devotion, and vision have made this text the most accepted medical reference for the patroller.

Components of OEC

A fundamental aim of the book is to present information in a systematic, logical format to facilitate understanding and attaining knowledge about important and sometimes complicated concepts. Basic science—including anatomy and physiology—is the first building block. After mastering this with its nomenclature, students learn patient assessment.

Because the outdoor care provider frequently operates in severe environmental conditions, the standard EMS approach to assessment reflects this—undressing the patient outdoors may be undesirable. The rescuer needs to actively conserve the patient's body temperature and transport the patient rapidly to an aid room or some other type of shelter. Although the EMS terminology of scene size-up, initial assessment, detailed physical examination, and ongoing assessment is used in this text, the term "rapid body survey" will be retained from the previous edition to indicate a head-to-toe, clothes-on, hands-on body survey done on every patient with

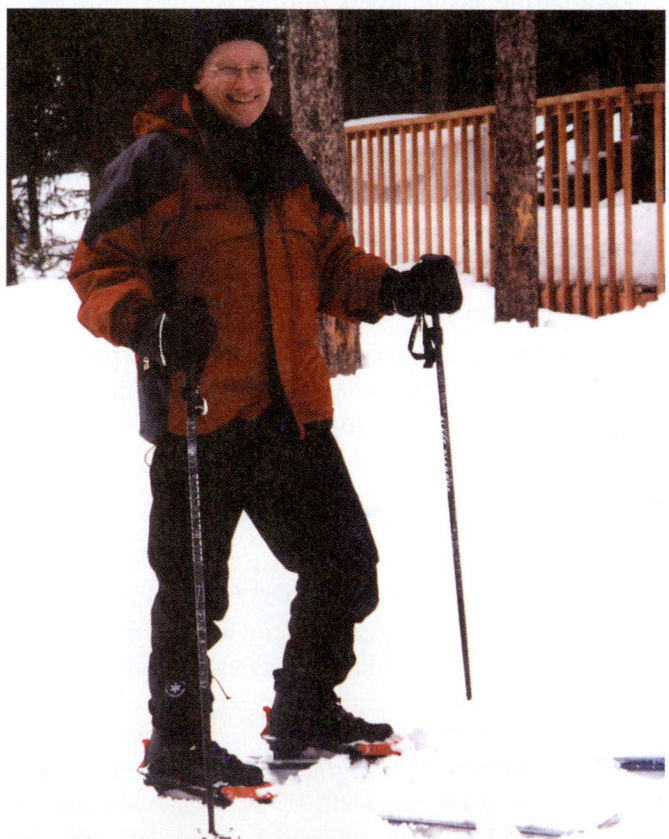

Figure 1-4   Dr. Warren D. Bowman, Jr., was an active patroller in Montana from 1964 to 1990. He is an active member of the American Alpine Club and founding member and past president of the Wilderness Medical Society.

altered vital signs, serious injuries, severe medical problems, and altered level of consciousness for any reason. This is done on-site before transport. In addition, *early* distinction between a conscious patient and a patient with an altered level of responsiveness is emphasized, and the assessment and care of each of these two types of patients is discussed in separate sections.

Once basics are learned, such as vital signs, ABCs (airway, breathing, circulation) and SAMPLE history, more complex issues are approached. These include shock, lifts and loads (including use of splints and backboards), and more complex issues with differing anatomic structures.

A new chapter on interfacing with emergency medical personnel shows the OEC technician how to communicate in the medical system ▶ **Figure 1-5** . Following evaluation and initial emergency care, the patient is frequently referred to a higher level of caregiver. Not only are communication skills important during the transfer of patients, but the ability to work together in patrol rooms or clinics with other medical personnel is essential. Establishing credibility as a patroller with local medical personnel ensures better patient care.

The ski industry is evolving into a full outdoor recreation industry. Now people on snowboards, telemark skis, and snowblades make up a large percentage of the former alpine ski population, giving rise to the all-encompassing and generic term "snowsports" ▶ **Figure 1-6** . Tubing parks and snow-biking areas exist at many winter resorts. Terrain parks, half pipes, shaped skis, and the opening of more off-area terrain are having an impact on traditional patroller training and activities. In summer, mountain biking and swimming at mountain resorts, as well as boating, rafting, and kayaking at nearby lakes and rivers have become a part of resort activities. These sports involve different injuries and patterns of injuries for the rescuer to assess and care for, and make such skills as water rescue and care for water emergencies much more important in OEC than they were formerly.

With the advent of many snowsports programs for physically challenged persons at North American winter resorts, the patroller needs new information and techniques. Understanding the injured or ill patient who is now able to participate in winter or summer outdoor recreation but has physical, mental, and/or emotional disabilities is discussed. The patroller may need to deal with a colostomy bag or evacuate a person who skis sitting down from a chairlift.

As the outdoor recreation industry attracts the younger enthusiast into the sport, the pediatric population has grown ▶ **Figure 1-7** . Children are arriving at ski

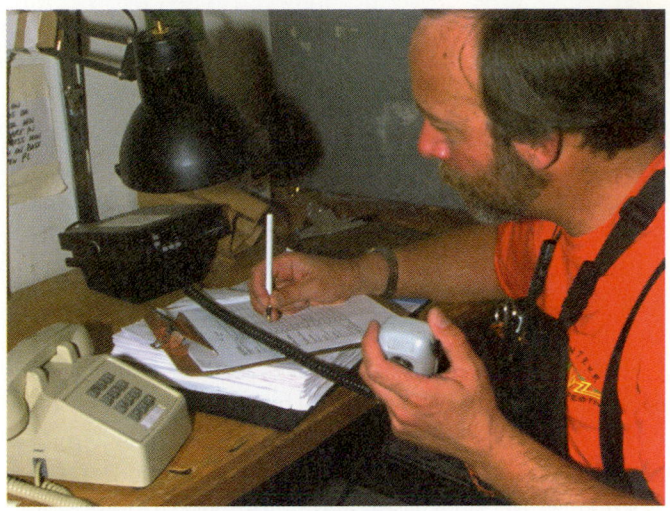

Figure 1-5 Trained dispatchers obtain information about the call and then send responders to the scene as needed.

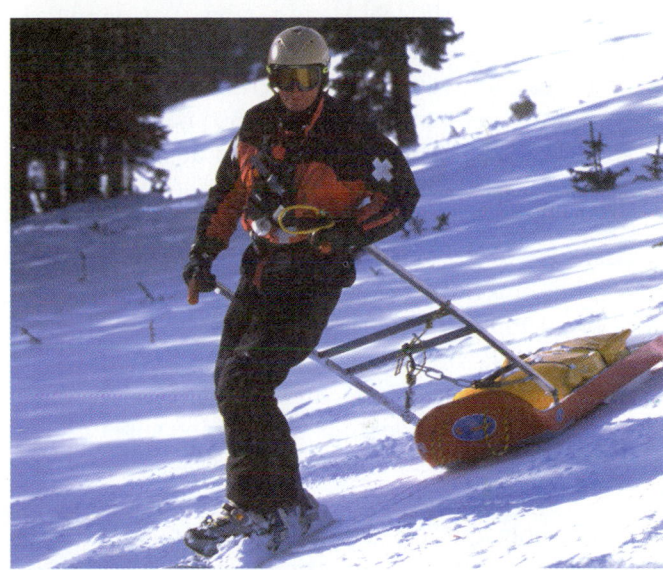

Figure 1-6 As the snowsports population changes, so does the equipment that rescuers use.

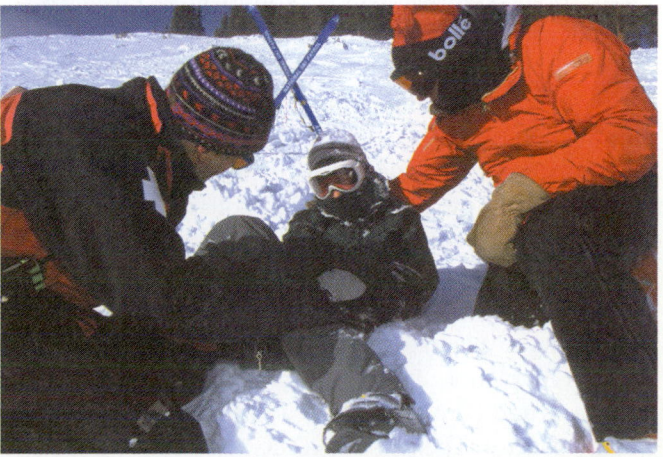

Figure 1-7 Providing health care for children in the outdoor environment requires a different mindset than with adults.

areas by the school bus load. Children are anatomically and physiologically different from adults and care may be psychologically more challenging than caring for adults.

Outdoor Emergency Care and the NSP

Continuous quality improvement (CQI) is a circular system of continuous internal and external reviews of all aspects of OEC training, evaluation, and patient care. The NSP has developed a hierarchy of personnel to facilitate the delivery of its educational programs. The NSP national medical director oversees the National Medical Advisory Committee. This committee is composed of experts, most of whom are physicians with expertise in the various aspects of outdoor medical care. They develop policy consistent with current prehospital emergency care trends within the EMS system.

Each division of the NSP has a medical advisor who also serves on the National Medical Advisory Committee. These individuals are a valuable resource for each geographic area and its special characteristics and needs. Every individual mountain resort is encouraged to have a local medical advisor who helps with local protocols and medical education for his or her patrol. The local physician patroller or advisor works in conjunction with local management to serve the local area's needs. Every ski patrol should seek a local medical director (advisor) to help develop and oversee local protocols.

The NSP's National Outdoor Emergency Care Committee oversees OEC technician training and continuing education. Made up of the division supervisors, this committee consists of teachers, physicians, administrators, and other laypersons who facilitate delivery of the OEC program. This committee develops courses to train instructors and examiners and regularly revises and promotes the teaching process using this text as its primary source of information. As an integral part of the program, the National OEC Committee has created various teaching aids and a study book to accompany the OEC curriculum. The OEC supervisors also manage the quality assurance programs within their divisions with regular coaching and mentoring instructors and instructor trainers during scheduled courses and with networking training sessions in the off-season.

NSP-certified OEC instructors teach OEC courses and continuing education programs in their local regions. Instructor trainers oversee instructors and help instructors to evaluate new OEC technicians before their course completion. Instructor trainers also monitor refreshers and continuing education programs to ensure quality control. The National OEC Committee directs the instructors, instructor trainers, and region administrators through various channels of quality management, administration, and program delivery, providing materials and feedback for improvements of the overall program (▼ Figure 1-8).

OEC is a part of the emergency medical care provided by EMS, advanced life support personnel, emergency department physicians, and other specialists who provide definitive care in the hospital. There are many professional associations that provide research, the establishment of standards for quality assurance, continuing education, and publications for the EMS system. As an OEC technician, you are frequently the first part of the professional continuum of care provided to ill and injured patients in the outdoor environment. The efforts of these people and groups help you to be a better emergency care provider.

With input from the National OEC Committee and the National Medical Advisory Committee, the NSP publishes a quarterly magazine, *Ski Patrol Magazine,* with specific OEC and medical articles, a national education newsletter called *Pointers,* and an *OEC Instructor's Bulletin* for all its certified instructors. Included in these publications is new information, teaching methods, changes in medical protocol, new medical information, and administrative direction.

Every NSP member must demonstrate competence in the knowledge and skill objectives for the OEC course as a basis for becoming a basic patroller (auxiliary or ski/snowboard). Besides the annual OEC refresher, the NSP has other continuing educational requirements. Refreshing Professional Rescuer CPR skills annually is mandatory. If resort management requires patrollers to use an automated external defibrillator, this skill must

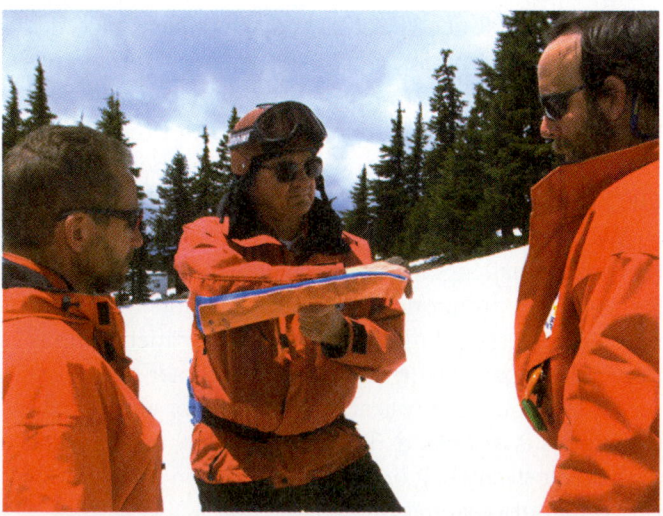

Figure 1-8 The OEC student has plenty of opportunity to interact with OEC instructors to ensure quality learning.

be refreshed as required. Once the season has begun in the outdoor environment, OEC continuing education scenarios are recommended for OEC technicians. As mentioned before, shadowing with more seasoned patrollers after you obtain your OEC training can be very educational. Lastly, the NSP recommends that each ski patrol, or other agency using the OEC standard of training, annually review any specific local protocols as directed by local medical authorities and/or mountain resort management.

Responsibility of OEC Technicians Working at Mountain Resorts

Much effort is required from you, the local patrol or agency, instructors, and examiners before you become an OEC technician. Whether you are a volunteer or a paid patroller, you are a professional. Your responsibility is to make sure patient care is given high priority without endangering your own safety or the safety of others.

People who engage in snowsports easily recognize the white or gold cross on the back of a patroller's jacket ▼ **Figure 1-9** . Another part of the responsibility to fellow patrollers, the patient, other health care professionals, and yourself is to maintain a professional appearance and manner at all times. Wear a clean, easily identifiable uniform consistent with all rescuers at your area. As a rescuer, take pride in your appearance, grooming, and hygiene. Professional appearance helps build confidence and eases a patient's anxiety ▶ **Figure 1-10** . Exhibiting a pleasant and professional demeanor, performing under pressure with composure

and self-confidence, and caring for people as you would like to be treated all are important.

Caring for patients in a professional manner reflects well on you, your patrol, your ski resort, your rescue unit, and the reputation of patrollers and rescuers in general. Keep in mind that in order for an area to need patrollers, it needs customers. People return to resorts where they feel safe, their emergency care needs have been met, and they have been treated well.

Watch rescuers who have been around a long time. They usually exhibit these characteristics; try to emulate them.

Rescuer Tips

Role of an OEC Technician

- Provide a high level of patient care without endangering personal safety or the safety of others.
- Maintain a professional appearance and manner at all times.
- Wear a clean, easily identifiable uniform.
- Exhibit a pleasant and professional demeanor.
- Treat patients and their families with understanding, compassion, and respect.
- Be nonjudgmental and overcome your instincts to react negatively or aggressively.
- Respect patient confidentiality.

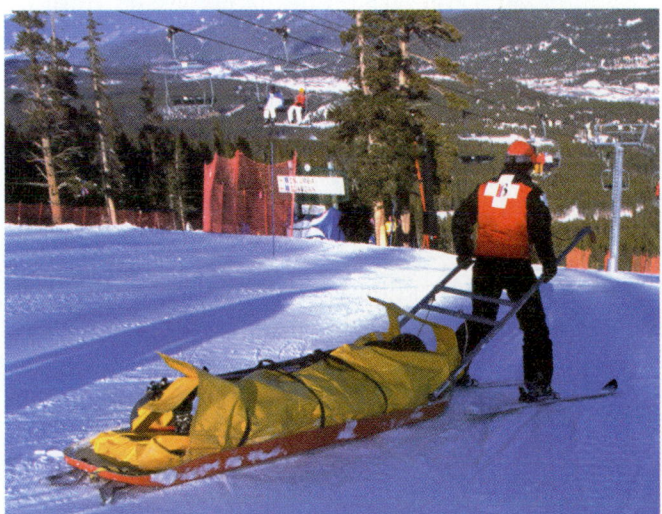

Figure 1-9 The ski patroller, who has successfully evaluated, treated, packaged, and loaded an injured person, is shown skiing down the slope.

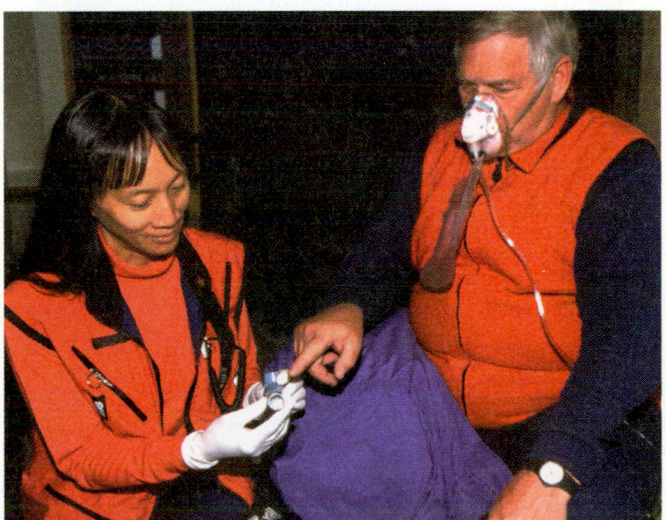

Figure 1-10 A professional appearance and manner help to build confidence and ease patient anxiety.

Emergency Care Responsibilities of the OEC Technician

As an OEC technician, you will be the first health care professional to assess and treat the patient in the outdoor environment. As such, you have certain roles and responsibilities (▼ Table 1-2). Often, patient outcomes are determined by the care that you provide in the field and your identification of patients who need prompt transport.

Patients and families who are under stress need to be treated with understanding, compassion, and respect. Most will reciprocate with cooperation and appreciation. However, some patients and families are uncooperative, demanding, ungrateful, or verbally abusive. When individuals are hurt, ill, anxious, frightened, under the influence of drugs or alcohol, or feel threatened, they or their family members will often react with inappropriate behavior, even toward those who are trying to help them. You must be nonjudgmental and overcome your instincts to react poorly or aggressively to such behavior. Every patient, regardless of his or her attitude, deserves respect, compassion, and understanding as you deliver the best care that you can provide.

Some patients may not appear to you to have an important problem. Remember, however, that the problem is important to the patient, and may interfere with the patient's ability to ski. In this case, simple transport to a base lodge or other shelter may be indicated.

Patient confidentiality must be respected. You must not discuss your findings or disclose information about the patient to anyone but those who are caring for the patient, other medical personnel to whom the care is transferred, or as required by law, ie, the police or social agencies. Be careful not to disclose the name or identity of patients you have treated. Newspaper reporters and radio and television announcers should not be given any information unless the patient permits this. The patient has the right to keep his or her medical problem a private matter.

You should become familiar with your local EMS system, the local clinic, hospital, and any other rescue

---

Table 1-2   Roles and Responsibilities of the OEC Technician

- Size up the scene and situation
- Ensure safety for all at the scene, including yourself
- Observe **body substance isolation** (BSI)
- Rapidly assess the patient's mental status
- Introduce yourself to a conscious patient and ask the patient whether you can help
- Rapidly assess the patient's ABCs
- Provide any essential immediate intervention
- If needed, radio for more help, equipment, or a higher level of medical care
- Perform a thorough, accurate patient assessment
- Obtain the SAMPLE history
- Provide prompt, efficient, prioritized patient care based on your assessment
- Discuss effectively any care or procedures you will perform with the patient
- Interact and communicate effectively with other responders and bystanders at the scene
- Identify "load and go" patients, rapidly package them, and initiate transport without delay
- As needed, apply bandages, splints, and backboards and other devices correctly without causing further harm
- Safely lift and move the patient onto a toboggan and secure him or her prior to transport
- Communicate effectively with the base aid facility for all necessary medical needs
- Continue to assess the patient, including obtaining vital signs frequently, during transport and while waiting for the ambulance in the patrol room
- Document all findings and accurately complete all required medical reports
- Obtain the names and addresses of all witnesses or bystanders involved with the incident
- Give a concise verbal report to the next level of medical care
- Protect the patient's privacy rights

groups that function in your area. Know what equipment these groups use and learn how it is used. Become acquainted with the functions of various staff members and the policies and procedures used in all emergency situations. This experience will help you recognize your place in the emergency care system, understand how your care influences the patient's recovery, and appreciate the importance and benefits of proper prehospital care. It will also show you the consequences of delay, inadequate care, or poor judgment.

Remember that the best, most efficient patient care is achieved through cooperation of all involved parties.

Medical, Legal, and Ethical Issues

This section will introduce you to some of the basic concepts and definitions of the law and how it applies to rescues. It will introduce you to the two main types of civil suits—the negligence suit and the intentional tort suit. It will explain some legal defenses to suits and how certain immunity laws may assist you. Most importantly, if you understand the law, this knowledge can help you to be alert and warn you of risky situations so that you may avoid them.

All rescuers know a basic rule of emergency care is to "do no further harm." You intend to save lives and rescue the injured and ill. Despite your good intentions and best efforts, mistakes happen. Mistakes can cause additional harm. Your intentional acts even when you mean no harm, may cause additional harm. When someone suffers additional harm, that person may be able to sue you, go to court, and collect money as his or her remedy.

When a person wrongfully intends to cause an injury, this is called an **intentional tort**. For example, when Bill hits John during an argument and John sustains a broken nose, this is an example of an intentional tort. Harm can result from good intentions as well. Should rescuer Bill force a bandage on Larry, after Larry clearly refuses emergency care as a competent adult, this is also an intentional tort. The additional harm may be only an insult or a violation of Larry's right to refuse treatment, but this is still an injury for which Larry could sue and be awarded money. Normally, people want emergency care. When someone does not want emergency care, we must be very careful to honor the request unless we know of a legal reason to properly override the refusal. Those exceptions will be discussed later in this chapter.

The unintentional tort or **negligence suit** can result when a person is harmed as a result of another's negligent actions, although the harm was unintentional. For example, rescuer Bill puts a quick splint on John, who

asks for help, but the splint is very loose and the knee is further injured during the toboggan ride to the patrol room. Rescuer Bill did not want or intend for this injury to happen. This tort or injury is called negligence, and the resulting legal action is called a negligence tort. As rescuers involved in emergency care, general rescue work, and also in the training of other rescuers, we need to focus on both intentional and negligence torts so we will be able to manage the risk and reduce or prevent such torts before they happen.

Can a rescuer be sued? Yes. That possibility is present in every activity of life. Compared to most of life's activities such as driving a car or repairing a vehicle, providing rescuer services (including patrolling) carries very little risk of being sued.

It is impossible for a rescuer to completely eliminate all risk of being sued. Our system of justice allows any person the right to file a suit (the right to be heard by the court) simply by paying the court fee and filing the papers in the proper form; therefore, a suit may be filed even when it is without merit. The focus of this section is on how the rescuer can avoid being successfully sued or if successfully sued, how the rescuer can keep from being hurt financially.

The rescuer can minimize the possibility of suit through "risk management." Learning and refreshing OEC skills and following the training standards, guidelines, or rules and regulations established by the NSP for its entire emergency care training activities are two ways to minimize the risk. The following are also ways to minimize the risk of a suit:

- Perform each act in the best and safest way
- Practice to become skillful in all areas of rescue responsibilities, eg, transport and toboggan handling to practicing the safe loading of patients into toboggans
- Act with reason
- Use good judgment
- Focus
- Plan the safest way to perform the activity

Also, and very, very importantly, if the requested duties are performed in the manner specified by area/resort management or rescue organization accordingly, they should be covered by the area, resort, or rescue organization's liability policy. In addition, purchasing personal insurance, educating yourself about the immunity provided by your state, and not acting when the situation is too risky are effective ways to manage risk.

Risk management should begin with understanding the elements of the suit we are trying to avoid. When a negligence suit is filed, the person suing (the **plaintiff**) must prove three things to win:

1. The person being sued had a duty to perform some act (a rescue or emergency care procedure).

2. There was a failure in the performance of that duty (negligence).

3. An injury was caused to the plaintiff by the negligent act, resulting in damages.

This is the basic format of each negligence suit. These three elements of the negligence suit will be discussed in more detail below.

Negligence

Duty to Rescue

The average citizen has no general duty to act or to go to the aid of another person unless that citizen has a legal relationship to the person (such as a child-parent or employer-employee relationship) or he or she was involved in the events that led to the injury of that person regardless of fault. When two skiers collide, most jurisdictions require both people to remain at the scene and render limited aid to the other regardless of who is at fault. Another skier passing the incident scene who is not involved usually has no legal duty to remain at the scene.

Patrollers in uniform are under a duty not to ski past an incident scene. They are not considered in the class of the average citizen, but they occupy a special legal status when they are on patrol or are seen by the public to be patrollers. This special status obligates them to perform the duty to perform a rescue or provide patient care. This duty may be imposed by state statute or it may be created by the implied or written contract between the resort and the guest. The writing that creates the rescuer's duty may be as simple as a lift ticket or it may be a lengthy written agreement signed between the resort and a tour group. Some states follow the law or doctrine of "public reliance" whenever a uniformed rescuer is in view of the public.

This legal doctrine of public reliance is very old. It is based on the following: people will tend to help those they see in trouble, even though there is no law that demands they go to their aid and it is human nature for people not to go to the aid of someone when trained rescuers are seen responding or in the area. The typical person by nature will pass a bad accident and not stop when there is a police car, fire truck, and

an ambulance on scene. This typical person would rely on the police, fire, and medical professionals to render aid. Based on this doctrine, if you wear the insignia of the local rescue squad or local ski patrol and it is visible to the public or if the public knows you are present at the area because the rescue/ski patrol presence is visible, the general public would rely on the rescue squad/patrol to act and the law requires the rescue squad/patrol to act. You may refuse to act only if there is a threat to your safety.

Do you have to respond to the rescue when you are not on duty? The answer is slightly more difficult depending on your particular state. Some states require certain individuals who are licensed by the state to render emergency care regardless of their on- or off-duty status. In effect, the state says you are always on duty. Other states require you to act when on duty but not generally when you are off duty unless, by your uniform or other insignia in view of the public, you appear to the public to be on duty. If you appear to be or show a sign of being on duty, you must respond. The law might consider a sign of being on duty to include something as small as a special license plate, window decal, and badge or insignia pin worn in public. If you walk to the patrol room wearing your patrol parka, you should expect to be recognized as being on duty regardless of your true status, and in those cases do not be surprised if by law you are expected to respond. Failure to respond in such a situation might be considered negligence. It is a good idea to have an understanding of your state's statutes in this situation.

Once a rescue or emergency care has begun, all states require you to continue your care until one of the following occurs:

- All the care needed is given and there is no legal duty to do anything else,

- The patient is transferred to another caregiver who has equal or higher training and certification, or

- The patient is delivered to a medical treatment facility.

Any failure to continue care is abandonment. **Abandonment** is the intentional stopping of care without legal excuse and is an intentional tort. Informed refusal by a competent person allows legal abandonment and will be discussed in detail at another point in the chapter. The rescuer or rescue unit that inappropriately abandons a patient is liable to the patient for all of the resulting harm caused by the abandonment. Most states also impose sanctions against the individual rescuer.

Duty to Train Safely

Duty and Training Rescuers

Trainers have a general duty not to injure trainees or expose them to unreasonable risks or dangers. Each trainee has a duty not to cause injury to himself or herself while training and to keep the trainer informed of his or her physical, mental, and emotional status.

The duty between trainers and candidates is complex. Training requires the trainee to be challenged, to grow, to be stretched, and to exceed the trainee's current skill and ability level. For growth to occur, trainers by necessity must require trainees to attempt to exceed their current level of skill. This always carries some risk and danger. Patrolling or service with a rescue unit, without regard to the training aspect, carries the inherent risk of injury, illness, or death for the rescuer or caregiver. Danger is part of being an active rescuer. It may be the danger of being exposed to an illness or the danger of being present in the slide area of a potential avalanche to perform a rescue. Learning to meet, manage, and safely conquer the dangerous situations of patrolling and finding reasonable ways to overcome the danger is a core component of training. Thus, danger in training is always present and must be recognized by each trainee and thoughtfully managed. Each trainee must realize and accept responsibility for his or her own personal risk management.

Who is in the best position to manage the danger, the trainer or the trainee? The answer depends on who is in the best position to avoid injury. The trainer and trainee must recognize one simple fact: only the person being trained can know, moment to moment, what physical, emotional, or mental changes are taking place in himself or herself. Only the person being trained can know and appreciate the effect that stress, illness, injury, drugs, or fatigue is having as the training progresses. Being aware of these factors is necessary for the trainee to avoid unacceptable risk of injury, and the communication of these factors to the trainer is vital. Each trainee must continually monitor himself or herself and, when necessary, be willing to warn the trainer about current status changes. Trainers should begin each session by emphasizing the following points.

- The trainee should acknowledge any physical, mental, or emotional status that could place him or her at risk.

- The trainee should immediately inform the trainer in the event he or she is not comfortable with any request made by the trainer.

- Both the trainer and the trainee must manage

Rescuer Safety

Each trainee has a duty not to cause injury to himself or herself while training and to keep the trainer informed of his or her physical, mental, and emotional status.

the risks of training, and no one should ever attempt any portion of training that is believed to be risky.

The trainer has a duty to assist the candidate in this risk management process, but when the trainee does not make a good decision, the trainer must be willing to step in and manage the risk. The trainer has the obvious duty to challenge the candidate to grow. The trainer has a higher duty to be vigilant for signs and symptoms that the trainee is about to enter the zone of unacceptable risk. What should happen when either the trainer or the trainee believes training is about to cross into a zone of unacceptable danger? Training should be stopped or altered!

Both the trainee and the trainer must be willing to stop or alter training to reduce risk. This is called risk management. Safety is the first and highest priority. A trainee may fail a test or not be allowed to advance with the rest of the class because a situation has been determined to be unsafe. Trainers using NSP education programs must recognize individuals have individual limits. Thus, the trainer may have to stop training even when the trainee wants or requests to continue. Training should be started or resumed only when both the trainer and trainee have considered all of the facts and are comfortable with the continuation of the training.

Negligence

Negligence is failing to provide care equal to the standard of care expected of the rescuer who is a reasonable person, fully trained, and is acting under similar circumstances. In a lawsuit, after proving the plaintiff was owed a duty by the rescuer, the plaintiff must then prove how the rescuer failed to perform the task up to the standard of quality expected of the reasonable rescuer. The "reasonable rescuer" is defined as a good rescuer who is not perfect but is fully trained. The jury or judge trying the case will determine if you meet this standard. How do you avoid being found negligent? Ask yourself as you perform any rescue task, "If I were a spectator observing this conduct, would I expect the reasonable rescuer to perform it this way?" If you are not confident in your abilities to provide the expected standard of care, you are in jeopardy of being found negligent.

Exceeding the Scope of Your Training
Negligence can occur when you are exceeding your training or going beyond what you are permitted to do under OEC training guidelines or the protocol laws of your state. Any time you render emergency care to another person, this has the remote potential of being declared the practice of medicine. Each state has laws that regulate what is considered the practice of medicine and what is considered emergency care. The authors of this manual have been careful to limit you to what is emergency care. However, the law of your state could outlaw, prohibit, or not allow an emergency care procedure, or could require you to be licensed to perform it. In those cases, your state law prevails over this manual and you must not cross into that restricted area of practice without proper certification.

Be careful to perform only the emergency care authorized by the organization responsible for each individual rescue event. Individuals with advanced training or licenses are advised to seek clarification from their area management or their licensor as to what advanced procedures or protocols they can and cannot follow in a particular venue or under the direction of a particular management.

Causing the Injury
The final element of a tort in a negligent act is the cause of the injury. If the negligence does not directly cause the injury, you will not be held responsible for the injury even if all of the other elements of the case are present and proven. If you ski a toboggan much too fast for the conditions, hold on with only one hand, wear improper boots and bindings, take an unnecessary jump, lose both skis, fall down, let go of the toboggan, most would agree that you were negligent, but these actions would not be enough to prove a suit of negligence if they did not result in the injury. If the toboggan picks up speed and slams into a tree, injuring the patient, this is a direct cause and you are liable for the loss.

This concludes the three elements necessary to prove liability in a civil, negligence suit. Once the plaintiff proves the three elements, the case is not over. One may avoid liability by various means that will be discussed in the following sections of this chapter. There is one defense that may allow you to escape

from the suit almost as soon as it has been filed and prior to the first taking of evidence. This defense is called immunity.

Immunity
Immunity will forgive your negligence or your error and stop the suit. Many states have an immunity law called the "Good Samaritan" law or act. This law is based on the philosophy that charitable deeds should not be punished. When a person voluntarily goes to the aid of another, the rescuer should not be held liable for errors and omissions that are made in giving good faith, emergency care. People should be encouraged, not discouraged, to go to the rescue of another person in need. The state trades or cancels the right of a person to hold the rescuer responsible for a bad outcome in exchange for immunity that encourages people to step forward and perform acts of rescue or first aid. These laws are great gifts but are usually strictly drawn or written and most often very strictly interpreted. They will not protect you if you are not clearly covered, if your conduct is intentional, or if your conduct is so wanton, gross, or willfully negligent that the law considers the act outside the immunity.

Immunity varies greatly from state to state. You must not only read the law very carefully, but also be familiar with the case law of your state to understand how the limitations may or may not apply to the rescuer. It might give immunity to a volunteer rescuer but exclude paid rescuers, or it may be limited to certain types of rescues. Your state's immunity may include special emergency care procedures that are authorized only for certain organizations or members with certain certifications. For example, some states grant immunity for administering epinephrine, using an automated external defibrillator, or giving glucose; other states withhold it. Be familiar with your state law on this issue. If you have exceeded your training or scope of authority, most states withdraw immunity.

Consent and Refusal
Every competent person has the ability (within certain limits) to decide how he or she wants to live within society. This right to decide the path of one's life includes the right not to be forced to live in a certain way or accept help from others. The basic civil right to be left alone even exists when it involves the right to be left alone to die. Thus, under most circumstances, before a rescuer begins treatment of any competent, conscious person, **consent** must be obtained from that person so the patroller does not violate the patient's right to be left alone.

Failing to obtain consent prior to treatment violates the inherent right of the injured person to be left alone. Failure to respect this right can be both a civil rights violation and a criminal offense. Touching someone who does not desire to be touched is battery. **Assault** is placing someone in a position in which he or she reasonably fears a battery will occur and consent is not given to being placed in that position. Assault and **assault and battery** are both intentional torts. Each is a civil wrong, a civil rights violation for which a person can be sued and be forced to pay damages to the wronged or injured person. If a rescuer forces emergency care on someone who does not want help and is competent to refuse the aid, the rescuer is viewed by the courts as causing the injury of insult or violation of the civil right to be left alone. The good intentions of the rescuer are not a defense.

If being sued does not make you hesitate—be warned. A person who competently refuses aid or is not asked if they wish aid and nonetheless receives it (whether forced or not) could prefer criminal charges against the aid provider. Battery could include a situation in which you failed to obtain consent, put on a quick splint for a broken leg, took a pulse, or administered oxygen to a person having difficulty breathing. To ensure that you have consent, simply ask, "May I help you?" and wait for the patient's positive response. Also, if the emergency care might require complex care and treatment, be sure to explain all that will be involved so that the patient can be shown to have given full and complete informed consent to the treatment. Obtaining a full and complete informed consent is accomplished in one of the following ways.

When in doubt, it is always best to proceed with treatment. When there is doubt as to the patient's competence, but there is evidence present that you can explain and document that makes you believe the patient is not mentally competent and there is risk of serious injury or death if treatment is not rendered, it is best to proceed with treatment. Here it is important to have other rescuers witness the event, if possible. This is the best course of action because providing treatment is a much more defensible position than failing to treat a person who is later found not to be competent. Failure to treat a person who is not competent is a form of negligence or abandonment.

Expressed Consent

Expressed consent (or actual consent) is the type of consent in which the patient expressly authorizes you to provide care or transport. It must be **informed con-**sent, which means that the patient has been told of the potential risks, benefits, and alternatives to treatment and has given consent to treatment. The legal basis for this doctrine rests on the assumption that the patient has a right to determine what is to be done with his or her body. The patient must be of legal age and able to make a rational decision.

A patient might agree to certain emergency medical care but not to other care. For example, a patient might agree to be removed from a car but refuse further care. An injured person might agree to emergency care at home but refuse to be transported to a medical facility. Informed consent is valid if given orally; however, it may be difficult to prove. Having the patient sign a consent form does not eliminate your responsibility to fully inform the patient.

The information needed on the consent or refusal form should include the full nature and extent of the injury to the extent you are able to know, what emergency care was given, and what treatment or referrals to medical treatment were made. If there is any refusal of emergency care or refusal to pursue future treatment, it becomes very important to indicate all problems you communicated to the patient that might result to the patient if treatment is not finished. This should be written in detail and signed by the patient.

Implied Consent

When a person is unconscious and unable to give consent, or when a person not competent to decide about treatment is ill or injured, the law assumes that the patient would consent to care and transport to a medical facility if he or she were conscious or competent. This is called **implied consent**. Implied consent is limited to true emergency situations and is appropriate when the patient is unconscious, delusional, unresponsive as a result of drug or alcohol use, or otherwise physically unable to give expressed consent. However, many things may be unclear about what represents a "serious threat to life." Legal proceedings would likely revolve around that question. This becomes a medicolegal judgment, which should be supported by the rescuer's best efforts to obtain consent. **Medicolegal** is a term that relates to medical jurisprudence (law) or forensic medicine. In most instances, the law allows the spouse, a close relative, or next of kin to give consent for an injured person who is unable to give consent. Refusal of your offer to render emergency care also may be implied. For example, a patient's action in pulling his or her arm from your splint may be an indication of refusal of consent.

Minors and Consent

Because a minor might not have the wisdom, maturity, or judgment to give valid consent, the law requires that a parent or legal guardian give consent for treatment or transport. However, in some states, a minor can give valid consent to receive medical care, depending on the minor's age and maturity. Many states also allow emancipated, married, or pregnant minors to be treated as adults for the purposes of consenting to medical treatment. You should obtain consent from a parent or legal guardian whenever possible; however, if a true emergency exists and the parent or legal guardian is not available, the consent to treat the minor is implied, just as with an adult.

A good solution to the problem of obtaining consent to treat minors at a ski resort or any recreational event or area is to have group leaders or chaperones bring signed consent-to-treat forms with them when they host a group of minors. This may be a good practice regardless of whether the parents are with the group or not. Reaching a parent by telephone or trying to find a parent on the ski slope can be difficult and frustrating for the patrol and prolong the painful wait for treatment for the child. Having the medical consent form handy is a quick and easy solution to immediate emergency care for minors. Remember, however, that you must never withhold lifesaving care.

Mentally Incompetent Adults

Assisting patients who are mentally ill, in behavioral (psychological) crisis, under the influence of drugs or alcohol, or developmentally delayed is complicated. An adult patient who is mentally incompetent is not able to give informed consent. From a legal perspective, this situation is similar to those involving minors. Consent for emergency care should be obtained from someone who is legally responsible, such as a guardian or conservator. In many cases, however, such permission will not be readily obtainable. Many states have protective custody statutes allowing such a person to be taken, under law enforcement authority, to a medical facility. Know the provisions in your area. Remember that when a true emergency exists, you can assume that implied consent exists.

The Right to Refuse Treatment

Mentally competent adults have the right to refuse treatment or withdraw from treatment at any time. However, these patients present you with a dilemma. Should you provide care against their will and risk being accused of battery? Should you leave them alone? If you leave patients alone, you risk being accused of negligence or abandonment if their condition becomes worse.

If a patient refuses treatment or transport, you must make sure that he or she understands, or is informed about, the potential risks, benefits, treatments, and alternatives to treatment. You must also fully inform the patient about the consequences of refusing treatment and encourage the patient to ask questions. Remember that competent adults who refuse specific kinds of treatment for religious reasons generally have a legal right to do so.

You may also be faced with a situation in which a parent refuses to permit treatment of an ill or injured child. In this situation, you must consider the emotional impact of the emergency on the parent's judgment. In this and virtually all cases of refusal, you can usually resolve the situation with patience and calm persuasion. You may also need the help of others, such as law enforcement officials.

There will be times when you are not able to persuade the patient, guardian, conservator, or parent of a minor or mentally incompetent patient to proceed with treatment. In this case, you must obtain the signature of the individual who is refusing treatment on an official release form that acknowledges refusal. You must be sure to document any assessment findings and emergency care that you provided. You must also obtain a signature from a witness to the refusal. You should then keep the refusal with the patient care report. In addition to the release form itself, you should write a note about the refusal on the patient care report. If the patient refuses to sign the release form, the best you can do is inform your medical director or risk manager and thoroughly document the situation and the refusal. Report to medical control or area management, and/or follow your local protocols with regard to this situation.

Chapter *Sweep*

Ready for Review

This text has been developed as the primary resource for Outdoor Emergency Care (OEC), the National Ski Patrol's course designed to train outdoor prehospital emergency care providers. OEC training is used by a wide variety of outdoor enthusiasts to provide emergency care in settings as diverse as ski areas, whitewater rafting, mountain bike events, and even the Winter and Summer Olympics. OEC training occupies a unique niche in emergency care somewhere between ambulance-based urban care and remote wilderness care. OEC technicians are trained in basic emergency skills and, for like topics, adhere to the same standards of training as outlined by the US Department of Transportation's (DOT) EMT-Basic National Standard Curriculum. OEC is a solid building block for higher levels of training within the EMS system.

This text has been prepared under the auspices of the NSP's National Medical Advisory Committee. It stresses a basic science background as a foundation for practical concepts and emergency care skills. Local management may specify and require additional skills. This text will be the basis of the core curriculum for an OEC course as well as a resource for other information that may be taught in a course.

OEC training is divided into four main categories: the care of life-threatening or potentially life-threatening conditions, the care of conditions that are not immediately life-threatening, skills that facilitate the delivery of care in the outdoor setting, and finally, the issues of local protocols. OEC is performance driven, and classes may occur outdoors in different settings. OEC training will include reading, demonstrations, and the use of summary skills sheets and case presentations and scenarios. OEC students will receive a 3-year certification upon successful completion of the written and practical exam. In order for OEC technicians to maintain certification, they are required to complete annual refreshers that cover one third of the course content.

This fourth edition of OEC builds on previous texts and incorporates many of the terms used in EMS systems today. New information is presented to stay current with the changing face of outdoor recreation, including adaptive skiers, interfacing with EMS, and the well-being of the rescuer. As before, quality improvement and quality management are important themes in OEC and procedures exist to incorporate them into instruction and evaluation.

As a trained OEC technician, you will have many responsibilities to fulfill in your quest to provide high quality emergency care to patients. These include, but are not limited to, ensuring safety for all at the scene, including yourself; rapidly assessing patients' conditions; performing needed medical interventions professionally; evacuating patients in a timely manner; and fulfilling any procedures and documents required by your management. You are directed to protect a patient's right to privacy at all times.

While providing emergency care to sick and injured patients is very altruistic, certain rules and limitations apply. The basic rule is to "do no further harm." Certain immunity laws provide some protection legally, but it is the responsibility of all rescuers to follow training standards and perform emergency care in the best and safest way. A sense of personal risk management should be used to evaluate and act in a way that reduces a rescuer's exposure to legal action. OEC technicians should be familiar with the terms negligence, abandonment, duty to act, and all forms of consent. Be aware that minors and unresponsive or incapacitated patients may require a different form of consent. Finally, any competent adult may refuse any or all emergency treatment at any time. It is an OEC technician's responsibility to honor these wishes and to treat all patients humanely and professionally.

Chapter *Sweep*

Vital Vocabulary

abandonment Failure to continue service or care of another that by law one is required to complete.

Americans with Disabilities Act (ADA) Comprehensive legislation that is designed to protect individuals with disabilities against discrimination.

assault Placing an individual in a position without consent in which the individual fears physical harm will occur.

assault and battery The illegal infliction of injury to a person by physical means, the act of which was initiated with a wrongful or evil intent.

automated external defibrillation (AED) A portable electrical device that is capable of analysis of heart rhythms by an on-board computer and making the medical decision to use or withhold the use of an electrical shock capable of stopping the uncontrolled fibrillation of the heart muscle. This device is designed to be used out of the hospital environment by lay persons with a minimum of training.

body substance isolation (BSI) The techniques and equipment for isolating the rescuer's body from contact with moist body substances of a patient.

consent Permission to render care.

continuous quality improvement (CQI) A system of internal and external reviews and audits of all aspects of the OEC program and the EMS system.

core curriculum The essential curriculum content that must be covered in every OEC course.

emergency medical services (EMS) A multidisciplinary system that represents the combined efforts of several professionals and agencies to provide prehospital emergency care to the sick and injured.

EMT-Basic An EMT who has training in basic emergency care skills, including automated external defibrillation, use of a definitive airway adjunct, and assisting patients with certain medications.

expressed consent A type of consent in which a patient gives express authorization for provision of care or transport.

first responder The first trained individual, such as a police officer, fire fighter, or other rescuer, to arrive at the scene of an emergency to provide initial medical assistance.

implied consent Type of consent in which a patient who is unable to give consent is given treatment under the legal assumption that he or she would want treatment.

informed consent Permission for treatment given by a competent patient after the potential risks, benefits, and alternatives to treatment have been explained.

intentional tort A wrong inflicted by one person against another person (a victim) after thoughtful consideration and directed by a conscious, reasonable mind. The wrong or violation must cause a physical, mental, or emotional injury to the victim, and if these elements are all present, the law gives the victim a remedy, usually in money.

medical director (advisor) The physician who oversees prehospital protocols at a local resort or who authorizes or delegates the authority to perform medical care in the field .

medicolegal A term relating to medical jurisprudence (law) or forensic medicine.

National Ski Patrol (NSP) A federally chartered education association servicing the snowsports and outdoor recreation communities by providing exceptional education programs.

negligence Lacking in due care or concern.

negligence suit A court action that decides the issue of who should be responsible for damage caused to a person (plaintiff) by someone (defendant) who commits a careless or reckless act. This suit allows the court to determine not only who is at fault, but also the amount of money required to be paid to restore or compensate the plaintiff.

OEC technician An individual who has training in basic emergency care skills, including using airway adjuncts, assisting patients with medications, splinting, providing emergency care for environmental illnesses and injuries, spinal injuries, and ski and other outdoor injuries, using special equipment, performing techniques used in difficult or prolonged transport, and in some cases, automated external defibrillation.

Outdoor Emergency Care (OEC) A comprehensive prehospital care education and training program for nonurban settings.

plaintiff The party that institutes a suit in a court.

public accommodation A legally recognized business, organization, group, or other legal entity that affords a service, trade, or work to the general public, or may be controlled by the federal government because of its connection with interstate commerce or trade.

quality control Ensuring that the appropriate emergency care standards of training are met by OEC technicians on each call; this is the responsibility of the medical director.

refresher An annual continuing education program designed by the NSP and required for its members to review one third of the entire OEC curriculum.

Winter Emergency Care (WEC) The original name of the OEC course. Also used to identify the core curriculum that targets the winter environment.

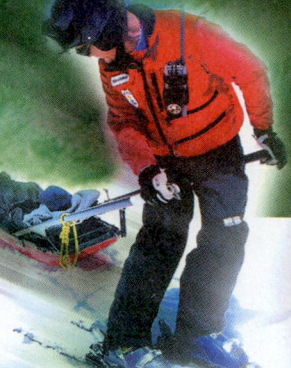

Assessment in Action

You are an OEC technician who patrols in the winter for a local resort. On a hot summer day, you are enjoying an afternoon off, when the doorbell rings. A process server hands you a summons.

She explains you are to report for depositions at a downtown law office in 2 weeks. Someone is suing two other patrollers and the ski resort where you patrol. The amount of money demanded in the suit gets your attention. The date of the incident was 2 years ago. You cannot recall the events and the name of the injured person is not familiar to you. You begin to worry, "Will I be sued?" You see the words "negligence" and "tort." What do they mean in this context? What should you know about civil suits as a patroller?

1. After a call to the ski area, you determine that the basis of the lawsuit is not an intentional tort. An intentional tort could occur if a:
   A. rescuer harms a patient while performing needed care improperly.
   B. patient refuses treatment and suffers further injury.
   C. patient accidentally injures a rescuer while he or she is performing needed care.
   D. rescuer causes harm during treatment to a patient who has refused care.

2. During the deposition, the plaintiff's attorney asks you if the patient had been abandoned. Legally, abandonment occurs when there is a failure to continue giving care. Which of the following situations could lead to a finding of abandonment?
   A. Discontinuing needed care without the consent of the patient
   B. Transferring a patient to another caregiver who has less training and certification
   C. Not delivering a patient to a medical treatment facility if a proper transfer of care has not occurred
   D. All of the above

3. The ski area's attorney advises you that as a volunteer rescuer, you are protected from a civil judgment by your state's "Good Samaritan" law. In what instances might protection be denied?
   A. You are a paid employee of the ski area.
   B. The patient died as a result of the original injuries.
   C. The patient has filed a suit against you.
   D. An error of omission has occurred during the act of providing emergency care.

4. If you are called upon to treat a minor and the patient's parent or legal guardian is not available to authorize such treatment, what type of consent allows you to treat this patient?
   A. Actual consent
   B. Implied consent
   C. Informed consent
   D. Expressed consent

5. A question during the deposition centers on the patroller's duty to provide care to the ski area's guests. Which of the following conditions may not constitute a duty to act? Mark all that apply.
   A. Skiing on your day off while wearing your aid belt with its distinctive white cross visible.
   B. Attaching a window decal to your car that identifies you as a member of a rescue organization.
   C. Bypassing the scene of an accident when other rescuers are present and caring for the injured.
   D. If providing care, you would expose yourself to an immediate threat to your own safety.

Challenging Questions

6. During the ensuing trial, a witness recounts that she heard the plaintiff tell one of the patrollers that he "only wanted a ride down" and refused to have a splint applied to his injured extremity. How might this apparent refusal impact a negligence lawsuit? What would be the course of action if the patient were visibly intoxicated or otherwise mentally impaired?

Points to Ponder

After a particularly busy, warm spring day at the ski area, the patrol director asks if you can step into her office. You chat about the spring break crowd and how this was perhaps the busiest day the ski area has had this season. The patrol director inquires about an incident that you responded to where the appropriate medical equipment was delayed and you chose to transport the patient without using a special splint even though your training standard requires its use. Could your act of omission result in a judgment against you and the ski area if a lawsuit were filed? What if you were a volunteer? Would the situation be different if the patient had refused medical treatment but demanded immediate transport to the base lodge? What would happen if the

refusal were not documented? What would happen if you treated a different patient with a similar injury using the splint?

Issues Legal Liability, Documentation, OEC Training Standards, Patient Care Standards

Online Outlook

The National Ski Patrol System, Inc. (NSP) is a federally chartered education association serving the snowsports and outdoor recreation communities by providing exceptional education programs. Learn more about the National Ski Patrol and the services it provides by completing Exercise 1 at **www.OECzone.com**.

The Well-Being of the Rescuer

Cognitive

🌲 **1.** List possible emotional reactions that the rescuer may experience when faced with trauma, illness, death, and dying (p 43).

🌲 **2.** Discuss the possible reactions that a family member may exhibit when confronted with death and dying (p 43).

3. State the steps in the rescuer's approach to the family confronted with death and dying (p 46).

4. State the possible reactions that the family of the rescuer may exhibit due to their outside involvement in EMS (p 53).

🌲 **5.** Recognize the signs and symptoms of critical incident stress (p 51).

🌲 **6.** State possible steps that the rescuer may take to help reduce/alleviate stress (p 52).

🌲 **7.** Explain the need to determine scene safety (p 54).

8. Discuss the importance of body substance isolation (BSI) (p 55).

9. Define the term "universal precautions" and describe when it is appropriate to use such measures (p 55).

10. Describe the steps the rescuer should take for personal protection from airborne and bloodborne pathogens (p 55).

11. Identify appropriate task-specific personal protective equipment (p 57).

12. Identify the benefits of an exposure control plan (p 55).

13. List the mechanisms of disease transmission (p 55).

14. List the components of postexposure management and reporting (p 59).

🌲 **15.** List the personal protective equipment necessary for each of the following situations (p 55):
- Hazardous materials
- Rescue operations
- Exposure to bloodborne pathogens
- Exposure to airborne pathogens

🌲 **16.** Discuss the ways in which the body produces, loses, and conserves heat, and how they are important in adjusting to cold and hot weather (p 28).

🌲 **17.** List the ways in which the body adapts to high altitude (p 27).

🌲 **18.** List the signs and symptoms due to rapid, short-term exposure to high altitude (p 28).

🌲 **19.** Discuss the principles and practical methods of dressing for cold and hot weather (p 31).

🌲 **20.** Discuss the importance of good nutrition and adequate fluid supply when working in the outdoor environment (p 39).

🌲 **21.** List the ways to secure safe water in the outdoors (p 41).

🌲 **22.** List the components of a good exercise program (p 42).

Affective

🌲 **23.** Explain the rationale for serving as an advocate for the use of appropriate protective equipment (p 55).

🌲 **24.** List the factors to be taken into consideration when it is necessary to adapt to the outdoor environment (p 24).

Psychomotor

🌲 **25.** Given a scenario with potential infectious exposure, the rescuer will use appropriate personal protective equipment. At the completion of the scenario, the rescuer will properly remove and discard the protective garments (p 57).

26. Given the above scenario, the rescuer will complete disinfection/cleaning and all reporting documentation (p 59, 77-78).

🌲 These are core concepts in initial patrol training.

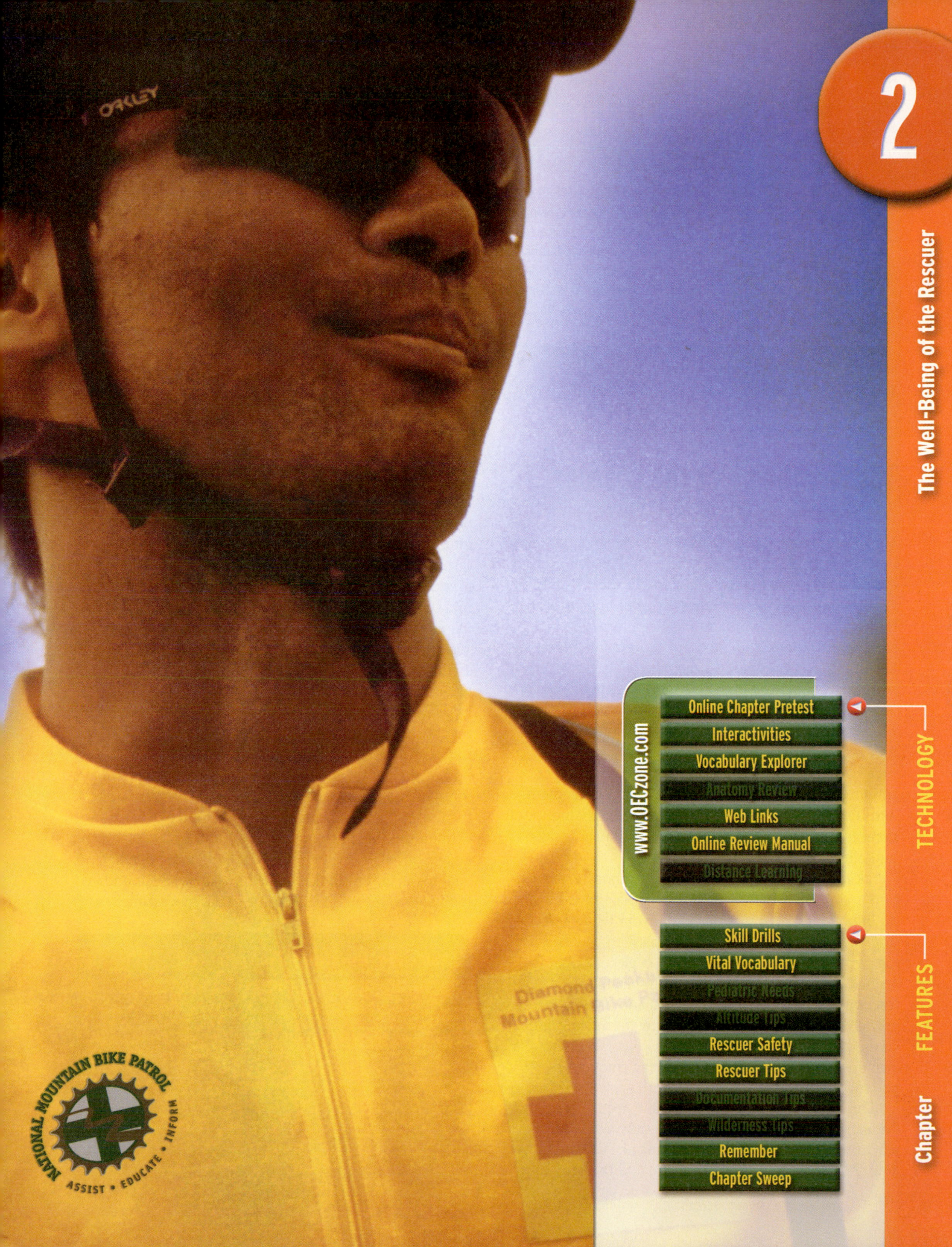

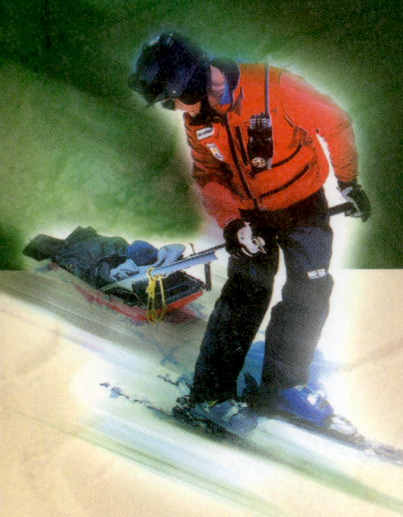

You are the rescuer

It is a cold day on a weekend in January. You have just finished sweeping the upper mountain at your ski area and are looking forward to starting home. Darkness is falling. A call comes over the radio that there is a teenaged skier missing. According to his companions, he skied off-area 3 hours ago heading for a steep drainage and was supposed to meet them an hour ago at the base lodge. The local search and rescue group is organizing an off-area rescue operation. Experienced rescuers will be needed to look for his ski tracks and follow them through very difficult terrain.

This chapter will help you become aware of some of the dangers inherent in these activities and help you answer the following questions:

1. How should you dress for this search?

2. What equipment and supplies should you take along? For yourself? For the lost skier?

The Well-Being of the Rescuer

Adapting to the Outdoor Environment

Most of us spend a large part of our lives in temperatures that can be regulated, where food, water, and clothing are easy to obtain, and where shelter is always available. As a result, our knowledge of how to adapt to the outdoor environment has been forgotten— sometimes at considerable cost. Equipment failure, becoming lost, or a natural calamity such as a severe storm may suddenly impose complete dependence on whatever personal resources are immediately at hand. Many people regard the outdoor environment as hostile, especially in severe weather, when in fact it is merely indifferent and impartial. Therefore, proper training and equipment, experience, good judgment, and the possession of at least a rudimentary amount of common sense can prepare anyone to function safely and effectively in the outdoors.

Because the main purpose of this textbook is to train you to give emergency care in the outdoor environment, an important task is to protect you, your fellow rescuers, and your patients from outdoor hazards. These hazards vary greatly, ranging from personal neglect to environmental and human-caused threats to health and safety. You will also learn about the mental and physical stresses that you must cope with when caring for the sick and injured. Death and dying challenge you to deal with the realities of human weaknesses and the emotions of the survivors.

This chapter examines the specific needs of the human body and how they can be satisfied in outdoor environments where the weather may be severe, oxygen low, food and water hard to obtain, and the need for

physical exertion extreme (▼ Table 2-1). The human body needs a constant supply of oxygen, a stable internal body (core) temperature, water, food, and a certain amount of self-confidence, faith, and the will to live. For comfort and optimum performance, there must be body integrity, ie, good physical condition and freedom from injury and illness. While each of these survival requirements is unique and complex, they are all interrelated. For example, because most deaths occurring outdoors in cold weather are due to injury, hypothermia, or both, it is most important to maintain body temperature and integrity. However, dehydration, starvation, and exhaustion make it difficult to maintain body temperature and also interfere with the rational thought and agility required to prevent emergencies. Insufficient oxygen becomes a contributing factor at extreme altitude or in the case of suffocation due to avalanche burial or carbon monoxide poisoning due to cooking in an unventilated shelter. And while abundant food and water are of little value to a hypothermic

Table 2-1 Survival Requirements

- Oxygen
- Stable body temperature
- Water
- Food
- Confidence, faith, and the will to live
- Body integrity

person dying from insufficient clothing or shelter, the lack of food and water will eventually be disastrous in an otherwise healthy and comfortable person.

Moreover, during a survival experience, lack of self-confidence, faith, and the will to live may engender a sense of panic and a defeatist attitude, which tend to prevent one from taking timely survival actions such as preparing a shelter or lighting a fire. Poor physical condition, injury, and illness interfere with the body's ability to maintain a stable body temperature by shivering or other muscular activity. These factors also hamper gathering wood, building shelter, and performing other necessary actions.

The essentials for hot weather survival are a stable core temperature and water. To stabilize your core temperature you must wear proper clothing, have adequate shelter to protect against heat *gain*, and be able to evaporate sweat and radiate heat from the skin to promote heat *loss*. A heart and circulatory system capable of sustaining increased circulation of hot blood to the skin is essential.

In addition, enough water must be available to maintain blood volume, sweating capacity, and urine output.

Oxygen

Air at sea level has a barometric pressure of 760 millimeters of mercury (mm Hg) and is composed of 21% oxygen and 78% nitrogen. The remaining 1% is made up of a small amount of carbon dioxide and trace amounts of rare gases such as argon and neon. From the standpoint of human survival and well-being, the most important physical property of oxygen is its **partial pressure**, which is the fraction of total air pressure due to oxygen. At sea level, this is 160 mm Hg (0.21×760 mm Hg). When we breathe, the inspired air travels to the most distant parts of the respiratory tract—the alveoli (the smallest air sacs of the lungs)—where the air is diluted by alveolar carbon dioxide and water vapor. This dilution lowers the partial pressure of oxygen (PO_2) from 160 to 104 mm Hg (▼ **Figure 2-1**).

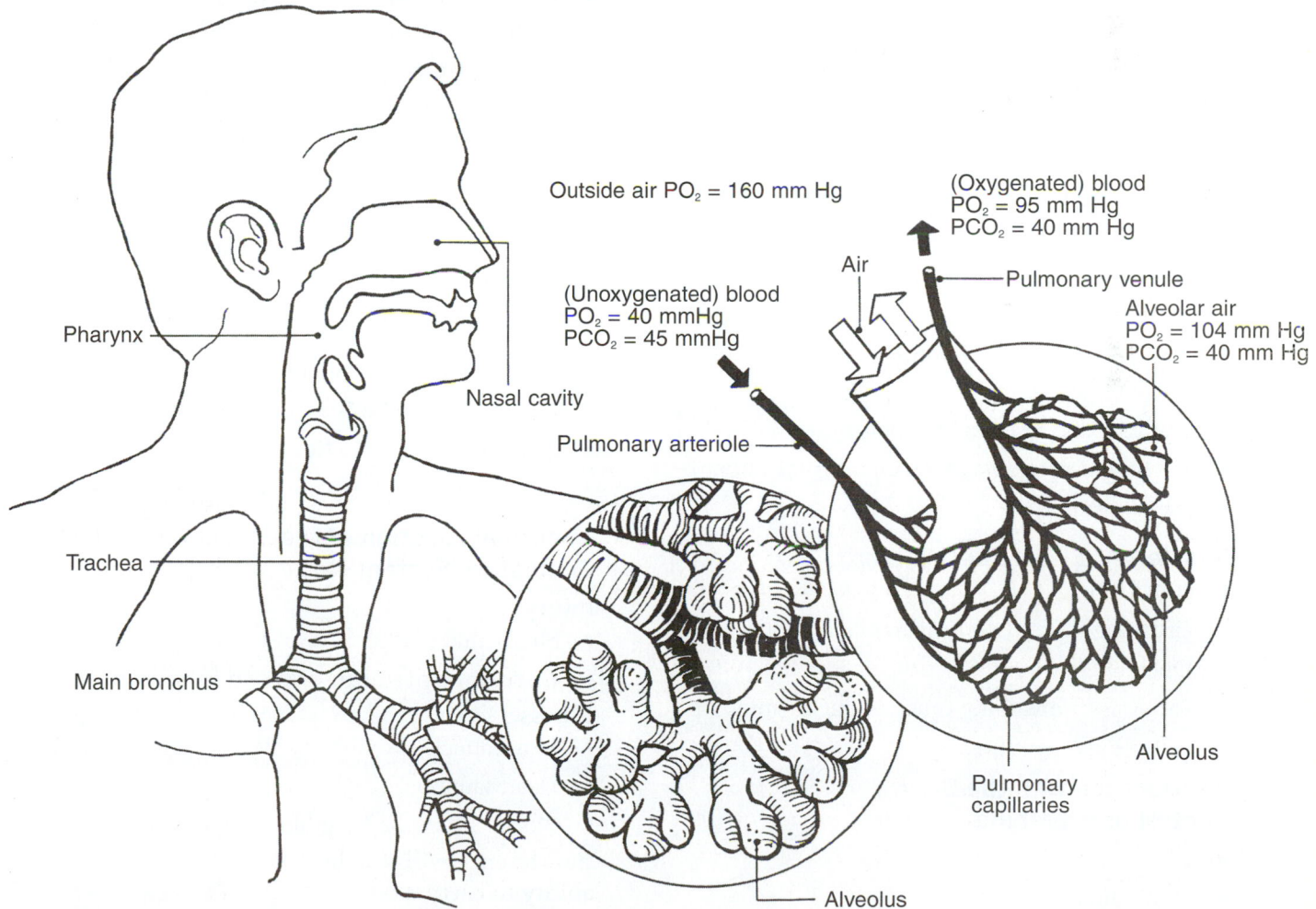

Outside air PO_2 = 160 mm Hg

(Oxygenated) blood
PO_2 = 95 mm Hg
PCO_2 = 40 mm Hg

Air

(Unoxygenated) blood
PO_2 = 40 mmHg
PCO_2 = 45 mmHg

Pulmonary venule

Alveolar air
PO_2 = 104 mm Hg
PCO_2 = 40 mm Hg

Pharynx

Nasal cavity

Pulmonary arteriole

Trachea

Main bronchus

Alveolus

Pulmonary capillaries

Alveolus

Figure 2-1 Changes in partial pressure of oxygen and carbon dioxide between outside air and blood.

A major function of blood circulation is to carry oxygen from the air *to* the body cells and to carry carbon dioxide back *from* the body cells to the air. The exchange of oxygen and carbon dioxide between air and blood occurs in the alveoli. The blood in the tiny alveolar vessels (capillaries) is separated from the alveolar air by two thin membranes: the walls of the capillaries and the walls of the alveoli, which together have a thickness of only a few microns (about 1/10,000″).

An important physical law of the behavior of gases states that any gas tends to diffuse from an area of higher pressure to an area of lower pressure. Thus, the higher partial pressure of oxygen (PO_2) in the alveolar air drives oxygen across the thin intervening membranes into the oxygen-poor capillary blood, increasing its PO_2 from 40 mm Hg to 104 mm Hg. Similarly, the slightly higher partial pressure (45 mm Hg) of carbon dioxide (PCO_2) in the capillary blood drives the carbon dioxide from the blood into the alveolar air ($PCO_2 = 40$ mm Hg), where it can be excreted through the lungs. As the newly oxygenated (arterial) blood circulates through the body, cells extract about 60% of its oxygen (equivalent to 64 mm Hg of PO_2), so that the PO_2 of deoxygenated (venous) blood falls to only 40 mm Hg.

If the circulatory and respiratory systems are normal, a sea level atmospheric PO_2 of 160 mm Hg is more than

---

Table 2-2 Common Causes of Interrupted Tissue Oxygen

Low Oxygen Supply in Outside Air
- High altitude
- Avalanche burial
- Poorly ventilated snow shelter or other confined space
- Malfunction of SCUBA gear
- Near drowning
- Replacement of oxygen by another gas such as carbon dioxide

Upper Airway Obstruction
- Blockage by tongue in an unconscious person
- Aspiration of food, vomitus, dentures, or other foreign material
- Swelling due to burn or other injury
- Swelling due to allergic reaction or infection
- Facial trauma

Interference with Chest Integrity or Function
- Crushing injury (rib fracture, flail chest)
- Open chest wound
- Paralysis of breathing muscles due to spinal cord injury

Interference with the Brain's Control of Breathing
- Head injury
- Meningitis
- Stroke
- Upper cervical spine injury

Interference With Lung Function
Sudden:
- Pneumonia, lung hemorrhage, or pulmonary edema fills up alveoli with blood, pus, or fluid
- Lung collapses because of pressure from blood, fluid, or air in the chest cavity
- Asthma or bronchitis partially plugs bronchi

Chronic:
- Fibrous tissue replaces normal lung tissue
- Emphysema destroys some alveoli and narrows bronchi
- Lung tumor replaces normal lung tissue

Lower Airway Obstruction
- Inhaled foreign body
- Swelling due to infection
- Inability to cough up blood, pus, or mucus

Abnormal Function of the Circulatory System
Injury
- Shock due to blood loss
- Direct injury to heart or blood vessels

Illness
- Heart attack
- Heart failure
- Blood clot in the lung blocking blood flow

Interference with the blood's ability to carry oxygen
- Anemia
- Carbon monoxide poisoning

adequate for normal body function. However, at high altitude where there is insufficient oxygen in the air, or with interruption of normal transport pathways due to injury or illness, serious problems may occur. ◄ Table 2-2 lists common causes of interrupted oxygen supply, which are discussed in detail in subsequent chapters of this textbook.

EFFECTS OF HIGH ALTITUDE ON THE BODY. As you ascend from sea level, the barometric pressure drops by 20 mm Hg for each 1,000′ (305 m) of elevation ◄ Figure 2-2 . At 10,000′ (3,048 m), the barometric pressure is two thirds that at sea level; at 18,000′ (5,486 m) it is only half. The percentage of oxygen in the air remains constant at 21%, but the partial pressure drops along with the barometric pressure.

If a person who is accustomed to low altitude is suddenly taken to high altitude without supplemental oxygen, the lowest alveolar PO_2 at which he or she can remain conscious is about 40 mm Hg, equivalent to an altitude of 18,000′. At altitudes of 25,000′ (7620 m) or higher, the alveolar PO_2 is so low that consciousness is immediately lost and death soon follows unless the person descends rapidly or receives supplemental oxygen.

Despite these limitations, there are permanent human habitations at close to 17,000′ (5,181 m) in the Chilean Andes and Tibet. Humans have climbed to the top of Mt Everest—29,028′ (8,847 m)—without supplemental oxygen. Such feats are possible because, if given enough time, the body is able to adjust to high altitude through **acclimatization**, a process that starts within several days of arrival at altitude but takes several weeks or longer to complete. During acclimatization:

• the rate and depth of breathing increases (**hyperventilation**), which

• removes carbon dioxide faster and adds oxygen rapidly enough to raise the alveolar PO_2. Then,

• the blood becomes more alkaline, which increases the hemoglobin's ability to take up oxygen.

• Later, the rate and depth of breathing are reset at a permanently higher level,

• the body produces more red blood cells to carry oxygen to the tissues, and

• the actions of the heart and skeletal muscles become more efficient.

People who live at high altitude develop larger chests and lungs, have higher pulmonary artery pressures, and have *thicker* blood than lowlanders because of the increased number of red blood cells.

▼ Figure 2-3 shows what happens to alveolar PO_2 and PCO_2 as you ascend to high altitude. At about 8,000′ (2,438 m), the PO_2 has fallen enough to stimulate an increase in breathing rate and depth, thus slowing the drop in PO_2 but increasing the drop in PCO_2 as the hyperventilation washes CO_2 out of the lungs. This process corresponds with the common observation that around 8,000′ you "start to feel the altitude."

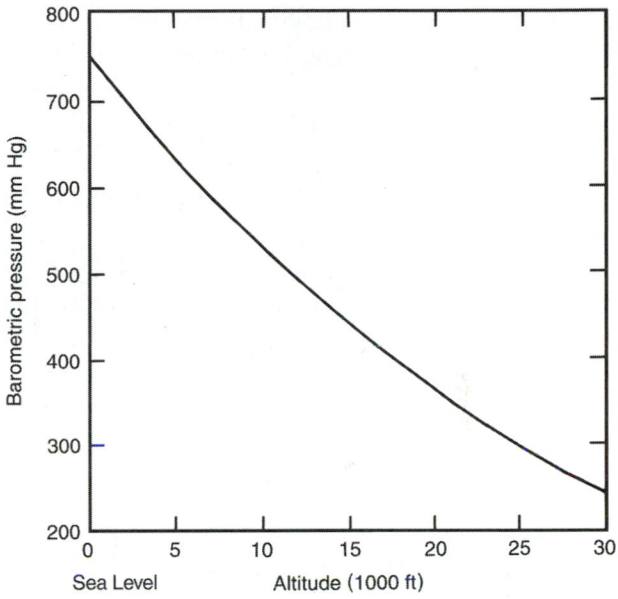

Figure 2-2 Relationship between barometric pressure and altitude. Reproduced with permission from Pugh, L.G.C.E., *Journal of Physiology*, London 1957; 135, 590-610.

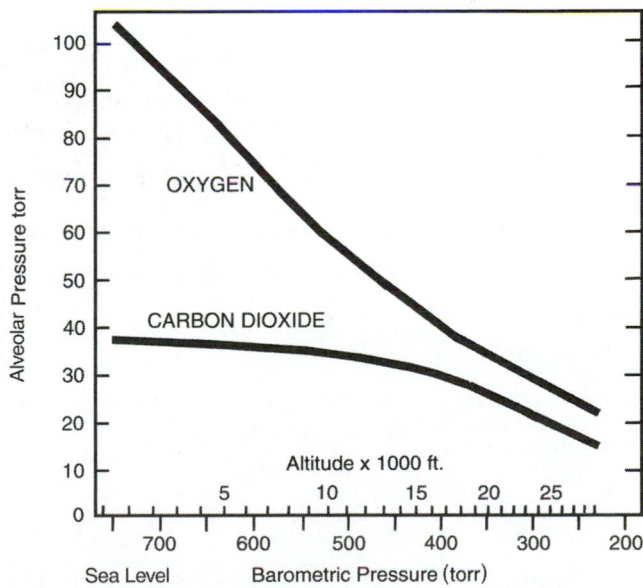

Figure 2-3 Changes in alveolar gases at altitude. Reproduced with permission from Houston C.S., *Going Higher*, 3rd ed. Boston, MA, Little, Brown and Co. 1987; 80.

Serious illnesses due to high altitude commonly begin to occur at 7,500' to 8,000' (2,286 to 2,438 m) but may develop at altitudes as low as 6,000' (1,829 m). They should be suspected in people who become ill within a day or two of arriving at these (or higher) altitudes, including anyone who becomes ill after flying from a low-altitude home to ski or snowboard at 8,000' or higher.

During the first day at high altitude, rest more than usual. Avoid strenuous exertion, get plenty of sleep, increase your fluid intake, and avoid alcohol for the first few days. Although **hypoxia** (lack of oxygen) is an important stress factor at high altitude, its effects are often hard to separate from those of hangovers, cold, high winds, dehydration, exhaustion, hypothermia, malnutrition, and other stress factors that may develop in the mountains.

A slow ascent to high altitude is the most effective way to ensure acclimatization. Schedule a rest day after ascending from sea level to 10,000' (3,048 m), and limit additional altitude gains to about 1,000' (305 m) per day. The average climber should "carry high and sleep low" when climbing, ie, ferry loads of supplies to a high cache and return to a lower camp for the night, because the altitude at which you sleep strongly affects acclimatization. Also, be sure to anticipate the possibility of extreme conditions and prepare for them by bringing adequate supplies of food, shelter-building equipment, and extra clothing.

Because of exertion, lower humidity, and an increased breathing rate, the amount of water lost through the skin and lungs increases at high altitude; therefore, water requirements are much higher than normal. The time it takes to melt enough snow for an adequate water supply is time well spent. Meals and snacks should be frequent, nourishing, and tasty. Clothing should be protective, and shelters should be warm, windproof, and easy to construct or assemble.

During rapid, short-term exposure to high altitude, the decrease in PO_2 can lead to the following signs and symptoms:

- fatigue
- weakness
- headache
- loss of appetite
- nausea
- vomiting
- insomnia
- shortness of breath on exertion

- waxing and waning of the breathing depth, with regular periods during which breathing ceases (Cheyne-Stokes respirations)

These generally occur to some extent in anyone who goes rapidly from sea level to 8,000' (2,438 m) or above.

Regulation of Body Temperature

The term **metabolism** refers to the sum of the living body's chemical reactions that produce or use energy. The term **basal metabolism** means the minimal amount of energy that must be produced to maintain basic body functions such as breathing, blood circulation, digestion, and stable body temperature. Through effective mechanisms of heat production and heat loss, humans and other warm-blooded creatures are able to maintain a relatively constant internal body temperature. Humans, unlike frogs, snakes, and other cold-blooded creatures, do not have to lie in the sun to warm up enough to move.

The human body, then, can be thought of as a heat-generating and heat losing machine whose relatively constant internal temperature is the result of opposing mechanisms that increase or decrease body heat production, body heat loss, and the addition of heat from the outside. Through these mechanisms, the body can almost always regulate its core temperature successfully despite seasonal outside temperatures that can range from subzero to well over 100° F (37° C). However, physiologic mechanisms that protect against excessive heat are better developed than those that protect against excessive cold.

When studying body temperature regulation, it is convenient to think of the body as a **shell**, which consists of the skin, muscles, and extremities, and a **core**, which includes the central nervous system, heart, lungs, liver, and other important internal organs (▶ **Figure 2-4**).

Basal body heat production, which averages 50 kilocalories (kcal or Calorie) per square meter of body surface per hour, is the result of never-ceasing internal metabolic processes. Additional heat production when needed to prevent body temperature from falling can be produced by the following:

- muscular activity such as shivering and exercise
- eating
- exposure to cold

Shivering can increase body heat production four to five times above basal level, vigorous exercise up to 10 times. Eating produces heat both by digestion of food and by metabolism of digested food. Cold exposure increases hunger and the release of hormones that stimulate heat production. The body can also draw heat from external sources such as the sun, a fire, a stove, and hot food and drink.

Body heat is lost to or gained from the external environment in five ways: conduction, convection, evaporation, radiation, and respiration.

CONDUCTION. Conduction is the direct transfer of heat by contact, either from the warm body to a cooler object or to the cool body from a warmer object. Contact with metal or other materials that conduct heat rapidly may cause frostbite at low temperatures or burns at high temperatures. You can decrease the speed of heat conduction from the body by adding clothing and increase it by removing clothing.

> ## Remember
>
> Body heat is lost to or gained from the external environment in five ways:
>
> - Conduction
> - Evaporation
> - Respiration
> - Convection
> - Radiation

CONVECTION. Convection refers to the transfer of heat when air (or water) of a different temperature from that of the body moves across the body's surface. When the air temperature is low and there is no shelter, exposure to high winds can cause rapid heat loss, a condition known as "windchill." As with conduction, you can decrease the speed of heat transfer by convection by adding insulating clothing (especially if it is windproof) and increase it by removing clothing. Rapidly moving cold water can cause even faster heat loss than rapidly moving cold air.

EVAPORATION. Evaporation is the loss of heat when water, perspiration, or another volatile liquid on the body's surface is converted to vapor. Because of the high heat of vaporization of water (586 kcal are required to vaporize 1 L of water), you can lose considerable heat through evaporation of sweat or other water from the skin. Evaporation is increased in the presence of wind and low relative humidity, is decreased in high relative humidity, and is a major source of beneficial heat loss in hot climates. In the desert, sweat may not be visible because it evaporates so quickly. Frostbite caused by conduction and evaporation can occur rapidly when very cold, volatile liquids with freezing points below that of water, such as gasoline, are spilled on the skin.

RADIATION. Radiation refers to the transfer of heat to or from the body by infrared waves. You can lose major amounts of heat by radiation from uncovered skin. This may be beneficial in hot climates, but when you are exposed to cold temperatures you need adequate clothing to prevent radiation heat loss. Warm headgear and protection for the neck are especially important because an uncovered head or neck is a major source of heat loss. Conversely, in hot climates you gain considerable heat by radiation unless you are protected from the sun by clothing or shelter.

RESPIRATION. Respiration contributes a small amount to heat loss when cool inhaled air is warmed to body

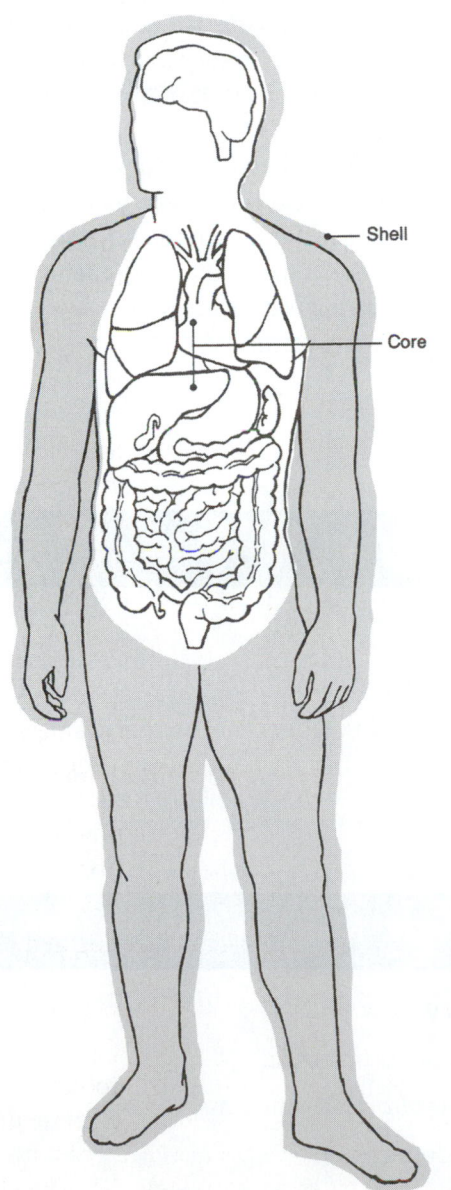

Figure 2-4   Shell and core concept in body temperature regulation.

temperature before being exhaled. The amount of heat lost depends on the outside air temperature and the rate and depth of breathing. You can also gain heat by inhaling hot air.

The body has both **voluntary** and **involuntary** methods of decreasing or increasing heat loss ▼ Tables 2-3 and 2-4 . The most important organ for stabilizing body temperature is the human brain. Behavioral changes such as adding or removing clothing, seeking shelter, lighting a fire, eating and drinking, and regulating the amount of heat produced by muscular activity are more important than the body's automatic adjustments to excessive heat or cold.

In a moderate, comfortable environment, the body's core temperature is kept stable by constant, small, involuntary adjustments in metabolic rate, muscular activity, perspiration, and skin circulation. When you feel chilled, your body augments heat production by increasing the metabolic rate slightly, by creating a compulsion to stamp your feet or move around, and eventually by shivering. At the same time, your body reduces heat loss by limiting perspiration and restricting blood circulation to the shell. If your body temperature continues to fall, you feel compelled to curl up into a ball to expose a smaller surface area to the environment. During this time, your brain should be telling you to decrease heat loss by putting on more clothing for insulation and wind protection, by stopping and seeking shelter, and to increase heat gain by building a fire and having something to eat. Note that some of the body's automatic adjustments to reduce heat loss tend to preserve the core temperature at the expense of the shell temperature.

When the body overheats, these mechanisms are reversed. Your body increases heat loss by increasing circulation to the skin and extremities and increasing perspiration. It also decreases heat production by resisting physical activity—making you feel sluggish and languid—so that heat-producing muscular activity decreases. Your brain should be telling you to seek shelter from the sun, remove clothing, and fan yourself.

The mechanisms of body temperature regulation work best if you are well fed and hydrated, properly rested, and in good physical condition through regular exercise. If these mechanisms fail to maintain body heat within the optimal range, injury can occur in the form of frostbite and hypothermia at one extreme or heat stroke at the other.

In summary, the body has three methods for avoiding dangerous degrees of cooling: it can increase internal heat production, add heat from the environment, or decrease heat loss. Of these, the most energy-efficient method is to *decrease body heat loss*. ▶ Table 2-5 summarizes the ways to do this.

ADJUSTING TO COLD WEATHER. Insulating garments prevent heat loss caused by conduction, convection,

---

Table 2-3 Methods of Decreasing Body Heat Loss

Involuntary	Voluntary
Decrease perspiration	Add clothing
Shunt blood away from the shell	Seek shelter from chilling mechanisms
	Decrease body surface area (by curling into a ball)

Table 2-4 Methods of Increasing Body Heat Loss

Involuntary	Voluntary
Increase perspiration	Expose more skin surface
Shunt blood to the shell	Seek shelter from warming mechanisms
	Remove clothing

and radiation. Because air conducts heat poorly, the best garments for cold climates are those made of materials that trap and maintain a layer of still, warm air around the body. The best garments also

- are lightweight,
- are easy to dry,
- wick water well (to remove perspiration from the skin), and
- retain insulating ability even when wet.

Remember that garments insulate in both directions and may slow rewarming by outside heat unless removed.

The preferred materials for insulating garments fall into two general groups: fibers woven into a fabric and fibers used as filler in quilted garments such as jackets and vests. Some fibers such as polyester can be both woven into a fabric and used as filler.

Blowing wind can turn a cold day even colder. As the wind velocity rises, the "effective" temperature drops. This concept, known as the "windchill," refers to the *rate* of heat loss rather than the actual temperature reached, as long as evaporation is not a factor. ▶ **Figure 2-5** illustrates the relationship between actual temperature, wind velocity, and effective temperature at the exposed human face, and underscores the necessity for windproof outer clothing and for seeking shelter during periods of cold and high wind.

Because a body in motion tends to create its own wind, a moving person is more susceptible to frostbite than a stationary one ▶ **Figure 2-6** . There is a marked danger of frostbite developing in 10 minutes at wind speeds easily attained by a snowmobiler or moving snow rider (even on a chair lift) when the temperature is −20° F (29° C). Inadequate clothing, especially facial protection, is a common cause of frostbite in persons riding chair

lifts in cold, windy weather. When the weather is cold, windy, and wet—such as during a severe snowstorm at 32° F (0° C)—conduction, convection, evaporation, and radiation combine to produce rapid heat loss. This environment can be very dangerous for anyone who is unprepared.

To reduce heat loss from radiation and convection, always wear a hat ▶ **Figure 2-7** . At 5° F (−15° C), up to 70% of your body heat can be lost through an uncovered head. This occurs partly because the head has a high blood supply (18% of the heart's total output) and does not reduce its blood flow in response to cold. With this in mind, remember the useful adage "If your feet are cold, put on your hat." In addition, because the large arteries that supply blood to the head lie close to the skin surface in the neck, protect your neck with a high jacket collar or neck gaiter.

Avoid heat loss from conduction by sitting on a toboggan, pack, or log rather than in the snow or on a cold rock or metal object ▶ **Figure 2-8** . Because bare fingers can freeze to metal objects such as ski bindings and crampons, wear thin gloves (glove liners) while adjusting them. Avoid skin contact with gasoline or other volatile liquids with freezing points lower than water, because they will cause instant frostbite through conduction and evaporation.

To reduce heat loss from conduction and evaporation, stay dry or dry off quickly when you become wet in cold weather. Ideally, your outer clothing should be windproof and shed snow and water; however, outer clothing should not be *completely* waterproof because your perspiration won't evaporate. Manufacturers who strive to create the ideal outer garment have a difficult task: to develop fabric that will allow water to pass from the inside out but not from the outside in.

Table 2-5 Practical Ways of Decreasing Heat Loss

- Wear garments made of proper insulating materials: wool, polypropylene, treated polyester, down, Dacron, polyester pile, fleece, foam, etc.

- Avoid cotton.

- Use the layering principle so you can add clothing to prevent chilling or remove clothing to prevent overheating and excessive sweating.

- Protect yourself from the wind.

- Use adequate coverings for body parts with a large surface-to-volume ratio (nose, ears, fingers, toes).

- Avoid getting wet.

- Avoid direct contact with cold substances.

- Avoid excessive respiratory heat loss.

- Avoid alcohol and nicotine.

- Use a personal flotation device or wet suit in water-related sports.

Wind mph	Temperature (° F)																	
Calm	40	35	30	25	20	15	10	5	0	−5	−10	−15	−20	−25	−30	−35	−40	−45
5	36	31	25	19	13	7	1	−5	−11	−16	−22	−28	−34	−40	−46	−52	−57	−63
10	34	27	21	15	9	3	−4	−10	−16	−22	−28	−35	−41	−47	−53	−59	−66	−72
15	32	25	19	13	6	0	−7	−13	−19	−26	−32	−39	−45	−51	−58	−64	−71	−77
20	30	24	17	11	4	−2	−9	−15	−22	−29	−35	−42	−48	−55	−61	−68	−74	−81
25	29	23	16	9	3	−4	−11	−17	−24	−31	−37	−44	−51	−58	−64	−71	−78	−84
30	28	22	15	8	1	−5	−12	−19	−26	−33	−39	−46	−53	−60	−67	−73	−80	−87
35	28	21	14	7	0	−7	−14	−21	−27	−34	−41	−48	−55	−62	−69	−76	−82	−89
40	27	20	13	6	−1	−8	−15	−22	−29	−36	−43	−50	−57	−64	−71	−78	−84	−91
45	26	19	12	5	−2	−9	−16	−23	−30	−37	−44	−51	−58	−65	−72	−79	−86	−93
50	26	19	12	4	−3	−10	−17	−24	−31	−38	−45	−52	−60	−67	−74	−81	−88	−95
55	25	18	11	4	−3	−11	−18	−25	−32	−39	−46	−54	−61	−68	−75	−82	−89	−97
60	25	17	10	3	−4	−11	−19	−26	−33	−40	−48	−55	−62	−69	−76	−84	−91	−98

Frostbite in >>   30 min   10 min   5 min

(**Figure 2-5**) Windchill chart.

Be sure to cover your head, ears, hands, and feet adequately. This counteracts the tendency of body parts with a high surface area-to-volume ratio to lose heat rapidly by conduction, convection, and radiation. Coverings should not be so tight that they restrict blood circulation. When socks and mittens get wet, dry them or replace them with dry ones.

To prevent heat loss through respiration, avoid overexertion and excessively heavy breathing. When temperatures are extremely cold, pull your jacket hood forward to form a "frost tunnel," or use a scarf, facemask, or neck gaiter over your mouth and nose.

You can increase heat production by increasing your level of muscular activity. If possible, walk around, stamp your feet, swing your arms, and wiggle your fingers and toes (▶ **Figure 2-9**). If such activities combined with adding more layers of clothing do not work, consider seeking shelter.

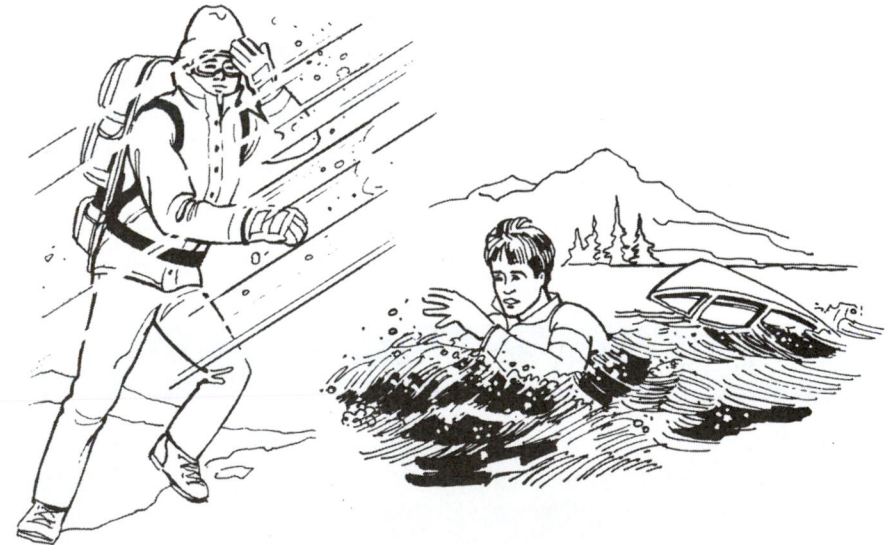

(**Figure 2-6**) The cold, windy, wet outdoor environment can be dangerous to those caught unprepared.

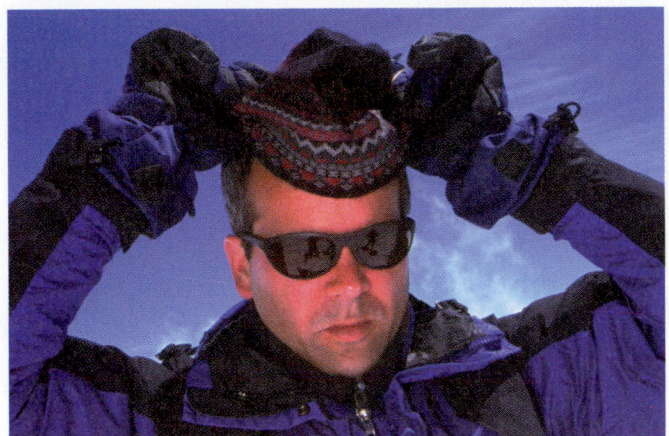

Figure 2-7 Wear a hat in cold weather.

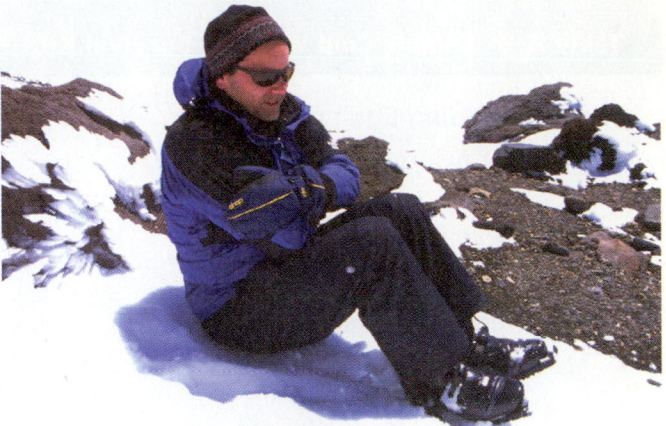

Another way to keep warm is to eat. Food fuels metabolism, and the process of digestion creates heat as well. In cold weather, meals should be regular and snacks frequent. Avoid alcohol because it lowers blood sugar levels, increases heat loss by dilating small blood vessels in the skin, and interferes with judgment. Also avoid nicotine, which constricts small blood vessels in the hands and feet, predisposing them to frostbite.

Know when to seek shelter! Rescuers should know the basics of emergency shelter construction and how to build a fire in adverse conditions ▶ **Figure 2-10** . Always carry emergency survival equipment during back-country outings ▶ **Table 2-6** .

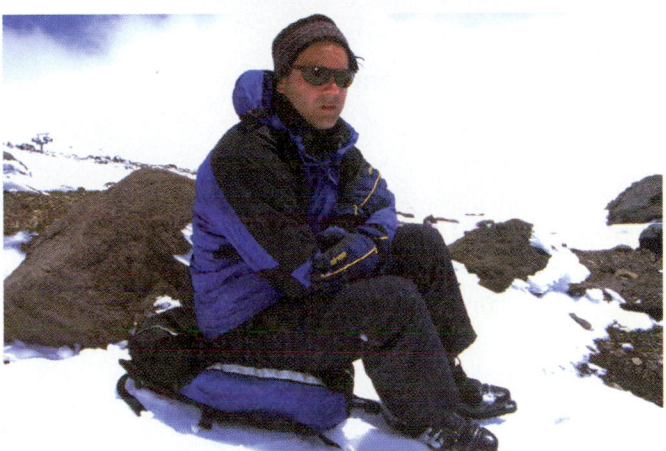

Figure 2-8 Avoid unnecessary contact with cold objects.

COLD WEATHER CLOTHING. Currently, the best and most practical insulating materials for cold weather clothing are the fabrics polyester, wool, polypropylene, and acrylic; and the fillers down, Dacron, polyester, polyester pile and fleece, and foam. Wool, although heavier and harder to dry than the newer

synthetics, is tough and durable, making it useful for clothing subject to heavy wear such as socks, mittens, and trousers. Popular types of polyester include treated polyester, hollow polyester, and pile and fleece. Certain microfibers provide good insulation with less bulk.

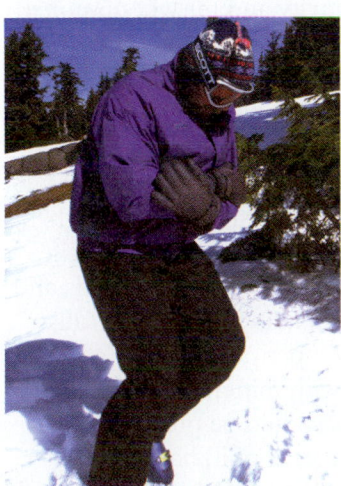

Figure 2-9 Muscular activity increases heat production.

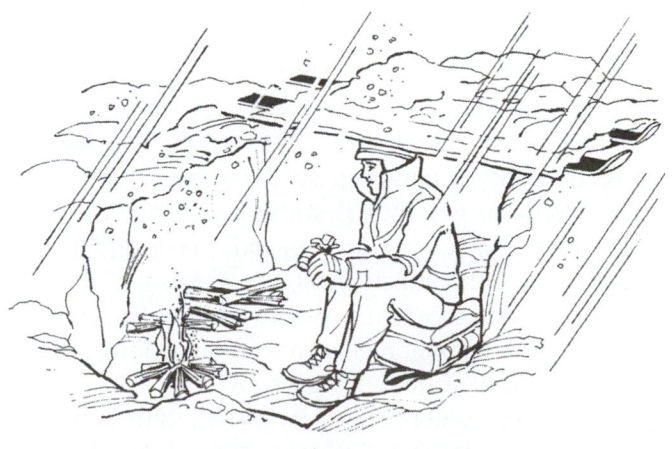

Figure 2-10 Know when to seek shelter.

Table 2-6 Sample Cold Weather Survival Kit

Shelter-Building Equipment
- Plastic or nylon tarp, 8′ × 10′
- Snow shovel, with scoop of Lexan or metal
- 1/8″ braided nylon cord, 50′
- Folding saw

Fire-Building Equipment
- Matches in waterproof container/lighter
- Firestarter
- Candle
- Sturdy hunting knife

Signaling Equipment
- Plastic whistle
- Signal mirror
- Card with ground-to-air signals
- Headlamp with spare batteries
- Coins for pay phone or cellular phone

Other
- Compass/global positioning system (GPS) instrument
- Map
- Emergency care kit
- Metal pot with bale
- Metal cup
- Toilet paper

- Sunglasses
- Sunscreen cream and lip balm, SPF 15 or greater
- Canteen (wide mouth) full of water
- Emergency food
- One extra layer, eg, pile jacket and pants
- Spare mittens and socks

Avalanche Terrain
- Transceiver
- Folding probe, or ski poles that fasten together to make probe

Optional
- Therm-A-Rest pad or piece of Ensolite
- Altimeter
- Flashlight
- Cigarette lighter
- Small ax
- Stove and fuel
- Snow saw (essential if above timberline)
- Sleeping bag rated for lower-than-expected temperatures
- GPS unit
- Water purification equipment (if there is no snow to melt)

Do *not* wear cotton in cold weather. Cotton garments, particularly denim and corduroy, insulate poorly, absorb water excessively, and dry slowly. Wet cotton has little or no insulating ability and increases heat loss through evaporation.

Regardless of the type or brand of garments in your outdoor ensemble, always **layer** your clothing to prevent both chilling and overheating ▶ **Figure 2-11** . Layering allows flexibility because you can add or subtract one or more layers as necessary and, with this in mind, three or four relatively light layers are more adjustable and flexible than one or two thick layers. Overheating is undesirable because it causes you to sweat. This increases heat loss through evaporation of sweat and reduction of the insulating ability of clothing by wetting it.

Be sure to consider the activity as well as the climate when selecting clothing. For example an alpine skier or snowboarder who spends considerable time riding chair

lifts and whose downhill speed generates significant windchill will need more layers of clothing, including quilted garments, than a nordic skier who generates more heat from muscular activity and for whom quilted garments may be too hot.

Cold weather clothing should be easy to adjust and easy to vent, and long underwear should fit snugly to wick perspiration efficiently. Outer layers should be generously sized so inner layers can expand to their full thickness. Shells, vests, and jackets should have high necks and full-length zippers that open from both the top and bottom. Shells should have adjustable cuffs and ventilation zippers, and wind pants should have full-length side zippers as well. Zipper pulls should have tabs so they can be worked with mittened fingers, and metal snaps and zipper pulls should be protected from bare skin by cloth flaps. Zippers should have a weather flap that closes with snaps or Velcro. Outermost

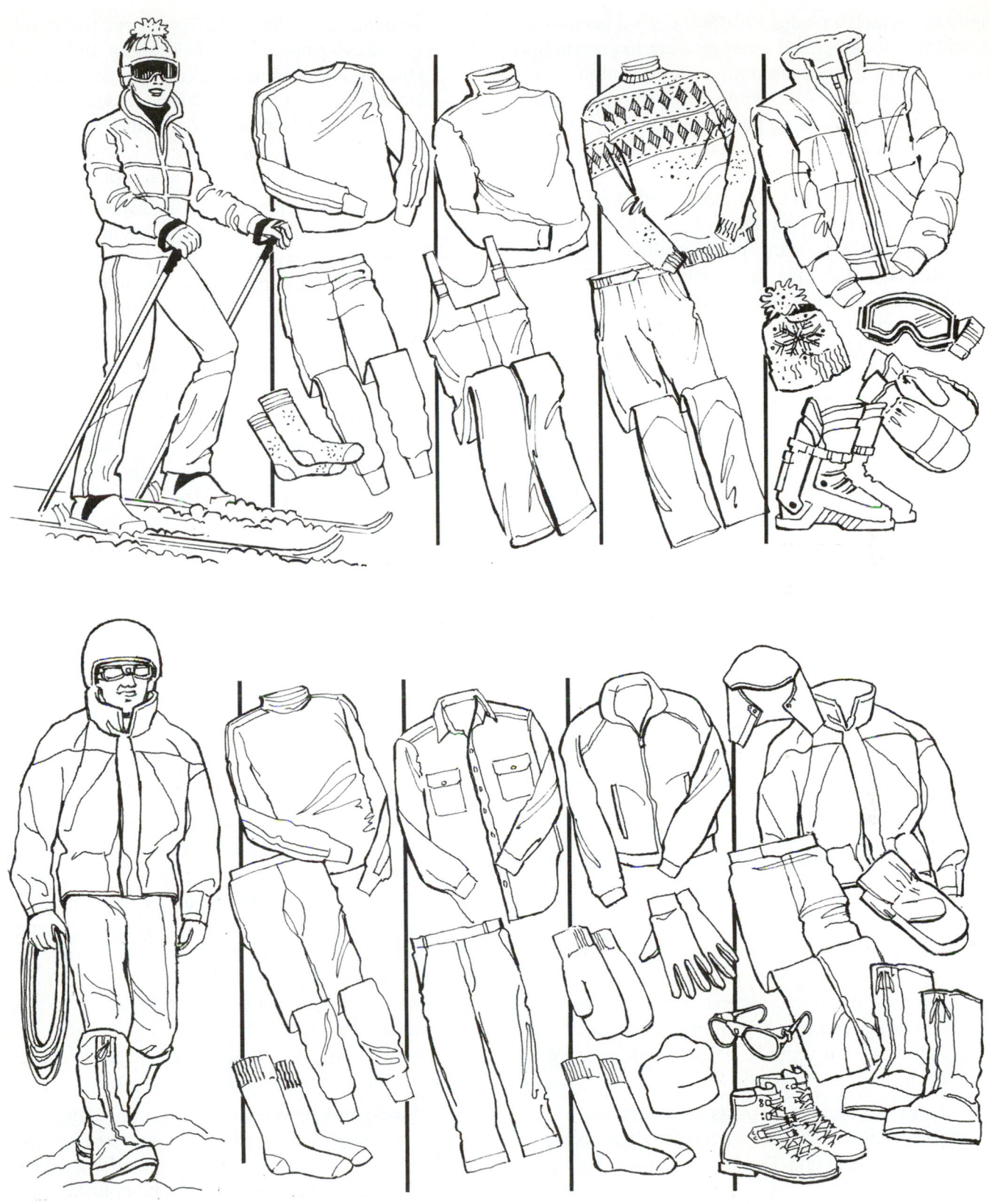

Figure 2-11   Alpine skiers, snowboarders, cross-country skiers, and mountaineers should apply the layering principle when selecting and using cold weather clothing.

clothing—which includes a parka and wind pants—should be windproof and water-resistant to prevent heat loss by conduction, convection, and evaporation. Vertical zippers are easier to pull down with one hand than to pull up—closing a pocket securely to protect its contents from loss may be more important than opening it easily.

The clothing selected for any cold weather activity should depend on the type and level of activity as well as the anticipated temperature range, amount and type of precipitation, and altitude. For example, in the Coastal Alpine Zone (Cascades, Sierra Nevada, Appalachians), where temperatures are moderate and rain is common even in winter, rescuers should wear clothing made of materials that function well when wet, are easy to dry, and repel water. In the High Alpine Zone (Rocky Mountains and other inland ranges), where temperatures are lower and you are less apt to get wet, materials with high insulating and windproofing value are more practical. To repeat, it is always wise to wear *layers* of clothing so you can add or subtract them to accommodate changes in your activity level, the weather, or your location. The four-layer system is widely used.

First layer

- **Long underwear:** Soft wool or synthetics are best. Some brands are available in light, medium, and expedition weights.
- **Socks:** Wool, wool-synthetic blends, and polypropylene are best. A good system is a pair of polypropylene socks next to the skin and one to two pairs of heavy wool or wool-synthetic outer socks.
- **Glove liners:** Light polypropylene or polyester/Lycra gloves are useful when performing delicate jobs in cold weather.

Second layer

- **Shirt:** Wool, fleece, wool synthetic, or polypropylene for very cold activities; acrylic, nylon, or a polyester blend for moderate activities. The shirt should open completely in front or at least have a half-zipper for ventilation. Large button or zip front pockets are useful.
- **Pants:** Wool or fleece pants for mountaineering, part-wool stretch bibs or pants for alpine skiing and snowboarding. Denim jeans should not be worn.
- **Boots:** Choice should depend on the type of activity and the expected temperature. Alpine ski boots need to be snug, should fit well, have an adjustable forward lean, canting capacity, and be warm. Hiking boots should be roomy enough to

accommodate a pair of polypropylene socks and one to two pairs of heavy wool socks, and large enough so toes are neither cramped nor likely to strike the end of the boot during downhill travel. Lace them firmly enough so that the heel does not move, but not so tight that circulation is restricted. Be sure you can wiggle your toes easily.

For moderate temperatures, lightweight combination fabric and leather boots are ideal for light-duty trail hiking, but for rugged, off-trail work, use sturdy full-thickness leather climbing boots that extend above the ankle and have rubber lug soles.

Double mountaineering boots work well for the colder temperatures of winter mountaineering. These consist of outer boots made of leather, plastic, or nylon, and inner boots insulated with felt or foam. Boots used for ice climbing and high-angle cramponing need to be stiffer. Boots with a removable felt inner liner work well for light snowshoeing and other types of nontechnical activities.

For ski touring, telemarking, and ski mountaineering, single and double ski boots are available.

Third Layer

- **Parka:** For alpine skiing or snowboarding, this can be a standard quilted or insulated ski/snowboard or mountain parka, but a pile or quilted jacket or vest in addition to a shell is more versatile. Hikers, climbers, and nordic skiers usually choose the latter combination for layerability. The shell should be windproof and water-resistant, have factory-sealed seams, and a hood with a drawstring closure that is large enough to go over a hat. Unless bibs are worn, the shell should be long enough to keep hips and waist warm and to avoid exposing bare skin when you bend over. It should have multiple pockets, including a pair of lined hand-warmer pockets that close with zippers, Velcro, or snaps. The pockets should be accessible when you are wearing an emergency care belt or a backpack with the waist belt fastened.
- **Wind pants or warm-up pants:** These types of pants must be worn in cold, windy weather, for digging a snow cave, and for caring for a patient in wet or deep snow. They can be unlined but should be made of windproof and water-resistant material.
- **Mittens or gloves:** Mittens are warmer than gloves but are less useful when delicate finger movements are required. Excellent three-layer

mitten and glove sets are available that include windproof shells with leather palms and two sets of removable pile liners. Another good option is to wear a glove liner inside a heavy wool or pile mitten inside a Gore-Tex shell. Depending on temperature, wind, and type of activity, you can wear any combination of the three layers. Shells should have "nose-warmers" of pile or mouton on the backs. They should also be long enough to cover your wrists and have palms of soft leather or sticky fabric so you can hold ice axes or ski poles securely.

- **Gaiters and over-boots:** Gaiters, which are nylon tubes long enough to cover the leg and upper boot, are designed to keep snow, sand, and gravel out of the boots. They open at the side or in front with a zipper or Velcro, usually have a strap that fits under the instep to keep them snug on the boot, and some type of fastener at the top to keep them up. Those with a front opening closed by a wide Velcro strap are easiest to get on and off. Shorter versions that extend to just above the ankle are adequate for summer mountaineering.

  Special insulated over-boots or lined gaiters are essential for high-altitude mountaineering or extremely cold conditions.

- **Hat:** An excellent and versatile choice (especially if you wear glasses) is a wool or pile ski cap you can pull down to cover your ears plus a neck gaiter you can pull up over your lower face. Alternatives are a hat with a facemask or balaclava feature, or a ski cap plus ski goggles and a partial facemask. A bill feature or tennis visor is useful for high-glare conditions, and "bomber" caps with bills and pull-down earflaps are also popular. Many backcountry travelers prefer Andean caps with earflaps. One variety is built like a stovepipe—for ventilation the top can be opened and closed with a drawstring.

Fourth Layer
- **In addition to the above three layers,** which are usually worn on the body, you should have a fourth layer easily accessible in your pack or the patrol locker room. This layer should consist of an insulated vest or jacket and a pair of pile or quilted pants.

ADJUSTING TO HOT WEATHER. Conditions that predispose humans to serious heat stress occur throughout most of the temperate zone during the summer months and in the tropics year-round. Because heat stress is a

Rescuer Tips

Key elements of adjusting to hot weather:
- Maintain physical fitness
- Maximize heat loss
- Minimize heat gain
- Minimize body heat production

function of both temperature and humidity, a moderately warm tropical environment with high humidity can be just as uncomfortable and dangerous as a hotter, drier desert environment.

In North America, you can experience serious heat stress while participating in marathon races in hot weather, during long climbs on sun-exposed mountain faces, and during desert treks and deep canyon hikes. Vehicle breakdowns in isolated desert locations can be very hazardous to unprepared occupants. Death can occur if the temperature of the body core rises above 105° F (41.6° C) for a long period of time.

The body adapts much better to heat (and altitude) than to cold. It adapts (acclimates) to heat by
- increasing the blood volume,
- dilating skin blood vessels, and
- improving heart efficiency so as to carry more heat from the body core to the skin surface.

The acclimated person starts to:
- perspire at a lower temperature,
- increase the sweat volume,
- decrease the amount of salt in the sweat.

All of these adaptations aid heat loss through evaporation of sweat and by radiation from the skin. Acclimatization requires a minimum of 7 days of constant exposure to heat, after which heat is much less debilitating.

On return to a cooler climate, these processes reverse, the most obvious sign being a temporary increase in urine output as the blood volume contracts and the kidneys excrete the excess liquid.

A high level of physical fitness, especially aerobic fitness, is more important in a hot environment than in a cold environment, because a good cardiovascular system is necessary to keep heat loss through the skin at a high level (see the Physical Conditioning section later in this chapter). However, even the most physically fit person should allow time to acclimate before engaging in prolonged, strenuous physical exercise in a hot environment.

MAXIMIZE HEAT LOSS. Exposing the maximum amount of bare skin to circulating air increases heat loss through conduction, convection, and radiation. This is best done in the shade to protect the skin from sunburn. In the sun, the use of topical sunscreens, while permitting more skin exposure, may impair heat loss from the skin by radiation and evaporation of perspiration. A good compromise, therefore, is to cover the face (especially the lips and undersurfaces of the nose and chin), ears, and hands with sunscreen and wear a long-sleeved shirt and long pants of thin, loose, and light-colored (preferably white) material. Avoid dark clothing because dark colors absorb more of the sun's rays than light colors and are therefore hotter. Always reapply a topical sunscreen several times a day.

Clothing should be loose and easily opened for ventilation; shirts should open fully in front. Although you should avoid wearing cotton in cold weather, it is an excellent choice for hot weather clothing because of its high thermal conductivity, poor insulating ability, and good wicking ability. Consider wearing clothing with mesh panels at the armpits, under the back and front yokes, and at the crotch. Wear a light-colored hat with a wide brim, or a Foreign Legion-style cap with a neck protector and ventilation holes in the crown. A baseball cap with a bandana tied around your neck is also a good combination. Avoid T-shirts because they have a Sun Protection Factor (SPF) of only 5 to 9. Special clothing is available made of fabric with an SPF of 30 or greater.

Drink adequate amounts of fluids, which means up to 1.1 qt (1 L) an hour during strenuous exercise, for a total of as many as 13 qt (12 L) a day ▼ **Figure 2-12**. Some of these fluids can contain electrolyte supplements. It is better to drink small amounts of fluid at frequent intervals than to drink a lot at one time. Among other things, frequent drinking helps you perspire freely because water can move from the stomach to sweat glands within 9 to 18 minutes. Always carry water or have it readily available, and be sure to wrap water containers in clothing or other insulation and bury them in a backpack to keep them cool.

In the desert, use the layering principle so you can take off layers of clothing during the heat of the day and add them at night when the dry desert air cools rapidly. Remember to bring a pile jacket, wind shell, and wind pants with you as part of your layering system.

MINIMIZE HEAT GAIN. In high temperatures always wear coverings to protect your head and body from the direct rays of the sun ▼ **Figure 2-13**. Erect a sun shelter with a tarp so you can seek shade during the hottest part of the day and during rest periods. Because desert air is much cooler a foot above or a few inches below the ground surface, sleep or rest on a platform or in a scooped-out depression rather than directly on the ground. Do not remain in a stranded vehicle during the day but lie under it or in a separate shelter nearby.

Avoid direct contact with the hot ground and other hot objects, particularly metal. Wear sturdy, above-the-ankle, full-leather, lug-sole boots, not only to protect your feet from the hot ground but also to shield them from sharp rocks and cactus spines. Gaiters are effective in keeping sand and rocks out of boots. Wear two pairs of socks: an inner pair of cotton for wicking and an outer pair of synthetic for insulation from the heat.

Protect your hands with wear-resistant cotton gloves, and in areas full of cacti, also carry a pair of leather gloves. In addition, wear high-quality sunglasses with side extensions to protect your eyes from glare and to block damaging ultraviolet rays.

MINIMIZE BODY HEAT PRODUCTION. Since active muscles produce large amounts of heat, avoid muscular exertion

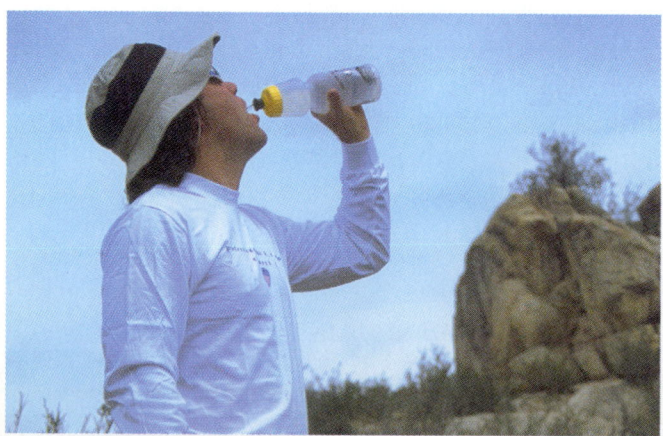

Figure 2-12 When in a hot environment, drink plenty of fluids. Rest in a shelter during the hottest times of the day.

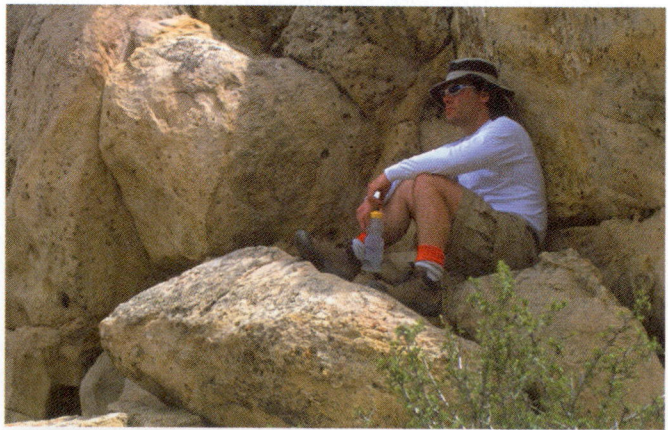

Figure 2-13 Be sure to wear proper protective clothing in hot weather.

Table 2-7 Avoiding Excess Body Heat

General

- Maintain good aerobic fitness
- Acclimatize
- Hydrate

Increasing Body Heat Loss

- Expose as much skin to the air as possible
- Wear loose, light-colored clothing of cotton or another suitable fabric
- Stay hydrated to promote perspiration

Reducing Heat Gain from the Environment

- Wear protective clothing
- Seek shade during the hottest part of the day
- Avoid touching hot objects
- Do not lie directly on the ground

Decreasing Body Heat Production

- Decrease muscular activity

during periods of high heat and high humidity, and do your traveling early or late in the day, or at night. ◄ **Table 2-7** lists ways to avoid excess body heat.

Food and Water

Good nutrition, which includes hydration, must be a concern to outdoor travelers, especially members of rescue groups who may engage in unplanned heavy physical activity for long periods in severe weather without adequate food or rest. Nutrition—along with physical fitness—is a bedrock of physical performance. Performance can be enhanced if the principles of good nutrition are applied before, during, and after an outdoor experience. The six groups of nutrients are carbohydrates, fats, proteins, vitamins, minerals, and water.

Poor nutrition and dehydration, which frequently go together, have similar effects: fatigue, decreased work capacity, lack of endurance, poor recovery from exercise, lack of cold or heat tolerance (with an increased susceptibility to hypothermia or heat illness), weight loss, depression, apathy, and discouragement. Coordination may also suffer because there may not be enough glycogen in muscle fibers to perform rapid corrective movements efficiently (see Physical Conditioning in the next section).

Your body's three sources of fuel—carbohydrates, fat, and protein—are used in increased quantities during stress, particularly if physical activity is involved. The quickest source of energy is glucose, taken from glycogen stored in the liver. However, this supply will last less than a day. Protein, drawn primarily from muscle, is a long-term source of glucose. Tissues can use fat for energy. The body also conserves water during periods of stress. Other nutrients that are susceptible to depletion are the vitamins and minerals that are not stored in the body in substantial quantities. These include water-soluble vitamins and most minerals.

Regular, well-balanced meals are essential to provide the nutrients that are necessary to keep your body fueled ◄ **Figure 2-14** . Vitamin pills or other preparations that provide a balanced mix of all the essential vitamins and minerals may be desirable to supplement a less than perfectly balanced diet.

If you expect to engage in strenuous physical activity, you should increase the percentage

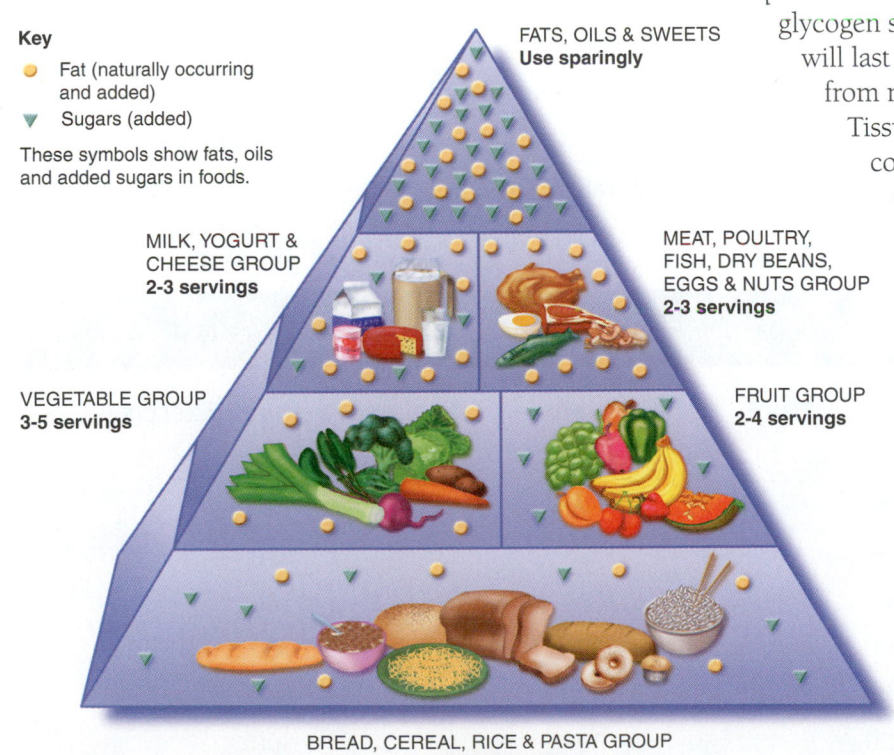

Key

- Fat (naturally occurring and added)
- Sugars (added)

These symbols show fats, oils and added sugars in foods.

FATS, OILS & SWEETS
Use sparingly

MILK, YOGURT & CHEESE GROUP
2-3 servings

MEAT, POULTRY, FISH, DRY BEANS, EGGS & NUTS GROUP
2-3 servings

VEGETABLE GROUP
3-5 servings

FRUIT GROUP
2-4 servings

BREAD, CEREAL, RICE & PASTA GROUP
6-11 servings

Figure 2-14 A healthy diet is illustrated by the USDA Food Guide Pyramid.

of carbohydrate in your diet to 60% to 80% of total calories for several days before as well as during the activity by eating large amounts of potatoes, rice, pasta, and other high carbohydrate foods. This diet can double glycogen stores in your muscles and increase endurance by as much as three times as compared to an ordinary diet. Furthermore, you should continue this diet for several days after the activity to replenish these glycogen stores. Conversely, a low-carbohydrate diet can decrease glycogen stores and reduce endurance by as much as half.

An average sedentary adult requires only 2,500 to 3,000 calories per day to sustain normal physical activity. A prolonged rescue effort or mountaineering expedition may require as many as 5,000 calories per day. In cold weather even more calories may be needed because moving about in heavy clothing, shoveling snow, and working and traveling in deep snow make a given task require up to 15% more energy than it would in warm weather.

Food carried for emergency purposes or as part of a search-and-rescue 72-hour pack should be tasty, light-weight, high in energy, rich in carbohydrates, resistant to spoilage, and should not require cooking or complicated preparation. Examples include cheese, sausage, candy bars, gorp ("good ol' raisins and peanuts"), bread, crackers, cookies, nuts, cocoa, instant breakfast drink, fruitcake, and dried fruit.

Here is an example of a backpacking menu that requires only the addition of hot or cold water:

- **Breakfast:** citrus beverage; granola or instant hot cereal with raisins, powdered milk, brown sugar, and spices such as nutmeg or cinnamon to taste; breakfast bars; hot tea or freeze-dried coffee; multivitamin pill.

- **Lunch:** bread, preferably a type that will not crumble in the pack, such as hard rolls, pita bread, bagels, or soft tortillas; sandwich fillers such as cheese, summer sausage, freeze-dried tuna salad or chicken salad; candy bars; powdered instant tea; powdered fruit or electrolyte drink.

- **Snacks** (to be eaten every 2 hours on the trail): dried fruit, candy, granola bars, cookies, and gorp.

- **Dinner:** hot, fruit-flavored gelatin drink; instant soup; commercial freeze-dried dinner; instant pudding; hot beverage (preferably decaffeinated).

The average *sedentary* person loses about 2.4 qt (2,300 mL) of water daily (▼ **Table 2-8**). Of this total, 1.5 qt (1,400 mL) is lost in the urine, 0.85 qt (800 mL) through the skin and lungs, and 3 oz (100 mL) in the stool. Therefore, to prevent dehydration, you need to drink at least 2.4 quarts of water daily. About half of this amount is provided by body metabolism and water contained in food. The other half must come from drinking water and other liquids.

Table 2-8 Water Balance in a Sedentary Person (in mL)

Gain	Loss
Water from metabolism: 300	Urine: 1,400
Water in food: 800	Skin and lungs: 800
Liquids: 1,200	Feces: 100
Total: 2,300	**Total: 2,300**

Table 2-9 Daily Loss of Water (in mL)*

Route of Water Loss	Normal Temperature	Hot Weather	Prolonged Heavy Exercise
Insensible Loss			
• Skin	350	350	350
• Respiratory tract	350	250	650
Urine	1,400	1,200	500
Sweat	100	1,400	5,000
Feces	100	100	100
Total	**2,300**	**3,300**	**6,600**

At high altitude, in hot weather, and during strenuous exercise, the amount of water lost through the skin and lungs increases greatly. These losses can total 1.1 qt (1,000 mL) per hour during nordic ski racing, up to 1.8 qt (1,600 mL) per hour during strenuous exercise in hot weather, and up to 3.3 qt (3,000 mL) per hour in highly trained, acclimatized soldiers exercising in the heat. ◄ Table 2-9 shows the routes and amounts of water loss in different situations.

In the outdoors, you must constantly make active efforts to prevent dehydration by both increasing your water intake and decreasing your water loss, especially at temperature extremes and at high altitude. Cold weather decreases the sense of thirst, which may lead to a state of chronic, mild dehydration. At temperatures below freezing and at elevations above the snow line, the lack of liquid water and the time and effort required to melt snow compound the problem. In desert areas, water may be almost impossible to obtain without a solar still ► Figure 2-15 .

Drink 4 to 6 qt (3.8 to 6 L) or more of water per day during heavy exertion in cold weather and at high altitude, and up to 1.1 qt (1 L) an hour during heavy exer-

tion in very hot weather. In the heat, when water is limited, decrease water loss by resting in the shade during the heat of the day and traveling at night. ▼ Table 2-10 lists what you need to have with you in the desert.

Although new snow is clean, assume that all liquid surface water is contaminated. Always purify surface water by boiling, filtration, or chemical disinfection. Remove obvious dirt first by straining the water through a clean cloth or coffee filter. The most effective treatment method is boiling. At altitudes lower than 18,000' (5,486 m), simply bringing water to a boil will kill almost all harmful viruses, bacteria, and protozoa. However, fuel limitations and the time involved may make boiling impractical. Many excellent brands of water filters are available, and most have pores small enough to remove protozoan cysts and bacteria (around 0.1 micron pore size). They will not remove viruses or smaller protozoan cysts (such as *Cryptosporidium*), which require smaller filter pore sizes.

Many products for chemical disinfection of water are available, most of which contain halogens (iodine or chlorine). One widely used example is tetraglycine hydroperiodide. Standard mountaineering and back-

Table 2-10 Sample Desert Survival Kit

Shelter-Building Equipment
- Plastic or nylon tarp, 8' × 10'
- ⅛" braided nylon cord, 50'
- Folding saw
- Short-handled folding shovel with steel blade
- Sturdy knife

Fire-Building Equipment
- Matches in a waterproof container
- Firestarter
- Candle

Signaling Equipment
- Plastic whistle
- Flashlight
- Signal mirror
- Coins for a pay phone
- Card with ground-to-air signals

Other
- Water, as much as you can carry (at least 5 qt in a nylon canteen)
- Water purification equipment
- Insect repellent
- Toilet paper
- Spare sunglasses
- Sunblock cream and lip balm
- Map
- Compass
- Headlamp
- Spare hat
- Metal pot with bale
- Metal cup
- Emergency care kit (see Appendix C)
- Heavy gloves
- Emergency food

Solar Still Equipment
(*one still per person;* ► Figure 2-15)
- One sheet of clear plastic, 6' × 6', reinforced in the center with an X of duct tape
- One piece of ¼" vinyl tubing, 6' to 8' long, with plug for exposed (outside) end
- 1-qt plastic bowl

Optional
- GPS unit

Additional for Vehicles
- 5 gal of water for each person
- CB radio
- Cellular phone

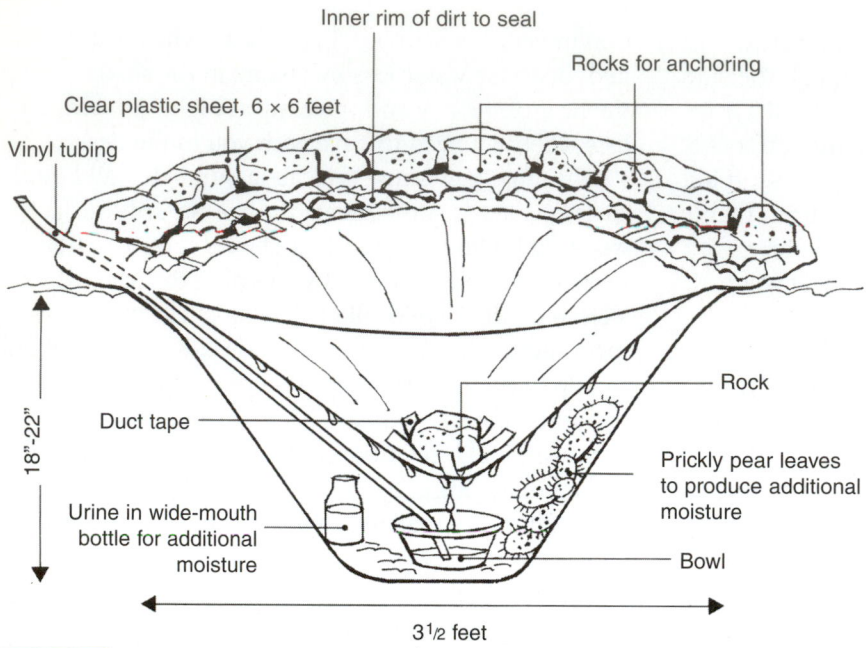

Inner rim of dirt to seal

Rocks for anchoring

Clear plastic sheet, 6 × 6 feet

Vinyl tubing

Rock

Duct tape

18"–22"

Prickly pear leaves to produce additional moisture

Urine in wide-mouth bottle for additional moisture

Bowl

3½ feet

Figure 2-15   A solar still.

The sun's heat causes water to evaporate from soil and vegetable matter, collect on the inside of the plastic sheet, and drip into the bowl. Don't open the still after it starts working, but remove water by sucking it up through the tubing. The still should be placed in the moistest possible area, such as a bend of a dry stream bed or behind the first or second row of sand dunes on a beach (not *in* a sand dune).

packing texts contain useful information about other available products. Halogenation is usually effective for bacteria, viruses, and *Giardia* (a protozoan found in wild animal and human feces that causes diarrhea and abdominal discomfort); it will not kill *Cryptosporidium*, another protozoan recently recognized to be a widespread surface-water contaminant. Infection with this organism can be fatal in those with impaired immunity, although it causes only mild to moderate diarrhea in healthy persons. Even backcountry water should be treated by boiling or with filtration (smaller than 0.1 micron pore size).

The time required to kill infectious organisms depends on the amount of sediment in the water, the water temperature, and the type and dose of chemical disinfectant, so follow the manufacturer's directions carefully and allow the water to stand the specified amount of time before drinking it. For extra safety or for heavily contaminated water, use both filtration and halogens. Many filters include a halogen.

Urine output is a good indicator of the state of hydration. Daily urine production should be light yellow and at least 1.1 to 1.6 qt (1 to 1.5 L). Although strenuous exercise may turn urine orange-brown and vitamin supplements containing riboflavin (vitamin B_2) will turn it bright yellow, you should always suspect dehydration when urine is dark.

Physical Conditioning

Physical fitness and conditioning are important to members of any outdoor recreational or rescue group because outdoor travel imposes unique physical demands and presents the possibility of severe, prolonged physical stress. Therefore, rescuers should achieve and maintain a superior level of physical fitness. Most rescuers participate in sports related to their rescue interests, such as climbing, recreational skiing, and kayaking—activities that require strength, suppleness, and durability for full enjoyment. Although the best training for any sport is to practice it, people with demanding urban jobs may have to substitute a carefully selected set of exercises they can perform regularly in their spare time and close to home.

Proper physical conditioning improves the strength of muscles and tendons, enhances coordination, flexibility, and endurance, and reduces the chance of injury. It allows you to exert yourself harder and longer without tiring and to recover more rapidly after rest. Conditioning also increases the margin of safety in a survival situation because your body is more prepared to meet the demands of the outdoor environment. In addition, proper conditioning slows aging and helps you maintain your normal weight. The fit rescuer performs better because the fit body functions better, is better able to avoid injury, and recovers faster if injured. The drop in US cardiovascular disease mortality in the last third of the 20th century was probably due in part to increased participation in active sports by people of all ages. Unfortunately, more recent sedentary lifestyles are leading to an increase in obesity, diabetes, and poor physical condition.

Fitness can be divided into two parts: motor fitness and cardiovascular fitness. Suitable programs should develop both types of fitness. **Motor fitness** refers to strength, power (the ability to exert force rapidly), endurance, balance, agility, and flexibility. **Cardiovascular fitness** refers to the ability of the heart and circulatory system to meet the active body's changing needs for blood. An important index of cardiovascular fitness is **aerobic capacity**—the body's ability to take, transport, and use oxygen. This is

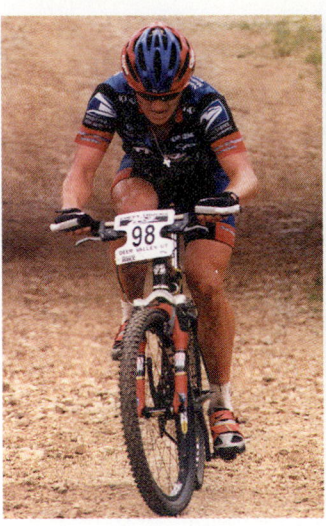
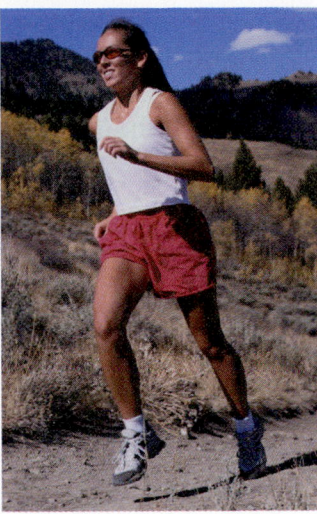

Figure 2-16 Two types of endurance athletes.

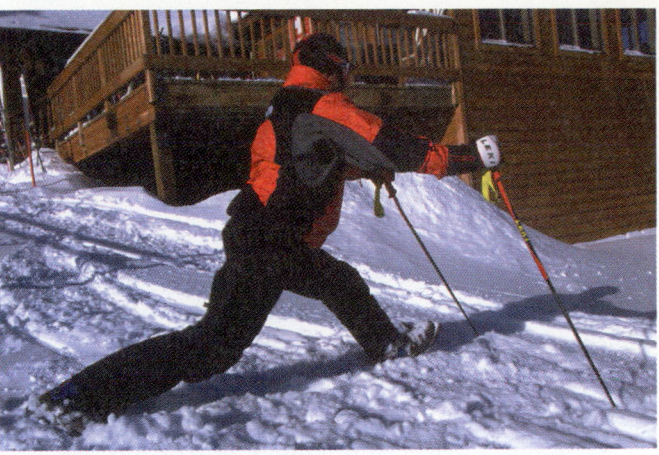

Figure 2-17 A good physical conditioning program includes a warm-up and cool-down period, stretching exercises, calisthenics, and aerobic exercise.

especially important in endurance activities such as cross-country skiing and long-distance running (▲ Figure 2-16). The greatest aerobic capacity is developed through training that uses the upper and lower extremities at the same time, such as swimming, speed hiking with poles on dry land, nordic skiing on snow, and using a nordic skiing simulator.

Although alpine skiers and snowboarders need considerable motor fitness, they also need cardiovascular fitness. Note that the limiting factor in the delivery of oxygen to the muscles during exercise is not lung capacity but rather the heart's ability to pump blood to the muscles. Good physical fitness generally leads to good psychological fitness, which enables a person to manage physical and mental stresses with increased confidence.

The training goal for any type of endurance sport is to maximize the body's aerobic capacity, which can be measured by pulmonary function tests. If you are interested in designing a training program for yourself, it is helpful to consult sports medicine specialists and skilled trainers, who can demonstrate exercises and recommend instruction books. A good general program (▲ Figure 2-17) should include the following components:

- A proper warm-up period that includes stretching exercises to develop flexibility
- Selected calisthenics to develop the upper and lower extremities, back, and trunk
- A period of aerobic exercise to build cardiovascular fitness and endurance
- A cool-down period

Emotional Aspects of Emergency Care

After completing your training and becoming an outdoor emergency care provider, you will be exposed to scenes and involved in activities like none you have experienced before. You will see patients who are in great pain, who are anxious and afraid, and who may be uncooperative, ungrateful, and even hysterical. At times, your care may be unappreciated or you may be criticized unjustly. Occasionally, you may see horribly disfiguring and gruesome injuries, and—rarely—a death. You will find these experiences hard to deal with at first, but try to remember that your reactions of alarm, concern, grief, and sorrow are normal. Every rescuer who must deal with such situations has these feelings. Although the struggle to remain calm in the face of disturbing events is a necessary one, it contributes to the emotional stress of the job. As you become more experienced, however, you will develop a professional approach that will help you deliver competent care and show concern without becoming emotionally involved to the point of being inefficient or ineffective.

Death and Dying

Today, life expectancy has dramatically increased; nearly two thirds of all deaths occur among those age 65 years and older. Sixty percent of all deaths today are attributed to heart disease. From the age of 1 year to the age of 34 years, trauma is the leading cause of death. Death today is likely to occur either quite suddenly or after a prolonged terminal illness. The environment of death has changed since our nation's earlier days; it no longer occurs in the home setting. The setting of death is somewhere else—in the hospital, a hospice, or a convalescent home, at the workplace, or on the highway. For this reason, we are less familiar with death than our ancestors were. We tend to deny death in America. Illness can be much more drawn-out and much more removed from daily life. Life support systems and impersonal care remove the whole experience of death from most people's awareness. The mobility of families also makes it less likely that there will be extended family support when death does occur.

Death was once both an expected and accepted fact in earlier American history. Life expectancy was brief (compared to today's), mortality rates (the ratio of number of deaths to a given population size) were high, and childbirth was hazardous, often resulting in the death of both the mother and the baby. Hardships of the times, both natural and human-made, were great. Children and adults died of disease, injuries, and the traumas of war. Most people had experienced the death of someone close to them. There were no funeral homes; mourning occurred at home in the family setting. The presence of a dead body was a natural event.

No matter what the frequency of response to emergency calls, death is something that every emergency caregiver will sometimes face. For some, it may be infrequent. Others, in urban settings, may see death many times in responding to motor vehicle crashes, drug overdoses, suicides, or homicides. Some rescuers may have to deal with mass casualties from lift incidents, airplane crashes, or hazardous materials accidents. In all these cases, coming to grips with your thoughts, understandings, and adjustment to death is not only important personally, but also a function of delivering emergency medical care.

Physical Signs of Death

Only a physician or other legally constituted authority can pronounce a patient dead. However, a properly performed examination can help the rescuer tell if death is obvious or likely, based on the presumptive and definite signs of death listed below. An important question that often arises is whether to begin basic life support in a person who may be dead. In the absence of physician orders such as do not resuscitate (DNR) orders, the general rule is: if the body is still warm and intact, initiate emergency medical care. An exception to this rule is cold temperature (hypothermia) emergencies. Hypothermia is a general cooling of the body in which the internal body temperature becomes abnormally low: 95° F (35° C). It is considered a serious condition and is often fatal. At 86° F (30° C),

> **Remember**
>
> **Definitive Signs of Death**
> - Obvious mortal damage
> - Dependent lividity
> - Rigor mortis
> - Putrefaction

the brain can survive without perfusion for about 10 minutes. When the core temperature drops to 82.4° F (28° C), the patient is in grave danger; however, individuals have survived a hypothermia accident with a temperature of 64.4° F (18° C). In cases of hypothermia, the patient should not be considered dead until he or she is warm and dead.

PRESUMPTIVE SIGNS OF DEATH. Most medicolegal authorities will consider the presumptive signs of death that are listed in ▶ Table 2-11 adequate, particularly when they follow a severe trauma or occur at the end stages of long-term illness such as cancer or other prolonged diseases. These signs would not be adequate in cases of sudden death due to hypothermia, acute poisoning, or cardiac arrest. Usually, in these cases, some combination of the signs is needed to declare death, not just one of them alone.

DEFINITIVE SIGNS OF DEATH. Definitive or conclusive signs of death that are obvious and clear to even nonmedical persons include the following:

- Obvious mortal damage, such as a body in parts (decapitation, severing of the trunk, massive open wounds of the head, chest, or abdomen).

- **Dependent lividity**, blood settling to the lowest point of the body, causing discoloration of the skin.

- **Rigor mortis**, the stiffening of body muscles caused by chemical changes within muscle tissue. It develops first in the face and jaw, gradually extending downward until the body is in full rigor. The rate of onset is affected by the body's ability to lose heat to its surroundings. A thin body loses heat faster than a fat body. A body on a tile floor loses heat faster than a body wrapped up in a blanket in a bed. Rigor mortis occurs some time between 2 and 12 hours after death.

- **Putrefaction**, decomposition of body tissues. Depending on temperature conditions, this occurs some time between 40 and 96 hours after death.

TABLE 2-11 Presumptive Signs of Death
• Unresponsiveness to painful stimuli
• Lack of a pulse or heartbeat
• Absence of breath sounds
• No deep tendon or corneal reflexes
• Absence of eye movement
• No systolic blood pressure
• Profound cyanosis
• Lowered or decreased body temperature

Medical Examiner Cases

Involvement of the medical examiner, or the coroner in some states, depends on the nature and scene of the death. In most states, when trauma is a factor or the death involves suspected criminal or unusual situations such as hanging or poisoning, the medical examiner must be notified (▼ **Figure 2-18**). Once it is determined that the medical examiner should be notified, the body must not be moved except under the direction of the medical examiner or his or her legal delegate, such as the police. When the medical examiner or coroner assumes responsibility of the scene, that responsibility supersedes all others at the scene, including the family's. The following are considered the medical examiner's cases:

- When the person is dead on arrival (DOA)
- Death without previous medical care or when the physician is unable to state the cause of death

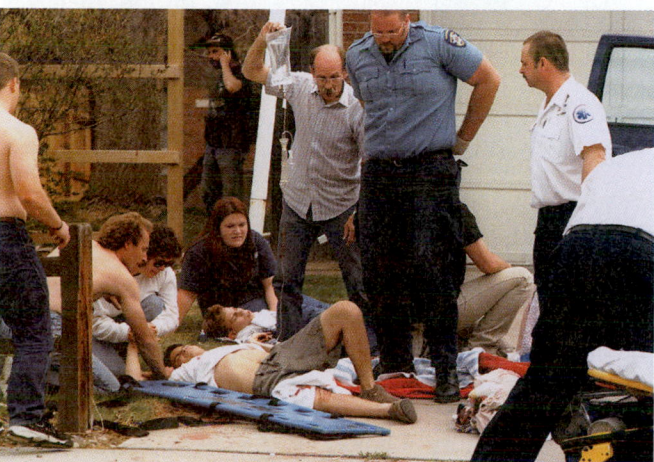

Figure 2-18 Involvement of the authorities is required when the cause of death is uncertain or is due to violence, accident, suicide, or foul play.

- Suicide (self-destruction)
- Violent death
- Poisoning, known or suspected
- Death resulting from accidents
- Suspicion of a criminal act

If emergency medical care has been initiated, keep thorough notes of what was done and found on both scene size-up and assessment. These records may be important during a subsequent investigation.

The Grieving Process

The death of a human being is one of the most difficult events for another human being to accept. If the survivor is a relative or close friend of the deceased, it is even more difficult. Emotional responses to the loss of a loved one or friend are appropriate and should be expected. In fact, it is expected that you will feel emotional about the death of a patient. Feelings and emotions are part of the grieving process. All of us experience these feelings after a stressful situation that causes us personal pain.

In 1969, Dr. Elisabeth Kubler-Ross published research revealing that people go through several stages of grieving. The stages of grieving are as follows:

1. **Denial.** Refusal to accept diagnosis or care, unrealistic demands for miracles, or persistent failure to understand why there is no improvement.

2. **Anger, hostility.** Projection of bad news onto the environment and commonly in all directions, at times almost at random. The person lashes out. Someone must be blamed, and those who are responsible must be punished. This is usually an ugly phase.

3. **Bargaining.** An attempt to secure a prize for good behavior or promise to change lifestyle. "I promise to be a 'perfect patient' if only I can live until 'x' event."

4. **Depression.** Open expression of grief, internalized anger, hopelessness, the desire to die. It rarely involves suicidal threats, complete withdrawal, or giving up long before the illness seems terminal. The patient is usually silent.

5. **Acceptance.** The simple "yes." Acceptance grows out of a person's conviction that all has been done and the person is ready to die.

Stages may follow one another or occur simultanously. They may last different amounts of time.

Even though the event (death) has not yet happened, the patient knows that it will happen. The patient has no control over this process. The patient will die whether or not he or she is ready to die. Furthermore, being ready to die does not mean that the patient will be happy about dying. You may encounter situations in which the patient is close to death, and you may need to provide reassurance and emotional care (▶ **Figure 2-19**).

What Can the Rescuer Do?

Do helpful things, and make simple suggestions. Ask whether there is anything that you can do that will be of help, such as calling a relative or religious advisor. Provide gentle and caring support. Reinforcing the reality of the situation is important. This can be accomplished by merely saying to a grieving person, "I am so sorry for your loss." Your actual words are not as important as your demeanor. The grieving person needs to grieve, so avoid statements that suggest a "silver lining behind the clouds" or make light of the situation (▼ **Table 2-12**). In many cases the person needs to talk and the best thing you can do is be willing to listen in a kind manner. You can ask, "Would you like to talk about how you're feeling?" Then, accept the response.

Always be honest with grieving persons, and do not give false hope. Be concerned about their privacy and their wishes, and let them know that you take their concerns seriously. Remember that anger is a stage of grieving, and the anger may be directed at you. The anger may seem irrational, but is real to a grieving person.

Approach to the Dying, Critically Ill, or Injured Patient

Individuals in the process of dying will feel threatened, partly because of their concerns about survival. These

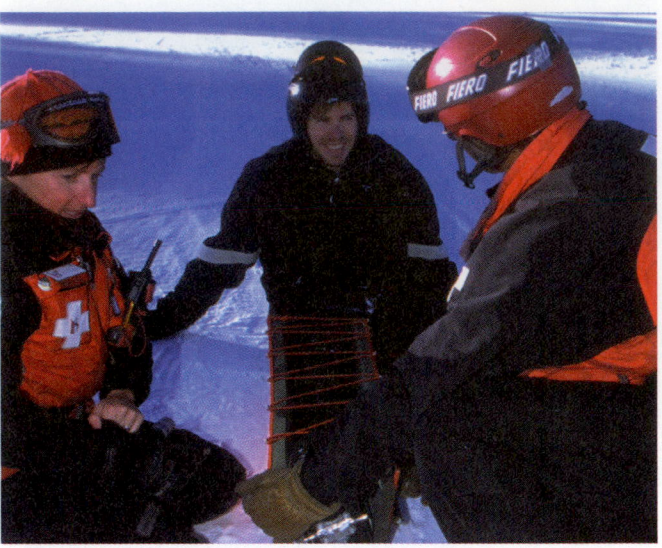

Figure 2-19   Explaining what is going on can help alleviate fear and confusion.

concerns may involve feelings of helplessness, disability, pain, and separation, and are related to the patient's sense of self and understanding of death.

ANXIETY. Anxiety is a response to the anticipation of danger. The source of the anxiety is often unknown; but in the case of seriously injured or ill patients, the source is usually recognizable. What may increase the anxiety are the unknowns of the current situation. Patients may ask the following:

- What will happen to me?
- What are you doing?
- Will I make it?
- What will my disabilities be?

TABLE 2-12 Responding to Grief	
Don't Say...	**Try Instead...**
Give it time. Things will get better.	I'm sorry.
You should not question God's will.	It is okay to be angry.
You have to get on with your life.	It must be hard to accept.
You have to keep on going.	That must be painful for you.
You can always have another child.	Tell me how you are feeling.
You're not the only one who suffers.	Let's spend some time together.
The living must go on.	If you want to cry, it's okay.
I know how you feel.	People really cared for…

Patients who are anxious may exhibit the following signs and symptoms:

- Upset
- Sweaty and cool (diaphoretic)
- Rapid breathing (hyperventilating)
- Fast pulse (tachycardic)
- Restless
- Tense
- Fearful
- Shaky (tremulous)

For the anxious patient, time seems to be extended; seconds seem like minutes, and minutes seem like hours.

PAIN AND FEAR. Pain and fear are very closely inter-related. Pain often is associated with illness or trauma. Fear is generally thought of in relation to the oncoming pain and the outcome of the damage. It is often helpful to encourage patients to express their pains and fears, since expression of them begins the process of adjustment to the pain and acceptance of the emergency medical care that may be necessary. Some individuals have difficulty in openly admitting their fear. The fear may be expressed as bad dreams, withdrawal, tension, restlessness, "butterflies" in the stomach, or nervousness. In some cases, it may be expressed as anger.

ANGER AND HOSTILITY. Anger may be expressed by very demanding and complaining behavior. Often, this may be related to the fear and anxiety of the emergency medical care that is being given. Sometimes, the fear is so acute that the patient may want to express anger toward you or others but is unable to do so because of the dependency factor. If you find that you are the target of the patient's anger, make sure that you are safe; do not take the anger or insults personally. Be tolerant, and do not become defensive.

The anger may also be expressed physically, and you may be the target of the displaced aggression. If the patient or a relative becomes so emotionally upset that you are physically assaulted or you believe that this could happen, back out of the situation. Such hostility must be contained. If emergency medical care is not possible under these circumstances, law enforcement intervention is required.

DEPRESSION. Almost all dying patients feel some degree of depression because of internalized anger and other factors. Some patients may have many dissatisfactions and regrets about their lives; others may be wrapped up in concerns about financial, legal, social, or family

Remember

Concerns of the dying, critically ill, or injured patient include:

- Anxiety
- Pain and fear
- Anger and hostility
- Depression
- Dependency
- Guilt
- Mental health problems
- Receiving unrelated bad news

problems. The patient should be encouraged to express his or her feelings. Assisting the patient and his or her family in resolving unsettled matters may decrease feelings of depression.

DEPENDENCY. When emergency medical care is given to any individual, a sense of dependency develops. Individuals who are placed in this position often feel helpless and may become resentful. The resentfulness may arouse feelings of inferiority, shame, or weakness.

GUILT. Many patients who are dying, their families, or the caregivers of those patients may feel guilty over what has happened to them. Occasionally family members and/or long-term caregivers may feel a degree of relief when an extended illness is finally over. That relief may later turn into guilt. Most of the time, however, no one can explain these feelings. The magnitude of the guilt may be very great. Sometimes, feelings of guilt can result in a delay in seeking emergency medical care.

MENTAL HEALTH PROBLEMS. Mental health problems such as disorientation, confusion, or delusions may develop in the dying patient. In these instances, the patient may display behavior inconsistent with normal patterns of thinking, feeling, or acting. Common characteristics of such behavior may include the following:

- Loss of contact with reality
- Distortion of perception
- Regression
- Diminished control of basic impulses and desires
- Abnormal mental content, including delusions and hallucinations

In some long-term situations, generalized personality deterioration may occur.

RECEIVING UNRELATED BAD NEWS. A patient who is in critical condition or is dying may not want to hear of unrelated bad news, such as the death of someone close to them. Such news may depress the patient or cause the patient to give up hope.

Caring for Critically Ill and Injured Patients

Patients need to know who you are and what you are doing. If the patient is conscious, ask if you can give care. Let the patient know that you are attending to his or her immediate needs and that these are your primary concerns at this moment. As soon as possible, explain to the patient what is going on. Confusion, anxiety, and other feelings of helplessness will be decreased if you keep the patient informed from the start.

Avoid Sad and Grim Comments

Rescuers, family, and bystanders must avoid grim comments about a patient's condition. Remarks such as "This is a bad one" or "The leg is badly damaged, and I think he will lose it" are inappropriate. These remarks may upset or increase anxiety in the patient and compromise possible recovery outcomes. This is especially true for the patient who may be able to hear and remember, but not to respond.

Orient the Patient

You should expect a patient to be disoriented in an emergency situation. The aura of the emergency situation—discomfort, lights, smells, unfamiliar surroundings, and strangers—is intense. The impact and effect of injuries or acute illness may cause the patient to be confused or unsettled. It is important to orient the patient to his or her surroundings. To orient the patient, use brief, concise statements such as "Mr. Smith, I am John Foxworth of the Winter Valley Ski Patrol. I am here to help you. I'm going to stabilize your injury and get you off the mountain."

Be Honest

In approaching any patient, you must decide how much each patient is able to understand and accept. You should be honest without additionally shocking the patient or giving information that is unnecessary or that may not be understood. Simply explain what you are doing, and allow the patient to be part of the care being given; this can relieve feelings of helplessness as well as some of the fear.

Acknowledge the Seriousness of the Condition

There may be occasions when a patient may refuse emergency medical care and insist that you do nothing

Rescuer Tips

Caring for Critically Ill and Injured Patients
- Avoid sad and grim comments
- Orient the patient
- Be honest
- Acknowledge the seriousness of the condition
- Allow for hope
- Locate and notify family members

or leave him or her alone. In these cases, it is important to impress on the patient the seriousness of the condition without causing undue alarm. Saying, "Everything will be okay," when it is obvious that it is not, is not being truthful. Generally, seriously ill or injured patients know that they are in trouble.

Allow for Hope

In trauma and acute medical conditions, patients may ask whether they are going to die. You may feel at a loss for words. You may also know, on the basis of past experience or in view of the seriousness of the present situation, that the prognosis is poor. But it is not up to you to tell the patient that he or she is dying. Statements such as "I don't know if you are going to die; let's fight this one out together" or "I am not going to give up on you, so do not give up on yourself" are helpful. These statements transmit a sense of trust and hope, and they let the patient know that you are doing everything possible to save his or her life. If there is the slightest chance of hope remaining, you want that message transmitted in your attitude and in the statements you make to the patient.

Locate and Notify Family Members

Many patients will be concerned and ask you to notify their family or others close to them. The patient may or may not be able to assist you in doing this. You should see to it that an appropriate and responsible person makes an effort to locate the desired persons. Assuring the patient that someone is going to do this may be a significant part of the patient's care.

Injured and Critically Ill Children

Injured and critically ill children who have life-threatening conditions should be cared for as any patient would be, insofar as an assessment of airway, breathing, and circulation (ABC) and immediate life threats are concerned. Due regard should be given to variations in height, weight, and size in providing emergency medical care. Because of the increased excitement and extraordinary nature of the emergency scene for a child, it is important that a relative or responsible adult accompany the child to relieve anxiety and assist in care as appropriate.

Dealing with the Death of a Child

The death of a child is a tragic and dreaded event. It is not unusual to think about the fact that the dead or dying child has a lot more to do and should have many more years to live. In our society, we assume that only old people are supposed to die. Children die less frequently now than they did in earlier times, so most people are unprepared for what they will feel when a child dies. You may think about your own children and those whom you know: nephews, nieces, grandchildren, and children of close friends. And you may think, "Why should this child, who is only 5 years old, die?" The situation may also make you reflect on the difficult questions of your own mortality.

The death of a child is never an easy subject to talk about, especially for the family. Although it is unusually stressful for the rescuer, you may be in the best position to help the family begin to cope with their loss until more definitive and professional help can be available. You can help the family through its initial period of grief and alert the family to the follow-up counseling and support services that are available.

Helping the Family

If the child is dead, acknowledging the fact of the death is important. This should be done in a private place. Reactions vary; in many cases the parents cannot believe that the death is real. Shock, disbelief, and denial are common. Some parents show little emotion at the initial news.

If it is possible, find a place where the mother and father can hold the child. This is important in the parents' grieving process; it helps to lessen the sense of disbelief and makes the death real. Even if the parents do not ask to see the child, you should tell them that they may. Your decision in permitting the parents to see the child may need some discretion. For example, in the case of a traumatic death in which there is significant disfigurement, that decision might have to be delayed. The delay may involve having support services available or contacting the family physician or others who can help the parents through this difficult situation. This may involve preparing the parents for what they will see and the changes brought on by rigor mortis, asphyxiation, and so forth.

Sometimes, you do not need to say much. In fact, silence can sometimes be more comforting than words. You can express your own sorrow. Do not overload grieving parents with a lot of information; at this point, they cannot handle it. Nonverbal communication, such as holding a hand or touching a shoulder, may also be valuable. Let the family's actions be your guide about what is appropriate. It is important that parents be encouraged to talk about their feelings.

Stressful Situations

Many situations, such as mass-casualty scenes, gruesome accidents, infant and child trauma, or the death of a coworker will be stressful for everyone involved ▼ **Figure 2-20** . During these situations, you must exercise extreme care in both your words and your actions. Be careful to present a professional demeanor in words and actions at the scene. Words that do not seem important, or that are said jokingly, may hurt someone. Conversations at the scene must be professional. You should not say, "Everything will be all right," or "There is nothing to worry about." A critically injured person knows that all is not well. What will reassure the patient is your calm and caring approach to the emergency situation. Briefly explain your plan of action to assist the patient in the crisis. Inform the patient that you need his or her help and the assistance of family members or bystanders to carry out the plan of action.

How a patient reacts to injury or illness may be influenced by certain personality traits. Some patients may become highly emotional over what may seem to be a minor problem. Others may show little or no

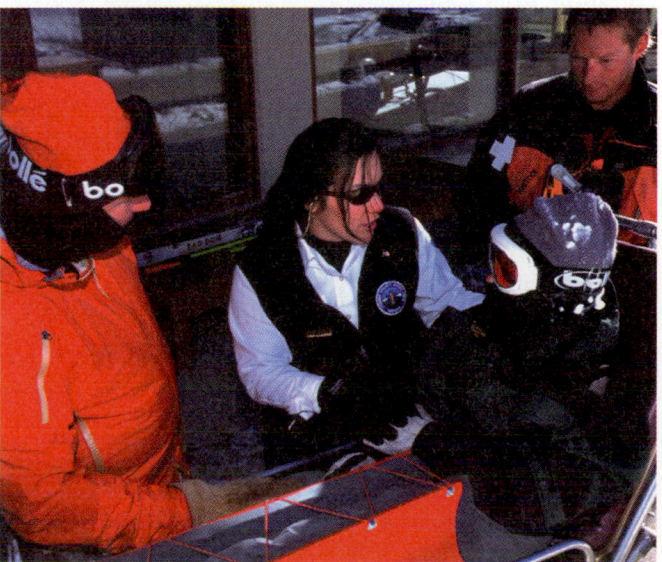

Figure 2-20 Exercise care in your words and actions in a stressful situation.

emotion, even after serious injury or illness. Many other factors influence how a patient reacts to the stress of an emergency care incident. Among these factors are the following:

- Socioeconomic background
- Fear of medical personnel
- Alcohol or substance abuse
- History of chronic disease
- Mental disorders
- Reaction to medication
- Age
- Nutritional status
- Feelings of guilt

You are not expected to always know why a patient is having an unusual emotional response. However, you can quickly and calmly assess the actions of the patient, family members, and bystanders. This assessment will help you to gain the confidence and cooperation of everyone at the scene. In addition, you should use a professional tone of voice and show courtesy, along with sincere concern and efficient action. These simple considerations will go far to relieve worry, fear, and insecurity. Calm reassurance will inspire confidence and cooperation. Compassion is important, but you must be careful. Your professional judgment takes priority over compassion. For example, suppose a screaming child with no obvious life-threatening injuries is covered with another patient's blood. This frightened child appeals to your compassion and thus gets your attention. In the meantime, an unconscious, nonbreathing adult nearby could die from lack of care.

Patients must be given the opportunity to express their fears and concerns. You can easily relieve many of these concerns at the scene. Usually, patients are concerned about the safety or well-being of others who are involved in the accident and about the damage or loss of personal property. Your responses must be discreet and diplomatic, giving reassurance when appropriate.

Some patients, especially children and the elderly, may be terrified or feel rejected when separated from family members. Other patients may not want family members to share their stress, see their injury, or witness their pain. It is usually best if parents go with their children and relatives accompany elderly patients
▶ **Figure 2-21** .

Religious customs or needs of the patient must also be respected. Some people will cling to religious medals or charms, especially if any attempt is made to remove them. Others will express a strong desire for religious

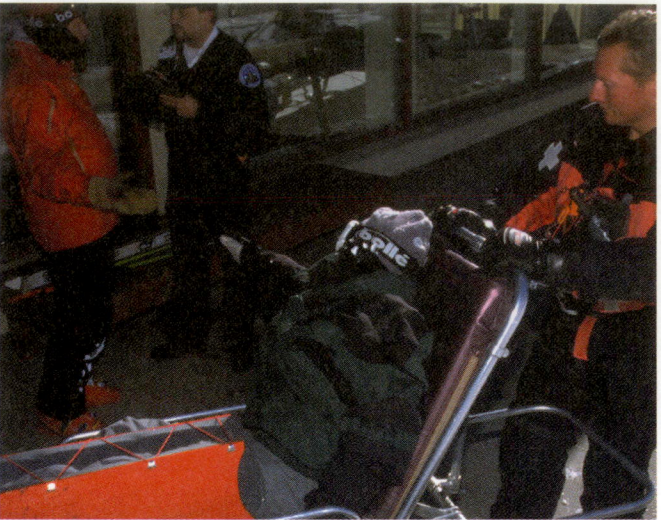

Figure 2-21 Children may be frightened when separated from family members.

counsel, baptism, or last rites if death is near. You must try to accommodate these requests. Some people have religious convictions that strongly oppose the use of drugs, blood, and blood products. If you obtain such information, it is imperative that you report it to the next level of care.

In the event of a death, you must handle the body with respect and dignity. It must be exposed as little as possible. Learn your local regulations and protocols about moving the body or changing its position, especially if you are at a possible crime scene. Even in these situations, cardiopulmonary resuscitation (CPR) and appropriate treatment must be given unless there are obvious signs of death.

Uncertain Situations

There will be times when you are unsure whether a true medical emergency exists. However, you should realize that the most minor symptoms may be early signs of severe illness or injury. Symptoms of many illnesses can be similar to those of substance abuse, hysteria, or other conditions. You must accept the patient's complaints and provide appropriate care until you are able to transfer care of the patient to a higher level (eg, paramedic, nurse, or physician). Your local protocols will direct your actions in these uncertain situations. When in doubt, err on the side of caution, and acquire the patient's consent and transport to the medical facility.

Stress Warning Signs

Emergency care is a high-stress job. Understanding the causes of stress and knowing how to deal with them are critical to your job performance, health, and interpersonal relationships. To prevent stress from affecting your life negatively, you need to understand what stress is, its physiologic effects, what you can do to minimize these effects, and how to deal with stress on an emotional level.

Stress is the impact of stressors on your physical and mental well-being. Stressors include emotional, physical, and environmental situations or conditions that may cause a variety of physiologic, physical, and psychological responses. The body's response to stress begins with an alarm response, followed by a stage of reaction and resistance, and then recovery or, if the stress is prolonged, exhaustion. This three-stage response is referred to as the <u>general adaptation syndrome</u>.

The physiologic responses involve the interaction of the endocrine and nervous systems, resulting in chemical and physical responses. This is commonly known as the *fight-or-flight response*. Positive stress, such as exercise, as well as negative forms of stress, such as shift work, long hours, or the frustration of losing a patient, all have the same physiologic manifestations. These include the following:

- Increased respirations and heart rate
- Increased blood pressure
- Dilated venous vessels near the skin surface (causes cool, clammy skin)
- Dilated pupils
- Tensed muscles
- Increased blood glucose levels
- Perspiration
- Decreased blood flow to the gastrointestinal tract

Stress may also have physical symptoms such as fatigue, changes in appetite, gastrointestinal problems, or headaches. Stress may cause insomnia or hypersomnia, irritability, inability to concentrate, and hyperactivity or underactivity. Additionally, stress may manifest itself in psychologic reactions such as fear, dull or nonresponsive behavior, depression, oversensitivity, anger, irritability, and frustration. Often, today's fast-paced lifestyles compound these effects by not allowing a person to rest and recover after periods of stress. Prolonged or excessive stress has been proven to be a strong contributor to heart disease, hypertension, cancer, alcoholism, and depression.

Many people are subject to cumulative stress, whereby insignificant stressors accumulate to a larger stress-related problem. In other cases, unusually

stressful incidents can cause acute severe stress, called *critical incident stress*. Such incidents include:

- Mass-casualty incidents
- Serious injury or traumatic death of a child
- Additional death or serious injury following an accident, as when a responding ski patroller runs into another skier.
- Death or serious injury of a coworker on the job

<u>Posttraumatic stress disorder (PTSD)</u> may develop after a person has experienced a psychologically distressing event. It is characterized by reexperiencing the event and overresponding to stimuli that recall the event. PTSD is sometimes referred to as "Vietnam veteran's disease" because of its classification as a mental disorder following the Vietnam conflict. Stressful events in prehospital care are sometimes psychologically overwhelming. Some of the symptoms include depression, startle reactions, flashback phenomena, and dissociative episodes (eg, amnesia of the event). Volunteer rescuers who are involved in a tragic event, who leave the area, return home and are not in contact during the next week or two with fellow rescuers involved in the incident, are especially vulnerable to this form of stress.

A rescuer need not suffer through the emotional aftermath of these difficult situations. A process called <u>critical incident stress management (CISM)</u> was developed to address this need (▼ **Figure 2-22**). This process confronts the responses to critical incidents and defuses them, directing the emergency services personnel toward physical and emotional equilibrium. CISM can occur formally, as a debriefing for those who

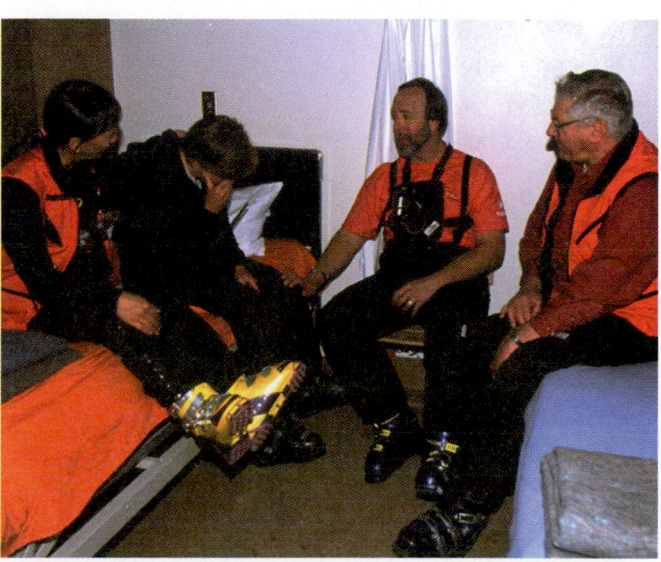

Figure 2-22 Critical incident stress management plays an important role in helping rescuers to relieve stress.

TABLE 2-13   Strategies to Manage Stress

- Change or eliminate stressors.
- Change partners to avoid a negative or hostile personality.
- Change work hours.
- Cut back on overtime.
- Change your attitude about the stressor.
- Stop wasting your energy complaining or worrying about things that you cannot change, such as:
  - Reckless skiers and snowriders
  - Injured children
  - Unpredictable weather
- Try to adopt a more relaxed, philosophical outlook.
- Expand your social support system apart from your coworkers.
- Sustain friends and interests outside emergency services.
- Minimize the physical response to stress by employing various techniques, including:
  - A deep breath to settle an anger response
  - Periodic stretching
  - Slow, deep breathing
  - Regular physical exercise
  - Progressive muscle relaxation

were on scene. A trained CISM team of peers and mental health professionals may facilitate this. Additionally, CISM can occur at an ongoing scene in the following circumstances:

- When rescuers are assessed for signs and symptoms of distress while resting
- Before re-entering the scene
- During a scene demobilization in which personnel are educated about the signs of critical incident stress and given a buffer period to collect themselves before leaving

The most common form of CISM is peer defusing, when a group informally discusses events that they experienced together.

Stress Management

There are many methods of handling stress. Some are positive and healthy; others are harmful or destructive. Americans consume more than 20 tons of aspirin per day, and doctors prescribe muscle relaxers, tranquilizers, and sedatives more than 90 million times per year to patients in the United States. Although these medications have legitimate uses, they do nothing to combat the stress that may cause the medical problems described previously.

The term "stress management" refers to the tactics that have been shown to alleviate or eliminate stress

reactions. These may involve changing a few habits, changing your attitude, and perseverance ▲ **Table 2-13**.

A clue to the management of stress comes from the fact that it is not the event itself but the individual's reaction to it that determines how much it will strain the body's resources. Remember that stress is defined as anything that you perceive as a threat to your equilibrium. Stress is an undeniable and unavoidable part of our everyday life. By understanding how it affects you physiologically, physically, and psychologically, you can more successfully manage it.

Supporting patients in emergency situations is difficult. It is stressful for them but also for you. You are vulnerable to all the stresses that go with being a rescuer. It is critical that you recognize the signs of stress so that it does not interfere with your emergency care work, job, or home life. The signs and symptoms of chronic stress may not be obvious at first. Rather, they may be subtle and not present all the time ▶ **Table 2-14**.

The following sections provide some suggestions for how to cope better with stress. Some of them may be useful in helping you to prevent problems from developing. Others may help you to solve problems, should they develop.

LIFESTYLE CHANGES. Your well-being is of primary importance to your job as an effective rescuer. The effectiveness and efficiency with which you do your job depend on your ability to stay in shape and avoid the

TABLE 2-14 Warning Signs of Stress

- Irritability toward coworkers, family, and friends
- Inability to concentrate
- Difficulty sleeping, increased sleeping, or nightmares
- Anxiety
- Indecisiveness
- Guilt
- Loss of appetite (gastrointestinal disturbances)
- Loss of interest in sexual activities
- Isolation
- Loss of interest in work
- Increased use of alcohol
- Recreational drug use

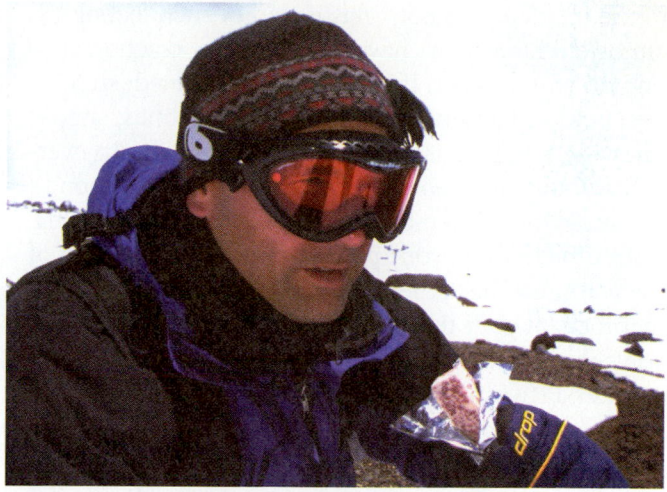

Figure 2-23   Carry a supply of high-energy food with you so that you can maintain your energy levels.

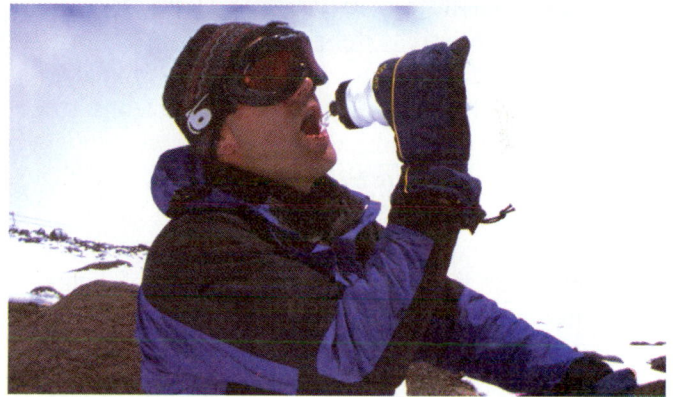

Figure 2-24   Maintain an adequate fluid intake by drinking plenty of water or other nonalcoholic, caffeine-free fluid.

risk of personal injury. <u>Burnout</u> is a condition of chronic fatigue and frustration that results from mounting stress over time. To avoid burnout, you need to be in good physical and mental health. Be aware of the potential hazards in rescue and emergency medical care. You must also learn how to avoid or prevent personal injury or illness.

NUTRITION. To perform efficiently, you must eat nutritious food and maintain hydration, as discussed previously in this chapter. Carry an individual supply of high-energy food to help you maintain your energy levels (▶ **Figure 2-23**). Try eating several small meals throughout the day to keep your energy resources at constant high levels. Remember, however, that overeating may reduce your physical and mental performance. After a large meal, the blood that is needed for the digestive process is not available for other activities.

EXERCISE AND RELAXATION. A regular program of exercise will enhance the benefits of maintaining good nutrition and adequate hydration (▶ **Figure 2-24**). When you are in good physical condition, you can handle job stress more easily. A regular program of exercise will increase your strength and endurance.

BALANCING WORK, FAMILY, AND HEALTH. As a rescuer, you may be called to assist the sick and injured any time of the day or night. Unfortunately, there is no rhyme or reason to the timing of illness and injury.

You may be called away from family and friends during social activities. You should never let this interfere excessively with your own needs. Find a balance between work and family; you owe it to yourself and to them. It is important to make sure that you have the time that you need to relax with family and friends.

It is also important to realize that coworkers, family, and friends often may not understand the stress involved in emergency care. As a result of a particularly trying experience, you might not feel like going out to a movie or attending a family event that has been planned for some time. In these situations, help from a critical incident stress debriefing team or other assistance program may help you in resolving these problems.

Critical Incident Stress Debriefing

You may be called to a situation so horrible that you find it difficult to respond as you were trained. You may have an immediate or delayed negative response to the incident. Do not be ashamed of such feelings; almost all responders have had the same reaction at one time or another. If you feel overwhelmed, step back and call additional resources. Sometimes, simply knowing that help is on the way can help you to overcome your fear or anxiety and enable you to respond to the situation. Remember that if you have these feelings from time to time, your partner and other members of the team may have them, too. Keep an eye on other members of your team. Confirm that they are under control and act appropriately during a major disaster.

After a stressful run or a disaster, there may be an emotional letdown. This letdown is often overlooked. However, it may be more important to deal with than the initial contact response. Critical incident stress debriefing is a way to deal with this emotional letdown phase. A critical incident is any event that causes anxiety and mental stress to emergency workers. <u>Critical incident stress debriefing (CISD)</u> is a program in which severely stressful job-related incidents are discussed. These discussions are conducted in strict confidence with other emergency workers who are trained in CISD (▼ **Figure 2-25**). The purpose of CISD is to relieve personal and group anxieties and stress. Never be ashamed to report your feelings, because such a debriefing can be vital to your emotional well-being. It should not be dismissed as trivial or nonessential.

CISD teams consist of peer counselors and mental health professionals who help you to deal with critical incident stress. Usually, CISD meetings are held within 24 to 72 hours of a major incident. CISD meetings may also have to be repeated at a later time. A CISD meeting is not an investigation or an interrogation. It is an opportunity to discuss your feelings, fears, and

reactions to the event. All information that is discussed in the meeting should remain confidential. The CISD leaders and mental health professionals will help you by listening and then offering suggestions on how to overcome the stress. CISD is designed to accelerate the normal recovery process following a critical incident. These meetings are helpful to all rescuers who are involved in an incident, whether or not they think they were stressed. A CISD meeting provides a means to quickly vent feelings in a nonthreatening atmosphere.

CISD programs are located throughout the United States. CISD teams usually can be located by calling telephone directory assistance in your area and asking for CISD. The International Critical Incident Stress Foundation, Inc. has an emergency access number: (410) 313-2473. For general information, call (410) 750-9600, or contact the foundation by e-mail at icisf@icisf.org.

A comprehensive CISM system includes the following 10 components:

- Preincident stress education
- On-scene peer support
- One-on-one support
- Disaster support services
- Defusings
- CISD
- Follow-up services
- Spouse and family support
- Community outreach programs
- Other health and welfare programs, such as wellness

Scene Safety and Personal Protection

The personal safety of all those involved in an emergency situation is very important. In fact, it is so important that the steps you take to preserve personal safety must become automatic. A second accident at the scene or an injury to a rescuer creates more problems, delays emergency medical care for patients, increases the burden on the other rescuers, and may result in unnecessary injury or death. Carelessness when exposed to body fluids, contaminated clothing, or contaminated emergency care equipment may cause serious and difficult to treat illnesses in yourself or others. Exposure to hazardous materials may cause serious illness and injury.

As you approach a scene, the first thing you should note is whether there is any danger to rescuers, the

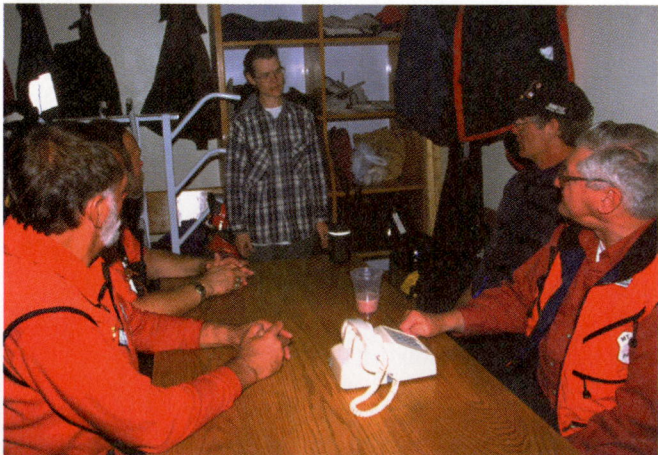

Figure 2-25 CISD sessions are conducted in strict confidence with other emergency workers who are trained in CISD.

patient(s), or others. In the outdoors in general, this includes severe weather, hazardous terrain (steep, slippery, icy, etc), rock fall, avalanche, swift water, flood, or fire. On highways, it includes such things as moving vehicles, slick roads, hazardous materials such as chemical spills, toxic fumes, explosions, or live electric wires. On ski slopes or snowboard slopes, you need to watch out for reckless skiers or snowboarders and snowmobiles or other over-snow vehicles. Note whether there is any danger of avalanche, or risk that the patient will slip or fall from an insecure location. When working at night, as in an off-area rescue, make sure you have plenty of headlamps or other light sources.

At an accident scene on snow, always place a pair of skis (yours or the patient's) upright in an X several yards above the accident. This will caution other skiers and snowboarders and help toboggan handlers locate the accident scene.

Communicable Diseases

As an emergency caregiver, you will occasionally see patients with infectious diseases, most of which can be transmitted from one person to another. These are called communicable diseases. Most of these diseases are much harder to catch than is commonly believed. In addition, there are many immunizations, protective techniques, and devices that can minimize the rescuer's risk of infection. When these protective measures are used, the risk of the health care provider contracting a serious communicable disease is negligible.

Routes of Transmission

While all infections result from an abnormal invasion of body spaces and tissues by germs, different germs use different means of attack. There are four basic mechanisms of transmission: direct contact (touching or contact with body substances) and indirect contact with living objects (vectors such as mosquitoes or ticks), inanimate objects (contaminated bedding and equipment), or airborne particles (aerosols).

Risk Reduction and Prevention

The **Occupational Safety and Health Administration (OSHA)** develops, publishes, and enforces guidelines for reducing risk in the workplace. In order to avoid infectious agents, emergency care workers must be trained in techniques for approaching the patient who may have a communicable disease and for avoiding all possibly infectious substances. Because there are so many different types of infectious diseases to be concerned about,

> ## Remember
>
> ### Infectious, contagious, or communicable
>
> Many people confuse the terms "infectious" and "contagious." In fact, all contagious diseases are infectious, but only some infectious diseases are contagious. For example, pneumonia caused by the pneumococcus bacteria is an *infectious* process, but it is not *contagious*. In other words, it will not be transmitted from one person to another. However, other infectious agents, such as the hepatitis B virus, are contagious because they can be transmitted from one person to another. An **infection** is an abnormal invasion of a host or host tissue by organisms such as bacteria, viruses, or parasites. A **pathogen** is a microorganism that is capable of causing disease in a host. A **host** is simply the organism or individual that is invaded. An **infectious disease**, then, is a disease that is caused by an infection. For example, Lyme disease is an infectious disease caused by the *Borrelia burgdorferi* bacterium, which lives in deer ticks. However, Lyme disease is not contagious. Again, a **contagious** or **communicable disease** can be transmitted from one person to another or from an animal to a person. The only way to get Lyme disease is to be bitten by a deer tick.

the Centers for Disease Control and Prevention (CDC) developed a set of **universal precautions**. These protective measures are designed to prevent caregivers from coming into direct contact with infectious agents spread by any method. The term "universal" is meant to remind you to apply precautions in all situations in which you have direct patient contact. It is impossible to tell whether an individual is free from a communicable disease in all situations, even if he or she appears healthy. Therefore, you should always take precautions.

Body Substance Isolation

The danger of exposure to infection by human immuno-deficiency virus (HIV), the hepatitis viruses, and other communicable diseases carried by blood and other body substances is a concern for emergency caregivers, but can be controlled by simple, common sense measures. Always follow **body substance isolation (BSI)** precautions to protect yourself and your patient. BSI is an infection control concept and practice that views *all* body substances as being potentially infectious. The most high-risk substances for bloodborne infection are:

- Human blood, including menstrual blood, blood products, or blood components
- Any body fluid visibly contaminated with blood

Rescuer Safety

Remember the following elements of BSI:

- Hand washing
- Gloves
- Eye protection
- Masks and gowns
- Patient care equipment
- Stretcher blankets, bed linens, and nondisposable clothing
- Resuscitation devices
- Disposal and cleanup

- Certain other body fluids, such as semen, vaginal secretions, amniotic fluid (from childbirth or miscarriage), cerebrospinal fluid (from an open head injury), synovial fluid (from an open dislocation), pleural or pericardial fluid (from an open chest injury), peritoneal fluid (from an open abdominal injury), breast milk, and saliva

- Any unknown or unidentified body fluid

- Clothing, bedding, and other absorbent materials soiled with any of the above. For example, hepatitis viruses can survive on the surface of clothing at room temperature for at least a week and thus can be spread by contact with dirty laundry.

Nasal secretions, sputum, sweat, tears, urine, and vomitus—if uncontaminated by blood, have not been shown to be dangerous. However, any body fluid can contain blood, which may or may not be visible. In addition, because you may not always be able to tell what type of fluid you are dealing with under emergency conditions, *you should avoid unprotected contact with all moist body substances*. Modes of transmission include the following:

- Blood or fluid splash
- Surface contamination
- Needle or other sharp object stick
- Oral contamination due to lack of or improper hand washing

HAND WASHING. Hand washing is perhaps one of the simplest yet most effective ways to control disease transmission (▶ **Figure 2-26**). Always wash your hands before and after contact with a patient, regardless of

whether you wear gloves. The longer the germs remain with you, the greater their chance of getting through your barriers. Wash your hands before performing a procedure, after glove removal, and between patients. Use a plain—not necessarily antiseptic—soap. If a glove breaks while you are caring for a patient, take both gloves off immediately and wash your hands before putting on a new pair of gloves. The proper procedure for hand washing is as follows:

1. Use soap and water.
2. Rub your hands together for 10 to 15 seconds to work up lather.
3. Rinse your hands, and dry them with a paper towel.
4. Use the paper towel to turn off the faucet.

In the outdoors, if your hands or any other body parts are exposed to contamination or contaminated clothing, immediately wash yourself with one of the following substances, listed in order of preference.

1. Soap and water
2. Waterless antiseptic hand cleaner
3. Plain water
4. Snow (▶ **Figure 2-27**)

Afterwards, wash thoroughly with soap and water as soon as you reach a facility where it is available.

If your mucous membranes (such as the eyes, nose, or mouth) are splashed by a body fluid, immediately flush the area with clean water.

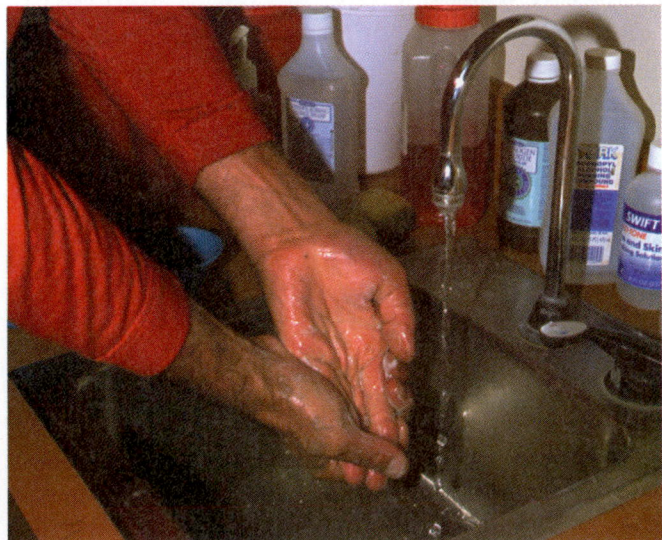

Figure 2-26 Wash your hands before and after patient contact.

GLOVES AND EYE PROTECTION. Gloves and eye protection are the minimum standard for all patient care if there is any possibility for exposure to blood or body fluids. Both vinyl and latex gloves provide adequate protection. However, some individuals are allergic to latex. Wear double gloves if there is substantial bleeding. You may also wear double gloves if you will be exposed to large volumes of other body fluids. Be sure to change gloves as you move from patient to patient. Do not use petroleum jelly with latex gloves, and always change latex gloves if they are exposed to motor oil, gasoline, or any petroleum-based product. For cleaning and disinfecting the patrol aid room, you should use heavy-duty utility gloves ▶ Figure 2-28 . *You should never use lightweight latex or vinyl gloves for cleaning.*

Removing used latex or vinyl gloves requires a methodical technique to avoid contaminating yourself with the materials on the surface of the golves ▶ Skill Drill 2-1 .

1. **Begin by partially removing one glove.** With the other gloved hand, pinch the first glove at the wrist—being certain to touch only the outside of the first glove—and start to roll it back off the hand, inside out. Leave the exterior of the fingers on that first glove exposed **(Step 1)**.

2. **Use the still-gloved fingers** of the first hand to pinch the wrist of the second glove and begin to pull it off, rolling it inside-out toward the fingertips as you did with the first glove **(Step 2)**.

3. **Continue pulling the second glove off** until you can pull the second hand free **(Step 3)**.

4. **With your now-ungloved second hand,** grasp the exposed inside of the first glove and pull it free of your first hand and over the now-loose second glove. Be sure that you touch only clean, interior surfaces with your ungloved hand **(Step 4)**.

EYE PROTECTION. Eye protection is important to prevent a blood or fluid splatter from reaching your eye ▼ Figure 2-29 . If this is a possibility, wearing safety or ski goggles is your best protection. However, you need

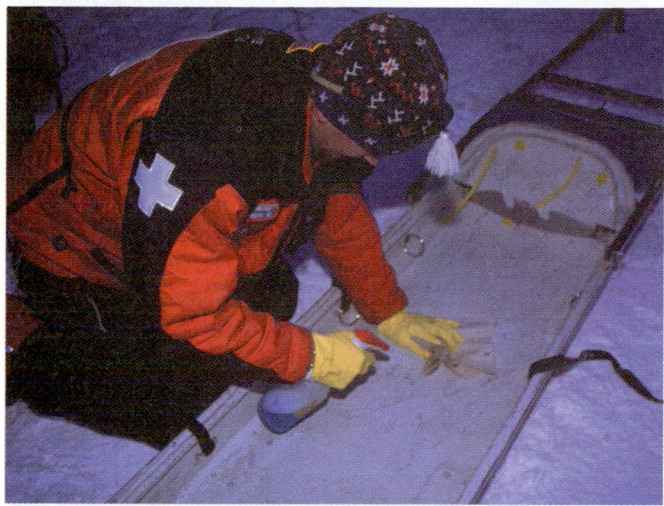
Figure 2-28 Use heavy-duty utility gloves to clean up spills of blood or other body fluids.

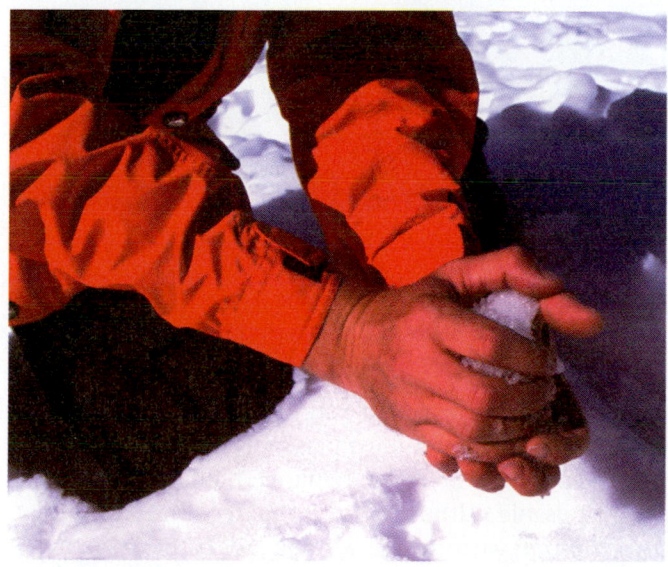
Figure 2-27 If nothing better is available, wash your hands in snow.

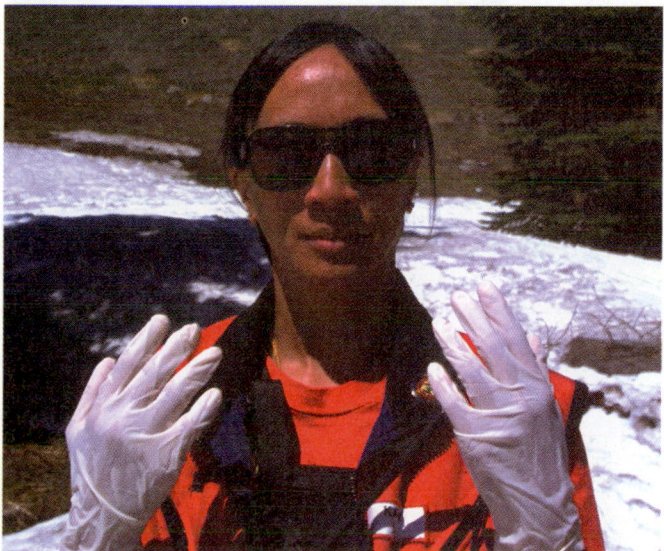
Figure 2-29 Wear eye protection to prevent blood splatter into your eyes.

Skill Drill 2-1   Proper Glove Removal Technique

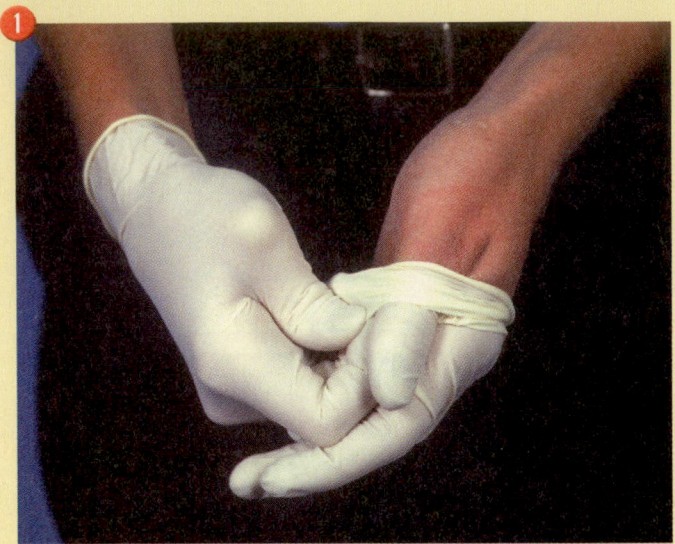

① Partially remove the first glove by pinching at the wrist. Be careful to touch only the outside of the glove.

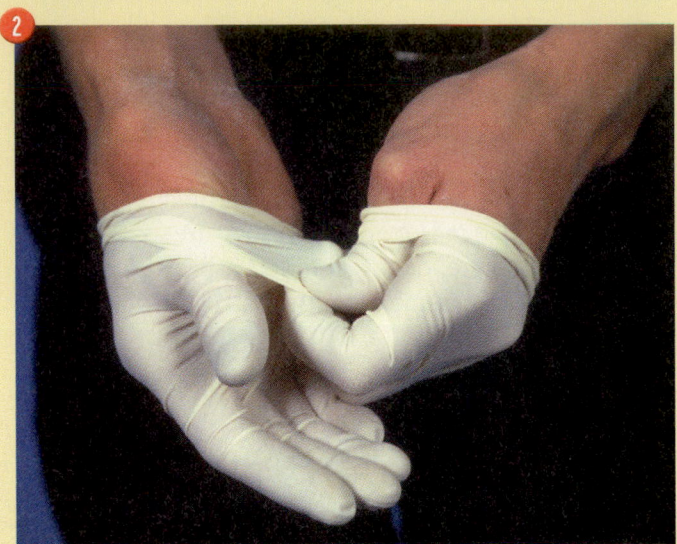

② Remove the second glove by pinching the exterior with the partially gloved hand.

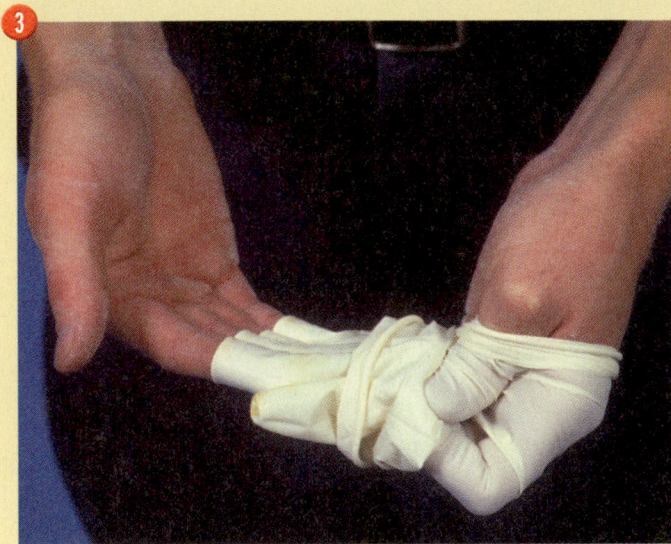

③ Pull the second glove inside out toward the fingertips.

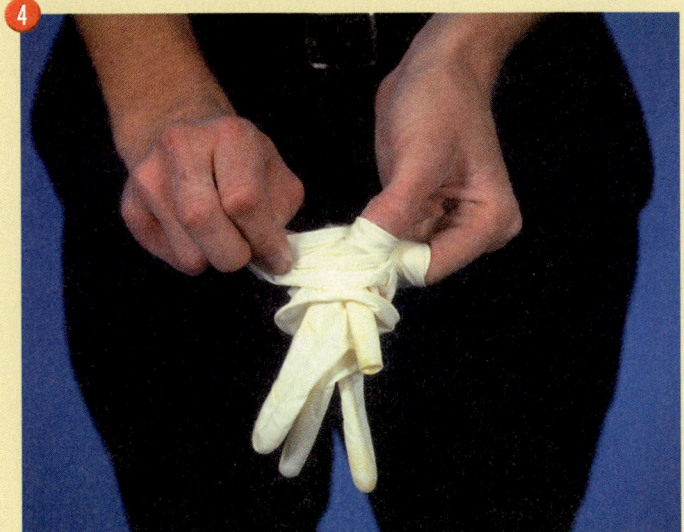

④ Grasp both gloves with your free hand touching only the clean, interior sufaces.

not wear goggles if you wear prescription glasses, but you must add removable eye shields when there is danger of splatter.

GOWNS AND MASKS. Occasionally, you may need to wear a mask and gown. A mask and gown provide protection from extensive blood or fluid splatter, as with major trauma or emergency childbirth. The best type of mask is a disposable surgical mask, some varieties of which include a plastic eye shield.

Gowns should be clean, reinforced, fluid-resistant, and disposable. Although gowns are recommended for the aid room, wearing a gown may not be practical in the field. The water-resistant parkas and overpants frequently worn by patrollers and other nonurban rescuers also offer good protection, although properly cleaning the clothing afterwards can be difficult. After care is provided, remove soiled gowns or other clothing as promptly as possible and wash your hands. Remember that the outside surfaces of these items are considered contaminated after they have been exposed to the patient. Gloves, masks, gowns, and all other items that have been exposed to blood or other body fluids must be disposed of (or cleaned, in the case of clothing) according to local guidelines. If you suspect that the patient has an airborne disease, place a surgical mask on the patient as well. If you suspect that the patient has tuberculosis, place a surgical mask on the patient and wear a High-Efficiency Particulate Air (HEPA) respirator yourself. You should not place a HEPA respirator on a patient because it is unnecessary and uncomfortable. A simple surgical mask will reduce the risk of transmission of germs from the patient into the air. Use of a HEPA respirator should comply with OSHA standards, which state that facial hair, such as long sideburns or a mustache, will prevent a proper fit.

If you are stuck by a needle or another sharp object while caring for a patient, get blood in your eye, or have any unprotected body fluid contact with a patient, immediately report this incident to your supervisor.

PATIENT CARE EQUIPMENT. When handling emergency care equipment that has been soiled by body fluids, make sure you do not expose your skin and mucous membranes and do not let it touch your clothing. Be sure that reusable equipment is not used for the care of another patient until it has been cleaned and disinfected. Discard disposable items properly.

Preferably, splints, backboards, and other reusable equipment are made of plastic or fiberglass so they will be easy to clean. If you already have equipment that is made of wood, make sure it is treated with polyurethane varnish or other nonabsorbent finish.

When giving rescue breathing or CPR, the device best equipped to protect you from the patient's saliva is a bag-valve-mask device, which does not require using your mouth to ventilate the patient. This device should be disposable. If it is not available, a disposable pocket mask or one with a disposable mouthpiece that contains a filter and one-way valve can be used. Two mouthpieces used in tandem are even safer. Devices to assist breathing are discussed in Chapter 6.

Because open fractures may contaminate splints and splint straps with blood, cover a bandaged extremity with a clear plastic bag before splinting it. You can use a 15-gal clear plastic garbage can liner to cover a lower extremity; use a smaller size for an upper extremity. Roll

the top of the bag down, insert the patient's hand or foot, then roll the bag back up the extremity like a long sock. You can then fasten all straps, including traction hitches, in place over the bag.

Your local hospital and EMS agency are possible sources of supply catalogs that contain disposable medical equipment and personal protective items that meet OSHA requirements. OSHA requires that all emergency caregivers be trained in the handling of bloodborne pathogens and in techniques of approaching the patient who has a communicable or infectious disease. Training must also be provided for such issues as blood and body fluid precautions, respiratory precautions, secretion precautions, and contamination precautions.

BED LINEN AND NONDISPOSABLE CLOTHING. Do not allow contaminated items such as bed linen and nondisposable clothing to contact your unprotected skin or clothing. Use rubber gloves when handling, transporting, and processing contaminated bed linen and nondisposable clothing items. In general, place them in a separate red plastic bag labeled with the biohazard warning symbol ▼ Figure 2-30 after use and keep them there until laundered. Your local hospital is a good source of information on where to have these items laundered and may even offer this service. Consult local regulations on handling contaminated laundry.

RESUSCITATION DEVICES. Use a bag-valve-mask device, pocket mask with removable mouthpiece (containing a filter and one-way valve, or mouth shield instead of performing direct mouth-to-mouth resuscitation. Resuscitation devices should be disposable if possible.

DISPOSAL AND CLEANUP. Consult local regulations on how to handle and dispose of infectious waste. In gen-

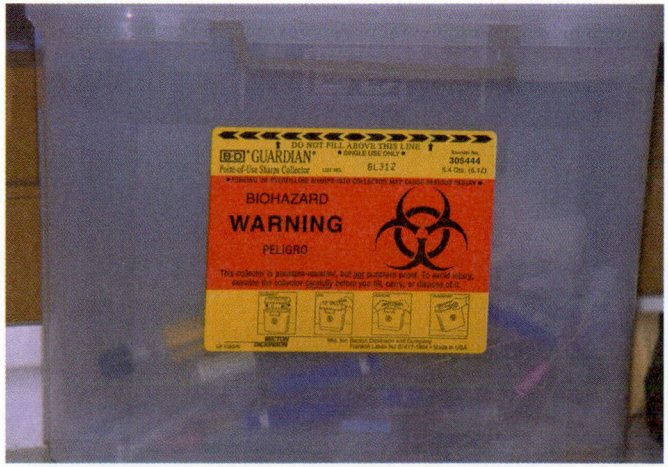

Figure 2-30   Biohazard warning symbol.

eral, you should handle this material with gloves, put it in a red plastic bag labeled with the biohazard warning symbol, keep it separated from ordinary waste, and dispose of it safely.

Clean up all spills of blood and other body fluids promptly, wearing rubber utility (household) gloves. Remove visible material with paper towels, wash the area with soap and water, and then scrub it thoroughly with a 1:10 solution of sodium hypochlorite (household bleach) in water.

Wear heavy-duty utility gloves while cleaning instruments and other medical equipment contaminated with blood or other body substances. Contaminated goggles and eyeglasses can be washed with soap and water. Disinfect reusable household gloves and equipment with one of the following substances, which have been shown to effectively inactivate HIV and the hepatitis viruses: 0.3% hydrogen peroxide, 25% ethyl alcohol, 35% isopropyl alcohol, 0.5% Lysol, 0.25% povidone iodine, 1:10 to 1:100 solution of sodium hypochlorite and water.

Many hospitals and commercial laundries wash all blood-contaminated bed linen and hospital gowns together, using two cycles: a cold-water cycle with bleach to remove blood, followed by a regular cycle depending on the type of fabric (usually a hot- or warm-water wash and a cold rinse). The laundry workers wear gowns, gloves, and goggles. Because bleach may ruin expensive garments such as parkas, wash these in cold water alone according to the label directions. If clothing is contaminated with "safe" blood (ie, your own), pretreat the bloody spots with hydrogen peroxide or unflavored meat tenderizer mixed with a small amount of water to make a paste, and then clean the clothing according to the label instructions.

Other Risks

LATEX ALLERGY. The widespread use of latex gloves has led to an increase in allergic reactions to latex. Seven percent to 10% of all health care workers have allergic reactions to latex, compared to less than 1% of the general population. This statistic probably reflects the increased exposure of health care workers.

Reactions can be mild or severe. Mild reactions include dermatitis due to direct contact with latex, and reactions due to airborne glove powder (hay fever-like symptoms, asthma). Severe reactions include anaphylactic shock (see Chapter 9).

If you suffer from latex allergy or suspect that an allergy is developing, be sure to consult an allergist.

Rescuers with mild latex allergy should avoid unnecessary exposure to gloves and other latex products; those with severe reactions should avoid all latex exposure.

Using a barrier cream or wearing a thin, cotton glove under the latex glove may be sufficient to control a mild allergic rash. In more severe cases, low-allergenic latex gloves or gloves made of vinyl, neoprene, styrene, or other nonlatex synthetic materials must be used. To prevent allergic respiratory tract reactions, individual patrols may wish to get rid of airborne glove powder by banning the use of powdered gloves by their patrollers.

HAZARDOUS MATERIALS (HazMat). According to OSHA, there are well over 500,000 existing chemical products in the United States, with hundreds of new ones being introduced each year. At any given time, 30 to 40 million workers are potentially exposed to one or more hazardous chemicals. Adverse effects of these chemicals include diseases of the heart, lungs, liver, and kidneys; cancer; sterility; burns; and dermatitis. Some chemicals can cause fires or explosions.

Exposure can occur through normal occupational activities as well as through accidents such as spills, vehicle crashes, and equipment failure. OSHA regulates almost all aspects of manufacturing, transport, use, and disposal of these chemicals. In addition, it is required that employers and employees be informed about and given training in self-protection against any hazardous materials to which they may be exposed in the workplace.

Since emergency care providers may be exposed to hazardous materials (HazMat) when they are called to care for accident victims, the identification and management of such risks is an important part of emergency care. Hazardous materials are identified by colored, diamond-shaped labels (▼ **Figure 2-31**). However, without

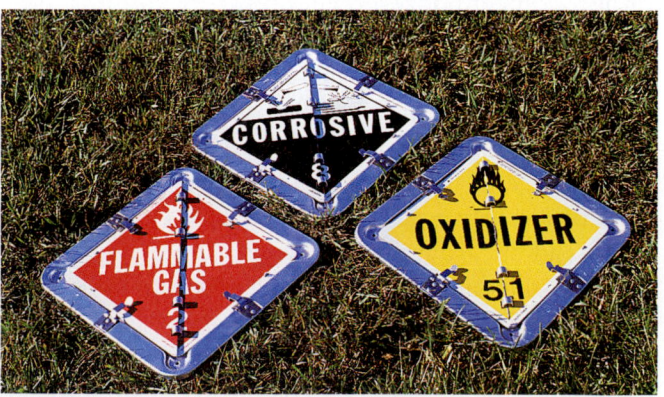

Figure 2-31 Hazardous materials safety placards are marked with colored diamond-shaped labels.

additional training, patrollers with OEC certification are not expected to do more than keep themselves and their companions out of danger, try to keep the incident from spreading, and care for patients who have self-evacuated or who can be reached safely.

Although HazMat exposure is uncommon among ski and snowboard patrollers and other nonurban rescuers, it is not absent. For example, ski areas and campgrounds use propane for heating buildings and chemicals for cleaning them. Gasoline, solvents, and lubricants are necessary wherever motorized vehicles and other equipment, such as ski lifts, are used. Vehicular accidents may produce spills.

As soon as you identify a HazMat incident, call 9-1-1 immediately and inform the dispatcher that there is a HazMat emergency so that specially trained technicians and specialists can respond. If you care for a patient, avoid contamination by wearing a hat, rubber gloves, goggles, a surgical mask, and fluid-resistant clothing. Do not attempt a HazMat rescue unless you have been properly trained. You may become a patient yourself.

Every ski patrol should contact the area manager for a copy of the written Hazardous Materials Communication program required by law. This lists the hazardous substances used or stored at the area, together with the manufacturer's Material Safety Data Sheet (MSDS) for each substance. The MSDS lists the known acute and chronic health effects of the substance, with instructions for handling, storage, decontamination, emergency care, and other important information.

Special training programs should be made available to patrollers and other rescuers who will have significant HazMat exposure.

Behavioral Emergencies: Methodology and Psychology of Dealing with the Injured and Ill

Most patients will be reasonable, cooperative, and grateful for your help. Any severe stress tends to cause regression to a more infantile and dependent state. Consequently, it is important to assume a calm demeanor of trustworthiness, competence, professionalism, kindness, and authority, even though you may feel uncertain and indecisive. Crouch or kneel so you are at eye level with the patient, make eye contact, introduce yourself as a trained rescuer and emergency care provider, and ask, "May I be of help?" or "May I help you?" In some cases, the patient will refuse help. A rational, informed adult with a normal mental status has a legal right to refuse care if he or she so desires.

Always document such a refusal, and have another rescuer or an onlooker witness the refusal. Be sure to explain what may happen if the individual refuses care, so he or she can make an "informed" refusal of care. Be sure to document this step as well. Members of ski and snowboard patrols and other rescue organizations often carry special forms for the injured or ill person or other responsible person to sign, acknowledging that care has been offered and refused.

Even if the person refuses help, stay with him or her until you are satisfied that everything is under control. A person with a significant injury or illness may soon realize that help will be needed after all. If a person who is irrational or has an altered mental status refuses help, you may have to provide necessary care despite the refusal. This should be documented and witnessed and you should also consider involving law enforcement personnel, if available, at this point.

Before caring for a child, you should always secure permission from the parent or other responsible adult if present. Because children are often more modest than adults, assessment may be difficult. It is especially important to position yourself at the child's eye level. Make eye contact, move slowly, use simple terms, and explain procedures, especially painful ones, before you carry them out. If parents or siblings are present, they may be able to help calm the child and explain what is happening.

Always think before speaking, since your statements can easily be misinterpreted by uncomfortable patients and their concerned friends and relatives at the scene. Explain each action to the patient *before* it takes place. Do not lie to the patient, particularly about a procedure that might be uncomfortable. Rescuers should never argue or criticize each other's actions within the hearing of the patient or bystanders (▼ **Figure 2-32**). Discuss

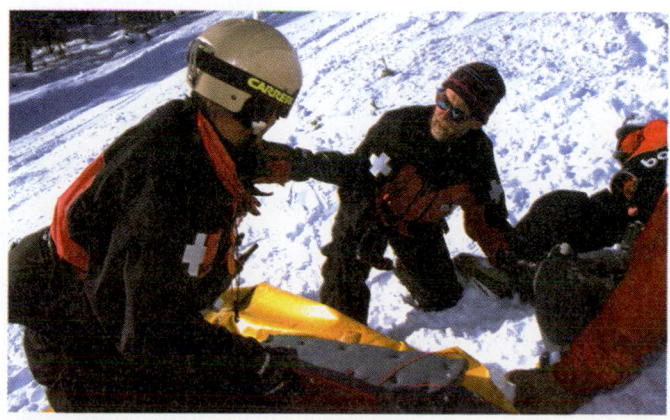

Figure 2-32   Do not be guilty of arguing or criticizing another rescuer's actions in front of the patient!

plans for emergency care and transport with your colleagues privately at first, involving the patient after you have outlined a plan.

Remember, *rescuers are not physicians.* It is inappropriate for you to offer detailed information on possible further treatment or outcome. In particular, avoid guessing how soon the patient will be well again. Do not make promises for others to keep. Prehospital emergency care is an inexact science: even the best assessment is imperfect; diagnostic facilities outside a medical center are relatively unsophisticated; and a serious injury or illness may not be obvious in the field. Remember that the patient may have more than one injury or illness. Avoid the temptation to attribute all signs and symptoms to the most obvious condition.

With this in mind, be aware that people who are under the influence of alcohol or other mind-altering substances are more prone to injury. They may deny using these substances, especially illegal drugs. In these patients, *it is important that you do not overlook injuries and unrelated illnesses and mistakenly attribute all signs and symptoms solely to the effects of the mind-altering substance.* These people and those who are senile or psychotic must sometimes be protected from injuring themselves or others. They may behave erratically and their normal judgment and usual protective reflexes may not be functioning. They may fall and injure themselves, wreck their vehicles, wander into danger, promote fights, and become belligerent and obnoxious. Occasionally, they may become violent and dangerous.

As the rescuer, you must remain calm, patient, nonjudgmental, nonthreatening, and reassuring. Approaching such a patient from the side may be preferable to a head-on approach, which may be misinterpreted as an act of aggression. Refrain from arguing and—except in an emergency and preferably with plenty of help and witnesses present—do not attempt to restrain the individual forcefully. Do not leave any patient with an altered mental status alone.

For an example of a type of adversarial reaction a patient may have, read Scenario 1 in Appendix A. It is based on an actual experience.

Immunizations

As a rescuer, you are at risk for acquiring an infectious or communicable disease. Using basic protective measures can minimize the risk. You are responsible for protecting yourself.

Prevention begins by maintaining your personal health. An annual physical examination is desirable. A history of all your childhood infectious diseases should be recorded and kept on file at home. Childhood infectious diseases include chickenpox, mumps, measles, rubella, and whooping cough. If you have not had one of these diseases, you must be immunized.

The CDC and OSHA have developed requirements for protection from bloodborne pathogens such as hepatitis B and HIV. An immunization program for hepatitis B should be in place in your patrol or rescue group. Immunizations should be kept up to date and recorded in your file. Recommended immunizations include the following:

- Tetanus-diphtheria boosters (every 10 years)
- Measles, mumps, rubella (MMR) vaccine
- Influenza vaccine (yearly)
- Hepatitis B vaccine

If you will be exposed to a patient who has a communicable disease, it is an advantage to have your health record available. If you have already had the disease or been vaccinated, the risk is low. However, you will not always know whether a patient has a communicable disease. Therefore, you should always follow BSI precautions if there is a possibility of exposure to blood or other body fluids.

Remember

If you are wearing gloves and touch body fluids, *everything else* you touch with the gloves becomes contaminated.

Chapter *Sweep*

Ready for Review

For basic survival, the body requires food, water, a constant supply of oxygen, and a core temperature regulated within the relatively narrow limits of 75° to 107° F or 24° to 42° C. For comfort and optimum performance, the body must be in top physical condition and free from disease or injury.

When signs of stress such as fatigue, anxiety, anger, feelings of hopelessness, worthlessness, or guilt, and other such indicators manifest themselves, behavioral problems can develop. Recognizing the signs of stress is important for all rescuers. CISD efforts, among other programs of support, are important in identifying potentially serious mental health problems, such as posttraumatic stress disorder, that can result from dealing with the overwhelming stress that sometimes develops in critical situations such as the death of patients. Posttraumatic stress disorder is a syndrome with onset following a traumatic, usually life-threatening event.

As a rescuer, you will arrive at scenes where potential danger to yourself is easily apparent. Every patient encounter should be considered to be potentially dangerous. Therefore, it is essential that you take all available precautions to minimize exposure and risk. Potential risks include scene hazards and infectious and communicable diseases.

Infectious diseases can be transmitted in one of four ways: direct transmission, vehicle-borne, vector-borne, and airborne. Even if you are exposed to an infectious disease, your risk of becoming ill is small. Whether or not an acute infection occurs depends on several factors, including the amount and type of infectious organism and your resistance to that infection. Most germs colonize the human body without causing any disease at all.

You can take several steps to protect yourself against exposure to infectious diseases, including keeping up to date with recommended vaccinations, using universal precautions and following BSI precautions at all times. Because it is often impossible to tell which patients have infectious diseases, you should avoid direct contact with the blood and body fluids of all patients. Use special caution if you have any open sores or cuts, no matter how small. If you think you may have been exposed to an infectious disease, see your physician (or your employer's designated physician) immediately.

You should know what to do if you are exposed to an airborne or bloodborne disease. The designated officer at the resort or organization where you work (paid or volunteer) will be able to help you follow the protocol set up in your area.

Infection control should be an important part of your daily routine. Be sure to follow the proper steps when dealing with potential exposure situations.

Scene hazards include potential exposure to terrain dangers, hazardous materials, electricity, and fire. Your safety is the most important consideration. Do not begin caring for patients until the scene has been made safe for you to enter.

Whenever you are in doubt about your safety do not put yourself at risk. If you see the potential for danger during a scene size-up, call for additional resources. Remember, your personal safety is of the utmost importance.

www.OECzone.com

Vital Vocabulary

acclimatization The process by which the body adjusts to a new environment.

aerobic capacity The body's ability to take, transport, and use oxygen.

basal metabolism Heat produced by constant internal metabolic processes (50 kcal per square meter of body surface per hour in an average person).

body substance isolation (BSI) An infection control concept and practice that assumes that all body fluids are potentially infectious.

burnout A condition of chronic fatigue and frustration that results from mounting stress over time.

cardiovascular fitness Conditioning the heart and circulatory system to meet an active body's changing needs for blood.

communicable disease Any disease that can be spread from person to person, or from animal to person.

conduction The transmission of heat, sound waves, nerve impulses, or electricity by contact.

contagious An infectious disease that is capable of being transmitted from one person to another.

convection Transmission of heat by a moving gas or liquid.

core The central nervous system, heart, lungs, liver, and other important internal organs of the body.

critical incident stress debriefing (CISD) A confidential group discussion of a severely stressful incident that usually occurs within 24 to 72 hours of the incident.

critical incident stress management (CISM) A process that confronts the responses to critical incidents and defuses them, directing the emergency services personnel toward physical and emotional equilibrium.

dependent lividity Blood settling to the lowest point of the body, causing discoloration of the skin.

evaporation Conversion of a liquid into a vapor.

general adaptation syndrome The body's three-stage response to stress. First, stress causes the body to trigger an alarm response, followed by a stage of reaction and resistance, and then recovery, or if the stress is prolonged, exhaustion.

host The organism or individual that is attacked by the infecting agent.

hyperventilation Deep, rapid breathing.

hypoxia Insufficient oxygen reaching the body tissues.

infection The abnormal invasion of a host or host tissues by organisms such as bacteria, viruses, or parasites, with or without signs or symptoms of disease.

infectious disease A disease that is caused by infection.

involuntary Not performed willingly; not subject to control.

layer A single thickness spread out or covering a surface.

metabolism The oxygen-requiring chemical reactions by which the body produces or uses energy.

motor fitness The possession of strength, power, balance, agility, flexibility, and endurance.

Occupational Safety and Health Administration (OSHA) The federal regulatory compliance agency that develops, publishes, and enforces guidelines concerning safety in the workplace.

partial pressure The percentage of total pressure accounted for by a specific gas, such as oxygen or carbon dioxide. For example, at sea level the partial pressure of oxygen is 160 mm Hg (21% of the total atmospheric pressure of 760 mm Hg).

pathogen A microorganism that is capable of causing disease in a susceptible host.

posttraumatic stress disorder (PTSD) A delayed stress reaction to a prior incident. This delayed reaction is the result of one or more unresolved issues concerning the incident that might have been alleviated with the use of critical incident stress management.

putrefaction Decomposition of body tissues.

radiation The process of emitting energy in the form of waves or particles.

respiration A general term for the process of exchanging oxygen and carbon dioxide between the atmosphere and the body cells. Frequently used as a synonym for breathing.

rigor mortis Stiffening of the body, is a definitive sign of death.

shell The skin, muscles, and extremities of the body.

universal precautions Protective measures that have traditionally been developed by the Centers for Disease Control and Prevention (CDC) for use in dealing with objects, blood, body fluids, or other potential exposure risks of communicable disease.

voluntary Spontaneous, arising from one's own free will.

Assessment in Action

It is a cold, clear, windy day with the temperature at about 25°F. You arrive at an emergency scene to find a man in his 20s lying in the snow next to a large rock. He is moaning and has a large rip in his right trouser leg.

His right thigh is bent at an abnormal angle and there is blood on the trousers and in the snow. Preliminary assessment indicates that he probably has an open fracture of his right femur (thigh bone). You know you must protect yourself from his blood and other body fluids and factor in the cold temperatures when doing your management and decision-making.

1. What BSI would be most appropriate in this situation?
   A. Gloves and mask
   B. Mask and goggles
   C. Gloves and goggles
   D. Mask and gown

2. The most effective way to prevent disease transmission is to:
   A. wear gloves.
   B. wear goggles.
   C. wash your hands.
   D. become immunized.

3. After the patient has been cared for and is in the toboggan ready for transport, what precautions do you take next?
   A. Leave the bloody snow for another team to treat.
   B. Pack around the patient with snow.
   C. Give the patient something warm to drink.
   D. Alert receiving facility of BSI risks.

4. Because of the temperatures, what considerations need to be made for the patient before transport?
   A. Protect patient from conductive heat loss.
   B. Administer oxygen.
   C. Use cotton layers to increase warmth.
   D. Keep injury accessible for observation.

5. Because of the temperatures, what considerations need to be made for the rescuer?
   A. Change rescuer responsibilities every few minutes.
   B. Insert warming packs in boots and gloves.
   C. Guard for evaporative heat loss caused by exertion and perspiration.
   D. Adequate layering.

6. What are the warning signs of stress in a rescuer?
   A. Improvement in job performance
   B. Physical changes, eg, fatigue, weakness, nausea, sweating
   C. Positive emotional status
   D. Cognitive skills maintained

7. When should you seek professional assistance for yourself and your coworkers?
   A. When you see radical changes in behavior and appearance
   B. When your coworker asks for help
   C. When there are no warning signs
   D. When your routine responsibilities stay the same

8. What can you do to reduce some of the emotional risks associated with being a rescuer?
   A. Avoid eating and drinking
   B. Seek professional assistance
   C. Maintain a high level of training and readiness
   D. Be tolerant and empathetic

9. A situation forcing you to deal with a horrible, gruesome injury can be stressful in itself. What are some concrete methods to help prevent susceptibility to physical illness during stressful times?
   A. Keep your mind on your work
   B. Go out with the guys on a regular basis
   C. Watch your diet and exercise regularly
   D. Volunteer for as much extra work as you can

Challenging Questions

10. How would the patient care differ for a similar situation that occurred during the heat of summer on a mountain bike trail in the desert?

11. How would the patient care differ for a similar situation that occurred in the wilderness in the fall with temperatures dropping each evening into the 30s and with transportation to definitive medical care not accessible until the following day?

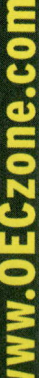

www.OECzone.com

Points to Ponder

You are stationed at the top of the course during a race. During the downhill, you receive a call that a racer has gone off the course and hit a tree. You start down immediately with a toboggan, headed for the accident site. When you arrive, you see a young male racer lying beside a large spruce tree; he is about the same age as your own son. He is not moving or speaking and his head is turned at an unusual angle. A crushed ski helmet is on the ground beside him. There is a large amount of blood in his hair and on the snow next to his head. You begin to assess him rapidly, noting that he is not breathing and has no carotid pulse. Your heart starts to pound, you become short of breath, and you feel that you may pass out.

Issues: Well-Being of the Rescuer, Patient Care Standards, Safety

Online Outlook

As a part of training you will begin to recognize and protect yourself from the environment and possible hazards. Nevertheless, injury and death to rescuers sometimes occur. Complete Exercise 2 at www.OECzone.com.

Interfacing with EMS and Other Medical Personnel

♠ These are core concepts in initial patrol training.

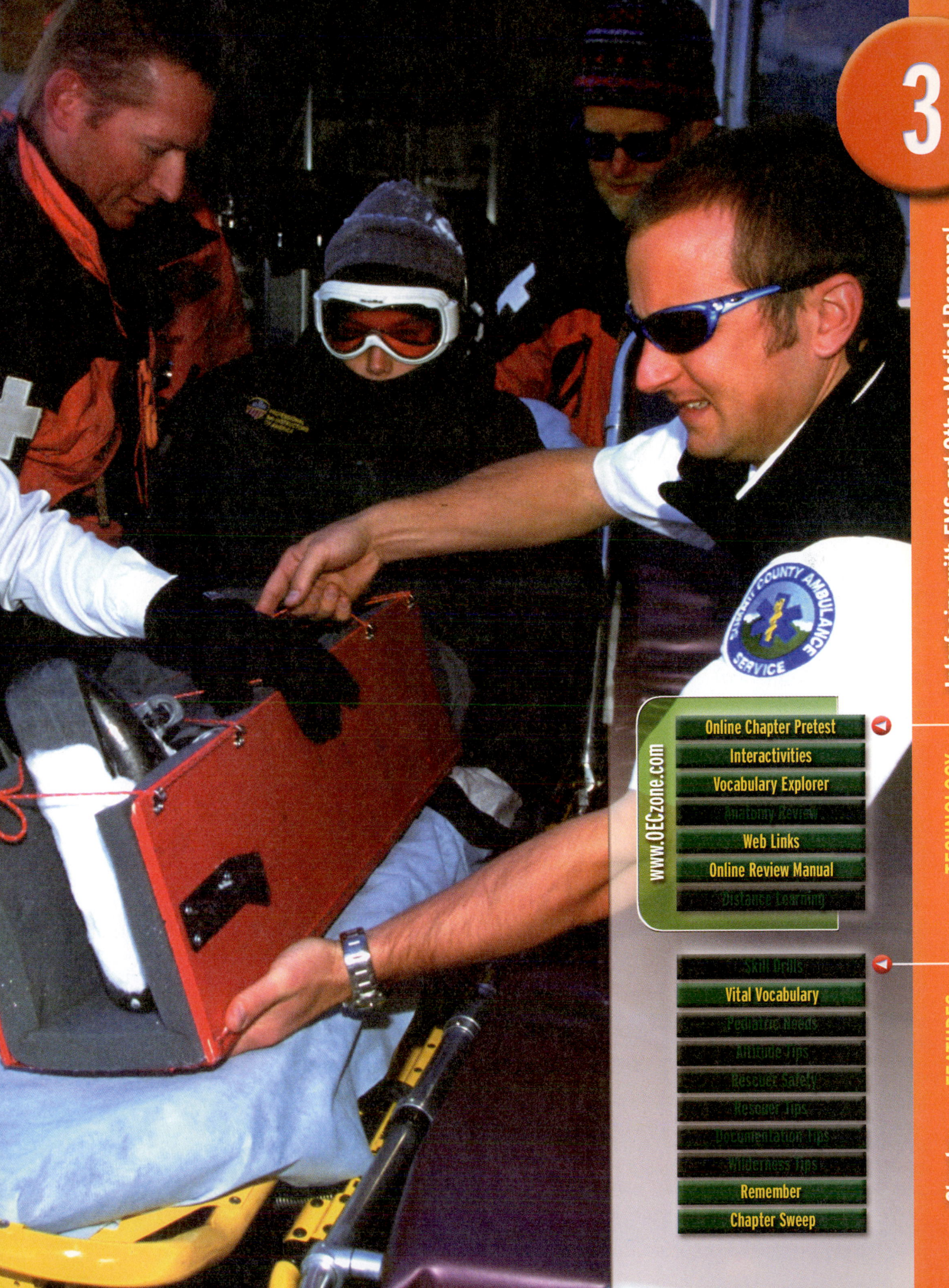

TECHNOLOGY

www.OECzone.com

- Online Chapter Pretest
- Interactivities
- Vocabulary Explorer
- Anatomy Review
- Web Links
- Online Review Manual
- Distance Learning

FEATURES

- Skill Drills
- Vital Vocabulary
- Pediatric Needs
- Altitude Tips
- Rescuer Safety
- Rescuer Tips
- Documentation Tips
- Wilderness Tips
- Remember
- Chapter Sweep

Chapter

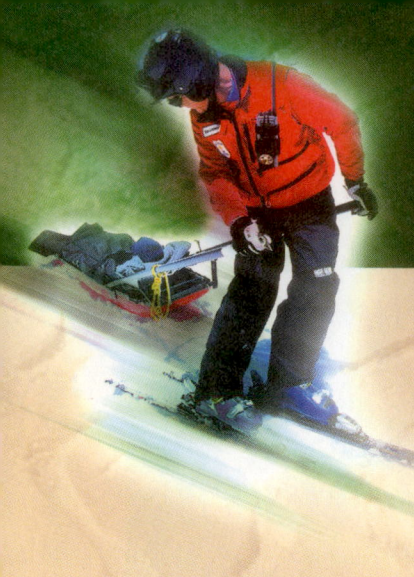

You are the rescuer

At the Junior Nationals Giant Slalom race, a competitor has had a nasty fall. The patrol responds and notes that her injuries appear limited to tenderness and deformity in the upper thigh. A traction splint is applied appropriately on the hill and she is transported down the mountain. Because the area is hosting a national competition, an ambulance is waiting at the base of the hill and the competitor's coach and family want her to be placed immediately in the ambulance and taken to the medical center. You are the lead patroller who is caring for the patient and you had made a decision on the race course to expedite her egress from the hill by placing the traction splint with her boot on. Now on arrival down the hill, she is beginning to complain of discomfort in her foot and cramps in her calf from the forward cant of the boot. The ambulance crew wants to take the patient the way she is and "deal with the boot on the way."

This chapter will help to introduce you to the relationships and good patient care that OEC technicians, emergency medical services (EMS), and other prehospital caregivers provide. It will also help you answer the following questions:

1. In the overall scheme of prehospital care, what are the primary roles and responsibilities of the OEC technician?

2. How can OEC technicians best interface with EMS personnel?

3. What are the differences between a standard of training and a standard of care?

Interfacing with EMS and Other Medical Personnel

The EMS System

Because they lack formal licensing within the local emergency medical services (EMS) system, ski patrollers are not a regulated part of the formal EMS system. Each state licensing scheme for EMS providers is a bit different, requiring somewhat different training, and perhaps providing for different levels of licensing and commensurately varying standards of care.

In order to fulfill its role as a nationwide educational program for patrollers and other outdoor rescuers with a single standard of training, it is critical that Outdoor Emergency Care not be regulated by individual state EMS systems. As outdoor rescuers, patrollers do not require state or local licensing.

Patrollers provide first response to emergency circumstances requiring initial emergency care and transport to enter the local EMS system. Typically, this involves the provision of limited emergency medical care (stabilization, transport, and transfer to EMS) within a limited geographic area (the ski area, touring center, race course, or other similarly limited geographic area). A ski area or touring center may elect to provide a higher level of care, and, if so, must do so in compliance with state and local EMS laws and rules. Many large resorts also routinely provide advanced life support (ALS) care or a clinic staffed with physicians.

Description of Emergency Medical Services System

The **emergency medical services** system in the United States began in the 1960s. At this time the President's Commission on Highway Safety published a report titled "Health, Medical Care and Transportation of the Injured," in which the Commission recommended a national program to reduce deaths and injuries resulting from motor vehicle accidents. In 1966, the National Academy of Science–National Research Council published "Accidental Death and Disability: the Neglected Disease of Modern Society," which described the very primitive state of prehospital care at that time and provided recommendations to address the deficiencies. In these early stages, health care officials were taking note of the effective prehospital care provided in a military setting, first in Korea and, at the time of the reports, in Vietnam.

In this climate of heightened awareness about prehospital care, Congress established the Department of Transportation (DOT) and adopted two laws: the National Traffic and Motor Vehicle Safety Act of 1966, and the Highway Safety Act of 1966. Formation of the DOT created the financial and legislative authority needed to establish EMS on a national scale. The new department of the federal government set standards for highway safety—including those related to EMS—which all states were required to meet.

Government provided the mandate, framework, and funding for the system that was going to become EMS, but it took a number of years for the demonstration projects, technology, think tanks, and politics to coalesce and begin to take shape. In 1973, the Emergency Medical System Act was passed. Its goal was to encourage the development of comprehensive regional EMS systems throughout the country. Within this act were the "Fifteen Essential Components of EMS" listed in ▼ Table 3-1 , which all federally funded systems were required to address.

These components persisted in one form or another as a measuring guide for EMS until 1996, when the National Highway Traffic Safety Administration (NHTSA) produced the consensus document, "1996 EMS Agenda for the Future." Contained within this document were the 14 "Essential Components of an EMS System" listed in ▼ Table 3-2 , which superceded and updated the original 15.

During this nascent period for EMS, issues of personnel and training were undergoing evolution, standardization, and formalization. No longer would a chauffeur's license suffice as the sole entry criteria for driving the hospital or local ambulance. The Highway Safety Act of 1966 contained funds to develop a curriculum for a training course for the new position of

Emergency Medical Technician-Ambulance (EMT-A). The American Academy of Orthopaedic Surgeons (AAOS) published the 70-hour EMT-A curriculum in 1969, and, thereafter, states increasingly required ambulance drivers to attain an EMT-A certification. In 1970, a national registry for those with EMT-A certification was established, although most states still require state certification as well. In 1972, the Department of Labor officially recognized the **emergency medical technician (EMT)** as a profession.

The education and role of paramedics developed somewhat independently of the programs for EMT-As. The use of paramedics in urban emergency care arose in the late 1960s out of specialized local training that sprang up in a few cities throughout the country to support prehospital cardiac programs. Fueled by issues of demand, technology, and an influx of Vietnam-seasoned military medics, paramedic certification grew in the 1970s at the same quickened pace of EMT-A certification. The two programs eventually started to mesh, and in the early 1980s, the DOT published its first EMT-Paramedic curriculum ▶ Figure 3-1 .

The current EMS system has evolved from these modest beginnings. EMS clearly provides a fundamental public safety role (on-scene medical stabilization and transport to definitive care) that could be filled by

Table 3-1 Fifteen Essential Components of EMS (1973)

1. Manpower
2. Training
3. Communications
4. Transportation
5. Facilities
6. Critical care units
7. Public safety agencies
8. Consumer participation
9. Access to care
10. Patient transfer
11. Coordinated patient record keeping
12. Public information and education
13. Review and evaluation
14. Disaster plan
15. Mutual aid

Table 3-2 Essential Components of an EMS System (1996)

1. Integration of health services
2. EMS research
3. Legislation and regulation
4. System finance
5. Human resources
6. Medical direction
7. Public education
8. Prevention
9. Public access
10. Communication
11. Clinical care
12. Information systems
13. Evaluation
14. Education

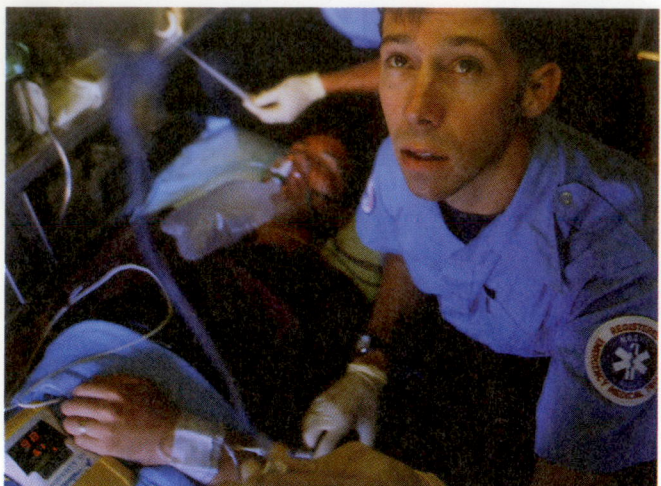

Figure 3-1 In the early 1980s, the DOT published its first EMT-Paramedic curriculum.

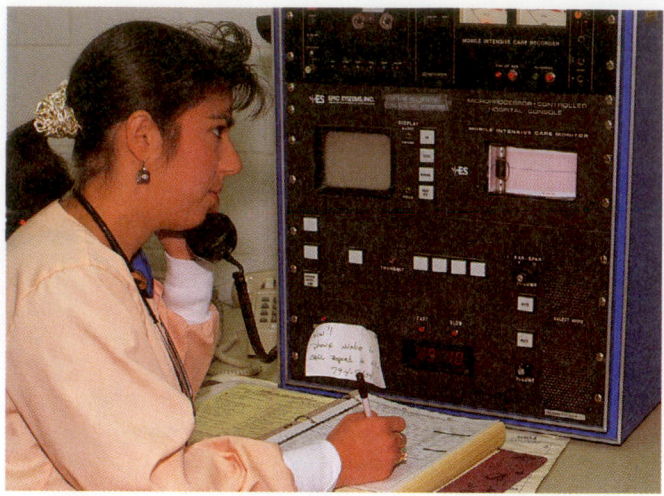

Figure 3-2 Direct contact with a medical control physician or facility is called "on-line" medical control.

no other agency. The crowning achievement of the EMS system is transferring the injured patient to the facility best suited to the medical care for his or her particular injuries or illness. At the state and regional levels, it provides a method for coordinating large-scale emergency services.

State EMS Offices

One of the goals of the federal EMS program was to establish an EMS "lead agency" in each state. Each state now has such an agency, with most located in the state's health department or an equivalent organization. The roles and responsibilities of this office vary but in most cases, the agency is charged with setting EMS standards for that state. The role of enforcing EMS-related statutes regarding ambulance licensure, certification of personnel, and even the designation of hospital specialty care centers may also be filled by state EMS agencies. In addition to the state office, regional EMS organizations are established in most states and have varying degrees of authority and responsibilities for certification, licensing, educational, and prevention issues within their regions.

State and Regional Protocols

EMS is largely protocol-driven with an established method of demonstrating basic competency at defined provider levels. When a system uses direct contact with a "medical control physician or facility," it is called "on-line" **medical control** (▲ Figure 3-2). In these systems, a physician or nurse at the "control facility" serves as the control point for the use of various prehospital interventions or drugs. Direct orders are then given to the EMS crew based on the situation report given to medical control by the crew. Usually, these orders will

follow a written guideline, standing orders, or protocol, particularly if nurses are used to staff the facility.

Other systems provide the EMS crews with a set of protocols that cover the usual encountered situations. The crew is preauthorized to use these protocols for their actions. No direct contact is required for most situations. This is called "off-line" medical control.

Many systems use a combination of the two methods, reserving on-line contact for particularly complicated cases. The provision of the protocols varies by region. In some locales, the sponsoring medical physician for the ambulance service has complete control over these protocols, usually within the bounds set by state EMS regulations for various levels of EMS providers. Other areas have state or regional protocols that all providers within its scope are obligated to use.

National Training Curriculums

The NHTSA is the lead agency that provides national curricula guidelines for EMS levels from first responder to paramedic. The details and requirements of each of these generally fall under specific state regulations. The programs are materially alike, however.

Training Levels

The First Responder curriculum provided by the NHTSA gives core knowledge, skills, and attitudes to function in the capacity of a first responder. The course provides 40 hours of instruction.

Advanced Levels of Care

An **EMT-Basic** (EMT-B) must generally complete about 110 hours of classroom instruction. All other levels require EMT-B training plus additional hours of training.

An <u>EMT-Intermediate</u> (EMT-I) must complete 300 to 400 hours of classroom instruction in addition to EMT-B training.

An <u>EMT-Paramedic</u> (EMT-P) must complete 1,000 to 1,200 hours of classroom instruction plus a riding internship of 480 hours.

Participation in the Local EMS System

If there are many unique features to every region's EMS environment, there is certainly one unifying feature: it is a politically charged venue wherever it exists. From hospital-based EMS to volunteer rural squads to big city private industry competing with fire unions for health care dollars, it is never a dull place to be.

EMS within communities is generally highly regulated as to what level of care is provided and as to who may provide it. Many of these regulations help to preserve good patient care by determining that it will be provided by units that meet the skill and resource capabilities demanded by the community; others run to a point that some would argue are protectionist of various providers.

As noted at the outset of this chapter, the ski area and backcountry rescue environment has not been significantly affected by the urban EMS system. The participation of ski patrollers is a tier of prehospital care that often occurs before participation of ambulance-based providers.

BLS versus ALS

Terms often used in EMS are <u>basic life support (BLS)</u> and <u>advanced life support (ALS)</u>. Strict definitions of these terms may vary. BLS is generally thought of as care that requires no cardiac monitoring, advanced airway skills, or IV medication skills; ALS includes these interventions and the use of additional specific medications.

Comparison of OEC with Urban EMS

The education of DOT/NHTSA first responders focuses on stabilization and transportation. In the outdoor setting, these solutions are substantially different from urban EMS and generally focus on getting patients to and into the EMS system.

The additional tier of care providers creates the possibility for communication problems. These problems range from minor transfer issues to conflicts that possibly jeopardize patient care. Different standards of care and different protocols can make patient transfer difficult. These elements create challenges in building trust, especially between the outdoor emergency care provider, the EMT-B or paramedic, the hospital emergency department, and definitive treatment providers.

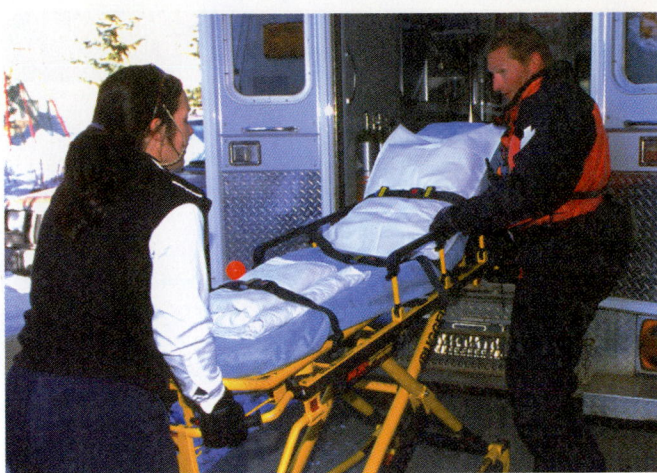

Figure 3-3 Providers need to consciously work together to communicate, share educational responsibilities, recognize strengths and weaknesses, and build trust.

In some systems, these care providers may never meet each other, let alone get to know and trust their respective skills. Despite this, all providers need to consciously work together to communicate, share educational responsibilities, recognize strengths and weaknesses, and build trust (▲ **Figure 3-3**).

The provision of outdoor emergency care is generally not regulated. While the federal government has played an increasing role in health care, very little of federal law has any direct application to outdoor emergency care, due to the absence of an ambulance in outdoor emergency locations serviced by ski patrollers and mountain rescue groups.

For the past 25 years, the DOT has promulgated regulations and curricula relating to the delivery of prehospital care by ambulance services. These rules were developed because of the high cost, both physical and economic, of highway motor vehicle accidents. Accordingly, the primary emphasis has been on organized EMS systems in the urban environment.

The DOT curriculum for first responders sets a standard of training that can be applied by analogy to the outdoor setting. Variations from the DOT curriculum are possible, but these must be justified by objective differences between the assumed urban environment of the DOT curriculum and the outdoor setting.

In tandem with federal rules, state laws and regulations regarding EMS systems have been directed at urban trauma, where it is assumed the care provider will have an ambulance nearby to store medical supplies and provide patient transportation. Licensing of EMS providers is focused on such urban EMS systems.

The National Ski Patrol has set a standard of training for the development and delivery of the Outdoor

Emergency Care program. The program is designed to allow consistent training of rescuers in the skills that they require throughout the country. OEC focuses on care in a unique outdoor environment, generally some distance from a higher level of care, using different transportation methods than a cot and an ambulance. The OEC program is based in part on the DOT standards and is designed to meet or exceed the DOT first responder curriculum in all applicable areas.

There are other emergency care programs, eg, Wilderness EMT and Wilderness First Responder. Notable among these is the Wilderness EMT program initially developed by Peter Goth, MD. A review of popular literature reveals many first aid handbooks and videos that devote some or all of their attention to the outdoor setting.

Each educational program establishes a standard of training, which may or may not conform to the standard of care required in a particular jurisdiction. This distinction between **standards of training** and **standards of care** is important to recognize. One hopes that the training for a particular group is directed at allowing that group to perform in accordance with the applicable standard of care for their activities. However, the final determination of the applicable standard of care is the judge who is reviewing a claim of improper care in a particular case.

The OEC Technician as a First Responder

What is a "**first responder**"? Basically, a first responder is defined as the first medically trained person that responds to a medical scene to provide aid or assistance ▶ **Figure 3-4** . The first responder uses a limited amount of equipment to perform the initial assessment and intervention.

The Role of a First Responder in the Outdoor Environment

The outdoors can provide the first responder with challenges not usually encountered in an urban setting. In addition to caring for unique injuries and illnesses, rescuers often serve in locations far from hospitals and fre-

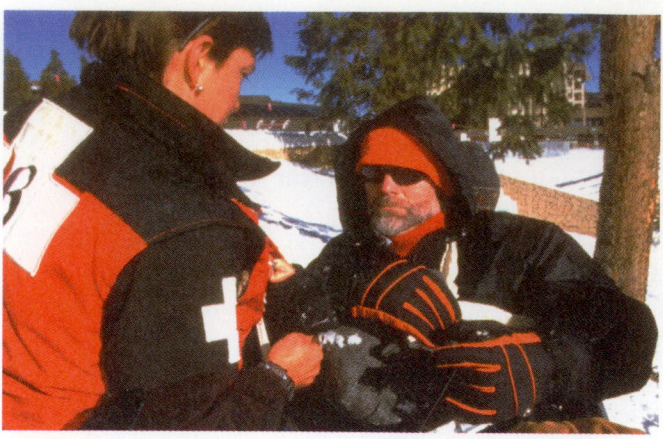

Figure 3-4 A first responder is the first medically trained person that responds to an incident scene to provide aid.

quently must provide care for an hour or more before patients can be turned over to the EMS system. Other outdoor rescuers can be many hours or even days from a physician or a hospital. Unlike urban EMTs, OEC technicians usually do not have a hospital emergency department a few minutes away and must know how to give care for a longer period of time before transferring the patient to the EMS system. Resources will typically be more primitive, if available at all. The environment itself may be an additional hindrance.

OEC technicians work in a wide variety of situations. Many are ski patrollers. Some ride mountain bikes, some are backcountry rangers, some serve on search-and-rescue teams, and others act as raft guides. This chapter will provide useful information to guide the OEC technician during interaction with other EMS providers.

The content will be presented in the context of an organized ski patrol, but other outdoor first responders can adapt these concepts to any situation they may encounter. Obviously, some ideas and procedures will be applicable and some will not, but it is important to remember that the only constant is the setting—the great outdoors! Outdoor rescuers need to be prepared to analyze and devise rational emergency care for unusual situations not specifically covered in training.

Role of Ski Patrollers as First Responders

The ski patroller clearly serves as the first responder to events that occur within the boundaries of the patrol's duties. The initial response is typically to assess the nature of the call and its severity, assess the need for immediate lifesaving intervention, to further communicate to other patrollers what additional resources will be required to safely treat and transport the patient and to anticipate whether urban EMS personnel or transport to definitive care may be required.

Ski Patrol First Response Systems

If one reviews Table 3-1, it is clear that most patrols satisfy a number of the requirements. Specifically, manpower, training, communications, transportation, access to care, patient transfer and disaster planning are all part of usual patrol operations. The modernized 1996 version (Table 3-2) of "Essential Components" finds the patrol with the following essential components: finance, human resources, medical direction, public education, prevention, public access, communication, clinical care, evaluation, and education.

Ski Area Policies and Protocols

One of the critical roles of ski area and touring center management is the development and consistent implementation of policies and procedures for taking care of the expected emergencies that occur at a ski area or touring center. Generally, such policies and procedures are developed by the local patrollers and/or area risk managers with the full knowledge and written consent of area management.

Some of the typical issues that are addressed in such policies include the spinal stabilization of the patient without symptoms, the protocol for the treatment and release of minors, release of patients with head injuries, handling the intoxicated patient and patients who wish to leave the aid room against patrol advice, protocols for written documentation, and procedures of dispensing over-the-counter medications to the public (analgesics).

Further standards and local protocols may need to be developed in conjunction with management with regard to cardiac arrest, use of an automated external defibrillator, use of ALS, and helicopter transport. These procedures can often be derived from existing local EMS protocol and should be developed in such a way to integrate the patrollers into the existing EMS system.

Clarifying and Standardizing Local Procedures

Ski area policies and procedures should include the process for calling and interfacing with the local EMS and medical resources. These must be arrived at in concert with all personnel who provide this care. Some may require only a verbal agreement among the parties, while others are best handled with a formal memorandum of agreement. It is important that each ski area evaluate the resources that are available in its immediate and extended community, and consider how these might need to be activated for a given situation.

For a given mountain resort, the most efficient situation might be to use the resort village's medical clinic for all situations not remedied by simple first aid ▲ **Figure 3-5** . Policies at remote ski resorts may require

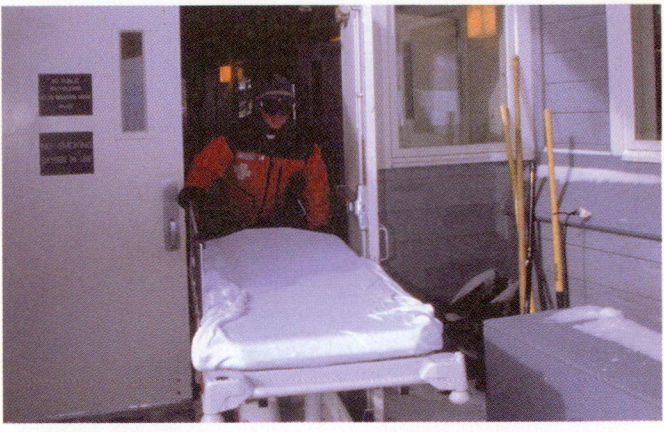

Figure 3-5 The most efficient situation might be to use a resort village's medical clinic for all situations not remedied by simple emergency care.

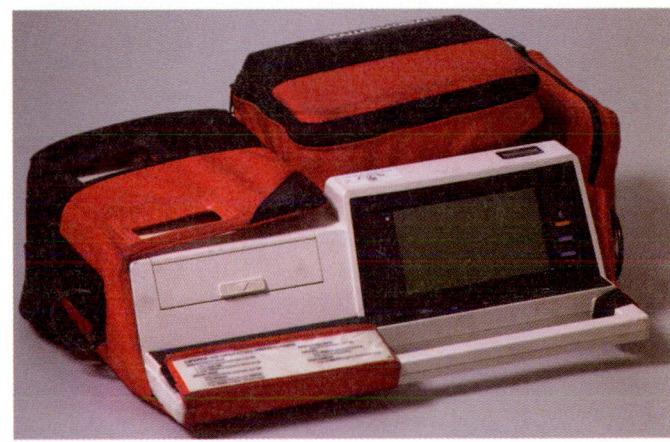

Figure 3-6 An automated external defibrillator.

handling a long ambulance ride to the nearest definitive care provider. The scope of activities performed by one patrol may therefore be quite different from others, and the proper development of local policies will carefully identify and deal with local geography and medical support issues.

At the forefront of an expanding scope of care at ski areas is the treatment of cardiac arrests. The automatic external defibrillator (AED) has been shown to be a lifesaving device that can be safely used by persons with minimal additional training beyond CPR ▲ **Figure 3-6** . It is to be found at a growing number of resorts, with many patrols having these devices at key locations for use by the patrol. The availability and use of the AED again stresses the need for clearly defined interactions with EMS. AEDs are properly used only in the context of a continuum of cardiac care. Patrols encountering a cardiac arrest patient must react according to a predefined plan that involves activation of EMS.

Procedures for requesting an ambulance should be clearly defined. There should also be a defined plan between patrol and EMS personnel for patient "handoff." Specifically, the patrol should understand its responsibilities to the patient and how that patient is transferred to EMS, which is usually the "higher level of care." When everyone understands each other's responsibilities, the transfer will go much more smoothly.

The EMS providers who are transporting the patient will want to independently confirm some of the historical and physical findings in the patrol report. EMS personnel, however, should rely on the patrol's expertise when independent confirmation may hurt the patient (eg, needlessly undoing an extremity splint).

Protocols regarding the use of helicopters for evacuation of patients from the patrol area of operation should be worked out in advance. The patrol should have an agreed upon plan with the medical evacuation service regarding "standby" (pre-alerts for potentially significant events), initiation and cancellation of a flight, and the operational parameters of the aircraft including hoist capabilities. Ground safety issues such as predefined landing zones, weather, and ground crew safety in approaching rotorwing aircraft must be a part of initial training in conjunction with the area operator.

Ski Patrol Medical Operations

Dispatch

Most areas designate one or more individuals as "dispatch." Depending on the area, this could range from an actual dispatch center to the working patrol director serving the function. Dispatch should serve as the point to which an initial accident report or injury is sent. Access to dispatch could come from patrollers with radios on the slope that have seen or have been notified of an incident, from the public via phones at the base of lifts or dedicated sites on the slope, and from area personnel in restaurants, shops, or lift facilities within the area. Increasingly, ski area guests are notifying dispatch by cell phones and newer "citizen band" handheld two-way radios.

Notification

Upon receipt of the call, dispatch, in consultation with the rescuers (or possibly other reporting parties or witnesses) on the scene, should process the call by evaluating its severity and by anticipating any special resources that may need to be activated. Information collected should include accurate descriptions of the location, the patient(s), the chief complaint(s) and/or the mechanism of injury, and any possible special needs of the patient(s). Notification is initially made to patrollers who are available in the call area. Patrollers

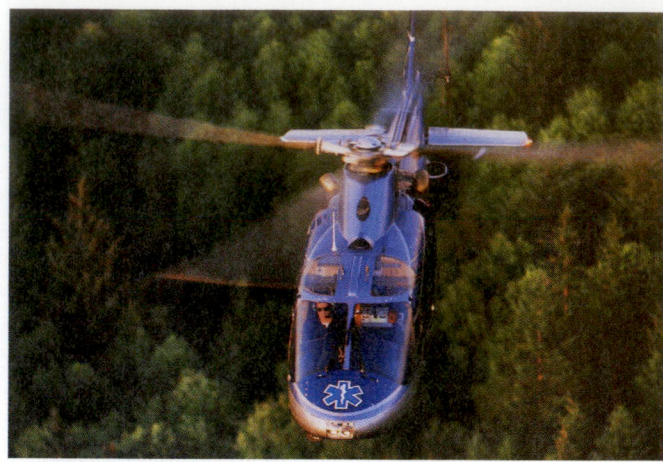

Figure 3-7 Dispatch may notify a helicopter medical evacuation service when the OEC technician is working on a patient with multiple injuries.

should be made aware of any special circumstances or dangers that may have been explicit or implicit in the original call.

At the time of the initial call and as updates are received, dispatch may alert EMS agencies or other special response groups if the need for these resources becomes likely or certain. Examples would be a report from a patroller on-scene that a skier has an obvious open fracture of the femur, from which would follow dispatch notification of local EMS to meet at the aid room for a required EMS transport to a hospital. Other such examples might include prenotification of a helicopter medical evacuation service when working on the slope on a critically injured patient with multiple injuries ▲ **Figure 3-7**.

Initial Assessment by a First Responder

The first rescuer on the scene needs to make a rapid scene survey and contact dispatch quickly. Dispatch needs to be told how many are injured, approximate age of the patient(s), types of injuries, specific needs in the field including oxygen or AED, if more help is needed, and what transportation is needed once the patient(s) are evacuated. The need for an ambulance, ALS, or a helicopter must be communicated in a timely manner. The on-scene rescuers update this information as new findings are made, or as changes in circumstance (both patient conditions and weather) occur. Good radio communication skills are paramount.

Initial Transport

At a ski area, transport is usually by toboggan ▶ **Figure 3-8**. During toboggan transport, reassessment of the patient (sometimes just maintaining voice contact) is important. If a serious condition warrants rapid

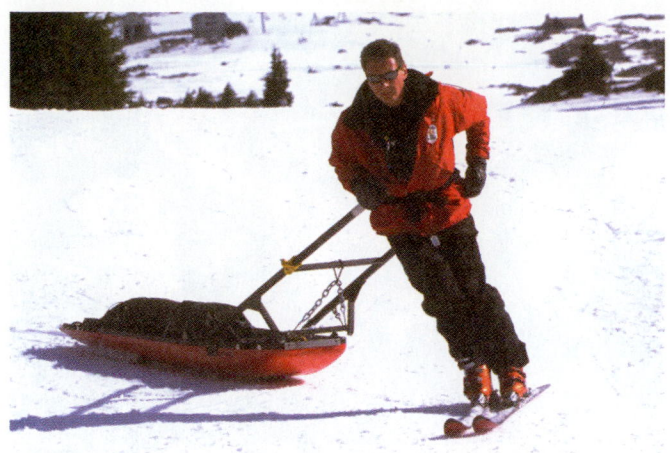

Figure 3-8 At a ski area, transport is usually by toboggan.

extrication, and a landing area is close, helicopter transport from the scene may be appropriate.

Follow-Up Assessment and Care in Patrol First Aid Facilities

Once the patient is in the aid room, a more thorough assessment may be done. This environment may allow the patient to relax somewhat. The detailed physical exam may reveal additional history or physical findings. Additional resources (personnel and equipment) are typically available to enhance patient care. This is a good time to reassess vital signs, adjust splints, remove boots, and replace wet clothing. It is important to continue to assess the patient's condition and reevaluate any treatments or interventions.

Resort Medical Clinics

Some areas have medical clinics on site. In general, the clinic will have been notified by dispatch of an incoming injury, and the patrol can deliver the patient to the receiving staff. Local policy will determine whether a written report needs to accompany the patient.

Transport Decisions

Some transport decisions are straightforward; others are difficult. Written policies regarding various frequently encountered scenarios provide for a smoother operation. Among other issues, such policies should address to whom an unemancipated minor with an injury may be released. It should also address the issue of EMS transport without parental consent. As always, such issues are highly dependent on the local area. It is obviously a much larger decision if the nearest EMS receiving facility is 45 miles away from the ski area and the minor's home than if the facility is local. Another

commonly encountered controversy is the asymptomatic or mildly symptomatic patient who has undergone spinal stabilization on the hill. Who can "clear" the spine? This should be clearly spelled out in policy. OEC technicians are not trained to clear spines.

Another arena of transport decisions is the type of transport requested and who makes that decision. This usually involves the use of ground versus air transport. Again, this is very much dependent on the area, local terrain, weather, and EMS issues. Nevertheless, the ski area policies should address such issues as the circumstances warranting consideration of air evacuation, identifying which service(s) will provide the transport, how and when such services are put on "alert" pending full information about the patient, whether high-angle rescue capabilities are required, and whether other specialized resources are needed.

Preparing the Patient for Transport

An important interface between the patrol and EMS is the preparation of the patient prior to EMS transport. This is a function that the patrol can perform for their patients to aid in the smooth, efficient transition toward definitive care of injury or illness. The preparation includes a review of all identified injuries to ensure that the on-the-slope impression is unchanged in the aid room.

With an extremity injury, there is usually no need to undo splints if there is no discomfort or problems, but a recheck of neurovascular integrity is always a good idea. The removal of wet clothing and general rewarming should now be pursued. It may be a good time to remove boots and protective gear such as helmets. Notification of the parents or guardian should take place, as well as any other medical history obtainable from that source if they are not on location.

Definitive information regarding medications or special needs and allergies should be obtained. This information should be transferred to EMS, preferably in writing. This is particularly important if longer transport times are anticipated. Patrollers should also collect and transfer all the patient's personal belongings, as this can be very important to the injured person. This responsibility should not be taken lightly.

Documentation

Documentation of prehospital care is an important part of the job of ambulance-based EMS. It helps those who were not at the scene to better understand the mechanisms of injury. In the case of medical illness, it gives physicians and nurses a reference point for the patient's condition at that time versus the condition on hospital

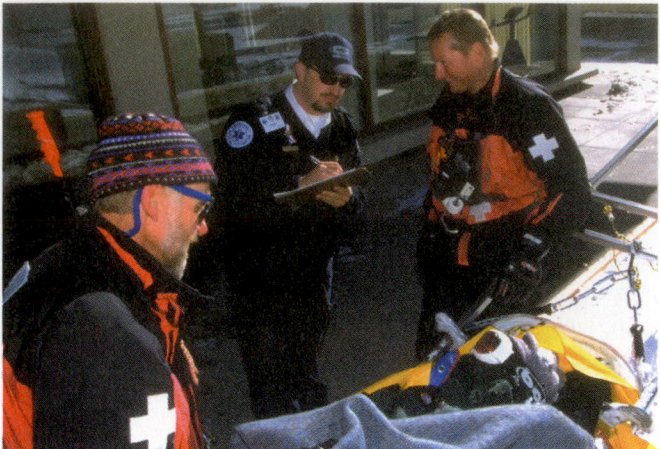

Figure 3-9 Documentation of prehospital care is an important part of the job.

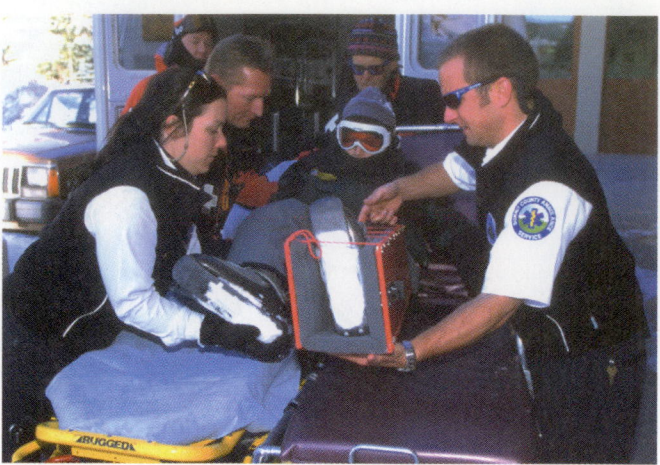

Figure 3-10 Work closely with the ambulance crew so the turnover of a patient is efficient and appropriate documentation is transferred.

arrival. Law enforcement or other authorities also on occasion use this documentation.

The documentation required of the patroller varies from area to area and is directed by area management. Area forms may be designed by the insurer for the area or a national body and are usually more of a risk management tool than a medical report. Unless local policy prohibits, a detailed report is desirable for all major events on the hill, and a copy should accompany the patient with EMS providers (▲ **Figure 3-9**).

Policies should exist for the documentation of unexpected events or outcomes. One such event is the "Refusal of Medical Advice" (RMA). This provides a record of instances in which a patient refuses the medical advice or medical care of the patrol. Another event that should be documented is any adverse patient outcomes that occurred while the patient was under the care of the patrol and the circumstances surrounding the event.

Significant breaches from local protocol should be documented. Sometimes this might represent an educational lapse, rarely someone overstepping the scope of his or her skills, and most often it probably represents an unusual event that required an unusual solution. All such events should be documented, and the patrol director, possibly with the help of the patrol physician, should address these individually with the parties involved in accordance with the policies of area management and its insurer. As the cornerstone of a quality management program, documentation provides tremendous opportunities for all patrol members to learn and examine how they might have reacted in a similar situation. Therefore, more often than not, these events are not disciplinary but an opportunity to improve quality.

Turnover to Ambulance Crew

The turnover of the patient to the ambulance should be a smooth and practiced operation (▲ **Figure 3-10**). Minimizing the turnover time helps all parties involved: the patient arrives at definitive care earlier, the ambulance crew turns around quicker for other 9-1-1 calls, and the patrol can return to patrolling.

An efficient turnover begins before the season starts, with meetings with the local EMS providers. Plans should be made regarding the needs and requirements of local EMS for "patient packaging." Conversely, local EMS needs to know about such issues as the types of splints used on the hill, policy on spinal stabilization, area AED programs, and a number of other issues that may be specific to outdoor care at any given area. It is important that such basic issues as ambulance access to ski area medical treatment facilities are worked out and the EMS crews and their dispatchers know those locations.

In general, the turnover of the patient involves a verbal report by the treating patroller to the receiving ambulance crew. Crucial information includes what is known about the mechanism of injury and how and in what shape the patrol found the patient. All interventions performed and the patient's response to them should be conveyed. Any other events witnessed by the patrol or bystanders located and interviewed by the patrol should be conveyed. Conveying a SAMPLE history is equally important. In the case of a minor, all releases and/or parental or guardian notifications should be passed on to EMS as well. If time permits, providing this in writing is preferred. Flow sheets of vital signs are especially helpful to give the ambulance crew. Remember to transfer the patient's possessions as well.

Ambulance Crew Expectations

The arriving ambulance crew will expect to receive a patient who was provided appropriate on-hill treatment and is ready for transport. In many jurisdictions, the crew will have the ability to provide additional treatments beyond that available by the patrol. Most notable may be their ability to provide IV analgesia. The crews may opt to establish an IV and give medication before transferring a skier with painful injuries to a stretcher. They should be entitled to expect the patrollers to assist them in this, at a minimum by providing the space in the aid room, and often as an active participant under the crew's direction.

Relationships with Ambulance Crew

Ambulance Crew Responsibilities and Protocols

EMS providers have responsibilities defined by state statutes and local protocols and/or on-line medical control. The crews may be able to respond in a manner entirely consistent with what the patrol wishes. For example, local medical control may require that crews always use a specific type of stabilization device or that distal pulses always be checked on an injured extremity.

Despite a patroller's common sense notion that such requirements may be unnecessary, in fact they may be highly desirable from the larger system perspective of the EMS medical director. The ambulance crew may be in charge of the patient's care for a prolonged period of time if the nearest receiving facility is far away.

It is important for the patroller to realize how hard it can be to carefully monitor a patient in a moving, noisy ambulance. An experienced provider knows that things can change and that a change for the worse that occurs half an hour before arrival at the hospital is something everyone tries to avoid. So, as a patroller trying to ensure the best care for the patient, it is important to also consider the perspective and training of the EMS crews. Facilitating the patient's exam and packaging is helpful for patient care.

Training of Ambulance Personnel

As stated earlier, an ambulance is typically staffed with one or more of the following levels of EMS providers: EMT-B, EMT-I, or EMT-P. State law, the level of certification, and local protocol will determine the additional skills and techniques that they may employ. The EMS provider's training is generally directed toward urban prehospital care based on a curriculum supported by the NHTSA.

Problem Resolution

As with any other activity with people interacting in a stressful environment, conflict will inevitably occur between patrollers and EMS providers. The best approach to this is to take preventive measures by preseason training and talk sessions in which potential conflict points are discussed and planned for ahead of time. If problems occur during the handoff of a patient, the first rule that all parties should follow is to focus on *what is best for the patient*. If this point cannot be agreed upon (and the debate may in fact be centering on differing views of this very issue), it comes time for someone to "give." The patroller must make a factually based determination of whether the actions of the EMS personnel are hurting the patient. If the answer is "no," it may be in the best interest of the patient to allow the EMS provider to continue treatment. If, however, you believe that the issue is one in which patient care or well-being is likely to be compromised, you should discuss this privately with the EMS providers. If it cannot be resolved at that level, you should involve your chain of command and/or contact the EMS chain of command.

EMS in OEC Training

Annual preseason preparations for the patrol should involve a training and social event in which all of the local EMS personnel and officers are invited to discuss the interface between the patrol and EMS ▼ Figure 3-11 . There should be training of EMS on the types of splints and rescue devices used on the hill. Chair evacuation and other evacuation activities should be discussed and (preferably) demonstrated. A mass-casualty plan should be in place to cover plausible mass-casualty emergencies. The patrol should use this as an opportunity to

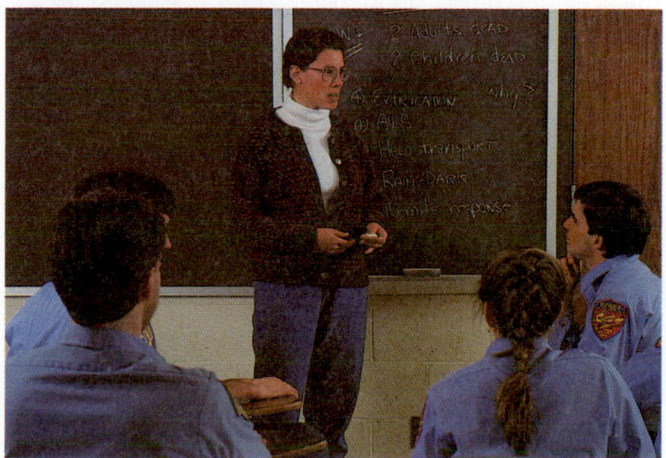

Figure 3-11 Annual preseason training and social events for the patrol and local EMS personnel and officers should occur to improve interface and total patient care.

showcase specific skills and the unique operating environment in which they are performed.

EMTs should demonstrate the loading and unloading of patients from ambulances and introduce the patrol to the equipment carried and capabilities of the crew and equipment. All of this should be done in a setting that allows socialization. Conflict resolution rarely comes in to play if you know someone by his or her first name.

Ambulance Service Medical Director

Every ambulance service will have a medical director who provides oversight and either a set of orders under which the EMS providers operate (off-line medical control) or who provides direct radio control of EMS actions (on-line medical control). It is important to involve the medical director(s) in the decision-making process of EMS and patrol interface, to be sure that things are consistent with the medical director's requirement of his or her crews. The medical director, if properly apprised of all of the issues surrounding the patrol's activities, can be a significant asset in smoothing the transition of patient care from the patrol to EMS.

Physician Involvement at Ski Areas

Physician involvement with patrols can happen in many ways, from the incidental offer of assistance on the hill to a formal relationship as a physician associated with the patrol or as a physician-patroller.

The offer of assistance to the patrol by a physician who encounters an accident scene while skiing is a situation often encountered at all areas. The usual scenario is that the physician identifies himself or herself to the patrol and offers assistance. By and large, at a simple ski hill accident, physician involvement is not necessary for the initial assessment, packaging, and transport of the patient. The patrol should therefore thank the physician for the courtesy but decline the offer.

Occasionally, a physician will try to take over an accident scene. In those rare situations, the patrol may have to be more forceful in declining the offer. It can be helpful in this situation to remind a physician that by providing treatment, he or she has accepted some responsibility for this patient. Often, the physician will realize that he or she is ill prepared to provide treatment and evacuation and will readily acquiesce. If the physician persists in participating in treatment, have him or her help you by holding traction or maintaining cervical spine stabilization ▶ **Figure 3-12** . Another rare situation may involve a patient who has an acute and life-threatening condition for which a physician's intervention

may be lifesaving. For example, a heli-skiing anesthesiologist may carry airway equipment in his or her backpack that can successfully resuscitate an avalanche victim. In such situations, the patrol should try to verify that the individual is a bona fide physician with appropriate expertise and monitor the situation carefully. These situations call for real-time decision-making that cannot be solved by checking credentials at the scene. It is important to remember that the ski area, and the ski patrollers as the area's agents, are ultimately responsible for patient care.

The means by which physicians may become involved with the patrol are varied and different areas have developed a variety of methods. A common situation is one in which "physician patrols" are established—usually a collection of physicians who are approved to serve as "hill docs." They make themselves available to the patrol by radio, phone, or beeper and are then called on an as-needed basis by the patrol, usually for serious injuries. The approval process for a physician to join is defined by area management but usually requires that the individual have outdoor experience as well as a medical background that is compatible with the treatment of the acutely ill or injured.

An alternative means of physician interaction with the patrol is to become a ski patrol member and perform regular duties with the patrol, with the added knowledge and skill set of a physician. Typically, this individual may provide a series of guidelines or protocols for various EMS agencies to use. It also may be the physician on duty at the resort's receiving facility. These relationships can be tremendously helpful as a resource to contact during difficult cases.

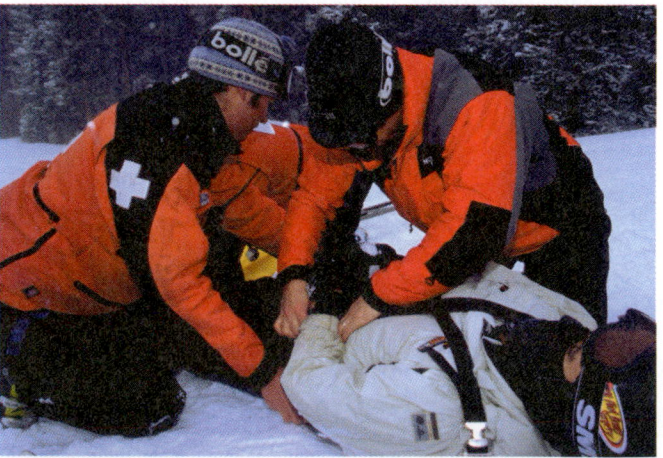

Figure 3-12   If a physician insists on helping, have him or her help with patient care. Often, they can help to stabilize the cervical spine or hold traction on a femur fracture.

Physicians on the Ski Hill

A physician who is "acclimated" to the outdoor environment is an asset to the patrol. It may be of benefit to review some of the issues that would lead other physicians less well equipped to effectively function in this environment (from Marc Bond, "The Role of the Physician-Patroller in the Outdoor Recreation Environment," *Ski Patrol Magazine,* March 1997).

Environment

Most physicians are used to providing care within a building where weather is not an issue. Additionally, patients are usually seen at waist level on a stretcher, having been prepared for an exam. Delays in care in the outdoors can lead to the secondary complication of hypothermia, a problem exacerbated by the usual (in-facility) practice of exposing the patient.

Technology

Much of medical practice is achieved with the aid of electronic devices, many of which are not available on the slope.

Personnel

The personnel in a physician's usual environment are part of a hierarchy with defined roles and responsibilities understood by each person. All perform their designated functions without question. The physician's interaction on the hill will be with a collection of individuals who may not recognize the physician's authority nor respond to his or her directions. Typically, the care on the hill is more cooperative and less well scripted than what might be found in the hospital. So, while the physician is recognized as having superior medical knowledge, this knowledge may be less important than a patroller's superior rescue skills.

Standard of care

A physician responding to any medical emergency may find that the standard of care judged applicable to the problem in court will be all relevant medical skills that could bear upon the problem. So, the physician should not be limited to those skills and diagnostics taught in outdoor emergency care, as he or she may ultimately be held to a higher standard of care. However, since the equipment necessary to perform most advanced interventions is not typically available on a ski slope or in the backcountry, a higher standard of care may not be possible. Conversely, a practitioner could go beyond simple first aid and engage in a procedure that might be more safely done at a nearby clinic (eg, reduction of large joint dislocation) and could be held liable for a bad outcome.

Licensure

A physician who is not licensed in the state in which he or she patrols would have to have a licensing board clarify whether this would constitute practice without a license.

Medical Malpractice

A physician engaged in activities on the hill may or may not be protected by Good Samaritan laws. In some states, Good Samaritan laws may not cover a physician who is performing an organized first responder role or has a legally defined "duty to act." The practitioner who wishes to work with the patrol should review the risk posed by looking at the number of skier visits and type of accidents seen by the patrol. The physician should then review this with a malpractice insurer as well with the area management to see whether coverage exists for his or her activities.

Medical Advice, Direction, and Control

Ski Patrol Medical Advisors and Medical Directors

There are various means by which a physician becomes associated with the OEC program. Each division of the National Ski Patrol has a Division Medical Advisor appointed by the Division Director. This physician also serves on the Medical Committee for the National Ski Patrol and helps guide overall medical policy.

Ski areas may elect to have a **medical director** to provide oversight for their patrol. The duties of a medical director vary from area to area but usually involve the provision of a set of guidelines for various treatment options on the hill and in the aid room. Most medical directors spend some time at the area, working with the patrol by teaching and by giving advice on medical issues.

Areas that have a number of physicians wishing to participate with the patrol may form a physician patrol. The physician patrol would generally be a schedule of physicians who could be expected to be at the area on a regular basis and can be called on to help with various emergencies and with decision-making processes, such as the discontinuation of spinal precautions. Another variation on this is areas that have a list of participating physicians who are approved to interact with the patrol or medical associates.

Area management must be fully informed and must approve of any arrangement for the use of physicians at the ski area.

Chapter *Sweep*

Ready for Review

Outdoor Emergency Care (OEC) is a program that provides a standard of training intended to prepare the student to understand the human body both in health and injury or illness and to quickly detect serious deviations from the normal. The OEC program contains baseline knowledge and skills derived from the US Department of Transportation's (DOT) national emergency medical technician (EMT) curriculum but is tailored for the nonurban environment. OEC is also designed to help rescuers interface with the EMS system in a timely and effective manner.

The OEC course provides a standard of training, **not** an *operational standard of care*. OEC technicians are trained to think while they are reacting to a situation and to make decisions based on their training and knowledge of emergency care objectives. OEC technicians are trained to be able to provide the best possible care in any given situation, not to make the situation fit the training. Rescuers need to rely on their experience and their knowledge of a situation and equipment as they make their emergency care decisions.

The OEC curriculum teaches accepted prehospital care techniques appropriate to the outdoor environment. Ski area management and other outdoor recreational organizations establish the standard of care and local protocols (standard routines) when it puts in place OEC technicians, rescuers with other medical training, specific equipment, physician advisors, base clinics, advanced life support, and other medical resources.

Vital Vocabulary

advanced life support (ALS) Advanced lifesaving procedures, some of which are now being provided by the OEC technician and the EMT-B.

basic life support (BLS) Noninvasive emergency lifesaving care that is used to treat airway obstruction, respiratory arrest, or cardiac arrest.

emergency medical services (EMS) A multidisciplinary system that represents the combined efforts of several professionals and agencies to provide prehospital emergency care and transport to the sick and injured.

emergency medical technician (EMT) An EMS professional who is trained and licensed by the state to provide emergency medical care in the field.

EMT-Basic An EMT who has training in basic emergency care skills, including automated external defibrillation, use of a definitive airway adjunct, and assisting patients with certain prescribed medications.

EMT-Intermediate An EMT who has extensive training in advanced life support, including intubation, IV (intravenous) therapy, pharmacology, cardiac monitoring, and other advanced assessment and treatment skills.

EMT-Paramedic An EMT who has extensive training in advanced life support including intubation, IV skills, pharmacology, cardiac life support and advanced assessment and treatment skills. Additionally, EMT-Paramedics are required to complete a lengthy supervised internship.

first responder The first medically trained individual, such as a patroller, search and rescue personnel, police officer, or other rescuer, to arrive at the scene of an emergency to provide initial medical assistance.

medical control Physicians' instructions that are given directly by radio (online/direct) or indirectly by protocol/guidelines (off-line/indirect), as authorized by the medical director of the service program.

medical director The physician who develops the protocols for a management group or authorizes the OEC technician or EMT to perform emergency medical care in the field.

standard of care What the specific area has chosen to use as its methods of providing the care to the ill and injured patients.

standard of training The tools to facilitate training OEC technicians to operate in a variety of situations, using an assortment of equipment.

www.OECzone.com

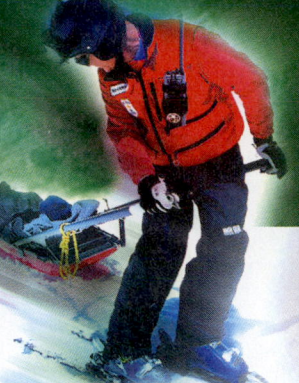

Assessment in Action

Your emergency care training for the outdoor, nonurban environment can involve you in close relationships with other organized units and trained individuals, each with their own established protocols and methods of operation.

As an OEC technician, it is important to recognize the most effective ways to interface with these operations, who is in charge, and how to provide the most efficient emergency and medical care to the patients.

1. You are a patroller at a small ski resort. You have an aid room at the base of the resort. The nearest volunteer ambulance is 30 minutes away in the nearest town. Who oversees the actions taken by the patroller?
   A. Local ambulance service
   B. Hospital medical advisor
   C. Patrol director
   D. Area management

2. You are a member of a volunteer and rescue team. As a result of an avalanche in the backcountry, you have been called on to participate in a search. To whom do you report and whose directions do you follow?
   A. Incident commander rescue leader
   B. Patrol director
   C. County sheriff
   D. Local ambulance service

3. You work for a patrol that has a medical clinic at the base of the resort. When you bring a patient from out of bounds with a suspected fractured femur off the slopes to the resort base, who takes charge?
   A. Patrol aid room staff
   B. Clinic medical staff
   C. Local ambulance service
   D. Search-and-rescue leader

4. There is an altercation in the bar at the resort base. Who would be your immediate interface?
   A. Area management
   B. Local law enforcement
   C. EMS system
   D. Sheriff's department

Challenging Questions

5. Characterize the various methods used to access the following systems in your patrol or community.
   A. Incident command system
   B. Local law enforcement
   C. Search-and-rescue interface
   D. Ambulance interface
   E. EMS system
   F. Medical direction
   G. Hospital interface

Points to Ponder

The patrol has brought a snowboarder to the aid room after he had a bad landing from a jump off a 20' cornice. There was a loss of responsiveness for 10 minutes. He was rapidly assessed on the hill, secured to a backboard with cervical spine precautions, and transported to the aid room with prenotification of EMS.

Your assessment finds him to be confused with a variable level of responsiveness and his neck and back are tender to palpation, but he moves all extremities. The chest, abdomen, and pelvis are absolutely nontender. The EMS crew arrives and they are from a neighboring jurisdiction with whom you have not worked before. They move directly to the patient, ask you no questions, and then begin taking off the straps securing him to the board. You are more than a little surprised! You ask them to explain what is going on and they state that since they are the "higher level of care," they are required to independently confirm all elements of the patient's exam. They also mention that they doubt that all of the spinal precautions are required based on what "they are seeing." What would you do next?

Issues Duty to Act, Patient Care, EMS Relationship, Legal Liability

Online Outlook

The Outdoor Emergency Care program is consistent with universally accepted standards of emergency and medical care that have been endorsed by many respected medical groups and widely accepted principles taught in national training programs in prehospital trauma life support (PHTLS), advanced trauma life support (ATLS), advanced cardiac life support (ACLS), and pediatric advanced life support (PALS), US Department of Transportation's (DOT) National Standard Curriculum for EMTs, and the American Society for Testing and Materials (ASTM). The principles in this text are modified only as appropriate to the outdoor, nonurban invironment. Improve your knowledge of the broad scope of emergency and prehospital care by completing Exercise 3 at www.OECzone.com.

www.OECzone.com

Human Anatomy and Physiology

Objectives

Cognitive

🌲 1. Identify and locate on the body the following topographic terms:
medial, lateral, proximal, distal, superior, inferior, anterior, posterior,
midline, right and left, midclavicular, bilateral, and midaxillary (p 86).

🌲 2. Describe the anatomy and function of the following major body
systems: respiratory, circulatory, musculoskeletal, nervous, and
endocrine (p 101).

Affective

None

Psychomotor

None

🌲 These are core concepts in initial patrol training.

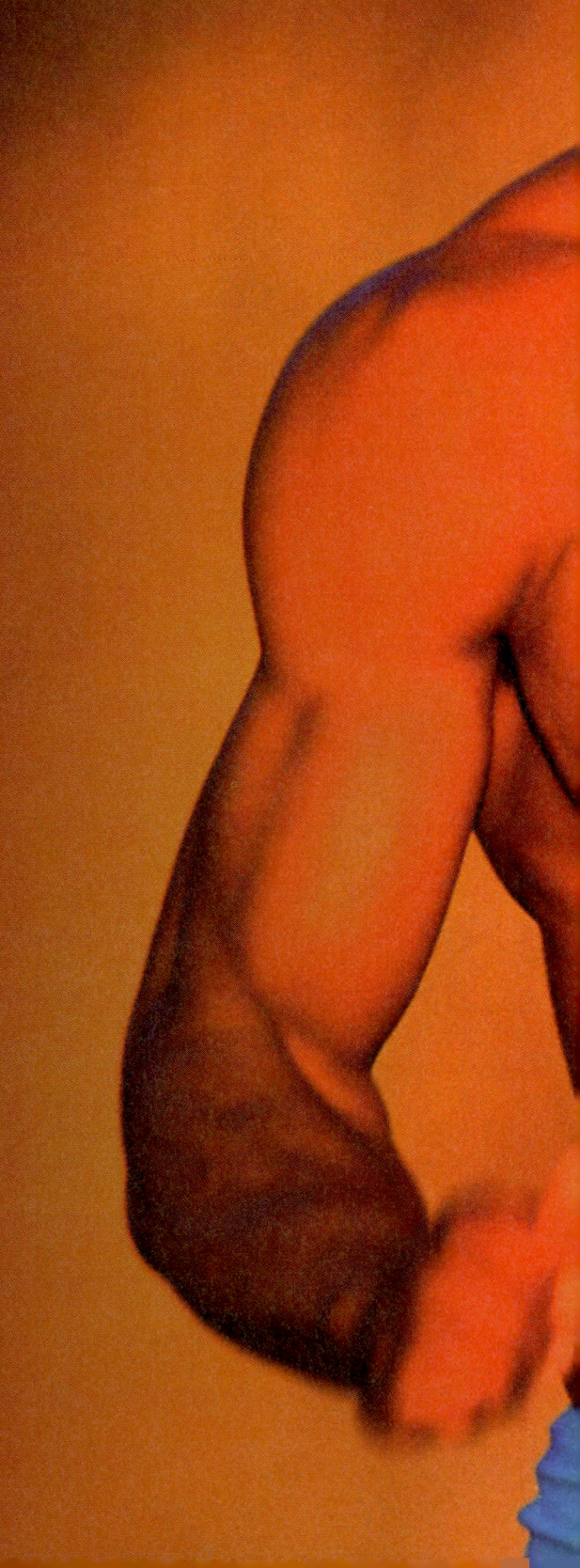

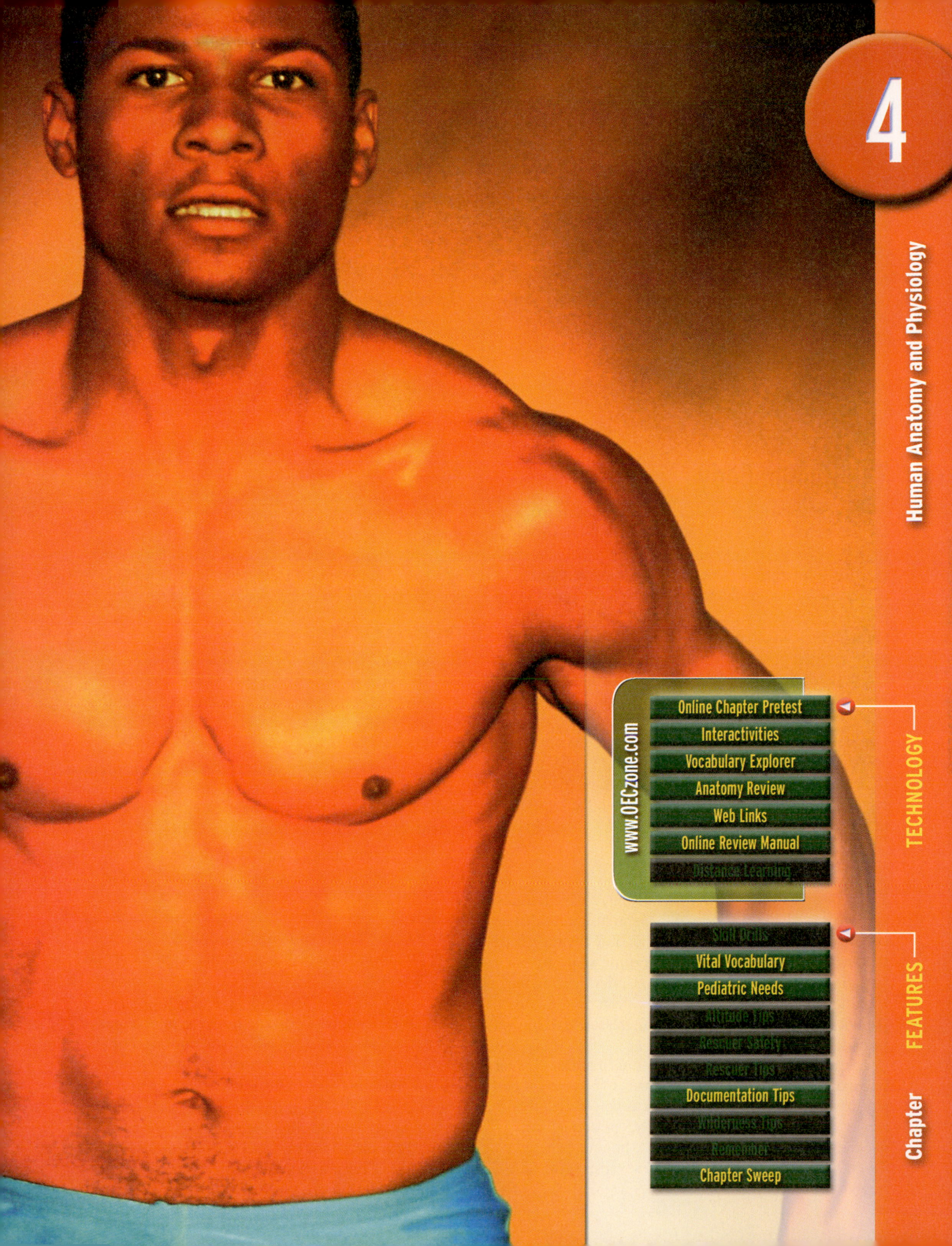

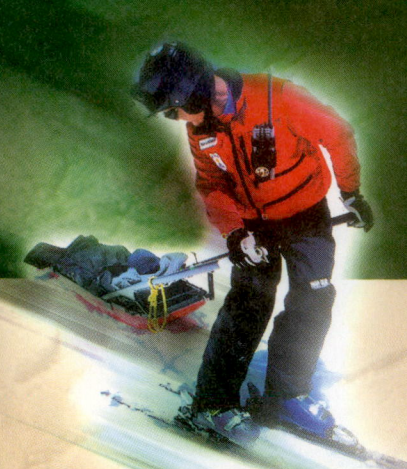

You have been dispatched to a black diamond mogul slope where you find a skier down with a ski pole impaled in his abdomen. As you palpate his abdomen and stabilize the pole, you wonder what internal organs have been damaged by the puncture injury, and to what extent.

This chapter provides essential information about the basic workings of the human body and will also help you answer the following questions:

1. How does each body system respond when another body system is damaged from illness or injury?

2. Why is it necessary for a rescuer to have a fundamental working understanding of medical terminology and human anatomy?

The Human Body

A working knowledge of human anatomy is important for you as a rescuer. Even though you will not make diagnoses, you can help hospital personnel by communicating information using the correct medical terms. All rescuers must be familiar with the language of topographic anatomy. By using the proper medical terms, you will be able to communicate correct information with the least possible confusion.

Using topographic anatomy is actually like using a road map. The terms that are introduced in this chapter will help you to identify the topographic (ie, on the surface) landmarks of the body. These landmarks are used as guides to locate the internal structures that lie under them. These terms also refer to the names of the major regions of the body and the way in which the locations of these regions are described in relation to one another.

Topographic Anatomy

The surface of the body has many definite visible features that serve as guides or landmarks to the structures that lie beneath them. You must be able to identify the superficial landmarks of the body—its **topographic anatomy**— to perform an accurate assessment. Understanding the terminology is also important so that you can describe patient findings correctly to assisting rescuers, ALS providers, and EMS personnel.

Learning the terms that are introduced in this chapter will make your job as a rescuer easier, since you will be able to correctly identify structures as you complete and report your assessment findings. EMS personnel will use these terms to ask you questions about a patient. Therefore, you must learn what these terms mean and how to use them.

The terms that are used to describe the topographic anatomy are applied to the body when it is in the **anatomic position**. This is a position of reference in which the patient stands facing you, arms at the side, with the palms of the hands forward.

The Planes of the Body

The anatomic planes of the body are imaginary straight lines that divide the body ▶ Table 4-1 . These planes help you to identify the location of internal structures and understand the relationships between and among the organs.

ANTERIOR AND POSTERIOR. Anterior refers to the front surface of the body, the side facing you in the anatomic position. **Posterior** refers to the back surface of the patient, or the side away from you.

MIDLINE. An imaginary vertical line drawn from the middle of the forehead, through the nose, to the umbilicus (navel), and then to the floor is called the **midline** of the body. This imaginary line divides the body into two halves that are mirror images. The nose, chin, umbilicus (navel), and spine are examples of midline structures.

MIDCLAVICULAR LINE. The **midclavicular line** is an imaginary line drawn vertically from the middle portion of the clavicle and parallel to the midline. For example, the nipples of the breasts are in the midclavicular line on either side of the body.

MIDAXILLARY LINE. The **midaxillary line** is an imaginary vertical line drawn through the middle of the axilla (armpit) parallel to the midline. This line is also in the middle of the anterior and posterior surfaces of the body.

Directional Terms

In this section, terms that indicate direction are introduced. These terms indicate distance and direction from the midline (▼ **Figure 4-1**), (▼ **Table 4-2**).

RIGHT AND LEFT. The terms "right" and "left" refer to the patient's right and left sides, not to your right and left sides.

SUPERIOR AND INFERIOR. The **superior** part of the body, or any body part, is the portion nearer to the head.

The part nearer to the feet is the **inferior** portion. These terms are also used to describe the relationship of one structure to another. For example, the nose is superior to the mouth and inferior to the forehead.

LATERAL AND MEDIAL. Parts of the body that lie farther from the midline are called **lateral** (outer) structures. The parts that lie closer to the midline are called **medial** (inner) structures. For example, the knee has medial (inner) and lateral (outer) aspects.

PROXIMAL AND DISTAL. The terms "proximal" and "distal" are used to describe the relationship of any two structures on an extremity. **Proximal** describes structures that are closer to the trunk. **Distal** describes structures that are farther from the trunk or nearer to the free end of the extremity. For example, the elbow is distal to the shoulder and proximal to the wrist and hand.

TABLE 4-1 Anatomic Planes of the Body	
Term	**Definition**
Anterior	Front
Posterior	Back
Midline	Line drawn from nose to the umbilicus
Midclavicular	In the middle of the clavicle, parallel to the midline
Midaxillary	In the middle of the armpit, parallel to the midline

TABLE 4-2 Directional Terms	
Term	**Definition**
Right	The patient's right
Left	The patient's left
Lateral	Farther from the midline
Medial	Closer to the midline
Superior	Closer to the head, higher
Inferior	Farther from the head, lower
Proximal	Closer to the midline (in an extremity, closer to the trunk)
Distal	Farther from the midline (in an extremity, closer to the free end)
Dorsal	Toward the spine
Ventral	Toward the abdomen
Palmar	The front region of the hand
Plantar	The bottom of the foot

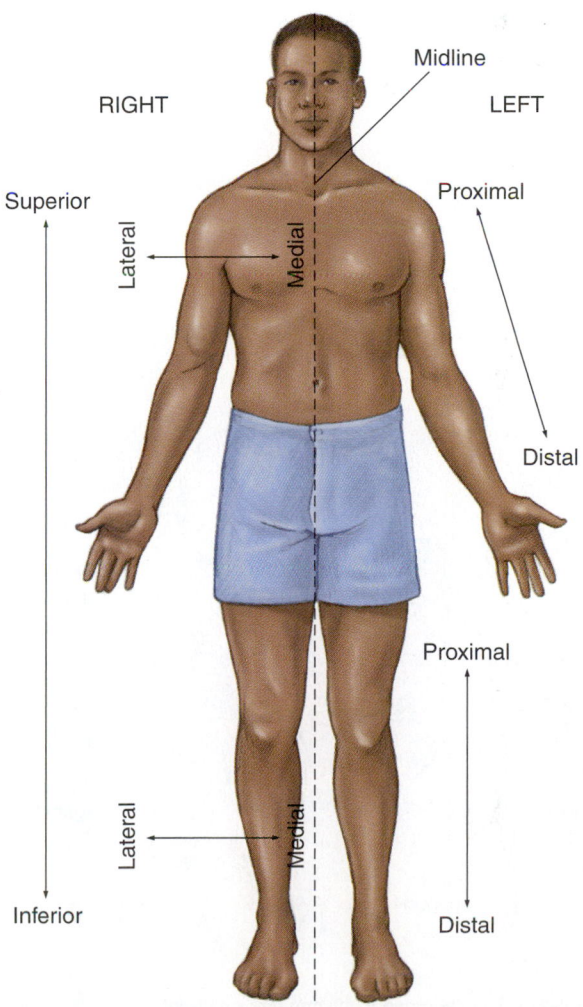

Figure 4-1   Directional terms indicate distance and direction from the midline.

SUPERFICIAL AND DEEP. <u>Superficial</u> means closer to or on the skin. <u>Deep</u> means farther inside the body and away from the skin.

VENTRAL AND DORSAL. <u>Ventral</u> refers to the anterior surface of the body. <u>Dorsal</u> refers to the posterior surface of the body, including the back of the hand.

PALMAR AND PLANTAR. The front region of the hand is referred to as the palm or <u>palmar</u> surface. The bottom of the foot is referred to as the <u>plantar</u> surface.

APEX. The <u>apex (plural: apices)</u> is the tip or the topmost portion of a structure. For example, the tips of the shoulders are the apices of the shoulders. The most superior portions of the lungs are the apices of the lungs. The exception to this is the heart.

Other Directional Terms

Many structures of the body occur bilaterally. A <u>bilateral</u> structure is a body part that appears on both sides of the midline. For example, the eyes, ears, hands, and feet are bilateral structures. This is also true for structures inside the body, such as the lungs and kidneys. Structures that appear on only one side of the body are said to occur unilaterally. For example, the spleen is on the left side of the body only, and the liver is on the right side.

As part of the assessment process, you will palpate the abdomen and report your findings. Therefore, it is important that you be able to describe the exact location of areas of the abdomen. The way to describe the sections of the abdominal cavity is by <u>quadrants</u>. Imagine two lines intersecting at the umbilicus, dividing the abdomen into four equal areas (▼ Figure 4-2). These are referred to as the right upper quadrant (RUQ), left upper quadrant (LUQ), right lower quadrant (RLQ), and left lower quadrant (LLQ). Remember that here, too, right and left refer to the patient's right and left, not yours.

It is important to learn all of these terms and concepts so that you can describe the location of any injury or assessment findings. When you use these terms properly, any other medical personnel who care for the patient will know immediately where to look and what to expect.

Anatomic Positions

You will use these terms to describe the position of the patient as you find him or her or as you transport the patient (▶ Figure 4-3).

PRONE AND SUPINE. These terms describe the position of the body. The body is in the **prone position** when lying face down; the body is in the **supine position** when lying face up.

FOWLER'S POSITION. A patient who is sitting up or semi-sitting with the knees bent is in **Fowler's position**.

SHOCK POSITION. In the **shock position**, or modified Trendelenburg's position, the head and **torso** (the trunk without the head and limbs) are supine, and the lower extremities are elevated 6″ to 12″. This helps to increase blood flow to the brain.

TRENDELENBURG'S POSITION. In **Trendelenburg's position**, the body is supine with the head lower than the feet.

RECOVERY POSITION. The **recovery position** is the preferred body position for an unresponsive patient with no spine injury. The patient lies on his or her side with the opposite knee flexed and the head cushioned on the hand. Also called the semiprone, rescue, stable side, or NATO position.

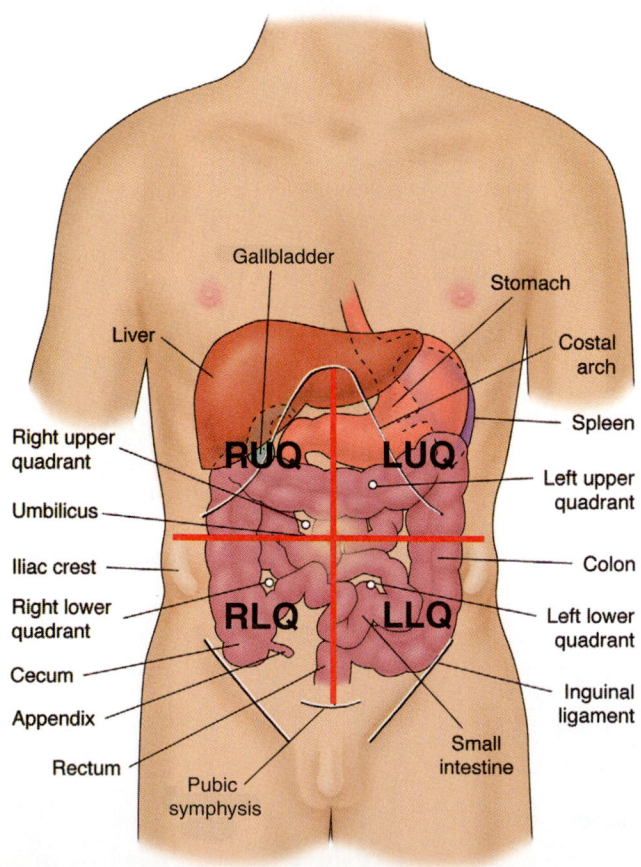

Gallbladder
Stomach
Liver
Costal arch
Spleen
Right upper quadrant
RUQ   LUQ
Left upper quadrant
Umbilicus
Iliac crest
Colon
Right lower quadrant
RLQ   LLQ
Left lower quadrant
Cecum
Appendix
Inguinal ligament
Rectum
Small intestine
Pubic symphysis

(**Figure 4-2**)   The abdomen is divided into quadrants.

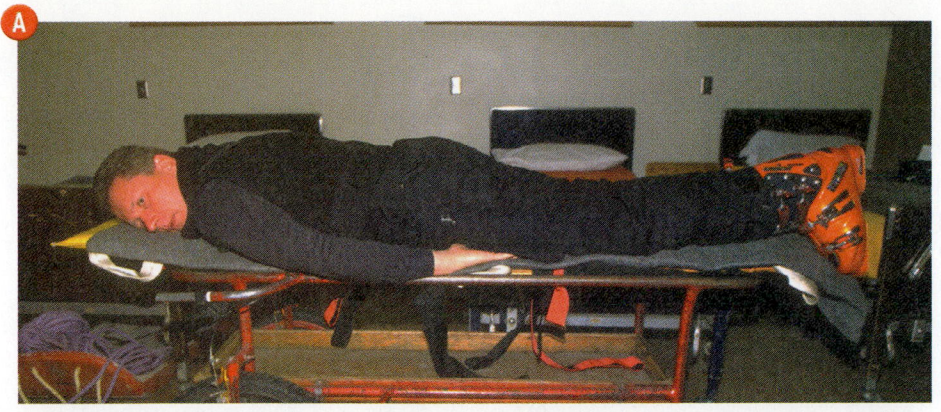

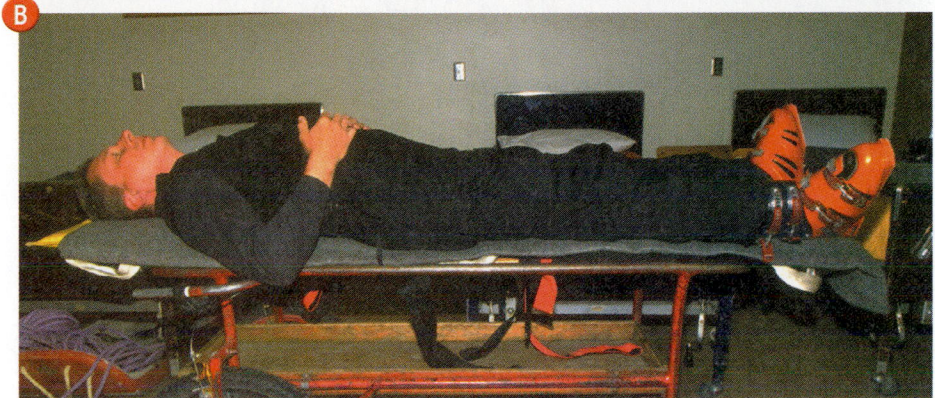

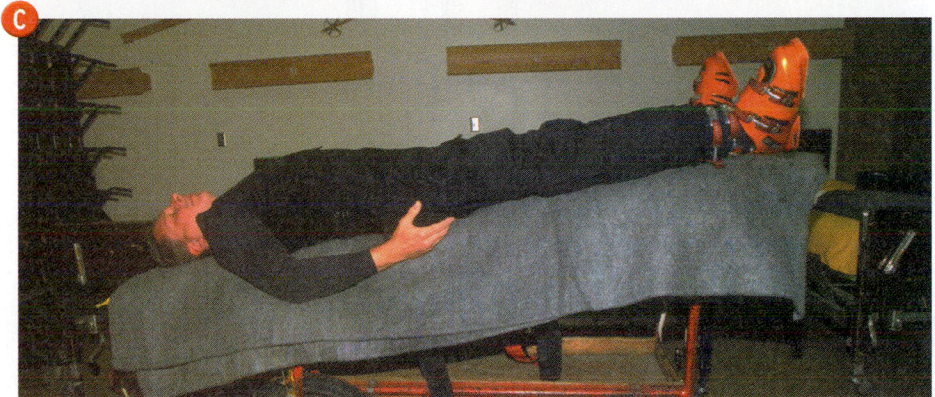

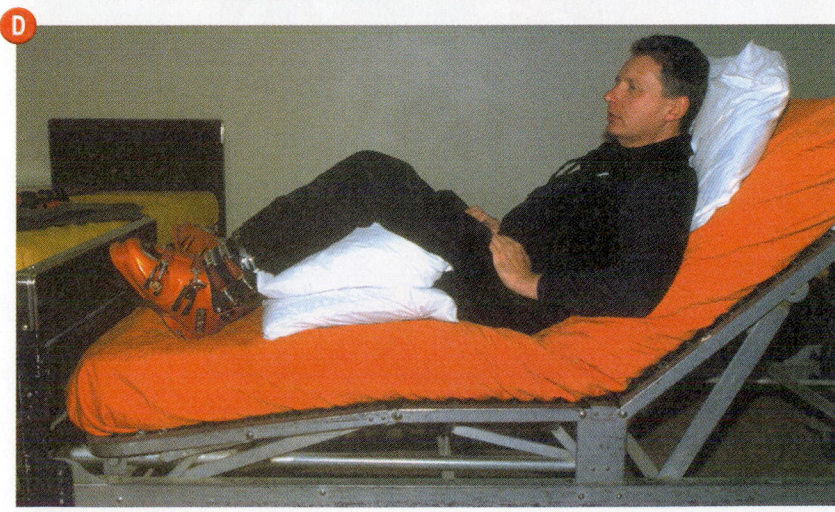

Figure 4-3   **A.** Prone. **B.** Supine.
C. Trendelenburg's position. **D.** Fowler's position.

The Skeletal System

The <u>skeleton</u> gives us our recognizable human form and protects our vital internal organs (▶ **Figure 4-4**). The brain lies within the skull. The heart, lungs, and great vessels are protected by the thorax, which is part of the torso. Much of the liver and spleen is protected by the lower ribs. The spinal cord is contained within and protected by a bony <u>spinal canal</u> formed by the vertebrae.

The 206 bones of the skeleton provide a framework for the attachment of muscles. The skeleton is also designed to allow motion of the body. Bones come into contact with one another at joints where, with the help of muscles, the body is able to bend and move.

The Skull

The <u>cranium</u> is composed of a number of thick bones that fuse together to form a shell above the eyes and ears that holds and protects the brain (▼ **Figure 4-5**). The brain connects to the spinal cord through a large opening at the base of the skull (the <u>foramen magnum</u>). The spinal cord is composed of virtually all the nerves that carry messages between the brain and the rest of the body.

The most posterior portion of the cranium is called the <u>occiput</u>. On each side of the cranium, the lateral portions are called the

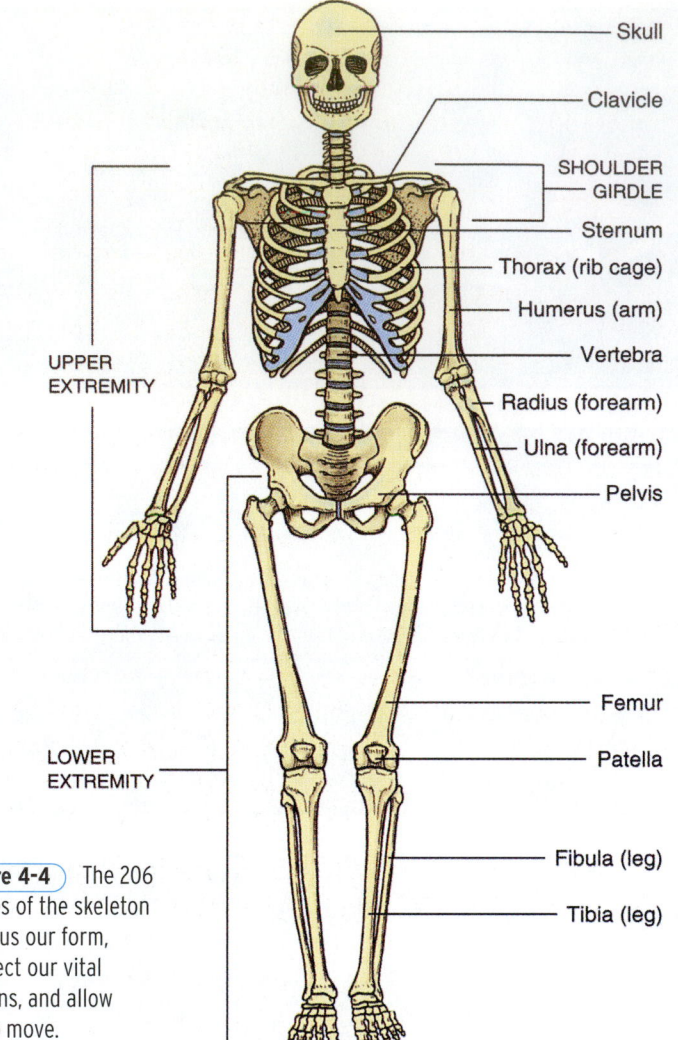

Figure 4-4 The 206 bones of the skeleton give us our form, protect our vital organs, and allow us to move.

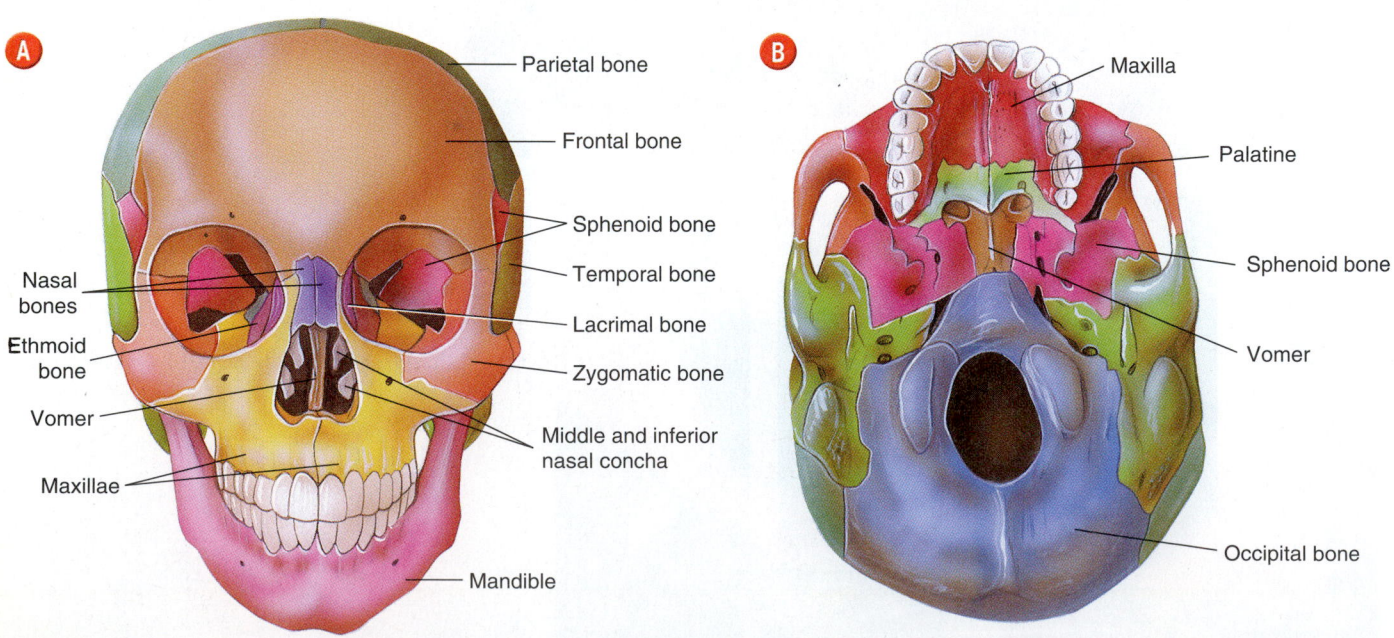

Figure 4-5 The skull. **A.** Front view. **B.** Bottom view.

temples or **temporal regions**. Between the temporal regions and the occiput lie the **parietal regions**. The forehead is called the frontal region. Just anterior to the ear, in the temporal region, you can feel the pulse of the superficial temporal artery. The thick skin covering the cranium and usually bearing hair is called the **scalp**.

The face is composed of the eyes, ears, nose, mouth, and cheeks. Six bones—the nasal bone, the two **maxillae** (upper jawbones), the two **zygomas** (cheek bones), and the **mandible** (lower jawbone)— are the major bones of the face.

The **orbit** (eye socket) is made up of two facial bones: the maxilla and the zygoma. The orbit also includes the frontal bone of the cranium. Together, these bones form a solid bony rim that protrudes around the eye to protect it. If you look at the face from the side, you can see that the eyeball sits back within the orbit. The nasal bone is very short, because most of the nose is made of flexible cartilage. In fact, only the proximal one third of the nose, the bridge, is formed by bone. Unlike the nose, the exposed portion of the ear is made up entirely of cartilage that is covered by skin. The external, visible part of the ear is called the **pinna**. The ear lobes are the fleshy parts at the bottom of each ear. About 1″ posterior to the external opening of the ear is a prominent bony mass at the base of the skull called the **mastoid process**.

The maxilla contains the upper teeth and forms the hard palate (roof of the mouth). The mandible is the only movable facial bone that has a joint (**temporo-mandibular joint**) where it meets with the temporal bone of the cranium just in front of each ear.

The Neck

The neck contains many important structures. It is supported by the cervical spine, or the first seven vertebrae in the spinal column (C1 through C7). The spinal cord exits from the foramen magnum and lies within the spinal canal formed by the vertebrae. The upper part of the esophagus and the **trachea** (windpipe) lie in the midline of the neck. The carotid arteries may be found on either side of the trachea, along with the jugular veins and several nerves.

Several useful landmarks can be palpated and seen in the neck (▼ **Figure 4-6**). The most obvious is the firm prominence in the center of the anterior surface commonly known as the **Adam's apple**. Specifically, this prominence is the upper part of the larynx, the **thyroid cartilage**. It is more prominent in men than in women. The other, lower portion is the **cricoid cartilage**, a firm ridge of cartilage inferior to the thyroid cartilage, which is somewhat more difficult to palpate. Between the thyroid cartilage and the cricoid cartilage in the midline of the neck is a soft depression, the **cricothyroid membrane**. This is a thin sheet of connective tissue (**fascia**) that joins the two cartilages. The cricothyroid membrane is covered at this point only by skin.

Inferior to the larynx, several additional firm ridges are palpable in the anterior midline. These ridges are the cartilage rings of the trachea. The trachea connects the larynx with the main air passages of the lungs (the bronchi). On either side of the lower larynx and the upper trachea lies the thyroid gland. Unless it is enlarged, this gland is usually not palpable.

Pulsations of the carotid arteries are easily palpable in a groove about ¹/₂″ lateral to the larynx. Lying immediately adjacent to these arteries, but not palpable, are the internal jugular veins and several important nerves. Lateral to these vessels and nerves lie the **sternocleido-mastoid muscles**, which allow movement of the head. These muscles originate from the mastoid process of the cranium and insert into the medial border of each collarbone and the **sternum** (breastbone) at the base of the neck.

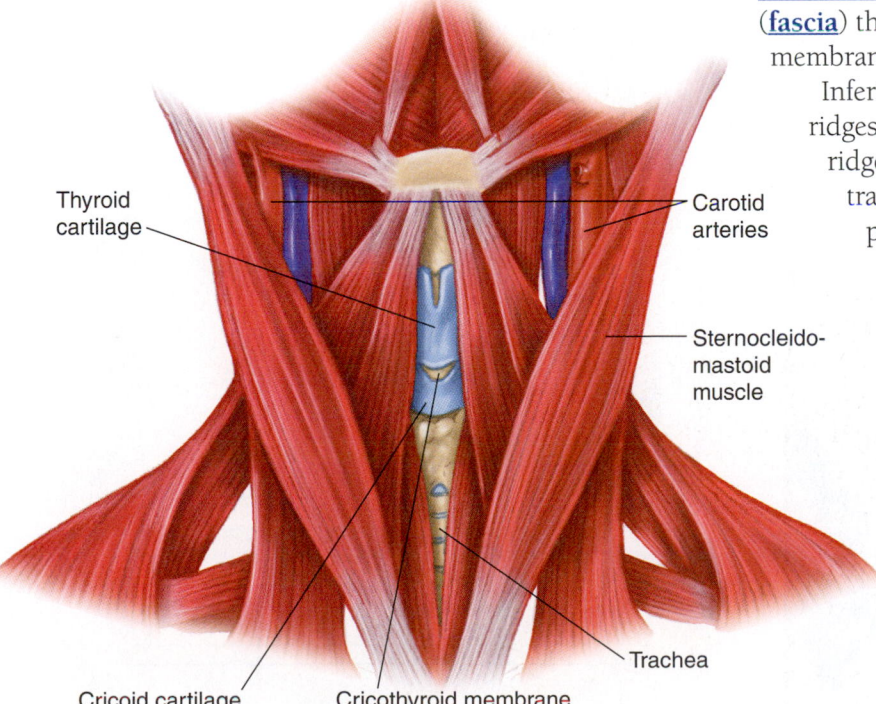

Thyroid cartilage

Carotid arteries

Sternocleido-mastoid muscle

Trachea

Cricoid cartilage   Cricothyroid membrane

Figure 4-6 The principal structures of the neck include the trachea, along with many blood vessels, muscles, and nerves.

A series of bony prominences lie posteriorly, in the midline of the neck. They are the spines of the cervical vertebrae. The lower cervical spines are more prominent than the upper ones, and they are more easily palpable when the neck is flexed. At the base of the neck posteriorly, the most prominent spine is the seventh cervical vertebra (▼ Figure 4-7).

The Spinal Column

The spinal column is the central supporting structure of the body and is composed of 33 bones, each called a vertebra. The **vertebrae** are named according to the section of the spine in which they lie and are numbered from top to bottom (▼ Figure 4-8). From the top down, the spine is divided into five sections:

- **Cervical spine**. The first seven vertebrae (C1 through C7), which lie in the neck, form the cervical spine. The skull rests on the first cervical vertebra (the atlas) and articulates with it.

- **Thoracic spine**. The next 12 vertebrae make up the thoracic spine. One pair of ribs is attached to each of the thoracic vertebrae.

- **Lumbar spine**. The next five vertebrae form the lumbar or dorsal spine.

- **Sacrum**. The five sacral vertebrae are fused together to form one bone called the sacrum. The sacrum is joined to the iliac bones of the pelvis with strong ligaments at the sacroiliac joints to form the pelvis.

- **Coccyx**. The last four vertebrae form the coccyx or tailbone.

The **spinal cord** is an extension of the brain, composed of virtually all the nerves that carry messages between the brain and the rest of the body. It exits through a large hole in the base of the skull called the foramen magnum and is contained within and protected by the vertebrae of the **spinal column**. The spinal column is virtually surrounded by muscles. However, the posterior spinous process of each vertebra can be felt as it lies just under the skin in the midline of the back.

The anterior part of each vertebra consists of a round, solid block of bone called the body. The posterior part of each vertebra forms a bony arch. This series of arches from one vertebra to the next forms a tunnel that runs the length of the spine, called the spinal canal. The bones of the spinal canal encase and protect the spinal cord (▶ Figure 4-9). Nerves branch from the spinal cord and exit from the spinal canal between each two vertebrae to form the motor and sensory nerves of the body.

The vertebrae are connected by ligaments, and between each two vertebrae is a cushion called the intervertebral disk. These ligaments and disks allow some motion so that the trunk can bend forward and

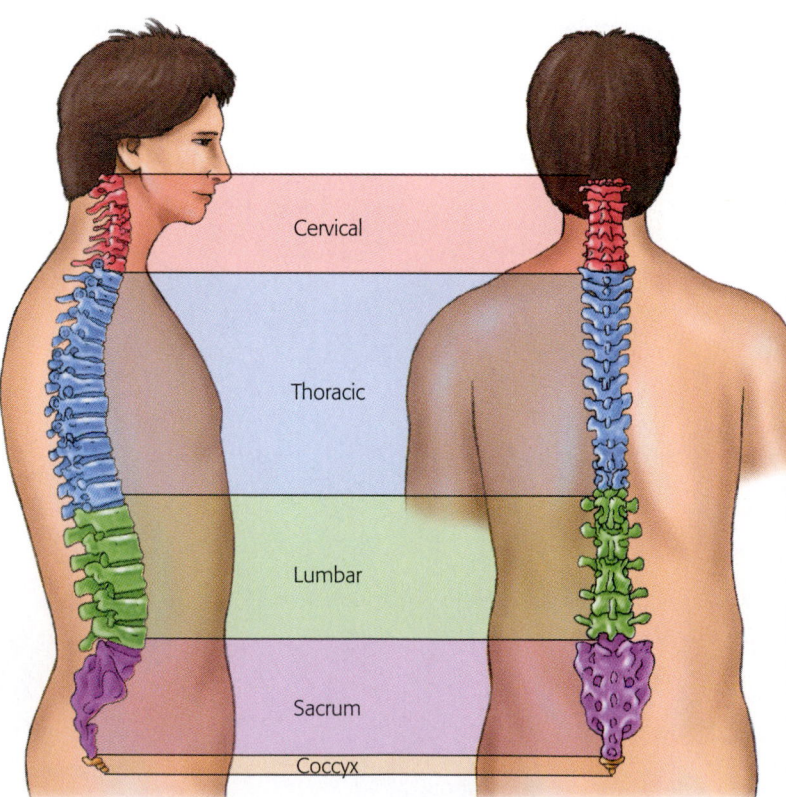

Cervical

Thoracic

Lumbar

Sacrum

Coccyx

Figure 4-7 The most prominent of the cervical vertebrae is the spine of C7.

Figure 4-8 The spinal column is composed of 33 bones divided into five sections.

back. However, they also limit motion of the vertebrae so that the spinal cord will not be injured. An injury to the spine may damage part of the spinal cord and its nerves that may not be protected by the vertebrae. Therefore, until the injury is stabilized, you must use extreme caution in caring for the patient to prevent injury to the spinal cord.

The Thorax

The **thorax** (chest) is the cavity that contains the heart, lungs, esophagus, and great vessels (the aorta and two venae cavae). It is formed by the 12 thoracic vertebrae (T1 through T12) and their 12 pairs of ribs. The **clavicle** (collarbone) overlies the superior boundaries of the thorax in front and articulates laterally with the **scapula** (shoulder blade), which lies in the muscular tissue of the thoracic wall. The inferior boundary of the thorax is the diaphragm, which separates the thorax from the abdomen.

ANTERIOR ASPECTS. The dimensions of the thorax are defined by the **thoracic cage** (bony rib cage) and its attachments (▼ Figure 4-10A). Anteriorly, in the midline of the chest is the sternum. The superior border of the sternum forms the easily palpable jugular notch. The sternum has three components: the manubrium, the body, and the xiphoid process. The upper quarter of the sternum is called the **manubrium**. The body comprises the rest of the sternum except for a narrow, cartilaginous tip inferiorly, which is called the

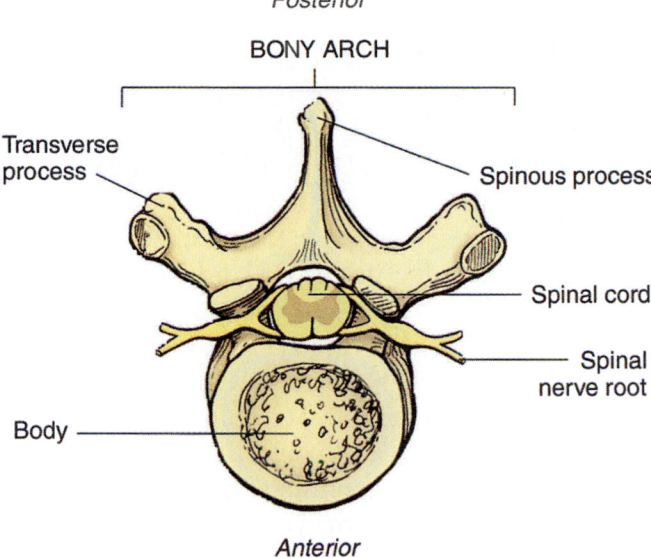

Figure 4-9 The bones of the spinal column encase and protect the spinal cord.

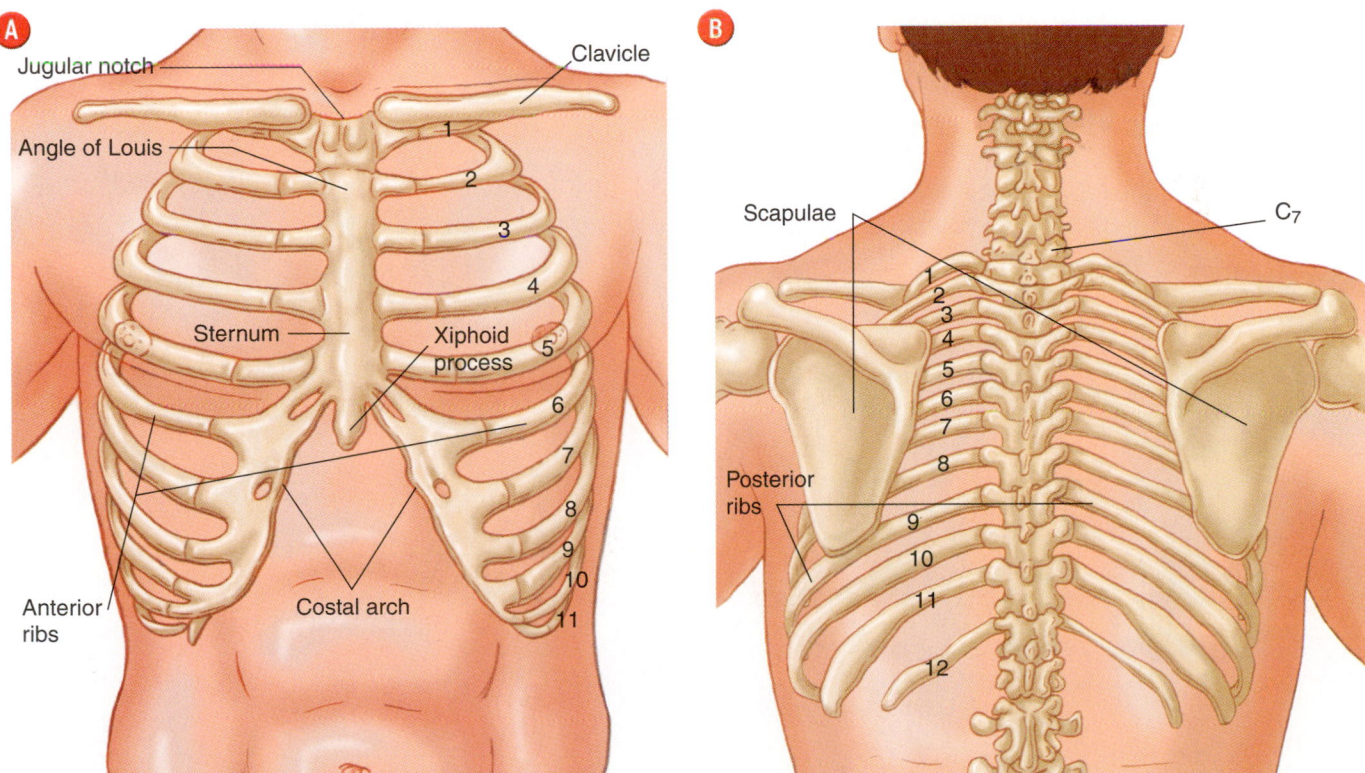

Figure 4-10 **A.** The anterior aspect of the thorax includes the following bony landmarks: the clavicle, the Angle of Louis, the sternum, the xiphoid process, and the anterior ribs. **B.** The posterior aspect of the thorax includes the following bony landmarks: the scapulae, the thoracic vertebrae, and the posterior ribs.

xiphoid process. The junction of the manubrium and the body forms a very prominent ridge on the sternum, called the angle of Louis. The **angle of Louis** lies at the level where the second rib is attached to the sternum; it provides a constant and reliable bony landmark on the anterior chest wall.

In the midline of the upper back, the spines of the 12 thoracic vertebrae can be palpated. Twelve **ribs** on each side form small joints with their respective thoracic vertebrae and extend around to the front to create the walls of the thoracic cage. The upper five ribs connect to the sternum through a short bridge of cartilage. The sixth through tenth ribs insert into the costal arch. The **costal arch** is a bridge of cartilage that connects the ends of the sixth through tenth ribs with the lower portion of the sternum. The eleventh and twelfth ribs are called **floating ribs**, because they do not attach to the sternum through the costal arch. The costal arch is easily palpable and represents the boundary between the lower border of the thorax and the upper border of the abdomen.

POSTERIOR ASPECTS. On the posterior chest wall, the scapulae overlie the thoracic wall and are surrounded by large muscles (◄ **Figure 4-10B**). When the patient is standing or sitting erect, the two scapulae should lie at approximately the same level, with their inferior tips at about the level of the seventh thoracic vertebra. In the lower part of the thorax on each side, an angle called the **costovertebral angle** is formed by the junction of the spine and the tenth rib. The kidneys lie deep in (beneath) the back muscles under the costovertebral angle.

DIAPHRAGM. The **diaphragm** is a muscular dome that forms the inferior boundary of the thorax, separating the chest from the abdominal cavity (▼ **Figure 4-11**). Its contraction, along with that of the chest wall muscles, assists with allowing air to be drawn into the lungs. Anteriorly, it attaches to the costal arch; posteriorly, it attaches to the **lumbar vertebrae**. The diaphragm cannot be seen or palpated.

ORGANS AND VASCULAR STRUCTURES. Within the thoracic cage, the largest structures are the heart and lungs (▼ **Figure 4-12**). The heart lies immediately under the sternum. It extends from the second to the sixth ribs anteriorly and from the fifth to the eighth thoracic vertebrae posteriorly. The inferior border of the heart extends into the left side of the chest. Diseased hearts may be larger or smaller. The major blood vessels that travel to and from the heart also lie in the chest cavity. On the right side of the spinal column, the superior and inferior venae cavae carry blood to the heart.

Just beneath the manubrium of the sternum, the arch of the aorta and the pulmonary artery exit the heart. The arch of the aorta passes to the left and

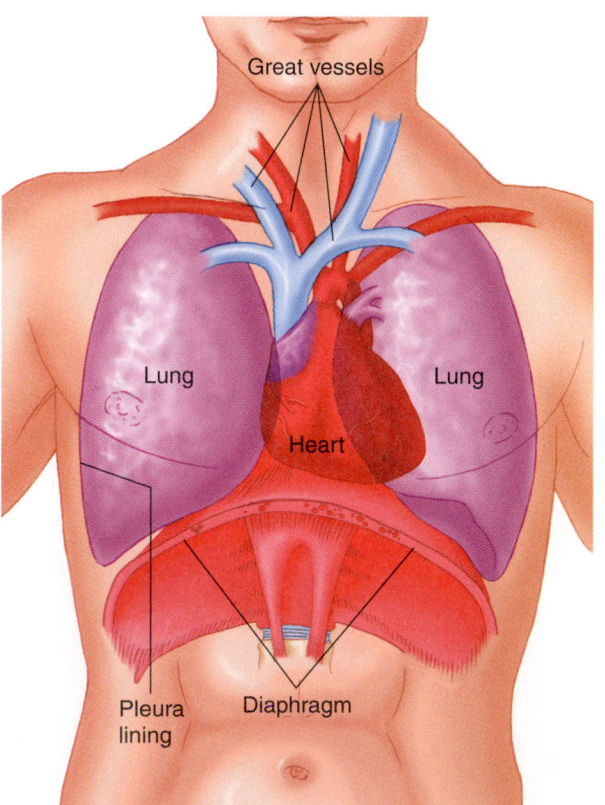

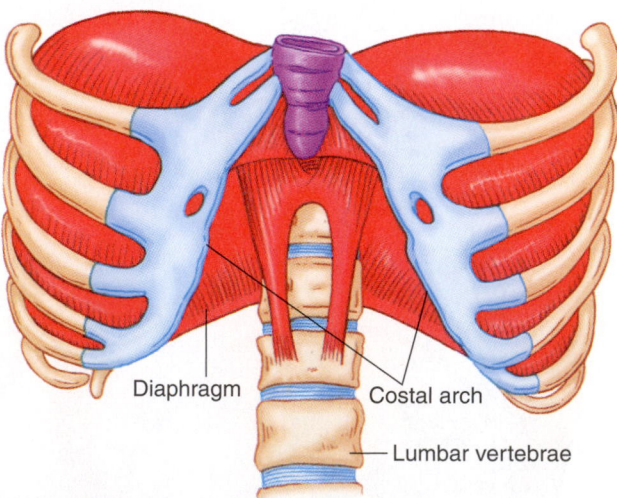

Figure 4-11 The diaphragm forms the undersurface of the thorax, separating the chest from the abdominal cavity.

Figure 4-12 The anterior aspect of the thorax shows the relative positions of the principal organs beneath the surface.

lies along the left side of the spinal column as it descends into the abdomen. The esophagus lies behind the great vessels and directly on the anterior aspect of the spinal column as it passes through the chest into the abdominal cavity.

All space within the chest that is not occupied by the heart, great vessels, and esophagus is occupied by the lungs. Anteriorly, the lungs extend down to the surface of the diaphragm at the level of the xiphoid process. Posteriorly, the lungs extend farther inferiorly to the surface of the diaphragm at the level of the twelfth thoracic vertebra.

ANATOMIC LANDMARKS. The major palpable landmarks in the chest are obviously the ribs. Most of them can be easily felt except for the first, which is hidden under and behind the clavicle. Between each rib is the "intercostal space." These spaces can be located by palpating the jugular notch and moving lateral (the first intercostal space). Counting the successive spaces between the ribs gives us the second, third, etc. Both clavicles and the sternum can be easily palpated. The jugular notch is the top portion of the sternum. Lateral to that is the first intercostal space. Inferiorly, the costal arch is readily palpable on both sides of the anterior chest wall. In the midline, the tip of the xiphoid process is a tender and easily palpated landmark.

> The foundation for good patient care is a strong working knowledge of human anatomy and physiology. Anatomy is the study of body structure. Physiology is the study of how the body functions.

The Abdomen

The **abdomen** is the second major body cavity; it contains the major organs of digestion and excretion. The diaphragm separates the thoracic cavity from the abdominal cavity. Anteriorly and posteriorly, thick muscular abdominal walls create the boundaries of this space. Inferiorly, the abdomen is separated from the pelvis by an imaginary plane that extends from the pubic symphysis through the sacrum (▼ Figure 4-13). Many organs lie in both the abdomen and the pelvis, depending on the posture of the patient.

The simplest and most common method of describing the portions of the abdomen is by quadrants, the four equal areas formed by two imaginary lines that intersect at right angles at the umbilicus. On the anterior abdominal wall, the quadrants thus formed are the right upper,

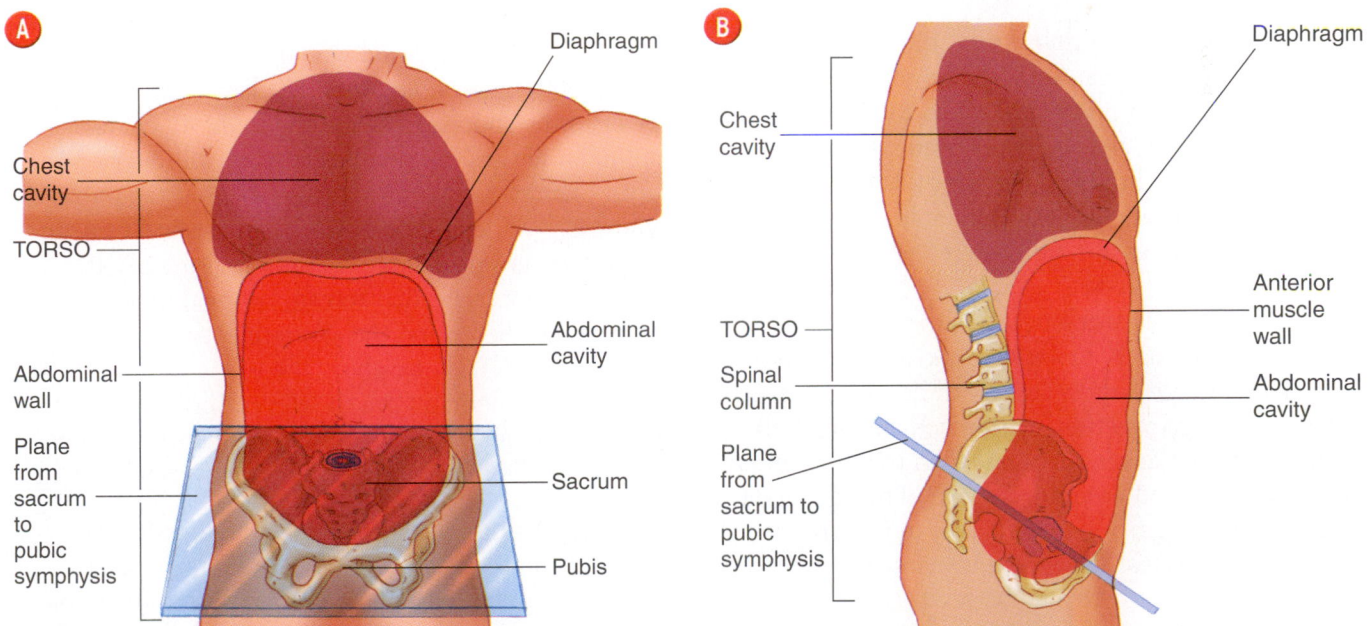

Figure 4-13   The boundaries of the abdomen are the anterior and posterior abdominal cavity walls, the diaphragm, and an imaginary plane from the pubic symphysis to the sacrum. **A.** Anterior view. **B.** Lateral view.

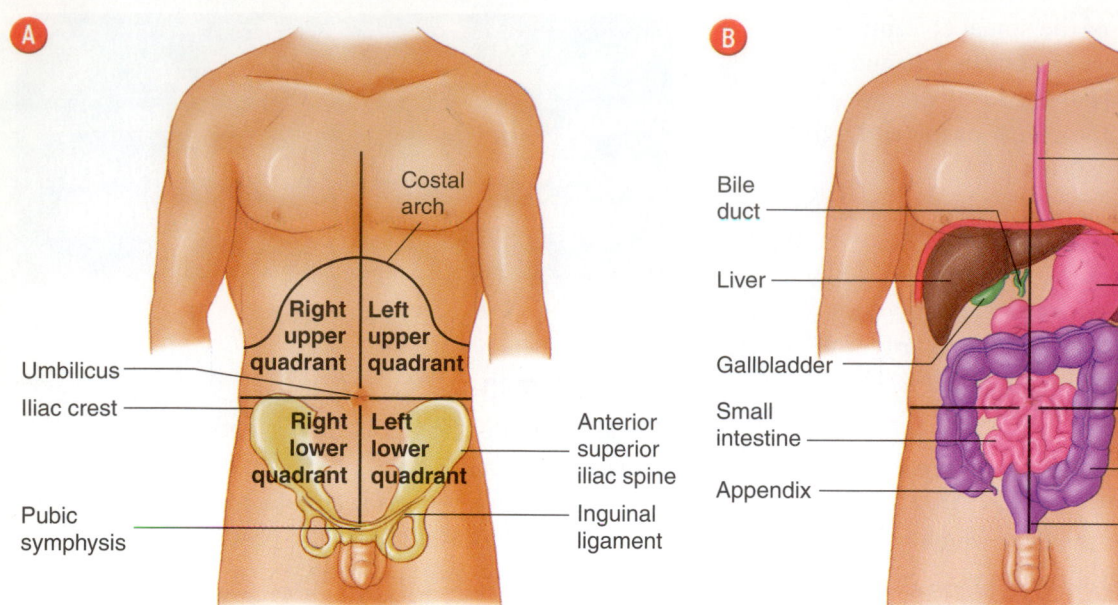

Figure 4-14 **A.** In the abdomen, quadrants are the easiest system for identifying areas. Major bony landmarks are also shown. **B.** Many of the organs in the abdomen lie in more than one quadrant.

right lower, left upper, and left lower (▲ **Figure 4-14**). The terms "right quadrant" and "left quadrant" refer to the patient's right and left as you face them, not to your right and left sides. Pain or injury in a given quadrant usually arises from or involves the organs that lie in that quadrant. This simple means of designation will allow you to identify injured or diseased organs that require emergency attention.

ORGANS AND VASCULAR STRUCTURES. In the right upper quadrant (RUQ), the major organs are the liver, the gallbladder, and a portion of the colon. Most of the liver lies in this quadrant, almost entirely under the protection of the eighth to twelfth ribs. The liver fills the entire anteroposterior depth of the abdomen in this quadrant. Therefore, injuries in this area are frequently associated with injuries of the liver.

In the left upper quadrant (LUQ), the principal organs are the stomach, the spleen, and a portion of the colon. The spleen is almost entirely under the protection of the left rib cage, whereas the stomach may sag well down into the left lower quadrant when full. The spleen lies in the lateral and posterior portion of this quadrant, under the diaphragm and immediately in front of the ninth to eleventh ribs. The spleen is frequently injured, especially when these ribs are fractured.

The right lower quadrant (RLQ) contains two portions of the large intestine: the **cecum**, the first portion into which the small intestine (ileum) opens, and the ascending colon. The **appendix** is a small

tubular structure that is attached to the lower border of the cecum. Appendicitis is the most frequent cause of tenderness and pain in this region. In the left lower quadrant (LLQ) lie the descending and the sigmoid portions of the colon.

Several organs lie in more than one quadrant. The small intestine, for instance, occupies the central part of the abdomen around the umbilicus, and parts of it lie in all four quadrants. The pancreas lies just behind the abdominal cavity on the posterior abdominal wall in both upper quadrants. The large intestine also traverses the abdomen, beginning in the RLQ and ending in the LLQ as it passes through all four quadrants. The urinary bladder lies just behind the pubic symphysis in the middle of the abdomen and therefore lies in both lower quadrants and also in the pelvis.

The kidneys are called **retroperitoneal** organs because they lie behind the abdominal cavity (▶ **Figure 4-15**). They are above the level of the umbilicus, extending from the eleventh rib to the third lumbar vertebra on each side. They are approximately 5″ long and lie just anterior to the costovertebral angle.

ANATOMIC LANDMARKS. The chief landmarks in the abdomen are the costal arch, the umbilicus, the anterior superior iliac spines, the iliac crest, and the pubic symphysis. The costal arch, as was noted earlier, is the fused cartilages of the sixth through the tenth ribs. It forms the superior arching boundary of the abdomen. The umbilicus, a constant structure, is in the same

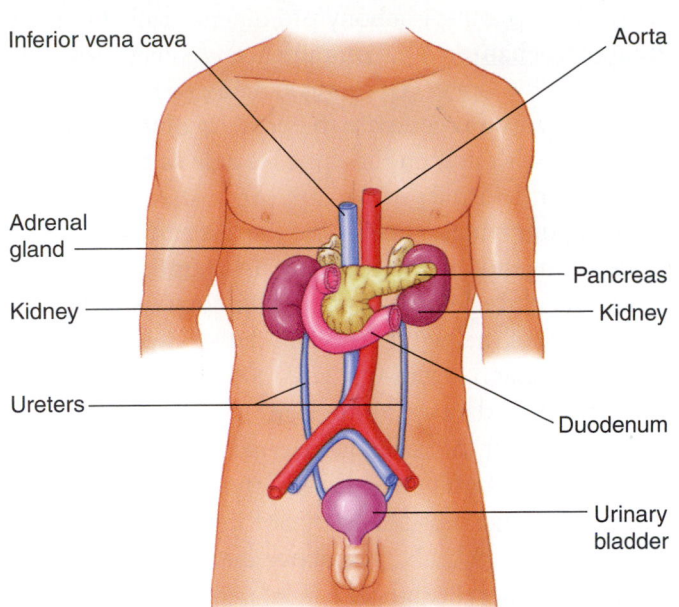

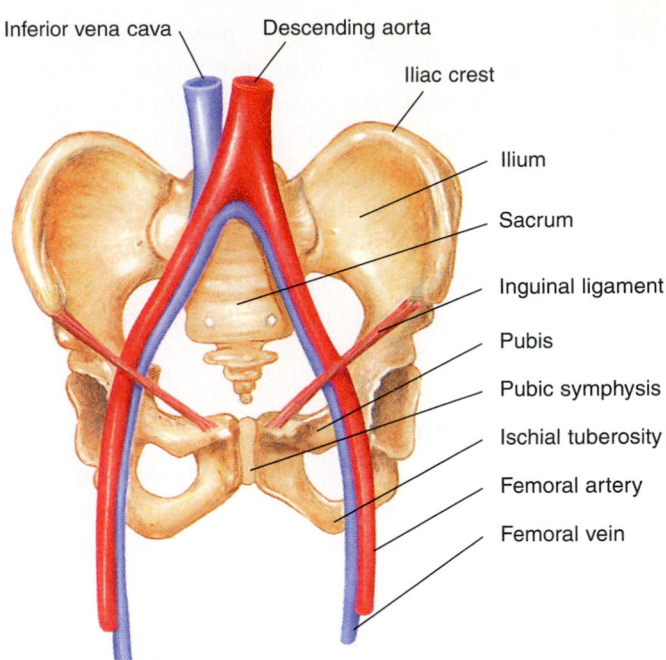

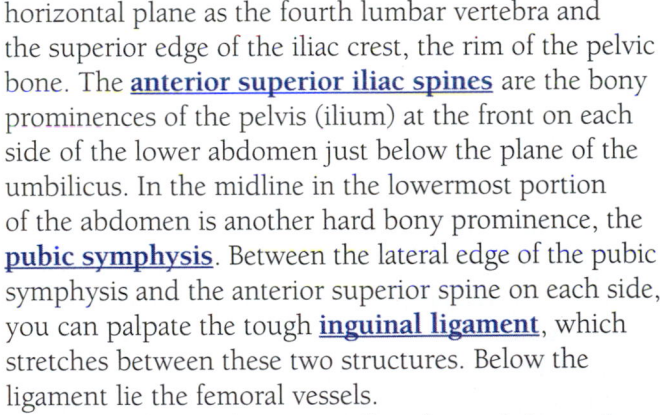

(Figure 4-15) The major organs of the retroperitoneal space lie behind the abdominal cavity, above the level of the umbilicus, and extend from the eleventh rib to the third lumbar vertebra. Note that the bladder, inferior vena cava, and aorta also lie in this plane.

(Figure 4-16) The pelvis is a closed bony ring that consists of the sacrum, ilium, and ischium.

horizontal plane as the fourth lumbar vertebra and the superior edge of the iliac crest, the rim of the pelvic bone. The **anterior superior iliac spines** are the bony prominences of the pelvis (ilium) at the front on each side of the lower abdomen just below the plane of the umbilicus. In the midline in the lowermost portion of the abdomen is another hard bony prominence, the **pubic symphysis**. Between the lateral edge of the pubic symphysis and the anterior superior spine on each side, you can palpate the tough **inguinal ligament**, which stretches between these two structures. Below the ligament lie the femoral vessels.

Posteriorly, you do not usually refer to abdominal quadrants. The posterior portion of the iliac crest can be palpated, as can the spines of the five lumbar vertebrae (Ll through L5) in the midline.

The Pelvis

The **pelvis** is a closed bony ring that consists of three bones: the sacrum and the two pelvic bones (▲ **Figure 4-16**). Much like the skull, each pelvic bone is formed by the fusion of three separate bones. These three bones are called the **ilium**, the **ischium**, and the **pubis**. These bones meet at three joints: the two posterior sacroiliac joints and the anterior midline pubic symphysis. All three joints allow very little

motion, as they are firmly held together by strong ligaments. On the lateral side of each pelvic bone—where the three component bones join—is the socket for the hip joint. This depression, in which the femoral head fits very snugly, is called the **acetabulum**.

The **pelvic cavity** is bounded superiorly by an imaginary plane that runs from the pubic symphysis to the top of the sacrum. Its lateral walls are formed by the inner borders of the pelvic bone, and its inferior boundary is the pelvic outlet, a layer of muscles with openings for the gastrointestinal tract (the rectum), the female reproductive system (the vagina), and the urinary tract (the urethra). In addition, the pelvis contains the final portions of the gastrointestinal tract (the rectosigmoid colon), the female reproductive organs, and the urinary bladder.

ANTERIOR ASPECTS. The prominent anterior bony landmarks of the pelvis are the pubic symphysis in the midline and the anterior superior iliac spines. The inguinal ligament attaches to these two bony prominences and can be palpated in a thin person. Just distal to the midpoint of the inguinal ligament, the femoral artery can be palpated as it enters the thigh. From the anterior superior iliac spine, the ilium extends laterally and posteriorly to form the rim of the pelvis. This bony ridge is called the **iliac crest**, or wing of the pelvis.

POSTERIOR ASPECTS. Posteriorly, the pelvis appears flat, and in the middle third, the firm bony sacrum can be palpated. Just lateral to the sacrum on either side is a joint with the iliac portion of the pelvic bone (the sacroiliac joint). In the sitting position, a bony prominence is easily felt below the middle of each buttock. These prominences are the ischial tuberosities. The sciatic nerve, which is the major nerve to the lower extremity, lies just lateral to the tuberosity as it enters the thigh.

The Lower Extremity

The main parts of the lower extremity are the thigh, the leg, and the foot (▼ **Figure 4-17**). Three joints connect the parts of the lower extremity: the hip, the knee, and the ankle. The joint between the thigh and pelvis is called the hip. The joint between the thigh and the leg is the knee. The joint between the leg and the foot is the ankle.

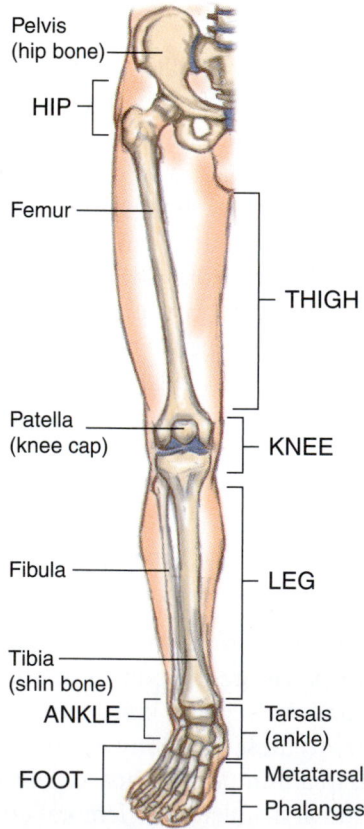

Pelvis
(hip bone)

HIP

Femur

THIGH

Patella
(knee cap)

KNEE

Fibula

LEG

Tibia
(shin bone)

ANKLE

Tarsals
(ankle)

FOOT

Metatarsals

Phalanges

Figure 4-17 The principal parts of the lower extremity include the thigh, leg, and foot. The principal parts of the leg include the tibia and fibula.

THIGH. On the proximal lateral side of the thigh, just below the hip joint, is a bony prominence called the **greater trochanter**. This prominence is sometimes called the "hip bone." During patient assessment, you should always compare the position of the greater trochanter with that on the opposite side as a guide to injury or deformity of the hip.

The **femur** (thigh bone) is the longest and one of the strongest bones in the body. The **femoral head** (at the top of the femur) forms the hip joint with the acetabulum of the pelvis. This ball-and-socket joint allows for flexion, extension, and motion toward (**adduction**) and away (**abduction**) from the midline. It also allows for internal and external rotation of the entire lower extremity. The shaft of the femur is surrounded by large muscles (the quadriceps in front and the hamstrings in back). Just above the knee, the medial and lateral femoral condyles can be palpated.

KNEE. Between the thigh and the leg is the largest joint in the body: the knee. The knee is essentially a hinge joint, allowing only flexion and extension between the distal femur and the proximal tibia. Adduction, abduction, and rotation of the knee are resisted by complex ligaments that are quite susceptible to injury. Anterior to the knee is a specialized bone called the **patella** (kneecap). It lies within the tendon of the quadriceps muscle and protects the front of the knee from injury.

LEG. The leg lies between the knee and the ankle joint and is composed of the **tibia** and the fibula. The tibia (shin bone) is the larger bone and lies in the front of the leg. You can palpate the entire length of the tibia on the anterior surface of the leg just under the skin. The **fibula** lies on the lateral side of the leg. You can palpate the head of the fibula on the lateral aspect of the knee joint. Its distal end forms the lateral malleolus of the ankle joint.

ANKLE AND FOOT. The ankle is a **hinge joint** that allows flexion and extension of the foot on the leg (▶ **Figure 4-18**). The end of the tibia forms the medial malleolus, and the end of the fibula forms the lateral malleolus. These two bony prominences form the socket of the ankle joint. Both are surface landmarks of the ankle joint and are easily palpated. The foot contains seven tarsal bones. The talus is one of the largest; the calcaneus, which forms the prominence of the heel, is the other large tarsal bone. The Achilles tendon inserts into the back of the calcaneus. Five metatarsal bones form the substance of the foot. The five toes are formed by 14 phalanges—two in the great toe and three in each of the smaller toes.

The Upper Extremity

The upper extremity extends from the shoulder girdle to the fingertips and is composed of the arm, elbow, forearm, wrist, hand, and fingers. The arm extends from the shoulder to the elbow.

SHOULDER GIRDLE. The proximal portion of the upper extremity is called the **shoulder girdle** and consists of three bones: the clavicle, the scapula, and the humerus (▼ **Figure 4-19**). The shoulder girdle is where the upper extremity attaches to the trunk. The upper extremity can move through a wide range of motion, allowing the hand to be placed in almost any position. This motion occurs at three joints within the shoulder girdle: the sternoclavicular joint, the acromioclavicular (A/C) joint, and the glenohumeral joint. Only slight motion occurs normally at the sternoclavicular and A/C joints. The ball-and-socket arrangement of the glenohumeral joint allows great freedom of motion in almost any direction.

The clavicle is a long, slender bone that lies just under the skin and provides support for the upper extremity. The clavicle is palpable through its entire length from the sternum to its attachment to the scapula. Its medial end is attached by very strong ligaments to the manubrium of the sternum to form the sternoclavicular joint. Its lateral end forms a joint with the acromion process of the scapula to create the A/C joint.

The scapula is a large, flat, triangular bone that overlies the posterior wall of the thorax and is surrounded by large muscles. Because of these muscles, only small parts of this bone are palpable. The scapula has two specially named regions that form joints with the clavicle and the humerus. The acromion process in the front forms part of the A/C joint. The glenoid fossa joins with the humeral head to form the glenohumeral joint. The spine and medial border of the scapula can be seen and palpated posteriorly. The acromion process forms the rounded edge of the shoulder girdle. You can feel this if you slowly move your finger along the clavicle and across the A/C joint.

ARM. The supporting bone of the arm is the **humerus**. Its long, straight shaft serves as an effective lever for heavy lifting. As in the thigh, there are few bony landmarks in the arm because it is covered by large muscles: the **biceps** in the front and the **triceps** in the back. The head of the humerus is covered by muscles that form the rounded prominence of the shoulder girdle laterally. The distal end articulates with both the radius and ulna at the elbow joint (▶ **Figure 4-20**).

The humerus joins with the radius and ulna to form the elbow, which is a relatively simple hinge joint. You can easily see and feel three prominences on the back of the elbow: the medial and lateral condyles of the humerus and the olecranon process of the ulna.

FOREARM. The forearm is composed of the radius and the ulna. The **ulna** is larger in the proximal forearm, and the **radius** is larger in the distal forearm.

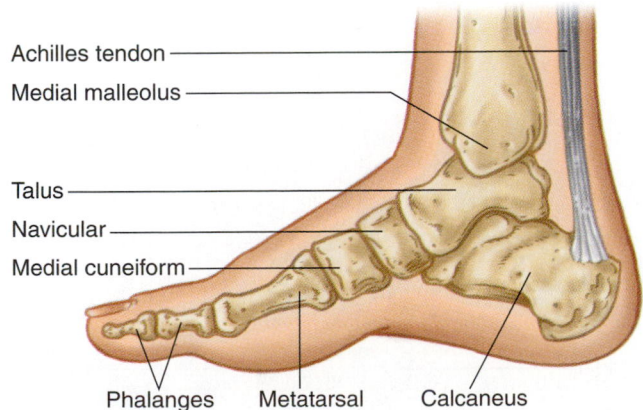

Achilles tendon
Medial malleolus
Talus
Navicular
Medial cuneiform
Phalanges   Metatarsal   Calcaneus

Figure 4-18   The surface landmarks of the foot and ankle include the medial malleolus, the calcaneus, and the phalanges.

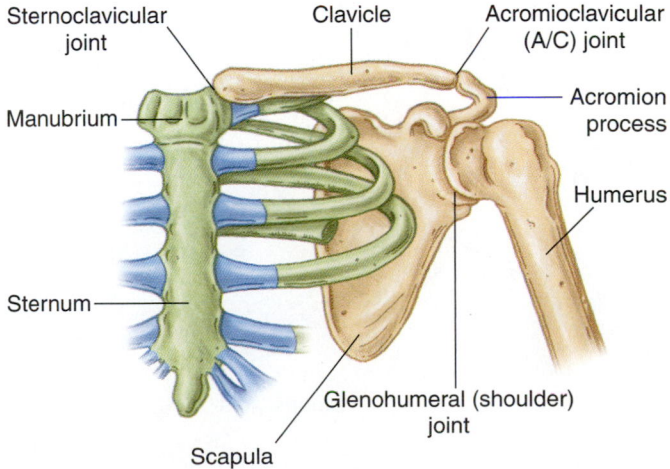

Sternoclavicular joint
Clavicle
Acromioclavicular (A/C) joint
Manubrium
Acromion process
Humerus
Sternum
Glenohumeral (shoulder) joint
Scapula

Figure 4-19   The bones of the shoulder girdle include the clavicle, the scapula, and the humerus.

The olecranon process of the ulna forms most of the elbow joint. The entire ulnar shaft from the tip of the olecranon process distally can be palpated, because it lies just under the skin on the back of the forearm. The radius is covered by muscles and cannot be palpated except in the lower third of the forearm, where it enlarges to form a major portion of the wrist joint. The radius rotates about the ulna, which allows the palm of the hand to turn up or down. At the wrist, the ends of the radius and ulna (the styloid processes) lie directly under the skin and can be easily palpated. The radial styloid is slightly longer than the ulnar styloid. The radius lies on the lateral, or thumb, side of the forearm, and the ulna is on the medial or little finger side.

WRIST AND HAND. The wrist is a modified ball-and-socket joint formed by the ends of the radius and ulna and several small wrist bones (▼ Figure 4-21). There are eight bones in the wrist, called carpal bones. Extending from the carpal bones are five metacarpals, which serve as a base for each of the five fingers or digits. The carpometacarpal joint (thumb joint) is a modified ball-and-socket joint that allows the thumb to rotate as well as to flex and extend. The other joints in the hand are simple hinge joints. In the thumb, there are two

bones beyond the metacarpal: the proximal and distal phalanges. The remaining four digits of the hand are named in order: the index, long, ring, and small finger. Each of these contains three phalanges.

Joints

Wherever two bones come in contact, a joint (articulation) is formed. A joint consists of the ends of the bones that make up the joint and the surrounding connecting and supporting tissue (► Figure 4-22). Most joints in the body are named by combining the names of the two bones that form that joint. For example, the sternoclavicular joint is the articulation between the sternum and the clavicle. Most joints allow motion—for example, the knee, hip, or elbow—whereas some bones fuse with one another at joints to form a solid, immobile, bony structure. For instance, the skull is composed of several bones that fuse as a child grows. An infant, whose skull bones are not yet fused, has fontanels (soft spots) between the bones. The fontanels close as the bones fuse together when the infant's skull reaches the adult size. Some joints have slight, limited motion in which the bone ends are held together by fibrous tissue. Such a joint is called a symphysis.

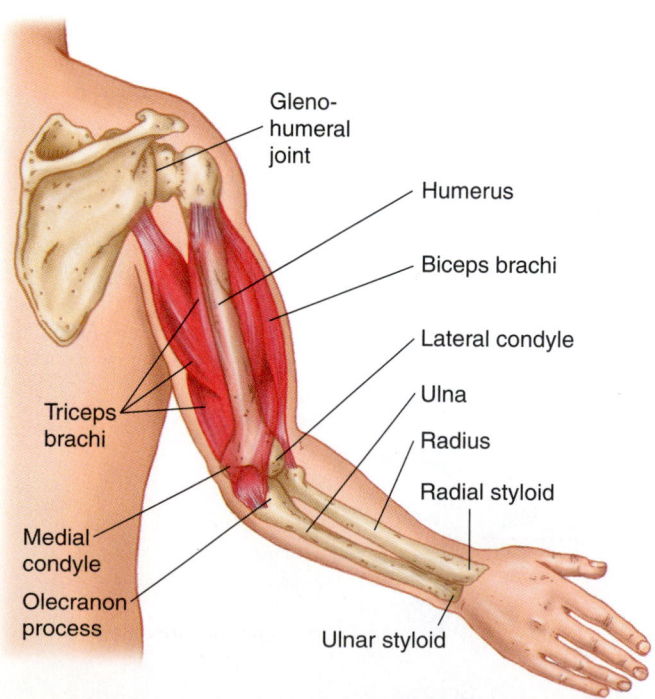

Figure 4-20   The principal bones in the arm and forearm include the humerus, the radius, and the ulna.

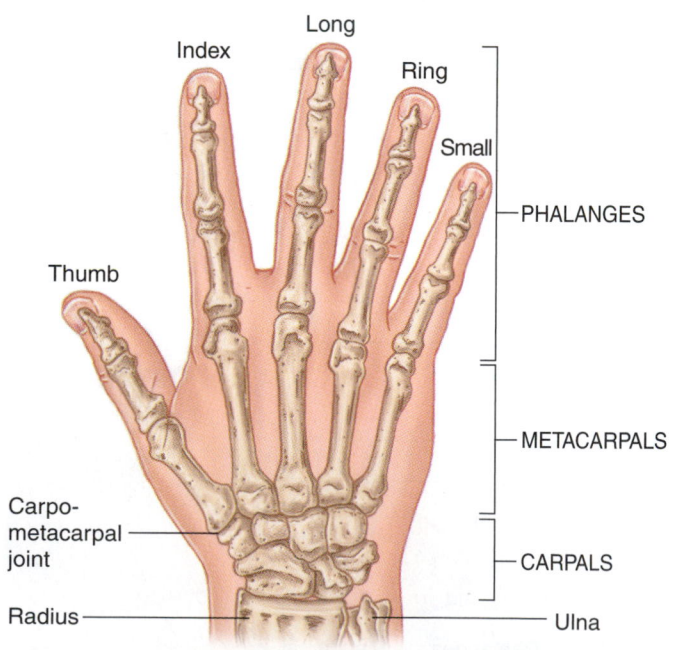

Figure 4-21   The principal bones in the wrist and hand include the carpals, the metacarpals, and the phalanges.

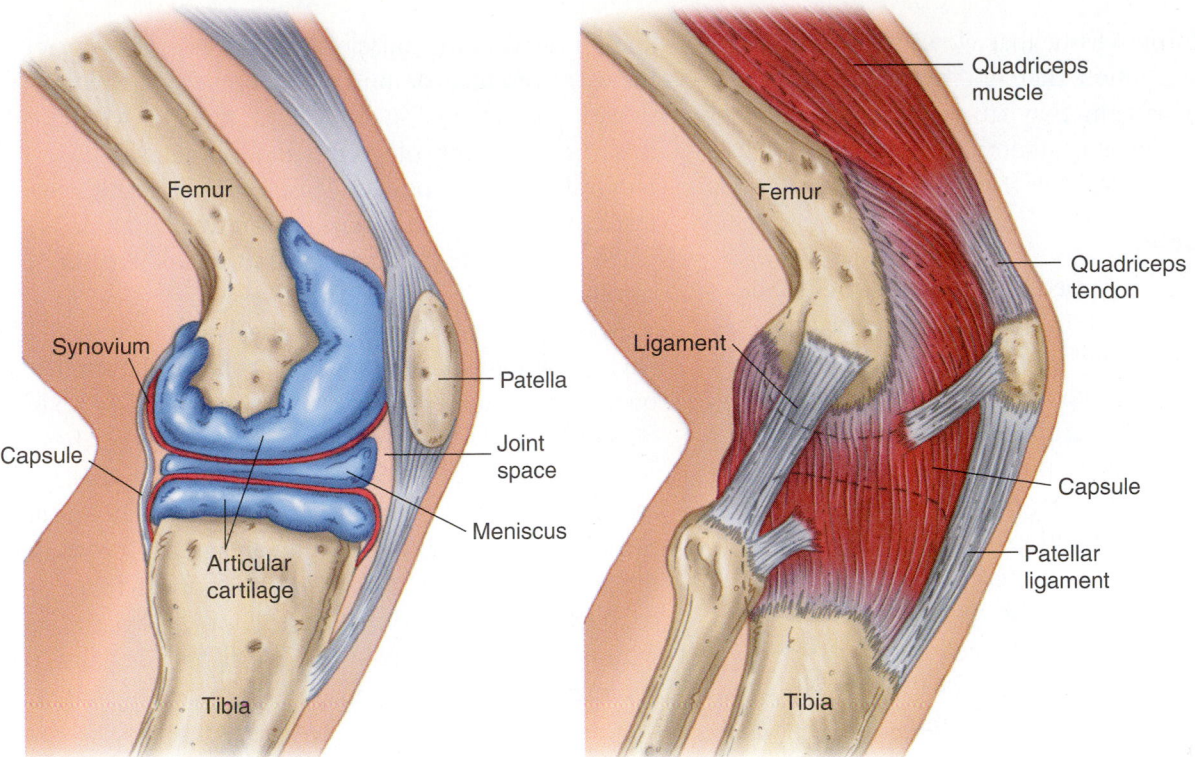

Figure 4-22   A joint consists of bone ends, the fibrous joint capsule, and ligaments. The degree to which a joint can move is determined by how the ligaments hold the bone ends and by the configuration of the bones themselves.

The bone ends of a joint are held together by a fibrous sac with a synovial lining, called the **joint capsule**. At certain points around the circumference of the joint, the capsule is lax and thin so that motion can occur. In other areas, it is quite thick and resists stretching or bending. These bands of tough, thick tissue are called **ligaments**. A joint such as the sacroiliac joint that is virtually surrounded by tough, thick ligaments will have little motion, whereas a joint such as the shoulder, with few ligaments, will be free to move in almost any direction (and will, as a result, be more prone to dislocation).

The degree of freedom of motion of a joint is determined by the extent to which the ligaments hold the bone ends together and also by the configuration of the bone ends themselves. The shoulder joint is a ball-and-socket joint, which allows rotation as well as bending (▶Figure 4-23). The finger joints and the elbow are hinge joints, with motion restricted to one plane (▶ Figure 4-24). They can only **flex** (bend) and **extend** (straighten). Rotation is not possible because of the shape of the joint surfaces and the strong restraining ligaments on both sides of the joint. Thus, although the amount of motion varies from joint to joint, all joints have a definite limit beyond which motion cannot

occur. When a joint is forced beyond this limit, damage to some structure must occur. Either the bones that form the joint will break, or the supporting capsule and ligaments will be disrupted.

The Musculoskeletal System

The human body is a well-designed system whose form, upright posture, and movement are provided by the **musculoskeletal system.** As its combination form suggests, the term musculoskeletal refers to the bones and voluntary muscles of the body. The musculoskeletal system also protects the vital internal organs of the body.

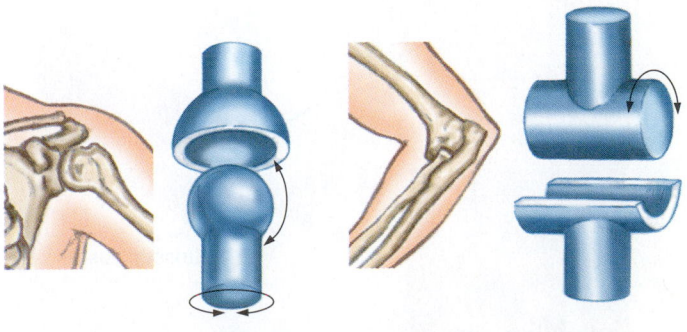

Figure 4-23   The shoulder is a ball-and-socket joint.

Figure 4-24   The elbow joints are hinge joints, which allow motion in only one plane.

Muscles are a form of tissue that allows body movement. Although there are more than 600 muscles in the musculoskeletal system, they are generally divided into three types: skeletal, smooth, and cardiac (▼ **Figure 4-25**).

Skeletal Muscle

Skeletal muscle, so named because it attaches to the bones of the skeleton, forms the major muscle mass of the body. It is also called **voluntary muscle**, because all skeletal muscle is under direct voluntary control of the brain and can be stimulated to contract or relax at will. Skeletal muscle is also called **striated muscle**, because when viewed under the microscope, it has characteristic stripes (striations). All body movement results from skeletal muscle contraction or relaxation. Usually, a specific motion is the result of several muscles contracting and relaxing simultaneously.

All skeletal muscles are supplied with arteries, veins, and nerves (▼ **Figure 4-26**). Arterial blood brings oxygen and nutrients to the muscle, and the veins carry away the waste products of muscular contraction (carbon dioxide and water). Muscles cannot function without this ongoing supply of oxygen and nutrients and removal of waste products. Muscle cramps result when insufficient oxygen or food is carried to the muscle or when acidic waste products accumulate and are not carried away.

Skeletal muscle is under the direct control of the nervous system and responds to a command from the brain to move a specific body part. Specific nerves pass directly from the brain to the spinal cord. There, they connect with other nerves that exit from the spinal cord and pass to each skeletal muscle. Electrical impulses are carried from the cells in the brain and spinal cord along the peripheral nerves to each muscle, signaling it to contract. When this normal nerve supply is lost through injury to the brain, spinal cord, or peripheral nerves, the voluntary control of the muscle is lost, and the muscle becomes paralyzed.

Most skeletal muscles attach directly to bone by tough, ropelike cords of fibrous tissue called **tendons**, which continue the fascia that covers all skeletal muscles. The fascia is much like the skin of a sausage in that it encases the muscle tissue. At either end of the muscle,

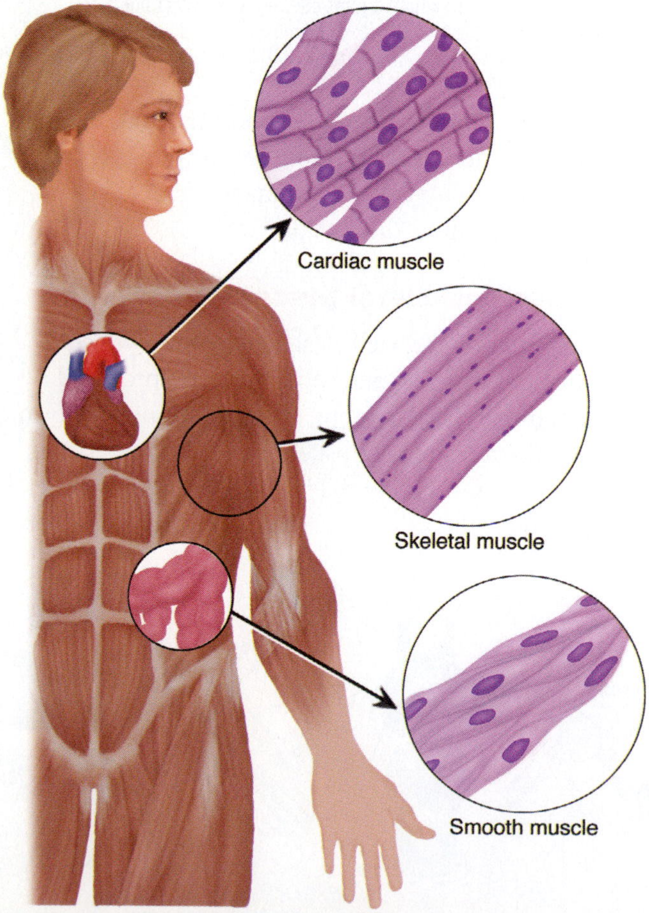

Cardiac muscle

Skeletal muscle

Smooth muscle

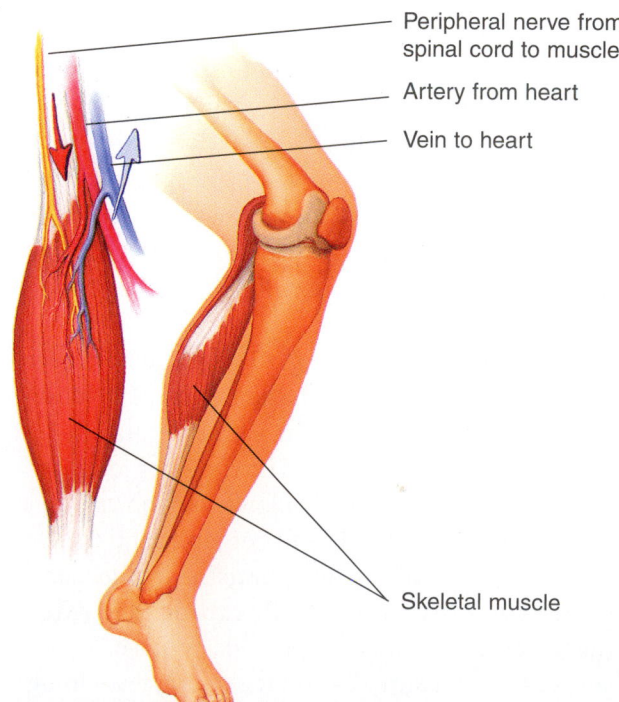

Peripheral nerve from spinal cord to muscle

Artery from heart

Vein to heart

Skeletal muscle

Figure 4-25   The three types of muscles are skeletal, smooth, and cardiac.

Figure 4-26   All skeletal muscles are supplied with arteries, veins, and nerves.

the fascia extends beyond the muscle to attach to a bone. This musculotendinous unit crosses a joint and is responsible for the motion of that joint. The proximal point of attachment of the musculotendinous unit is its origin, and the distal bony attachment is called the insertion of the muscle. When a muscle contracts, a line of force is created between the origin and the insertion, which pulls the points of origin and insertion closer together (▼ Figure 4-27). This motion occurs at the joint between the two bones.

Smooth Muscle

Smooth muscle carries out much of the automatic work of the body; therefore, it is also called involuntary muscle. Smooth muscle is found in the walls of most tubular structures of the body, such as the gastrointestinal tract, the urinary system, the blood vessels, and the bronchi of the lungs. Contraction and relaxation of smooth muscle propel or control the flow of the contents of these structures along their course. For example, the rhythmic contraction and relaxation

of the smooth muscles of the wall of the intestine propel ingested food through it, and smooth muscle in the walls of a blood vessel can alter the diameter of the vessel to control the amount of blood flowing through it (▼ Figure 4-28).

Smooth muscle responds only to primitive stimuli such as stretching, heat, or the need to relieve waste. An individual cannot exert any voluntary control over this type of muscle.

Cardiac Muscle

The heart is a large muscle composed of a pair of pumps of unequal force: one of lower pressure and one of higher pressure. The heart must function continuously from birth to death. It is a specially adapted involuntary muscle with a very rich blood supply and its own electrical system, which makes it different from both skeletal and smooth muscle. Another difference is that cardiac muscle has the property of "automaticity," which means that the heart muscle can set its own rhythm and rate without influence from the brain. This property is unique to heart muscle. Cardiac muscle can tolerate an interruption of its blood supply for only a few seconds. It requires a continuous supply of oxygen and glucose for normal function. Because of its special structure and function, cardiac muscle is placed in a separate category.

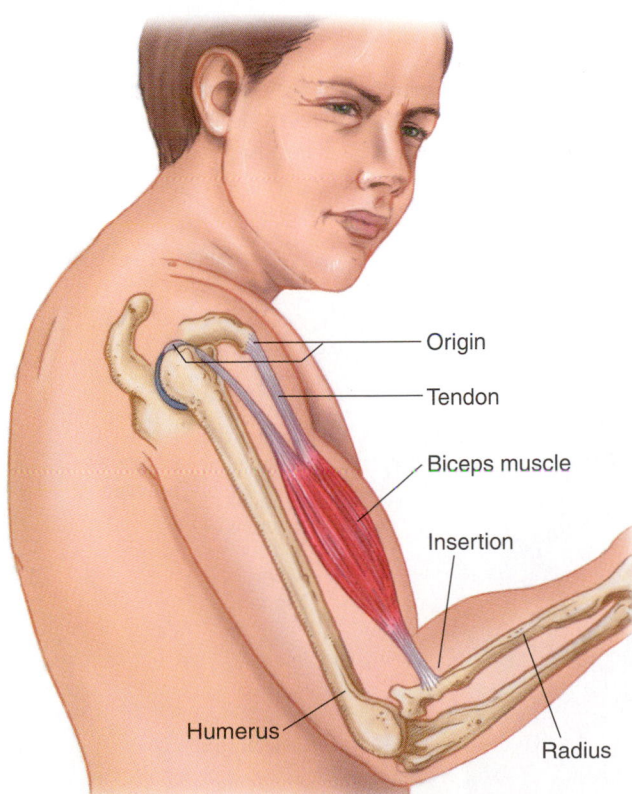

Figure 4-27   The biceps muscle causes the elbow to bend when it contracts. Note the points of tendon origin and insertion. As the muscle contracts and shortens, these points are pulled closer together, with motion occurring at the elbow joint.

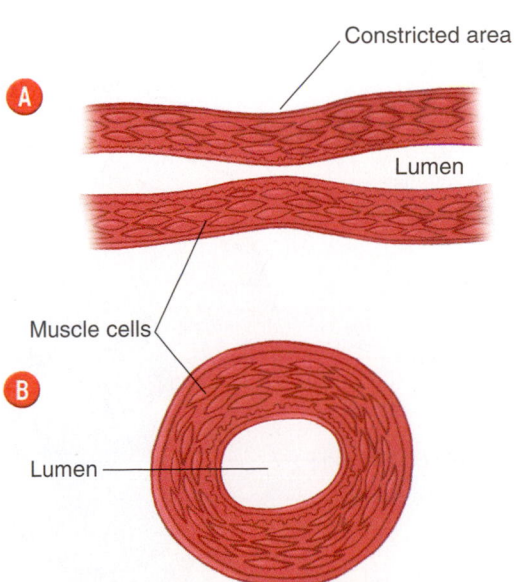

Figure 4-28   **A.** Smooth muscle lines the walls of the tubular structures of the body. **B.** Contraction of the muscles narrows the diameter of the structure, and relaxation allows the diameter to increase in size.

The Respiratory System

The **respiratory system** consists of all the structures of the body that contribute to respiration, or the process of breathing (▼ **Figure 4-29**). It includes the nose, mouth, throat, larynx, trachea, and **bronchi**, which are all air passages or airways. The system also includes the lungs, where oxygen is passed into the blood and where carbon dioxide is removed from the blood to be exhaled. Finally, the respiratory system includes the diaphragm, the muscles of the chest wall, and the accessory muscles of breathing, which permit normal respiratory movement. In this text, the term "airway" usually refers to the upper airway or the passage above the larynx (voice box).

The function of the respiratory system is to provide the body with oxygen and eliminate carbon dioxide. The exchange of oxygen and carbon dioxide takes place in the lungs and in the tissues. It is a complicated process that occurs automatically unless the airways or the lungs become diseased or damaged.

The Upper Airway

The structures of the upper airway are located anteriorly and at the midline. The upper airway includes the nose, nasal cavity, mouth, and pharynx. The nose and mouth lead to the **oropharynx** (throat). The nostrils lead to the **nasopharynx** (above the roof of the mouth, or soft palate), and the mouth leads to the oropharynx. The lining of the nasopharynx gives off watery secretions and helps to moisten the air as we breathe. Air enters through the mouth more rapidly and directly. As a result, it is less moist than air that enters through the nose.

Two passageways are located at the bottom of the pharynx: the esophagus behind and the trachea (windpipe) in front. Food and liquids enter the pharynx and pass into the esophagus, which carries them to the stomach. Air and other gases enter the trachea and go to the lungs.

Protecting the opening of the trachea is a thin, leaf-shaped valve called the **epiglottis.** This valve allows air to pass into the trachea but prevents food or liquid from entering the airway under normal circumstances.

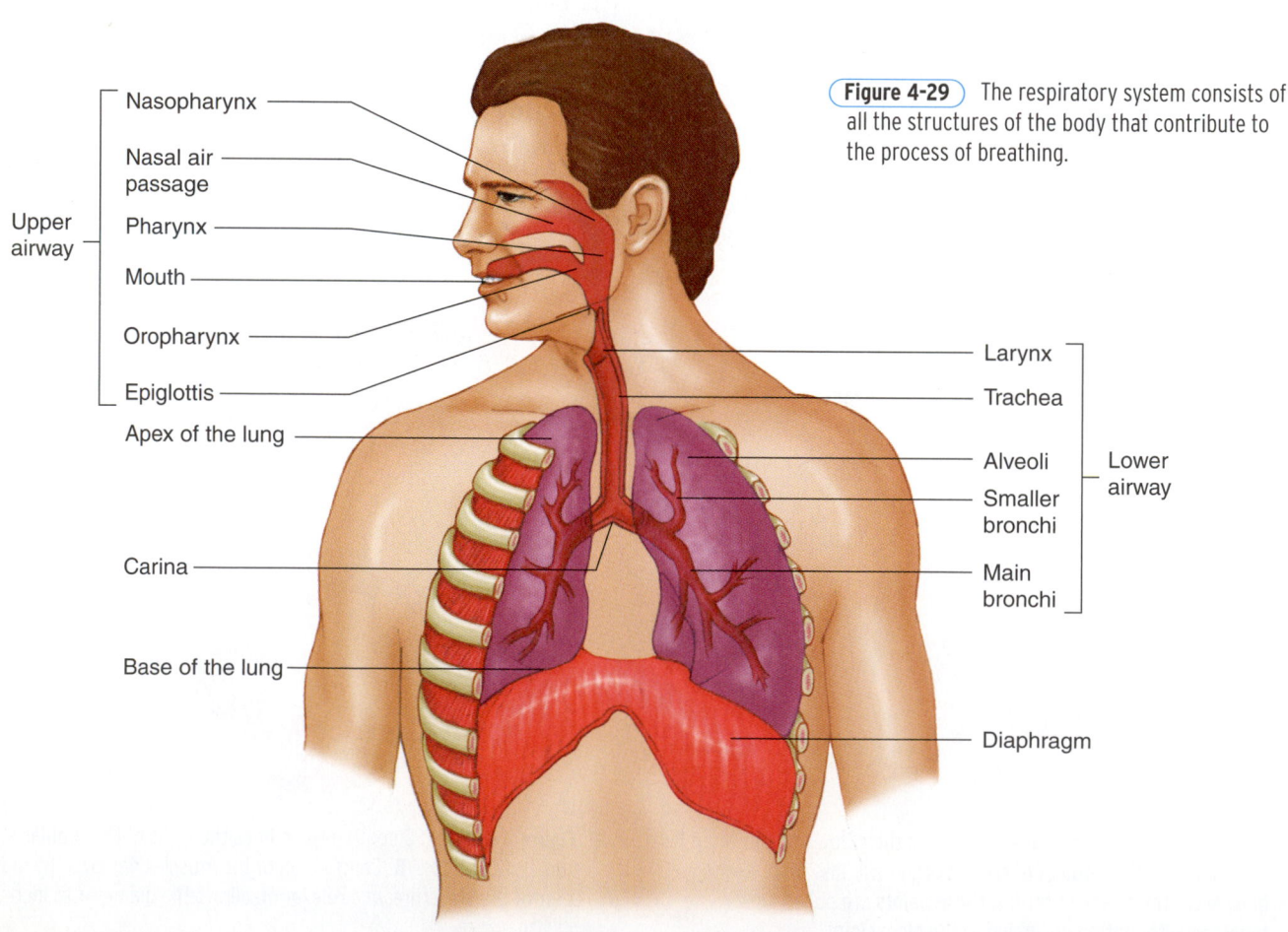

Figure 4-29 The respiratory system consists of all the structures of the body that contribute to the process of breathing.

Nasopharynx

Nasal air passage

Upper airway

Pharynx

Mouth

Oropharynx

Epiglottis

Apex of the lung

Carina

Base of the lung

Larynx

Trachea

Alveoli

Smaller bronchi

Main bronchi

Lower airway

Diaphragm

Air moves past the epiglottis into the larynx and the trachea.

The Lower Airway

The first part of the lower airway is the larynx, a rather complex arrangement of tiny bones, cartilage, muscles, and the two vocal cords. The larynx does not tolerate any foreign solid or liquid material. A violent episode of coughing and spasm of the vocal cords will result from contact with solids or liquids.

The Adam's apple, or thyroid cartilage, is easily seen in the middle of the front of the neck. The thyroid cartilage is actually the anterior part of the larynx. Tiny muscles open and close the vocal cords and control tension on them. Sounds are created as air is forced past the vocal cords, making them vibrate. These vibrations make the sound. The pitch of the sound changes as the cords open and close. You can feel the vibrations if you place your fingers lightly on the larynx as you speak or sing. The vibrations of air are shaped by the tongue and muscles of the mouth to form understandable sounds. Immediately below the thyroid cartilage is the palpable cricoid cartilage.

Between these two prominences lies the cricothyroid membrane, which can be felt as a depression in the midline of the neck just inferior to the thyroid cartilage. Below the cricoid cartilage is the trachea. The trachea is approximately 5″ long and is a semirigid, enclosed air tube made up of rings of cartilage that are open in the back. This enables food to pass through the esophagus, which lies right behind the trachea. The rings of cartilage keep the trachea from collapsing when air moves into and out of the lungs. The trachea ends at the carina and divides into smaller tubes. These tubes are the right and left main bronchi, which enter the lungs. Each main bronchus immediately branches within the lung into smaller and smaller airways. Within the right lung, three major bronchi are formed. Within the left, there are only two. Each bronchus supplies air to one lobe of the lung.

Lungs

The two lungs are held in place within the chest by the trachea, the arteries and veins that run to and from the heart, and the pulmonary ligaments. Each lung is divided into lobes. The right lung has three lobes: the upper, middle, and lower lobes. The left lung has an upper lobe and a lower lobe. Each lobe is divided further into segments. Also within each lung, the main bronchi divide until they end in very fine airways called **bronchioles**. The bronchioles end in about 700 million tiny grapelike sacs called **alveoli** (▼ Figure 4-30).

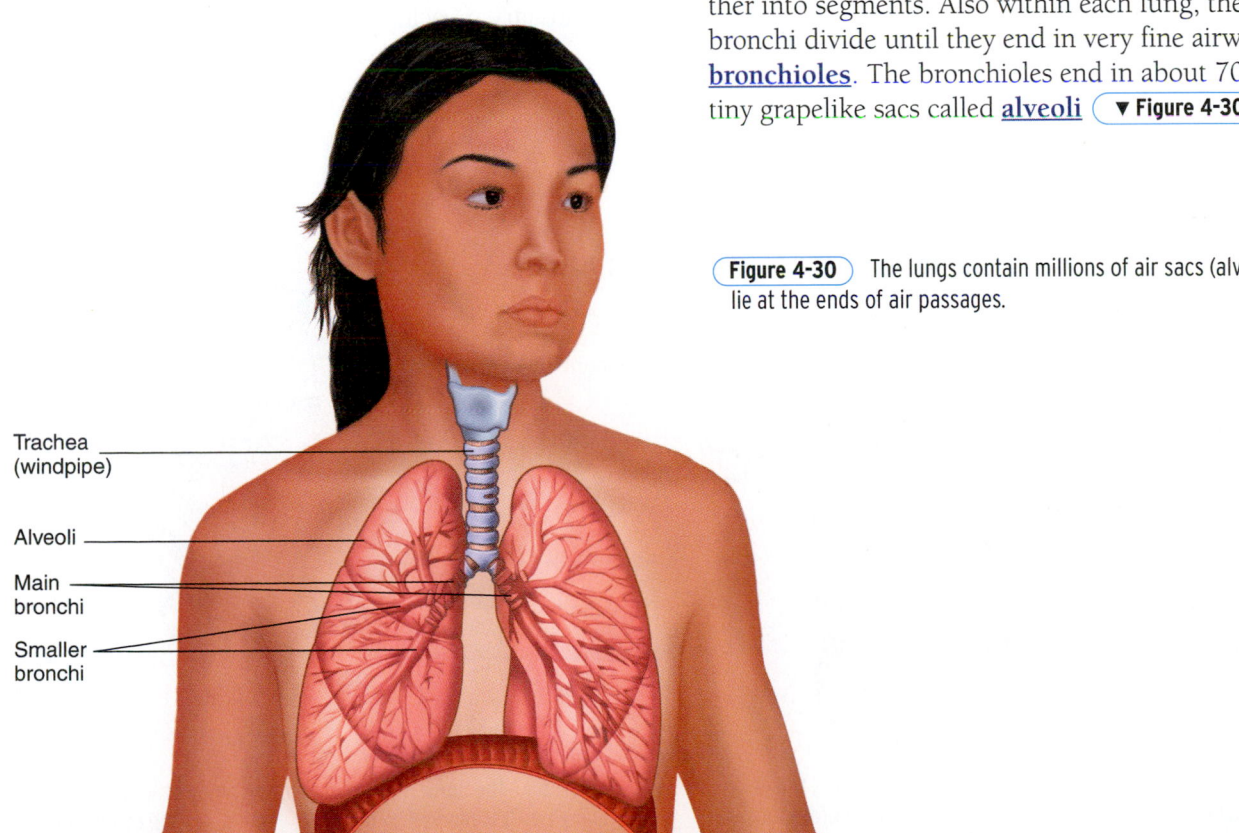

(Figure 4-30) The lungs contain millions of air sacs (alveoli), which lie at the ends of air passages.

Trachea (windpipe)

Alveoli

Main bronchi

Smaller bronchi

The exchange of oxygen and carbon dioxide occurs within these alveoli. The walls of the alveoli contain a network of tiny blood vessels (pulmonary capillaries) that carry the carbon dioxide from the body to the lungs and the oxygen from the lungs to the body.

The lungs cannot expand and contract themselves because they have no muscle. There is, however, a very definite mechanism to ensure that they follow the motion of the chest wall and expand or contract with it. Covering each lung is a layer of very smooth, glistening tissue called **pleura** (▼ Figure 4-31). Another layer of pleura lines the inside of the chest cavity. The two layers are called parietal pleura (lining the chest wall) and visceral pleura (covering the lungs).

Between the parietal pleura and the visceral pleura is the **pleural space**, called a "potential" space rather than an actual space in the usual sense because normally these layers are in close contact everywhere. In fact, the layers are sealed tightly against one another by a thin film of fluid. When the chest wall expands, the lung is pulled with it and made to expand by the force exerted through these closely applied pleural surfaces.

Diaphragm

The diaphragm is unique because it has characteristics of both voluntary (skeletal) and involuntary (smooth) muscle. It is a dome-shaped muscle that divides the thorax from the abdomen and is pierced by the great vessels and the esophagus (▼ Figure 4-32). Under the microscope, it has striations like skeletal muscle. Also, it is attached to the costal arch and the lumbar vertebrae like other skeletal muscles. Thus, in many ways, it looks like a voluntary muscle; however, we do not have complete voluntary control over its function. It acts like a voluntary muscle whenever we take a deep breath, cough, or hold our breath. We control these variations in the way we breathe.

However, unlike other skeletal or voluntary muscles, the diaphragm performs an automatic function. Breathing continues while we sleep and at all other times. Even though we can hold our breath or temporarily breathe faster or slower, we cannot continue these variations in breathing pattern indefinitely. Ultimately, when the concentration of carbon dioxide is close to being disturbed, automatic regulation of breathing resumes. Therefore, although the diaphragm looks like voluntary skeletal muscle and is attached to the skeleton, it behaves, for the most part, like an involuntary muscle.

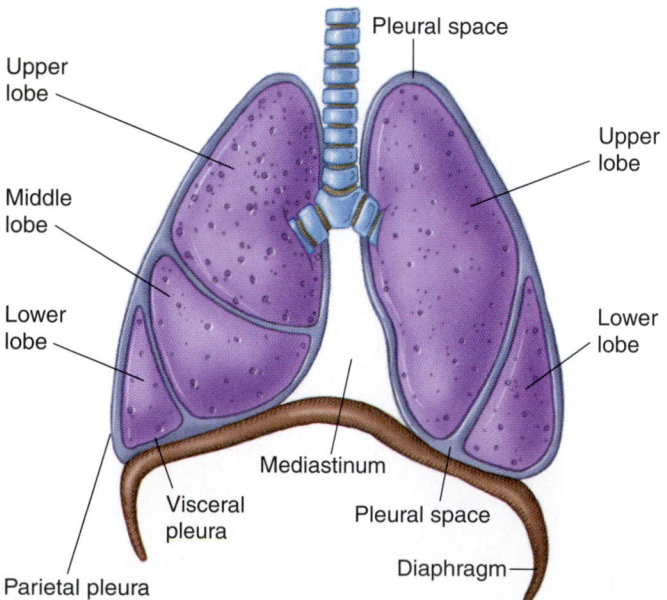

Figure 4-31 The pleura lining the chest wall and covering the lungs is an essential part of the breathing mechanism. The pleural space is not an actual space until blood or air leaks into it, causing the pleural surfaces to separate.

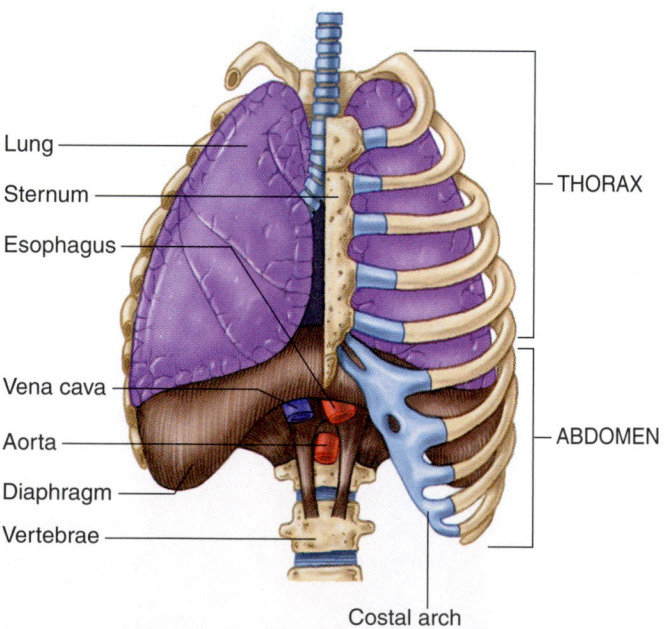

Figure 4-32 The dome-shaped diaphragm divides the thorax from the abdomen. It is pierced by the great vessels and the esophagus.

During **inhalation**, the diaphragm and **intercostal muscles** (the muscles between the ribs) contract. When the diaphragm contracts, it moves down slightly and enlarges the thoracic cage from top to bottom. When the intercostal muscles contract, they raise the ribs up and out. These actions combine to enlarge the chest cavity in all dimensions. Pressure within the cavity falls, and air rushes into the lungs.

During **exhalation**, the diaphragm and the intercostal muscles relax. Unlike inhalation, exhalation does not normally require muscular effort. As these muscles relax, all dimensions of the thorax decrease, and the ribs and muscles assume a normal resting position. When the volume of the chest cavity decreases, air in the lungs is compressed into a smaller space. Pressure is increased, and air is pushed out through the trachea.

Respiratory Physiology

Each living cell in the body requires a regular supply of oxygen. Some cells need a constant supply of oxygen to survive. For example, cells in the heart may be damaged if the oxygen supply is interrupted for more than a few seconds. Brain cells and cells in the nervous system may die after as few as 4 to 6 minutes without

> Techniques designed to support the integrity and function of the primary organ systems (circulatory, respiratory, and nervous systems) make up a major part of emergency care.

oxygen. Dead brain and nerve cells can never be replaced. Permanent changes in the body, such as brain damage, result from the damage caused by a lack of oxygen. Other cells in the body are not as vitally dependent on a constant oxygen supply. They can tolerate short periods without oxygen and still survive. Normally, the air that we breathe contains 21% oxygen and 78% nitrogen. Small amounts of other gases make up the remaining 1%.

THE EXCHANGE OF OXYGEN AND CARBON DIOXIDE. As blood travels through the body, it gives its oxygen and nutrients to various tissues and cells. Oxygen passes from the blood through the capillaries to tissue cells. In the reverse process, carbon dioxide and cell waste pass from tissue cells through capillaries to the blood ▼ Figure 4-33 .

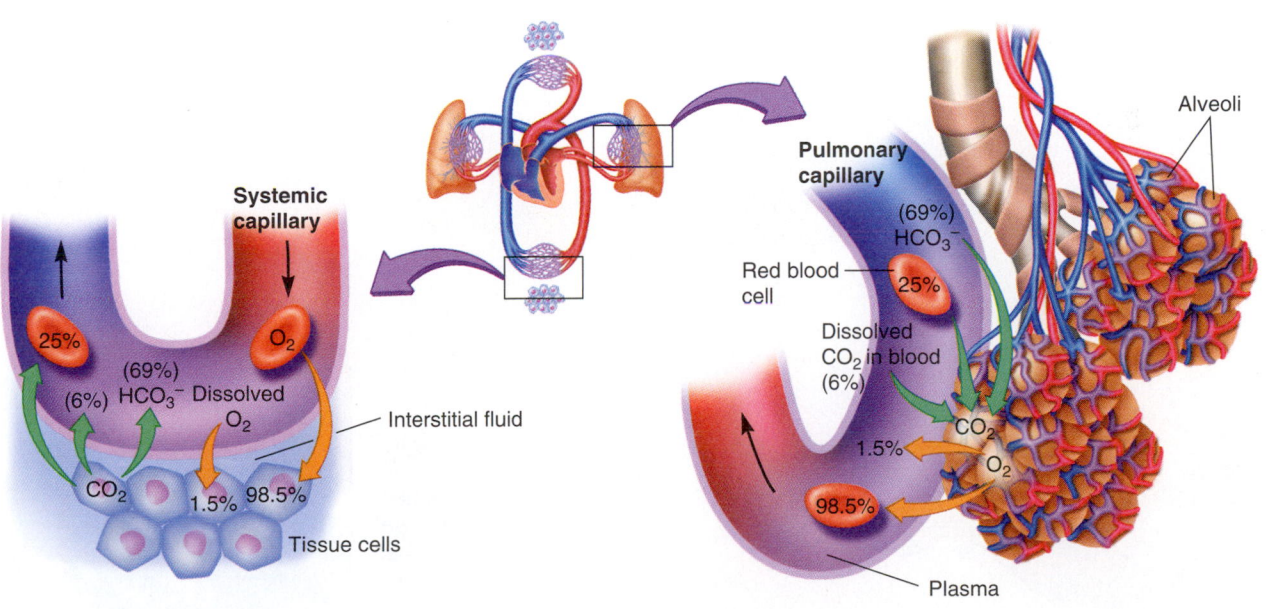

Figure 4-33 In the capillaries of the lungs, oxygen passes from the blood to the tissue cells, and carbon dioxide and waste pass from the tissue cells to the blood.

Each time we take a breath, the alveoli receive a supply of oxygen-rich air. The oxygen then passes into a fine network of pulmonary capillaries, which are in close contact with the alveoli. In fact, the capillaries in the lungs are located in the walls of the alveoli. The walls of the capillaries and the alveoli are extremely thin. Thus, the air in the alveoli and the blood in the capillaries are separated by two very thin layers of tissue.

Pediatric Needs

The anatomy of the respiratory system in children is proportionally smaller and less rigid than that in an adult ▼ **Figure 4-34**. A child's nose and mouth are much smaller than those of an adult. The larynx, cricoid cartilage, and trachea are smaller, softer, and more flexible as well. This makes the mechanics of breathing much more delicate. A child's pharynx is also smaller and less deeply curved. The tongue takes up proportionally more space in a child's mouth than in an adult's mouth.

These anatomic differences are important for your assessment. For example, the smaller larynx of a child becomes obstructed more easily. The chest wall in children is softer. Therefore, children depend more heavily on the diaphragm for breathing. You will notice that the abdomen moves in and out considerably with each breath, especially in an infant. Infants younger than age 1 month do not know how to breathe through the mouth. Therefore, as you assess an infant or a child, you must carefully consider these differences.

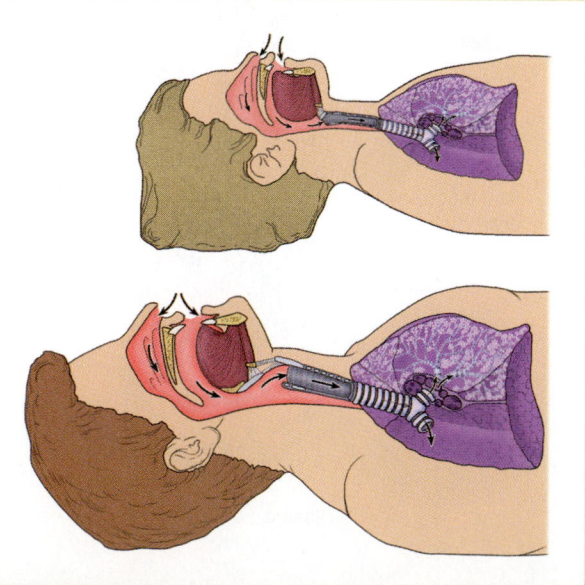

Figure 4-34 The respiratory system of a child is proportionally smaller and less rigid than that of an adult.

Oxygen and carbon dioxide pass rapidly across these thin tissue layers through diffusion. Diffusion is a passive process in which molecules move from an area with higher concentration of molecules to an area of lower concentration. For example, a gas such as hydrogen sulfide moves from an area of high concentration (a rotten egg) by spontaneous movement of the gas molecules until the odor fills the room. There are more oxygen molecules in the alveoli than in the blood. Therefore, the oxygen molecules move from the alveoli into the blood. Because there are more carbon dioxide molecules in the blood than in the inhaled air, carbon dioxide moves from the blood into the alveoli.

The blood does not use all the inhaled oxygen as it passes through the body. Exhaled air contains 16% oxygen and 3% to 5% carbon dioxide; the rest is nitrogen ▼ **Figure 4-35**. This 16% concentration of oxygen is adequate to support artificial ventilation. So as you provide artificial ventilations to a patient who is not breathing, that patient is receiving 16% concentration of oxygen with each ventilation.

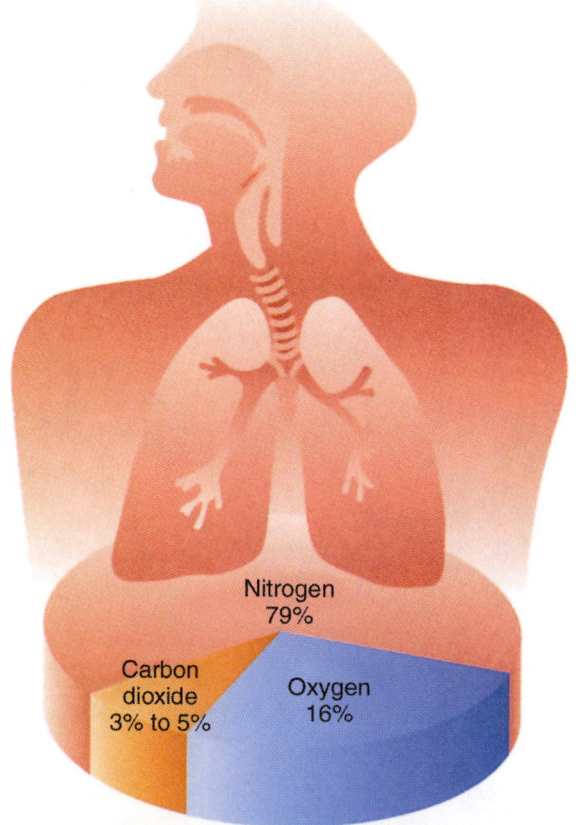

Components of Exhaled Air

Figure 4-35 The components of exhaled air include oxygen, carbon dioxide, and nitrogen.

THE CONTROL OF BREATHING. The brain—or more specifically, an area of the brain stem—controls breathing. This area is in one of the best-protected parts of the nervous system—deep within the skull. The nerves in this area act as sensors of the level of carbon dioxide in the blood. The brain automatically controls breathing if the levels of carbon dioxide or oxygen in the arterial blood are too high or too low. In fact, adjustments can be made in just one breath. For these reasons, you cannot hold your breath indefinitely or breathe rapidly and deeply indefinitely.

When the level of carbon dioxide becomes too high, the brain stem sends nerve impulses down the spinal cord that cause the diaphragm and the intercostal muscles to contract. This increases our breathing, or respirations. The higher the level of carbon dioxide in the blood, the stronger is the impulse to cause breathing.

Once the carbon dioxide levels become acceptable, the strength and frequency of respiration decrease.

We also have a "backup system" to control respiration called the **hypoxic drive**. When oxygen levels fall, this system will also stimulate breathing. There are areas in the brain, the walls of the aorta, and the carotid arteries that act as oxygen sensors. These sensors are easily satisfied by minimal levels of oxygen in the arterial blood. Therefore, our backup system, the hypoxic drive, is much less sensitive and less powerful than the carbon dioxide sensors in the brain stem.

CHARACTERISTICS OF NORMAL BREATHING. You can think of a "normal" breathing pattern as a bellows system. Normal breathing should appear easy, not labored. As with a bellows that is used to move air to start a fire, breathing should be a smooth flow of air moving into and out of the lungs. Normal breathing has the following characteristics:

- A normal rate and depth (tidal volume)
- A regular rhythm or pattern of inhalation and exhalation
- Good audible breath sounds on both sides of the chest
- Regular rise and fall movement on both sides of the chest
- Movement of the abdomen

INADEQUATE BREATHING PATTERNS IN ADULTS. An adult who is awake, alert, and talking to you has no immediate airway or breathing problems. However, you should keep supplemental oxygen on hand to assist with breathing if it should become necessary. An adult who is not breathing well will appear to be working hard to breathe. This type of breathing pattern is called **labored breathing**. Labored breathing requires effort and may involve the accessory muscles. The person may also be breathing either much slower (fewer than 8 breaths/min) or much faster (more than 24 breaths/min) than normal. An adult who is breathing normally will have respirations of 12 to 20 breaths/min ▼ Table 4-3.

Pediatric Needs

Normal breathing patterns in infants and children are essentially the same as those in adults. However, infants and children breathe faster than adults. An infant who is breathing normally will have respirations of 25 to 50 breaths/min. A child will have respirations of 15 to 30 breaths/min. Like adults, infants and children who are breathing normally will have smooth, regular inhalation and exhalation, equal breath sounds, and regular rise and fall movement on both sides of the chest.

Breathing problems in infants and children often appear the same as breathing problems in adults. Signs such as increased respirations, an irregular breathing pattern, unequal breath sounds, and unequal chest expansion indicate breathing problems in both adults and children. Other signs that an infant or child is not breathing normally include the following:

- Muscle retractions, in which the muscles of the chest and neck are working extra hard in breathing
- Nasal flaring in children, in which the nostrils flare out as the child breathes
- Seesaw respirations in infants, in which the chest and abdominal muscles alternately contract to look like a seesaw

Exhalation becomes active when infants and children have trouble breathing. Normally, inhalation alone is the active, muscular part of breathing, as described earlier. However, with labored breathing, both inhalation and exhalation are hard work. With labored breathing, exhalation is not passive. Instead, air is forced out of the lungs during exhalation, and the child will often begin to wheeze. This type of labored breathing involves the use of the accessory muscles of breathing.

TABLE 4-3 Normal Respiration Rate Ranges	
Adults	12 to 20 breaths/min
Children	15 to 30 breaths/min
Infants	25 to 50 breaths/min

With a normal breathing pattern, the accessory muscles are not being used. With inadequate breathing, a person, especially a child, may use the accessory muscles of the chest, neck, and abdomen. Other signs that a person is not breathing normally include the following:

- Muscle retractions above the clavicles, between the ribs, and below the rib cage, especially in children
- Pale or cyanotic (blue) skin
- Cool, damp (clammy) skin
- Tripod position (discussed in Chapter 5)

A patient may also appear to be breathing after the heart has stopped. These occasional, gasping breaths are called **agonal respirations**. Agonal respirations occur when the respiratory center in the brain continues to send signals to the breathing muscles. These respirations are not adequate, since they are slow and generally shallow. You should follow CPR protocols when patients present with agonal respirations.

The Circulatory System

The **circulatory system** is a complex arrangement of connected tubes, including the arteries, arterioles, capillaries, venules, and veins (▼ **Figure 4-36**). The circulatory system is entirely closed, with capillaries connecting arterioles and venules. There are two circuits in the body: the systemic circulation in the body and the pulmonary circulation in the lungs. The systemic circulation, the circuit in the body, carries oxygen-rich

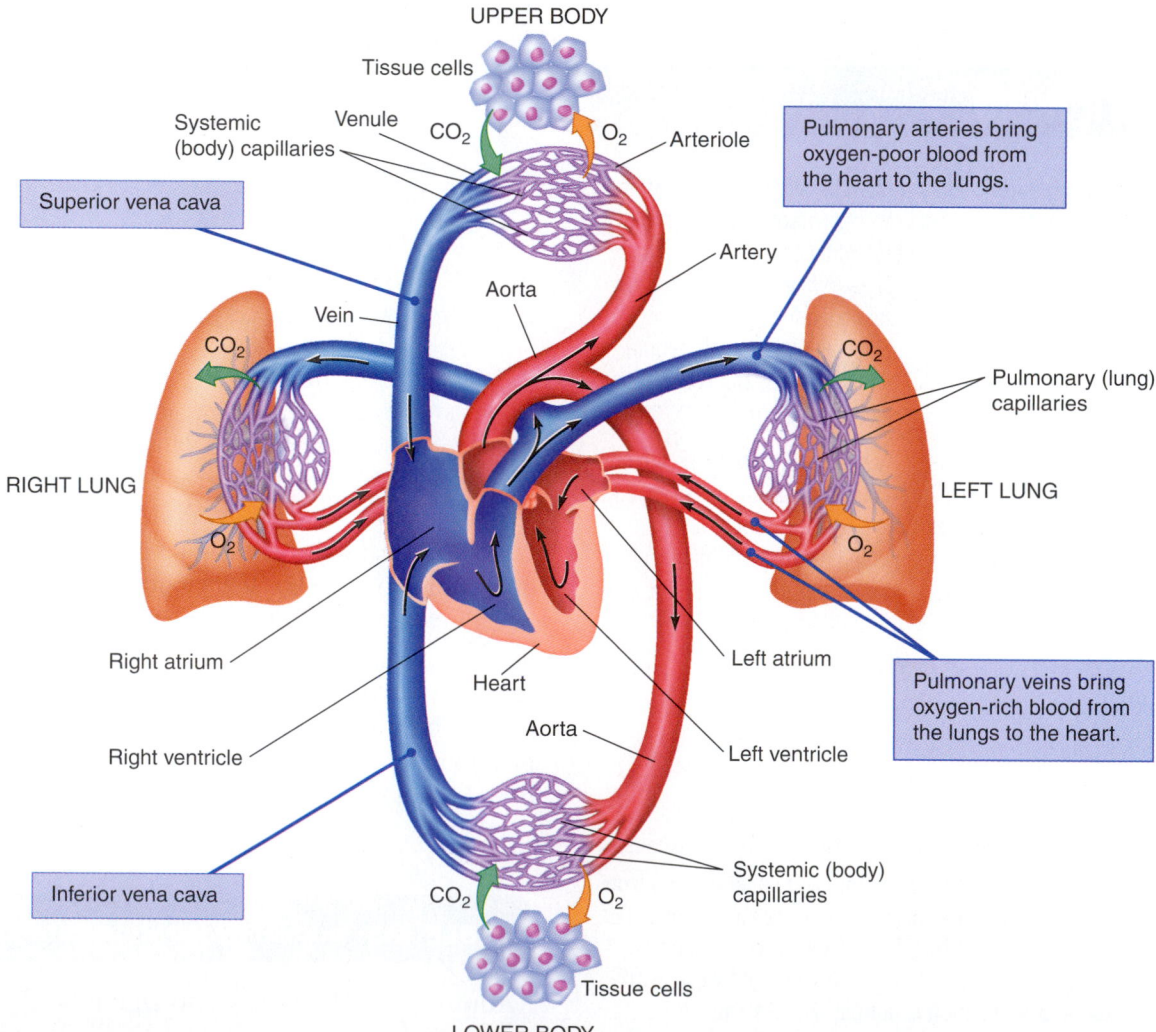

Figure 4-36 The circulatory system includes the heart, arteries, veins, and interconnecting capillaries. The capillaries are the smallest vessels and connect with the venules and arterioles. At the center of the system, and providing its driving force, is the heart. Blood circulates through the body under pressure generated by the two sides of the heart.

blood from the left ventricle through the body and back to the right atrium. In the systemic circulation, as blood passes through the tissues and organs, it gives up oxygen and nutrients and absorbs cellular wastes and carbon dioxide. The cellular wastes are eliminated in passages through the liver and the kidneys. The **pulmonary circulation**, the circuit in the lungs, carries oxygen-poor blood from the right ventricle through the lungs and back to the left atrium. In the pulmonary circulation, as blood passes through the lungs, it is refreshed with oxygen and gives up carbon dioxide.

Heart

The **heart** is a hollow muscular organ approximately the size of an adult's clenched fist. It is made of a unique, adapted tissue called cardiac muscle or **myocardium** and actually works as two paired pumps, the one on the left side being more muscular. A wall called the septum divides the heart down the middle into right and left sides. Each side of the heart is divided again into an upper chamber (**atrium**) and a lower chamber (**ventricle**).

The heart is an involuntary muscle. As such, it is under the control of the autonomic nervous system. However, it has its own electrical system and continues to function even without its central nervous system control. It is distinct from skeletal or smooth muscle in its requirement for a continuous supply of oxygen and nutrients.

The heart must function continuously from birth to death and has developed special adaptations to meet the needs of this continuous function. It can tolerate a serious interruption of its own blood supply for only a very few seconds before the signs of a heart attack develop. Thus, its blood supply is as rich and well distributed as possible.

HOW THE HEART WORKS. The heart receives the first blood distribution from the aorta. The two main coronary arteries have their openings immediately above the aortic valve at the beginning of the aorta where the pressures are highest (◄ **Figure 4-37**).

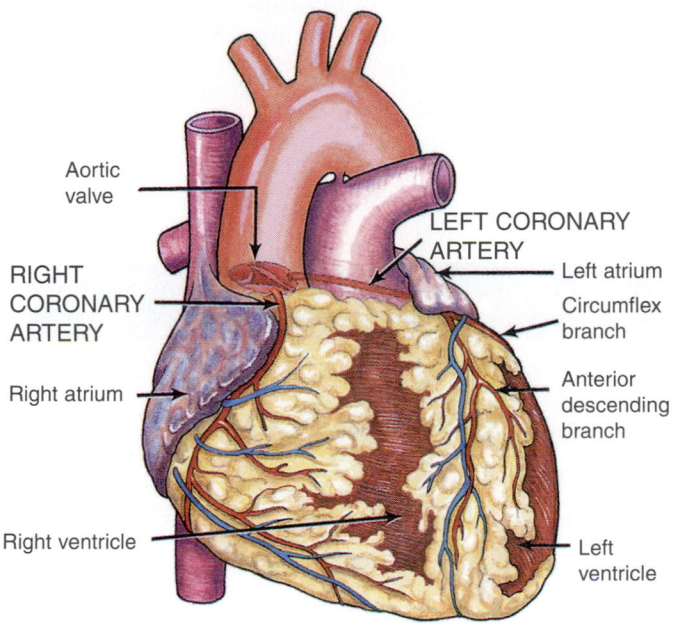

Figure 4-37 The two main coronary arteries supply the heart with blood.

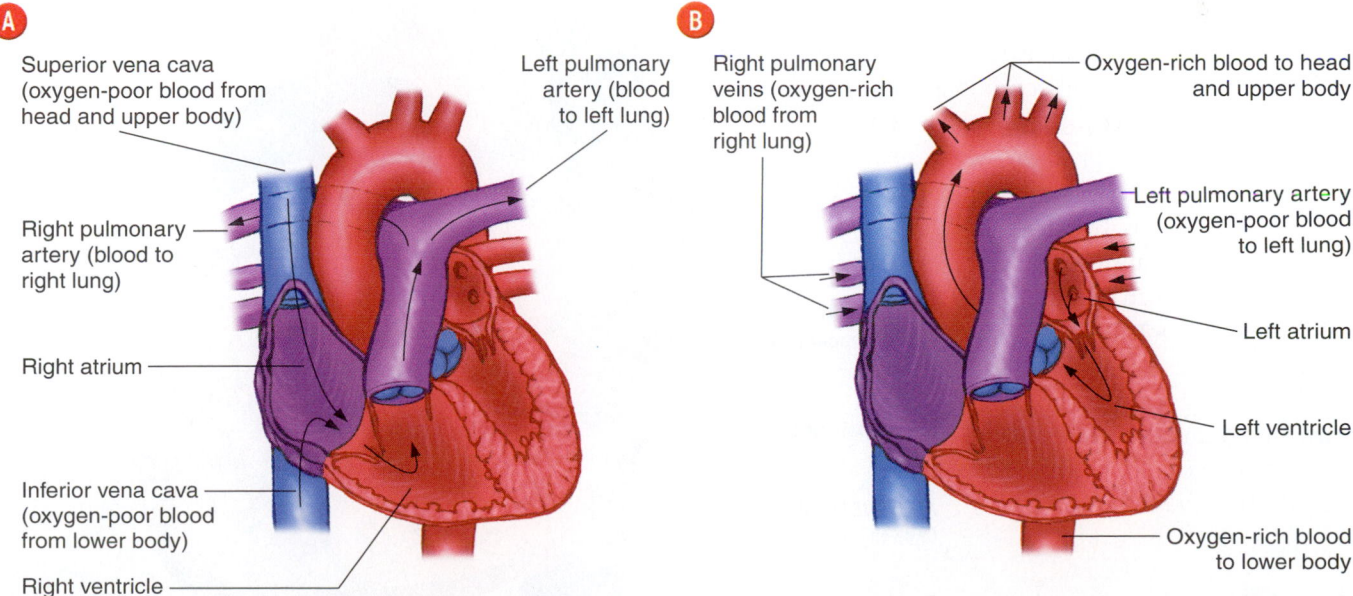

Figure 4-38 **A.** The right side, or lower pressure side, of the heart pumps blood from the body to the lungs. **B.** The left side, or higher pressure side, of the heart pumps oxygen-rich blood to all parts of the body.

The right side of the heart receives blood from the veins of the body (◄ **Figure 4-38A**). The blood enters from the **superior and inferior venae cavae** into the right atrium, then fills the right ventricle passing through a valve that closes to prevent backflow after the right atrial muscle contracts. Contraction of the right ventricle causes blood to flow into the **pulmonary artery** and the pulmonary circulation.

The left side receives oxygenated blood from the lungs through the **pulmonary veins** into the left atrium where it passes through a valve into the left ventricle (◄ **Figure 4-38B**). Contraction of this most muscular of the pumping chambers pumps the blood into the aorta and then to the arteries of the body.

The exit of each of the four heart chambers is governed by a one-way valve. The valves prevent the backflow of blood and keep it moving through the circulatory system in the proper direction. When a valve controlling the filling of a heart chamber is open, the other valve allowing it to empty is shut and vice versa. Normally, blood moves in only one direction through the entire system.

When a ventricle contracts, the valve to the artery opens, and the valve between the ventricle and atrium closes. Blood is forced from the ventricle out into the pulmonary artery or aorta. At the end of contraction, the ventricle relaxes. Backpressure causes the valve to the artery to close, and the entry valve to the ventricle opens as the ventricle relaxes. Blood then flows from the atrium into the ventricle. When the ventricle is stimulated to contract, the cycle is repeated.

NORMAL HEARTBEAT. In the normal adult, the heartbeat may range from 50 to 180 beats/min, depending on the level of activity. A very well-conditioned athlete may have a normal resting **heart rate** (**pulse**) of 50 to 60 beats/min. During vigorous physical activity, the heart rate may rise normally to as fast as 180 beats/min. The usual adult resting heart rate is between 60 and 100 beats/min (► **Table 4-4**). At each beat, 70 to 80 mL of blood is ejected from the adult heart. In one minute, the entire blood volume of 5 to 6 L is circulated through all the vessels.

ELECTRICAL CONDUCTION SYSTEM. A network of specialized tissue that is capable of conducting electrical current runs throughout the heart (▼ **Figure 4-39**). The flow of electrical current through this network causes smooth, coordinated contractions of the heart. These contractions produce the pumping action of the heart. Each mechanical contraction of the heart is associated with two electrical processes. The first is depolarization, during which the electrical charges on the surface of the muscle cell change from positive to negative. The second is repolarization, during which the heart returns to its resting state and the positive charge is restored to the surface.

When the heart is working normally, the electrical impulse begins high in the atria at the sinoatrial (SA)

TABLE 4-4 Normal Heart Rates	
Adults	60 to 100 beats/min
Children	80 to 100 beats/min
Toddlers	100 to 120 beats/min
Newborns	120 to 140 beats/min

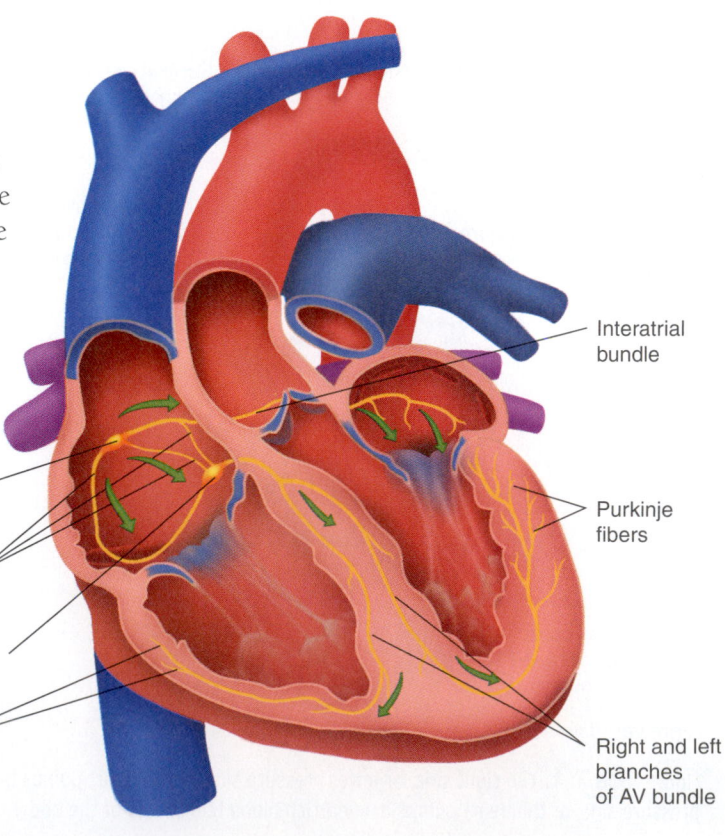

SINOATRIAL (SA) NODE (pacemaker)

Internodal bundles

ATRIOVENTRICULAR (AV) NODE

Purkinje fibers

Interatrial bundle

Purkinje fibers

Right and left branches of AV bundle

Figure 4-39 Electrical current flows through the heart to produce its pumping action.

node, then travels to the atrioventricular (AV) node, and moves through the Purkinje fibers to the ventricles. This movement produces a smooth flow of electricity through the heart, which depolarizes the muscle and produces a coordinated pumping contraction. The heart's electrical system becomes disturbed if part of the heart is oxygen deficient, is injured, or dies. As a result, the heart may not continue to beat properly. Blood pressure decreases, and a patient may lose consciousness.

Arteries

The **arteries** carry blood from the heart to all body tissues (▶ **Figure 4-40**). They branch into smaller arteries and then into arterioles. The arterioles, in turn, branch into smaller vessels until they connect to the vast network of capillaries. The walls of an artery are made of fine, circular muscle tissue. Some arteries even have elastic tissue.

Arteries contract to accommodate loss of blood volume and also to increase blood pressure. Blood is supplied to tissues as they need it. For example, the digestive system is supplied with more blood after you eat a meal. The leg muscles are more heavily supplied when jogging. Some tissues need a constant blood supply, especially the heart, the kidneys, and the brain. Other tissues, such as the muscles in the extremities, the skin, and intestines, can function with less blood when at rest.

The **aorta** is the principal artery leaving the left side of the heart; it carries freshly oxygenated blood to the body. This blood vessel is found just in front of the spine in the chest and abdominal cavities. The aorta has many branches that supply the heart, head, neck, arms, and abdominal and thoracic organs before it ends in the lower abdomen. It divides at the level of the umbilicus into the two common iliac arteries that lead to the lower extremities. All of the aorta's branches ultimately become arterioles leading into the body's capillary network.

The pulmonary artery begins at the right side of the heart and carries oxygen-poor blood to the lungs. It divides into finer and finer branches until it meets with the pulmonary capillary system located in the thin walls of the alveoli. These arteries are the only ones in the body that carry oxygen-poor blood.

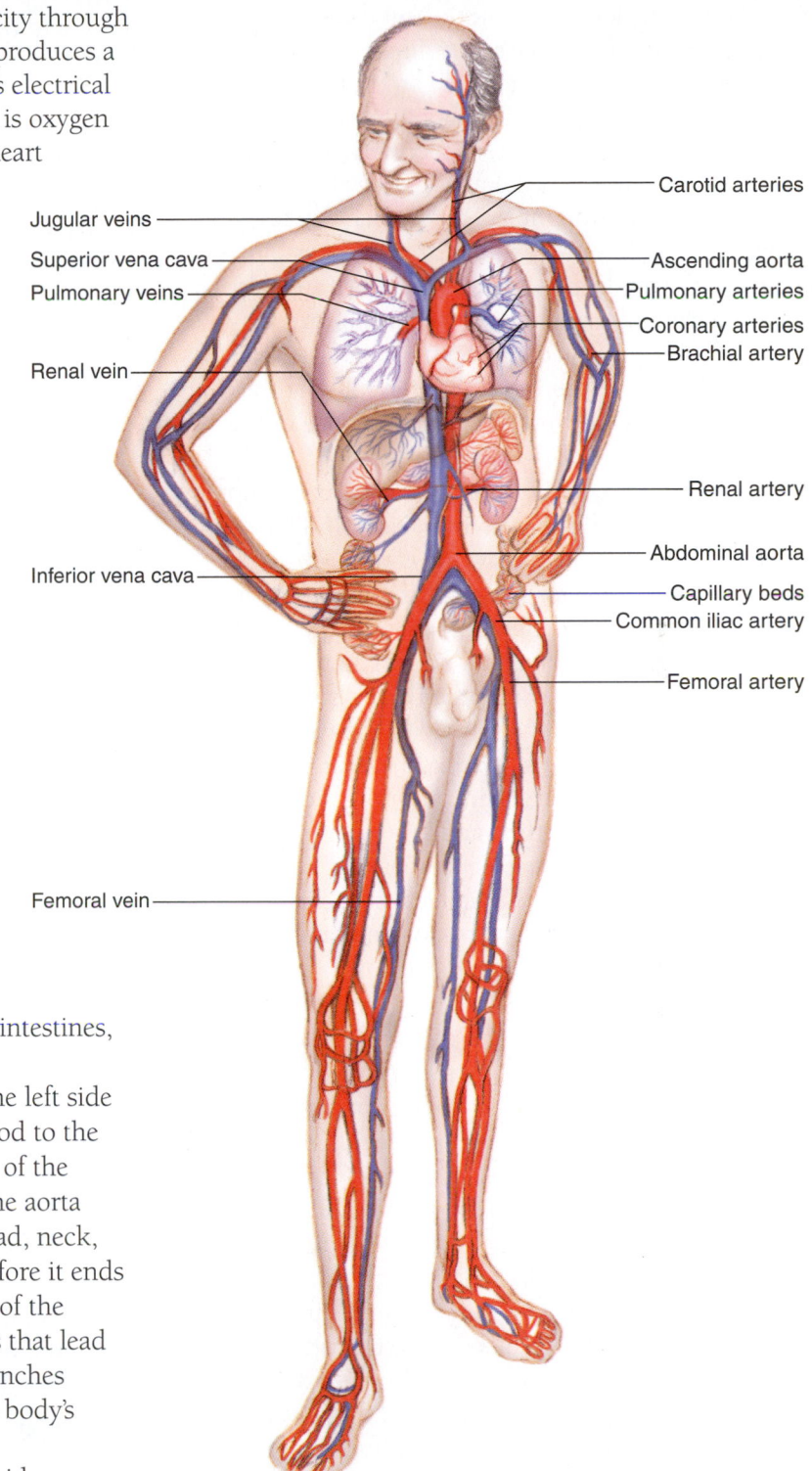

Jugular veins

Superior vena cava

Pulmonary veins

Renal vein

Inferior vena cava

Femoral vein

Carotid arteries

Ascending aorta

Pulmonary arteries

Coronary arteries

Brachial artery

Renal artery

Abdominal aorta

Capillary beds

Common iliac artery

Femoral artery

Figure 4-40   The principal arteries supply blood to a vast network of smaller arteries and arterioles, which nourish the tissue cells via the capillaries. Venules deliver oxygen-poor blood to the veins that return blood to the heart.

The <u>carotid artery</u> is the major artery that supplies blood to the head and brain. The carotid arteries are located on both sides of the neck. You can easily feel the carotid pulse if you place your fingers at the anterior lateral part of the neck. Since the carotid artery is rather close to the heart, you can feel its pulse even after the pulse in the distal extremities is too weak to feel.

The <u>femoral artery</u> is the major artery that supplies blood to the lower extremities. It is palpable in the groin. It divides at the level of the knee and supplies blood to the leg. At the ankle, two of these branches are palpable. You can feel a pulse at the <u>posterior tibial artery</u>, which is behind the medial prominence of the ankle (medial malleolus). You can also feel a pulse at the <u>dorsalis pedis artery</u> on the anterior surface of the foot (dorsum of the foot).

The <u>brachial artery</u> is the major vessel in the upper extremity that supplies blood to the arm. It divides into two major branches just below the elbow. This is the artery that is used in assessing blood pressure with a blood pressure cuff and stethoscope.

The <u>radial artery</u> is the major artery in the forearm and is palpable at the wrist on the thumb side (radial side). The <u>ulnar artery</u> is also palpable at the wrist on the opposite side (ulnar side, at the base of the fifth finger), although its pulse is not as strong. Both of these arteries supply blood to the hand.

Arteries branch into smaller arteries and then into arterioles. <u>Arterioles</u> are the smallest branches of an artery leading to the vast network of capillaries.

Capillaries

In the body, there are billions of cells and billions of capillaries. <u>Capillary vessels</u> are fine end-divisions of the arterial system that allow contact between cells of the body tissues and the plasma and the red blood cells. At this level, each individual cell of the body lives. Oxygen and other nutrients pass from blood cells and plasma in the capillaries to the individual tissue cells through the very thin wall of the capillary. Carbon dioxide and other metabolic waste products pass in a reverse direction from the tissue cells to the blood to be carried away. Blood in arteries is characteristically bright red, because its hemoglobin is rich in oxygen. Blood in the veins is dark bluish red, because it has passed through a capillary bed and given up some of its oxygen to the cells. Capillaries connect directly at one end with the flow-regulating arterioles and at the other with the venules.

Veins

Oxygen-poor blood from the capillary system next moves to the venules, which are the smallest branches of the veins. The <u>veins</u> then return blood to the heart.

Once blood passes through the network of capillaries and moves through the venules, it returns to the heart via a network of larger and larger veins. Veins have much thinner walls than arteries and are generally larger in diameter. The veins become larger and larger and ultimately form two major vessels. These major vessels, part of the great vessels, are located in the midline, just to the left of the spine, and channel blood from the body and collect it just before it enters the heart.

The superior vena cava carries blood returning from the head, neck, shoulders, upper chest, and upper extremities. Blood from the lower chest, abdomen, pelvis, and lower extremities passes through the inferior vena cava. The superior and inferior venae cava join at the right atrium of the heart. The right ventricle receives blood from the right atrium and pumps it through the pulmonary arteries into the lungs.

The pulmonary veins carry oxygen-rich blood from the lungs to the left atrium. The oxygenated blood from the lungs enters the four pulmonary veins that unite at the left atrium. It then passes to the left ventricle and is pumped to the body again.

Components of Blood

Blood is a complex, thick, red fluid composed of plasma, red blood cells called erythrocytes, white blood cells called leukocytes, and platelets (▶ **Figure 4-41**).

- <u>Plasma</u> is a sticky, yellow fluid that carries the blood cells and nutrients. It also transports cellular waste material to the organs of excretion. It contains most of the compounds needed to produce a blood clot.

- The iron-containing hemoglobin molecules in <u>red blood cells</u> (erythrocytes) give color to the blood and carry oxygen.

- <u>White blood cells</u> (leukocytes) play a role in the body's immune defense mechanisms against infection.

- <u>Platelets</u> are tiny, disk-shaped elements that are much smaller than the cells. They are essential in the initial formation of a blood clot, the mechanism that stops bleeding.

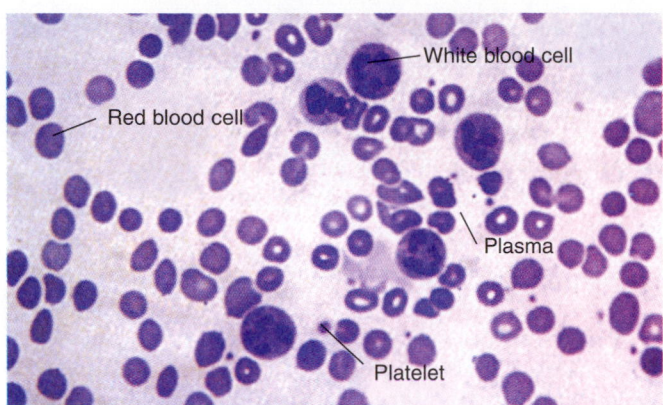

Figure 4-41 The components of blood include red blood cells, white blood cells, platelets, and plasma.

Blood under pressure will gush or spurt intermittently from an artery and is bright red. From a vein, it will flow in a steady stream and is dark bluish-red. From capillaries, it will ooze at many tiny individual points. Clotting normally takes from 6 to 10 minutes.

Physiology of the Circulatory System

The **pulse**, which is palpated most easily at the neck, wrist, or groin, is created by the forceful pumping of blood out the left ventricle and into the major arteries. It is present throughout the entire arterial system. It can be felt most easily where the larger arteries are near the skin. The central pulses are the carotid pulse, which can be felt at the upper portion of the neck, and the femoral pulse, which is felt in the groin. The peripheral pulses are the radial pulse, which is felt at the wrist at the base of the thumb; the brachial pulse, which is felt on the medial aspect of the arm, midway between the elbow and shoulder; the posterior tibial pulse, which is felt posterior to the medial malleolus; and the dorsalis pedis pulse, which is felt on the top of the foot ▶ **Figure 4-42**.

Blood pressure is the pressure that the blood exerts against the walls of the arteries as it passes through them. When the cardiac muscle of the left ventricle contracts, it pumps blood from the ventricle into the aorta. This muscular contraction phase is called **systole**. When the muscle of the ventricle relaxes, the ventricle fills with blood. This phase is called **diastole**. The pulsed, forceful ejection of blood from the left ventricle of the heart into the aorta is transmitted through the arteries as a pulsatile pressure wave. This pressure wave keeps the blood moving through the body. The high and low points of the wave can be measured with a sphygmomanometer (blood pressure cuff) and are expressed numerically

in millimeters of mercury (mm Hg). The high point is called the **systolic blood pressure** (measured as the heart muscle is contracting). The low point is called the **diastolic blood pressure** (measured when the heart muscle is in its relaxation phase).

The average adult has approximately 6 L of blood in the vascular system. Children have less, 2 to 3 L, depending on their age and size. Infants have only about 300 mL. The loss of an amount of blood that may be negligible for an adult could be fatal for an infant.

NORMAL CIRCULATION IN ADULTS. In all healthy people, the circulatory system is automatically adjusted and readjusted constantly so that 100% of the capacity of the arteries, veins, and capillaries holds 100% of the blood at that moment. Never are all the vessels fully dilated or constricted. The size of arteries and veins is controlled by the nervous system, according to the amount of blood that is available and many other factors to keep blood pressure normal at all times. Under the condition of normal pressure, with a system that can hold just 100% of the blood available, all parts of the system will have adequate blood supply all of the time.

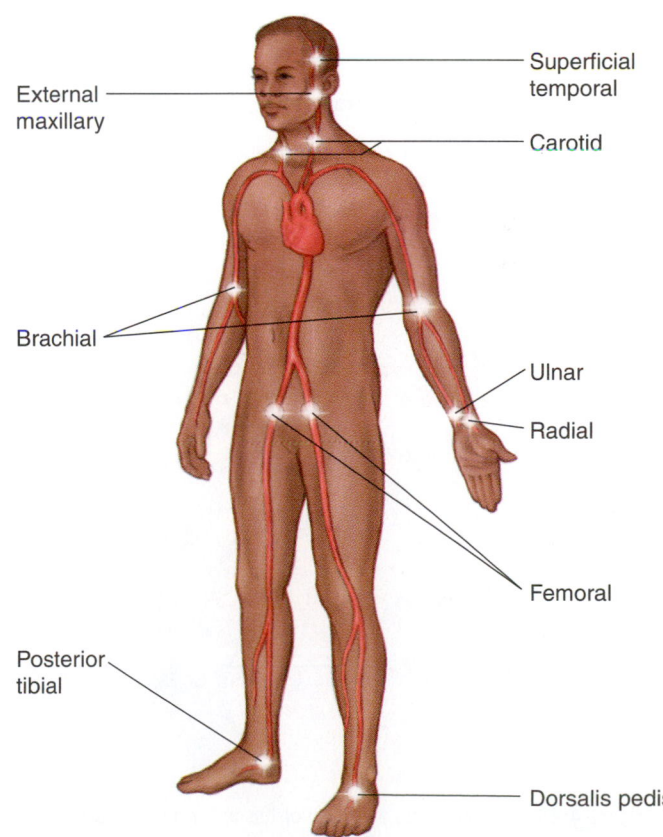

Figure 4-42 The central and peripheral pulses can be felt where the large arteries are near the skin.

Perfusion is the circulation of blood within an organ or tissue in adequate amounts to meet the cells' current needs. Blood enters an organ or tissue through the arteries and leaves it through the veins (▼ Figure 4-43). Loss of normal blood pressure is an indication that the blood is no longer circulating efficiently to every organ in the body. There are many reasons for loss of blood pressure. The result in each case is the same: organs, tissues, and cells are no longer adequately perfused or supplied with oxygen and food, and wastes can accumulate. Under these conditions, cells, tissues, and whole organs may die. The state of inadequate circulation, when it involves the entire body, is called shock or hypoperfusion.

INADEQUATE CIRCULATION IN ADULTS. When a patient loses a small amount of blood, the arteries, veins, and heart automatically adjust to the smaller new volume. The adjustment occurs in an effort to maintain adequate pressure throughout the circulatory system and thereby maintain circulation for every organ. The adjustment occurs very rapidly after the loss, usually within minutes. Specifically, the vessels constrict to

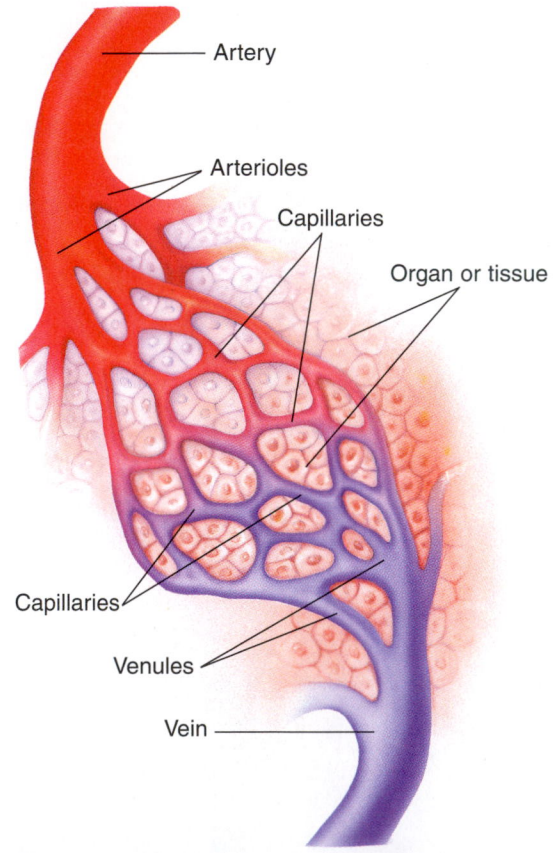

Artery

Arterioles

Capillaries

Organ or tissue

Capillaries

Venules

Vein

Figure 4-43 Blood enters an organ or tissue through the arteries and leaves through the veins. This process, called perfusion, provides adequate blood flow to the tissues to meet the cells' needs.

provide a smaller bed for the reduced volume of blood to fill. And the heart pumps more rapidly to circulate the remaining blood more efficiently. As the blood pressure falls, the pulse increases to attempt to keep the cardiac output constant at 5 to 6 L per minute. If the loss of blood is too great, the adjustment fails, and the patient goes into shock.

The Nervous System

The **nervous system** controls virtually all activities of the body, both voluntary and involuntary. The **somatic nervous system** is the part of the nervous system that regulates activities over which there is voluntary control. Such activities include walking, talking, and writing. The **autonomic nervous system** controls the many involuntary body functions, which occur without voluntary control. These activities include body functions such as digestion, dilation and constriction of blood vessels, sweating, and all other involuntary actions that are necessary for basic body functions. Anatomically, the nervous system is divided into two parts: the central nervous system and the peripheral nervous system. Thus, the nervous system as a whole can be divided anatomically into the central and peripheral nervous systems, and functionally into somatic (voluntary) and autonomic (involuntary) components.

The Central Nervous System

The **central nervous system** is made up of the brain and the spinal cord. From a practical point of view, the central nervous system can be considered the part of the nervous system that is covered and protected by bones. The brain is covered by the skull, and the spinal cord is covered by the spinal column. The major parts of most nerve cells (the nucleus and the cell body) lie within the central nervous system.

BRAIN. The **brain** is the controlling organ of the body. It is the center of consciousness. It is responsible for all our voluntary body activities, the perception of our surroundings, and the control of our reactions to the environment. In addition, the brain enables us to experience all the fine shadings of thought and feeling that make us individuals. The brain is subdivided into several areas, all of which have specific functions. Three major subdivisions of the brain are the cerebrum, the cerebellum, and the brain stem (▶ Figure 4-44).

The **cerebrum**, which is the largest part of the brain and is sometimes called the "gray matter," makes up

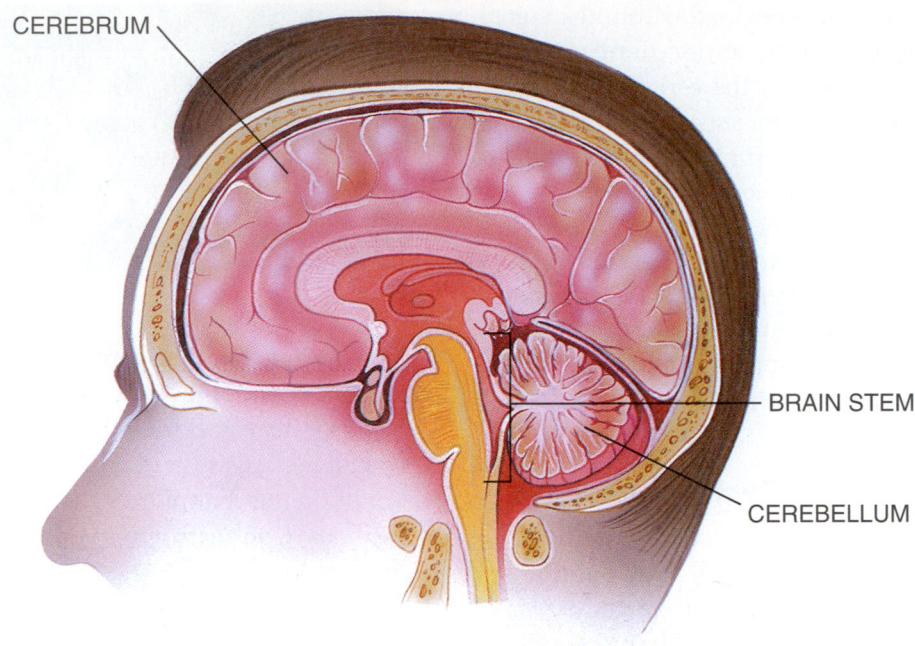

CEREBRUM

BRAIN STEM

CEREBELLUM

Figure 4-44 The brain lies well protected within the skull. Its principal subdivisions are the cerebrum, the cerebellum, and the brain stem.

about three fourths of the volume of the brain. It is divided into the left and right cerebral hemispheres. Each hemisphere is composed of four lobes: frontal, parietal, temporal, and occipital. The cerebrum on one side of the brain controls activities on the opposite side of the body. Each lobe of the cerebrum is responsible for a specific function. For example, one group of brain cells in the frontal lobe is responsible for the activity of all the voluntary muscles of the body. Brain cells in this area generate impulses that are sent along nerve fibers that extend from each cell into the spinal cord. Another area in the parietal lobe has cells that receive sensory impulses from the peripheral nerves of the body. Other parts of the cerebrum are responsible for other body functions. For instance, the occipital region, on the back of the cerebrum, receives visual impulses for the eyes; other areas control hearing, balance, and speech. Still other parts of the cerebrum are responsible for emotions and other characteristics of an individual's personality.

The **cerebellum**, which is located underneath the great mass of cerebral tissue, is sometimes called the "little brain." The major function of this area is to coordinate the various activities of the brain, particularly body movements. Without the cerebellum, very specialized muscular activities such as writing or sewing would be impossible.

The **brain stem** is so called because the brain appears to be sitting on this portion of the central nervous system as a plant sits on its stem. The brain stem is the most primitive part of the central nervous system. It lies deep within the cranium and is the best-protected part of the central nervous system. The brain stem is the controlling center for virtually all body functions that are absolutely necessary for life. Cells in this part of the brain control cardiac, respiratory, and other basic body functions.

The brain has many other anatomic areas, all of which have specific and important functions. The brain receives a vast amount of information from the environment, sorts it all out, and directs the body to respond appropriately. Many of the responses involve voluntary muscle action; others are automatic and involuntary.

SPINAL CORD. The spinal cord is the other major portion of the central nervous system ▶ Figure 4-45. Like the brain, the spinal cord contains nerve cell bodies, but the major portion of the spinal cord is made up of nerve fibers that extend from the cells of the brain. These nerve fibers transmit information to and from the brain. All the fibers join together just below the brain stem to form the spinal cord. The spinal cord exits through a large opening at the base of the skull called the foramen magnum. It is encased within the spinal canal down to the level of the second lumbar vertebra. The spinal canal is created by the vertebrae, stacked one on another. Each vertebra surrounds the cord, and together the vertebrae form the bony spinal canal.

The principal function of the spinal cord is to transmit messages between the brain and the body. These messages are passed along the nerve fibers as electrical impulses, just as messages are passed along a telephone cable. The nerve fibers are arranged in specific bundles within the spinal cord to carry the messages from one specific area of the body to the brain and back.

The Peripheral Nervous System

Many of the cells in the central nervous system have long fibers that extend from the cell body out through openings in the bony covering of the spinal canal to form a cable of nerve fibers that link the central nervous system to the various organs of the body. These cables of nerve fibers make up the **peripheral**

> The basic unit of all living matter is the cell. Individual cells join to form tissues, tissues join to form organs, and organs join to form organ systems.

nervous system. The three major types of nerves are sensory nerves, motor nerves, and connecting nerves. **Sensory nerves** carry information from the body to the central nervous system. **Motor nerves** carry information from the central nervous system to the muscles of the body. **Connecting nerves** do just what their name implies: they connect the sensory and motor nerves.

The peripheral nervous system is composed of 31 pairs of peripheral nerves called spinal nerves and 12 pairs called cranial nerves. At each vertebral level from the first cervical to the fifth sacral, on each side of the spinal cord, a spinal nerve exits the spinal cord and passes through an opening in the bony canal. This spinal nerve is composed of nerve fibers from nerve cells that originate within the spinal cord. The nerve fibers conduct sensory impulses from the skin and other organs to the spinal cord. They also conduct motor impulses from the spinal cord to the muscles that are present in that segment of the body. For example, between the seventh and eighth ribs, the spinal nerve carries sensory fibers from the skin between those two ribs and also has motor nerve fibers to innervate the intercostal muscle between the seventh and eighth ribs. This specific arrangement of nerve fibers becomes more complex and confusing in both the cervical and lumbar regions because of the large number of muscles in the arms and legs that must be supplied with nerve fibers. The spinal nerves combine to form a complex nerve network (called a plexus) in these two areas: the brachial plexus for the upper extremity and the lumbosacral plexus for the lower extremity.

The 12 pairs of peripheral nerves that exit the brain through holes in the skull are called the **cranial nerves**. For the most part, they are very specialized nerves that provide specific functions. For example, the facial (seventh cranial) nerves send motor impulses to many of the facial muscles.

SENSORY NERVES. Sensory nerves of the body are quite complex. There are many different types of sensory cells

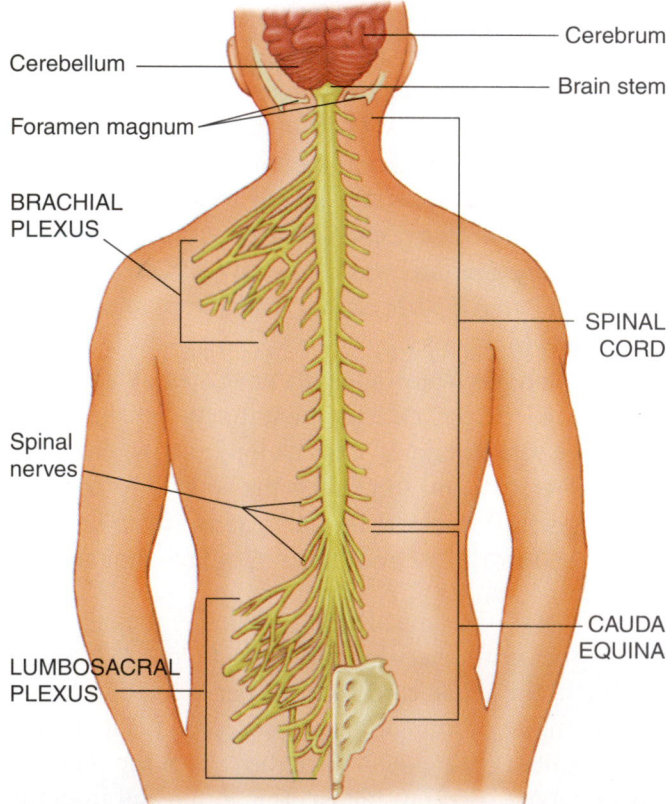

Cerebellum

Foramen magnum

BRACHIAL
PLEXUS

Spinal
nerves

LUMBOSACRAL
PLEXUS

Cerebrum

Brain stem

SPINAL
CORD

CAUDA
EQUINA

Figure 4-45   The spinal cord is a continuation of the brain stem. It exits the skull at the foramen magnum and extends down to the level of the second lumbar vertebra.

in the nervous system. One type forms the retina of the eye; others are responsible for the hearing and balancing mechanisms in the ear. Other sensory cells are located within the skin, muscles, joints, lungs, and other organs of the body. When a sensory cell is stimulated, it transmits its own special message to the brain. There are special sensory nerves to detect heat, cold, position, motion, pressure, pain, balance, light, taste, and smell, as well as other sensations. Specialized nerve endings are adapted for each cell so that it perceives only one type of sensation and it transmits only that message.

The sensory impulses constantly provide information to the brain about what the different parts of our body are doing in relation to our surroundings. Thus, the brain is continuously made aware of its surroundings. The cranial nerves supply sensations directly to the brain. Visual sensations (what we see) reach the brain directly by way of the optic nerve (the second cranial nerve) in each eye. The nerve endings for the optic nerve lie in the retina of the eye. The nerve endings are stimulated by light, and the impulses are carried along the nerve that passes through a hole in the back of the eye socket and carries impulses to the occipital portion of the brain.

When sensory nerve endings in the extremities are stimulated, the impulses are transmitted along a peripheral nerve to the spinal cord. The cell body of the peripheral nerve lies in the spinal cord. The impulse is then transmitted from that cell body to another nerve ending in the spinal cord. The impulse is then sent up the spinal cord to the sensory area in the parietal lobe of the brain, where the sensory information can be interpreted and acted on by the brain.

MOTOR NERVES. Each muscle in the body has its own motor nerve. The cell body for each motor nerve lies in the spinal cord, and a fiber from the cell body extends as part of the peripheral nerve to its specific muscle. Electrical impulses that are produced by the cell body in the spinal cord are transmitted along the motor nerve to the muscle and cause it to contract. The cell body in the spinal cord is stimulated by an impulse produced in the motor strip of the cerebral cortex. This impulse is transmitted along the spinal cord to the cell body of the motor nerve.

CONNECTING NERVES. Within the brain and the spinal cord are cells with short fibers that connect the sensory nerves with the motor nerves. In the spinal cord, they connect the sensory and motor nerves directly,

bypassing the brain. These connecting nerves allow sensory and motor impulses to be transmitted from one nerve to another within the central nervous system.

The connecting nerves in the spinal cord complete a reflex arc between the sensory and motor nerves of the limbs. An irritating stimulus to the sensory nerve, such as heat, will be transmitted from the sensory nerve along the connecting nerve directly to the motor nerve. This will stimulate the sensory nerve. The muscle responds promptly, withdrawing the limb from the irritating stimulus even before this information can be transmitted to the brain. When a physician taps your knee with a rubber hammer, he or she is testing to see whether your reflex arc is intact.

The Skin

The **skin**, the largest single organ in the body, serves three major functions: to protect the body in the environment, to regulate the temperature of the body, and to transmit information from the environment to the brain.

The protective functions of the skin are numerous. Over 70% of the body is composed of water. The water contains a delicate balance of chemical substances in solution. The skin is watertight and serves to keep this balanced internal solution intact. The skin also protects the body from the invasion of infectious organisms: bacteria, viruses, and fungi. These organisms are everywhere and are routinely found lying on the skin surface and deep in its grooves and glands. However, they never penetrate the skin unless it is broken by injury; thus, the skin provides a constant protection against outside invaders.

The energy of the body is derived from **metabolism** (chemical reactions) that must take place within a very narrow temperature range. If the body temperature is too low, these reactions cannot proceed, metabolism ceases, and the body dies. If the temperature becomes too high, the rate of metabolism increases. Dangerously high temperatures producing too high a metabolic rate can result in permanent tissue damage and death.

Functions of the Skin

The major organ for regulation of body temperature is the skin. Blood vessels in the skin constrict when the body is in a cold environment and dilate when the body is in a warm environment. In a cold environment, constriction of the blood vessels shunts the blood away from the skin to decrease the amount of heat radiated from the body surface. When the outside environment is hot, the vessels in the skin dilate, the skin becomes flushed or red, and heat radiates from the body surface.

Also, in the hot environment, sweat is secreted to the skin surface from the sweat glands. Evaporation of the sweat requires energy. This energy, as body heat, is taken from the body during the evaporation process, which causes the body temperature to fall. Sweating alone will not reduce body temperature; evaporation of the sweat must also occur.

Information from the environment is carried to the brain through a rich supply of sensory nerves that originate in the skin. Nerve endings that lie in the skin are adapted to perceive and transmit information about heat, cold, external pressure, pain, and the position of the body in space. The skin thus recognizes any changes in the environment. The skin also reacts to pressure, pain, and pleasurable stimuli.

Anatomy of the Skin

The skin is divided into two parts: the superficial epidermis, which is composed of several layers of cells, and the deeper dermis, which contains the specialized skin structures. Below the skin lies the subcutaneous tissue layer (▼ **Figure 4-46**). The cells of the epidermis are sealed to form a watertight protective covering for the body.

The **epidermis** is actually composed of several layers of cells. At the base of the epidermis is the germinal layer, which continuously produces new cells that gradually rise to the surface. On the way to the surface, these cells die and form the watertight covering. The epidermal cells are held together securely by an oily substance called sebum, which is secreted by the **sebaceous glands** of the dermis. The outermost cells of the epidermis are constantly rubbed away and then replaced by new cells produced by the germinal

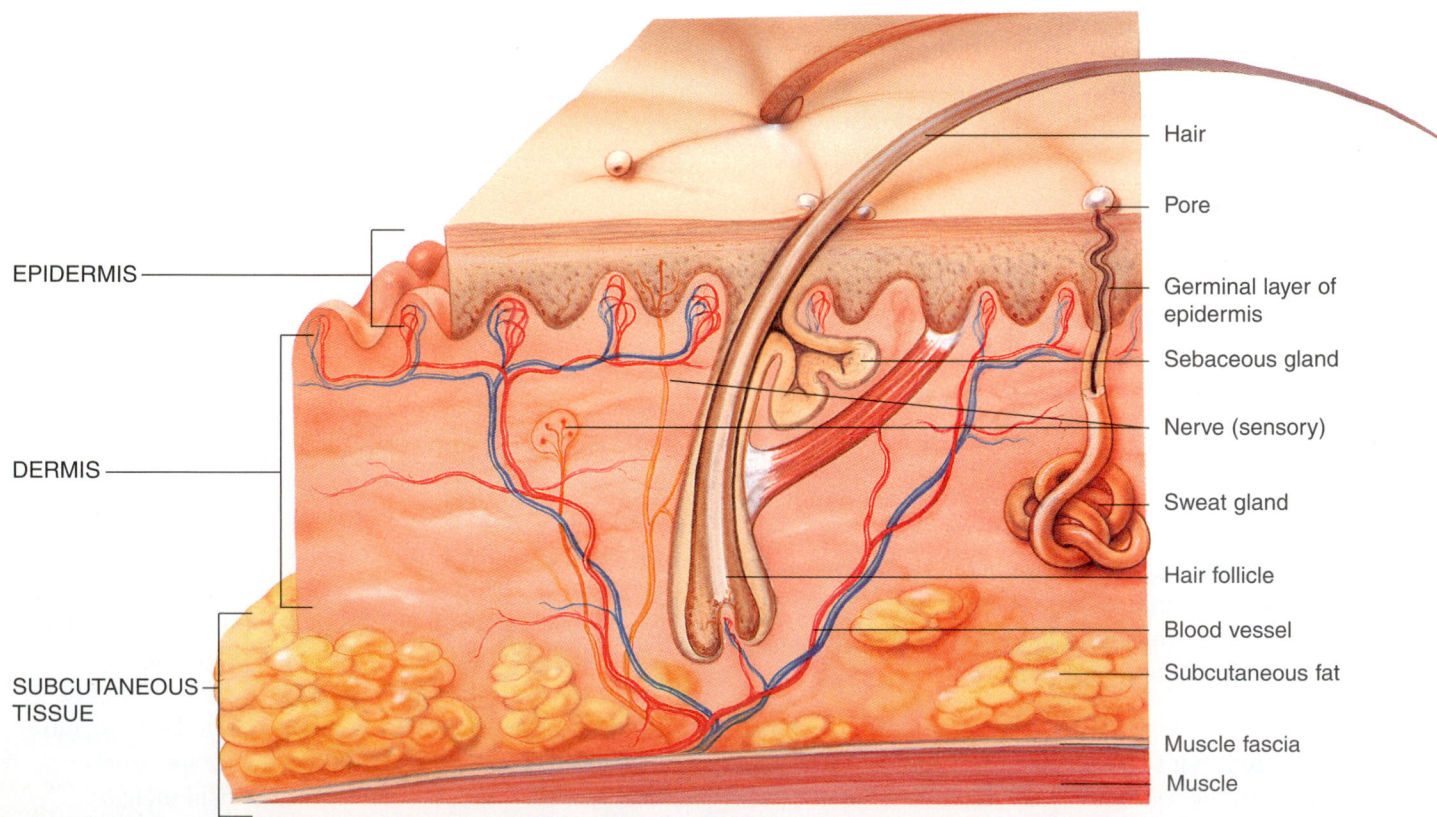

EPIDERMIS

DERMIS

SUBCUTANEOUS TISSUE

Hair
Pore
Germinal layer of epidermis
Sebaceous gland
Nerve (sensory)
Sweat gland
Hair follicle
Blood vessel
Subcutaneous fat
Muscle fascia
Muscle

Figure 4-46 The skin has two principal layers: the epidermis and the dermis. Below the skin is a layer of subcutaneous tissue.

layer. The deeper cells in the germinal layer also contain pigment granules that (along with the blood vessels lying in the dermis) produce skin color.

The epidermis varies in thickness in different areas of the body. On the soles of the feet, the back, and the scalp, it is quite thick, but in some areas of the body, the epidermis is only two or three cell layers thick. The watertight seal provided by the epidermis prevents the invasion of bacteria and other organisms.

The deeper part of the skin, the **dermis**, is separated from the epidermis by the layer of germinal cells. Within the dermis lie many of the special structures of the skin: sweat glands, sebaceous (oil) glands, hair follicles, blood vessels, and specialized nerve endings.

Sweat glands produce sweat for cooling the body. The sweat is discharged onto the surface of the skin through small pores, or ducts, that pass through the epidermis onto the skin surface. The sebaceous glands produce sebum, the oily material that seals the surface epidermal cells. The sebaceous glands lie next to hair follicles and secrete sebum along the hair follicle to the skin surface. In addition to providing waterproofing for the skin, sebum keeps the skin supple so that it does not crack.

Hair follicles are the small organs that produce hair. There is one follicle for each hair connected with a sebaceous gland and also with a tiny muscle. The muscle pulls the hair into an erect position when the individual is cold or frightened. All hair grows continuously and is either cut off or worn away by clothing.

Blood vessels provide nutrients and oxygen to the skin. The blood vessels lie in the dermis. Small branches extend up to the germinal layer. There are no blood vessels in the epidermis. A complex array of nerve endings also lie in the dermis. These specialized nerve endings are sensitive to environmental stimuli; they respond to these stimuli and send impulses along the nerves to the brain.

Beneath the skin, immediately under the dermis and attached to it, lies the **subcutaneous tissue**. The subcutaneous tissue is composed largely of fat. The fat serves as an insulator for the body and as a reservoir to store energy. The amount of subcutaneous tissue varies greatly from individual to individual. Beneath the subcutaneous tissue lie the muscles and the skeleton.

The skin covers all of the external surface of the body. The various orifices (openings to the body)—including the mouth, nose, anus, and vagina—are not covered by skin. Orifices are lined with mucous membranes.

Mucous membranes are quite similar to skin in that they provide a protective barrier against bacterial invasion. Mucous membranes differ from skin in that they secrete **mucus**, a watery substance that lubricates the openings. Thus, mucous membranes are moist, whereas the skin is dry. A mucous membrane lines the entire gastrointestinal tract from the mouth to the anus.

The Endocrine System

The brain controls the body through both the nervous system and the endocrine system. The **endocrine system** is a complex message and control system that integrates many body functions. It releases substances called hormones, either by target organs or into the bloodstream (▼ **Figure 4-47**). Adrenaline and insulin are examples of hormones. Each endocrine gland produces one or more hormones. Each hormone has a specific effect on some organ, tissue, or process (▶ **Table 4-5**). The brain controls the release of hormones by the endocrine glands with other (stimulating or inhibiting) hormones. The final effect influences the endocrine glands and the brain. As a result, we have a tightly controlled system with primary and secondary feedback

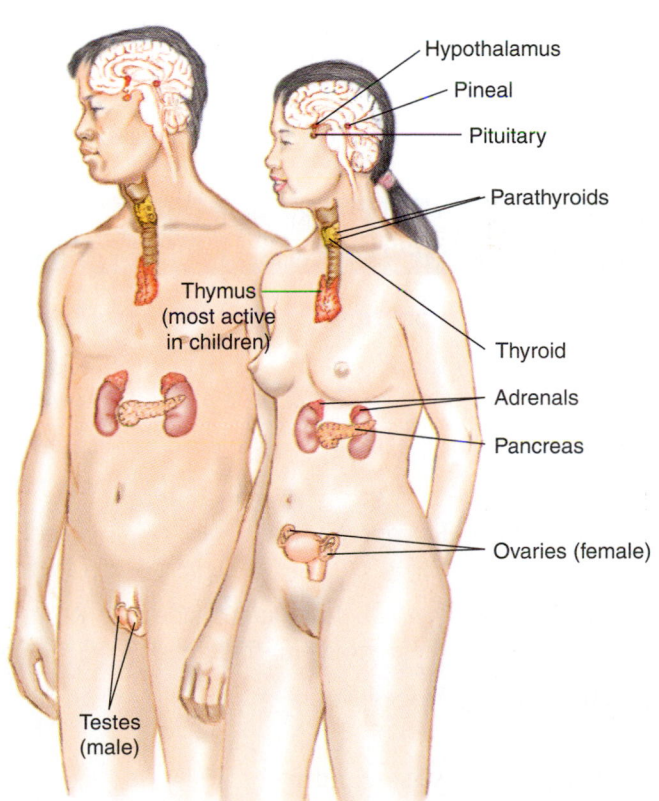

Figure 4-47 The endocrine system controls the release of hormones in the body.

loops to keep body systems in balance ▶ Figure 4-48 . For example, when we are frightened, the brain stimulates the adrenal gland through a hormone to release adrenaline (epinephrine). Release of adrenaline increases our blood pressure and heart rate. The resulting increase in blood pressure and heart rate decreases the amount of hormone released by the adrenal gland. The brain then reduces the amount of stimulation to the adrenal gland. Thus, a new steady state is achieved at heightened levels of alertness. Insulin is another hormone that is intimately involved in the control of the blood glucose and metabolism of food.

Excesses or deficiencies in hormones cause various diseases. With endocrine diseases, specific body functions are increased, decreased, or absent. Diabetes mellitus is a common problem. Because production of the hormone insulin is deficient, the body is unable to use glucose normally. This disease also damages the small blood vessels in the body. The tissue damage that results is as much a part of diabetes as is the difficulty in regulating the amount of glucose in the blood.

The Digestive System

The digestive system is composed of the gastrointestinal tract (stomach and intestines), mouth, salivary glands, pharynx, esophagus, liver, gallbladder, pancreas, rectum, and anus. The function of this system is **digestion**:

the processing of food that nourishes the individual cells of the body.

How Digestion Works

Digestion of food, from the time it is taken into the mouth until essential compounds are extracted and delivered by the circulatory system to nourish all of the cells in the body, is a complicated chemical process. In succession, different secretions, primarily enzymes, are added to the food by the salivary glands, the stomach, the liver, the pancreas, and the small intestine to convert the food into basic sugars, fatty acids, and amino acids. These basic products of digestion are carried across the wall of the intestine and transported through the portal vein to the liver. In the liver, the products are processed further and then stored or transported to the heart through veins draining the liver. The heart then pumps the blood with these nutrients throughout the arteries and then to the capillaries, where the nutrients pass through the capillary walls to nourish the body's individual cells.

In normal routine activity, without any food or fluid ingestion at all, between 8 to 10 L of fluid are secreted daily into the gastrointestinal tract. This fluid comes from the salivary glands, stomach, liver, pancreas, and small intestine. In a normal adult, about 7% of the body weight is delivered as fluid daily to the gastrointestinal tract. If significant vomiting or diarrhea occurs for more

TABLE 4-5 Endocrine Glands

Gland	Location	Function	Hormones Produced
Adrenal	Kidneys	Regulate salt, sugar, and sexual function	Adrenaline (epinephrine) and others
Ovary	Female pelvis (2 glands)	Regulate sexual function, characteristics, and reproduction	Estrogen and others
Pancreas	Retroperitoneal space	Regulate glucose metabolism and other functions	Insulin and others
Parathyroid	Neck (behind and beside the thyroid) (3–5 glands)	Regulate serum calcium	Parathyroid hormone
Pituitary	Base of skull	Regulate all other endocrine glands	Multiple, very important hormones
Testes	Male scrotum (2 glands)	Regulate sexual function, characteristics, and reproduction	Testosterone and others
Thyroid	Neck (over the larynx)	Regulate metabolism	Thyroxine and others

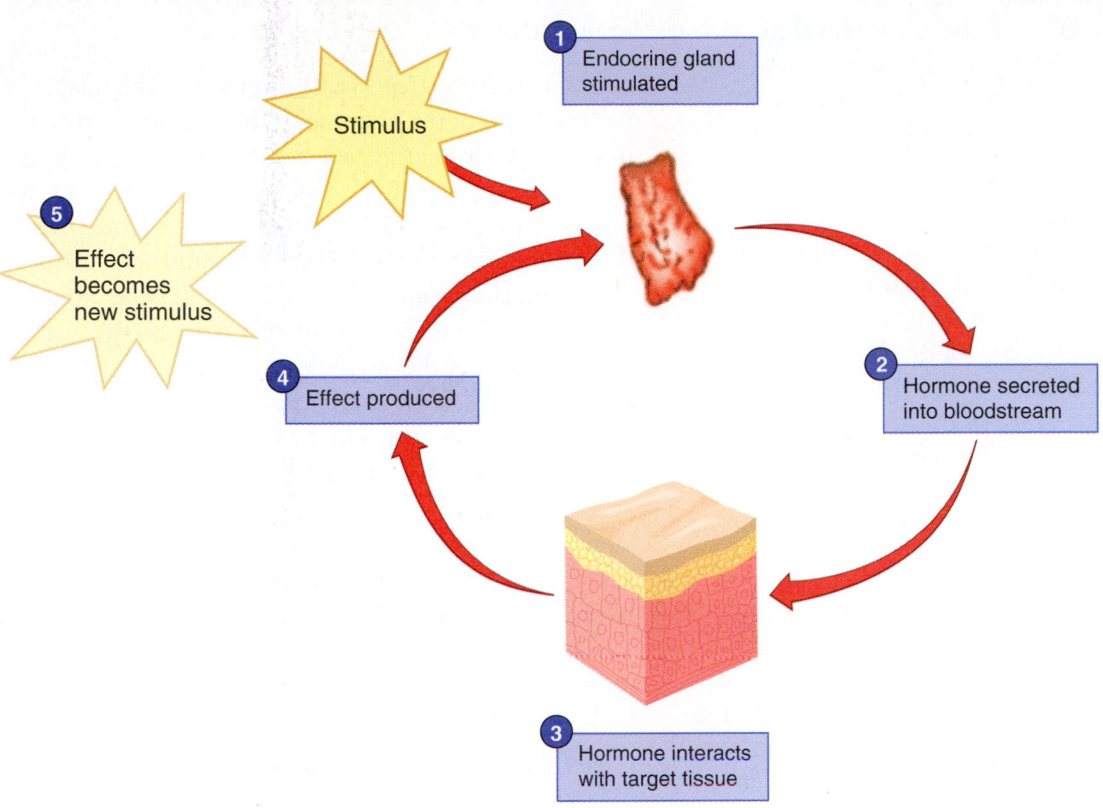

Figure 4-48 The endocrine system is tightly controlled with primary and secondary feedback loops to keep body systems in balance.

than 2 or 3 days, the patient will lose a very substantial portion of body composition and become severely ill.

Anatomy of the Digestive System

MOUTH. The mouth consists of the lips, cheeks, gums, teeth, and tongue. A mucous membrane lines the mouth. The roof of the mouth is formed by the hard and soft palates. The hard palate is a bony plate lying anteriorly; the soft palate is a fold of mucous membrane and muscle that extends posteriorly from the hard palate into the throat. The soft palate is designed to hold food that is being chewed within the mouth and to help initiate swallowing.

SALIVARY GLANDS. There are two **salivary glands** located under the tongue, one on each side of the lower jaw, and one inside each cheek. They produce nearly 1.5 L of saliva daily. Saliva is approximately 98% water. The remaining 2% is composed of mucus, salts, and organic compounds. Saliva serves as a binder for the chewed food that is being swallowed and as a lubricant within the mouth.

OROPHARYNX. The oropharynx is a tubular structure about 5" long that extends vertically from the back of the mouth to the esophagus and trachea. An automatic movement of the pharynx during swallowing lifts the larynx to permit the epiglottis to close over it so that liquids and solids are moved into the esophagus and away from the trachea.

ESOPHAGUS. The **esophagus** is a collapsible tube about 10" long that extends from the end of the pharynx to the stomach and lies just anterior to the spinal column in the chest. Contractions of the muscle in the wall of the esophagus propel food through it to the stomach. Liquids will pass with very little assistance.

STOMACH. The **stomach** is located in the left upper quadrant of the abdominal cavity, largely protected by the lower left ribs. Muscular contractions in the wall of the stomach and gastric juice, which contains much mucus, convert ingested food to a thoroughly mixed semisolid mass. The stomach produces approximately 1.5 L of gastric juice daily for this process. The principal function of the stomach is to receive food in large quantities intermittently, store it, and provide for its movement into the small bowel in regular, small amounts. In 1 to 3 hours, the semisolid food mass derived from one meal is propelled by muscular contraction into the **duodenum**, the first part of the small intestine.

PANCREAS. The **pancreas**, a flat, solid organ, lies below and behind the liver and stomach and behind the peritoneum. It is firmly fixed in position, deep within the abdomen, and is not easily damaged. It contains two kinds of glands. One set of glands secretes nearly 2 L of pancreatic juice daily. This juice contains many enzymes that aid in the digestion of fat, starch, and protein. Pancreatic juice flows directly into the duodenum through the pancreatic ducts. The other gland is the islets of Langerhans, which produces insulin. Insulin regulates the amount of glucose in the blood.

LIVER. The **liver** is a large, solid organ that takes up most of the area immediately beneath the diaphragm in the right upper quadrant. It is the largest solid organ in the abdomen and has several functions. Poisonous substances produced by digestion are brought to the liver and rendered harmless. Factors that are necessary for blood clotting and for the production of normal plasma are formed here. Between 0.5 and 1 L of bile is made by the liver daily to assist in the normal digestion of fat. The liver is the principal organ for the storage of sugar or starch for immediate use by the body for energy. It also produces many of the factors that aid in the proper regulation of immune responses. Anatomically, the liver is a large mass of blood vessels and cells, packed tightly together. It is fragile and, because of its size, relatively easily injured. Blood flow in the liver is high, because all of the blood that is pumped to the gastrointestinal tract passes into the liver, through the portal vein, before it returns to the heart. In addition, the liver has a generous arterial blood supply of its own. Ordinarily, approximately 25% of the cardiac output of blood (1.5 L) passes through the liver each minute.

BILE DUCTS. The liver is connected to the intestine by the **bile ducts**. The **gallbladder** is an outpouching from the bile ducts that serves as a reservoir and concentrating organ for bile produced in the liver. Together, the bile ducts and gallbladder form the biliary system. The gallbladder discharges stored and concentrated bile into the duodenum through the common bile duct. The presence of food in the duodenum triggers a contraction of the gallbladder

to empty it. The gallbladder usually contains about 60 to 90 mL of bile.

SMALL INTESTINE. The **small intestine** is the major hollow organ of the abdomen. The cells lining the small intestine produce enzymes and mucus to aid in digestion. Enzymes from the pancreas and the small intestine carry out the final processes of digestion. More than 90% of the products of digestion (amino acids, fatty acids, and simple sugars), together with water, ingested vitamins, and minerals are absorbed across the wall of the lower end of the small intestine into veins to be transported to the liver. The small intestine is composed of the duodenum, the jejunum, and the ileum. The duodenum, which is about 12″ long, is the part of the small intestine that receives food from the stomach. Here, food is mixed with secretions from the pancreas and liver for further digestion. Bile, produced by the liver and stored in the gallbladder, is emptied as needed into the duodenum. It is greenish black, but through changes during digestion, it gives feces its typical brown color. Its major function is in the digestion of fat. The jejunum and ileum together measure more than 20′ on average to make up the rest of the small intestine.

LARGE INTESTINE. The **large intestine**, another major hollow organ, consists of the cecum, the colon, and the rectum. About 5′ long, it encircles the outer border of the abdomen around the small bowel. The major function of the colon, the portion of the large intestine that extends from the cecum to the rectum, is to absorb the final 5% to 10% of digested food and water from the intestine to form solid stool, which is stored in the rectum and passed out of the body through the anus.

APPENDIX. The appendix is a tube 3″ to 4″ long that opens into the cecum (the first part of the large intestine) in the right lower quadrant of the abdomen. It may easily become obstructed and, as a result, inflamed and infected. Appendicitis, which is the term for this inflammation, is one of the major causes of severe abdominal distress. The appendix has no known function.

RECTUM. The lowermost end of the colon is the **rectum**. It is a large, hollow organ that is adapted to store quantities of feces until they are expelled. At its terminal end is the **anus**, a 2″ canal lined with skin. The rectum and anus are supplied with a complex series of circular muscles called sphincters that control, both voluntarily and automatically, the escape of liquids, gases, and solids from the digestive tract.

The Urinary System

The <u>urinary system</u> controls the discharge of certain waste materials filtered from the blood by the kidneys. In the urinary system, the kidneys are solid organs; the ureters, bladder, and urethra are hollow organs (▼ Figure 4-49). Ordinarily, we consider the urinary and genital systems together, because they share many organs.

The body has two <u>kidneys</u> that lie on the posterior muscular wall of the abdomen behind the peritoneum in the retroperitoneal space. These organs rid the blood of toxic waste products and control its balance of water and salt. Blood flow in the kidneys is high. Nearly 20% of the output of blood from the heart passes through the kidneys each minute. Large vessels attach the kidneys directly to the aorta and the inferior vena cava. Waste products and water are constantly

> **Develop the habit of always thinking of how peculiarities of human anatomy and physiology and mechanisms of injury can help predict the locations and types of injuries.**

filtered from the blood to form urine. The kidneys continuously concentrate this filtered urine by reabsorbing the water as it passes through a system of specialized tubes within them. The tubes finally unite to form the <u>renal pelvis</u>, a cone-shaped collecting area that connects the ureter and the kidney. Normally, each kidney drains its urine into one ureter through which the urine passes to the bladder.

A <u>ureter</u> passes from the renal pelvis of each kidney along the surface of the posterior abdominal wall behind the peritoneum to drain into the urinary bladder. The ureters are small (0.2″ in diameter), hollow, muscular tubes. <u>Peristalsis</u>, a wave-like contraction of smooth muscle, occurs in these tubes to move the urine to the bladder.

The <u>urinary bladder</u> is located immediately behind the pubic symphysis in the pelvic cavity and is composed of smooth muscle with a specialized lining membrane. The two ureters enter posteriorly at its base on either side. The bladder empties to the outside of the body through the <u>urethra</u>. In the male, the urethra passes from the anterior base of the bladder through the penis. In the female, the urethra opens just above the opening of the vagina. The normal adult forms 1.5 to 2 L of urine every day. This waste is extracted and concentrated from the 1,500 L of blood that circulate through the kidneys daily.

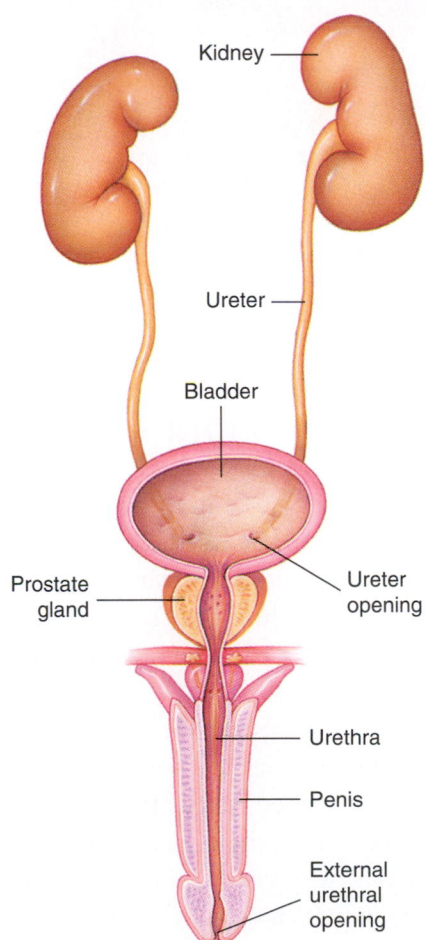

Kidney

Ureter

Bladder

Prostate gland

Ureter opening

Urethra

Penis

External urethral opening

(Figure 4-49) The urinary system lies in the retroperitoneal space behind the organs of the digestive system. The urinary system in males and females includes the kidneys, ureters, urinary bladder, and urethra. This diagram shows the male urinary system.

The Genital System

The <u>genital system</u> controls the reproductive processes by which life is created. The male genitalia, except for the prostate gland and the seminal vesicles, lie outside the pelvic cavity. The female genitalia are contained entirely within the pelvis. The male and female reproductive organs have certain similarities and, of course, basic differences. They allow the production of sperm and egg cells and appropriate hormones and the act of sexual intercourse and reproduction.

FRONT VIEW

SIDE VIEW

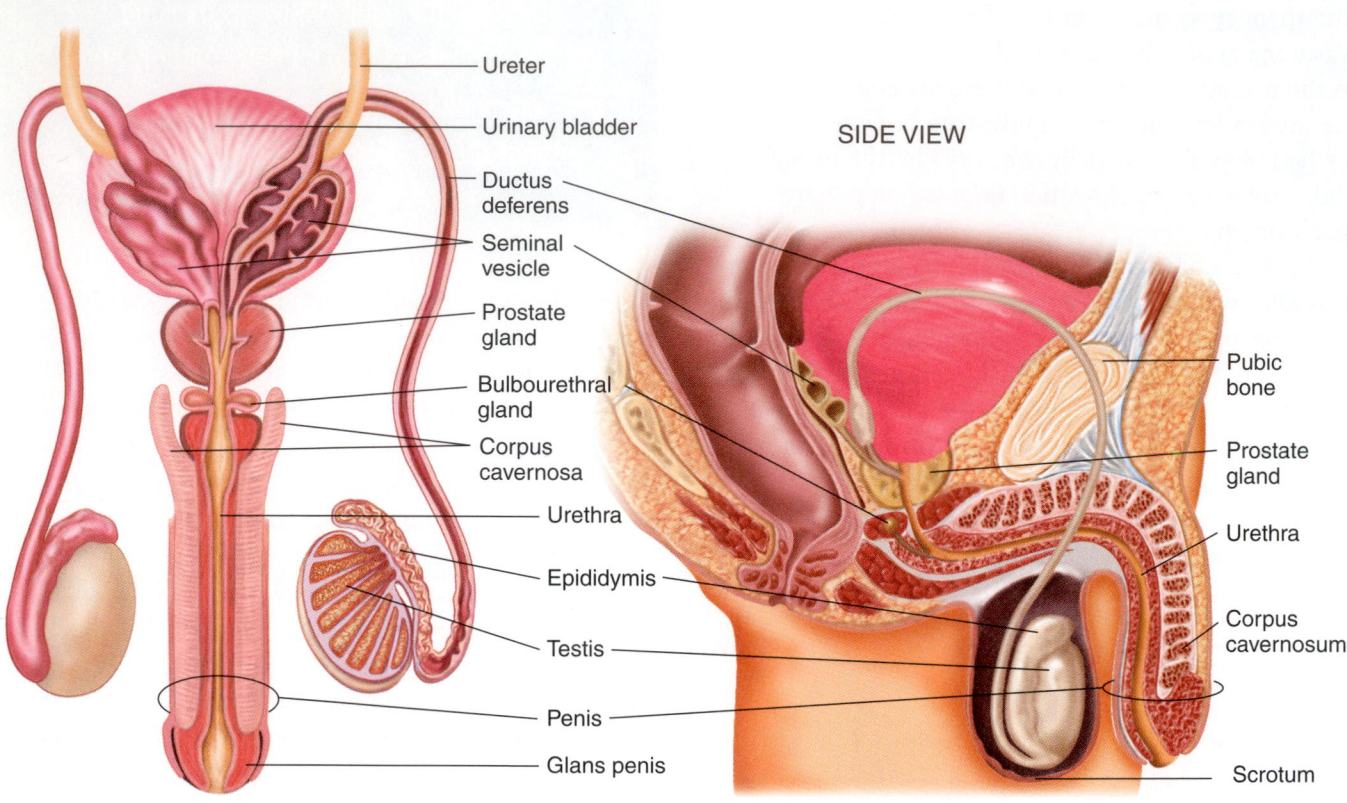

- Ureter
- Urinary bladder
- Ductus deferens
- Seminal vesicle
- Prostate gland
- Bulbourethral gland
- Corpus cavernosa
- Urethra
- Epididymis
- Testis
- Penis
- Glans penis

- Pubic bone
- Prostate gland
- Urethra
- Corpus cavernosum
- Scrotum

Figure 4-50   The male reproductive system consists of the testicles, vasa deferentia, seminal vesicles, prostate gland, urethra, and penis.

The Male Reproductive System and Organs

The male reproductive system consists of the testicles, vasa deferentia, seminal vesicles, prostate gland, urethra, and penis (▲ Figure 4-50). Each **testicle** contains specialized cells and ducts; some of these produce male hormones, and others develop sperm. The hormones are absorbed directly into the bloodstream from the testicles. The **vasa deferentia (or vas deferens)** are ducts that travel from the testicles up beneath the skin of the abdominal wall for a short distance. They then pass through an opening into the abdominal cavity and into the prostate gland to connect with the urethra. The vasa deferentia carry the sperm from the testicles to the urethra. The **seminal vesicles** are small storage sacs for sperm and seminal fluid. The vesicles also empty into the urethra, at the prostate.

Semen, also called seminal fluid, contains sperm cells that are carried up each vas from each testicle

to be mixed with fluid from the seminal vesicles and prostate gland. The **prostate gland** surrounds the urethra where it emerges from the urinary bladder. Fluids from the prostate gland and from the seminal vesicles mix during sexual intercourse. During intercourse, special mechanisms in the nervous system prevent the passage of urine into the urethra. Only seminal fluid, prostatic fluid, and sperm pass from the penis into the vagina during ejaculation.

The penis contains a special type of tissue called erectile tissue. This specialized tissue is largely vascular and, when filled with blood, causes the penis to distend into a state of erection. As the vessels fill under pressure from the circulatory system, the penis becomes a large, rigid organ that can enter the vagina. Certain spinal injuries and some diseases can cause a painful continuous erection called **priapism**.

FRONT VIEW   SIDE VIEW

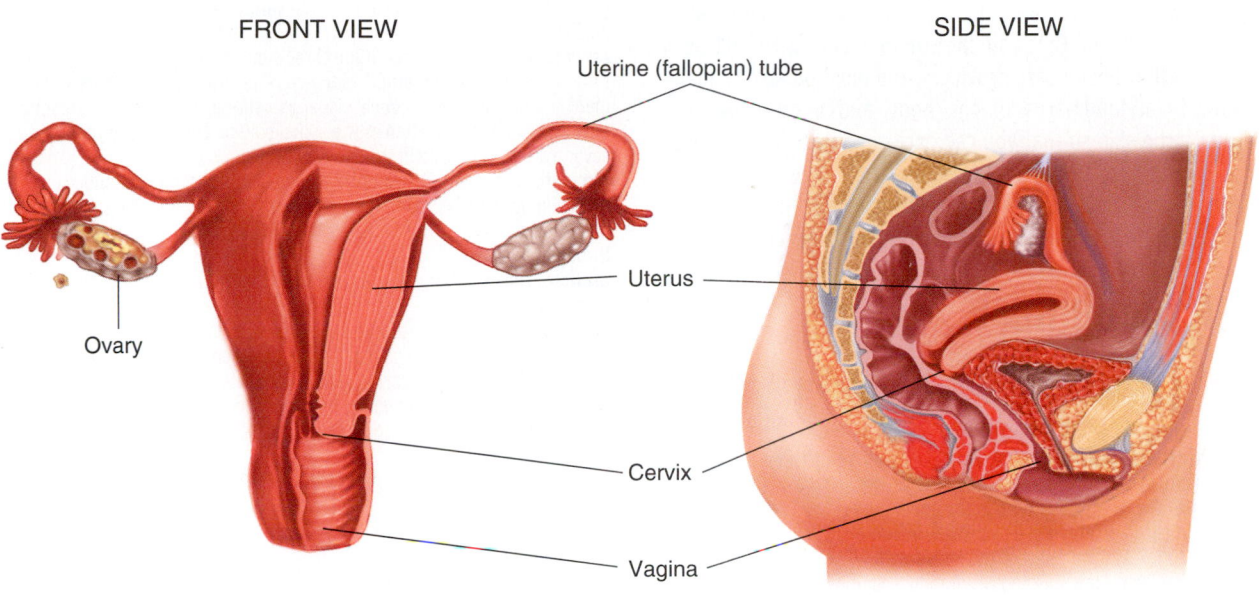

Uterine (fallopian) tube

Uterus

Ovary

Cervix

Vagina

Figure 4-51   The female reproductive system consists of the ovaries, fallopian tubes, uterus, cervix, and vagina.

The Female Reproductive System and Organs

The female reproductive organs include the ovaries, fallopian tubes, uterus, cervix, and vagina (▲ Figure 4-51). The **ovaries**, like the testicles, produce sex hormones and specialized cells for reproduction. The female sex hormones are absorbed directly into the bloodstream. A specialized ovum, or egg cell, is produced regularly during the adult female's reproductive years. The ovaries release a mature egg approximately every 28 days. This egg travels through the fallopian tubes to the uterus.

The **fallopian tubes** connect with the uterus and carry the ovum into the cavity of this organ. The uterus is pear-shaped and hollow, with muscular walls. The narrow opening from the uterus to the vagina is the cervix. The **vagina** (birth canal) is a muscular distensible tube that connects the uterus with the vulva (the external female genitalia). The vagina receives the penis during sexual intercourse, when semen is deposited in it. The sperm in the semen may pass into the uterus and fertilize an egg, causing pregnancy. Should the pregnancy come to completion at the end of 9 months, the baby will pass through the vagina and be born. The vagina also channels the menstrual flow from the uterus out of the body.

Chapter *Sweep*

Ready for Review

To do your work as a rescuer, you must have a working knowledge of human anatomy so that you can communicate with EMS personnel and other health care providers. You must be able to identify superficial landmarks of the body and know what lies underneath the skin so that you can perform an accurate assessment. EMS and hospital personnel will use these terms to ask you questions about a patient; therefore, it is critical for the well-being of your patient that you learn them and can use them correctly.

Vital Vocabulary

abdomen The body cavity that contains the major organs of digestion and excretion.

abduction Motion of a limb away from the midline.

acetabulum The depression on the lateral pelvis where its three component bones join, in which the femoral head fits snugly.

Adam's apple The firm prominence in the upper part of the larynx formed by the thyroid cartilage. It is more prominent in men than in women.

adduction Motion of a limb toward the midline.

agonal respirations Slow, gasping respiration, sometimes seen in dying patients.

alveoli The air sacs of the lungs in which the exchange of oxygen and carbon dioxide takes place.

anatomic position The position of reference in which the patient stands facing you, arms at the side, with the palms of the hands forward.

angle of Louis A ridge on the sternum that lies at the level where the second rib is attached to the sternum; provides a constant and reliable bony landmark on the anterior chest wall.

anterior The front surface of the body; the side facing you in the standard anatomic position.

anterior superior iliac spines The bony prominences of the pelvis (ilium) at the front on each side of the lower abdomen just below the plane of the umbilicus.

anus The terminal end of the rectum.

aorta The principal artery leaving the left side of the heart and carrying freshly oxygenated blood to the body.

apex (plural: apices) The tip or the topmost portion of a structure.

appendix A small tubular structure that is attached to the lower border of the cecum in the right lower quadrant of the abdomen.

arteries Tubular vessels that carry blood away from the heart.

arteriole The smallest branch of an artery leading to the vast network of capillaries.

atrium Upper chamber of the heart.

autonomic nervous system The part of the nervous system that regulates functions, such as digestion and sweating, that are not controlled voluntarily.

ball-and-socket joint Joint that allows rotation as well as bending.

biceps The large muscle that covers the front of the humerus.

bilateral A body part that appears on both sides of the midline.

bile ducts Ducts that convey bile between the liver and the intestine.

blood pressure The pressure that the blood exerts against the walls of the arteries as it passes through them.

brachial artery The major vessel in the upper extremity that supplies blood to the arm.

brain The controlling organ of the body and center of consciousness; functions include perception, control of reactions to the environment, emotional responses, and judgment.

brain stem The area of the brain that lies deep with the cranium and controls functions that are necessary for life, such as respirations.

bronchi The tubular air passages of the lungs.

bronchioles The smallest of the bronchi.

capillary vessels The fine end-divisions of the arterial system that allow contact between cells of the body tissues and the plasma and red blood cells.

carotid artery The major artery that supplies blood to the head and brain.

carpometacarpal joint The joint between the wrist and the metacarpal bones; the thumb joint.

cecum The first part of the large intestine, into which the ileum opens.

central nervous system The brain and spinal cord.

cerebellum One of the three major subdivisions of the brain, sometimes called the "little brain"; coordinates the various activities of the brain, particularly body movements.

cerebrum The largest part of the three subdivisions of the brain, sometimes called the "gray matter"; made up of several lobes that control movement, hearing, balance, speech, visual perception, emotions, and personality.

cervical spine The portion of the spinal column consisting of the first seven vertebrae that lie in the neck.

circulatory system The complex arrangement of connected tubes, including the arteries, arterioles, capillaries, venules, and veins, that moves blood, oxygen, nutrients, carbon dioxide, and cellular waste throughout the body.

clavicle The collarbone; it is lateral to the sternum and medial to the scapula.

coccyx The last four vertebrae of the spine; the tailbone.

connecting nerves Nerves that connect the sensory and motor nerves.

costal arch A bridge of cartilage that connects the ends of the sixth through tenth ribs with the lower portion of the sternum.

costovertebral angle An angle that is formed by the junction of the spine and the tenth rib.

cranial nerves Specialized nerves that arise directly from the brain, and provide specific functions.

cranium The area of the head above the ears and eyes; the skull. The cranium contains the brain.

cricoid cartilage A firm ridge of cartilage that forms the lower part of the larynx.

cricothyroid membrane A thin sheet of fascia that connects the thyroid and cricoid cartilages that make up the larynx.

deep Farther inside the body and away from the skin.

dermis The inner layer of the skin, containing hair follicles, sweat glands, nerve endings, and blood vessels.

diaphragm A muscular dome that forms the undersurface of the thorax, separating the chest from the abdominal cavity. Contraction of the diaphragm (and the chest wall muscles) brings air into the lungs. Relaxation allows air to be expelled from the lungs.

diastole The relaxation, or period of relaxation, of the heart, especially of the ventricles.

diastolic blood pressure The lowest point of the blood pressure curve.

digestion The processing of food that nourishes the individual cells of the body.

distal Structures that are farther from the trunk or nearer to the free end of the extremity.

dorsal The posterior surface of the body, including the back of the hand.

dorsalis pedis artery The artery on the anterior surface of the foot.

duodenum The first part of the small intestine, which connects the stomach to the jejunum.

endocrine system The complex message and control system that integrates many body functions, including the release of hormones.

epidermis The outer layer of skin, which is made up of cells that are sealed together to form a watertight protective covering for the body.

epiglottis A thin, leaf-shaped valve that allows air to pass into the trachea but prevents food or liquid from entering.

esophagus A collapsible tube that extends from the pharynx to the stomach; contractions of the muscle in the wall of the esophagus propel food and liquids through it to the stomach.

exhalation Breathing air out of the lungs.

extend To straighten.

fallopian tube Long, slender tube that extends from the uterus to the region of the ovary on the same side, and through which the ovum passes from ovary to uterus.

fascia A sheet or band of tough fibrous connective tissue; lies deep under the skin and forms an outer layer for the muscles.

femoral artery The principal artery of the thigh that supplies blood to the lower extremities.

femoral head The proximal end of the femur, articulating with the acetabulum to form the hip joint.

femur The thigh bone; the longest and one of the strongest bones in the body.

fibula The lateral of the two bones of the lower leg.

flex To bend.

floating ribs The eleventh and twelfth ribs, which do not attach to the sternum through the costal arch.

foramen magnum A large opening at the base of the skull through which the brain connects to the spinal cord.

Fowler's position The position in which the patient is sitting up or semisitting with the knees bent.

gallbladder A sac on the undersurface of the liver that collects bile from the liver and discharges it into the duodenum through the common bile duct.

genital system The male and female reproductive systems.

greater trochanter A bony prominence on the proximal lateral side of the thigh, just below the hip joint.

hair follicles The small organs in the skin that produce hair.

heart A hollow muscular organ that receives blood from the veins and propels it into the arteries.

heart rate (pulse) The wave of pressure that is created by the heart's contracting and forcing blood out the left ventricle and into the major arteries.

hinge joint A joint that can bend and straighten but cannot rotate; these joints restrict motion to one plane.

humerus The supporting bone of the arm.

hypoxic drive A "backup system" to control respiration; senses drops in the oxygen level in the blood.

iliac crest The rim, or wing, of the pelvic bone.

ilium One of three bones that fuse to form the pelvic ring.

inferior The part of the body, or any body part, nearer to the feet.

inferior vena cava One of the two largest veins in the body; carries blood from the lower extremities and the pelvic and abdominal organs into the heart.

inguinal ligament The tough, fibrous ligament that stretches between the lateral edge of the pubic symphysis and the anterior superior iliac spine.

inhalation Breathing air into the lungs.

intercostal muscles The muscles between the ribs.

involuntary muscle Muscle that continues to contract, rhythmically, regardless of the conscious will of the individual.

ischium One of three bones that fuse to form the pelvic ring.

joint (articulation) The place where two bones come into contact.

joint capsule The fibrous sac with synovial lining that encloses a joint.

kidneys Two retroperitoneal organs that excrete the end products of metabolism as urine and regulate the body's salt and water content.

labored breathing Breathing that is abnormal and associated with obvious patient distress.

large intestine The portion of the digestive tube that encircles the abdomen around the small bowel, consisting of the cecum, the colon, and the rectum.

lateral Parts of the body that lie farther from the midline; also called outer structures.

ligament A band of the fibrous tissue that connects bones to bones. It supports and strengthens a joint.

liver A large solid organ that lies in the right upper quadrant immediately below the diaphragm; it produces bile, stores sugar for immediate use by the body, and produces many substances that help regulate immune responses.

lumbar spine The lower part of the back, formed by the lowest five non-fused vertebrae; also called the dorsal spine.

lumbar vertebrae Vertebrae of the lumbar spine.

mandible The bone of the lower jaw.

manubrium The upper quarter of the sternum.

mastoid process A prominent bony mass at the base of the skull behind the ear.

maxillae The upper jawbones that assist in the formation of the orbit, the nasal cavity, and the palate, and lodge the upper teeth.

medial Parts of the body that lie closer to the midline; also called inner structures.

metabolism Chemical reactions that provide the body's energy; the process by which energy is made available for the uses of the organism.

midaxillary line An imaginary vertical line drawn through the middle of the axilla (armpit), parallel to the midline.

midclavicular line An imaginary vertical line drawn through the middle portion of the clavicle and parallel to the midline.

midline An imaginary vertical line drawn from the middle of the forehead through the nose and the umbilicus (navel) to the floor.

motor nerves Nerves that carry information from the central nervous system to the muscles of the body.

mucous membranes The lining of body cavities and passages that communicate directly or indirectly with the environment outside the body.

mucus A watery substance secreted by the mucous membranes that lubricates the body openings.

musculoskeletal system The bones and voluntary muscles of the body.

myocardium The heart muscle.

nasopharynx The part of the pharynx that lies above the level of the roof of the mouth, or soft palate.

nervous system The system that controls virtually all activities of the body, both voluntary and involuntary.

occiput The most posterior portion of the cranium.

olecranon process The bony projection of the ulna at the elbow to which the triceps muscle tendon is attached.

orbit The eye socket, made up of the maxilla and zygoma.

oropharynx A tubular structure that extends vertically from the back of the mouth to the esophagus and trachea.

ovary A female gland that produces sex hormones and ova (eggs).

palmar The front region of the hand.

pancreas A flat, solid organ that lies below and behind the liver and the stomach; it is a major source of digestive enzymes and produces the hormone insulin.

parietal regions The areas between the temporal and occiput regions of the cranium.

patella The kneecap; a specialized bone that lies within the tendon of the quadriceps muscle.

pelvic cavity The cavity in the lowest part of the trunk. Continuous with the abdominal cavity, it contains the bladder, rectum, and female reproductive organs.

pelvis A cone-shaped bony ring made up of the right and left pelvic bones joined in front at the pubis and in back to the sacrum at the sacroiliac joints. Each pelvic bone is made up of three fused bones: the ilium, ischium, and pubic bones. The pelvis contains the pelvic cavity.

perfusion The circulation of blood within an organ or tissue in adequate amounts to meet the cells' current needs.

peripheral nervous system The part of the nervous system that consists of 31 pairs of spinal nerves and 12 pairs of cranial nerves. These peripheral nerves may be sensory nerves, motor nerves, or connecting nerves.

peristalsis The wave-like contraction of smooth muscle by which the ureters or other tubular organs propel their contents.

pinna The external, visible part of the ear.

plantar The bottom of the foot.

plasma A sticky, yellow fluid that carries the blood cells and nutrients and transports cellular waste material to the organs of excretion.

platelets Tiny, disk-shaped elements that are much smaller than the cells; they are essential in the initial formation of a blood clot.

pleura The serous membrane covering the lungs and lining the thoracic cavity, completely enclosing a potential space known as the pleural space.

pleural space The potential space between the parietal pleura and the visceral pleura. It is described as "potential" because under normal conditions, the lungs fill this space.

posterior The back surface of the body; the side away from you in the standard anatomic position.

posterior tibial artery The artery just posterior to the medial malleolus; it supplies blood to the foot.

priapism A continuous and painful erection of the penis caused by certain spinal injuries and some diseases.

prone position The position in which the body is lying face down.

prostate gland A small gland that surrounds the male urethra where it emerges from the urinary bladder; it secretes a fluid that is part of the ejaculatory fluid.

proximal Structures that are closer to the trunk.

pubic symphysis A hard bony prominence that is found in the midline in the lowermost portion of the abdomen.

pubis One of three bones that fuse to form the pelvic ring.

www.OECzone.com

Chapter *Sweep* Continued.

pulmonary artery The major artery leading from the right ventricle of the heart to the lungs; it carries oxygen-poor blood.

pulmonary circulation The closed circuit of the circulatory system that includes the lungs. Blood is pumped from the right side of the heart through the lungs and back to the left side of the heart.

pulmonary veins The four veins that return oxygenated blood from the lungs to the left atrium of the heart.

pulse The wave of pressure created as the heart contracts and forces blood out the left ventricle and into the major arteries.

quadrants The way to describe the sections of the abdominal cavity. Imagine two lines intersecting at the umbilicus dividing the abdomen into four equal areas.

radial artery The major artery in the forearm; it is palpable at the wrist on the thumb side.

radius The bone on the thumb side of the forearm.

recovery position The preferred body position for an unresponsive patient with no spine injury. The patient lies on his or her side with the opposite knee flexed and the head cushioned on the hand. Also called the semiprone, rescue, stable side, or NATO position.

rectum The lowermost end of the colon.

red blood cells Cells that carry oxygen to the body's tissues; also called erythrocytes.

renal pelvis A cone-shaped collecting area that connects the ureter and the kidney.

respiratory system All the structures of the body that contribute to the process of breathing, consisting of the upper and lower airways and their component parts.

retroperitoneal Behind the abdominal cavity.

rib One of 12 paired, curved bones that form and support the chest wall.

sacrum One of three bones (sacrum and two pelvic bones) that make up the pelvic ring; consists of five fused sacral vertebrae.

salivary glands The glands that produce saliva to keep the mouth and pharynx moist.

scalp The thick skin covering the cranium, which usually bears hair.

scapula The shoulder blade.

sebaceous glands Glands in the dermis that produce an oily substance called sebum, which discharges along the shafts of the hairs.

semen Seminal fluid ejaculated from the penis and containing sperm.

seminal vesicles Storage sacs for sperm and seminal fluid, which empty into the urethra at the prostate.

sensory nerves The nerves that carry sensations of touch, taste, heat, cold, pain, or other modalities from the body to the central nervous system.

shock position The position that has the head and torso (trunk) supine and the lower extremities elevated 6" to 12". This helps to increase blood flow to the brain; also referred to as the *modified Trendelenburg's position*.

shoulder girdle The proximal portion of the upper extremity, made up of the clavicle, the scapula, and the humerus.

skeletal muscle Muscle that is attached to bones and usually crosses at least one joint; striated, or voluntary, muscle.

skeleton The framework that gives us our recognizable human form; also designed to allow motion of the body and protection of vital organs.

skin The outer covering of the body, made up of the outer epidermis and the inner dermis.

small intestine The portion of the digestive tube between the stomach and the cecum, consisting of the duodenum, jejunum, and ileum.

smooth muscle Nonstriated, involuntary muscle; it constitutes the bulk of the gastrointestinal tract and is present in nearly every organ to regulate automatic activity.

somatic nervous system The part of the nervous system that regulates activities over which there is voluntary control.

spinal canal The tunnel in which the spinal cord lies; formed by the successive vertebral arches.

spinal column The bony column, composed of 33 vertebrae, that forms the main support for the body and protects the spinal cord.

spinal cord An extension of the brain, composed of virtually all the nerves carrying messages between the brain and the rest of the body. It lies inside of, and is protected by, the spinal canal.

sternocleidomastoid muscles The muscles on either side of the neck that allow movement of the head.

sternum The breastbone.

stomach The saclike organ between the esophagus and the duodenum where food is mixed with gastric juice to form a semifluid substance that is passed on to the intestines for further digestion.

striated muscle Muscle that has characteristic stripes, or striations, under the microscope; voluntary, or skeletal, muscle.

styloid process A long, pointed process of a bone.

subcutaneous tissue Tissue, largely fat, that lies directly under the dermis and serves as an insulator of the body.

superficial Closer to or on the skin.

superior The part of the body, or any body part, nearer to the head.

superior vena cava One of the two largest veins in the body; carries blood from the upper extremities, head, neck, and chest into the heart.

supine position The position in which the body is lying face up.

sweat glands The glands within the dermis that secrete sweat.

symphysis The joint that is held together with fibrous tissue allowing slight, limited motion.

systole The contraction, or period of contraction, of the heart, especially that of the ventricles.

systolic blood pressure The highest point of the blood pressure curve.

temporal regions The lateral portions on each side of the cranium.

temporomandibular joint The joint where the mandible meets with the temporal bone of the cranium just in front of each ear.

tendon A tough fibrous cord that attaches a muscle to a bone.

testicle A male genital gland that contains specialized cells that produce hormones and sperm.

thoracic cage The chest or rib cage.

thoracic spine The 12 vertebrae that lie between the cervical vertebrae and the lumbar vertebrae. One pair of ribs is attached to each of the thoracic vertebrae.

thorax The chest cavity that contains the heart, lungs, esophagus, and great vessels (the aorta and the two venae cavae).

thyroid cartilage A firm prominence of cartilage that forms the upper part of the larynx; the Adam's apple.

tibia The shin bone, the larger of the two bones of the lower leg.

topographic anatomy The superficial landmarks of the body that serve as guides to the structures that lie beneath them.

torso The trunk without the head and limbs.

trachea The windpipe; the main trunk for air passing to and from the lungs.

Trendelenburg's position The position in which the body is supine with the head lower than the feet.

triceps The largest muscle that covers the back of the humerus.

ulna The inner bone of the forearm, on the side opposite the thumb.

ulnar artery One of the major arteries of the forearm; it can be palpated at the wrist on the ulnar side (at the base of the fifth finger).

ureter A small, hollow tube that carries urine from the kidneys to the bladder.

urethra The canal that conveys urine from the bladder to outside the body.

urinary bladder A sac behind the pubic symphysis made of smooth muscle that collects and stores urine.

urinary system The organs that control the discharge of certain waste materials filtered from the blood and excreted as urine.

vagina A muscular distensible tube that connects the uterus with the vulva (the external female genitalia); also called the birth canal.

vasa deferentia (vas deferens) The spermatic duct of the testicles.

veins Tubular vessels that carry blood from the tissues back to the heart.

ventral The anterior surface of the body.

ventricle Lower chamber of the heart.

vertebrae The 33 bones that make up the spinal column.

voluntary muscle Muscle that is under direct voluntary control of the brain and can be contracted or relaxed at will; skeletal, or striated, muscle.

white blood cells Blood cells that play a role in the body's immune defense mechanisms against infection; also called leukocytes.

xiphoid process The narrow, cartilaginous lower tip of the sternum.

zygomas The quadrangular bones of the cheek, articulating with the frontal bone, the maxillae, the zygomatic processes of the temporal bone, and the great wings of the sphenoid bone.

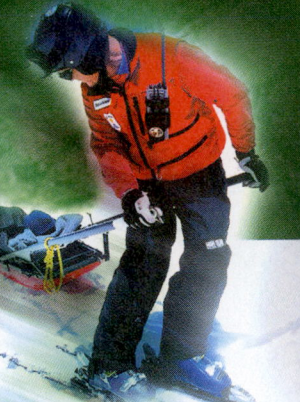

Assessment in Action

You are dispatched to a curve in a ski race course where you find a responsive 19-year-old woman off the course next to a tree. She has deformity and swelling of the left arm just above the elbow, is short of breath, and complains bitterly when you palpate her right costal margin and the RUQ of her abdomen.

1. Which organs/structures lie directly under the right costal margin?
   A. Liver and lung
   B. Spleen and lung
   C. Spleen and liver
   D. Cecum and lung

2. On the basis of this injury and the possible damage to organs directly underneath, you would most likely suspect that the patient is at risk for developing difficulty breathing and:
   A. a bowel obstruction.
   B. vomiting and diarrhea.
   C. lower extremity paralysis.
   D. severe internal bleeding.

3. Using anatomic terms, the injury to the elbow was located:
   A. proximal to the shoulder.
   B. in the distal humerus.
   C. in the proximal humerus.
   D. distal to the elbow.

4. Using anatomic terms, the right costal margin is:
   A. lateral to the sternum, inferior to the right nipple.
   B. superior to the right nipple, medial to the sternum.
   C. superior to the RUQ, medial to the sternum.
   D. inferior to the umbilicus, lateral to the sternum.

5. Because of the injured left arm, which of the following actions is also likely?
   A. Cannot raise her shoulder
   B. May have pain in her clavicle
   C. Cannot flex her elbow
   D. May have associated pain in her hand

A 30-year-old man fell from his bike onto his left side during a downhill race. The fall was hard enough to fracture two ribs anteriorly.

6. Besides his lung, what other organ has a high likelihood of being injured in this area?
   A. Liver
   B. Heart
   C. Pancreas
   D. Spleen

7. A forward fall (outside edge) onto the shoulder cap usually results in injury to the:
   A. Scapula
   B. Midshaft humerus
   C. A/C joint
   D. Third and fourth ribs

8. Complications following a pelvis fracture most frequently involve hypovolemic shock and:
   A. ileus.
   B. puncture injury to adjacent structures.
   C. nausea and vomiting.
   D. priapism.

Challenging Questions

9. The alveoli are surrounded by a network of tiny blood vessels. These vessels are called pulmonary capillaries. If a blow to the chest caused internal hemorrhage from these capillaries, what external sign might the patient exhibit that would suggest the injury?

10. Injury to the kidney might not be discovered outside the hospital. However, if the injury is enough to cause blood to collect in the renal pelvis and bladder, how might the injury be recognized?

Points to Ponder

A 24-year-old female snowboarder enters the aid room complaining of acute abdominal pain. The woman describes a burning pain in her lower abdomen. She relates that her menses are due any day. The boarder points to the pain being just superior to her pubis. When you palpate the lower quadrants, she complains of pain on both sides. Would you expose the area for observation? What organ(s) may be involved? What other questions regarding her symptoms would you ask?

Issues Patient Respect, Personal Bias and Prejudice, Appropriate Discussions in Front of Nonemergency Care Personnel

Online Outlook

As an OEC technician, you must have a good understanding of basic human anatomy and physiology. Improve your knowledge by completing Exercise 4 under "Self Study" at www.OECzone.com.

www.OECzone.com

Baseline Vital Signs and SAMPLE History

Objectives

Cognitive

♣ 1. Identify the components of vital signs (p 136).

♣ 2. Describe the methods to obtain a breathing rate (p 137).

3. Identify the attributes that should be obtained when assessing breathing (p 137).

4. Differentiate between shallow, labored, and noisy breathing (p 137).

♣ 5. Describe the methods to obtain a pulse rate (p 139).

♣ 6. Identify the information obtained when assessing a patient's pulse (p 139).

7. Differentiate between a strong, weak, regular, and irregular pulse (p 140).

8. Describe the methods to assess skin color, temperature, and condition (capillary refill in infants and children) (p 140).

9. Identify normal and abnormal skin colors (p 140).

10. Differentiate between pale, blue, red, and yellow skin color (p 141).

11. Identify the normal and abnormal skin temperature (p 141).

12. Differentiate between hot, cool, and cold skin temperature (p 141).

13. Identify normal and abnormal skin conditions (p 141).

♣ 14. Identify normal and abnormal capillary refill (p 141).

♣ 15. Describe the methods to assess the pupils (p 147).

16. Identify normal and abnormal pupil size (p 147).

17. Differentiate between dilated (big) and constricted (small) pupil size (p 147).

18. Differentiate between reactive and nonreactive pupils and equal and unequal pupils (p 147).

♣ 19. Describe the methods to assess blood pressure (p 143).

20. Define systolic pressure (p 143).

21. Define diastolic pressure (p 143).

22. Explain the difference between auscultation and palpation for obtaining a blood pressure (p 143).

♣ 23. Identify the components of the SAMPLE history (p 149).

24. Differentiate between a sign and a symptom (p 135).

♣ 25. State the importance of accurately reporting and recording the baseline vital signs (p 136).

♣ 26. Discuss the need to search for additional medical identification (p 149).

Affective

♣ 27. Explain the value of performing the baseline vital signs (p 136).

28. Recognize and respond to the feelings patients experience during assessment (p 134).

29. Defend the need for obtaining and recording an accurate set of vital signs (p 136).

30. Explain the rationale of recording additional sets of vital signs (p 148).

♣ 31. Explain the importance of obtaining a SAMPLE history (p 149).

Psychomotor

32. Demonstrate the skills involved in assessment of breathing (p 136).

♣ 33. Demonstrate the skills associated with obtaining a pulse (p 139).

♣ 34. Demonstrate the skills associated with assessing the skin color, temperature, condition, and capillary refill (p 140).

35. Demonstrate the skills associated with assessing the pupils (p 148).

♣ 36. Demonstrate the skills associated with obtaining blood pressure (p 143).

♣ 37. Demonstrate the skills that should be used to obtain information from the patient, family, or bystanders at the scene (p 134).

♣ These are core concepts in initial patrol training.

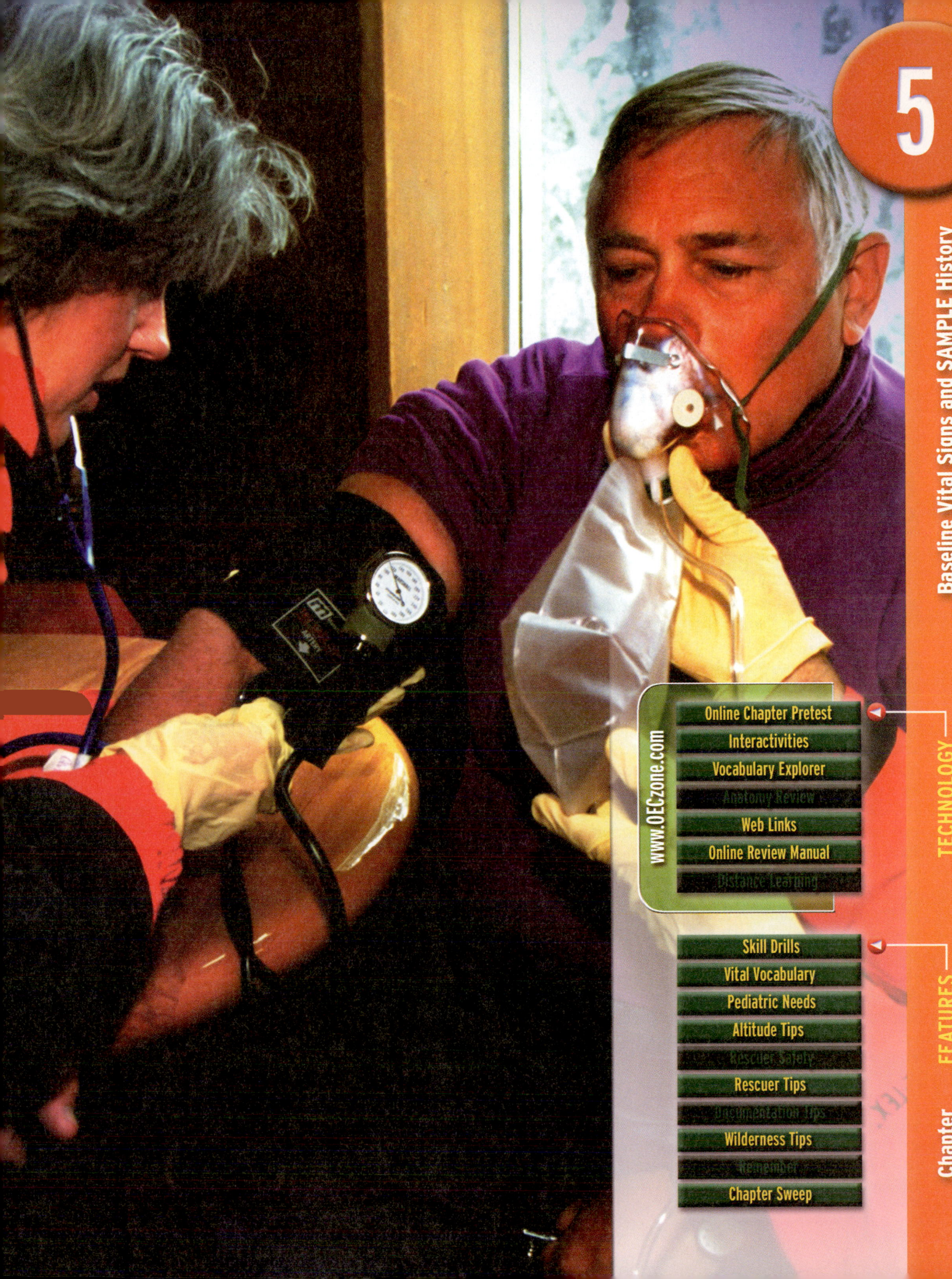

5

Baseline Vital Signs and SAMPLE History

TECHNOLOGY

www.OECzone.com

Online Chapter Pretest
Interactivities
Vocabulary Explorer
Anatomy Review
Web Links
Online Review Manual
Distance Learning

Chapter   FEATURES

Skill Drills
Vital Vocabulary
Pediatric Needs
Altitude Tips
Rescuer Safety
Rescuer Tips
Documentation Tips
Wilderness Tips
Remember
Chapter Sweep

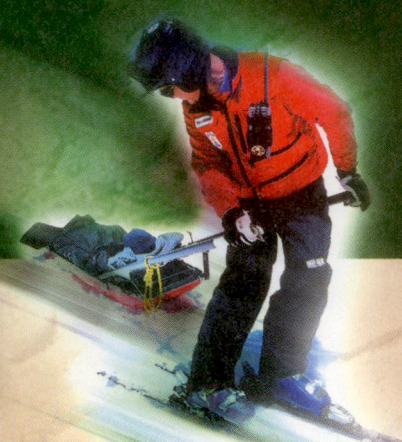

You are the rescuer

On the ski slope, the patroller in charge asks for another check of the patient's vital signs. Because of the patient's injury and the outdoor temperature, another rescuer questions the request as he asks, "Do you really want me to recheck them again so soon? I just checked them 5 minutes ago." A "Yes, please" reply gets him started on his task.

This chapter introduces the essential care concept relative to obtaining and evaluating a patient's baseline vital signs and the SAMPLE history. It will also help you answer the following questions:

1. Why are serial vital signs necessary when caring for seriously ill or injured patients?

2. How can the SAMPLE history and vital signs that are obtained in the field setting be of value to subsequent caregivers?

Baseline Vital Signs and SAMPLE History

As a rescuer, you must perform a quick but thorough assessment to identify a patient's needs and to provide proper emergency medical care. Patient assessment includes many steps and is the most complex skill that you will learn in the OEC course. To make the task easier, it is helpful to identify and discuss the key components and skills of patient assessment before you learn the entire process.

As you begin your assessment, you must gather and record some key information about the patient. You will also need to obtain and evaluate the patient's vital signs. The injuries, illnesses, or symptoms and the history of what occurred before and since you arrived are key pieces of information that you will have to obtain by asking a series of questions. You must also learn about the patient's past medical history and overall health.

This chapter begins by defining the chief complaint and signs and symptoms. It then explains what key information about the patient you need to obtain at the start of the assessment and why you need it. It also describes each of the vital signs and provides a step-by-step explanation of how to obtain each. Both normal and abnormal vital signs are discussed. The chapter ends with a description of the SAMPLE history.

Gathering Key Patient Information

During the assessment, you will be using your eyes, ears, nose, hands, and a few basic medical instruments to obtain information about your patient. You will need to know which questions to ask and how to ask them

▼ Figure 5-1). By using your deductive powers, you will be able to interpret the meaning and implications of your findings and the information that you have gathered. When assessing the patient, you will have to look, listen, feel, and think. Your scene size-up or the information that is given to you by a bystander or relative when you arrive at the scene should make it immediately apparent whether you were called to the scene because of an accident with injuries or an acute medical problem.

First, find out the patient's name. You will need to know the patient's name so that you can properly address the patient. Unless an adult patient is a close friend or relative of yours, you should address him or her as "Mr.," "Ms.," "Miss," or "Mrs.," followed by the

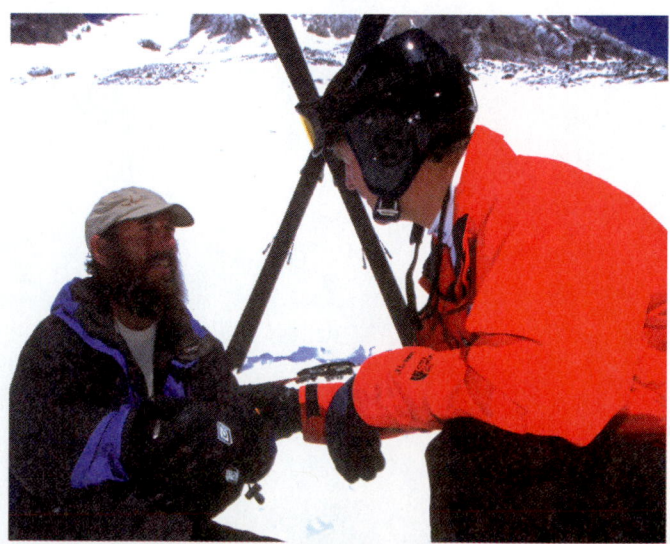

Figure 5-1 You must know how to gather information about the scene and the patient by using your senses and by asking relevant questions.

Pediatric Needs

Place yourself at eye level when interacting with children. A towering stance can be very frightening.

patient's last name. You may ask the patient how he or she wishes to be called and address the patient in that manner. This is especially important when relating to someone who may be frightened, hurt, and cold. If the patient's name is difficult to pronounce, you can simply say "Sir" or "Ma'am" instead, to convey a similar respectful and professional manner.

You should try to address children by their first name, especially the name they are customarily called, such as "Johnny," "Betty," or "Joey." Even infants and toddlers who do not yet respond verbally can recognize their name and may be less anxious when it is used.

If an unaccompanied patient is disoriented or unconscious, you should look in his or her wallet or purse for a driver's license or other piece of identification that will tell you the patient's name. At the same time, you should check for any hospital identification or medical alert card. *Always* look for patient identification in the presence of another rescuer at the scene.

Age and gender are also important considerations in assessing a patient. Some conditions and illnesses are found predominantly in younger patients; others are commonly found only in older patients. Some conditions are prevalent in a certain age group in adult men but in a different age group in women. Some are more prevalent in one gender, and some are limited exclusively to either male or female patients. In addition, the normal range of some of the vital signs will be different for different age groups of children, adults, and elderly patients.

Chief Complaint

If information regarding the mechanism of injury can be relayed in the first dispatch, it may direct the rescuer to the patient's **chief complaint**. In the most literal definition, chief complaints are the major signs and symptoms that the patient reports when asked, "What seems to be the matter?" or "What's wrong?" A patient who responds "My chest hurts" is stating the chief complaint. What you see must also be considered in determining the chief complaint. If the patient's response demonstrates that he or she is having significant difficulty breathing, "difficulty breathing" should be included in the chief complaint as if the patient had

reported it verbally. In some protocols, a chief complaint also includes any significant gross, apparent injuries.

The problems or feelings the patients report to you, such as, "I feel dizzy," "My leg hurts," or "Ow, that hurts a lot!" are called **symptoms** (▼ **Figure 5-2A**). These cannot be felt or observed by others. The severity of a symptom is subjective because it is based on the patient's interpretation and tolerance. **Signs** are objective conditions that can be seen, heard, felt, smelled, or measured by you or others (▼ **Figure 5-2B**). Wounds, external bleeding, marked deformities, respirations, and pulse are all signs.

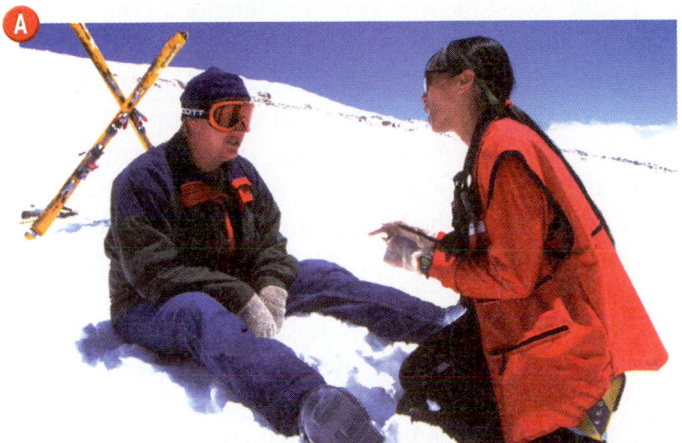

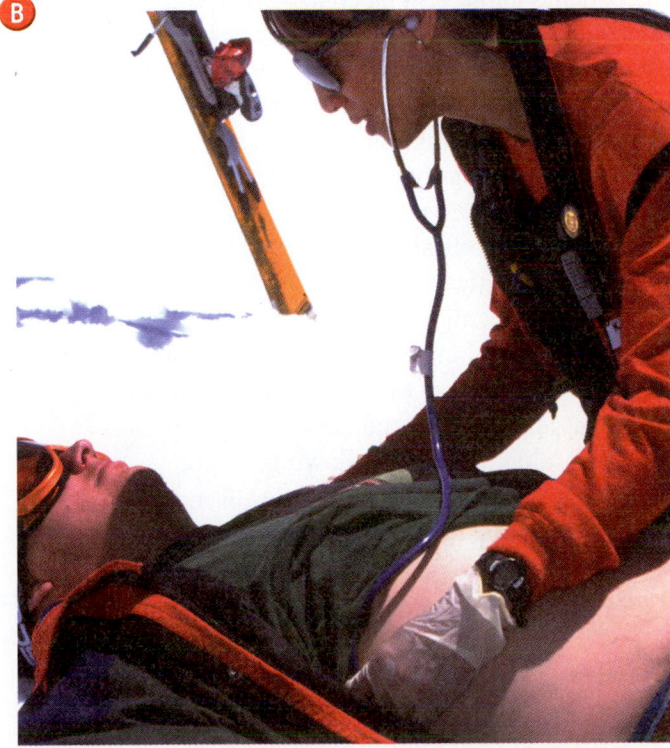

Figure 5-2 **A.** A symptom is a condition that the patient feels and tells you about. **B.** A sign is a condition that you can observe about the patient.

Signs and symptoms that occurred before you arrived, such as dizziness that resulted in a loss of consciousness, may be reported by the patient or others at the scene. Because signs and symptoms are essential to understanding the sequence of events and may include signs that are no longer present, they are important parts of the patient history. You should always report how and/or when the signs and symptoms began. This information is important because the reason that signs and symptoms develop often differs, depending on the situation.

Baseline Vital Signs

The initial assessment is a rapid evaluation of the patient's general condition to identify any potentially life-threatening conditions. The brain and other vital organs require constant oxygen. Significant problems with breathing or circulation must be considered potentially life-threatening conditions. A critical problem or deficit in any of the body's other vital systems or functions will progressively affect and be reflected by changes in the respiratory, circulatory, and central nervous systems. Therefore, the status of these systems serves as your guideline for evaluating and measuring the patient's general condition.

Vital signs are the key signs that are used to evaluate the patient's initial general condition. The first set of vital signs that you obtain is called the *baseline vital signs*. By periodically reassessing the vital signs and comparing the findings with the baseline set, you will be able to identify any significant trends in the patient's condition, particularly whether the patient's condition is becoming worse ▶ Figure 5-3 .

Because key indicators include a quantitative (numeric) objective measurement, you will always include the patient's respirations, pulse, and blood pressure when taking and evaluating the vital signs. Other key indications of the patient's respiratory, cardiovascular, and central nervous system status include evaluation of the following:

- Skin temperature and condition in adults
- Capillary refill in children
- Pupillary reaction
- Level of consciousness

Respirations

A patient who is breathing without assistance is said to have spontaneous respirations or spontaneous ventilations. Each complete breath includes two distinct phases: inspiration and expiration. During inspiration

Rescuer Tips

Obtaining the respirations or pulse rate

When obtaining a patient's respirations or pulse rate, count the number of breaths or beats in a 30-second period and then multiply by 2. This method produces a significantly more reliable figure than you would get if you counted for only 15 seconds and multiplied by 4. With either method, the result will always be an even number.

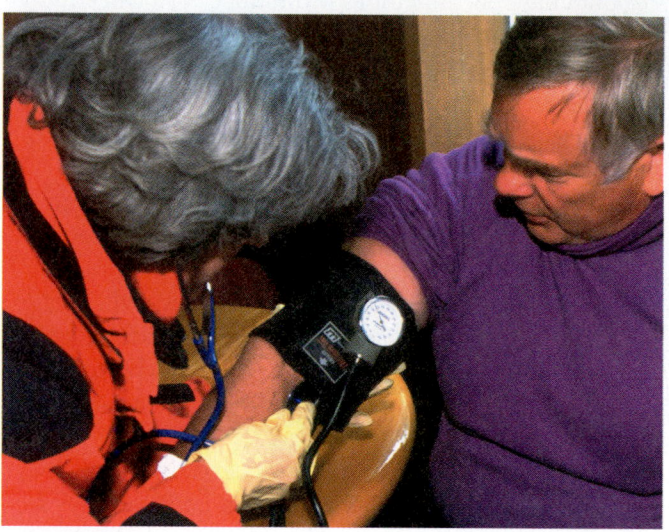

Figure 5-3 Baseline vital signs are key signs that are used to establish the patient's initial condition and should be obtained in any serious injury.

(inhalation), the chest rises up and out, drawing oxygenated air into the lungs. During expiration (exhalation), the chest returns to its original position, releasing air with an increased carbon dioxide level out of the lungs. Inhalation and exhalation times occur in a 1:3 ratio; the active inhalation phase lasts one third the amount of time of the passive exhalation phase.

Breathing is a continuous process in which each breath regularly follows the last with no notable interruption. Breathing is normally a spontaneous automatic process that occurs without conscious thought, visible effort, marked sounds, or pain. You will assess breathing by watching the patient's chest rise and fall, feeling for air through the mouth and nose during exhalation, and listening to breath sounds with a stethoscope over each lung. Chest rise and breath sounds should be equal on both sides of the chest. A conscious patient who is speaking has spontaneous respirations.

If a patient has a significant mechanism of injury, abnormal pulse, or abnormal breathing, do a rapid assessment of vital signs without removing any clothes.

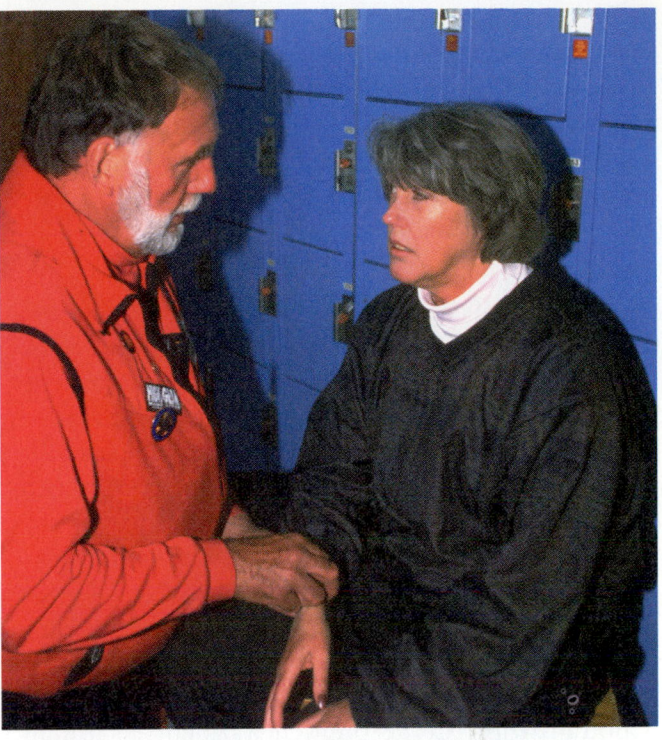

Figure 5-4 Assess respirations in a conscious patient by first taking a radial pulse and then, without releasing the patient's wrist, counting the chest rise and fall for 30 seconds.

When assessing respirations, you must determine the rate, quality (character), and depth of the patient's breathing.

RATE. Respirations are determined by counting the number of breaths in a 30-second period and multiplying by 2. The result equals the number of breaths per minute. For accuracy, you should count each breath at the same point in its cycle. This is most easily done by counting each peak chest rise. Although you can see peak chest rise, it is easier to place your hand on the patient's chest and feel it. However, be aware that a conscious patient who knows that you are evaluating his or her breathing will often override the automatic rate and depth by breathing more slowly and deeply. To prevent this from happening, you should check respirations in a conscious, alert patient without making the patient aware of what you are evaluating. This can be easily done by first taking a radial pulse and then, without releasing the wrist or otherwise suggesting a change, counting the chest rise that you see or feel as the patient's forearm rises and falls with the movement of the chest ▶ **Figure 5-4** . If the patient coughs, yawns, sighs, or talks during the 30-second period, you should wait a few seconds and start again. ▼ **Table 5-1** shows the normal range of respiratory rates of patients who are at rest.

QUALITY. You can determine the quality or character of respirations as you are counting. ▶ **Table 5-2** shows four ways in which the quality or character can be described.

TABLE 5-1 Normal Ranges for Respirations	
Age	**Range**
Adults	12 to 20 breaths/min
Children	15 to 30 breaths/min
Infants	25 to 50 breaths/min

TABLE 5-2 Characteristics of Respirations	
Normal	Breathing is neither shallow nor deep
	Equal chest rise and fall
	No use of accessory muscles
Shallow	Slight chest or abdominal wall motion
Labored	Increased breathing effort
	Use of accessory muscles
	Possible gasping
	Nasal flaring, supraclavicular and intercostal retractions in infants and children
Noisy	Increase in sound of breathing, including snoring, wheezing, gurgling, crowing, grunting, and stridor

RHYTHM. While counting the patient's respirations, you should also note the rhythm. If the time from one peak chest rise to the next is fairly consistent, respirations are considered regular. If respirations vary or change frequently, they are considered irregular. When you document the vital signs, be sure to note whether the patient's respirations were regular or irregular.

EFFORT. Normally, breathing is an effortless process that does not affect a patient's speech, posture, or positioning. Speech is a good indicator of whether a conscious patient is having difficulty breathing. A patient who can speak smoothly without unusual extra pauses is breathing normally. However, a patient who can speak only one word at a time or must stop every two to three words to catch his or her breath is having significant difficulty breathing. Patients who are having marked difficulty breathing will instinctively assume a posture in which it is easier for them to breathe. There are two common postures that indicate that the patient is trying to increase airflow. The first is called the **tripod position**. In this position, a patient sits leaning forward on outstretched arms with the head and chin thrust slightly forward and is having sufficient difficulty breathing that a significant conscious effort is required (▼ **Figure 5-5**). The second is most commonly seen in children—the **sniffing position**. The patient sits upright with the head and chin thrust slightly forward and the patient appears to be sniffing.

Breathing that becomes progressively more difficult requires progressively more effort. When you can see

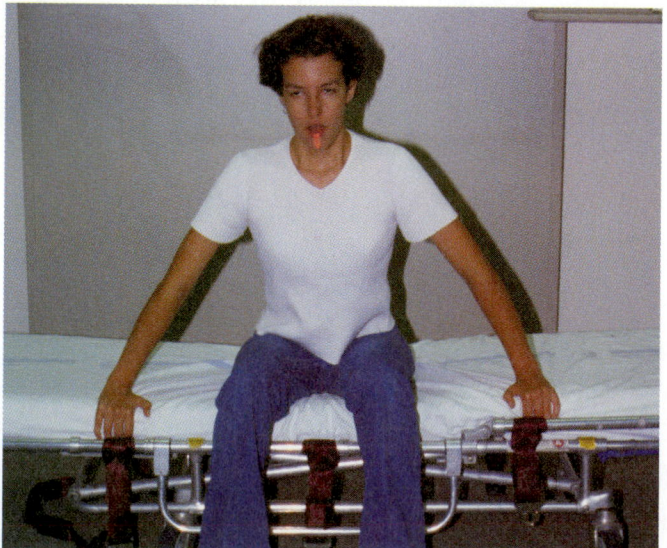

Figure 5-5   A patient in the tripod position will sit leaning forward on outstretched arms with the head and chin thrust forward slightly.

Pediatric Needs

Chest rise in a small child is less marked than that in an adult. However, a small child's abdomen moves more with each breath than an adult's does. Place your hands on the outer margin of the lower anterior chest to feel the chest wall and abdominal movement, and determine whether the depth is normal, shallow, or deep. In a patient of any age, if it is difficult to gauge the depth of breathing from the chest movement, note instead the amount of air that you feel is exhaled with each breath. This also is useful in patients with heavy clothing.

that effort, the patient's breathing is described as **labored breathing**.

Initially, labored breathing is characterized by the patient's position, concentration on breathing, and the increased effort and depth of each breath. As breathing becomes more labored, accessory muscles in the chest and neck are used, and the patient may make grunting sounds with each breath. In infants and small children, nasal flaring and supraclavicular and intercostal retractions (indentation above the clavicles and in the spaces between the ribs) are commonly associated with labored breathing. Sometimes, the patient may be gasping.

Infants and small children will continue to have labored breathing for a sustained period, will then often become exhausted, and finally will no longer have the strength to maintain the necessary energy to breathe. In infants and small children, cardiac arrest is generally caused by respiratory arrest.

NOISY BREATHING. Normal breathing is silent or, in a very quiet environment, accompanied only by the sounds of air movement at the mouth and nose. Through a stethoscope, normal breath sounds include only the sound of air movement through the bronchi accompanied by a soft, low-pitched murmur. Breathing accompanied by other sounds indicates a significant respiratory problem. When the airway is partially obstructed by a foreign body or swelling, you may hear **stridor**, a harsh, high-pitched, crowing sound. If you can hear bubbling or gurgling, the patient probably has fluid in the airway. You may hear other sounds, including wheezes, snoring, gurgling, or bubbling. The presence of any of these indicates that a serious respiratory problem exists. With a complete airway obstruction, the patient will not be able to move any air and will no longer be able to cough or talk.

A patient who coughs up thick, yellowish or greenish sputum (matter from the lungs) most likely has an advanced respiratory infection. A patient with a chest injury may cough up blood or a frothy whitish or pinkish foam-like sputum. A patient with congestive heart failure may also cough up a frothy sputum. The presence of either substance, regardless of its cause, indicates that an urgent, potentially critical cardiovascular and respiratory problem exists. The patient's condition may deteriorate rapidly to a point at which the patient can no longer breathe.

DEPTH. The amount of air that the patient is exchanging depends on both the rate and the **tidal volume**, the amount of air that is exchanged with each breath. The depth of the breath determines whether the tidal volume is normal, less than normal, or more than normal. Respirations are described as shallow when the movement of the chest wall and air that you feel exhaled with each breath is less than normal. Deep respirations occur when chest movement and exhaled air are significantly greater than normal. You should document when the patient's respirations are shallow or deep; however, you do not have to record a normal depth of breathing.

Pulse

With each heartbeat, the ventricles contract, forcefully ejecting blood from the heart and propelling it into the arteries. The **pulse** is the pressure wave that occurs as each heartbeat causes a surge in the blood circulating through the arteries. The pulse is most easily felt at a pulse point where a major artery lies near the surface and can be pressed gently against a bone or solid organ. To *palpate* (feel) the pulse, hold together your index and long fingers and place their tips over a pulse point, pressing gently against the artery until you feel intermittent pulsations. Sometimes, you may have to slide your fingertips a little to each side and press again until you feel a pulse. When palpating a pulse, do not allow your thumb to touch the patient. If you do so, you may mistake the strong pulsing circulation in your thumb for the patient's pulse.

In responsive patients who are older than 1 year, you should palpate the radial pulse at the wrist ▶ **Figure 5-6A** . In unresponsive patients older than 1 year, you should palpate the carotid pulse in the neck ▶ **Figure 5-6B** . When palpating the carotid pulse, you should place the fingertips of your index and long fingers along the carotid artery in the groove between the trachea and the neck muscle. Use caution when palpating the carotid pulse in a responsive patient, especially an elderly patient. Only gentle pressure on one side of the neck

should be used. Never press on the carotid arteries on both sides of the neck at the same time. Doing so can cut off circulation to the brain.

In infants, both the radial and carotid pulses are difficult to locate. Because of the infant's soft, immature trachea, palpating the carotid pulse is not recommended. Palpate the brachial pulse, located at the underside of the upper arm, in children younger than 1 year ▼ **Figure 5-7** . With the infant lying supine,

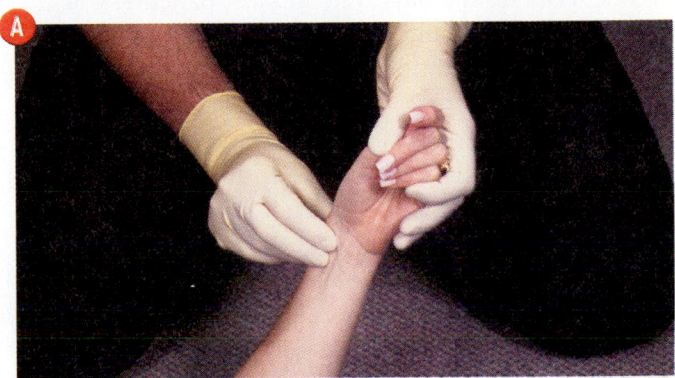

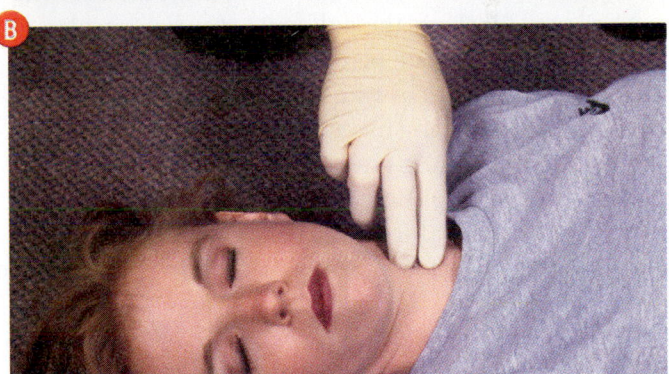

Figure 5-6   **A.** To palpate the radial pulse, place the tips of your first two fingers over the radial artery, pressing gently until you feel intermittent pulsations. **B.** To palpate the carotid pulse, place the tips of your first two fingers over the carotid artery, pressing gently until you feel intermittent pulsations.

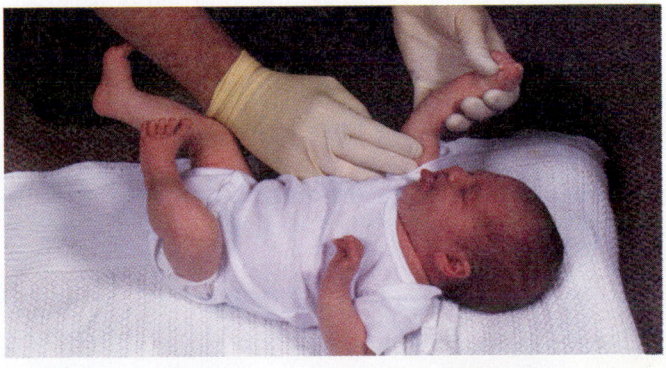

Figure 5-7   To palpate the brachial pulse in an infant, press firmly along the brachial artery at the underside of the upper arm.

you can access the brachial pulse by elevating the arm over the infant's head. Because most infants have chubby arms, you need to press your adjacent fingertips firmly along the brachial artery, which lies parallel to the long axis of the upper arm, to be able to palpate the pulse.

Your first consideration when taking a pulse is to determine whether the patient has a palpable pulse or is pulseless. When taking the pulse, you should assess and report its rate, strength, and regularity.

RATE. To obtain the pulse rate in most patients, you should count the number of pulses felt in a 30-second period and then multiply by 2. A pulse that is weak and difficult to palpate, irregular, or extremely slow should be palpated and counted for a full minute. A pulse rate is counted as beats per minute; however, in reporting the pulse rate, it is not necessary to state or write "beats per minute" after the number.

The pulse rate in most adults (at rest) averages around 72 beats/min. However, pulse rate can vary significantly from person to person. In the well-conditioned athlete or in individuals taking heart medications such as beta-blockers, the pulse rate may be considerably lower. A pulse rate between 60 and 100 beats/min is considered normal in adults. The average pulse rate in children is generally higher. (▼ **Table 5-3**) shows the normal ranges of pulse rates.

In assessing the pulse rate in an adult patient, a rate that is greater than 100 beats/min is described as **tachycardia**, and a rate of less than 60 beats/min is described as **bradycardia**.

STRENGTH. You should always report the pulse's strength whenever reporting or recording the pulse. The pulse is generally palpated at the radial or carotid arteries in adults and at the brachial artery in infants, because it is normally strong and easily palpable at these locations. Therefore, if the pulse feels of normal strength, you should describe it as being strong. You should describe a stronger than normal pulse

as "bounding" and a pulse that is weak and difficult to feel as "weak" or "thready." With a little experience, you will be able to make the necessary distinctions easily.

REGULARITY. When assessing the quality of the pulse, you must also determine whether it is regular or irregular. When the interval between each ventricular contraction of the heart is short, the pulse is rapid. When the interval is longer, the pulse is slower. No matter what the rate, the interval between each contraction should be the same, and the pulse that results should occur at a constant, regular rhythm. You should note and document this rhythm as regular.

The rhythm is considered irregular if the heart periodically has a premature or late beat or if a pulse beat is missed. Some individuals have a chronically irregular pulse; however, if an irregular pulse is found in a patient with signs and symptoms that suggest a cardiovascular problem, the patient likely needs advanced cardiac assessment and life support. Therefore, depending on your protocols, you should call for ALS backup, arrange for an intercept, or initiate prompt transport to definitive care.

The Skin

The condition of the patient's skin can tell you a lot about the patient's peripheral circulation and perfusion, blood oxygen levels, and body temperature. When assessing the skin, you should evaluate its color, temperature, and moisture.

COLOR. Assessing the skin helps you to determine the adequacy of perfusion. **Perfusion** is the circulation of blood within an organ or tissue. Adequate perfusion meets the cells' current needs; inadequate perfusion will cause cells and tissues to die.

Many blood vessels lie near the surface of the skin. The skin's color is determined by the blood circulating through these vessels and the amount and type of pigment that is present in the skin. Blood is red when it is adequately saturated with oxygen. As a result, skin in lightly pigmented individuals is pinkish. The pigmentation in most individuals will not hide changes in the skin's underlying color, regardless of the individual's race. In patients with deeply pigmented skin, changes in color may be apparent only in certain areas, such as the fingernail beds, the mucous membranes in the mouth, the lips, the underside of the arm and palm (which are usually less pigmented), and the **conjunctiva** of the eyes. The conjunctiva is the delicate membrane lining the eyelids and it covers the exposed surface of the eye. In addition, the palms of the hands and soles of the feet should be assessed in infants and children.

TABLE 5-3 Normal Ranges for Pulse Rate	
Age	Range, beats/min
Adults	60 to 100
Children	80 to 120
Toddlers	90 to 150
Newborns	120 to 160

Poor peripheral circulation will cause the skin to appear pale, white, ashen, or gray, possibly with a waxy translucent appearance like a white candle. Abnormally cold or frozen skin may also appear this way. When the blood is not properly saturated with oxygen, it appears bluish. Therefore, in a patient with insufficient air exchange and low levels of oxygen in the blood, the blood and vessels become bluish, and the lips, mucous membranes, nail beds, and skin over the blood vessels appear blue or gray. This condition is called **cyanosis**
▼ Figure 5-8 .

High blood pressure may cause the skin to be abnormally flushed and red. In some patients with extremely high blood pressure, all the visible blood vessels will be so full that the skin will appear to be a dark reddish-purple. A patient with carbon monoxide poisoning or a significant fever, heatstroke, sunburn, mild thermal burns, or other conditions in which the body is unable to properly dissipate heat will also appear to have red skin.

Changes in skin color may also result from chronic illness. Liver disease or dysfunction may cause **jaundice**, resulting in the patient's skin and **sclera** turning yellow. The sclera is the normally white portion of the eye.

TEMPERATURE. Normally, the skin is warm to the touch. When the patient has a significant fever, sunburn, or hyperthermia, the skin feels hot to the touch. The skin will feel cool when the patient is in early shock, has mild hypothermia, or has inadequate perfusion. The skin will feel cold when the patient is in profound shock, has hypothermia, or has frostbite.

Body temperature is normally measured with a thermometer in the hospital. However, in the field, feeling the patient's forehead with the back of your hand is usually adequate to determine whether the patient's temperature is elevated or depressed ▼ Figure 5-9 .

MOISTURE. Dry skin is normal. Skin that is wet, moist (often called diaphoretic), or excessively dry and hot suggests a problem. In the early stages of shock, the skin will become slightly moist. Skin that is only slightly moist but not covered excessively with sweat is described as clammy, damp, or moist. When the skin is bathed in sweat, such as after strenuous exercise or when the patient is in shock, the skin is described as wet or **diaphoretic**.

Because the skin's color, temperature, and moisture are often related signs, you should consider them together. When recording or reporting your assessment of the skin, you should first describe the color, then the temperature, and last, whether the skin is dry, moist, or wet. For example, you could say or write, "Skin: pale, cool, and clammy."

Capillary Refill

Capillary refill is a test that evaluates the ability of the circulatory system to restore blood to the capillary system. When evaluated in an uninjured limb, capillary refill reflects the patient's perfusion. Capillary refill time is often affected by the patient's body temperature, position, and medications. A cold environment and a patient's age can affect the reliability of this test. To test capillary refill, place your thumb on the patient's fingernail with your fingers on the underside of the patient's finger, and gently compress
► Figure 5-10A . The blood will be forced from the capillaries in the nail bed. When you remove the pressure applied against the tip of the patient's finger, the nail bed will remain blanched and white for a brief period.

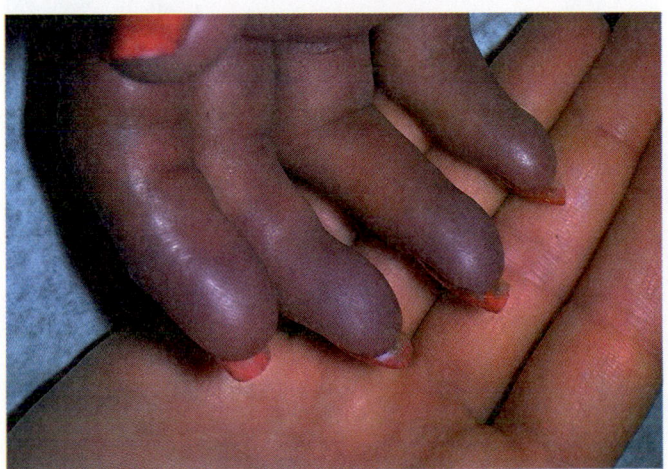

Figure 5-8 Cyanosis occurs when the patient has low levels of oxygen in the blood.

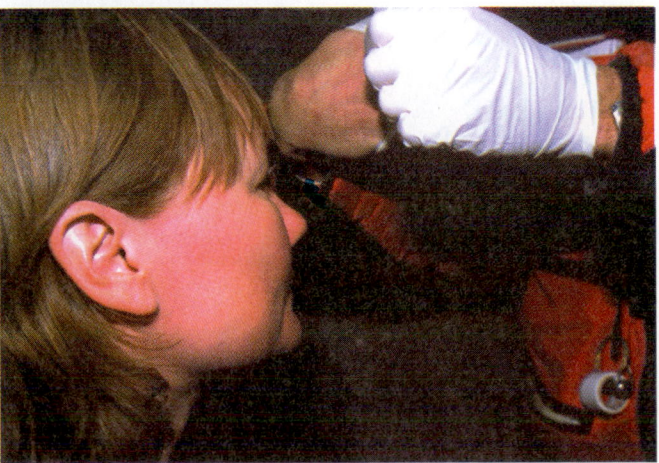

Figure 5-9 Assess skin temperature by feeling the patient's forehead with the back of your hand.

As the underlying capillaries refill with blood, the nail bed will be restored to its normal pink color.

Under ideal or normal conditions, capillary refill should be both prompt and pink. With adequate perfusion, the color in the nail bed should be restored to its normal pink within 2 seconds, or about the time it takes to say "capillary refill" at a normal rate of speech (▼ **Figure 5-10B**). You should report and document the capillary refill as normal, "CRT=2" or "CRT>2." You should suspect poor peripheral circulation when capillary refill takes more than 2 seconds or the nail bed remains blanched. In this instance, you should report and document the capillary refill as delayed.

A bluish color may indicate that the capillaries are refilling with blood drawn from the veins rather than with fresh, oxygenated blood from the arteries, making the test invalid. You should also consider the capillary refill test invalid if the patient is in or has been exposed to a cold environment or if the patient is elderly. In both situations, delayed capillary refill is normal.

To assess capillary refill in infants and children younger than 6 years, press on the skin or nail bed, and determine how long it takes for the pink color to return. As with adults, normal capillary refill takes less than 2 seconds.

Blood Pressure

Adequate blood pressure is necessary to maintain proper circulation and perfusion of the vital organ cells. **Blood pressure (BP)** is the pressure of circulating blood against the walls of the arteries. A decrease in the blood pressure may indicate one of the following:

Wilderness Tips

Patients with cold extremities will exhibit delayed capillary refill. This is a normal sign.

- Loss of blood or its fluid components
- Loss of vascular tone and sufficient arterial constriction to maintain the necessary pressure even without any actual fluid or blood loss
- A cardiac pumping problem

When any of these conditions occurs and results in a drop in circulation, the body's compensatory mechanisms are activated, the heart and pulse rates increase, and the blood vessels constrict. Normal blood pressure is maintained, and by decreasing the blood flow to the skin and extremities, available blood volume is temporarily redirected to the vital organs so that they remain adequately perfused. However, as shock progresses, and the body's defense mechanisms can no longer keep up, the blood pressure will fall. *Decreased blood pressure is a late sign of shock and indicates that the critical decompensated phase has begun.* Any patient with a markedly low blood pressure has inadequate pressure to maintain proper perfusion of all the vital organs and needs to have his or her blood pressure and perfusion restored immediately to a normal level. In this case, the patient will require rapid transport to definitive care.

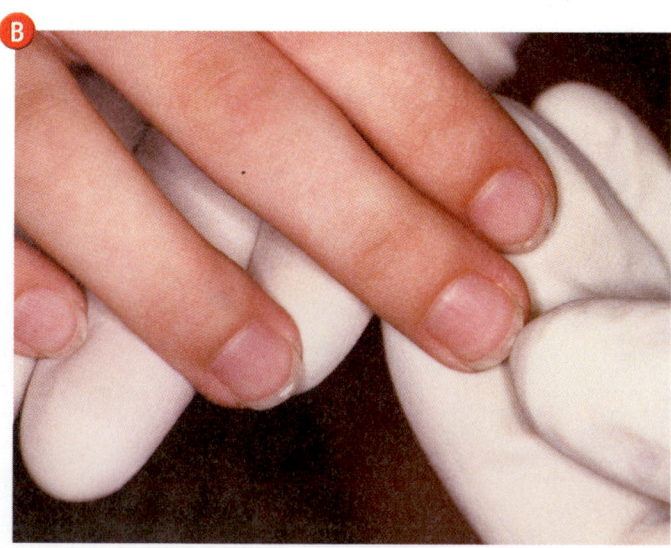

Figure 5-10 **A.** To test capillary refill, gently compress the fingertip until it blanches. **B.** Release the fingertip, and count until it returns to its normal pink color.

When the blood pressure becomes elevated, the body's defenses act to reduce it. Some individuals have chronically high blood pressure from progressive narrowing of the arteries that occurs with age, and during an acute episode, their blood pressure may increase to even higher levels. Head injury or a number of other conditions may also cause blood pressure to rise to very high levels. Abnormally high blood pressure may result in a rupture or other critical damage in the arterial system.

You should measure blood pressure in all patients older than 3 years who have had a serious injury.

Blood pressure contains two key separate components: systolic pressure and diastolic pressure. **Systolic pressure** is the increased pressure that is caused along the artery with each contraction (systole) of the ventricle and the pulse wave that it produces. **Diastolic pressure** is the residual pressure that remains in the arteries during the relaxing phase of the heart's cycle (diastole), when the left ventricle is at rest. Systolic pressure represents the maximum pressure to which the arteries are subjected, and the diastolic pressure represents the minimum amount of pressure that is always present in the arteries.

Early blood pressure gauges contained a column of mercury and a linear scale that was graduated in millimeters. Even though different gauges are used today, the blood pressure is still measured in millimeters of mercury (mm Hg). Blood pressure is reported as a fraction in the form systolic pressure over diastolic pressure. Therefore, if the patient's systolic pressure is 120 and the diastolic pressure is 78, you would record it as "BP 120/78 mm Hg." You would report the patient's blood pressure verbally as "BP is 120 over 78."

EQUIPMENT FOR MEASURING BLOOD PRESSURE. You will use a sphygmomanometer (blood pressure cuff) to apply pressure against the artery when measuring the blood pressure. The sphygmomanometer contains the following components:

- A wide outer cuff designed to be fastened snugly around the entire arm or leg
- An inflatable wide bladder sewn into a portion of the cuff
- A ball-pump with a one-way valve that allows air to enter and a turn-valve that can be closed or, when opened, will allow air to be released at a controlled speed from the cuff
- A pressure gauge calibrated in millimeters of mercury, which indicates the pressure that exists in the cuff that is being applied against the underlying artery

Altitude Tips

Recent ascent to altitude will affect baseline vital signs. Patients will normally show an increase in respiratory rate and depth, a mild increase in blood pressure, and a moderate increase in pulse rate. As acclimatization occurs, these signs will revert to more normal levels.

There are at least three sizes of blood pressure cuffs: adult, thigh, and pediatric ▼ Figure 5-11 . The normal size cuff is designed to wrap around the arm one to one and a half times and take up two thirds the length from the armpit to the crease in the elbow of most adults. Use a thigh cuff with patients who are obese or have exceptionally well-developed arm muscles or to take the blood pressure of the thigh in patients who have injuries in both arms. Use a small pediatric cuff with children and exceptionally small adults.

You must be sure to select the appropriately sized cuff. A cuff that is too small may result in falsely high readings; a cuff that is too large may result in falsely low readings.

AUSCULTATION. Auscultation is the method of listening to sounds within organs with a stethoscope. You will usually measure blood pressure by auscultation ▶ Skill Drill 5-1 . Follow these steps:

1. **With the patient's arm extended** with the palm up, place the cuff so that it lies across the upper arm and is located with its distal edge about 1″ above the crease at the inside of the patient's elbow. Make sure the center of the inflatable bladder, which is usually marked by an arrow on the cuff, lies over the brachial artery. Next, wrap

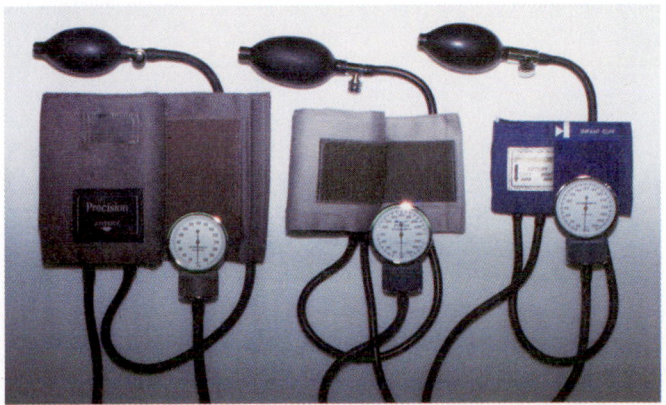

Figure 5-11 Three sizes of blood pressure cuffs: thigh, adult, and pediatric.

Skill Drill 5-1   Obtaining a Blood Pressure by Auscultation or Palpation

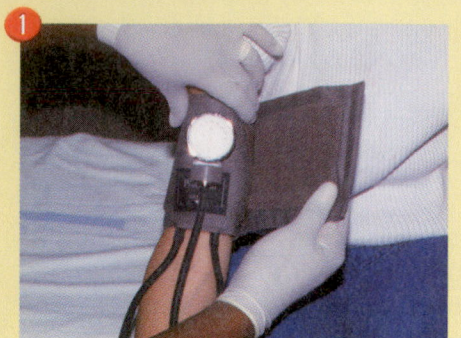

Apply the cuff snugly.

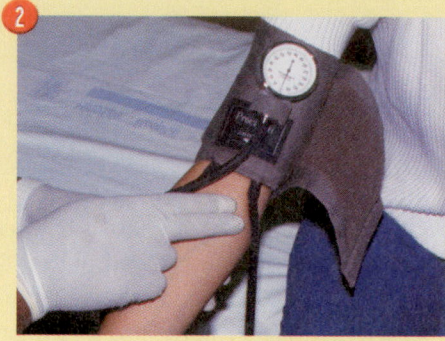

Palpate the brachial artery.

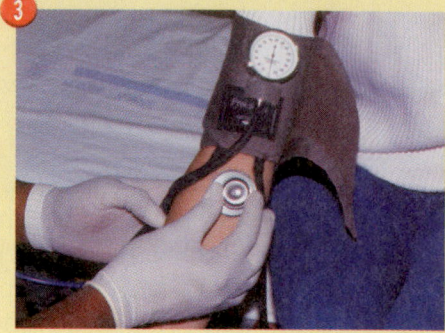

Place the stethoscope and grasp the ball-pump and turn-valve.

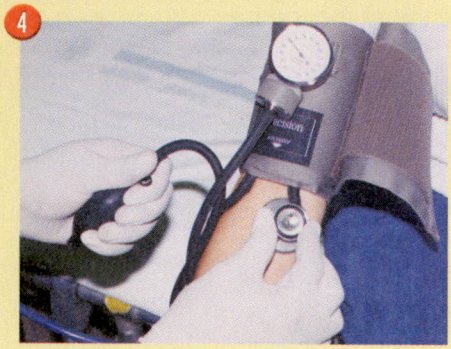

Close the valve and pump to 20 mm Hg above the point at which you stop hearing pulse sounds. Note the systolic and diastolic pressures as you let air escape slowly.

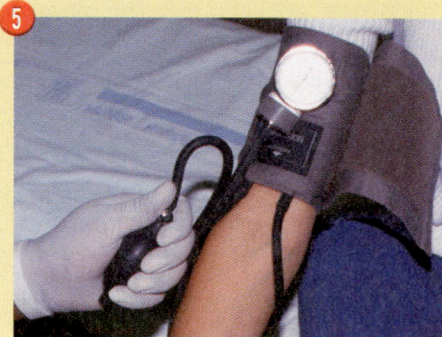

Open the valve and quickly release the remaining air.

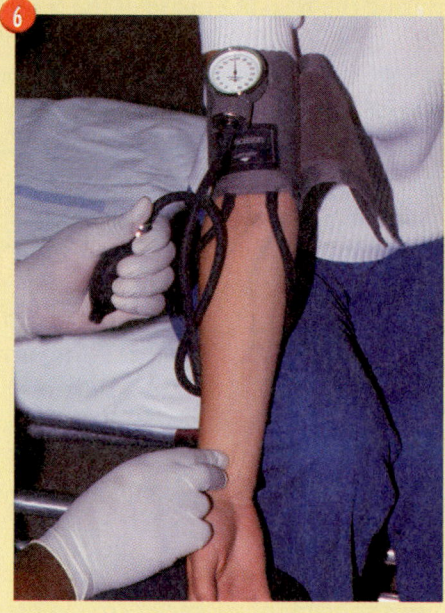

When using the palpation method, you should place your fingertips on the radial artery so that you feel the radial pulse.

the ends so that the cuff surrounds the upper arm snugly but not tightly. Secure the cuff with the Velcro fastener attached to it, making sure to rub your hand over the entire area where the two sides of the Velcro fastener are in contact. Once the cuff has been properly secured around the upper arm, the arm should be held at about the same level as the heart (Step 1).

2. **Palpate the brachial artery** (in the antecubital fossa, the anterior aspect of the elbow) to determine where to place the stethoscope (Step 2).

3. **Place the diaphragm of the stethoscope over the artery,** and hold it firmly pressed against the artery with the fingers of your nondominant hand. Hold the rubber ball-pump in the palm of your other hand and the turn-valve between your thumb and first finger (Step 3).

4. **Close the valve tightly, and pump the ball-pump** until you no longer hear pulse sounds. Continue pumping to increase the cuff's pressure by an additional 20 mm Hg. Next, slowly turn the valve, opening it until air is steadily escaping from the

cuff and you see the needle of the gauge slowly drop. Watch the gauge, and listen carefully. Note the patient's systolic pressure as the reading on the gauge at which the "taps" or "thumps" of the pulse waves can first be heard clearly. As the pressure in the cuff is progressively reduced, pulse sounds will continue for a time, then suddenly disappear. Note the patient's diastolic pressure as the reading on the gauge at which the sounds stopped **(Step 4).**

5. As soon as the pulse sounds stop, **open the valve, and release the remaining air quickly.** Once you have finished measuring the blood pressure, you should document your findings and the time at which the blood pressure was taken. Blood pressure is most often measured by auscultation with the patient in a sitting or semisitting position. Be sure to note whether a different method or position was used. Occasionally, when a patient's blood pressure is very low, you will continue to hear pulse sounds from the reading at which they started all the way until the gauge has reached 0. When this occurs, you should record the diastolic pressure as "0" or "all the way down" to indicate that it was not measurable by stethoscope **(Step 5).**

PALPATION. The auscultation method will be difficult or impossible to use in a very noisy environment and may produce inaccurate findings. The palpation method, which is examination by touch that does not depend on your ability to hear sounds, should be used in these cases (◄ **Skill Drill 5-1, Step 6**).

To measure blood pressure by palpation, secure the appropriately sized cuff around the patient's upper arm in the manner previously described. With your non-dominant hand, palpate the patient's radial pulse on the same arm as the cuff, without moving your fingertips once you have located it, until you have completed taking the blood pressure. While holding the ball-pump in your other hand, close the turn-valve and rapidly inflate the cuff to 200 mm Hg. As the cuff inflates, you will no longer feel the pulse under your fingertips. Open the turn-valve so that air slowly escapes from the cuff, and carefully observe the gauge. When you can again feel the radial pulse under your fingertips, you should note the reading on the gauge as the patient's systolic blood pressure. You will not be able to determine the diastolic pressure with this method. Next, open the turn-valve further, and completely deflate the cuff. Document your findings including the time, and note that the pressure was taken by palpation. On your patient care report, you can record the blood pressure as "120/P."

Wilderness Tips

In the absence of a BP cuff, a rescuer can generally assume the following minimum systolic blood pressures by palpating specific pulses:

Artery	Systolic BP
Radial Pulse	80 mm Hg
Femoral Pulse	70 mm Hg
Carotid Pulse	60 mm Hg

NORMAL BLOOD PRESSURE. Blood pressure levels vary with age and gender. (▼ **Table 5-4**) serves as a guideline for normal blood pressure ranges.

A patient has **hypotension** when the blood pressure is lower than the normal range and **hypertension** when the blood pressure is higher than the normal range.

Typically, you will see children less frequently than adults; therefore, you might not remember the normal ranges for the various age groups. You might wish to carry a chart with you that lists normal blood pressure ranges and other vital signs.

CRITICAL HYPOTENSION. You must assume that a patient who has a critically low blood pressure can no longer compensate sufficiently to maintain adequate perfusion. (▼ **Table 5-5**) shows the point at which blood pressure is considered to be critically low.

TABLE 5-4   Normal Ranges for Blood Pressure

Age	Range
Adults	100 to 140 mm Hg (systolic)
	60 to 90 mm Hg (diastolic)
Children (ages 1 to 8 years)	80 to 110 mm Hg (systolic)
Infants (newborn to to age 1 year)	60 mm Hg (systolic)

TABLE 5-5   Minimum Acceptable Systolic Blood Pressures

Adults/Adolescents	100 mm Hg or less
Children	70 mm Hg or less

Rescuer Tips

AVPU scale

The **AVPU scale** is a rapid method of assessing the patient's level of responsiveness using one of the following four terms:

A **A**wake and **A**lert

V Responsive to **V**erbal Stimulus

P Responsive to **P**ain

U **U**nresponsive

You should determine whether a patient is awake and alert. A patient who is not awake and alert but who is aroused and responds to your voice by opening his or her eyes, moaning, speaking, or moving is responding to verbal stimulus. A patient who does not respond to your normal speaking voice but who responds to your yelled voice is responding to loud verbal stimulus. Be sure to note how the patient responded. Tap a patient who is hearing impaired with your fingers repeatedly. If the patient responds, note that the patient is hearing impaired but responds to being tapped.

To determine whether a patient who does not respond to verbal stimuli will respond to a painful stimulus, you should gently but firmly pinch the patient's skin ▶ Figure 5-12 . A patient who moans or withdraws is responding to painful stimulus. Be sure to note the type and location of the stimulus and how the patient responded.

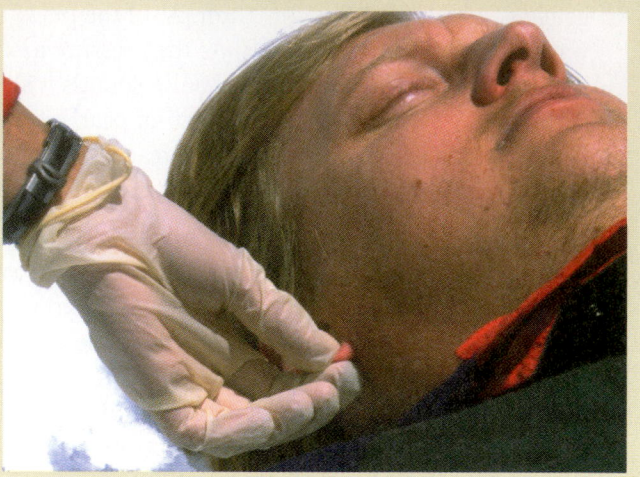

Figure 5-12   To assess whether a patient will respond to a painful stimulus, gently but firmly pinch the patient's skin. This can be done at the neck or on the earlobe.

If the patient does not respond to a painful stimulus on one side, try to elicit a response on the other side. Note that a patient who remains flaccid without moving or making a sound is unresponsive.

In assessing the patient's general circulation, the blood pressure, pulse, skin temperature, and capillary refill should *not* be assessed in an injured limb. However, once you have obtained these vital signs from an uninjured limb, you might wish to compare the distal skin temperature, quality of the distal pulse, and/or capillary refill time in the injured limb with those found on the uninjured side. This information is useful in evaluating whether the injury may have compromised the circulation in the injured limb.

Level of Responsiveness

The patient's level of responsiveness (LOR) is considered a vital sign because the status of the central nervous system is reflected by it. However, in the early assessment, you need to ascertain only the apparent gross level of responsiveness by determining whether the patient is awake and alert with an unaltered LOR, conscious but with an altered LOR, or unconscious.

As you assess a patient, you must determine the appropriateness of a response by how well it demon-strates the patient's understanding and mental activity, not how well it reflects your definition of socially acceptable behavior.

When a patient is less than completely responsive, the body's defense mechanisms may no longer be able to compensate adequately, possibly indicating that inadequate perfusion and oxygenation or a chemical or neurologic problem is adversely affecting the brain and its ability to function. A lowered level of responsiveness can also be caused by medications, drugs, alcohol, or poisoning.

Your assessment of a patient who is unresponsive when you arrive should be focused initially on airway, breathing, and circulation, and then on identifying other emergency care that the patient may need. Sustained unresponsiveness should warn you that a critical respiratory, circulatory, or central nervous system problem or deficit may exist, and you must assume that the patient has a potentially critical injury or potentially life-threatening condition. Therefore, after rapidly assessing the patient and providing emergency treatment, you should package the patient and provide rapid transport to the hospital.

The Glasgow Coma Scale is a method of assessing a patient's level of consciousness by scoring the patient's response to eye opening, motor response, and verbal response (▼ **Figure 5-13**). This was primarily developed for the clinical setting, but is occasionally used in the field.

PUPILS. The diameter and reactivity to light of the patient's pupils reflect the status of the brain's perfusion, oxygenation, and condition. The pupil is a circular opening in the center of the pigmented iris of the eye. The pupils are normally round and of approximately equal size and serve as optical diaphragms, adjusting their size depending on the available light. In normal room light, the pupil appears to be midsize. With less light, the pupils dilate, allowing more light

to enter the eye, making it possible to see even in dim light. With high light levels or when a bright light is suddenly introduced, the pupils instantly constrict, allowing less light to enter, protecting the sensitive receptors in the inner eye from damage (▼ **Figure 5-14A**). When a brighter light is introduced into one eye (or higher levels of light enter one eye only), both pupils should constrict equally to the appropriate size for the pupil receiving the most light.

In the absence of any light, the pupils will become fully relaxed and dilated (▼ **Figure 5-14B**). When light is introduced, each eye sends sensory signals to the brain indicating the level of light it is receiving. Pupil size is regulated by a series of continuous motor commands that the brain automatically sends through the oculomotor nerves to each eye, causing both pupils to constrict to the same appropriate size. Normally, pupil size changes instantly to any change in light level.

GLASGOW COMA SCALE

Eye Opening

Spontaneous	4
To Voice	3
To Pain	2
None	1

Verbal Response

Oriented	5
Confused	4
Inappropriate Words	3
Incomprehensible Words	2
None	1

Motor Response

Obeys Command	6
Localizes Pain	5
Withdraws (pain)	4
Flexion (pain)	3
Extension (pain)	2
None	1

Glasgow Coma Score Total	**15**

Figure 5-13   The Glasgow Coma Scale.

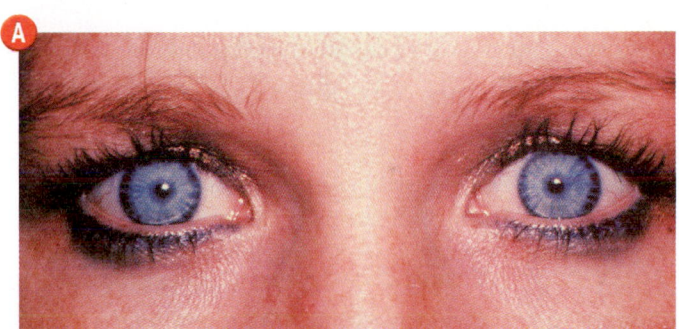
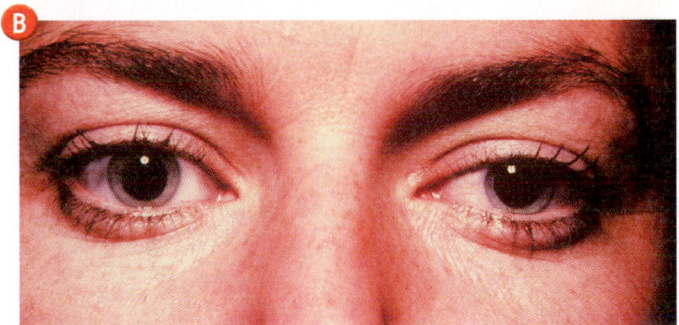
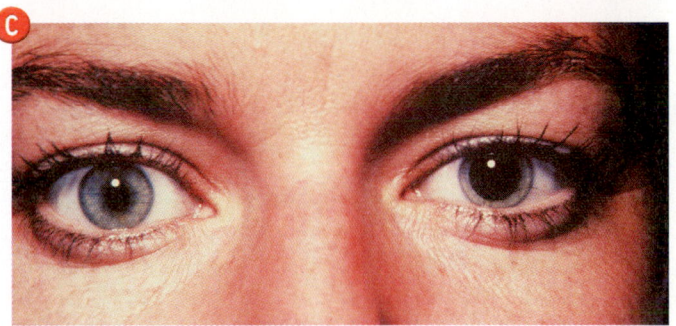

Figure 5-14   **A.** Constricted pupils. **B.** Dilated pupils. **C.** Unequal pupils.

You must assume the patient has depressed brain function as a result of either central nervous system depression or injury if the pupils react in any of the following ways:

- Become fixed with no reaction to light
- Dilate with introduction of a bright light and constrict when the light is removed
- React sluggishly instead of briskly
- Become unequal in size ◄ **Figure 5-14C**
- Become unequal in size when a bright light is introduced into or removed from one eye

Depressed brain function can be produced by the following situations:

- Injury of the brain or brain stem
- Trauma or stroke
- Brain tumor
- Inadequate oxygenation or perfusion
- Drugs or toxins (central nervous system depressants)

Opiates, and/or narcotic pain medications, which are one category of central nervous system depressants, cause the pupils to constrict so significantly, regardless of light, that they become so small as to be described as pinpoint. Intracranial pressure from intracranial bleeding may cause sufficient pressure against the oculomotor nerve on one side that the motor commands can no longer pass from the brain to that eye. When this occurs, the eye no longer receives commands to constrict, and its pupil becomes fully dilated and fixed. This is described as a blown pupil.

Pupils may be dilated, may be unequal as a result of medication placed into one or both eyes or from an injury or condition of the eye, or may not be reacting appropriately.

The letters PEARRL serve as a useful guide in assessing the pupils. They stand for the following:

P = **P**upils

E = **E**qual

A = **A**nd

R = **R**ound

R = **R**egular in size

L = react to **L**ight

You can report patients with normal pupils as "Pupils are equal, round, and regular in size, and react properly to light" or "pupils = PEARRL." Describe any abnormal findings using the longer form, such as "Pupils are equal and round, the left pupil is fixed and dilated, the right pupil is regular in size and reacts to light."

Reassessment of the Vital Signs

The vital signs that you obtain serve two important functions. The first set establishes an important initial measurement of the patient's respiratory and cardio-vascular systems and the quality of perfusion and oxygenation of the brain and other vital organs. The initial vital signs serve as a key baseline.

Throughout your care of the patient, you should monitor the patient's vital signs for any changes from your initial findings. You should reassess and record vital signs at least every 15 minutes in a stable patient and at least every 5 minutes in an unstable patient. You should also reassess and record vital signs following all medical interventions. This ongoing comparative assessment is an important indicator of whether your interventions have restored the patient's vital functions to an acceptable range or are at least preventing further deterioration. Reassessment also indicates whether you should consider more aggressive intervention whenever deterioration continues.

Obtaining a SAMPLE History

Once you have provided emergency care and are ready to further examine the patient, you should try to obtain a key brief history, or **SAMPLE history**. As part of the assessment of every patient, you should ask the following questions, using the word SAMPLE as a guideline:

- **S**igns and **S**ymptoms of the episode: What signs and symptoms occurred at onset of the incident? Does the patient report pain?

- **A**llergies: Is the patient allergic to any medication, food, or other substance? What reactions did the patient have to any of them? If the patient has no known allergies, you should note this on the run report as "no known allergies" or "nka."

- **M**edications: What medications was the patient prescribed? What dosage was prescribed? How often is the patient supposed to take the medication? What prescription and over-the-counter medications has the patient taken in the last 12 hours? How much was taken and when?

- **P**ertinent past history: Does the patient have any history of medical, surgical, or trauma occurrences? Has the patient had a recent accident, fall, or blow to the head?

You should reassess and record vital signs at least every 15 minutes in a stable patient and at least every 5 minutes in an unstable patient. Remember, your primary concern in the outdoor environment is expedient transport.

- **L**ast oral intake: When did the patient last eat or drink? What did the patient eat or drink and how much was consumed? Did the patient take any drugs or drink alcohol? Has there been any other oral intake in the last 4 hours?

- **E**vents leading to the injury or illness: What are the key events that led up to this incident? What occurred between the onset of the incident and your arrival? What was the patient doing when this illness started? What was the patient doing when this injury happened?

With practice, you will be able to obtain, document, and report a meaningful brief history. Be sure to ask the patient and bystanders for information. If the patient is unconscious, look for a medical identification tag or for a medical information card in the patient's wallet or purse. *Always* look for patient identification in the presence of another rescuer at the scene.

Chapter *Sweep*

Ready for Review

Whenever you are called to the scene of an illness or injury, you should find out the patient's chief complaint. Your assessment of the patient should include rapidly evaluating the patient's general condition and identifying any potentially life-threatening injuries or conditions. Baseline vital signs are the key signs that you will use to evaluate the patient's general condition. You will be assessing the patient's respirations, pulse, skin, blood pressure, level of consciousness, and pupils.

After you have initially assessed the patient and obtained the baseline vital signs, you should reassess the patient for any changes from your initial findings.

In addition to determining the chief complaint and assessing the patient's general condition, you should try to obtain a SAMPLE history from the patient or bystanders. By asking several important questions, you will be able to determine the patient's signs and symptoms, allergies, medications, pertinent past history, last oral intake, and the events leading up to the incident.

Vital Vocabulary

auscultation A method of listening to sounds within an organ with a stethoscope.

AVPU scale A method of assessing level of consciousness by determining whether the patient is awake and alert, responsive to verbal stimulus or pain, or unresponsive; used principally in the initial assessment.

blood pressure (BP) The pressure of circulating blood against the walls of the arteries.

bradycardia Slow heart rate, less than 60 beats/min.

capillary refill A test that evaluates the ability of the circulatory system to restore blood to the capillary system.

chief complaint The reason a patient called for help. Also, the patient's response to questions such as "What's wrong?" or "What happened?"

conjunctiva The delicate membrane lining the eyelids and covering the exposed surface of the eye.

cyanosis A bluish-gray skin color that is caused by reduced levels of oxygen in the blood.

diaphoretic Characterized by profuse sweating.

diastolic pressure The pressure that remains in the arteries during the relaxing phase of the heart's cycle (diastole) when the left ventricle is at rest.

Glasgow Coma Scale A method of assessing a patient's level of consciousness by scoring the patient's response to eye opening, motor response, and verbal response.

hypertension Blood pressure that is higher than the normal range.

hypotension Blood pressure that is lower than the normal range.

jaundice A yellow skin or sclera color that is caused by liver disease or dysfunction.

labored breathing Breathing that requires visibly increased effort; characterized by grunting, stridor, and use of accessory muscles.

perfusion Circulation of blood within an organ or tissue.

pulse The pressure wave that occurs as each heartbeat causes a surge in the blood circulating through the arteries.

SAMPLE history A brief history of a patient's condition to determine signs and symptoms, allergies, medications, pertinent past history, last oral intake, and events leading to the injury or illness.

sclera The white portion of the eye.

sign An objective finding that can be seen, heard, felt, smelled, or measured.

sniffing position An upright position in which the patient's head and chin are thrust slightly forward and the patient appears to be sniffing; most commonly seen in children.

spontaneous respirations Breathing in a patient that occurs with no assistance.

stridor A harsh, high-pitched, crowing inspiratory sound, such as the sound often heard in acute laryngeal (upper airway) obstruction.

symptom A subjective finding that the patient feels but that can be identified only by the patient.

systolic pressure The increased pressure along an artery with each contraction (systole) of the ventricle.

tachycardia Rapid heart rhythm, more than 100 beats/min.

tidal volume The amount of air that is exchanged with each breath.

tripod position An upright position where the patient leans forward onto outstretched arms and thrusts the head and chin slightly forward.

vital signs The key signs that are used to evaluate the patient's overall condition, including respirations, pulse, blood pressure, level of consciousness, and skin characteristics.

www.OECzone.com

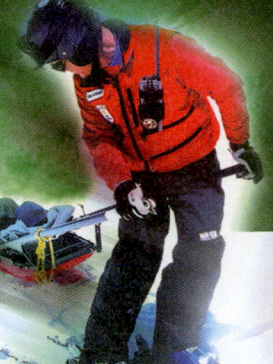

Assessment in Action

A 36-year-old patient complains that she "does not feel well." She is alert and oriented but you note that she is sitting in a tripod position. She appears pale but her lips are gray and her skin is pale, cool, and clammy.

She has no allergies but has a history of asthma and is on a Proventil inhaler. She has a blood pressure of 162/98 mm Hg, a pulse rate of 102 beats/min, and respirations of 28 breaths/min.

1. The A in SAMPLE History refers to:
   A. age.
   B. affect.
   C. attitude.
   D. allergies.

2. The tripod position usually suggests that the patient may have:
   A. difficulty sitting up.
   B. difficulty lying down.
   C. difficulty breathing.
   D. weakness or dizziness.

3. In this patient, which of the following assessment signs suggests poor perfusion?
   A. BP of 162/98
   B. Gray lips
   C. Pulse 102
   D. Tripod position

4. When getting a history, you note that she can only talk in two- to three-word sentences. Other signs of difficulty breathing you should be looking for include:
   A. accessory muscle use.
   B. difficulty sitting up.
   C. extremity paralysis.
   D. flushed face.

5. Of all the signs of difficulty breathing, which are specific for a child?
   A. Cyanosis
   B. Nasal flaring
   C. Mottled skin
   D. Fever

6. Finding the brachial pulse in an infant may be made easier by:
   A. placing the infant in a sitting position.
   B. lowering the infant's arm.
   C. raising the infant's arm.
   D. tilting the infant's head down.

7. This patient's BP is a little high. One thing that can cause a false high blood pressure is:
   A. a cuff that is too small.
   B. a cuff that is too large.
   C. using the bell of the stethoscope.
   D. using the diaphragm of the stethoscope.

8. This patient is alert, oriented, and squeezes your hands when asked. Her Glasgow Coma Scale score would be:
   A. 0   C. 10
   B. 3   D. 15

Challenging Questions

9. If a patient can talk in a complete sentence, what assumption can be made about tidal volume?

10. When a patient is verbally unresponsive, why should a painful stimulus be tried on both sides of the body?

Points to Ponder

The sheriff's department dispatches the local search and rescue unit to an out-of-bounds patient complaining of abdominal pain. After locating the incident scene, you are required to hike back uphill to assess the patient. Your partner complains about having to traverse uphill with a toboggan loaded with extra equipment. Your partner mumbles, "Let's leave him here until spring!" Hoping to keep your partner quiet, you suggest he take a set of vital signs. Your partner then replies that if the patient had stayed in bounds, no one would have to be here. How and when would you deal with your partner?

Issues Patient Respect, Personal Biases and Prejudices, Appropriate Discussions in Front of Non-Prehospital Care Personnel.

Online Outlook

If time permits, you should attempt to learn the patient's SAMPLE history. Improve your ability to identify SAMPLE information by completing Exercise 5 at www.OECzone.com.

www.OECzone.com

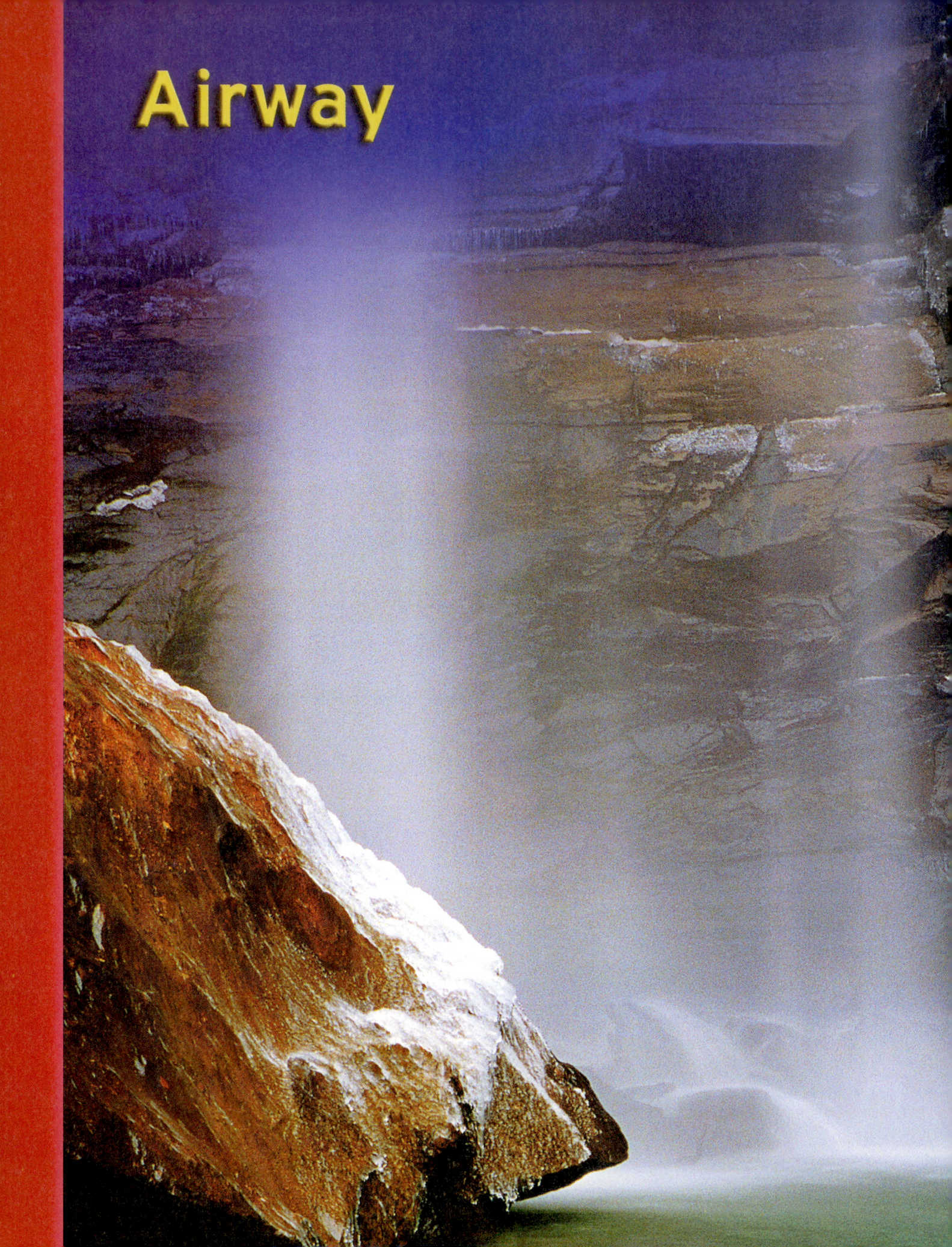

Airway

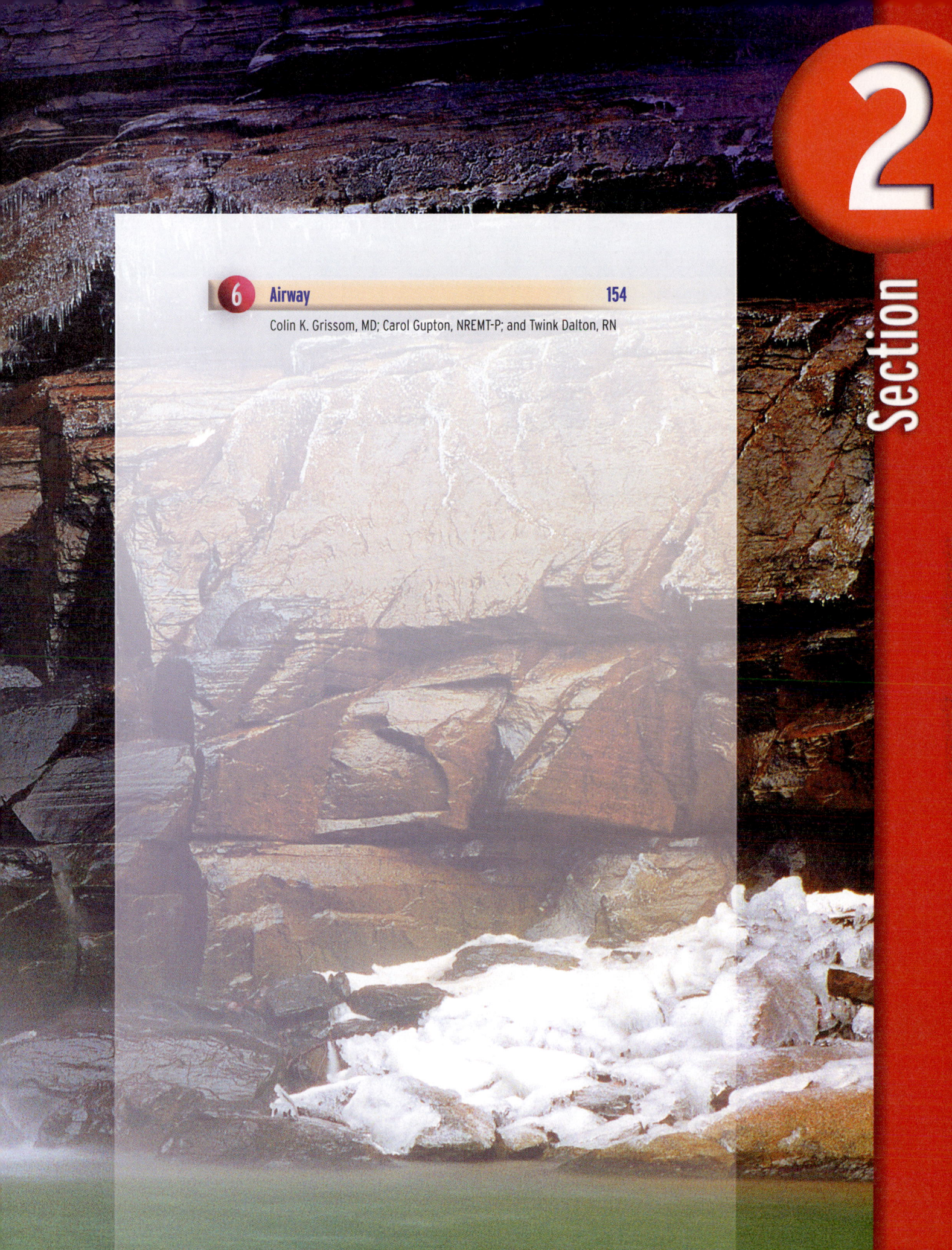

Airway

Objectives

Cognitive

1. Name and label the major structures of the respiratory system on a diagram (p 157).
2. List the signs of adequate breathing (p 162).
3. List the signs of inadequate breathing (p 162).
4. Describe the steps in performing the head tilt-chin lift maneuver (p 165).
5. Relate mechanism of injury to opening the airway (p 163).
6. Describe the steps in performing the jaw-thrust maneuver (p 165).
7. State the importance of having a suction unit ready for immediate use when providing emergency care (p 169).
8. Describe the techniques of suctioning (p 170).
9. Describe how to artificially ventilate a patient with a pocket mask (p 179).
10. Describe the steps in performing the skill of artificially ventilating a patient with a bag-valve-mask device while using the jaw-thrust maneuver (p 181).
11. List the parts of a bag-valve-mask system (p 180).
12. Describe the steps in performing the skill of artificially ventilating a patient with a bag-valve-mask device for one and two rescuers (p 181).
13. Describe the signs of adequate artificial ventilation using the bag-valve-mask device (p 182).
14. Describe the signs of inadequate artificial ventilation using the bag-valve-mask device (p 182).
15. Describe the steps in ventilating a patient with a flow-restricted, oxygen-powered ventilation device (p 183).
16. List the steps in performing the actions taken when providing mouth-to-mouth and mouth-to-stoma artificial ventilation (p 185).
17. Describe how to measure and insert an oropharyngeal (oral) airway (p 167).
18. Describe how to measure and insert a nasopharyngeal (nasal) airway (p 168).
19. Describe how to perform the Sellick maneuver (cricoid pressure) (p 183).
20. Define the components of an oxygen delivery system (p 172).
21. Identify a nonrebreathing face mask and state the oxygen flow requirements needed for its use (p 177).
22. Describe the indications for using a nasal cannula versus a nonrebreathing face mask (p 177).
23. Identify a nasal cannula and state the flow requirements needed for its use (p 177).

Affective

24. Explain the rationale for basic life support, artificial ventilation, and airway protective skills taking priority over most other basic life support skills (p 156).
25. Explain the rationale for providing adequate oxygenation through high inspired oxygen concentrations to patients who, in the past, may have received low concentrations (p 180).

Psychomotor

26. Demonstrate the steps in performing the head tilt-chin lift maneuver (p 165).
27. Demonstrate the steps in performing the jaw-thrust maneuver (p 165).
28. Demonstrate the techniques of suctioning (p 170).
29. Demonstrate the steps in providing mouth-to-mouth artificial ventilation with body substance isolation (barrier shields) (p 179).
30. Demonstrate how to use a pocket mask to artificially ventilate a patient (p 179).
31. Demonstrate the assembly of a bag-valve-mask unit (p 180).
32. Demonstrate the steps in performing the skill of artificially ventilating a patient with a bag-valve-mask device for one and two rescuers (p 181).
33. Demonstrate the steps in performing the skill of artificially ventilating a patient with a bag-valve-mask device while using the jaw-thrust maneuver (p 181).
34. Demonstrate artificial ventilation of a patient with a flow-restricted, oxygen-powered ventilation device (p 184).
35. Demonstrate how to artificially ventilate a patient with a stoma (p 185).
36. Demonstrate how to insert an oropharyngeal (oral) airway (p 167).
37. Demonstrate how to insert a nasopharyngeal (nasal) airway (p 168).
38. Demonstrate the correct operation of oxygen tanks and regulators (p 172).
39. Demonstrate the use of a nonbreathing face mask and state the oxygen flow requirements needed for its use (p 177).
40. Demonstrate the use of a nasal cannula and state the flow requirements needed for its use (p 177).
41. Demonstrate how to artificially ventilate the infant and child patient (p 179).
42. Demonstrate oxygen administration for the infant and child patient (p. 181)

🌲 These are core concepts in initial patrol training.

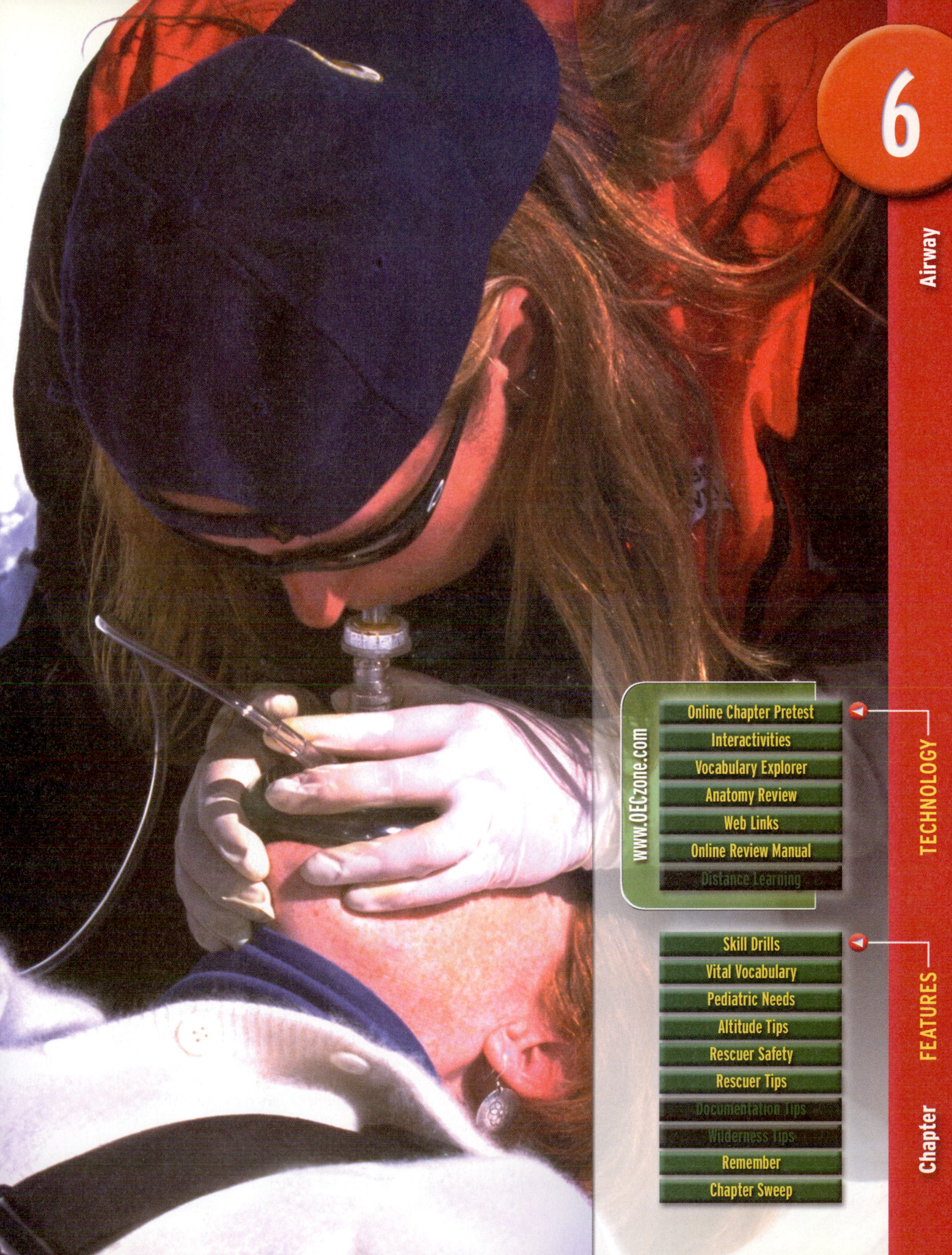

www.OECzone.com

Chapter

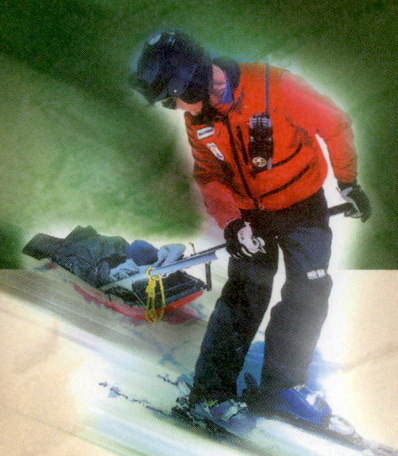

"Patrol 3, respond to the mid-mountain restaurant for a girl having difficulty breathing."
You arrive to find a very pale, frightened-looking girl sitting upright at a bench on the
outdoor deck struggling to breathe.

Airway and breathing problems are important for the outdoor rescuer to recognize and treat appropriately because they may be life threatening. In the ABCs, assessment of the airway and breathing come first.

1. Why does airway and breathing assessment and care have such a prominent position in the realm of a rescuer's scope of practice?

2. Is it necessary that you be familiar with all the airway equipment available at your aid room, or just that which you personally like to use?

Airway

The single most important step in caring for any patient is to make sure that he or she can breathe. The patient who cannot breathe properly is not delivering oxygen to body tissues and cells, which need a constant supply of oxygen to survive. Severe airway and breathing problems may deprive the heart of oxygen and result in an abnormal heart rhythm or cardiac arrest.

Oxygen reaches body tissues and cells through two separate but related processes: breathing and circulation. As we inhale, oxygen moves from the atmosphere into our lungs, then passes from the air sacs in the lungs into the capillaries to oxygenate the blood. The blood, enriched with oxygen, travels through the body by the pumping action of the heart. At the same time, carbon dioxide, produced by cells in the tissues of the body, moves from the blood into the air sacs. The carbon dioxide then leaves our bodies as we exhale.

As a rescuer, you must be able to locate the parts of the respiratory system, understand how the system works, and be able to recognize which patients are breathing adequately and which ones are breathing inadequately. This will enable you to determine how best to treat your patient.

This chapter will review the anatomy and physiology of the respiratory system, that is, the parts of the system and how they work. It will then describe how to assess patients quickly and carefully to determine their airway and ventilation status. The equipment, procedures, and guidelines that you will need to manage a patient's airway and breathing are described in detail. You will learn several ways to open a patient's airway and specific techniques for removing foreign objects or fluids that may be blocking the airway. Because artificial airway equipment can have serious results if used improperly, the chapter will thoroughly discuss airway adjuncts, oxygen therapy devices, and artificial ventilation methods.

Anatomy of the Respiratory System

The respiratory system consists of all the structures in the body that make up the airway and help us breathe, or ventilate ▶ Figure 6-1 . Structures that help us breathe include the diaphragm, the muscles of the chest wall, accessory muscles of breathing, and the nerves from the brain and spinal cord to those muscles. **Ventilation** is the exchange of air between the lungs and environment. The diaphragm and muscles of the chest wall are responsible for the regular rise and fall of the chest that accompany normal breathing.

Structures of the Airway

The **airway** is divided into both upper and lower airways. The upper airway consists of the nose, mouth, throat (pharynx), and a structure called the epiglottis. The epiglottis is a leaf-shaped structure above the larynx that prevents food and liquid from entering the larynx during swallowing. The portion of the throat behind the nose is the nasopharynx; the portion behind the mouth is the oropharynx.

The lower airway consists of the larynx, trachea, main bronchi, smaller bronchi, and the alveoli, small sacs where the actual exchange of oxygen and carbon dioxide occur.

The lower airway begins with the larynx (voice box/vocal cords). The cricoid cartilage is a firm cartilage ring that forms the lower part of the larynx. The trachea is directly connected to the larynx. The main bronchi and smaller bronchioles branch off from the trachea, extending into each lung. Eventually the smaller bronchioles end in the alveoli.

The chest (thoracic cage) contains the lungs, one in each half ▶ Figure 6-2 . The lungs hang freely within the chest cavity. Between the lungs is a space called the

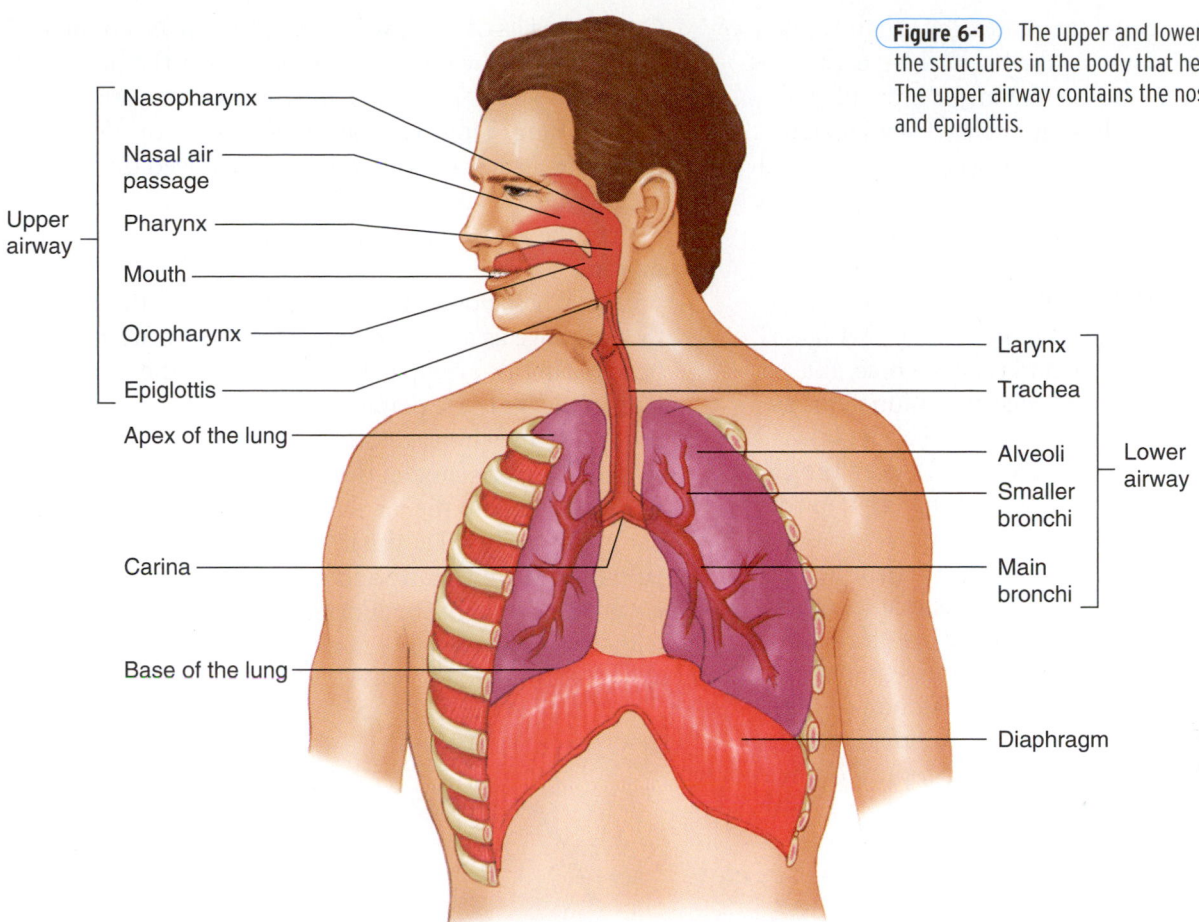

Figure 6-1 The upper and lower airways contain the structures in the body that help us to breathe. The upper airway contains the nose, mouth, throat, and epiglottis.

Nasopharynx

Nasal air passage

Pharynx

Mouth

Oropharynx

Epiglottis

Upper airway

Apex of the lung

Carina

Base of the lung

Larynx

Trachea

Alveoli

Smaller bronchi

Main bronchi

Lower airway

Diaphragm

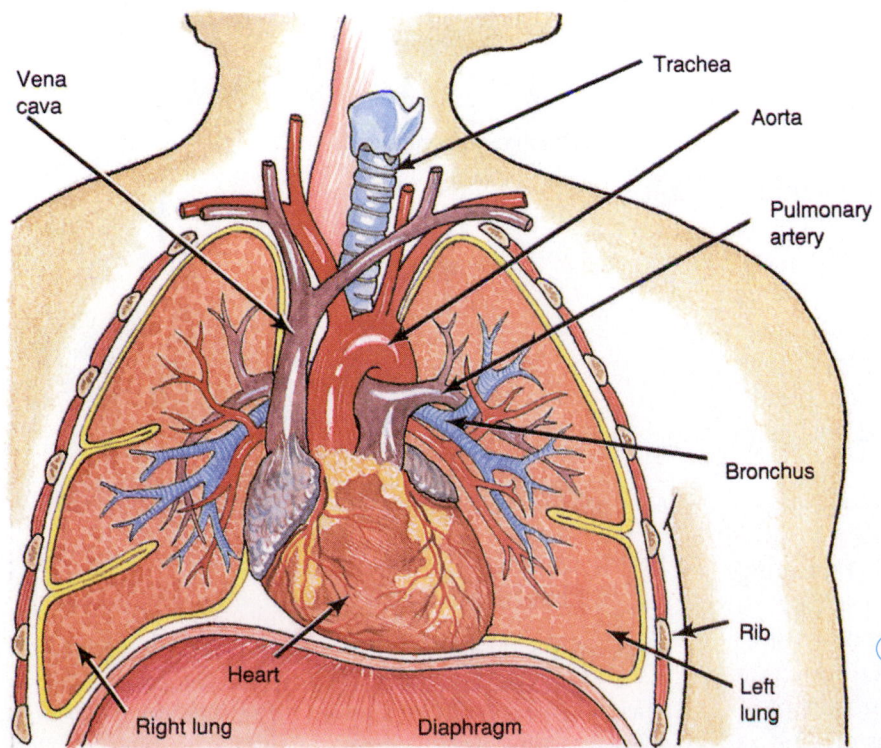

Vena cava

Trachea

Aorta

Pulmonary artery

Bronchus

Rib

Left lung

Heart

Right lung

Diaphragm

Figure 6-2 The thoracic cage contains important anatomic structures for respiration, including the lungs, the heart, the great vessels (the vena cava and aorta), the trachea, and the major bronchi.

mediastinum, which is surrounded by tough connective tissue. This space contains the heart, the great vessels, the esophagus, the trachea, the major bronchi, and many nerves. The mediastinum effectively separates the right lung space from the left lung space. The boundaries of the thorax are the rib cage anteriorly, superiorly, and posteriorly and the diaphragm inferiorly.

Structures of Breathing

The diaphragm is a skeletal muscle because it is attached to the costal arch and the vertebrae. It is considered a specialized muscle because it functions as both a voluntary and an involuntary muscle. It acts as a voluntary muscle whenever we take a deep breath, cough, or hold our breath—actions that we control. However, unlike other skeletal or voluntary muscles, the diaphragm also performs an automatic function. Breathing continues while we sleep and at all other times. Even though we can hold our breath or temporarily breathe more slowly, we cannot continue this indefinitely. When the concentration of carbon dioxide rises within the blood, the automatic regulation of breathing resumes under the control of the brain stem.

The lungs, because they have no muscle tissue, cannot move on their own. They need the help of other structures to be able to expand and contract as we inhale and exhale. Therefore, the ability of the lungs to function properly is partially dependent on the movement of the chest and supporting structures. These structures include the thorax, the thoracic cage (chest), the diaphragm, the intercostal muscles, and the accessory muscles of breathing.

Inhalation

The active, muscular part of breathing is called **inhalation**. As we inhale, air enters the body through the trachea. This air travels to and from the lungs, filling and emptying the alveoli. During inhalation, the diaphragm and intercostal muscles contract. When the diaphragm contracts, it moves down slightly and enlarges the thoracic cage from top to bottom. When the intercostal muscles contract, they raise the ribs up and out. As we inhale, the combined actions of these structures enlarge the thorax in all directions. Take a deep breath to see how your chest expands.

The air pressure outside the body is called the atmospheric pressure. As we inhale and the thoracic cage expands, the air pressure within the thorax decreases, creating a slight vacuum. This drives air in through the trachea and fills the lungs. When the air pressure outside equals the air pressure inside, air stops moving.

Gases, such as oxygen, will move from an area of high pressure to an area of lower pressure until the pressures are equal. At this point, the air stops moving, and we stop inhaling. **Tidal volume**, a measure of the depth of breathing, is the amount of air that is moved during one breath. Minute volume is tidal volume times respiratory rate, or the amount of air moved through the lungs in 1 minute.

It may help you to understand this if you think of the thoracic cage as a bell jar in which balloons are suspended. In this example, the balloons are the lungs. The base of the jar is the diaphragm, which moves up and down slightly with each breath. The ribs, which are the sides of the jar, maintain the shape of the chest. The only opening into the jar is a small tube at the top, similar to the trachea. During inhalation, the bottom of the jar moves down slightly and decreases pressure in the jar, creating a slight vacuum. As a result, the balloons fill with air (▼ Figure 6-3).

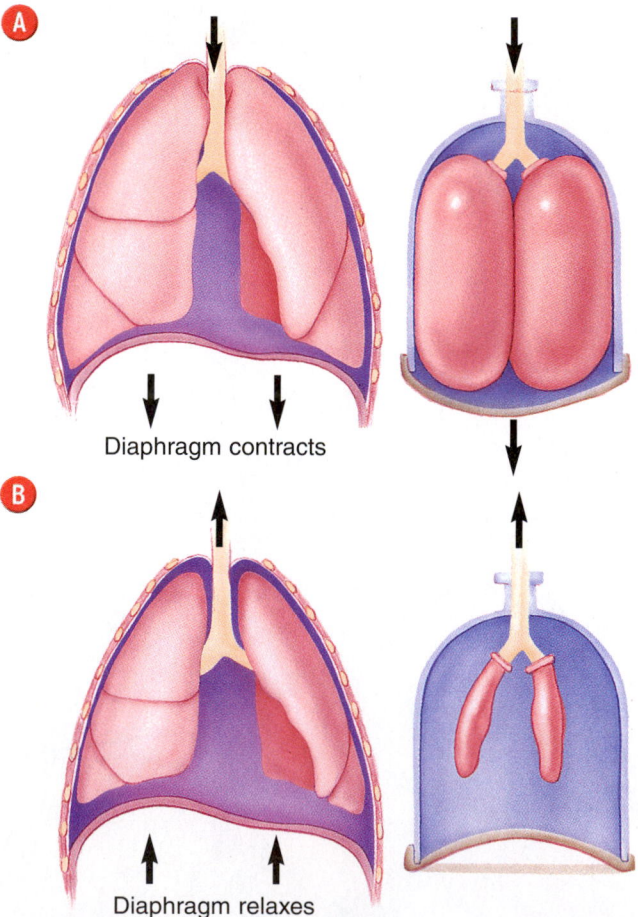

Diaphragm contracts

Diaphragm relaxes

Figure 6-3   The mechanisms of respiration can be compared with that of a bell jar. **A.** Inhalation and chest expansion, anatomic (left) and bell jar (right). **B.** Exhalation and chest contraction, anatomic (left) and bell jar (right).

Exhalation

Unlike inhalation, exhalation does not normally require muscular effort. During **exhalation**, the diaphragm and the intercostal muscles relax. In response, the thorax decreases in size, and the ribs and muscles assume a normal resting position. When the size of the thoracic cage decreases, air in the lungs is compressed into a smaller space. The air pressure within the thorax then becomes higher than the pressure outside, and air is pushed out through the trachea.

Let's return to the example of the bell jar. During exhalation, the bottom of the jar (the diaphragm) moves up, returning to its normal resting position. This movement increases air pressure within the jar. With this increase in pressure, the sides of the jar contract, and the balloons empty.

Remember that air will reach the lungs only if it travels through the trachea. This is why clearing and maintaining an open airway are so important. Clearing the airway means removing obstructing material, tissue, or fluids from the nose, mouth, or throat. Maintaining the airway means keeping the airway open so that air can enter and leave the lungs freely (▼ Figure 6-4).

Air may also pass into the chest cavity through another opening in the throat or chest wall as a result of trauma, keeping air from reaching the alveoli. In Chapter 22, Chest Injuries, you will learn how to recognize and manage these conditions.

Physiology of the Respiratory System

All living cells need energy to survive. Cells take energy from nutrients through a series of chemical processes. The name given to these processes as a whole is **metabolism**. During metabolism, each cell combines nutrients and oxygen and produces energy and waste products, primarily water and carbon dioxide.

Each living cell in the body requires a supply of oxygen and a regular means of getting rid of waste (carbon dioxide). The body provides these through respiration. Some cells need a constant supply of oxygen to survive. Other cells in the body can tolerate short periods without oxygen and still survive. For example, after 4 to 6 minutes without oxygen, brain cells and cells in the nervous system may be severely and permanently damaged and may even die (▼ Figure 6-5). Dead brain cells can never be replaced. However, cells in the kidney may be without oxygen for 45 minutes or more and still survive. This is why certain organ transplants are possible.

Normally, the air that we breathe contains 21% oxygen and 78% nitrogen. Small amounts of other gases make up the remaining 1%.

The Exchange of Oxygen and Carbon Dioxide

As blood travels through the body, it supplies oxygen and nutrients to various tissues and cells. Oxygen

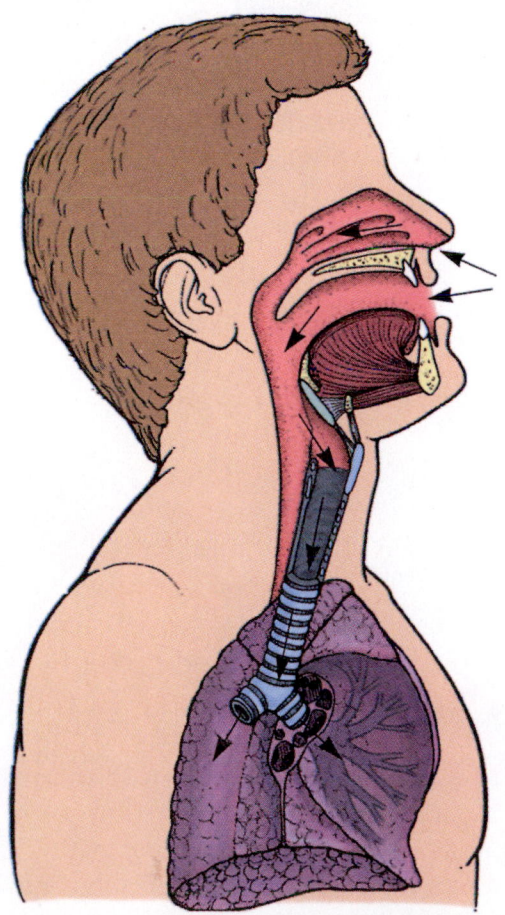

Figure 6-4 Air reaches the lungs only if it travels through the trachea. Maintaining the airway means keeping the airway open so that air can enter and leave the lungs freely.

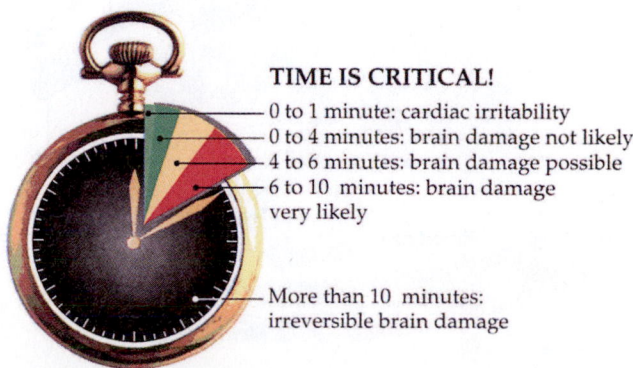

Figure 6-5 Cells need a constant supply of oxygen to survive. Some cells may be severely and permanently damaged after 4 to 6 minutes without oxygen following respiratory and cardiac arrest.

passes from the blood through the capillaries to tissue cells, while carbon dioxide and cell waste pass in the opposite direction: from tissue cells through capillaries to the blood (▼ **Figure 6-6**).

Each time we inhale, the alveoli receive a supply of oxygen-rich air. The alveoli are surrounded by a network of tiny pulmonary capillaries. These capillaries are, in fact, located in the walls of the alveoli. This means that the air in the alveoli and the blood in the capillaries are separated only by two very thin layers of wall tissue. Each time we exhale, the carbon dioxide from the bloodstream travels across the same two layers of tissue to the alveoli and is expelled into the atmosphere.

Oxygen and carbon dioxide pass rapidly across the walls of the alveoli and the capillaries through diffusion. **Diffusion** is a passive process in which molecules move from an area with higher concentration of molecules to an area of lower concentration. For example, when we walk into a kitchen and it smells like a rotten egg, that is because the molecules of hydrogen sulfide gas have moved spontaneously from an area of high concentration near the egg to fill the whole space. Molecules of oxygen move from the alveoli into the blood because there are fewer oxygen molecules in the blood. In the same way, molecules of carbon dioxide move from the blood into the alveoli because there are fewer carbon dioxide molecules in the alveoli (▶ **Figure 6-7**).

The alveoli produce a chemical, called surfactant, which lines the inside of the alveoli and creates surface tension to hold the alveoli open. This allows carbon

dioxide to diffuse from the capillary blood into the alveoli, and allows oxygen to diffuse from the alveoli into the capillary blood. Anything that removes surfactant (such as water from a drowning) will cause the alveoli to collapse, interfere with diffusion of oxygen and carbon dioxide, and result in acute respiratory distress.

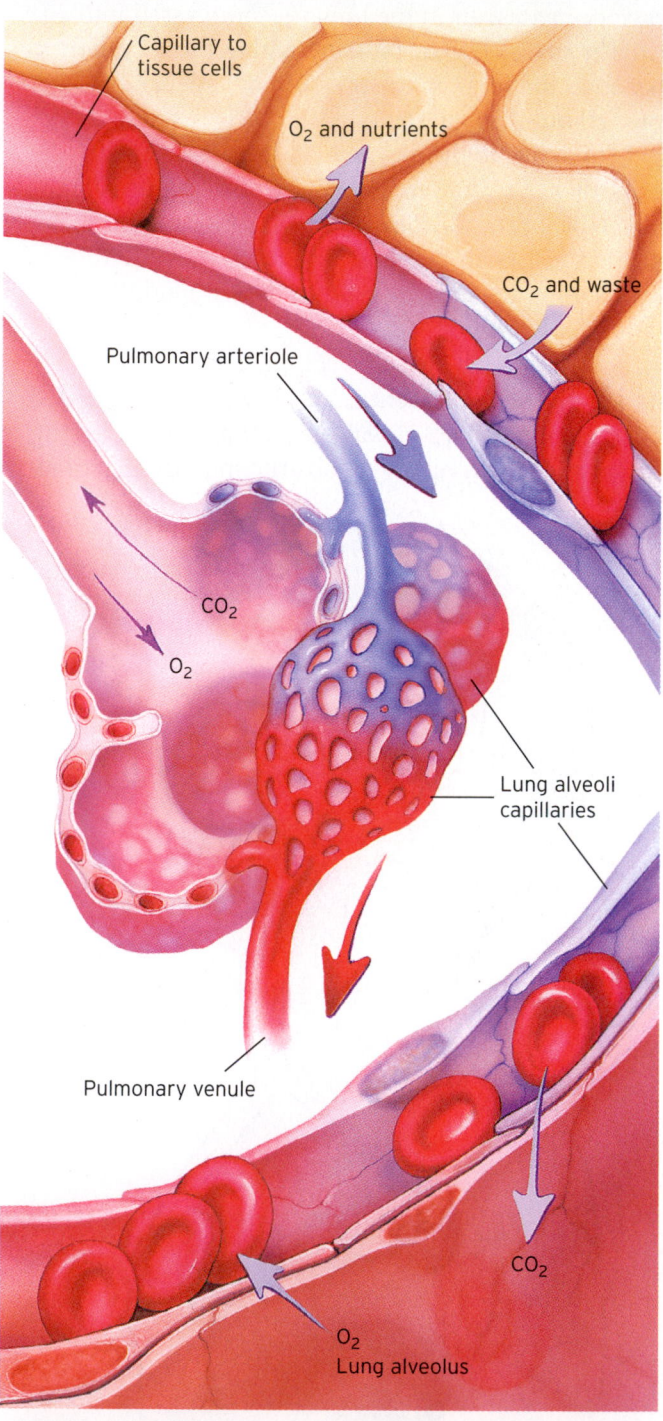

Figure 6-7 With diffusion, molecules of oxygen move from the alveoli into the blood, because there are fewer oxygen molecules in the blood. Similarly, molecules of carbon dioxide move from the blood into the alveoli, because there are fewer carbon dioxide molecules in the alveoli.

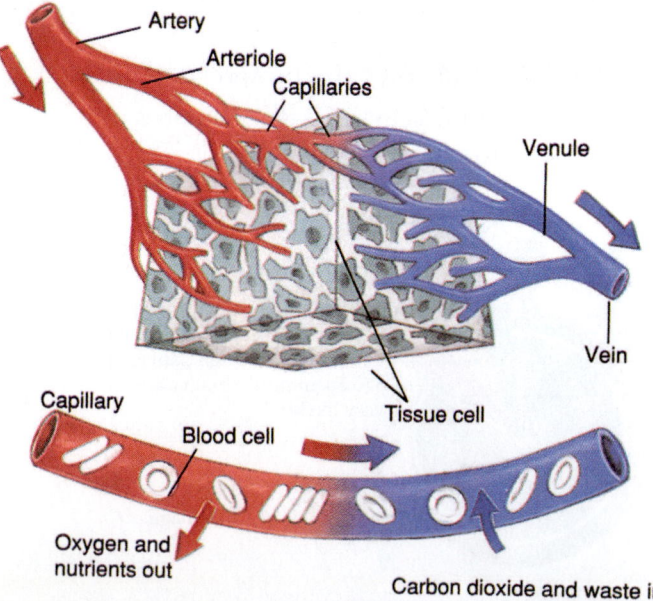

Figure 6-6 Oxygen passes from the blood through capillaries to tissue cells. Carbon dioxide passes from tissue cells through capillaries to the blood.

The blood does not use all the inhaled oxygen as it passes through the body. So the air that we exhale contains 16% oxygen and 3% to 5% carbon dioxide; the rest is nitrogen (▼ **Figure 6-8**). Therefore, when you provide artificial ventilations to a patient who is not breathing, that patient is receiving a 16% concentration of oxygen with each of your exhaled breaths.

The Control of Breathing

The area of the brain stem that controls breathing is deep within the skull, in one of the best-protected parts of the nervous system. The nerves in this area act as sensors, reacting primarily to the level of carbon dioxide in the arterial blood. If the levels of carbon dioxide are too high or too low, the brain automatically adjusts breathing. This happens very quickly, in just one breath. Again, this is why you cannot hold your breath indefinitely or breathe rapidly and deeply for very long. In a healthy person, the stimulus to breathe is referred to as the normal respiratory drive.

When the level of carbon dioxide becomes too high, the brain stem sends nerve impulses down the spinal cord that cause the diaphragm and the intercostal muscles to contract. This increases our breathing, or respirations. The higher the level of carbon dioxide in the blood, the stronger the impulses to cause breathing. Once the carbon dioxide returns to an acceptable level, the strength and frequency of respiration decrease.

We also have a "backup system" to control respiration, called the **hypoxic drive**. This system stimulates breathing when oxygen levels fall (hypoxia). Although the brain stem senses low oxygen and increases breathing, the primary receptors for the hypoxic drive are located in the carotid bodies, a group of nerves at the bifurcation of the common carotid artery in the neck. The hypoxic drive is important at high altitudes where the lower oxygen pressures in inhaled air result in lower oxygen in the blood and stimulate the brain stem and carotid bodies to increase breathing.

HYPOXIA. **Hypoxia** is an extremely dangerous condition in which the body's tissues and cells do not have enough oxygen. Hypoxia develops quickly in the vital organs of patients who are not breathing adequately, as well as in those who are not breathing at all. Inadequate breathing means that the person cannot move enough air into the lungs with each breath to meet the body's needs.

Patients who are breathing inadequately will show varying signs and symptoms of inadequate breathing (hypoxia). The onset and the degree of tissue damage will depend on the quality of ventilations. The signs of hypoxia may include mental status changes, the use of accessory muscles for breathing, difficulty breathing, possibly chest pain, and, late in the process, cyanosis. Early signs include nervousness, irritability, apprehension, fast heart rate (tachycardia), and fear. Conscious patients will complain of shortness of breath and may not be able to talk in complete sentences. The best time to give a patient oxygen is before any signs and symptoms appear.

The following conditions are commonly associated with hypoxia:

- **Aspiration.** Contents from the stomach are inhaled into the lung. This may occur with vomiting, trauma, or in a patient with a depressed level of consciousness (such as in a head injury or stroke).

- **Pulmonary edema.** Fluid accumulates in the lungs, making the transfer of oxygen to the blood from the alveoli less efficient. Pulmonary edema can occur in the setting of chronic heart failure, acute myocardial infarction (heart

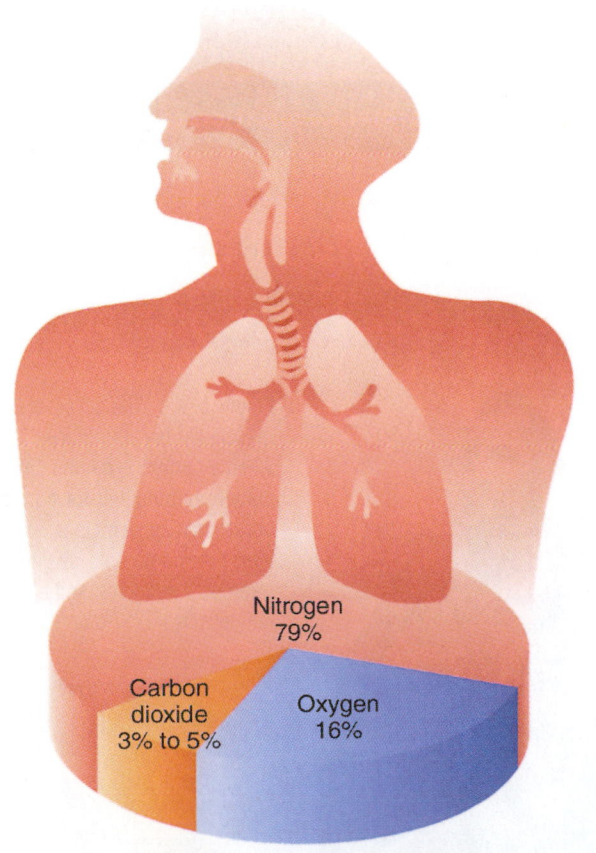

Nitrogen 79%

Carbon dioxide 3% to 5%

Oxygen 16%

Components of Exhaled Air

Figure 6-8 Exhaled air contains 16% oxygen and 3% to 5% carbon dioxide; 79% is nitrogen.

attack), cardiac arrest, or after rapid ascent to high altitude (high altitude pulmonary edema).

- **Blunt chest injury.** May cause bruising of the lung (pulmonary contusion), or collapse of the lung (pneumothorax), or fractured ribs (flail chest) that interfere with gas exchange.

- **Penetrating chest injury.** May cause bleeding in the lung or collapse of a lung (pneumothorax) that interferes with gas exchange.

- **Shock (hypoperfusion).** Shock often occurs as a result of injuries involving substantial blood loss. With the loss of red blood cells, not enough oxygen is available to the tissues.

- **Inhalation of smoke and/or toxic fumes.** These substances cause pulmonary edema and destroy lung tissue, causing problems with gas exchange.

- **Asthma.** Narrowing of respiratory passages and buildup of mucus causes air trapping and poor gas exchange.

- **Chronic obstructive pulmonary disease (chronic bronchitis and emphysema).** Chronic irritation of the lungs and air passages produces alveolar damage and poor gas exchange.

- **Pneumonia.** Infection in the lung causes inflammation that interferes with gas exchange.

All hypoxic patients, whatever the cause of their condition, should be treated with high-flow supplemental oxygen. The method of oxygen delivery will vary, depending on the cause and the severity of the hypoxia.

Patient Assessment

Recognizing Adequate Breathing

Earlier, we compared breathing to an expandable bell jar with a movable bottom. You can also think of a normal breathing pattern as a bellows system. Breathing should appear easy, not labored. As with a bellows used to move air to start a fire, breathing should be a smooth flow of air moving into and out of the lungs. Signs of normal (adequate) breathing for adult patients are listed below:

- A normal rate and depth (between 12 and 20 breaths/min) for adults

- A regular pattern of inhalation and exhalation

- Clear and equal lung sounds on both sides of the chest (**bilateral**)

- Regular and equal chest rise and fall (chest expansion)

- Adequate depth (tidal volume)

Recognizing Inadequate Breathing

An adult who is awake, alert, and talking to you has no immediate airway or breathing problems. However, you should always have supplemental oxygen close at hand to assist with breathing if this becomes necessary. An adult who is breathing normally will have respirations of 12 to 20 breaths/min (▼ Table 6-1). The adult patient who is breathing either much slower (fewer than 8 breaths/min) or much faster (more than 24 breaths/min) should be evaluated for inadequate breathing.

A patient with inadequate breathing may appear to be working hard to breathe. This type of breathing pattern is called **labored breathing**. It requires effort and, especially among children, may involve the accessory muscles. Accessory muscles are secondary muscles of respiration. They include the accessory muscles of inspiration: the neck muscles (sternocleido-mastoid and scalene), the intercostal muscles between the ribs, and the accessory muscles of expiration: the abdominal muscles (▼ Figure 6-9). These muscles are

TABLE 6-1 Normal Respiration Rate Ranges	
Adults	12 to 20 breaths/min
Children	15 to 30 breaths/min
Infants	25 to 50 breaths/min

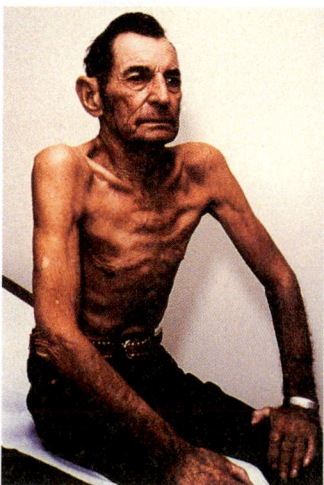

Figure 6-9 The accessory muscles of breathing are used when a patient is having difficulty breathing, not for normal breathing. These include the sternocleidomastoid, scalene, intercostal muscles, and abdominal muscles.

Altitude Tips

Patients at high altitude can exhibit abnormal respiratory rhythms, especially during sleep. Frequently, these patterns will be described as *periodic* or *Cheyne-Stokes* breathing. Cheyne-Stokes respirations can also occur in healthy, uninjured people during sleep at high altitudes.

not used in normal breathing. More information about recognizing labored breathing and respiratory distress in children may be found in Chapter 30, Pediatric Outdoor Emergency Care. Signs of inadequate breathing in adult patients are as follows:

- Respiratory rate of less than 8 breaths/min or greater than 24 breaths/min

- Accessory muscle use

- Skin pulling in around the ribs during inspiration (**retractions**)

- Pale, cyanotic, or cool (clammy) skin

- Irregular (uneven) pattern of inhalation and exhalation

- Lung sounds that are decreased, unequal, or "wet"

- Labored breathing

- Shallow and/or uneven chest rise and fall

- Two- or three-word sentences spoken

Cheyne-Stokes breathing

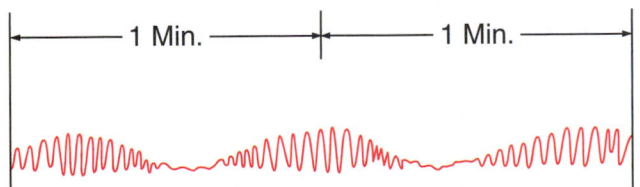

Inspiration/expiration

Figure 6-10 Cheyne-Stokes breathing shows irregular respirations followed by a period of apnea.

You should also be aware that a patient may appear to be breathing after the heart has stopped. These occasional, gasping breaths are called **agonal respirations**. They occur when the respiratory center in the brain continues to send signals to the breathing muscles. These respirations are not adequate, since they are slow and generally shallow. You will need to provide CPR to patients with agonal respirations.

Some patients may have irregular respiratory breathing patterns that are related to a specific patient condition. An example of this is Cheyne-Stokes respirations, which are often seen in patients with stroke and patients with serious head injuries (▼ **Figure 6-10**). Cheyne-Stokes respirations are an irregular respiratory pattern in which the patient breathes with an increasing rate and depth of respiration that is followed by a period of **apnea**, or lack of spontaneous breathing, followed again by the pattern of increasing rate and depth. Serious head injuries may also cause changes in the normal respiratory rate and pattern of breathing. The changes may be noted as irregular respirations that may or may not have an identifiable pattern. Cheyne-Stokes respirations can also occur in normal people during sleep at high altitudes.

Patients with inadequate breathing have inadequate minute volume and need to be treated immediately. This is most easily recognized in patients who are unable to speak in complete sentences when at rest. Emergency medical care includes airway management, supplemental oxygen, and ventilatory support.

Opening the Airway

Emergency medical care begins with ensuring an open airway. The patient's airway and breathing status are the first steps in your initial assessment for a very good reason: unless you can immediately open and maintain an airway, you will not be able to deliver appropriate patient care.

When you respond to a call and find an unconscious patient, you need to assess and determine immediately whether the patient has an open airway and breathing is adequate. In order to open the airway and to assess breathing, the patient needs to be in the supine position. If your patient is found in the prone (lying face down) position, he or she must be properly positioned to allow for assessment of airway and breathing and to begin CPR should it be necessary. The patient should be log rolled as a unit so the head,

SkillDrill 6-1   Positioning an Unconscious Patient

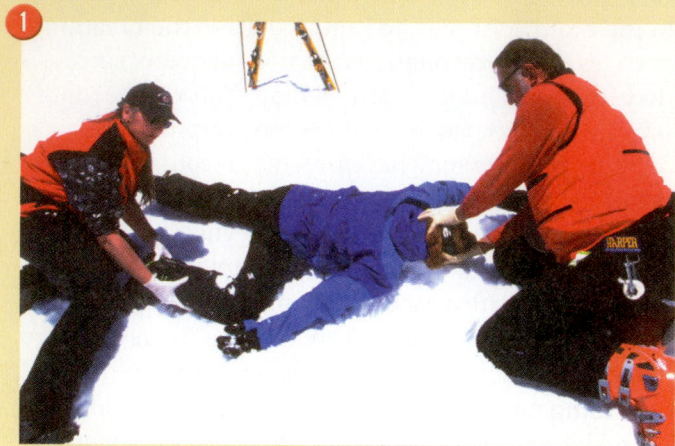

Support the head while your partner straightens the patient's legs.

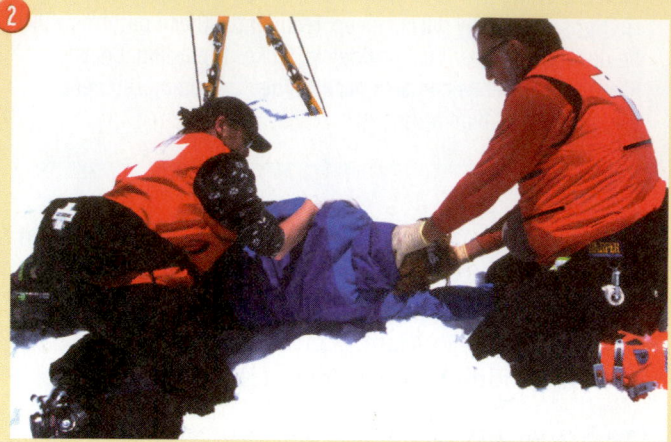

Have your partner place his or her hand on the patient's far shoulder and hip.

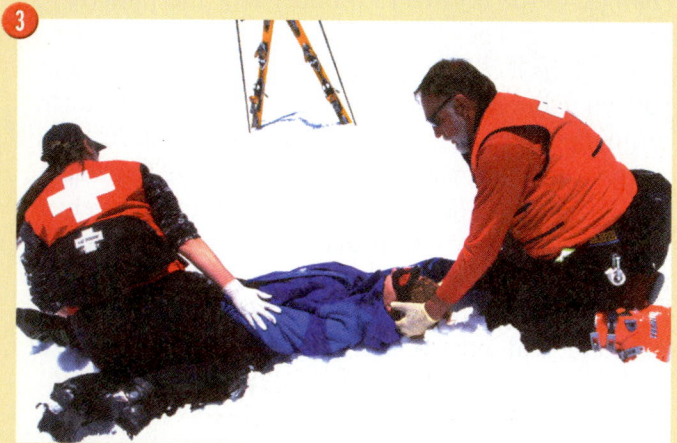

Roll the patient as a unit with the person at the head calling the count to begin the move.

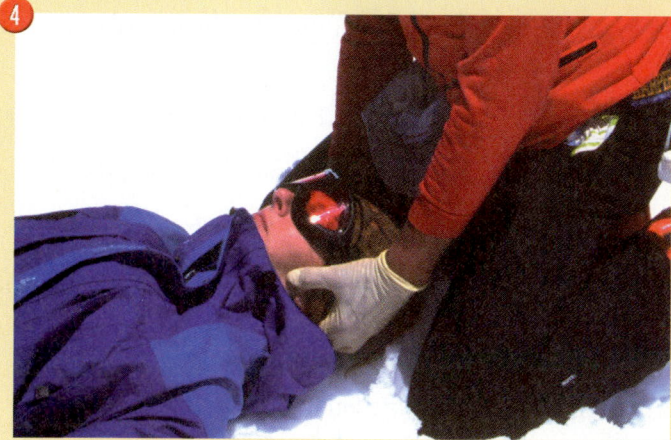

Open and assess the patient's airway and breathing status.

neck, and spine all move together without any twisting ▲ Skill Drill 6-1 .

1. **Kneel beside the patient.** Have your partner kneel far enough away so that the patient, when rolled toward you, does not come to rest in your lap. Rapidly straighten the patient's legs and move the nearer arm across the patient's chest to minimize movement. Place your hands behind the back of the patient's head and neck to provide in-line stabilization of the cervical spine **(Step 1)**.

2. **Have your partner** place his or her hands on the patient's far shoulder and hip **(Step 2)**.

3. **As you call the count** to control movement, have your partner turn the patient toward you by pulling on the far shoulder and hip. Control the head and neck so that they move as a unit with the rest of the torso. In this way, the head and neck stay in the same vertical plane as the back. This single motion will minimize aggravation of any spinal injury. At this point, you should apply a cervical collar. Replace the patient's farther arm back at his or her side **(Step 3)**.

4. **Once the patient is positioned,** maintain an open airway and check for breathing **(Step 4).**

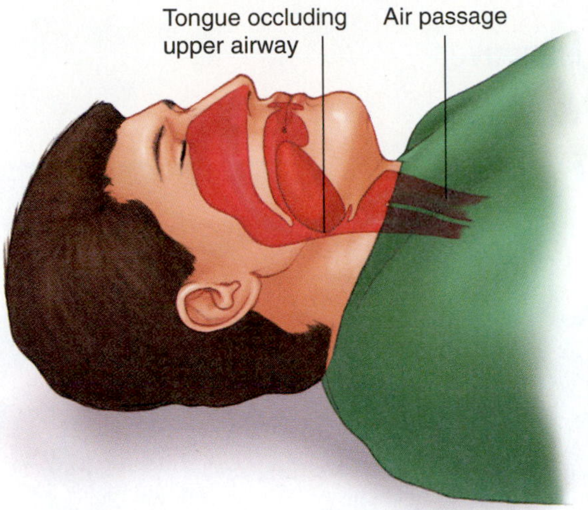

Tongue occluding upper airway   Air passage

Figure 6-11 The most common airway obstruction is the patient's own tongue, which falls back into the throat when the muscles of the throat and tongue relax.

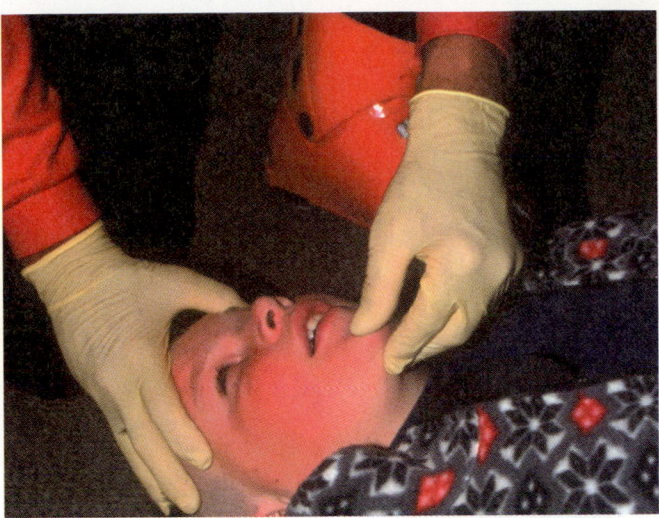

Figure 6-12 The head tilt-chin lift maneuver is a simple technique for opening the airway in a patient without a suspected cervical spine injury.

In an unconscious patient, the most common airway obstruction is the patient's own tongue, which falls back into the throat when the muscles of the throat and tongue relax (▲ **Figure 6-11**). Dentures (false teeth), blood, vomitus, mucus, food, or other foreign objects may also create a blockage. Therefore, you should always have a suction device available to help clear and maintain a patent airway.

Head Tilt-Chin Lift Maneuver

Opening the airway to relieve an obstruction can often be done quickly and easily by simply tilting the patient's head back and lifting the chin in what is known as the **head tilt-chin lift maneuver**. For patients who have not sustained trauma, this simple maneuver is sometimes all that is needed for the patient to resume breathing.

To perform the head tilt-chin lift maneuver, follow these steps:

1. With the patient in a supine position, position yourself beside the patient's head.

2. Place one hand on the patient's forehead, and apply firm backward pressure with your palm to tilt the patient's head back. This extension of the neck will move the tongue forward, away from the back of the throat, and clear the airway if the tongue is blocking it.

3. Place the tips of the fingers of your other hand under the lower jaw near the bony part of the chin. Do not compress the soft tissue under the chin, as this may block the airway.

4. Lift the chin upward, bringing the entire lower jaw with it, helping to tilt the head back. Do not use your thumb to lift the chin. Lift so that the teeth are nearly brought together, but avoid closing the mouth completely. Continue to hold the forehead to maintain the backward tilt of the head (▲ **Figure 6-12**).

Jaw-Thrust Maneuver

The head tilt-chin lift will open the airway in most patients. If you suspect a cervical spine injury, use the jaw-thrust maneuver. The **jaw-thrust maneuver** is a technique to open the airway by placing the fingers behind the angle of the jaw and lifting the jaw upward. You can easily seal a mask around the mouth while doing the jaw-thrust maneuver. This is the method of choice for patients with suspected cervical spine injury. See Chapter 26, Head and Spine Injuries, for a more detailed discussion of these types of injuries.

Perform the jaw-thrust maneuver in an adult in the following manner (▶ **Skill Drill 6-2**):

1. **Kneel above the patient's head.** Place your fingers behind the angles of the lower jaw, and forcefully move the jaw upward. Use your thumbs to help position the lower jaw to allow breathing through the mouth as well as the nose **(Step 1)**.

2. The completed maneuver should open the airway with the mouth slightly open and the jaw jutting forward **(Step 2)**.

SkillDrill 6-2   Performing the Jaw-Thrust Maneuver

1

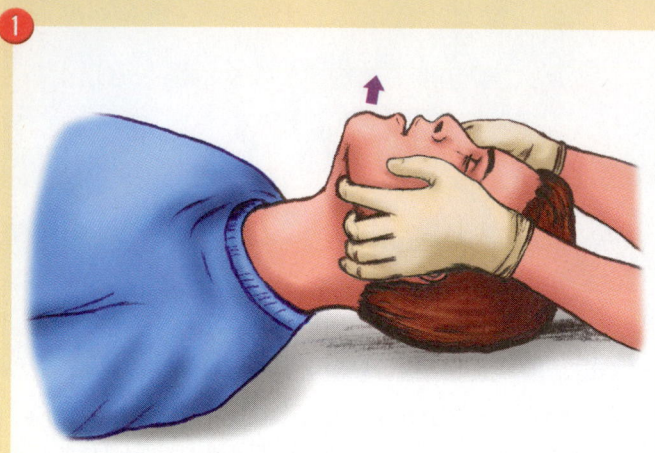

Kneeling above the patient's head, place your fingers behind the angles of the lower jaw, and forcefully move the jaw upward. Use your thumbs to help position the lower jaw.

2

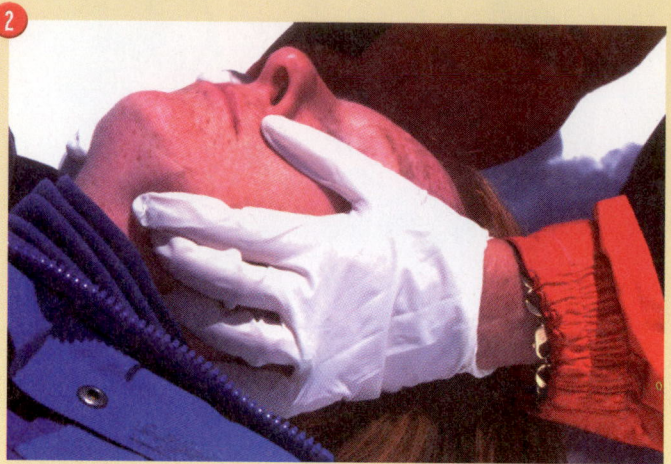

The completed maneuver should look like this.

Once the airway has been opened, the patient may start to breathe on his or her own. Assess whether breathing has returned by using the look, listen, and feel technique (▶ **Figure 6-13**).

With complete airway obstruction, there will be no movement of air. However, you may see the chest and abdomen rise and fall considerably with the patient's frantic attempts to breathe. This is why the presence of chest wall movement alone does not indicate breathing is present. Regular chest wall movement indicates a respiratory effort is present. Observing chest and abdominal movement is often difficult with a fully clothed patient. You may see little, if any, chest movement even with normal breathing. This is particularly true in some patients with chronic lung disease. You must begin artificial ventilation immediately if you use the three-part approach—look, listen, and feel—and discover that there is no movement of air.

Basic Airway Adjuncts

The primary function of an airway adjunct is to prevent obstruction of the upper airway by the tongue and allow the passage of air and oxygen to the lungs.

Oropharyngeal Airways

An **oropharyngeal (oral) airway** has two principal purposes. The first is to keep the tongue from blocking the upper airway. The second is to make it easier to suction the airway if necessary. Both functions are made possible by an opening down the center or along either side of the oropharyngeal airway (▶ **Figure 6-14**). This type of airway is often used in conjunction with bag-valve-mask (BVM) ventilation.

An oropharyngeal airway should be inserted promptly in unconscious patients who have no gag reflex. These patients may or may not be breathing on their own. The **gag reflex** is a protective reflex

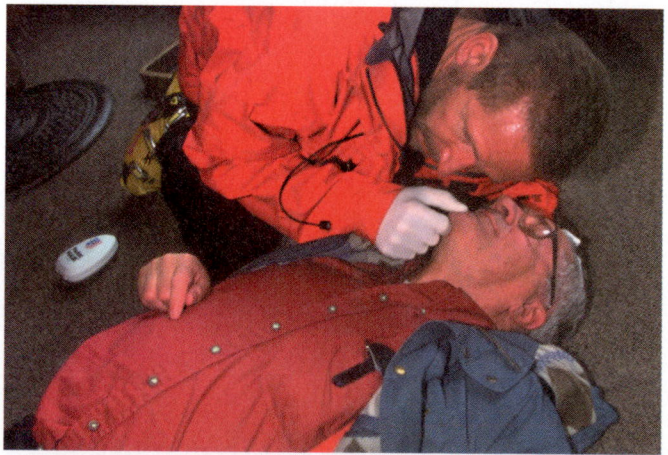

Figure 6-13   The look, listen, and feel technique is used to assess whether breathing has spontaneously returned.

Skill Drill 6-3   Inserting an Oral Airway

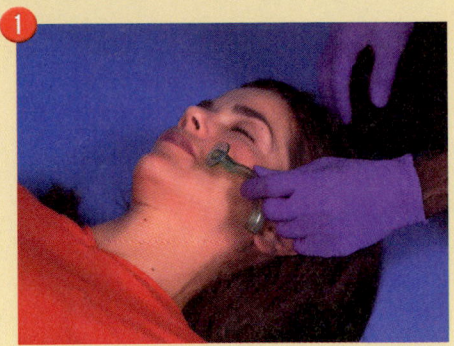

Size the airway by measuring from the patient's earlobe to the corner of the mouth.

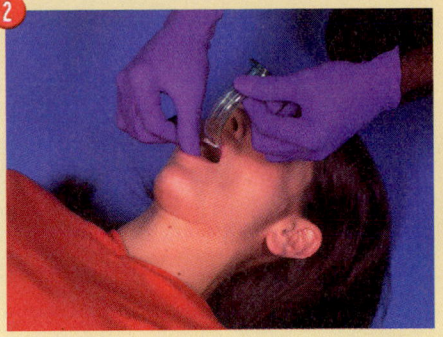

Open the patient's mouth with the cross-finger technique. Hold the airway upside down with your other hand. Insert the airway with the tip facing the roof of the mouth.

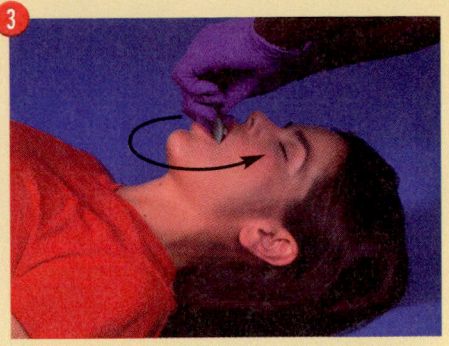

Rotate the airway 180°. Insert the airway until the flange (the trumpet-shaped flare) rests on the patient's lips and teeth. In this position, the airway will hold the tongue forward.

mechanism that prevents food and other particles from entering the airway. If you try to insert an oral airway in a patient with a gag reflex, the result may be vomiting or a spasm of the vocal cords. An oral airway is also a safe, effective way to help maintain the airway of the patient with a possible spinal injury. The use of an oral airway may make manual airway maneuvers such as the head tilt-chin lift and the jaw thrust easier to maintain.

You must be very clear on when and how this device is used. (▲ Skill Drill 6-3) shows the steps for inserting an oral airway. If the oropharyngeal airway is not the proper size or is inserted incorrectly, it could actually push the tongue back into the pharynx, blocking the airway. The following steps should be used when inserting an oropharyngeal airway:

1. **To select the proper size,** measure from the patient's earlobe to the corner of the mouth on the side of the face **(Step 1)**.

2. **Open the patient's mouth** with the cross-finger technique. Hold the airway upside down with your other hand. Insert the airway with the tip facing the roof of the mouth **(Step 2)**.

3. **Rotate the airway 180°. When inserted properly,** the airway will rest in the mouth with the curvature of the airway following the contour of the tongue. The flange should rest against the lips or teeth, with the other end opening into the pharynx **(Step 3)**.

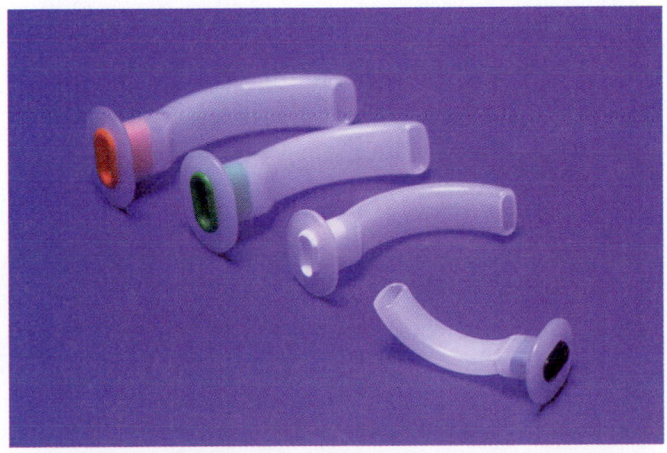

Figure 6-14 An oral airway is used for unconscious patients who have no gag reflex. It works to keep the tongue from blocking the airway and to make suctioning the airway easier.

Take care to avoid injuring the hard palate as you insert the airway. Roughness can cause bleeding, which may aggravate airway problems or even cause vomiting.

Skill Drill 6-4 Inserting an Oral Airway With a 90° Rotation

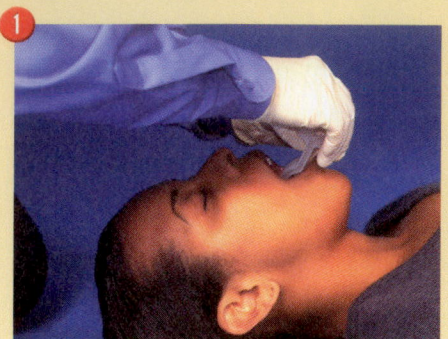

1 Depress the patient's tongue so it remains forward.

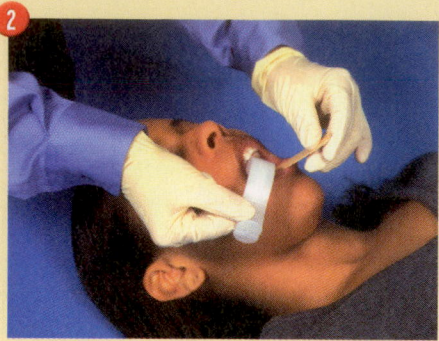

2 Insert the oral airway sideways from the corner of the patient's mouth, until the flange reaches the teeth.

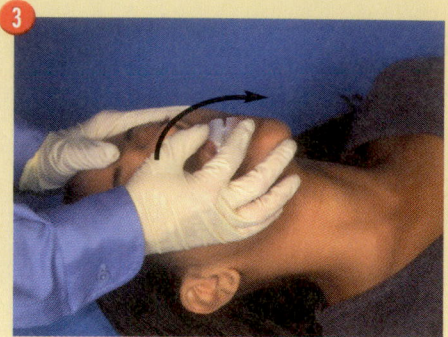

3 Rotate the oral airway at a 90° angle. Remove the tongue blade as you exert gentle backward pressure on the oral airway, until it rests securely in place against the lips and teeth.

If you encounter difficulty while inserting the oral airway, an alternative method may be used by following these steps (▲ Skill Drill 6-4):

1. **Use a tongue blade** to depress the tongue, ensuring that the tongue remains forward **(Step 1)**.

2. **Insert the oral airway sideways** from the corner of the mouth, until the flange reaches the teeth **(Step 2)**.

3. **Rotate the oral airway** at a 90° angle, removing the tongue blade as you exert gentle backward pressure on the oral airway, until it rests securely in place against the lips and teeth **(Step 3)**.

In some instances, a patient may become responsive and regain the gag reflex after you have inserted an oral airway. If this occurs, gently remove the airway by pulling it out, following the normal curvature of the mouth and throat. Be prepared for the patient to vomit.

Pediatric Needs

In children, the alternative method of inserting an oral airway, using a tongue blade to hold the tongue down while inserting the airway, is the only acceptable method. Because the airways of children are undeveloped, rotating an oropharyngeal airway in the posterior pharynx may cause damage. For more discussion on pediatric airways, see Chapter 30.

Have suction available, and log roll the patient onto his or her side to allow any fluids to drain out.

Nasopharyngeal Airways

A nasopharyngeal (nasal or trumpet) airway is usually used with a patient who has an intact gag reflex and is not able to maintain an airway (▶ Figure 6-15). Patients with an altered mental status or those who have just had a seizure may also benefit from this type of airway. You should have established protocols covering the use of nasopharyngeal airways for severe head or face traumas. Extreme care must be used with such trauma patients. If the airway is accidentally pushed through the hole caused by a fracture of the base of the skull, it may penetrate through the cranium and into the brain.

This type of airway is usually better tolerated by patients who have an intact gag reflex. It is not as likely as the oropharyngeal airway to cause vomiting. You should coat the airway well with a water-soluble lubricant before it is inserted. Be aware that slight bleeding may occur even when the airway is inserted properly. However, you should never force the airway into place.

Follow these steps to ensure correct placement of the nasopharyngeal airway (▶ Skill Drill 6-5):

1. **Before inserting the airway,** be sure you have selected the proper size. Measure from the tip of the patient's nose to the earlobe.

Skill Drill 6-5   Inserting a Nasal Airway

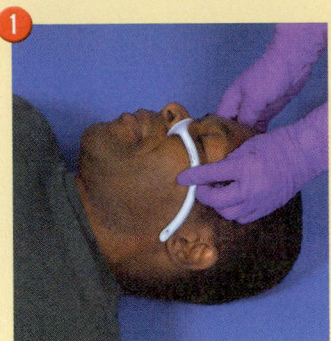

Size the airway by measuring from the tip of the nose to the patient's earlobe. Coat the tip with a water-soluble lubricant.

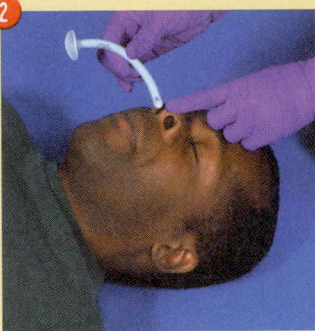

Insert the lubricated airway into the larger nostril with the curvature following the floor of the nose and the bevel toward the septum.

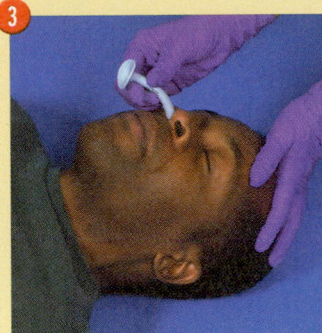

Gently advance the airway.

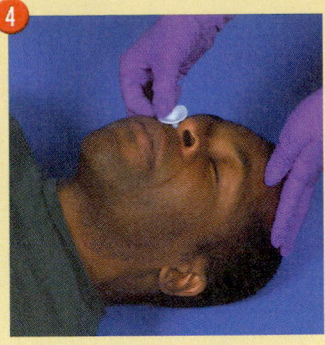

Continue until the flange rests against the skin. If you feel any resistance or obstruction, remove the airway and insert it into the other nostril.

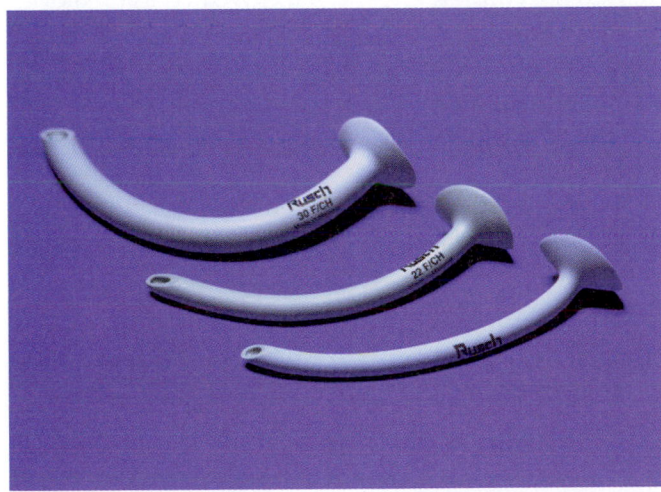

Figure 6-15   A nasal airway is better tolerated by patients who have an intact gag reflex.

In almost all individuals, one nostril is larger than the other (Step 1).

2. **The airway should be placed** in the larger nostril, with the curvature of the device following the curve of the floor of the nose (Step 2).

3. **Advance the airway gently** (Step 3).

4. **When completely inserted,** the flange rests against the nostril. The other end of the airway opens into the posterior pharynx (Step 4).

If the patient becomes intolerant of the nasal airway, you may have to remove it. Gently withdraw the airway from the nasal passage.

Disadvantages of the nasal airway include the following:

- May be contraindicated in severe head or facial trauma
- May traumatize delicate nasal membranes, causing bleeding
- May not be able to insert if the patient has a history of fractured nasal bones

Suctioning

You must keep the airway clear so that you can ventilate the patient properly. If the airway is not clear, you will force the material into the lungs and possibly cause a complete airway obstruction. Therefore, suctioning is

Rescuer Safety

A mask and goggles should be worn whenever airway management involves suctioning. Body fluids can become aerosolized, and exposure to the mucous membranes of the OEC technician's mouth, nose, and eyes can easily occur.

Skill Drill 6-6   Suctioning a Patient's Airway

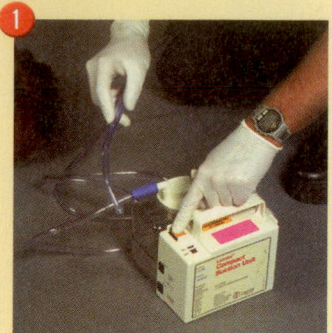

Make sure the suctioning unit is properly assembled and turn on the suction unit.

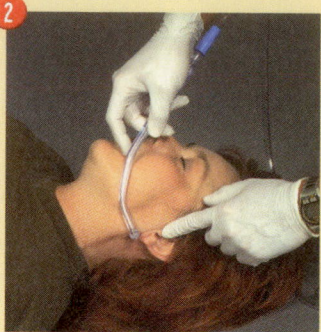

Measure the catheter from the corner of the patient's mouth to the earlobe.

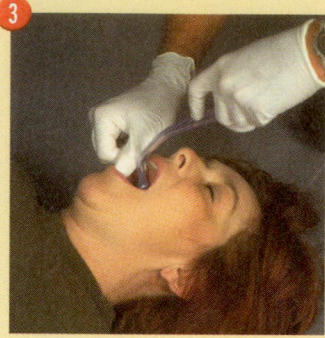

Open the patient's mouth and insert the catheter to the depth measured.

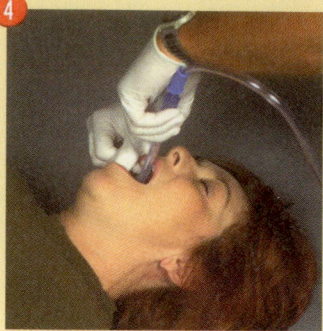

Apply suction in a circular motion as you withdraw the catheter. Do not suction an adult for more than 15 seconds.

your next priority. If you have any doubt about the situation, remember this rule: If you hear gurgling, the patient needs suctioning!

Suctioning Equipment

Portable, hand-operated, and fixed (mounted) suctioning equipment is essential for resuscitation ▶ Figure 6-16 . A portable suctioning unit must provide enough vacuum pressure and flow to allow you to suction the mouth and oropharynx effectively. Hand-operated suctioning units with disposable chambers are reliable, effective, and relatively inexpensive. A fixed suctioning unit should generate air flow of more than 40 L/min and a vacuum of more than 300 mm Hg when the tubing is clamped.

A suctioning unit should be fitted with the following:

- Wide-bore, thick-walled, nonkinking tubing
- Plastic, semirigid pharyngeal suction tips, called **tonsil tips** or Yankauer tips
- Nonrigid plastic catheters, called French or whistle-tip catheters
- A nonbreakable, disposable collection bottle
- A supply of water for rinsing the tips

You should make sure that the suction yoke, the collection bottle, water for rinsing, and the suction tube are easily accessible at the patient's head.

A **catheter** is a hollow, cylindrical structure that drains or delivers fluids. Tonsil tips are the best kind of catheter for suctioning the pharynx in adults and the preferred method for infants and children. These plastic

tips have a large diameter and are somewhat rigid, so they do not collapse. Tips with a curved contour allow for easy, rapid placement in the pharynx ▶ Figure 6-17 . Be careful not to touch the back of the airway. This can activate the gag reflex, cause vomiting, and increase the possibility of **aspiration** (introducing foreign material into the lung).

You should use extreme caution when suctioning a conscious or semiconscious patient. Put the tip in only as far as you can visualize. Be aware that suctioning may induce vomiting in these patients.

To properly suction a patient ▲ Skill Drill 6-6 :

1. **Turn on the assembled suction unit** (Step 1).

2. **Insert the catheter** to the correct depth by measuring the catheter from the corner of the patient's mouth to the edge of the earlobe (Step 2).

3. **Before applying suction,** open the patient's mouth using the cross-finger technique or by pulling the jaw, and insert the tip of the catheter to the depth measured (Step 3).

4. **Apply suction** in a circular motion as you withdraw the catheter. Do not suction an adult for more than 15 seconds (Step 4).

Soft plastic, nonrigid catheters, sometimes called French or whistle-tip catheters, are used to suction the nose and liquid secretions in the back of the mouth and in situations in which you cannot use a rigid catheter, such as for a patient with a **stoma**, an opening in the neck that connects the trachea directly to the skin

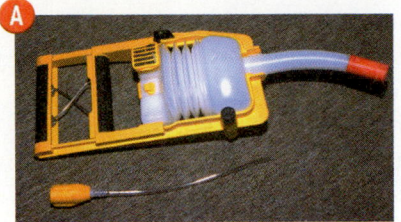

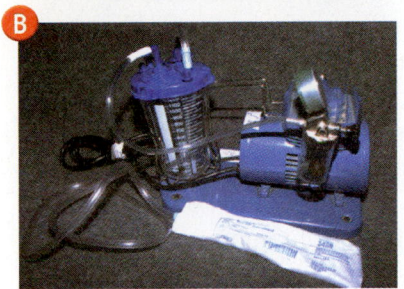

Remember

Suctioning Time Limits

Adult	15 seconds
Child	10 seconds
Infant	5 seconds

► **Figure 6-18**). For example, a patient could break off a tooth on a rigid catheter, whereas a flexible catheter may be worked along the cheeks without injury. Before you insert any catheter, make sure to measure for the proper size. Use the same technique as you would use when measuring for an oropharyngeal or nasopharyngeal airway. Never insert a catheter past the base of the tongue, as this may result in gagging and vomiting.

You should clean and decontaminate your suctioning equipment after each use according to the manufacturer's guidelines. You should also inspect this equipment regularly to make sure it is in proper working condition. Switch on the suction, clamp the tubing, and make sure that the unit generates a vacuum of more than 300 mm Hg. Check that a battery-charged unit has charged batteries.

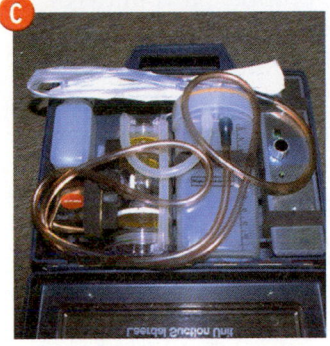
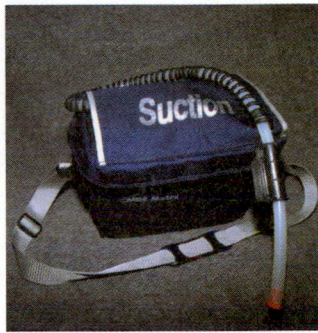

Figure 6-16) Suctioning equipment is essential for resuscitation. **A.** Hand operated. **B.** Fixed unit. **C.** Portable unit.

Techniques of Suctioning

Follow these steps to operate the suction unit:

1. Check the unit for proper assembly of all its parts. Turn on the suctioning unit. Select and attach the appropriate catheter to the tubing. Use a bulb suction or soft catheter set at the low to medium setting when suctioning the nose.

2. Measure the catheter to ensure that you do not allow it to be inserted too deeply.

3. Open the patient's mouth using the cross-finger technique or the jaw-thrust maneuver. Insert the suction tip along the roof of the mouth until you reach the pharynx. Do not use suction unless it is absolutely necessary. Insert the tip only to the base of the tongue.

4. After the tip is in place, apply suction as you withdraw the suction tip from the pharynx and mouth. Move the suction tip from side to side.

Never suction for more than 15 seconds at one time for adult patients, 10 seconds for children, and 5 seconds for infants. Suctioning removes oxygen from the airway

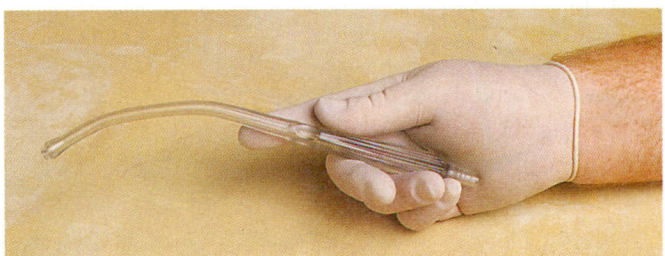

Figure 6-17) Tonsil-tip catheters are the best for suctioning, as they have wide diameter tips and are somewhat rigid.

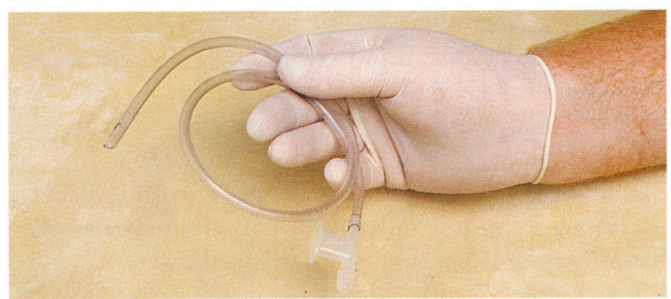

Figure 6-18) French, or whistle-tip, catheters are used in situations in which rigid catheters cannot be used, such as with a patient who has a stoma or if the patient's teeth are clenched.

along with obstructive material. Rinse the catheter and tubing with water to prevent clogging of the tube with dried vomitus or other secretions. Repeat suctioning only after the patient has been ventilated and re-oxygenated.

At times, a patient may have secretions or vomitus that cannot be suctioned quickly and easily. There are also some suction units that are unable to effectively remove solid objects such as teeth, foreign bodies, and food. In these instances, you should remove the catheter from the patient's mouth, log roll the patient to the side, and then clear the mouth carefully with your gloved finger. A patient may also produce frothy secretions as quickly as you can suction them from the airway. In this situation, you might need to alternate hyperventilation with suctioning. However, note that hyperventilation is not appropriate if vomitus or other particles are present.

Maintaining the Airway

The recovery position is used to help maintain a clear airway in a patient who has not had traumatic injuries and is breathing on his or her own with a normal rate and adequate tidal volume (depth of breathing). Take the following steps to put the patient in the recovery position:

1. Roll the patient onto his or her left side with the opposite knee flexed so that the head, shoulders, and torso move at the same time without twisting.

2. Place the patient's extended arm and other hand under his or her cheek (▶ Figure 6-19).

Once patients have resumed spontaneous breathing after being resuscitated, the recovery position will prevent the aspiration of vomitus. However, this position is not appropriate for patients with suspected spinal trauma, nor is it adequate for patients who are unconscious and require airway management. You must reposition such patients to provide access to the airway.

Supplemental Oxygen

You should always give supplemental oxygen to patients who are breathing inadequately because they are not getting enough oxygen to their lungs.

Some tissues and organs, such as the heart, the central nervous system, lungs, kidneys, and liver, need a constant supply of oxygen to function normally. **Never withhold oxygen from any patient who may benefit from it, even if you must assist ventilations.**

Use high-concentration oxygen in any cardiac and/or respiratory arrest situation, whether the patient is an infant or an adult.

Supplemental Oxygen Equipment

In addition to knowing when and how to give supplemental oxygen, you must understand how oxygen is stored and the various hazards associated with its use.

OXYGEN CYLINDERS. The oxygen that you will give to patients is usually supplied as a compressed gas in green, seamless steel or aluminum cylinders. Some bottles may be silver or chrome with a green area around the valve stem on top. Newer bottles are often made of lightweight aluminum or spun steel; older bottles are much heavier.

Check to make sure that the cylinder is labeled for medical oxygen. You should look for letters and numbers stamped into the metal on the collar of the cylinder (▼ Figure 6-20). Of particular importance are the month and year stamps, which indicate when the bottle was last tested.

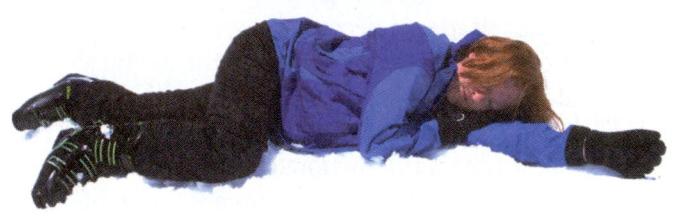

Figure 6-19   In the recovery position, the patient is rolled in a semiprone position.

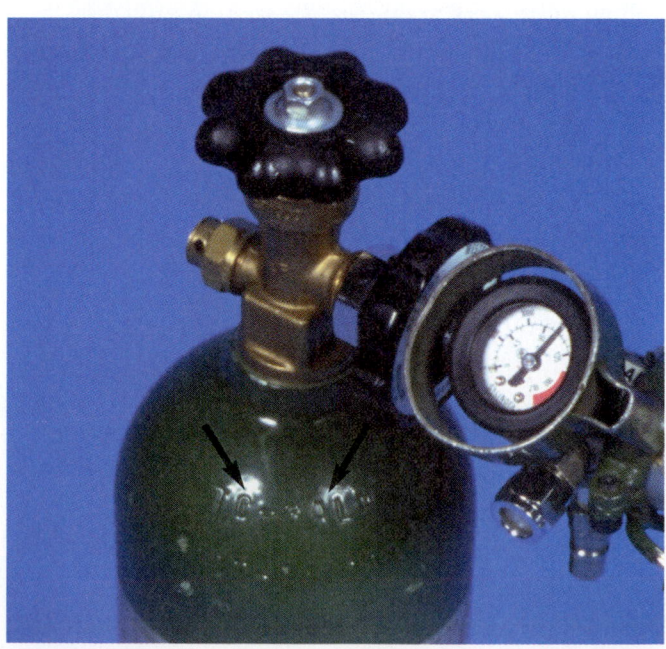

Figure 6-20   Oxygen tanks for medical use will have a series of letters and numbers stamped into the metal on the collar of the cylinder.

Oxygen cylinders are available in several sizes. The two sizes that you will most often use are the D (or super D) and M cylinders (▼ **Figure 6-21**). The D (or super D) cylinder is the most practical for field use. M tanks are useful as stationary units in aid rooms and other permanent emergency care facilities. Other sizes that you will see are A, E, G, H, and K (▼ **Table 6-2**).

The length of time you can use an oxygen cylinder depends on the pressure in the cylinder and the flow rate. A method of calculating cylinder duration is shown in (▼ **Table 6-3**).

SAFETY CONSIDERATIONS. Compressed gas cylinders must be handled very carefully because their contents are under pressure. Cylinders are fitted with pressure regulators to make sure that patients receive the right amount and type of gas. Make sure that the correct pressure regulator is firmly attached before you transport the cylinders. A puncture or hole in the tank can cause the cylinder to become a deadly missile. Do not handle a cylinder by the neck assembly alone. Cylinders should be secured with mounting brackets when they are stored. Oxygen cylinders that are in use during transport should be positioned and secured to prevent the tank from falling or from damage occurring to the valve-gauge assembly.

TABLE 6-2 Oxygen Cylinder Sizes

Size	Volume, L
D	350
Super D	500
E	625
M	3,000
G	5,300
H, A, K	6,900

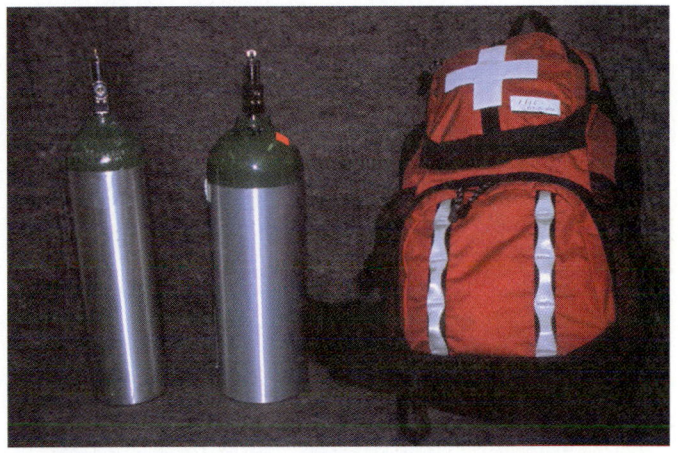

Figure 6-21 The cylinders that are most commonly used by outdoor rescuers are D (left) and super D (right) size cylinders.

TABLE 6-3 Oxygen Cylinders: Duration of Flow

Formula:

$$\frac{(\text{Gauge pressure in psi} - \text{the safe residual pressure}) \times \text{constant}}{\text{Flow rate in L/min}} = \text{duration of flow in minutes}$$

RESIDUAL PRESSURE = 200 psi

CYLINDER CONSTANT

D = 0.16	G = 2.41
E = 0.28	H = 3.14
M = 1.56	K = 3.14

Determine the life of a D cylinder that has a pressure of 2,000 psi and a flow rate of 6 L/min.

$$\frac{(2{,}000-200) \times 0.16}{6} = \frac{288}{6} = 48 \text{ min}$$

PIN-INDEXING SYSTEM. The compressed gas industry has established a **pin-indexing system** for portable cylinders to prevent an oxygen regulator from being connected to a carbon dioxide cylinder, a carbon dioxide regulator from being connected to an oxygen cylinder, and so on. In preparing to administer oxygen, always check to be sure that the pinholes on the cylinder exactly match the corresponding pins on the regulator.

The pin-indexing system features a series of pins on a yoke that must be matched with the holes on the valve stem of the gas cylinder. The arrangement of the pins and holes varies for different gases according to accepted national standards (▼ **Figure 6-22**). Other gases that are supplied in portable cylinders, such as acetylene, carbon dioxide, and nitrogen, use regulators and flowmeters that are very similar to those used with oxygen. Each cylinder of a specific gas has a given pattern and a given number of pins. These safety measures make it impossible for you to attach a cylinder of nitrous oxide to an oxygen regulator. The oxygen regulator will not fit.

The outlet valves on D size or smaller cylinders are designed to accept yoke-type pressure-reducing gauges, which conform to the pin-indexing system (▼ **Figure 6-23**). The safety system for large cylinders is known as the **American Standard System**. In this system, cylinders larger than D sizes are equipped with threaded gas outlet valves. The inside and outside thread sizes of these outlets vary depending on the gas in the cylinder. The cylinder will not accept a regulator valve unless it is properly threaded to fit that regulator.

The purpose of these safety devices is the same as in the pin-indexing system: to prevent the accidental attachment of a regulator to a wrong cylinder.

PRESSURE REGULATORS. The pressure of gas in a full oxygen cylinder is approximately 2,000 psi. This is far too much pressure to be safe or useful for your purposes. Pressure regulators reduce the pressure to a more useful range, usually 40 to 70 psi. Most pressure regulators that are in use today reduce the pressure in a single stage, although multistage regulators do exist. A two-stage regulator will reduce the pressure first to 700 psi and then to 40 to 70 psi.

After the pressure is reduced to a workable level, the final attachment for delivering the gas to the patient is usually one of the following:

- A quick-connect female fitting that will accept a quick-connect male plug from a pressure hose or ventilator or resuscitator

- A flowmeter that will permit the regulated release of gas measured in liters per minute

HUMIDIFICATION. Humidified oxygen is usually indicated only for long-term oxygen therapies. Dry oxygen is not considered harmful for short-term use. Therefore, many prehospital care providers do not use humidified oxygen in the outdoor setting. Always refer to medical control or local protocols for guidance involving patient treatment issues.

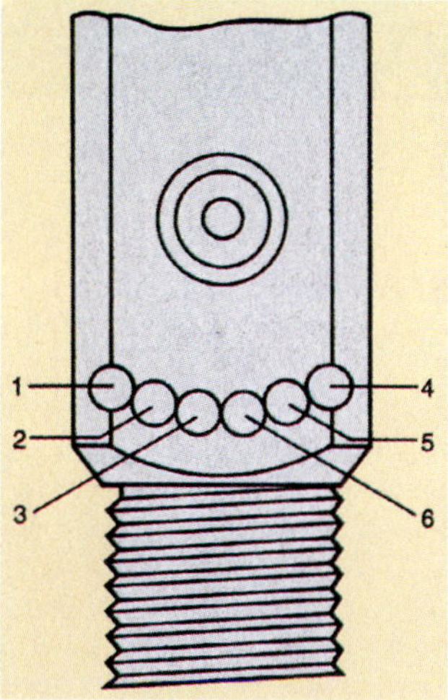

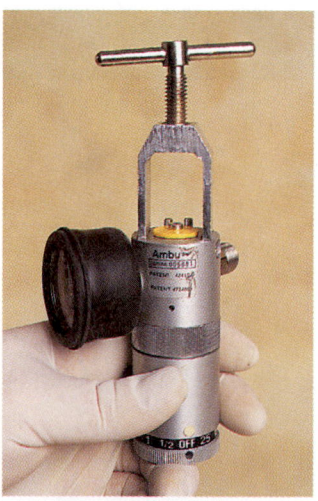

Figure 6-22 The locations of the pin-indexing safety system holes in a cylinder valve face. Each cylinder of a specific gas has a given pattern and a given number of pins.

Figure 6-23 A yoke-type pressure-reducing gauge is used with a small oxygen cylinder.

Wilderness Tips

Using oxygen in the outdoor setting can have additional challenges. Planning and preparation will help minimize these impacts.

Determine your duration of flow, as previously outlined, for various delivery rates. During long evacuations, use this information when treating a patient with oxygen.

Warm oxygen can help prevent further heat loss.

Request additional oxygen cylinders to ensure uninterrupted O_2 therapy.

FLOWMETERS. Flowmeters are usually permanently attached to pressure regulators on emergency medical equipment. The two types of flowmeters that are commonly used are pressure-compensated flowmeters and Bourdon-gauge flowmeters.

A pressure-compensated flowmeter incorporates a float ball within a tapered calibrated tube. The float rises or falls according to the gas flow within the tube. The flow of gas is controlled by a needle valve located downstream from the float ball. This type of flowmeter is affected by gravity and must always be maintained in an upright position for an accurate flow reading.

The Bourdon-gauge flowmeter is commonly used because it is not affected by gravity and can be used in any position. It is actually a pressure gauge that is calibrated to record flow rate (▼ **Figure 6-24**). The major disadvantage of this flowmeter is that it does not compensate for backpressure. Therefore, it will usually record a higher flow rate when there is any obstruction to gas flow downstream.

Operating Procedures

Before placing an oxygen cylinder into service (▶ **Skill Drill 6-7**):

1. **Inspect the cylinder** and its markings. If the cylinder was commercially filled, it will have a plastic seal around the valve stem covering the opening in the stem. Remove the seal, and inspect the opening to make sure that it is free of dirt and other debris. The valve stem should not be sealed or covered with adhesive tape or any petroleum-based substances. These can contaminate the oxygen and can contribute to spontaneous combustion when mixed with the pressurized oxygen.

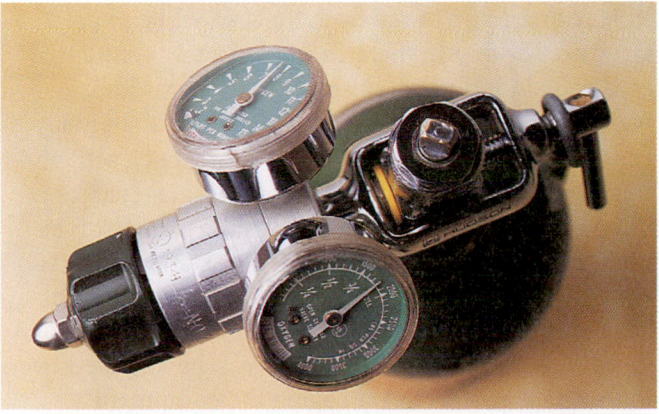

Figure 6-24 The Bourdon-gauge flowmeter is not affected by gravity and can be used in any position.

"Crack" the cylinder by quickly opening and then reclosing the valve to help make sure that dirt particles and other possible contaminants do not enter the oxygen flow. *Never face the tank toward yourself or others when cracking the cylinder.* Open the tank by attaching a tank key to the valve and rotating the valve counterclockwise. You should be able to hear clearly the rush of oxygen coming from the tank. Close the tank by rotating the valve clockwise **(Step 1)**.

2. **Attach the regulator/flowmeter** to the valve stem after clearing the opening. On one side of the valve stem, you will find three holes. The larger one, on top, is a true opening through which the oxygen flows. The two smaller holes below it do not extend to the inside of the tank. They provide stability to the regulator. Following the design of a pin-indexing system, these two holes are very precisely located in positions that are unique to oxygen cylinders.

   Above the pins on the inside of the collar is the actual port through which oxygen flows from the cylinder to the regulator. A metal or plastic O-ring is placed around the oxygen port to optimize the airtight seal between the collar of the regulator and the valve stem **(Step 2)**.

3. **Place the regulator collar** over the cylinder valve, with the oxygen port and pin-indexing pins on the side of the valve stem that has the three holes. Open the screw bolt just enough to allow the collar to fit freely over the valve stem. Move the regulator so that the oxygen port and the pins fit into the correct holes on the valve stem. The screw bolt on the opposite side should be aligned with the dimpled depression. As you hold the regulator securely against the valve stem, tighten the screw bolt until the regulator is firmly attached to the cylinder. At this point, you should not see any open spaces between the sides of the valve stem and the interior walls of the collar **(Step 3)**.

4. **With the regulator firmly attached,** open the cylinder and read the pressure level on the regulator gauge. Most portable cylinders have a maximum pressure of approximately 2,000 psi. Most prehospital care services consider a cylinder with less than 500 to 1000 psi to be too low to keep in service. Learn your area's policies in this regard and follow them.

Skill Drill 6-7   Placing an Oxygen Cylinder Into Service

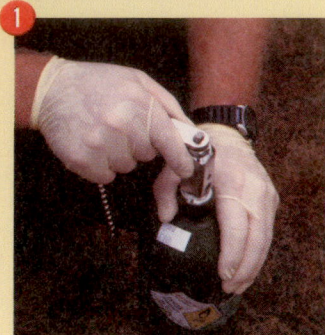
Using an oxygen wrench, turn the valve counterclockwise to "crack" the cylinder.

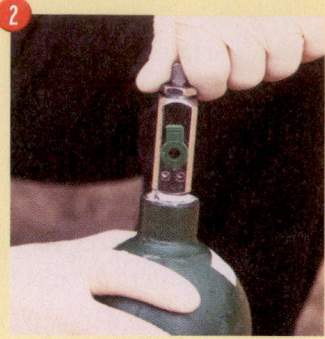
Attach the regulator/flowmeter to the valve stem using the two pin-indexing holes and make sure that the washer is in place over the larger hole.

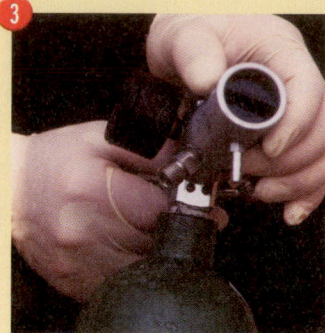
Align the regulator so that the pins fit snugly into the correct holes on the valve stem and hand tighten the regulator.

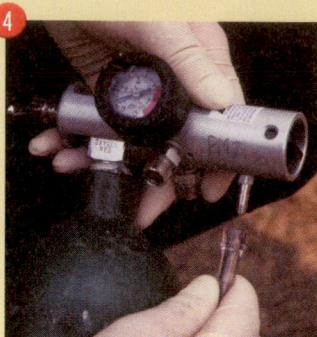
Attach the oxygen connective tubing to the flowmeter, if it is not permanently attached.

The flowmeter will have either a second gauge or a selector dial that indicates the oxygen flow rate. Several popular types of devices are widely used. Attach the selected oxygen device to the flowmeter by connecting the universal oxygen connective tubing to the "Christmas tree" nipple on the flowmeter. Most oxygen delivery devices come with this tubing permanently attached. Some oxygen masks do not. You must add this tubing to the oxygen delivery device if it is not attached (Step 4).

Open the flowmeter to the desired flow rate. Flow rates will vary based on the oxygen delivery device being used. Remember that you must be completely familiar with the equipment before attempting to use it on a patient. Once the oxygen is flowing at the desired rate, apply the oxygen device to the patient and make any necessary adjustments. Monitor the patient's reaction to the oxygen and to the oxygen device, and periodically recheck the regulator gauge to make sure there is sufficient oxygen in the cylinder. Disconnect the tubing from the flowmeter nipple and turn off the cylinder valve when oxygen therapy is complete, or when the patient has been transferred to the ambulance and has been switched to the ambulance's oxygen system. In a few seconds, the sound of oxygen flowing from the nipple will cease. This indi-cates that all the pressurized oxygen has been removed from the flowmeter. Turn off the flowmeter. The gauge on the regulator should read zero with the tank valve closed. This confirms that there is no pressure left above the valve stem. As long as there is a pressure reading on the regulator gauge, it is not safe to remove the regulator from the valve stem.

Hazards of Supplemental Oxygen

Oxygen does not burn or explode. However, it does support combustion. The more oxygen is around, the faster the combustion process. A small spark, even a glowing cigarette, can become a flame in an oxygen-rich atmosphere. Therefore, you must keep any possible source of fire away from the area while oxygen is in use. Make sure the area is adequately ventilated, especially in industrial settings where hazardous materials may be present and where sparks are easily generated. Be extremely cautious in any enclosed environment in which oxygen is being administered, as an oxygen-rich environment increases the chance of fire if a spark or flame is introduced. A bystander who is smoking or sparks from a vehicle extrication are possible ignition sources. Never leave an oxygen cylinder standing unattended. The oxygen can be knocked over, injuring the patient or damaging the equipment.

Oxygen Delivery Equipment

In general, the oxygen delivery equipment that is used in the field should be limited to nonrebreathing masks, bag-valve-mask (BVM) devices, and nasal cannulas, depending on local protocol. However, you may encounter other devices during transports between medical facilities.

Nonrebreathing Mask

The <u>nonrebreathing mask</u> is the preferred way of giving oxygen in the prehospital setting. With a good mask-to-face seal, it is capable of providing up to 90% inspired oxygen.

The nonrebreathing mask is a combination mask and reservoir bag system. The mask is similar to a simple face mask. Oxygen fills a reservoir bag that is attached to the mask by a one-way valve. The system is called a nonrebreathing mask because the exhaled gas escapes through flapper valve ports at the cheek areas of the mask (▼ **Figure 6-25**). The valve also prevents the patient from rebreathing exhaled gases as the gas in the reservoir bag flows into the mask during inhalation.

In this system, you must be sure that the reservoir bag is full before the mask is placed on the patient. Adjust the flow rate so that the bag does not fully collapse when the patient inhales. This is about two thirds of the bag volume, or 10 to 15 L/min. Use a smaller reservoir bag with infants and children, as they will inhale a smaller volume.

Nasal Cannula

A <u>nasal cannula</u> delivers oxygen through two small, tubelike prongs that fit into the patient's nostrils

(▼ **Figure 6-26**). This device can provide 24% to 44% inspired oxygen when the flowmeter is set at 1 to 6 L/min. For the comfort of your patient, flow rates greater than 6 L/min are not recommended because the nasal passages become irritated and dry.

The nasal cannula delivers dry oxygen directly into the nostrils. Therefore, when you anticipate a long transport time, you should consult medical control about humidification.

A nasal cannula has limited use in the prehospital care setting. For example, a patient who breathes through the mouth or who has a nasal obstruction will get little or no benefit from a nasal cannula. You may consider using this device with patients whom you believe to be stable and not hypoxic, but *always* use a nonrebreathing mask with patients in unstable condition who are breathing on their own. Always try to give high-flow oxygen through a nonrebreathing

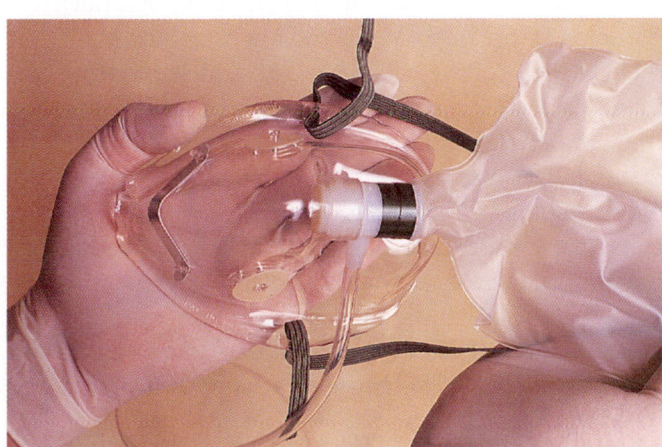

Figure 6-25 The nonrebreathing mask contains flapper valve ports at the cheek areas of the mask to prevent the patient from rebreathing exhaled air.

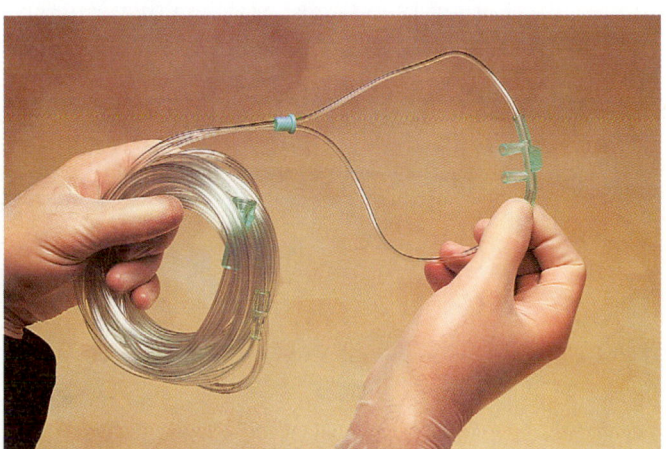

Figure 6-26 The nasal cannula delivers oxygen directly through the nostrils.

mask if you suspect that a patient may have hypoxia, coaching him or her as necessary. If the patient will not tolerate a nonrebreathing mask, you will have to use a nasal cannula, which some patients find more comfortable. As always, a good assessment of your patient will guide your decision.

Pulse Oximetry

Pulse oximetry is a recent assessment tool used to evaluate the effectiveness of oxygenation. The pulse oximeter is a photoelectric device that monitors the oxygen saturation of hemoglobin (the iron-containing portion of the red blood cell to which oxygen attaches) in the capillary beds. Parts that make up the pulse oximeter include a monitor and sensing probe (▼ Figure 6-27). The sensing probe clips onto a finger or ear lobe. The light source must have unobstructed access to a capillary bed, so fingernail polish should be removed. Results appear as a percentage on the display screen. Normally, pulse oximetry values will be greater than 95% on room air at sea level. At higher elevations, however, the normal range of oxygen saturation decreases (▶ Table 6-4).

The goal of any oxygen therapy is to increase oxygen saturation to normal levels. This device is a useful assessment tool to determine the effectiveness of oxygen therapy, bronchodilator therapy, and use of the BVM device in certain conditions. However, the pulse oximeter does *not* take the place of good assessment skills and should *not* prevent the application of oxygen to any patient who complains of difficulty breathing regardless of the pulse oximetry value.

Because the device presumes adequate perfusion and numbers of red blood cells, anything that causes vasoconstriction (such as hypoperfusion or cold

TABLE 6-4 Normal Oxygen Saturation Ranges		
Altitude	Barometric Pressure (mm Hg)	Unacclimatized Oxygen Saturation (SpO$_2$ %) for 20- to 40-year-olds
Sea Level	760	greater than 95%
5,000'	635	91% to 97%
9,000'	545	87% to 95%
12,000'	485	81% to 89%

extremities) or loss of red blood cells (such as bleeding or anemia) will result in inaccurate or misleading values. The device also presumes that oxygen is saturating hemoglobin. Therefore, any chemical that displaces oxygen (such as carbon monoxide) will cause misleading values.

The pulse oximeter is a useful tool as long as the rescuer remembers that the device is only a tool, not a substitute for a good assessment. The rescuer should recognize that the pulse oximeter may not be accurate when hypoperfusion is present such as when the extremities are cold or the patient is in shock. The pulse oximeter also will not differentiate between oxygen and carbon monoxide bound to hemoglobin in red blood cells and will therefore read an inaccurately high oxygen saturation in patients with smoke inhalation or carbon monoxide poisoning.

Assisted and Artificial Ventilation

Obviously, a patient who is not breathing needs artificial ventilation and supplemental oxygen. But the same is true of patients who are breathing inadequately, that is, fewer than 8 breaths/min or more than 24 breaths/min. The literature varies regarding the number of breaths/min that is considered inadequate; however, most sources state that fewer than 8 breaths/min or more than 24 to 30 breaths/min is considered inadequate. Keep in mind that fast, shallow breathing can be as dangerous as very slow breathing. Fast, shallow breathing moves air primarily in the larger airway passages (dead air space) and does not allow for adequate exchange of air and carbon dioxide in the alveoli. Patients with inadequate breathing require assisted ventilations.

Always institute body substance isolation (BSI) when providing supplemental oxygen to a patient because these procedures generally put you in contact with the person's saliva or vomit.

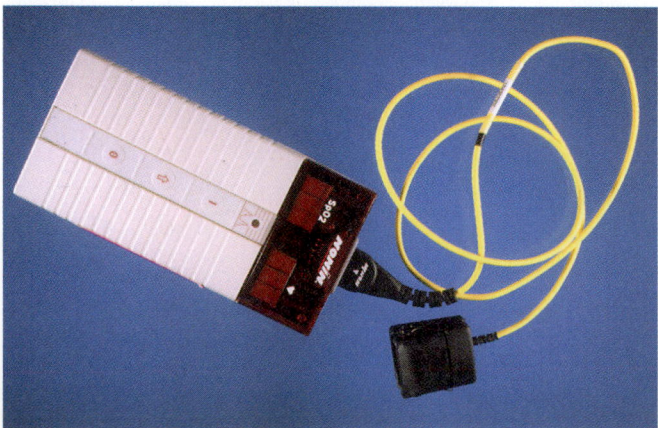

Figure 6-27   The pulse oximeter is a device that measures the saturation of oxygen in the blood.

Once you determine that a patient is not breathing or needs assisted ventilations, you should begin artificial ventilation immediately. With a patient who is not breathing, there are several ways to do this, some of which require equipment. The methods that a rescuer may use to provide artificial ventilation include the one- or two-person BVM device, mouth-to-mask ventilation, and the flow-restricted, oxygen-powered ventilation device. Note, however, that ventilation with a flow-restricted, oxygen-powered ventilation device and mouth-to-mask ventilation are now being used less often than in the past.

Mouth-to-Mouth and Mouth-to-Mask Ventilation

As you learned in your CPR course, mouth-to-mouth ventilations are now routinely done with a barrier device, such as a mask. A **barrier device** is a protective item that features a plastic barrier placed on a patient's face with a one-way valve to prevent the back flow of secretions, vomitus, and gases. Barrier devices provide adequate BSI. Mouth-to-mouth ventilations without a barrier device should be provided only in extreme conditions. Performing mouth-to-mask ventilations with a pocket mask with a one-way valve is a safer method of ventilation to prevent possible disease transmission ▼ **Figure 6-28**).

A mask with an oxygen inlet provides oxygen during mouth-to-mask ventilation to supplement the air from your own lungs. Remember that the gas you exhale contains 16% oxygen, more than enough to maintain the patient's life. With the mouth-to-mask system, however, the patient gets the additional benefit of significant oxygen enrichment with inspired air. This system also frees both your hands to help keep the airway open and helps you to provide a better seal between the mask and the face.

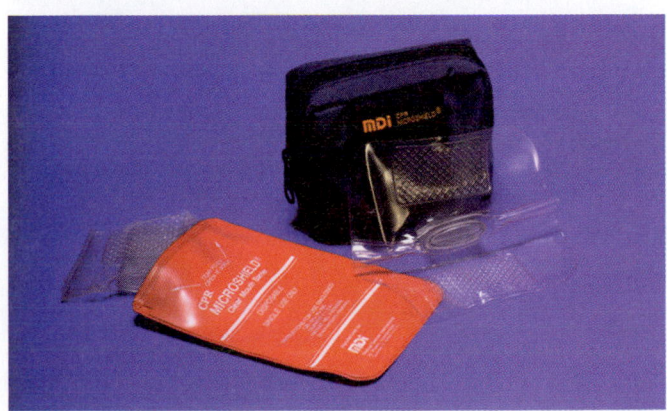

Figure 6-28) Barrier devices such as a plastic shield or a pocket mask with a one-way valve provide adequate BSI.

The mask may be shaped like a triangle or a doughnut, with the apex (top) placed across the bridge of the nose. The base (bottom) of the mask is placed in the groove between the lower lip and the chin. In the center of the mask is a chimney with a 15-mL connector.

Follow these steps to use mouth-to-mask ventilation ▶ **Skill Drill 6-8**):

1. **Kneel at the patient's head.** Open the airway using the head tilt-chin lift maneuver or the jaw-thrust maneuver if indicated. Connect the one-way valve to the face mask. Place the mask on the patient's face. Make sure the top is over the bridge of the nose and the bottom is in the groove between the lower lip and the chin. Grasp the patient's lower jaw with your first three fingers on each hand. Place your thumbs on the dome of the mask. Make an airtight seal by applying firm pressure between the thumbs and the fingers. Maintain an upward and forward pull on the lower jaw with your fingers to keep the airway open **(Step 1)**.

2. **Take a deep breath and exhale** through the open port of the one-way valve. Breathe slowly into the patient's mask for 2 seconds **(Step 2)**.

3. **Remove your mouth,** and watch for the patient's chest to fall during passive exhalation **(Step 3)**.

You know that you are providing adequate ventilations if you see the patient's chest rise and fall. Feel for resistance of the patient's lungs as they expand. You should also hear and feel air escape as the patient exhales. Make sure that you are providing the correct number of breaths per minute for the patient's age.

To increase the oxygen concentration, administer high-flow oxygen at 15 L/min through the oxygen inlet valve. This, when combined with your exhaled breath, will deliver approximately 55% oxygen to the patient.

SkillDrill 6-8   Performing Mouth-to-Mask Ventilation

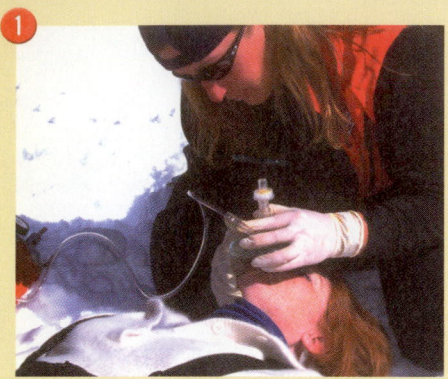

1 Once the patient's head is properly positioned, place the mask on the patient's face. Seal the mask to the face using both hands.

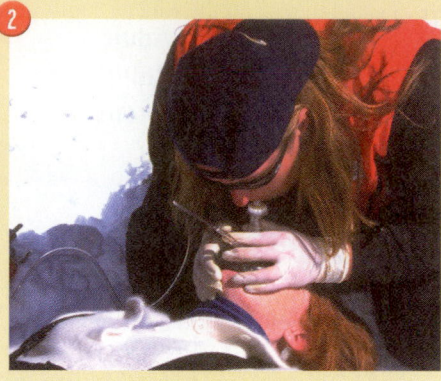

2 Exhale slowly into the open port of the one-way valve for 2 seconds as you watch for chest rise.

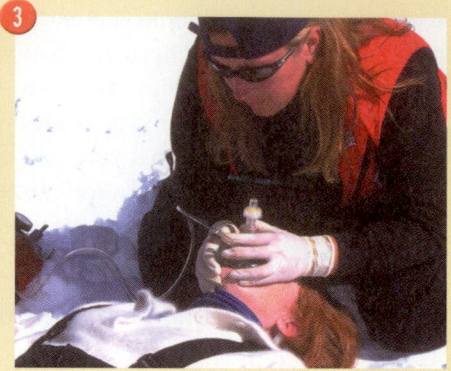

3 Watch the patient's chest fall during exhalation.

The mask also works well for patients breathing on their own who need supplemental oxygen but not full ventilatory assistance. The mask may have an elastic strap for use with these patients.

The Bag-Valve-Mask Device

Both mouth-to-mouth and mouth-to-mask ventilations can provide large volumes of inspired air—up to 4 L per breath, more than a patient needs. But with mouth-to-mouth ventilation, the concentration of oxygen delivered to the patient is only 16%. With mouth-to-mask ventilation connected to high-flow oxygen, the concentration of oxygen, at best, is only 55%.

At the same oxygen flow rate (10 to 15 L/min) as the mask alone, a **bag-valve-mask (BVM) device** with an oxygen reservoir can deliver nearly 100% oxygen (▶ Figure 6-29). Most BVM devices on the market today include modifications or accessories (reservoirs) that permit the delivery of oxygen concentrations approaching 100%. However, the device can deliver only as much volume as you can squeeze out of the bag by hand. The BVM device provides less tidal volume than mouth-to-mask ventilation; however, it delivers a much higher oxygen concentration. The BVM device is the most common method used to ventilate patients in the field. An experienced rescuer will be able to supply adequate tidal volumes with a BVM device. Be sure to practice on ventilation manikins several times before using a BVM device on a patient.

A BVM device should be used when you need to deliver high concentrations of oxygen to patients who

are not ventilating adequately. The device is also used for patients in respiratory arrest, cardiopulmonary arrest, and respiratory failure. The BVM device may be used with or without oxygen. However, the most efficient use is with supplemental oxygen and a reservoir. You should use an oral or nasal airway adjunct in conjunction with the BVM device.

COMPONENTS. All adult BVM devices should have the following components:

- A disposable self-refilling bag
- No pop-off valve, or if one is present, the capability of disabling the pop-off valve

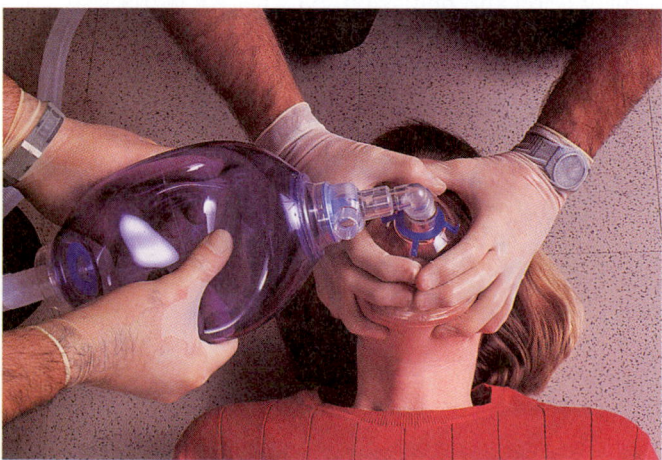

Figure 6-29 A BVM device with an oxygen reservoir can deliver nearly 100% oxygen if a good seal between the mouth and mask is achieved and if supplemental oxygen is used.

- An outlet valve that is a true valve for nonre-breathing
- An oxygen reservoir that allows for high oxygen concentration delivery
- A one-way, no-jam inlet valve system that provides an oxygen inlet flow at a maximum of 30 L/min with standard 15/22-mm fittings for face mask and endotracheal (or other advanced airway adjunct) connection
- A transparent face mask
- Ability to perform under extreme environmental conditions, including extreme heat or cold

The total amount of gas in the reservoir bag of an adult BVM device is usually 1,200 to 1,600 mL. The pediatric bag contains 500 to 700 mL, and the infant bag holds 150 to 240 mL.

The volume of air (oxygen) to deliver to the patient is based upon one key observation—chest rise and fall. In most situations, you will be using the BVM device attached to high-flow oxygen (15 L/min or more). When using the BVM device with high-flow oxygen on an adult patient, you should squeeze the bag enough to deliver a volume of 400 to 600 mL (approximately 6 to 7 mL/kg) over 2 seconds. When oxygen is not available, higher tidal volume amounts are required—700 to 1,000 mL (approximately 10 mL/kg) over 2 seconds. By delivering smaller tidal volumes when the BVM device is used with oxygen, the risk of gastric distention (and associated complications of vomiting and aspiration) is reduced.

There are two issues to consider with this approach. It is not practical for the rescuer to accurately measure tidal volumes in milliliters per kilogram for each patient ventilated in the field. There is also a significant risk of hypoxia when ventilating with smaller volumes. For these reasons, the key is to watch for good chest rise

and fall—let this observation be your key for the amount to deliver.

TECHNIQUE. Whenever possible, two rescuers should work together to provide BVM device ventilation. One rescuer can maintain a good mask seal by securing the mask to the patient's face with two hands while the other rescuer squeezes the bag. Ventilation using a BVM device is a challenging skill: it may be very difficult for one rescuer to maintain a proper seal between the mask and the face with one hand while squeezing the bag well enough to deliver adequate air to the patient. This skill can be difficult to maintain if you do not have many opportunities to practice the skill. Effective one-person BVM device ventilation requires considerable experience.

Follow these steps to use the two-person BVM device technique:

1. Kneel above the patient's head. If possible, your partner should be at the side of the head to bag the patient while you hold a seal between the mask and the patient's face with two hands. (This assumes that you have enough personnel to do everything else that needs to be done at the same time, such as chest compressions, putting the stretcher in place, or helping to lift the patient onto the stretcher.)

2. Maintain the patient's neck in an extended position unless you suspect a cervical spine injury. In that case, you should immobilize the patient's head and neck and use the jaw-thrust maneuver. Have your partner hold the head, or, if you are alone, use your knees to immobilize the head.

3. Open the patient's mouth, and suction as needed. Insert an oropharyngeal or nasopharyngeal airway to maintain an open airway.

4. Select the proper mask size.

5. Place the mask on the patient's face. Make sure the top is over the bridge of the nose and the

Indications That Artificial Ventilation Is Adequate

Equal chest rise and fall with ventilation

Ventilations delivered at the appropriate rate

- 12/min for adults
- 20/min for infants and children

Heart rate returns to normal range

Skin color ranges from pallor or cyanosis to pink or normal

Indications That Artificial Ventilation Is Inadequate

Minimal or no chest rise and fall

Ventilations are delivered too fast or too slow for patient's age

Heart rate does not return to normal range

bottom is in the groove between the lower lip and the chin. If the mask has a large, round cuff around the ventilation port, center the port over the patient's mouth. Inflate the collar to obtain a better fit and seal to the face.

6. Bring the lower jaw up to the mask with your ring finger and little finger. This will help to maintain an open airway. If you think the patient may have a spinal injury, make sure your partner immobilizes the cervical spine as you move the lower jaw.

7. Hold the mask in position by placing the thumbs over the top part of the mask and the index and middle fingers over the bottom half. Make sure you do not grab the fleshy part of the neck, as you may compress structures and create an airway obstruction.

8. Connect the bag to the mask if you have not already done so.

9. Hold the mask in place while your partner squeezes the bag with two hands until the patient's chest rises. Continue squeezing the bag once every 5 seconds for adults and once every 3 seconds for infants and children (▼ **Figure 6-30**).

10. If you are alone, hold your index finger over the lower part of the mask, and secure the upper part of the mask with your thumb. This is known as the C-clamp and will maintain the seal. Use the head tilt-chin lift maneuver to make sure the neck is extended. Squeeze the bag in a rhythmic manner once every 5 seconds with your other hand. Continue squeezing the bag once every 5 seconds for adults and once every 3 seconds for infants and children (▼ **Figure 6-31**).

When using the device to assist respirations, you should squeeze the bag as the patient tries to breathe in, ideally achieving a more normal rate and depth of respiration.

As you are assisting ventilations with a BVM device, you should evaluate how well the patient is breathing. You will know that artificial ventilation is not adequate

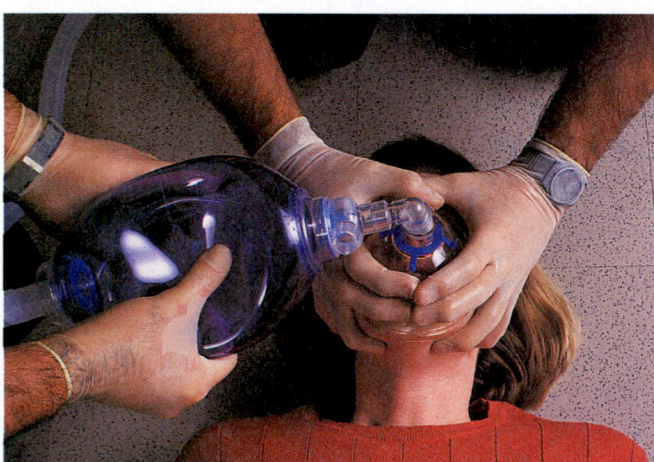

Figure 6-30 With two-person BVM device ventilation, you should hold the mask in place while your partner squeezes the bag with two hands until the patient's chest rises.

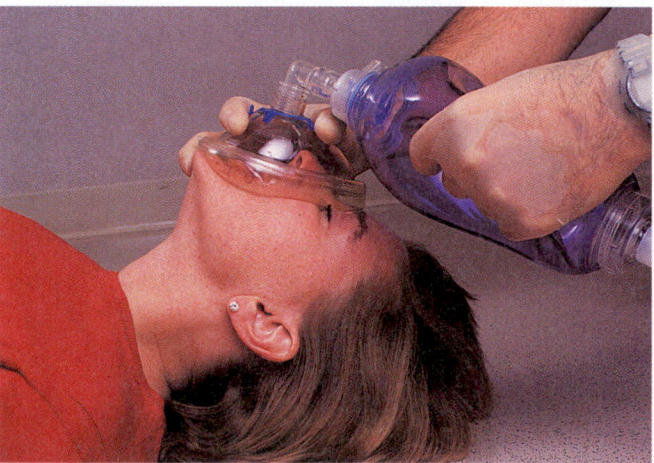

Figure 6-31 Maintain the seal of the mask to the face using the C-clamp if you must ventilate alone.

if the patient's chest does not rise and fall with each ventilation, the breathing rate is too slow or too fast, or the heart rate does not return to normal. If the patient's chest does not rise and fall, you may need to reposition the head, use an airway adjunct, or use **cricoid pressure**.

When using a BVM device or any other ventilation device, be alert for **gastric distention**, inflation of the stomach with air. To prevent or alleviate distention, use the **Sellick maneuver**. To perform the Sellick maneuver, have an additional rescuer apply cricoid pressure on the patient by placing the thumb and index finger on either side of the cricoid cartilage (at the inferior border of the larynx) and pressing down. By occluding the esophagus, this will: 1) inhibit the flow of air into the stomach, thus reducing gastric distention, and 2) reduce the chance of aspiration by helping block the flow of gastric contents up the esophagus. Cricoid pressure should only be performed on unconscious patients.

If the patient's stomach seems to be rising and falling, you should reposition the head and use cricoid pressure. In a patient with possible spinal injury, you should reposition the jaw rather than the head. If too much air is escaping from under the mask, reposition the mask for a better seal. If the patient's chest still does not rise and fall after you have made these corrections, check for an airway obstruction. If an obstruction is not present, you should attempt ventilations with another airway device.

Advanced airway techniques are beneficial when a good seal is difficult to maintain, the patient has a cervical spine injury, or the patient's condition warrants.

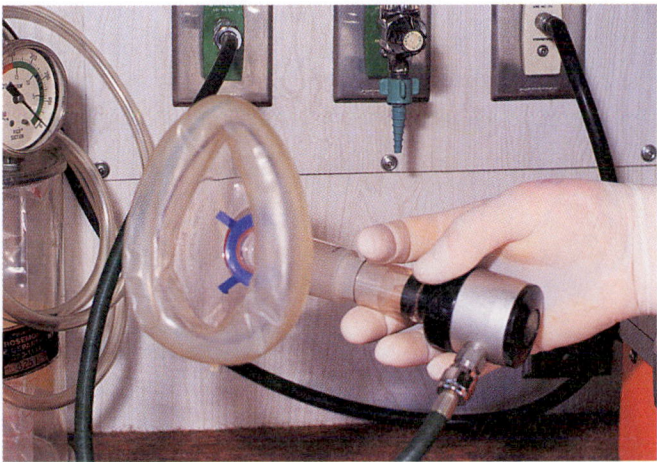

Figure 6-32 A flow-restricted oxygen-powered ventilation device can provide up to 100% oxygen.

A BVM device should be used when you need to deliver high oxygen concentrations to patients who are not ventilating adequately.

The BVM device can readily be used in conjunction with an endotracheal tube or with other airway adjunct devices such as the Esophageal Tracheal Combitube, the Pharyngeotracheal Lumen Airway, the Laryngeal Mask Airway, and the Trach-light.

Flow-Restricted, Oxygen-Powered Ventilation Devices

Another method of providing artificial ventilation is with flow-restricted, oxygen-powered ventilation devices. These devices are widely available and have been used in prehospital care for several years. However, recent findings suggest that they should not be used routinely due to the high incidence of gastric distention and possible damage to structures within the chest cavity. Flow-restricted, oxygen-powered devices *should not* be used on infants and children or on patients with suspected cervical spine or chest injury. *Cricoid pressure must be maintained whenever flow-restricted, oxygen-powered ventilation devices are used to ventilate a patient.* This will help to reduce the amount of gastric distention, the most common and significant side effect of the device.

COMPONENTS. Flow-restricted, oxygen-powered ventilation devices should have the following components ◄ Figure 6-32):

- A peak flow rate of 100% oxygen at up to 40 L/min

- An inspiratory pressure safety release valve that opens at approximately 60 cm of water and vents any remaining volume to the atmosphere or stops the flow of oxygen

- An audible alarm that sounds whenever you exceed the relief valve pressure

- The ability to operate satisfactorily under normal and varying environmental conditions

- A trigger (or lever) positioned so that both your hands can remain on the mask to provide an airtight seal while supporting and tilting the patient's head and keeping the jaw elevated

Learning how to use these devices correctly requires proper training and considerable practice. As with BVM devices, you must make sure there is an airtight fit between the patient's face and mask. The amount of pressure that is necessary to ventilate a patient adequately will vary according to the size of the patient, the patient's lung volume, and the condition of the lungs. A patient with chronic obstructive pulmonary disease (COPD) will need greater pressure to receive a given volume than would be necessary for a patient with normal lungs. Pressures that are too great can cause a **pneumothorax** (a partial or complete accumulation of air in the pleural space. Flow-restricted, oxygen-powered ventilation devices are not recommended for use on patients with COPD, chest injury, or on infants and children. Although these devices are simple to operate, *special training and authorization are required.*

Special Considerations

Gastric Distention

Gastric distention occurs when artificial ventilation fills the stomach with air. Although it most commonly affects children, it also affects adults. Gastric distention is most likely to occur when you blow or ventilate too forcefully or too often in artificial ventilation or when the airway is obstructed as a result of a foreign body or improper head position. For this reason, you are instructed to give slow, gentle breaths during artificial ventilation over 2 seconds in the adult patient. Slight gastric distention is not of concern; however, severe inflation of the stomach is dangerous because it may cause vomiting and increase the risk of aspiration during CPR. Gastric distention can also significantly reduce the lung volume by elevating the diaphragm. Gastric distention is a common side effect of flow-restricted, oxygen-powered ventilation devices—a key reason why this device is not highly recommended.

If the patient's stomach becomes distended as a result of rescue breathing, you should recheck and reposition the airway, apply cricoid pressure, and then watch for rise and fall of the chest wall as you perform rescue breathing. Continue slow rescue breathing without attempting to expel the stomach contents. Applying manual pressure over the patient's upper abdomen will likely result in vomiting. If vomiting does occur, turn the patient's entire body to the side, suction and/or wipe out the mouth with your gloved hand, and return the body back to a supine position so that you can continue CPR.

Stomas and Tracheostomy Tubes

BVM device ventilation must also be used for patients who have had a laryngectomy (surgical removal of the larynx). These patients have a permanent tracheal **stoma** (an opening in the neck that connects the trachea directly to the skin) (▼ **Figure 6-33**). It may be seen as an opening at the center, at the front and base of the neck. Many of these patients will have other openings in the neck, according to the type of operation performed. You should ignore any opening other than the midline tracheal stoma. The midline opening is the only one that can be used to put air into the patient's lungs.

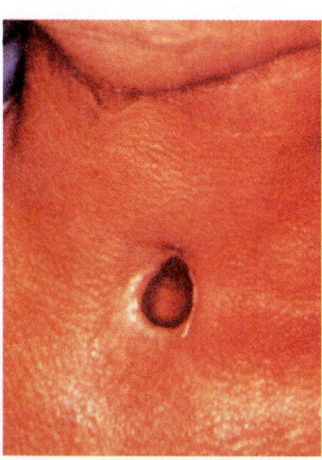

Figure 6-33   A tracheal stoma typically lies in the midline of the neck. The midline opening is the only one that can be used to deliver oxygen to the patient's lungs.

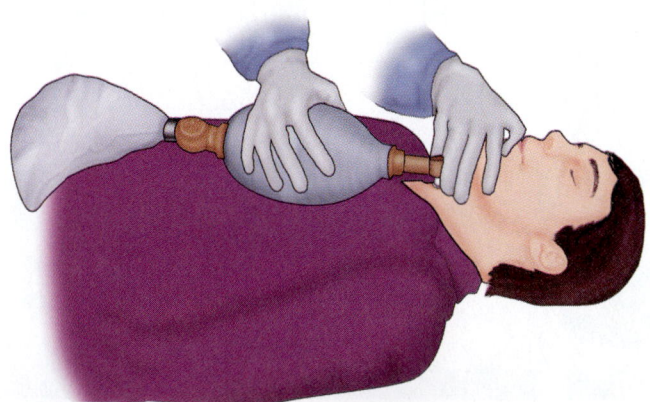

Figure 6-34   Use a BVM device to ventilate a patient with a tracheostomy tube.

Neither the head tilt-chin lift nor the jaw-thrust maneuver is required for ventilating a patient with a stoma. If the patient has a tracheostomy tube, you should ventilate through the tube with a BVM device and 100% oxygen ◀ **Figure 6-34** . If the patient has a stoma and no tube is in place, use an infant or child mask with your BVM device to make a seal over the stoma. Seal the patient's mouth and nose with one hand to prevent a leak of air up the trachea when you ventilate through a stoma. Release the seal of the patient's mouth and nose for exhalation. This allows the air to exhale through the upper airway.

If you are unable to ventilate a patient who has a stoma, try suctioning the stoma and the mouth with a French or soft tip catheter before giving the patient artificial ventilation through the mouth and nose. If you seal the stoma during ventilations, the ability to artificially ventilate the patient in this way may be improved, or it may help to clear any obstructions.

Foreign Body Airway Obstruction

A foreign body that *completely* blocks the airway in a patient is a true emergency that will result in death if not treated immediately. In an adult, sudden foreign body airway obstruction usually occurs during a meal. In a child, it occurs while eating, playing with small toys, or crawling around the house. An otherwise healthy child who has sudden difficulty breathing has probably aspirated a foreign object.

By far, the most common airway obstruction in an unconscious patient is the tongue, which relaxes back into the throat. There are other causes of airway obstruction that do not involve foreign bodies in the airway. These include swelling (from infection or acute allergic reactions) and trauma (tissue damage from injury). With airway obstruction from medical conditions such as infection and acute allergic reactions, repeated attempts to clear the airway as if there were a foreign body will be unsuccessful and potentially dangerous. These patients require specific emergency medical care for their condition and rapid transport to the hospital.

Recognition

Early recognition of airway obstruction is crucial for the rescuer to be able to provide emergency medical care effectively. Obstruction from a foreign body can

In general, and depending on the number of rescuers and equipment available, the order of preference in using adjunct devices is: mouth-to-pocket mask, two-rescuer BVM, flow-restricted, oxygen powered ventilation device, one-rescuer BVM.

result in either a **partial airway obstruction** or a **complete airway obstruction**.

Patients with a partial airway obstruction are still able to exchange air, but will have varying degrees of respiratory distress. Great care must be taken to prevent a partial airway obstruction from becoming a complete airway obstruction. The patient will usually have noisy breathing and may be coughing. You should assess the patient and determine whether the patient has **good air exchange** or **poor air exchange**.

With good air exchange, the patient can cough forcefully, although you may hear wheezing between coughs. As long as the patient can breathe, cough forcefully, or talk, you should not interfere with the patient's efforts to expel the foreign object on his or her own. Continue to monitor the patient closely and encourage the patient to continue coughing. Abdominal thrusts are usually not effective for dislodging a partial obstruction. Attempts to remove the object manually could force the object farther down into the airway and cause a complete obstruction. Continually reassess the patient's condition and be prepared to provide treatment if the air exchange becomes poor or a partial obstruction becomes a complete obstruction.

With poor air exchange, the patient has a weak, ineffective (not forceful) cough and may have increased difficulty breathing, stridor (a high-pitched noise heard primarily on inspiration), and cyanosis. You must quickly recognize this situation and provide care. *For patients with partial airway obstruction with poor air exchange, treat immediately as if there is a complete airway obstruction.*

Patients with complete airway obstruction cannot breathe, talk, or cough. One sure sign of a complete obstruction is the sudden inability to speak or cough during or immediately after eating. The person may clutch or grasp his or her throat (universal distress signal), begin to turn cyanotic, and have extreme

Rescuer Tips

Possible Causes of Airway Obstruction

Relaxation of the tongue in an unconscious patient

Aspirated vomitus (stomach contents)

Foreign objects—food, small toys, dentures

Blood clots, bone fragments, or damaged tissue
after an injury

Airway tissue swelling—infection, allergic reaction, asthma

difficulty breathing ▼ Figure 6-35 . There is little or no
air movement. Ask the conscious patient, "Are you
choking?" If the patient nods "yes," provide immediate
treatment. If the obstruction is not cleared quickly, the
amount of oxygen in the patient's blood will decrease
dramatically. If not treated, the patient will become
unconscious and then die.

Some patients with a complete airway obstruction
will be unconscious during your initial assessment. You
may not know that an airway obstruction is the cause of
their condition. There are many other causes of unconsciousness and respiratory failure, including stroke,
heart attack, seizures, and drug overdoses. A complete
and thorough patient assessment by you, therefore, is
key in providing appropriate emergency medical care.

Any person found unconscious must be managed as
if he or she has a compromised airway. You must first
open the airway and provide artificial ventilation if the
patient is not breathing ▼ Figure 6-36 . If, after
opening the airway, you are unable to ventilate the
patient after several attempts (no chest rise and fall),
you feel resistance when ventilating, or pressure is felt
(poor chest compliance), consider the possibility of an
airway obstruction. **Chest compliance** is the ability of
the chest to expand when air is drawn in on inhalation; poor chest compliance is the inability of the
chest to fully expand on inhalation.

Emergency Medical Care for Foreign Body Airway Obstruction

Perform the head tilt–chin lift maneuver to clear an
obstruction that is caused by the tongue and throat
muscles relaxing back into the airway in any person
who is found unconscious, has inadequate breathing
or is not breathing, and is not suspected of having
spinal trauma. If spinal trauma is suspected, you
should open the airway with a jaw-thrust maneuver.
Large pieces of vomited food, mucus, loose dentures,
or blood clots in the mouth should be swept forward
and out of the mouth with your gloved index finger.

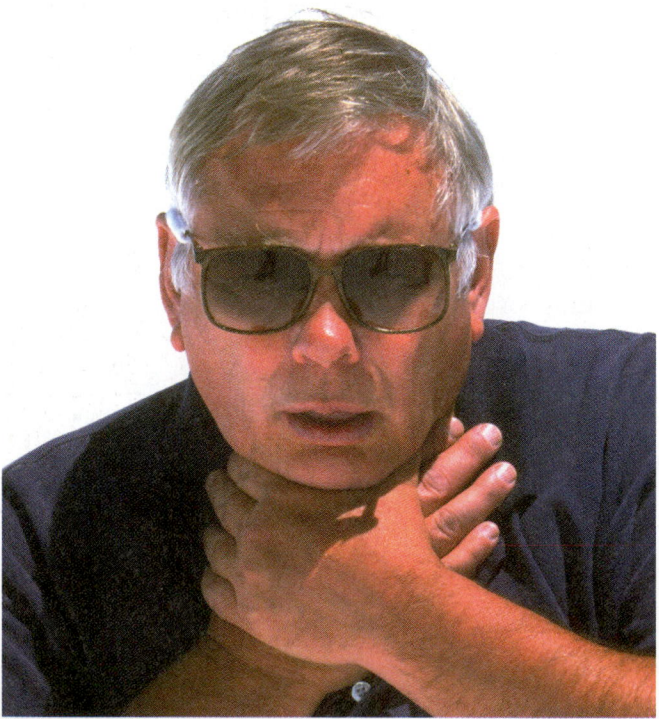

Figure 6-35   The universal sign of choking is a person who grasps
his or her throat, turns cyanotic, and has difficulty breathing.

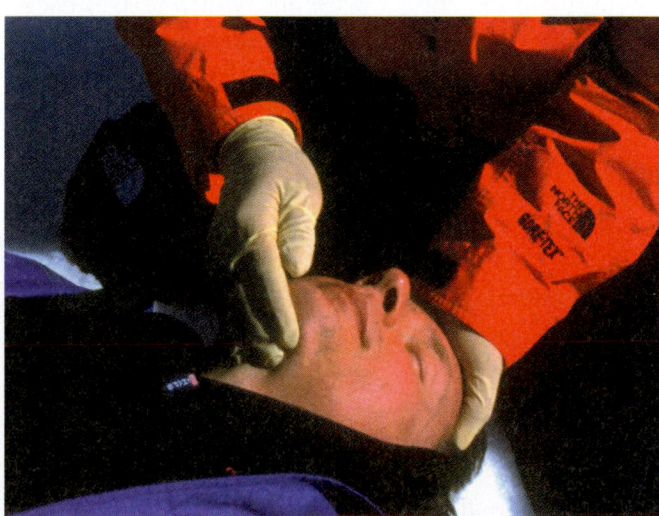

Figure 6-36   Securing and maintaining the airway and ensuring
adequate breathing are the first, most important steps in caring for
an unconscious patient.

Once available, suctioning should be used to maintain a clear airway.

The **Heimlich maneuver** (quick, repetitive upper abdominal thrusts) is the most effective method of dislodging and forcing an object out of the airway. Residual air, which is always present in the lungs, is compressed upward and used to expel the object. You should use the Heimlich maneuver followed by finger sweeps and attempts to ventilate in the adult patient with a complete airway obstruction. Specific techniques for the removal of foreign body airway obstruction in infants and children are reviewed in detail in Chapter 30.

If you are unable to clear a complete airway obstruction with your initial attempts, begin rapid transport and continue your efforts at relief of the obstruction with abdominal thrusts, finger sweeps, and attempts at ventilation en route to the hospital.

Remember to treat patients with a partial airway obstruction with *poor air exchange* as if they had a complete obstruction.

Patients with a partial airway obstruction with good air exchange should be monitored closely for change to a complete obstruction. If the patient is unable to clear the obstruction and remains conscious, support (or let the patient control) the airway position that is most efficient and comfortable. Provide supplemental oxygen and transport to the hospital.

Dental Appliances

Many dental appliances can cause an airway obstruction. If a dental appliance, such as a crown or bridge, dentures, or even a piece or section of braces, has become loose, you should manually remove it before providing ventilations. Simple manual removal may relieve the obstruction and allow the patient to breathe on his or her own.

Providing BVM device or mouth-to-mask ventilations is usually much easier when dentures can be left in place. Leaving the dentures in place provides more "structure" to the face and will generally assist you in being able to provide a good face-to-mask seal. However, loose dentures make it much more difficult to perform artificial ventilation by any method and can easily obstruct the airway. Therefore, dentures and dental appliances that do not stay in place should be removed. Dentures and appliances may become loose or be completely out of place following an accident or as you are providing care. Periodically reassess the patient's airway to make sure the devices are firmly in place.

Facial Bleeding

Airway problems can be especially challenging in patients with serious facial injuries (▼ Figure 6-37). Because the blood supply in the face is so rich, injuries to the face can result in severe tissue swelling and bleeding into the airway. Control bleeding with direct pressure and suction as necessary. Facial injuries are discussed in detail in Chapter 21.

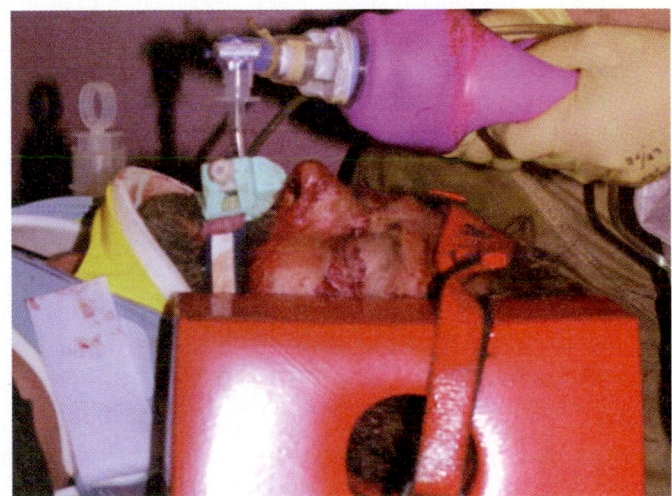

Figure 6-37 Airway problems can be especially challenging in patients with serious facial injuries.

Chapter *Sweep*

Ready for Review

The respiratory system includes the diaphragm, the muscles of the chest wall, and the accessory muscles of breathing. The term "airway" usually means the upper airway, which includes the respiratory structures above the vocal cords. Clearing the airway means removing obstructing material; maintaining the airway means keeping it open. Patients who are breathing inadequately show signs of hypoxia, a dangerous condition in which the body's tissues and cells do not have enough oxygen. Adequate breathing features a normal rate of 12 to 20 breaths/min, a regular pattern of inhalation and exhalation, bilateral clear and equal lung sounds, and regular and equal chest rise and fall. Patients with inadequate breathing need to be treated immediately. Prehospital care includes airway management, supplemental oxygen, and ventilatory support.

Basic techniques for opening the airway include the head tilt-chin lift maneuver and the jaw-thrust maneuver. One basic airway adjunct is the oropharyngeal or oral airway, which keeps the tongue from blocking the airway in unconscious patients with no gag reflex. If the oral airway is not the proper size or is inserted incorrectly, it can actually push the tongue back into the pharynx, causing an obstruction. Another basic airway adjunct is the nasopharyngeal or nasal airway, which is usually used with patients who have a gag reflex.

Suctioning is the next priority after opening the airway. Semirigid tonsil tips are the best catheters to use when suctioning the pharynx; soft plastic catheters are used to suction the nose and liquid secretions in the back of the mouth. The recovery position is used to help maintain the airway in patients without traumatic injuries who are breathing on their own.

You should always give supplemental oxygen to patients who are not breathing on their own or who have inadequate breathing. Handle compressed gas cylinders very carefully; their contents are under pressure. Always make sure the correct pressure regulator is firmly attached before transporting a cylinder. The pin-indexing safety system features a series of pins on a yoke that must be matched with the holes on the valve stem of the gas cylinder. Pressure regulators reduce the pressure of gas in an oxygen cylinder to between 40 and 70 psi. Pressure-compensated flowmeters and Bourdon-gauge flowmeters permit the regulated release of gas measured in liters per minute. When oxygen therapy is complete, disconnect the tubing from the flowmeter nipple and turn off the cylinder valve, then turn off the flowmeter. As long as there is a pressure reading on the regulator gauge, it is not safe to remove the regulator from the valve stem. Keep any possible source of fire away from the area while oxygen is in use.

Nasal cannulas and the far more effective nonrebreathing masks are used most often to deliver oxygen in the field; always try to use the latter with patients whom you suspect may have hypoxia. Nonrebreathing masks can provide more than 90% inspired oxygen. Pulse oximetry, an assessment tool to evaluate the effectiveness of oxygenation, does not take the place of a good assessment. This measurement depends on adequate perfusion to the capillary beds and is inaccurate when the patient is cold, in shock, or exposed to carbon monoxide.

The methods of providing artificial ventilation include a one- and two-person BVM device, mouth-to-mask ventilation, and a flow-restricted, oxygen-powered ventilation device. The flow-restricted, oxygen-powered ventilation device, however, is not a recommended ventilation device by most standards. Combined with your own exhaled breath, mouth-to-mask ventilation will give your patient up to 55% oxygen; a BVM device with an oxygen reservoir can deliver nearly 100% oxygen.

When you are providing artificial ventilations, remember that ventilating or blowing too forcefully can cause gastric distention. Slow, gentle breaths during artificial ventilation and use of cricoid pressure can help to prevent gastric distention. Also consider patients who have a tracheal stoma or a tracheostomy tube. You will need to ventilate these patients through the tube or the stoma.

Foreign body airway obstruction usually occurs during a meal in an adult, or while a child is eating, playing with small objects, or crawling about the house. The earlier you recognize any airway obstruction, the better. You must learn to recognize the difference between airway obstruction caused by a foreign object and that caused by a medical condition.

A complete airway obstruction can be removed by the Heimlich maneuver, finger sweeps, manual removal of the object, and attempts to ventilate. Treat patients with a partial airway obstruction with poor air exchange as if they had a complete obstruction. Patients with partial airway obstruction and good air exchange should be closely monitored.

Check for loose dental appliances in a patient before assisting ventilations. Loose appliances should be removed to prevent them from obstructing the airway.

www.OECzone.com

Vital Vocabulary

agonal respirations Occasional, gasping breaths that occur after the heart has stopped.

airway The upper airway tract or the passage above the larynx, which includes the nose, mouth, and throat. The lower airway includes the larynx, trachea, bronchi, and alveoli.

American Standard System A safety system for oxygen cylinders larger than size D, designed to prevent the accidental attachment of a regulator to a cylinder containing the wrong type of gas.

apnea Periods of not breathing.

aspiration The introduction of vomit or other foreign material into the lungs.

bag-valve-mask (BVM) device A device with a face mask attached to a ventilation bag containing a reservoir and connected to oxygen; delivers more than 90% supplemental oxygen.

barrier device A protective item, such as a pocket mask with a valve, that limits exposure to a patient's body fluids.

bilateral A body part or condition that appears on both sides of the midline.

catheter A hollow, cylindrical structure that drains or delivers fluids.

chest compliance The ability of the chest to fully expand when air is drawn in on inhalation.

complete airway obstruction Occurs when a foreign body completely obstructs the patient's airway. Patients cannot breathe, talk, or cough.

cricoid pressure Pressure on the cricoid cartilage; applied to inhibit gastric distention and aspiration of vomitus in the unconscious patient.

diffusion A process in which molecules move from an area of higher concentration of molecules to an area of lower concentration.

exhalation The part of the breathing process in which the diaphragm and the intercostal muscles relax, forcing air out of the lungs.

gag reflex A normal reflex mechanism that causes retching; activated by touching the soft palate or the back of the throat.

gastric distention A condition in which air fills the stomach as a result of high volume and pressure during artificial ventilation.

good air exchange A term used to distinguish the degree of distress in a patient with a partial airway obstruction. With good air exchange, the patient is still conscious and able to cough forcefully, although wheezing may be heard.

head tilt-chin lift maneuver A combination of two movements to open the airway by tilting the forehead back and lifting the chin; used for non-trauma patients.

Heimlich maneuver A technique for relieving upper-airway obstruction due to a foreign body by giving quick, repetitive upper abdominal thrusts.

hypoxia A dangerous condition in which the body tissues and cells do not have enough oxygen.

hypoxic drive Backup system to control respirations when oxygen levels fall.

inhalation The active, muscular part of breathing that draws air into the airway and lungs.

jaw-thrust maneuver Technique to open the airway by placing the fingers behind the angle of the jaw and bringing the jaw forward; used when a patient may have a cervical spine injury.

labored breathing Breathing that requires more than normal effort; may be slower or much faster than normal.

metabolism The chemical processes that provide the cells with energy from nutrients.

nasal cannula An oxygen delivery device in which oxygen flows through two small, tubelike prongs that fit into the patient's nostrils.

nasopharyngeal (nasal or trumpet) airway Airway adjunct inserted into the nostril of a conscious patient who is not able to maintain a natural airway.

nonrebreathing mask A combination mask and reservoir bag system that is the preferred way to give oxygen in the prehospital setting; delivers up to 90% inspired oxygen.

oropharyngeal (oral) airway Airway adjunct inserted into the mouth to keep the tongue from blocking the upper airway and to make suctioning the airway easier.

partial airway obstruction Condition in which an obstruction leaves the patient able to exchange some air, but also causes some degree of respiratory distress.

pin-indexing system A system established for portable cylinders to ensure that a regulator is not connected to a cylinder containing the wrong type of gas.

pneumothorax A partial or complete accumulation of air in the pleural space.

poor air exchange A term used to distinguish the degree of distress in a patient with a partial airway obstruction. With poor air exchange, the patient has a weak, ineffective cough, increased difficulty breathing, possible cyanosis, and may produce a high-pitched noise on inhalation (stridor).

pulse oximetry An assessment method that measures oxygen saturation of hemoglobin in the capillary beds.

recovery position A side-lying position used to maintain a clear airway in patients without injuries.

retractions Movements in which the skin pulls in around the ribs during inspiration.

Sellick maneuver A technique that is used to prevent gastric distention in which pressure is applied on the cricoid cartilage.

stoma Opening in the neck that connects the trachea directly to the skin.

tidal volume The amount of air moved during one breath.

tonsil tip A large, semirigid suction tip recommended for suctioning the pharynx; also called a Yankauer tip.

ventilation Exchange of air between the lungs and the air of the environment, either spontaneously by the patient or with assistance from a rescuer.

www.OECzone.com

Assessment in Action

You are a rescuer responding to an avalanche scene where there is a known burial victim. You arrive to find a rescuer at the scene performing ventilations on the victim who has just been extricated from the avalanche debris.

The patient is cold and pale. You expose the patient's chest by unzipping his jacket and note abdominal distention with each breath but no chest rise and fall. Because of this, you suspect there is little air getting into his lungs and gastric distention is present. Your partner immediately gets out the suction, oral airway, and BVM devices. You ask the rescuer to stop rescue breathing so you can assess the patient. You note that the man's face is pale and his skin is cold. You remember that dusky skin indicates poor oxygenation. Your partner checks the airway and begins to suction while you check for a pulse. There is a weak carotid pulse. The first rescuer on scene tells you that the skier was caught in the avalanche while skiing above a cliff band, and was likely carried over the rock by the avalanche. You observe contusions on his forehead and scalp and suspect head and spinal trauma. Your partner inserts an oral airway and begins to ventilate the patient at a rate of about 20 breaths/min. Because of suspected spinal trauma your partner stabilizes the patient's head between his knees while he ventilates. Because of the high risk of aspiration from gastric distention you apply cricoid pressure while monitoring his pulse. There is good chest rise and fall. After about 30 seconds of ventilation, his carotid pulse is stronger. While your partner continues to manage his airway, spinal immobilization equipment is readied, and with help, the patient is loaded into the toboggan for transport to a helicopter down the slope.

1. Which of the following techniques for opening the airway would have been appropriate in this situation?
   A. Head tilt-chin lift
   B. Jaw-thrust
   C. Jaw thrust-head tilt

2. Without knowing what type of gastric contents were present, which suction device would you initially have ready for this situation?
   A. French or whistle-tip catheter
   B. Tonsil tip or Yankauer tip catheter

3. How long should suction be applied at any one time?
   A. 15 seconds
   B. 30 seconds
   C. 45 seconds
   D. 60 seconds

4. What is the proper way to measure an oral airway?
   A. From the earlobe to the nose
   B. From the angle of the jaw to the nose
   C. From the earlobe to the corner of the mouth
   D. From the angle of the jaw to the corner of the mouth

5. An oral airway was used in this situation. What is its primary function?
   A. Prevents regurgitation
   B. Determines responsiveness
   C. Keeps the tongue forward
   D. Keeps the jaw forward

6. If the patient had started to gag when the oral airway was inserted, what would have been an appropriate action to take?
   A. Insert a nasopharyngeal airway.
   B. Start to ventilate with the BVM device.
   C. Wait for the spasm to relax and try again.
   D. Remove the oral airway.

7. What were the signs that ventilations were successful in this patient?
   A. There was good chest rise and fall.
   B. His skin was cool.
   C. You were able to insert an oral airway.
   D. His abdominal wall was distended.

8. The rescuer was attempting rescue breathing but there was no rise and fall of the chest wall. In this situation, what measures should have been done to correct that?
   A. Hyperextend the head.
   B. Perform the head tilt-chin lift maneuver.
   C. Perform the jaw-thrust maneuver.
   D. Place him in the recovery position.

Challenging Questions

9. This patient initially presented with a weak carotid pulse. After about 30 seconds of ventilations, his pulse got stronger. Why?

10. Why is suspected cervical spine injury such a threat to a patient's ability to breathe?

On a particularly cold morning, you receive a call from the base of a lift on the backside of the mountain. On arrival you find a 35-year-old man sitting on a bench next to the lift operator's shack. He is hunched over, breathing fast, and can only speak in short three- and four-word bursts when you question him.

He manages to tell you that he started having trouble breathing while riding up the lifts on the front side of the mountain this morning. After one run down the backside of the mountain he now has markedly worse shortness of breath and chest tightness. He asked the lift operator to call you. As he continues, you find that he is allergic to penicillin, uses a Ventolin inhaler, and has a history of hypertension and asthma. Your partner obtains his vital signs, which show a blood pressure of 152/90 mm Hg, a regular pulse of 122 beats/min, and shallow respirations of 34 breaths/min.

1. Of the following interventions, which would be the most appropriate at this time?
   A. Initiate CPR immediately.
   B. Open and assess the patient's airway.
   C. Insert a properly sized oropharyngeal airway.
   D. Apply oxygen using a nonrebreathing mask.

2. What signs/symptoms tell you his respirations are inadequate?
   A. Inability to talk in complete sentences
   B. Rapid respiratory rate
   C. Complaint of chest tightening
   D. All of the above

3. What is important about this patient's history?
   A. Ventolin inhaler and asthma
   B. His age
   C. Allergy to penicillin
   D. Hypertensive with no medication for the condition

Challenging Question

4. What is important about evacuation and transportation in the outdoor environment for this patient?

Points to Ponder

You are working as a ski patroller at a downhill ski race and respond to a racer who has had a bad fall at the base of the mountain. You find her unresponsive but breathing and with a pulse. You have her head stabilized and have administered supplemental oxygen using a nonrebreathing mask. The patient gagged but did not awaken when you tried to place an oropharyngeal airway, so you placed a nasopharyngeal airway. You quickly package the patient in the toboggan and transport her to a waiting ambulance not far away. The paramedic from the ambulance crew decides to intubate the patient for airway protection prior to transport. You offer your assistance and he tells you to just "back off." The patient is transferred into the ambulance just after intubation. Later, you learn that the patient died and that the endotracheal tube had been removed before she got to the hospital. You wonder if the patient was improperly intubated. Should you tell someone about this problem and your suspicions? Why?

Issues Scene Safety, Best Patient Care, Relationships with Other Emergency Services, Reporting Channels.

Online Outlook

The respiratory system is a very important part of the body. It delivers oxygen to the lungs and allows carbon dioxide to be removed. To learn more about the anatomy and physiology of the respiratory system, complete Exercise 6 at www.OECzone.com.

www.OECzone.com

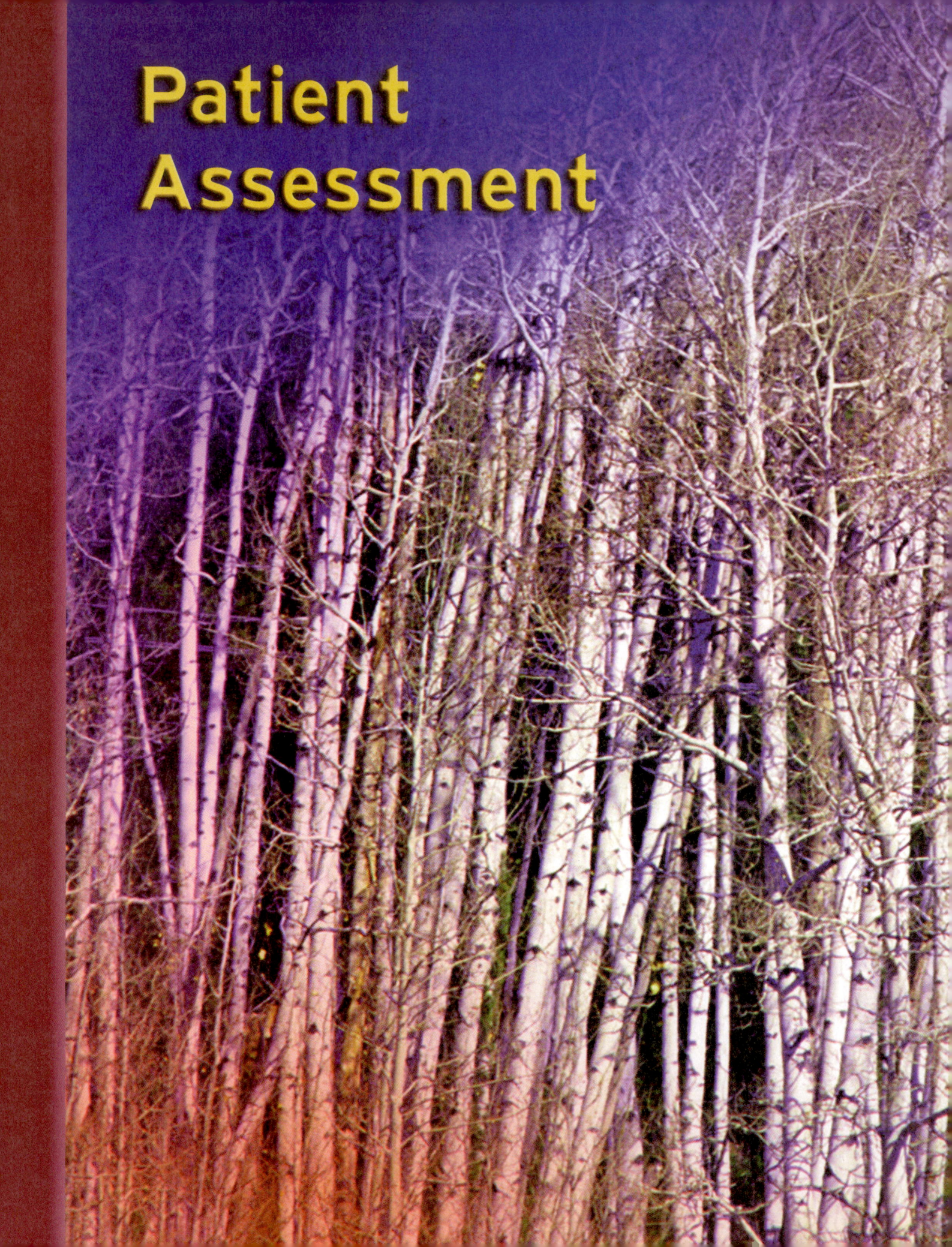

Patient Assessment

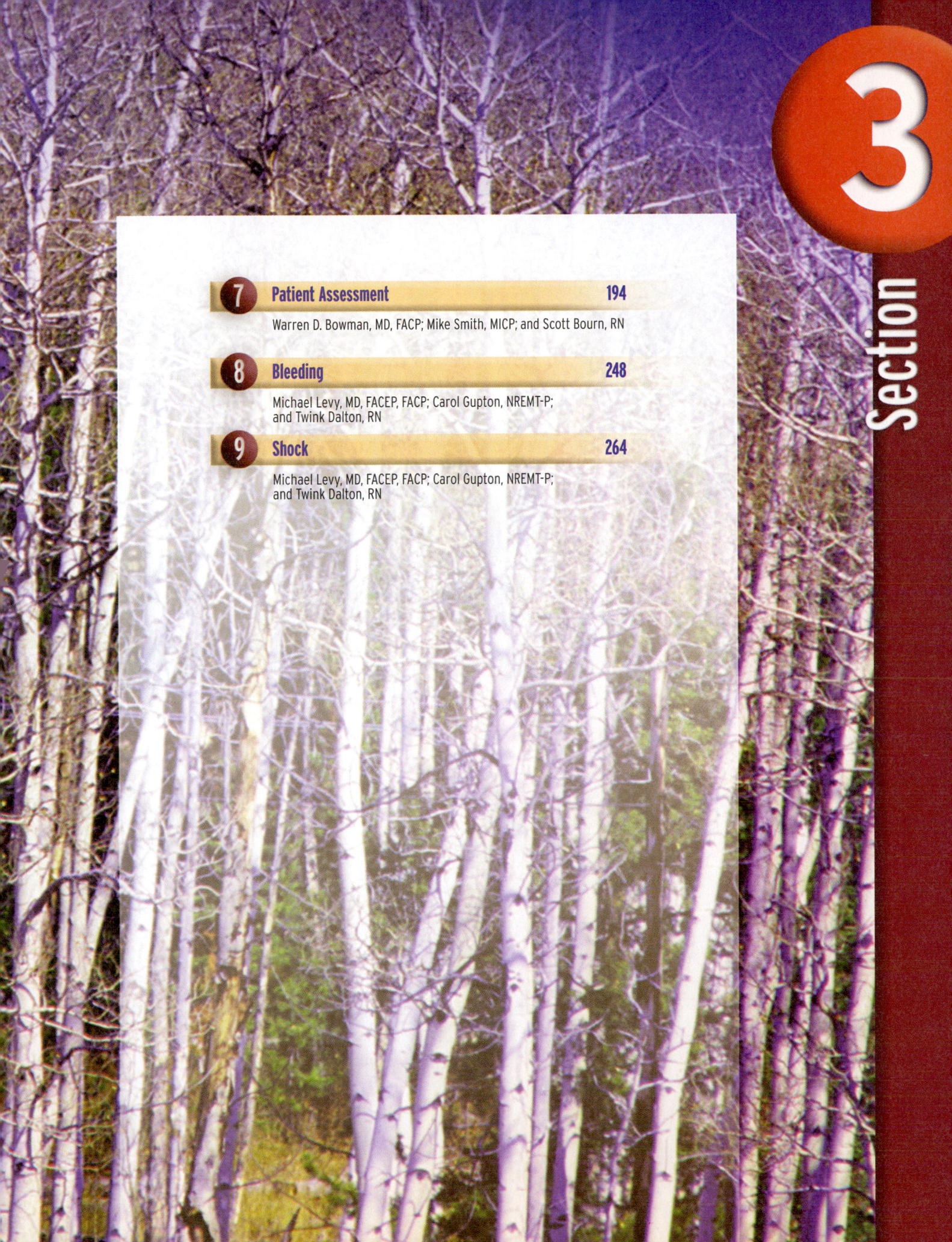

3

Section

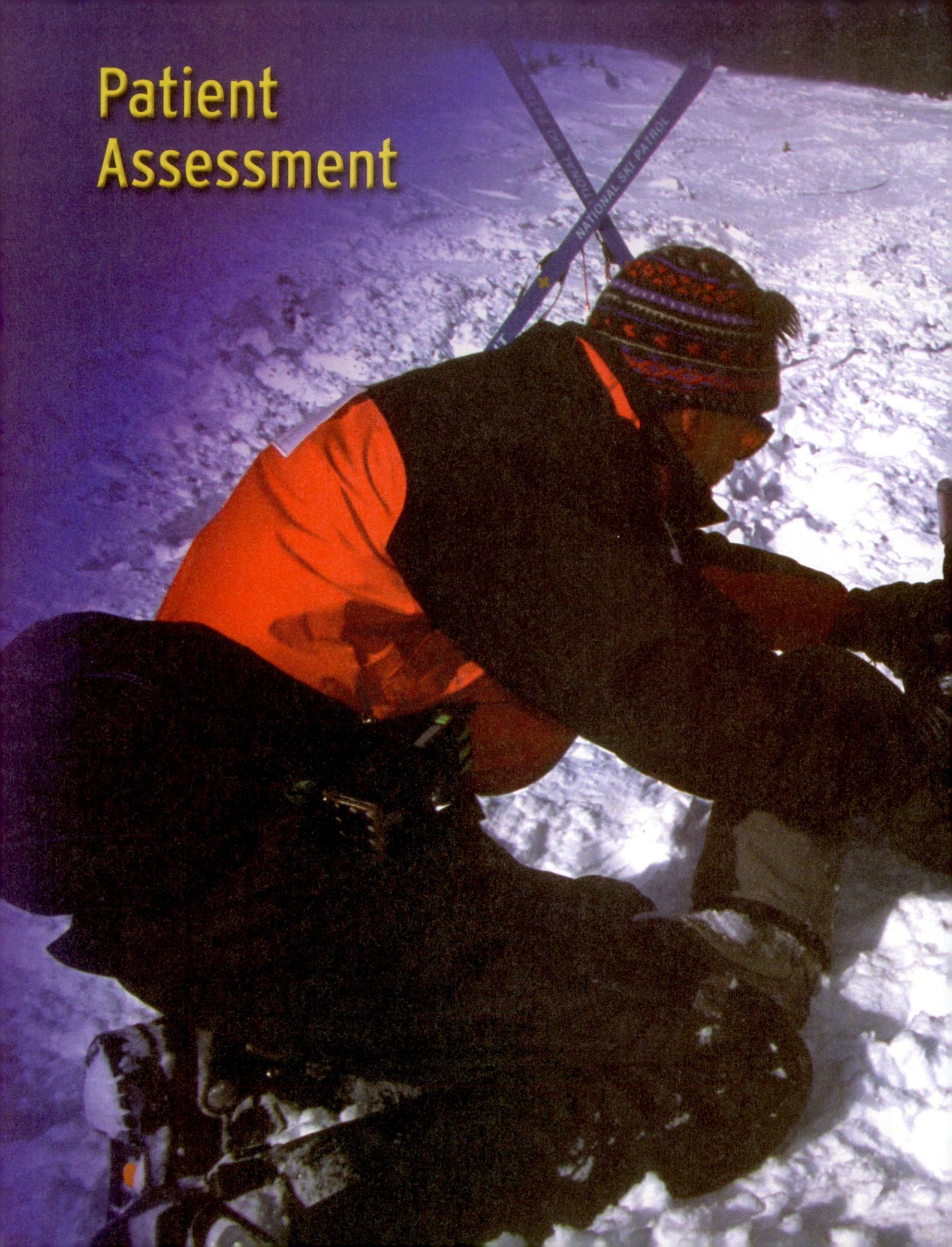

Patient Assessment

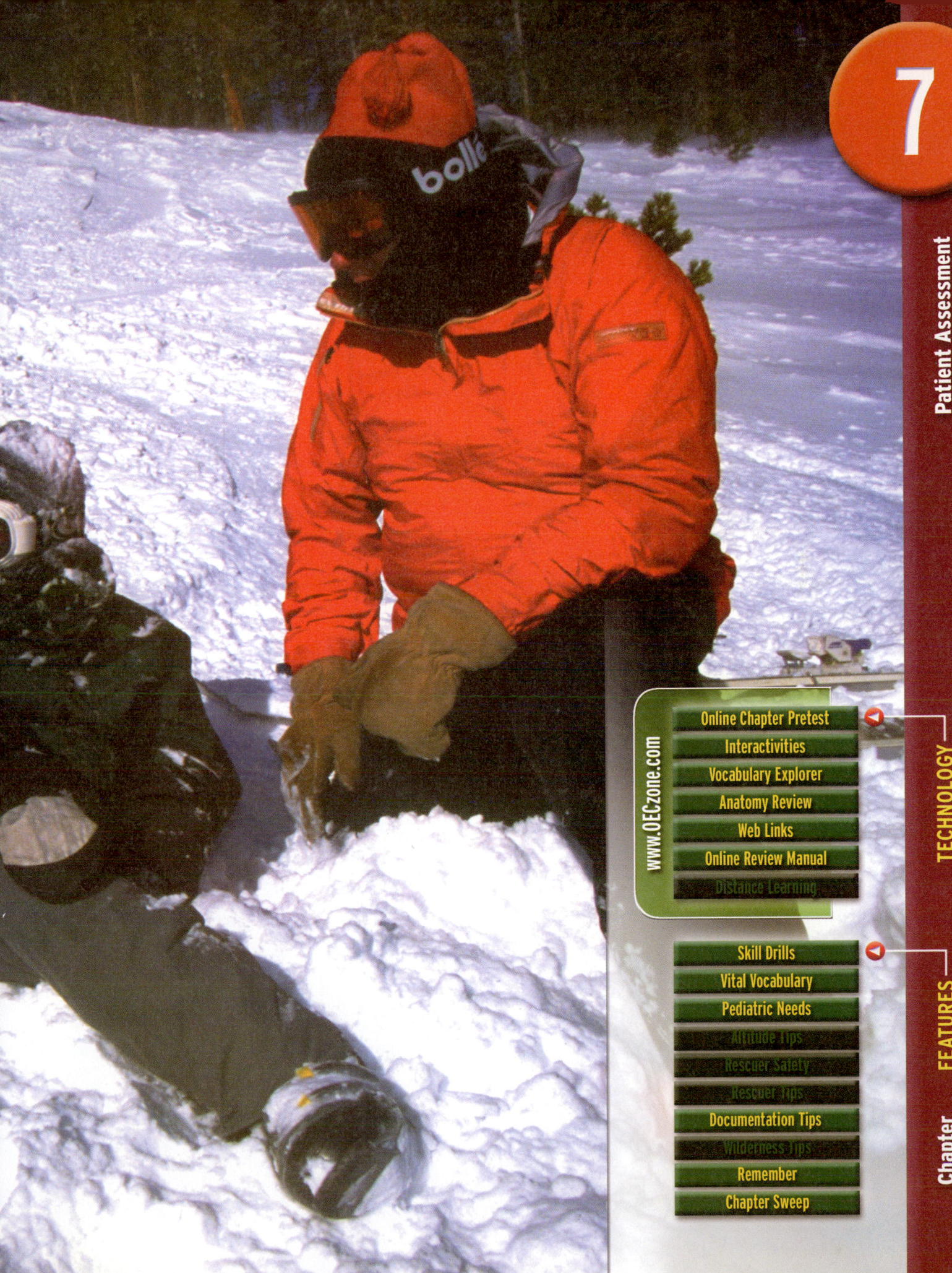

Patient Assessment

Scene Size-Up

Cognitive

🌲 **1.** Recognize actual and potential hazards (p 202).

🌲 **2.** Describe common hazards found at the scene of a trauma and a medical patient (p 202).

🌲 **3.** Determine if the scene is safe to enter (p 202).

🌲 **4.** Discuss common mechanisms of injury/nature of illness (p 200).

🌲 **5.** Discuss the reason for identifying the total number of patients at the scene (p 202).

🌲 **6.** Explain the reason for identifying the need for additional help or assistance (p 202).

🌲 **7.** Explain how you can determine that the patient is obviously responsive or possibly has altered responsiveness (p 202).

Affective

🌲 **8.** Explain the rationale for rescuers to evaluate scene safety before approaching the scene (p 202).

9. Serve as a model for others explaining how patient situations affect your evaluation of mechanism of injury or nature of illness (p 202).

Initial Assessment

Cognitive

🌲 **1.** Summarize the reasons for forming a general impression of the patient (p 204).

🌲 **2.** Discuss methods of assessing and managing the airway in the adult, child, and infant patient (p 206).

🌲 **3.** State reasons for management of the cervical spine once the patient has been determined to be a trauma patient.

🌲 **4.** Describe methods used for determining whether a patient is breathing and whether breathing is adequate (p 207).

5. State what care should be provided to the adult, child, and infant patient with and without adequate breathing (p 208).

🌲 **6.** Describe the methods used to assess circulation (p 209).

🌲 **7.** Differentiate between assessing circulation in an adult, child, and infant patient (p 209).

🌲 **8.** State what care should be provided to the adult, child, and infant patient with an abnormal or absent pulse (p 209).

🌲 **9.** Discuss the need for assessing the patient for external bleeding (p 209).

10. Describe normal and abnormal findings when assessing skin color, temperature, and moisture (p 237).

🌲 **11.** Explain the reasons for prioritizing a patient for care and transport (p 210).

Affective

🌲 **12.** Explain the importance of forming a general impression of the patient (p 204).

🌲 **13.** Explain the value of performing an initial assessment (p 204).

Psychomotor

🌲 **14.** Demonstrate the techniques for assessing responsiveness (p 204).

🌲 **15.** Demonstrate the techniques for assessing and stabilizing the ABCs (p 206).

16. Demonstrate the techniques for assessing the patient with external bleeding (p 209).

🌲 **17.** Demonstrate the techniques for assessing the patient's skin color, temperature, moisture, and capillary refill (p 218-219).

🌲 **18.** Demonstrate the ability to prioritize patients (p 210).

Rapid History and Physical Exam: Unresponsive Patients

Cognitive

🌲 **1.** Discuss the method of assessing altered responsiveness (p 211).

🌲 **2.** Describe the unique needs for assessing an individual who is unresponsive (p 211).

🌲 **3.** Describe the indications for doing a rapid body survey (p 211).

🌲 **4.** Discuss the various rapid transport protocols for your location or organization (p 215).

Affective

🌲 **5.** Explain the indications and value of performing a rapid body survey on site (p 211).

Psychomotor

🌲 **6.** Demonstrate the performance of a rapid body survey (p 211).

🌲 **7.** Demonstrate the patient care skills that should be used to assist an unresponsive patient (p 211).

Focused History and Physical Exam: Responsive Trauma Patients

Cognitive

🌲 1. Discuss the significance of the mechanism of injury (p 216).

🌲 2. Differentiate when the assessment may be altered in order to provide patient care (p 216).

🌲 3. Discuss the reason for performing a focused trauma history and physical exam (p 216).

Affective

4. Recognize and respect the feelings that patients might experience during assessment (p 216).

Psychomotor

🌲 5. Demonstrate the trauma assessment that should be used to assess a responsive patient based on mechanism of injury (p 219).

Focused History and Physical Exam: Responsive Medical Patients

Cognitive

🌲 1. Describe the unique needs for assessing an individual with a specific chief complaint with no known prior history (p 222).

Affective

2. Attend to the feelings that these patients might be experiencing (p 224).

Psychomotor

🌲 3. Demonstrate the patient care skills that should be used to assist a responsive patient with a medical illness (p 226).

Detailed Physical Exam

Cognitive

🌲 1. Discuss the components of the detailed physical exam (p 233).

🌲 2. State the areas of the body that are evaluated during the detailed physical exam (p 233).

🌲 3. Explain what additional care should be provided while performing the detailed physical exam (p 232).

Affective

4. Explain the rationale for the feelings that these patients might be experiencing (p 230).

Psychomotor

🌲 5. Demonstrate the skills involved in performing the detailed physical exam (p 233).

Ongoing Assessment

Cognitive

🌲 1. Discuss the reason for repeating the initial assessment as part of the ongoing assessment (p 242).

🌲 2. Describe the components of the ongoing assessment (p 242).

🌲 3. Describe monitoring of the assessment components (p 242).

Affective

🌲 4. Explain the value of performing an ongoing assessment (p 242).

🌲 5. Explain the value of trending assessment components to other health professionals who assume care of the patient (p 242).

Psychomotor

🌲 6. Demonstrate the skills involved in performing the ongoing assessment (p 242).

🌲 These are core concepts in initial patrol training.

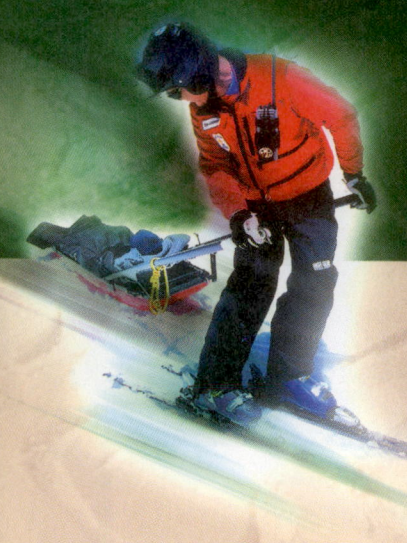

You are the rescuer

You are responding to a radio report of a male skier lying motionless in the snow on upper Big Pine run. Another skier reported this to the lift operator, who called the patrol; no other information is available. Fortunately, you have just gotten off Big Pine lift and are able to reach the site in 2 minutes. As you approach, you note that the skier is lying on his back at the side of the run where there is little danger from or to other skiers. One ski is off, the other is attached to a boot that is turned to an unusual angle. You stop several yards above the skier, remove your skis, plant them in an X in the snow, and approach him. He is not moving but appears to be breathing. There is no obvious blood on the snow or his clothing. You kneel at his side, palpate the carotid pulse, and ask "Sir, are you okay?"

Good patient care is directly linked to good patient assessment. This chapter will cover this most essential of all rescuer skills as well as help you answer the following questions:

1. Why is patient assessment considered one of the cornerstones of prehospital care?

2. Is there a difference between assessment of a trauma patient and a patient with a medical condition? If so, what is it?

About This Chapter

The first step in providing emergency care to someone who is injured or ill is to identify the problem. To identify the type and extent of the problem, prehospital emergency care providers use a type of examination referred to as patient assessment. This chapter will provide a clear and comprehensive approach to patient assessment. The Patient Assessment Flowchart is repeated at every section to show you "at a glance" where you are in the patient assessment process.

The chapter has been divided into four major sections. The second section, Initial Assessment, comprises three subsections, making seven divisions in all.

Scene size-up
Initial assessment (in the field)
• Assessment of unresponsive patients
• Assessment of responsive trauma patients
• Assessment of responsive medical patients
Rapid or focused history and physical exam
Detailed physical examination (in a warm environment)
Ongoing assessment

Each division is color coded and numbered for easy reference.

Patient Assessment

Patient assessment consists of a series of actions that must be performed correctly and in the proper order each time. The nature of these actions and their proper order has been perfected through many years of experience by expert health care workers. These actions form the core of every course in emergency care and are remarkably similar from one course to another. However, because patrollers and other outdoor emergency caregivers operate in a unique environment, the sequences and details of assessment as described in this textbook differ somewhat from those described in first responder and EMT textbooks.

The goals of assessment are as follows:

1. Detect life-threatening conditions rapidly and care for them immediately.

2. Determine whether you need to attend to any other problems.

3. Evaluate and facilitate the rapid transport of the patient to enter the EMS system or to get to definitive medical care.

4. Perform a complete assessment and note all significant findings.

5. Do nothing that would make the patient worse.

As a rescuer, you must learn the techniques of assessment thoroughly and practice them often so you can perform them accurately and in the right order, despite distractions or a hostile environment. When mistakes in emergency care are made, they usually result from failure to conduct a thorough or systematic assessment rather

Patient Assessment

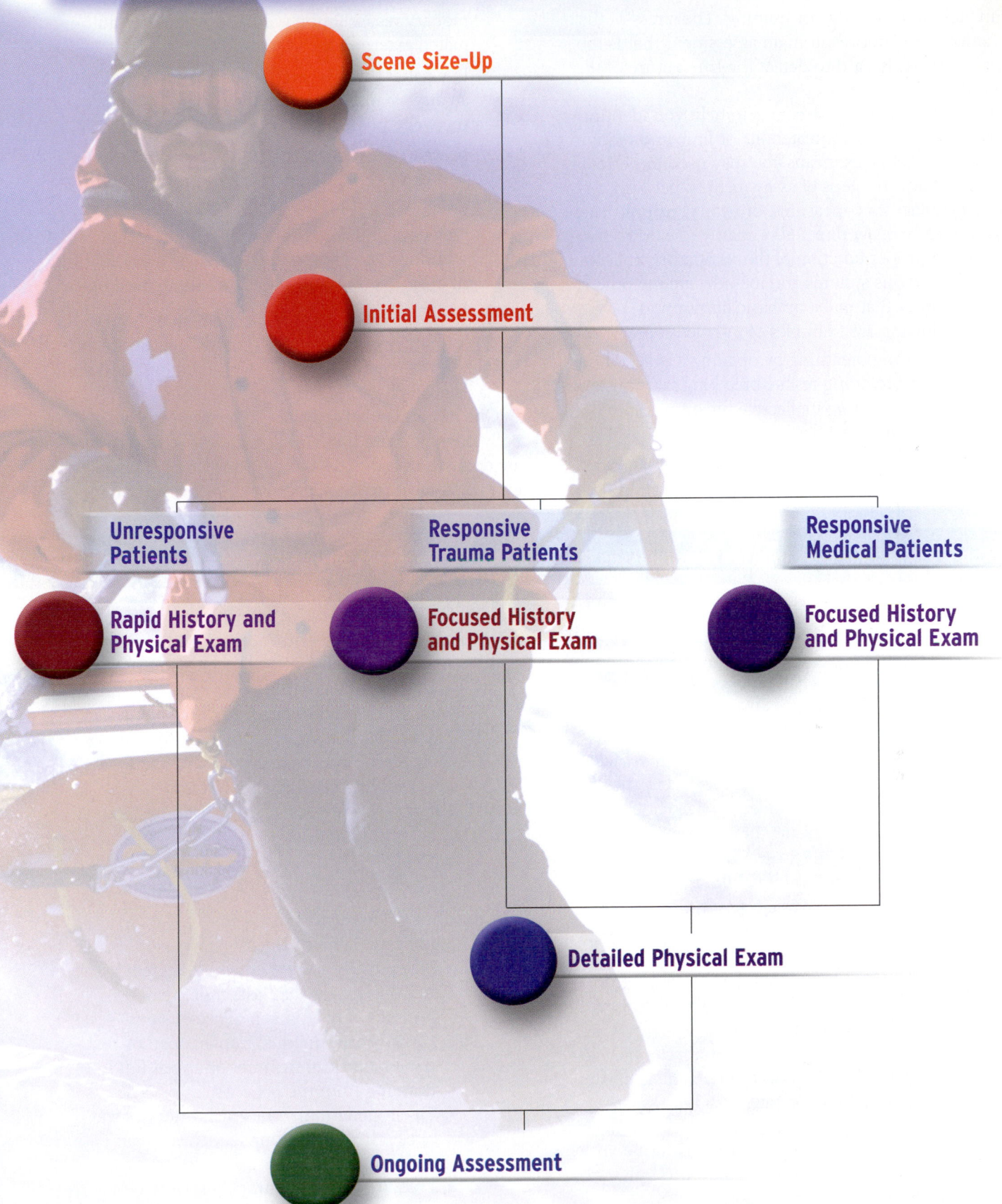

Scene Size-Up

Initial Assessment

Unresponsive Patients

Responsive Trauma Patients

Responsive Medical Patients

Rapid History and Physical Exam

Focused History and Physical Exam

Focused History and Physical Exam

Detailed Physical Exam

Ongoing Assessment

than lack of knowledge or training. The stress of the situation must not result in an assessment that is too hurried or haphazard to detect the true nature of the problem.

One purpose of assessment is to help you identify those conditions that threaten life or limb and require immediate care. This means you may need to periodically interrupt the steps of assessment to perform certain emergency care measures, or **interventions**. These urgent measures are directed primarily toward reestablishing the proper function of the respiratory, circulatory, and nervous systems and include, among others, the techniques that make up basic life support.

The following are examples of interventions:

1. Supporting breathing by opening a blocked airway, providing rescue breathing, administering oxygen, assisting ineffective breathing, and sealing an open chest wound.

2. Supporting circulation by controlling hemorrhage, caring for shock, providing cardiopul-

monary resuscitation (CPR), and using an automated external defibrillator (AED).

3. In a patient with altered responsiveness, inserting an airway and/or placing the patient in the **recovery position**.

4. In a patient with a suspected neck or back injury, stabilizing the neck and back to prevent motion that might injure the spinal cord.

5. Providing initial care for serious injuries, eg, splinting a fractured femur, bandaging and splinting an open fracture, and stabilizing an impaled object.

Assessment incorporates the **mechanism of injury (MOI)** or **nature of illness (NOI)**, an initial assessment, a rapid body survey, a focused history and physical exam, and a detailed physical exam.

One recommended sequence for conducting a total body physical exam is advised, regardless of whether you are doing the rapid body survey or the detailed physical exam, and whether the patient is responsive or unrespon-

Table 7-1 Significant Injuries and Illnesses Requiring Rapid Transport and EMS Interface

1. Significant **Mechanism of Injury (MOI)**
   A. Fall from a height 2½ to 3 times the patient's height (or less if horizontal motion was involved; eg, a moving chair-lift)
   B. Involvement in a moderate- to high-speed vehicle accident with an auto, motorcycle, bicycle, snowmobile, or all-terrain vehicle
      - Accident in which another occupant of the vehicle was killed
      - Auto accident in which the passenger was unrestrained (no seat belt or air bag; in the case of a young child, no child seat)
      - Patient who was ejected from a vehicle or in a vehicle that rolled over during a crash
      - Passenger who was in a car whose front end or front axle was displaced rearward 20″ or more by a crash
      - Accident involving a motorcycle, bicycle, snowmobile, or all-terrain vehicle crash, especially if the patient did not wear a helmet
   C. Pedestrian or bicyclist who was hit by an automobile traveling 25 mph (40 kph) or faster

   D. Patient who collided at high speed with another skier or snowboarder or an immobile object such as a tree or lift tower while skiing or snowboarding
   E. Gunshot wound to head, neck, or trunk
   F. Extrication that takes more than 30 minutes
   G. Patient who was buried in an avalanche or involved in a cave-in or explosion
   H. Patient who was struck by a rock, tree, or other falling object
   I. Exposure to electricity, either AC or DC, that results in thermal or neurologic emergencies

2. Significant **Threat to Life**
   A. Significant **Type of Injury**
      - Head injury accompanied by altered responsiveness that lasts more than 5 minutes, any lapses in consciousness, convulsions, unequal pupils, open or depressed skull fracture, or spinal fluid draining from the patient's ear or nose
      - Open, penetrating, or crush injury of the neck, chest (including flail chest), abdomen, or pelvis
      - Fracture of the femur, pelvis, or two or more extremities
      - Two or more dislocations

sive. There are certain variations, depending on which type of assessment you are conducting and the patient's level of responsiveness, and these will be clearly noted.

In addition to using your eyes, ears, hands, and nose, you must use your brain to make accurate observations, ask appropriate questions, evaluate the information gathered, pursue promising leads, and take appropriate action. Although assessment is relatively easy to learn and perform under classroom conditions, *it may be very difficult to conduct under severe environmental conditions.* For example, cold and wind may numb your fingers and make it unwise to undress the patient, or you may need to assess the patient in a confined area such as in a tree well or on a narrow ledge.

Two types of body assessment performed in the outdoor environment vary slightly from the EMT protocol. The **rapid body survey** is part of the rapid history and physical exam and is accomplished in the outdoor elements. Also, the detailed physical exam typically is not performed in the field but only when shelter is reached.

Transport Decisions

Most seriously injured patients have about 1 hour before their condition begins to deteriorate rapidly. This critical period, known as the **Golden Hour**, is a window of time in which the level of care the patient receives determines the patient's chances of survival. After the first hour, for every 30 minutes that pass without hospital care, the patient's chances of survival are cut in half. Therefore, a patient with a serious or life-threatening injury or illness (▼ **Table 7-1**) should be kept in the field only long enough for the initial assessment and necessary interventions to be performed.

Do not delay transporting the patient to a location where you can interface with the EMS system and obtain advanced life support or emergency department care. Start arrangements for transport and EMS interface during the scene size-up or early initial assessment, as soon as you recognize the serious nature of the patient's condition.

- Traumatic amputation of an extremity other than a digit
- Any injury accompanied by an abnormal pulse or respirations, shock, or uncontrolled, severe bleeding
- Moderate to critical burns (see Chapter 19 for burn classifications)
- Suspected internal injuries with or without obvious bleeding

B. Significant **Nature of Illness (NOI)**
- Patient unresponsive or with altered responsiveness
- Stroke
- Respiratory or cardiorespiratory arrest
- Chest pain of uncertain cause that recurs frequently or lasts more than 15 minutes
- Abnormal pulse or respirations; labored breathing resulting from any cause other than a temporary asthma attack
- Venomous animal or insect bite (black widow spider, brown recluse spider, snake, etc)
- Near-drowning
- Severe allergic reaction, such as anaphylactic shock
- Suspected poisoning or overdose
- Complicated emergency childbirth

- Severe, unrelieved pain
- High fever that lasts more than a few hours and does not improve with non-prescription medications
- High fever accompanied by stiff neck
- Intractable vomiting or diarrhea, especially if it is accompanied by the inability to keep food or fluids down for more than 12 hours
- Vomiting blood or passing bloody stools or urine

3. Significant **Threat to Limb** (generally not life-threatening but may result in serious disability)
   A. Any dislocation other than that of a digit
   B. Neck, back, or extremity injury with altered circulation, motion, and/or sensation (CMS)
   C. Major eye injuries
   D. Crushing injury of an extremity
   E. Fractures or fracture-dislocations near the elbow or knee

4. Possible **Threat to Life or Limb**
   A. Ongoing assessment detects significant abnormal changes in responsiveness, pulse, or respirations
   B. Any patient who, in the opinion of an experienced rescuer, looks seriously injured or ill

Scene Size-up

When approaching the scene, the rescuer forms an immediate first impression of what is occurring, which is called the **scene size-up**. The scene size-up should take less time to register than to read about here (▶ **Table 7-2**).

The scene size-up begins to take form when you receive information via the initial radio call or other notification and continues from when you catch sight of the patient until you arrive at his or her side. It consists of the following essential information, which your brain registers almost simultaneously.

1. Is there any danger to the rescuer(s), patient(s), or others at the scene? Possible danger includes the following:
   - Environmental hazards such as blizzard conditions, steep terrain, falling rocks, snow avalanche, flooding, or swift water
   - Traffic from over-the-snow or other vehicles, reckless skiers, or snowboarders
   - Live wires, lightning strikes, and other electrical hazards
   - Hazardous materials such as chemical spills, toxic fumes, etc.
   - Structural collapses in natural or man-made disasters
   - Falling from an insecure location
   - Dangerous animals in the immediate area

2. How many patients are there? Will **triage** be required?

3. Will you have difficulty reaching the patient(s)? Can you reach the patient(s) with emergency care equipment? With transport equipment such as a toboggan or litter?

4. Will you need to disentangle or extricate the patient(s) from an awkward or difficult location?

5. Will you need additional help?

6. What has most likely occurred, as indicated by the patient's location, position, and other objective factors? Does the patient have an injury or an illness? What is the probable mechanism of injury or nature of illness?

7. Is the patient obviously responsive or possibly unresponsive?

8. Is the patient obviously breathing? Talking?

9. Is there obvious bleeding?

10. Do you have a "poor" general impression (ie, does the patient appear to be critically injured or ill)?

TABLE 7-2 Scene Size-Up
Body Substance Isolation
Scene Safety
Determine Mechanism of Injury/Nature of Illness
Determine Number of Patients
Request Additional Assistance
Consider C-Spine Immobilization

If the scene appears to be hazardous, never underestimate the importance of scene safety. If there is any risk to the rescuer, do not enter the hazardous area.

Making a scene safe may be as simple as posting a guard or as complicated as using resources of many different rescuers or agencies.

Be sure to adhere to **body substance isolation (BSI)** techniques throughout every emergency care situation to reduce exposure to potentially dangerous body substances (▼ **Figure 7-1**).

When more than one rescuer is present at the scene, someone should be put in charge. The leader usually is either the first person at the scene or the most experienced person present. If enough help is available, the leader should avoid direct participation and concentrate on managing the scene, assigning and overseeing assessment and emergency care, calling for additional help or equipment as needed, arranging for EMS interface, and seeing that a log of events and vital signs is kept.

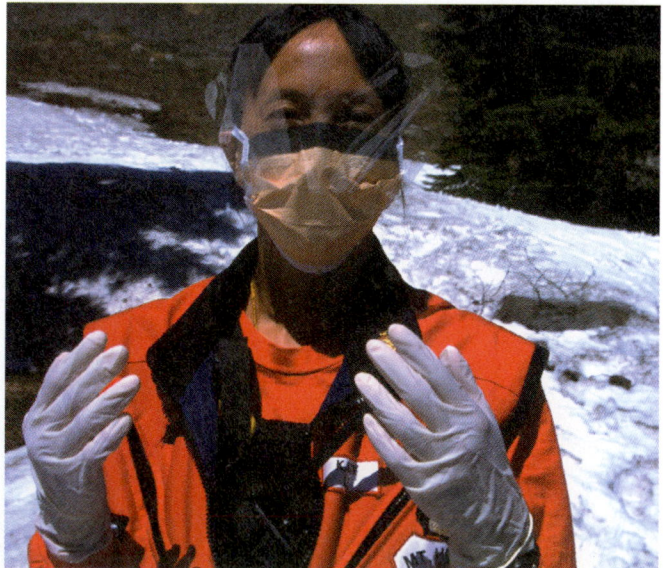

Figure 7-1 Proper protective equipment is vital when you are called to a scene in which there is a lot of blood or other body fluids.

Patient Assessment

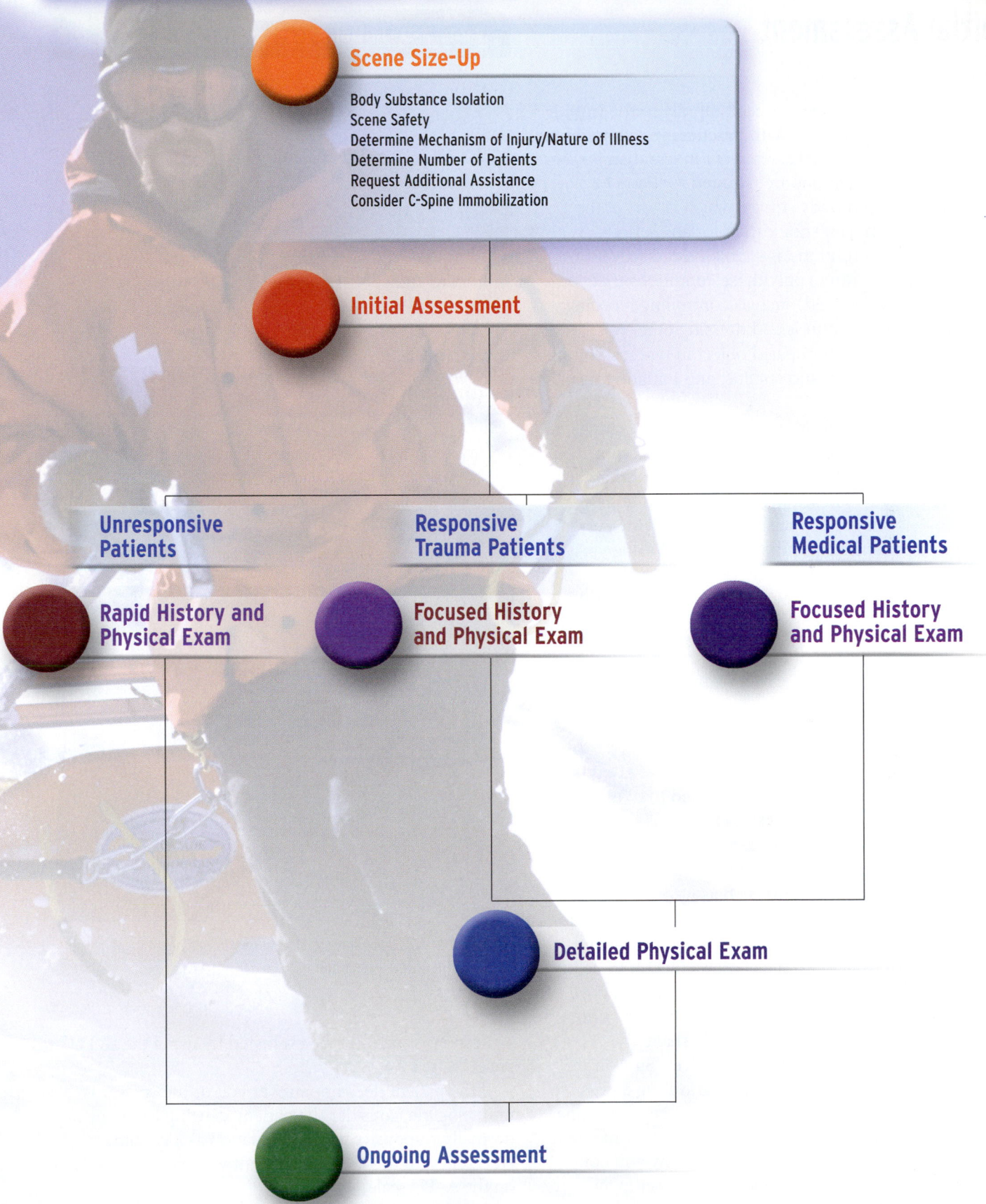

Scene Size-Up

Body Substance Isolation
Scene Safety
Determine Mechanism of Injury/Nature of Illness
Determine Number of Patients
Request Additional Assistance
Consider C-Spine Immobilization

Initial Assessment

Unresponsive Patients

Responsive Trauma Patients

Responsive Medical Patients

Rapid History and Physical Exam

Focused History and Physical Exam

Focused History and Physical Exam

Detailed Physical Exam

Ongoing Assessment

Initial Assessment

General Impression

After sizing up the scene, proceed rapidly to the **initial assessment** (▶ **Table 7-3**). With practice, you should be able to perform the initial assessment in less than 90 seconds, unless interventions are required (▼ **Figure 7-2**).

During the rapid body survey, which is part of the initial assessment, you should care for any serious or life-threatening conditions as soon as you discover them. However, address only those conditions that you can deal with in the field, such as controlling bleeding; sealing open chest wounds and dressing other open wounds; stabilizing an impaled object in place; splinting fractures, dislocations, and sprains; and initiating treatment of shock.

In cold weather, cut or open the patient's clothing only as a last resort, using trauma shears or a seam ripper. When the skin of the chest, neck, or abdomen must be assessed, expose only one small part at a time, by pulling clothing up or pushing it down. However, in the injured patient, inspect both outer and undergarments as thoroughly as possible for evidence of bleeding. Certain injuries such as open fractures and severely bleeding wounds must be exposed before you can care for them.

Assess Responsiveness

For brevity and clarity, in this chapter the term **unresponsive** will be used to indicate a patient who is not fully alert, that is, a patient who scores V, P, or U on the **AVPU** scale. **Responsiveness** is preferred to terms such as "consciousness" or "mental status," because it is more objective, documents what the examiner actually observes, and does not include any assumptions or connotations. For example, terms such as *mental status, consciousness, confusion, stupor, unconsciousness,* and *coma* are not strict medical terms. They have psychological and philosophic overtones that make them difficult to define.

Shortly after reaching the patient, you should have a good idea whether the patient is responsive or unresponsive. If you are not certain, gently shake the patient's shoulder and ask in a firm voice, "Sir (Ma'am or Miss), are you okay?" To avoid aggravating a possible spine injury while doing this, protect the cervical spine. Steady the patient's head by placing your other hand on his or her forehead. Beyond this point, how you conduct the assessment will *depend on the answer to this question.*

Table 7-3   Initial Assessment
Form General Impression of the Patient
Assess Responsiveness
Assess the Airway, Breathing, and Circulation (ABCs)
Stabilize ABCs
Identify Priority Patients
Initiate Transport Decision

Remember

The assessment techniques described in this chapter are for adult patients; children and infants require different techniques that will be identified in Pediatric Needs boxes.

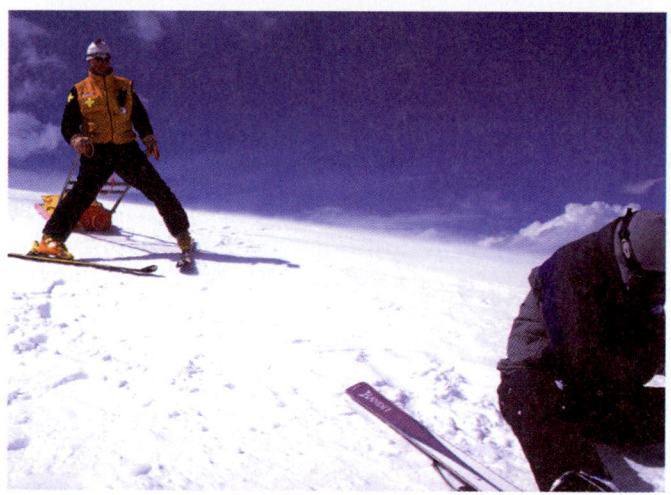

Figure 7-2 As you approach the patient, form a general impression of his or her overall condition.

Responsiveness can be evaluated by using the AVPU scale (▶ **Table 7-4**).

If the patient does not answer you or the answer is unintelligible, consider the patient as being less than normally responsive and the situation as a genuine emergency. In this case, the patient will score V, P, or U on the AVPU scale.

Patient Assessment

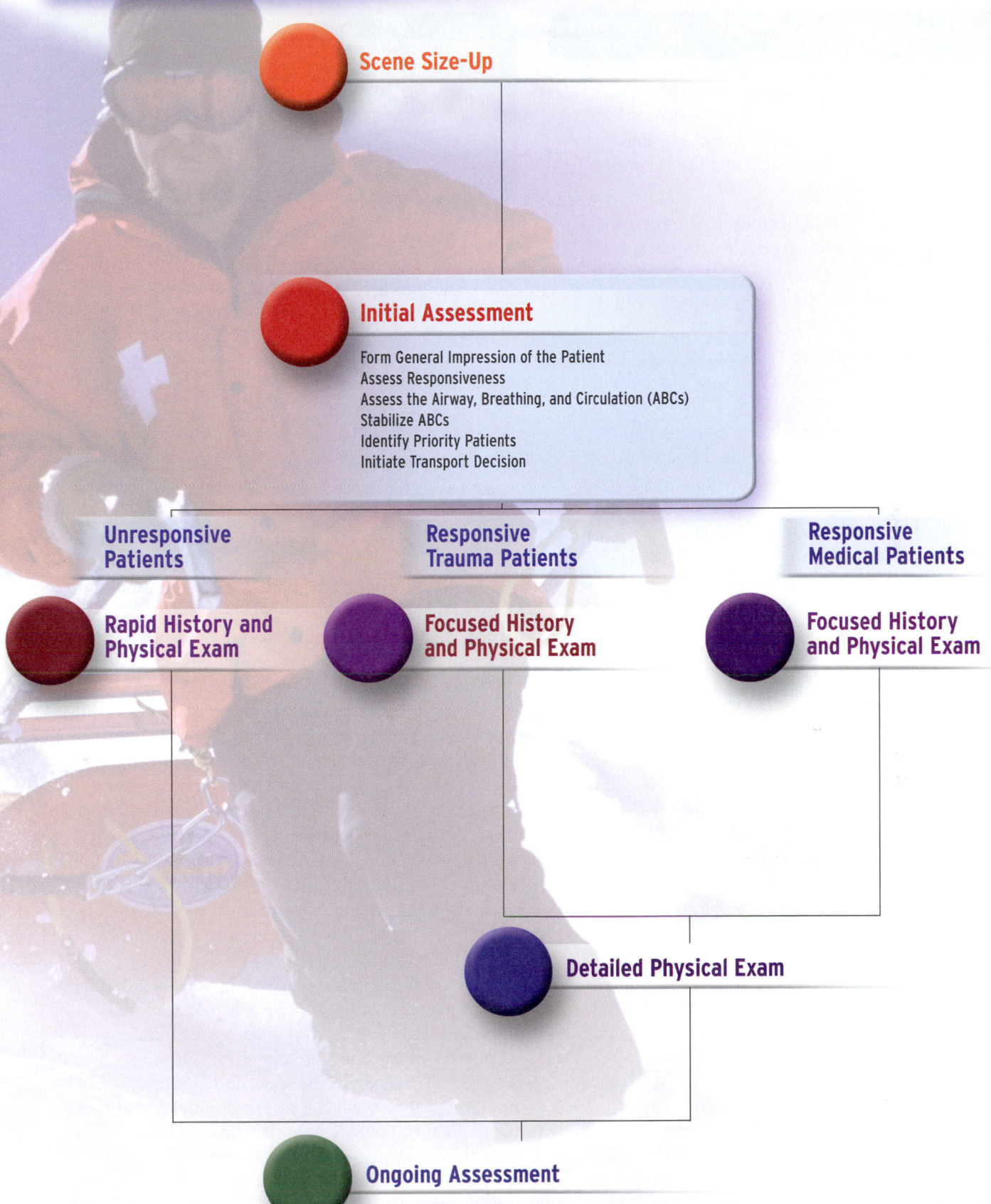

Scene Size-Up

Initial Assessment

Form General Impression of the Patient
Assess Responsiveness
Assess the Airway, Breathing, and Circulation (ABCs)
Stabilize ABCs
Identify Priority Patients
Initiate Transport Decision

Unresponsive Patients

Responsive Trauma Patients

Responsive Medical Patients

Rapid History and Physical Exam

Focused History and Physical Exam

Focused History and Physical Exam

Detailed Physical Exam

Ongoing Assessment

Table 7-4 AVPU Scale

<u>A</u>lert: The patient's eyes open spontaneously as you approach, and the patient appears aware of and responsive to the environment. The patient appears to follow commands, and the eyes visually track people and objects.

Responsive to <u>V</u>erbal Stimulus: The patient's eyes do not open spontaneously. However, the patient's eyes do open to verbal stimuli, and the patient is able to respond in some meaningful way when spoken to.

Responsive to <u>P</u>ain: The patient does not respond to your questions but moves or cries out in response to a painful stimulus. This response is tested by gently but firmly pinching the patient's earlobe, by pressing down on the bone above the eye, or by pinching the muscles of the neck. The sternal rub, although advocated in CPR training, is not recommended because it may provide an inaccurate finding in patients with cervical spine injuries. The use of ammonia "smelling salts" also is not recommended. An appropriate response is moaning or pushing away or withdrawing from the pinch. Use of extremely painful stimuli is never appropriate.

<u>U</u>nresponsive: The patient does not respond to any stimulus.

Although a person can fake altered responsiveness, this distinction should be made by definitive caregivers at a hospital or physician's office, not by you—the prehospital caregiver.

To be considered responsive, a patient must have some function of the circulatory, respiratory, and nervous systems. Consequently, you may not need to conduct the exhaustive type of assessment you would if the patient were unresponsive.

You must remember, however, that even if the patient is responsive, problems with vital systems may be present or developing as a result of bleeding, the early stages of heart attack or shock, or some other significant condition. These situations are true emergencies, and you can care for them better if you suspect them and discover them early.

Airway obstruction in an unresponsive patient is most commonly due to relaxation of the tongue muscles back into the throat.

It is best to perform a complete initial assessment, and include a rapid body survey if the patient appears seriously injured or ill, there is a significant mechanism of injury or nature of illness, the pulse or respirations are abnormal, or the patient presents a poor general first impression.

Assess and Stabilize the Airway

As you move through the steps of assessment, you must always be alert for signs of respiratory compromise or airway obstruction. Regardless of the cause, airway obstruction may result in inadequate or absent air flow into and out of the lungs, which may cause permanent damage to the brain, heart, and lungs and may even result in death.

You should immediately assess the patency of the airway in an unresponsive patient or a patient with a decreased level of consciousness.

Although you can usually open the airway, it is difficult to assess and care for a patient who is not in the **supine** position. Therefore, you'll need to turn, or log roll, an unresponsive patient who is prone or semiprone to a supine position. Because of the strong possibility that a neck or back injury might be aggravated in a patient who is unresponsive because of trauma, you usually should wait to turn a patient who is breathing normally until enough help arrives to use safe turning techniques. Proper lifting and moving techniques are covered in Chapter 27.

It is very dangerous to delay resuscitative efforts in a patient who is breathing abnormally and does not improve rapidly with airway-opening techniques or is in respiratory or cardiorespiratory arrest. Therefore, if you are the only rescuer on the scene and competent help is not immediately available, you must quickly and single-handedly turn the patient to the supine position using special techniques (▶ **Table 7-5**).

In the unresponsive patient, the muscles of the upper airway may relax, allowing the tongue to fall back and close the airway by obstructing the pharynx. Because

Table 7-5 Turning Priorities in a Prone or Semiprone Patient

Normal Breathing	**Neck or Back Injury Unlikely** Turn the patient to the supine position using the one-rescuer turning technique. **Neck or Back Injury Likely** If there is time, wait for help and turn the patient using the multiple-rescuer turning technique; otherwise, use the one-rescuer technique.
Abnormal Breathing	**Neck or Back Injury Unlikely or Likely** Immediately open the airway, then turn the patient to the supine position using the one-rescuer turning technique.

the tongue is attached to the lower jaw, any movement that brings the lower jaw forward will move the tongue forward and away from the pharynx.

In a situation in which trauma was unlikely, the preferred method for opening the airway in an unresponsive patient is the simple and effective head tilt-chin lift technique. If you suspect a neck injury, try the chin-lift technique without the head tilt. If this does not open the airway (or if the head tilt-chin lift technique did not work), use the jaw-thrust maneuver. This technique is very effective but is more difficult than the head tilt-chin lift technique. If the patient needs CPR, the jaw-thrust technique will slow this procedure, especially if the patient is lying on the ground rather than on a cot or hospital litter.

When you practice the jaw-thrust technique on a volunteer, it may be painful and difficult for the "patient." Remember that the jaw muscles of an unresponsive patient are relaxed, making the maneuver much easier.

Techniques for opening the airway are discussed in Chapter 6.

Assess and Stabilize Breathing

Once the airway is open, assess the patient's breathing by *observing* whether his or her chest rises and falls, *listening* for the escape of air (by placing your ear next to the patient's mouth and nose), and *feeling* for the flow of air (▶ **Figure 7-3**). If the patient is breathing effectively, assess the respirations per minute, and continue to monitor breathing.

Watch for vomiting. Test the patient's gag reflex by gently and carefully touching the back of the tongue or back of the throat with a tongue blade. If the patient does not gag, insert an oral (oropharyngeal) or nasal (nasopharyngeal) airway to help keep the airway open (▶ **Figure 7-4**).

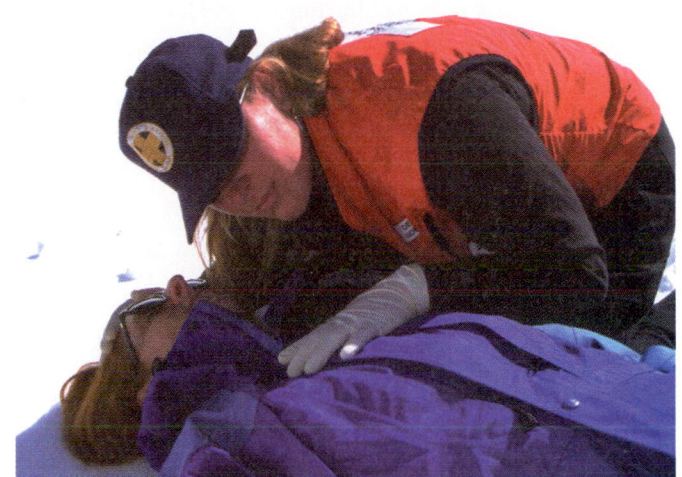

Figure 7-3 Assessing breathing.

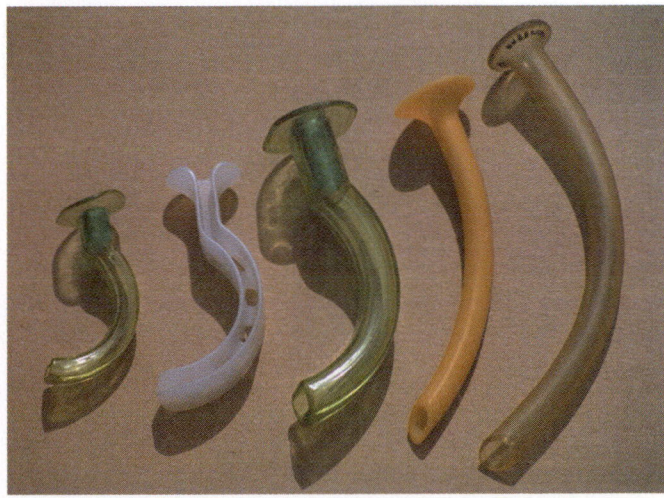

Figure 7-4 Oropharyngeal and nasopharyngeal airways.

TABLE 7-6	Determining the Quality of Breathing
Normal	• Breathing is neither shallow nor deep • Average chest wall motion • No use of accessory muscles
Shallow	• Slight chest or abdominal wall motion
Labored	• Increased breathing effort • Grunting, stridor • Use of accessory muscles • Gasping for air • Nasal flaring, supraclavicular and intercostal retractions (in infants and children)
Noisy	• Increase in sound of breathing, including snoring, wheezing, gurgling, and crowing

TABLE 7-7	Normal Respiratory Rates (breaths/min)
Adults	12 to 20
Children	18 to 34
Infants	30 to 60

TABLE 7-8	Average Pulse Rates (beats/min)
Adults	60 to 100
Children	70 to 140
Toddlers	90 to 150
Infants	100 to 160

If the patient is breathing ineffectively or not at all, begin rescue breathing or use an adjunct device such as a bag-valve-mask (BVM) device to ventilate the patient, adding oxygen as soon as it is available.

If the patient is unresponsive but is breathing spontaneously and has a pulse, you should place an oral airway unless the patient has a gag reflex. A patient with a gag reflex will not tolerate the placement of a nasopharyngeal or oropharyngeal airway. As soon as it is available, start high-flow oxygen at 12 to 15 L/min, using a nonrebreathing mask. Evaluate the quality of breathing and the pulse (▲ Table 7-6, 7-7, 7-8).

Important clues to look for in the unresponsive, breathing patient with a pulse include determining whether breathing and pulse are normal or abnormal. Abnormal (ineffective) breathing is too slow, too fast, or too shallow; an abnormal pulse is too slow, too fast, weak, or irregular.

Concerns Related to Rescue Breathing

Rescue breathing has been performed traditionally by the *mouth-to-mouth* technique, which is effective because the air that one person exhales into another person's lungs retains sufficient oxygen to support life (16%), at least at low-to-moderate altitudes of below 10,000′ (3,047 m). However, the acquired immunodeficiency syndrome (AIDS) epidemic has raised concerns

about using the direct mouth-to-mouth technique. Transmission of hepatitis, tuberculosis, and other contagious diseases also is a danger.

Although none of these diseases is known to have been transmitted via rescue breathing to date, AIDS and hepatitis viruses have been found in human saliva. Therefore, using your unprotected mouth to perform rescue breathing is discouraged unless there is no alternative. Mouth-to-mouth rescue breathing is described here because rescue breathing may be necessary at times when a barrier device (mask or mouth shield) is not available, as in emergency resuscitation of a family member.

Rescuers should carry pocket masks, or at least mouth shields, at all times and use them whenever they provide emergency mouth-to-mouth rescue breathing or CPR (▶ Figure 7-5). In the field, you can carry these devices in an emergency care belt or vest or in an emergency care kit; in town, the devices easily fit into a purse, briefcase, or coat pocket. Large devices for assisting ventilation, such as BVM devices, can be carried in emergency care kits, backpacks, and toboggans.

All masks and shields should be made of clear plastic that does not become rigid or brittle in the cold, and they should have valves and filters to protect you from the patient's saliva.

Pediatric Needs

You can feel the pulse of a child at the carotid artery, as in an adult. However, palpating this pulse in an infant may present a problem. Because an infant's neck is often very short and fat, and its pulse is often quite fast, you may have a hard time finding the carotid pulse. Therefore, in infants younger than 1 year, you should palpate the brachial artery to assess the pulse. Normal pulse rates for children are shown in (▼ Table 7-9).

TABLE 7-9 Normal Pulse Rates in Infants and Children	
Age	**Range (beats/min)**
Newborn: birth to 1 month	120 to 160
Infant: 1 month to 1 year	100 to 160
Toddler: 1 to 3 years	90 to 150
Preschool-age: 3 to 6 years	80 to 140
School-age: 6 to 12 years	70 to 120
Adolescent: 12 to 18 years	60 to 100
Older than 18 years	Adult normal ranges (60 to 100)

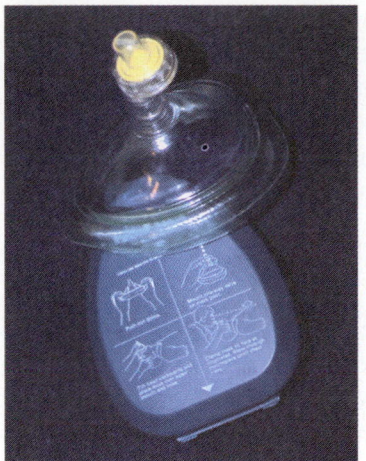

Figure 7-5 Pocket mask.

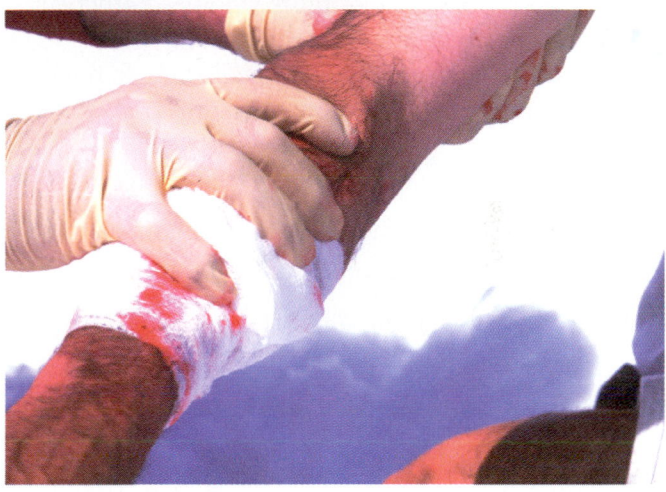

Figure 7-6 Direct pressure.

Assess and Stabilize Circulation

After the patient has begun to breathe again, assess his or her circulation by determining whether he or she has a carotid pulse. Because serious complications can occur when external chest compressions are performed on a patient with a pulse, you must be careful not to miss a weak or slow pulse. If there is any question about the status of the patient's pulse, continue checking the pulse for several more seconds. Check for up to 45 seconds in a patient with **hypothermia**, because the pulse may be very slow and weak.

If the patient has a pulse but is not breathing spontaneously, continue rescue breathing at a rate of one breath every 5 seconds, that is, 12 breaths/min for an adult (count "one and two and three and four and breathe and one and two…"). Each breath should last 2 seconds.

If there is no pulse, the patient is in *cardiac arrest* and you should immediately begin external chest compressions along with rescue breathing ("full" CPR). Call for

an AED as soon as possible. Various locally available CPR classes teach how to perform single-rescuer and multiple-rescuer CPR.

As soon as it is available, give high-flow oxygen to any patients who are receiving rescue breathing or CPR. Techniques for oxygen delivery are described in Chapter 6.

Assess and Manage Hemorrhage

Severe bleeding (**hemorrhage**), in which blood is spurting or flowing rapidly from a wound, is almost as life threatening as cardiac or respiratory arrest because a patient can bleed to death within minutes from an injury to a large artery.

If the patient's clothing is covering a wound that is bleeding severely, immediately cut away the material or rip along a seam to expose the area. Control the bleeding as rapidly and effectively as possible by applying direct pressure (▲ Figure 7-6). Techniques of controlling hemorrhage are covered in Chapter 8.

If you are alone and other urgent steps need to be taken, substitute a pressure dressing for direct pressure. If another rescuer is present, one of you can control bleeding while the other performs the rest of the initial assessment. However, because a little blood frequently looks like a lot of blood, especially on snow, you should avoid delaying other, more important resuscitative measures to stop minor bleeding that isn't life threatening.

Identify Priority Patients

Once you have completed the initial assessment, you have to make some decisions about patient care. You should have already addressed life-threatening injuries and/or illnesses as they were found. Next, you must identify priority patients, or those who need other interventions and/or immediate transport.

Patients with one or more of the following findings are considered high priority and should be transported immediately:

- Poor general impression
- Unresponsive with no gag or cough reflexes
- Responsive but unable to follow commands
- Difficulty breathing
- Pale skin or other signs of poor perfusion
- Complicated childbirth
- Uncontrolled bleeding
- Severe pain in any area of the body
- Severe chest pain, especially when the systolic blood pressure is less than 100 mm Hg
- Inability to move any part of the body

Correct identification of high-priority patients is an essential aspect of the initial assessment and helps to improve patient outcome. Many locales have specific guidelines for transporting critical patients. Some states even have regulations that guide patient care from the initial response through a final destination.

Initiate Transport Decision

As part of the initial assessment, you should consider what options are available to transport patients to an appropriate destination. Weather, local resources, and their status will affect the options you may use. In some instances, a local protocol will affect your decision. Many times, a multiple response involving more than one agency with different types of vehicles will be required. All of these factors should be considered beforehand with guidelines and operating procedures developed and understood. The goal is to get the patient to definitive care in a timely manner. In the case of a person suffering from an injury that is uncomplicated and stable, you may be able to delay the transport decision until after the patient has been evacuated to an aid room or triage station.

On the other hand, a critically injured patient may require a call for an ambulance or a helicopter. This call should be made as soon as you recognize the need for immediate hospital treatment. The key is good preplanning with the available resources and a simple and concise plan. Develop a precise decision process and identify which rescuers or staff can make those decisions. Communicate your transport needs as early as possible and update the dispatcher(s) as needed. Maximize the efficient use of transport resources (ambulances, helicopters, fire rescuer trucks, etc.). In many areas, resources are limited and having an ambulance wait for you to evacuate a patient or even obtain consent for transport is poor form. There may be another patient somewhere else who is a higher priority. Remember that some patients have only that Golden Hour and, for a successful outcome, you will need to make transport decisions early.

Assessment of Unresponsive Patients

With unresponsive patients, perform assessment with the goal of evacuating the patient to definitive care as quickly as possible ▶ Table 7-10 as part of the **rapid history and physical exam**. As part of the initial assessment, first radio for help, telephone 9-1-1 or another appropriate emergency number, or shout for help and ask that preparations for rapid transport be started. Then, unless the patient is obviously breathing normally, immediately open the airway using the jaw-thrust maneuver and determine the presence or absence of breathing. Continue to focus your attention on the basic life support interventions—maintaining the airway, immobilizing the spine, assisting with ventilations, administering supplemental oxygen, controlling bleeding, providing CPR if necessary, and providing immediate transport to an appropriate facility. These priorities reflect the importance of the ABC approach to the initial assessment.

Rapid Body Survey

Make sure the patient's body temperature is being maintained. In cold or windy weather, this usually requires placing windproof insulating material such as spare clothing over and under the patient. If the patient is very cold—and you will not become overly chilled yourself—you can put your parka, jacket, or vest over the patient while waiting for the toboggan with its blankets or sleeping bag. In hot weather, protect the patient from direct sunlight by using a tarp, clothing, or natural materials to make a sun shield.

If a patient is unresponsive because of trauma or an unknown cause, always assume a spine injury, especially to the cervical spine. Because such injuries can result in spinal cord damage with the danger of permanent disability, you must stabilize the cervical spine as soon as possible and maintain stabilization during the rest of the assessment and transport.

Keep the patient in the supine position and stabilize the cervical spine manually by firmly holding the head and neck in the neutral (anatomic) position between your hands: eyes forward, nose in line with the navel, and no flexion, extension, or rotation of the head or neck ▶ Figure 7-7. For a discussion of the technique of moving the head and neck into the neutral position, see *Long Backboard Application Technique* in Chapter 26.

Rapidly assess (examine) the patient's entire body from the head down, in the following order: head, neck,

TABLE 7-10 Rapid History and Physical Exam: Unresponsive Patients
Rapid Body Survey
Baseline Vital Signs
SAMPLE History (from family, friends, or bystanders)
Rapid Transport from Outdoor Environment

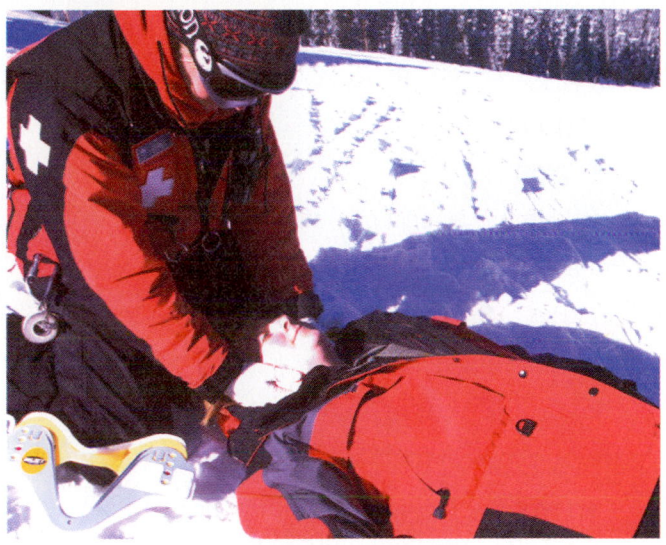

Figure 7-7 Manually stabilizing the head and neck.

chest, abdomen, pelvis, lower extremities, upper extremities, and back. The mnemonic **DCAP-BTLS** is widely used in the EMS system and is useful in helping you remember general things to look for during the rapid body survey:

Deformities

Contusions

Abrasions

Punctures, **P**enetrations

Burns, **B**leeding

Tenderness

Lacerations

Swellings

The rapid body survey, conducted at the site, is a hands-on, clothes-on assessment of every unresponsive

Table 7-11 Some Causes of Unresponsiveness

Resulting from Injury

Airway obstruction

Head injury

Shock from bleeding

Resulting from Illness

Stroke

Heart attack

Shock from causes other than bleeding

Aftermath of seizure

Severe infection:

- Sepsis

- Meningitis, encephalitis, brain abscess

Brain tumor

Toxic and metabolic conditions:

- Poisoning

- Alcohol or drug overdose (legal or illegal)

- Hypoglycemia

- Hypoxia, including asphyxia, heart failure, lung failure, high-altitude illness

- Diabetic coma

- Kidney or liver failure

Resulting from Environment

Near-drowning

Hypothermia

Hyperthermia

Electrical injury

patient as well as any responsive patient who appears seriously injured or ill, has a significant mechanism of injury or nature of illness, or has an abnormal pulse or respirations (◄ **Table 7-11**). The rapid body survey also should be conducted if the patient presents a poor general impression. Thorough assessment requires removing at least some clothing, but this may be impractical as well as dangerous in a cold, windy environment. Do not remove or cut open any of the patient's clothes at this time, although jackets and shirts can be pulled up and trousers or skirts pulled down as necessary.

Any problem found during the rapid body survey must be corrected immediately. If no major problem is found, then the rapid body survey should continue.

As you prepare for the rapid body survey, also called the rapid trauma assessment for responsive trauma patients with a significant mechanism of injury, consider your transport decision and request all backup that is appropriate for your environment. Remember to continue spinal immobilization while you check the patient's ABCs for any changes in status since the initial assessment. Follow the steps in (► **Skill Drill 7-1**):

1. **Assess the head,** looking and feeling for DCAP-BTLS and crepitus **(Step 1)**.

2. **Assess the neck,** looking and feeling for DCAP-BTLS, jugular vein distention, and crepitus **(Step 2)**.

3. **Assess the chest,** looking and feeling for DCAP-BTLS, paradoxical motion, and crepitus. You should also assess for breath sounds **(Step 3)**.

4. **Assess the abdomen,** looking and feeling for DCAP-BTLS, rigidity (firm or soft), and distention **(Step 4)**.

5. **Assess the pelvis,** looking and feeling for DCAP-BTLS. If there is no pain, gently compress the pelvis downward or inward to determine tenderness or instability **(Step 5)**.

6. **Assess the lower extremities,** looking and feeling for DCAP-BTLS. Also assess and compare bilaterally for distal circulation, motor function, and sensation **(Step 6)**.

7. **Assess the upper extremities,** looking and feeling for DCAP-BTLS. Also assess and compare bilaterally for distal circulation, motor function, and sensation **(Step 7)**.

8. **Assess the back,** rolling the patient with spinal precaution, to assess the posterior aspects of the body, looking and feeling for DCAP-BTLS **(Step 8)**.

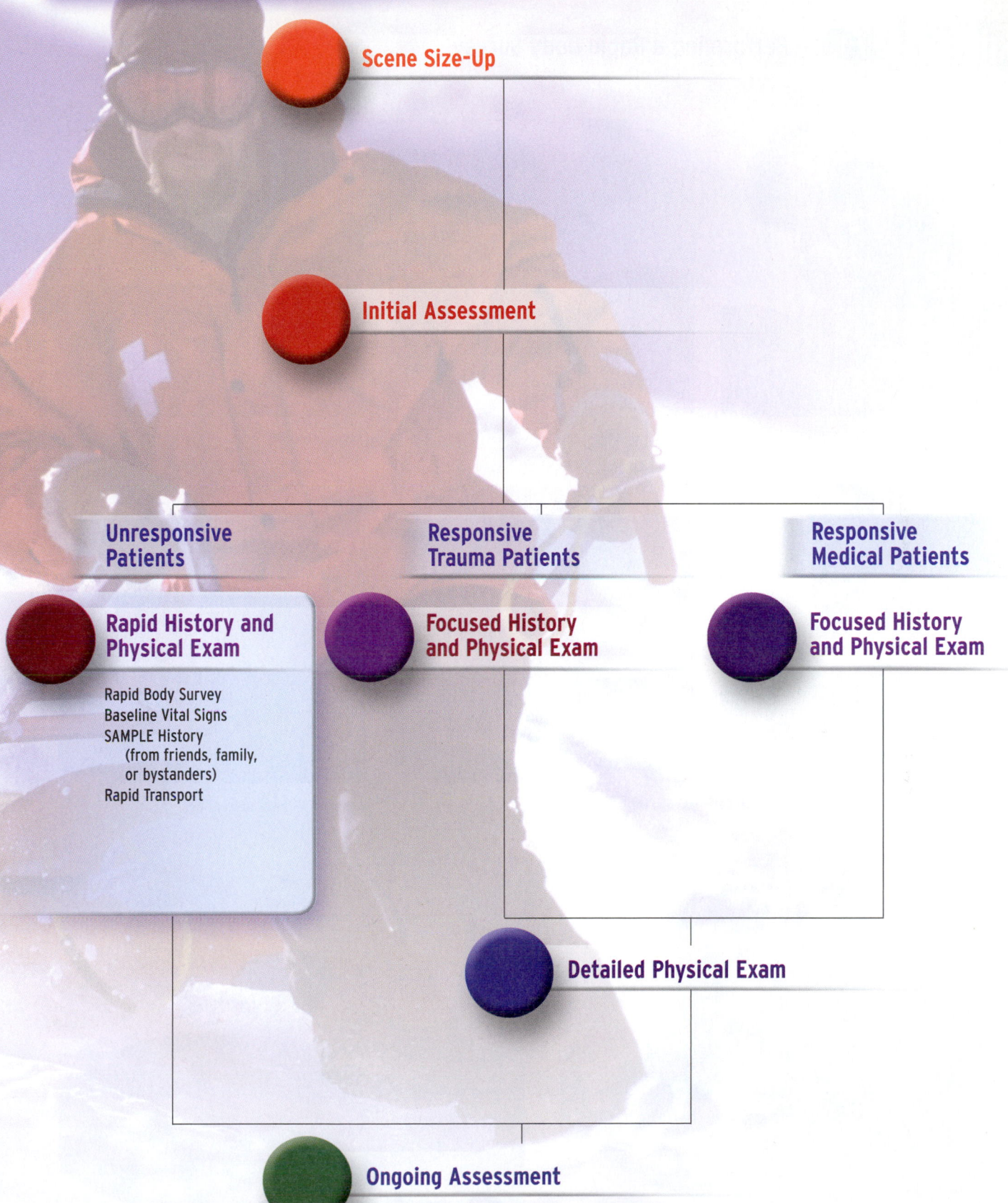

Scene Size-Up

Initial Assessment

Unresponsive Patients

Responsive Trauma Patients

Responsive Medical Patients

Rapid History and Physical Exam

Rapid Body Survey
Baseline Vital Signs
SAMPLE History
(from friends, family,
or bystanders)
Rapid Transport

Focused History and Physical Exam

Focused History and Physical Exam

Detailed Physical Exam

Ongoing Assessment

SkillDrill 7-1   Performing a Rapid Body Survey

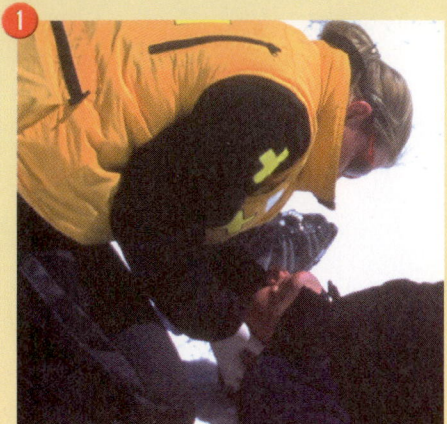

Assess the head.

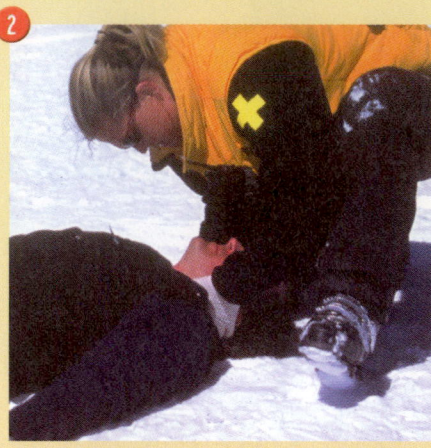

Assess the neck.

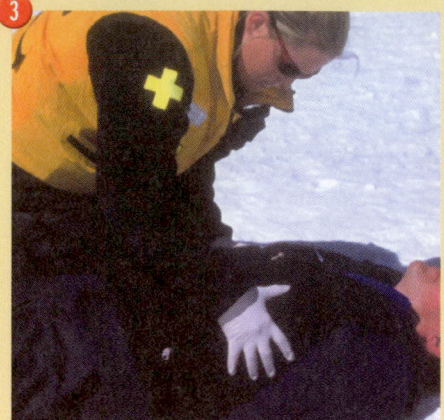

Assess the chest.

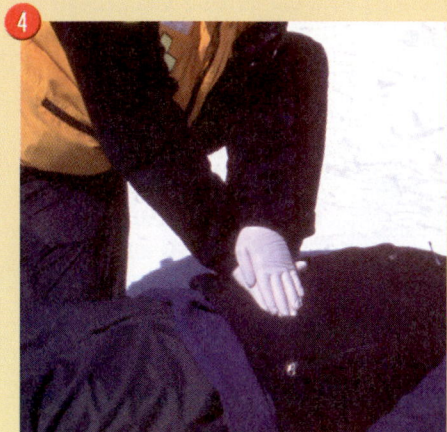

Assess the abdomen.

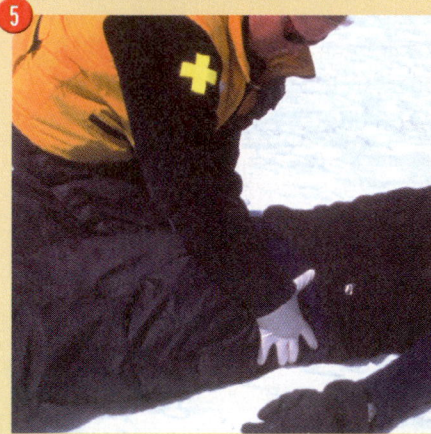

Assess the pelvis.

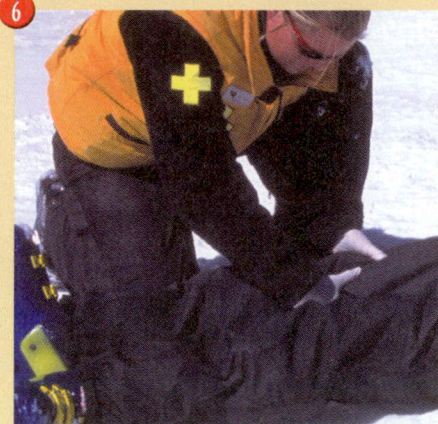

Assess the lower extremities.

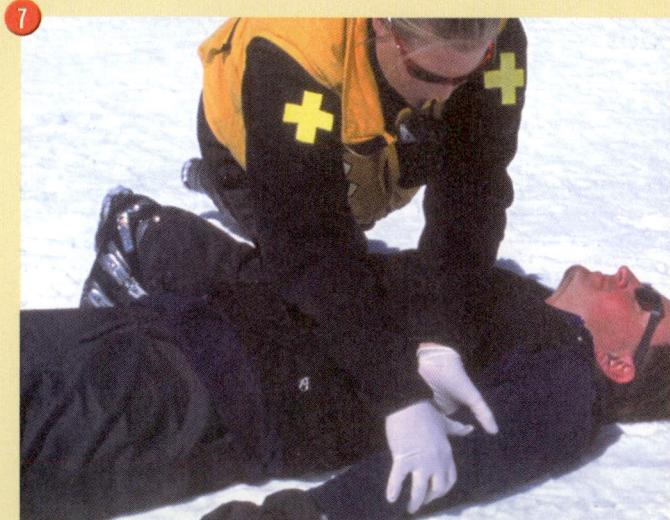

Assess the upper extremities.

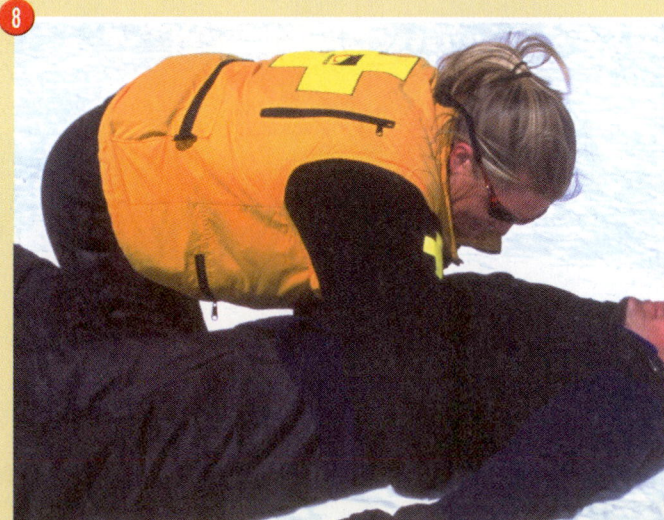

Assess the back.

Baseline Vital Signs and SAMPLE History

After you have completed the rapid body survey, it is time to obtain baseline vital signs and a **SAMPLE history**.

The baseline vital signs provide useful information about the overall functions of the patient's heart and lungs. After you have obtained the baseline vital signs, you should obtain a brief history from available witnesses, companions, or family members. Ask a witness what happened. The answer will help you determine whether the patient has an injury or illness. If the patient is injured, ask the witness about the mechanism of injury to help you anticipate what you found during the rapid body survey. However, never delay transport of an unresponsive patient to take a history from family members at the scene.

The mnemonic SAMPLE, defined as follows and widely used in the EMS system, will help you remember what the history should include:

- **S: S**igns and **S**ymptoms. Did the patient complain of or did the witness notice anything new or unusual before or during the current incident?

- **A: A**llergies. Does the patient have any allergies to insect stings, foods, medicines, plants, etc.? If so, has he or she been exposed to any of these substances recently? Look for a medical alert bracelet or necklace.

- **M: M**edications. Is the patient taking any medicines (prescription or nonprescription) or drugs (legal or illegal) regularly and/or recently? If so, for what condition(s)? Commonly taken medications include blood pressure medication, asthma inhalers, heart medication, pills or insulin shots for diabetes, arthritis medication, headache pills, thyroid pills, and birth control pills.

- **P: P**ertinent **P**ast History. Does the patient have any chronic medical conditions such as arthritis, diabetes, stroke, epilepsy, or heart disease? Have any of these conditions been causing trouble recently? Have there been problems in the past similar to the current one? Have there been any significant past injuries or operations? Is the patient currently under a doctor's care?

- **L: L**ast Oral Intake. When did the patient last eat or drink or, in the case of vomiting, when was he or she last able to hold anything down? This information is especially important in a patient with diabetes.

- **E: E**vents. Did anything unusual or significant occur leading up to the incident? Finally, ask if there is anything **E**lse you should know about the patient.

Documenting your baseline findings is important for tracking trends in the patient's condition and helping EMS and emergency department staff provide definitive treatment. Your report for the unresponsive patient should include documentation of the following:

- Findings from the initial assessment (ABCs)

- Baseline vital signs (pulse, blood pressure, respirations, temperature) and SAMPLE history (from bystanders)

- Skin color, temperature, and moisture

If an unresponsive patient must be transported rapidly to definitive medical care, there may not be time to do the detailed physical exam described later in this chapter. However, once you've transported the patient to the aid room or other suitable shelter, if time permits, begin to conduct the detailed physical exam. Unless the injury or illness is clearly minor, you should conduct this exam for every patient, removing clothing as needed to identify the nature or extent of the problem.

Rapid Transport Decisions

Rapid transport off the slope or out of the outdoor environment should have been initiated when the patient was originally assessed as unresponsive during the initial assessment. The request for rapid transport would have been relayed with the initial call for equipment, assistance, EMS requirements, and transport needs.

Assessment of the Responsive Trauma Patient

This section discusses assessment of the responsive trauma patient (▶ **Table 7-12**).

Reconsider the Mechanism of Injury

As part of the scene size-up, you evaluated the mechanism of injury before you began treatment. At this point in the assessment process, you should look at the mechanism again to ensure that you have not missed important information. Understanding the mechanism of injury helps you to understand the severity of the patient's problem and provide invaluable information to hospital staff as well. Some patients have experienced a significant mechanism of injury; others clearly have not.

The rapid body survey, (also called the rapid trauma assessment) using the simple mnemonic "DCAP-BTLS" should be performed on any responsive patient with significant mechanisms of injury to identify life-threatening injuries. The purpose of this assessment is to zero in on the patient's problems, and identify potentially life-threatening conditions, which will direct your physical exam. Remember, you can use a responsive patient as a resource; you should ask him or her about symptoms throughout your assessment.

With any responsive patient with no significant mechanism of injury, you will not need to perform such a complete exam.

Proper use of the mechanism of injury to predict possible injuries requires exploring and documenting exactly *what* happened, *how* it happened, *when* it happened, *why* it happened, *where* the resulting damage is, and *how bad* it seems to be. You should try to reconstruct the events leading up to the injury in a chronologic order.

Approach the patient, make eye contact, and introduce yourself as a person trained in emergency care by giving your name and the name of your organization (eg, a ski patrol or mountain rescue group, etc). Next, ask the patient's name and whether you can be of help. If the patient accepts your help, put on protective gloves and follow other BSI precautions regardless of whether moist body substances are visible.

Next, if there is any obvious, severe bleeding, control it immediately. After the hemorrhage is controlled, or in the patient who has no obvious, severe bleeding, ask, "What's wrong?" or "What's happened to you?" The answer to this type of question is called the **chief complaint**.

Table 7-12 Responsive Trauma Patient

Trauma—Significant Mechanism of Injury

- Rapid Trauma Assessment (Rapid Body Survey)
- Baseline Vital Signs and SAMPLE History
- Rapid Transport

Trauma—No Significant Mechanism of Injury

- Focused Physical Exam: Based on Chief Complaint
- Baseline Vital Signs and SAMPLE History
- Reevaluate transport

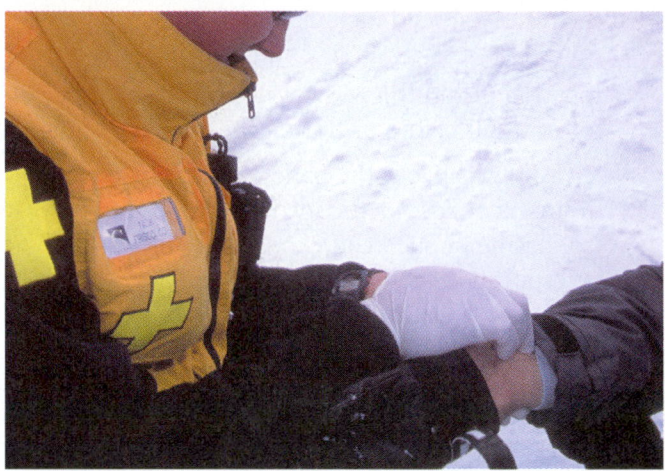

Figure 7-8 Assessing the radial pulse.

If possible, kneel or sit so that you are at eye level with the patient. Address the patient by name; if the patient is your age or younger, you can use the first name. An older person should be addressed more formally (for instance, address the patient as "Mr. Smith" or "Ms. Jones").

Early in the assessment, you should be able to determine whether the patient is injured or ill. However, you should never forget that a patient may be *both* injured and ill!

Focused History and Physical Exam

Continue to maintain eye contact as you question and examine the patient so you can detect his or her reactions, such as a grimace because of pain. Ask appropriate questions and follow leads to identify the patient's main problem(s) (▲ **Figure 7-8**).

Patient Assessment

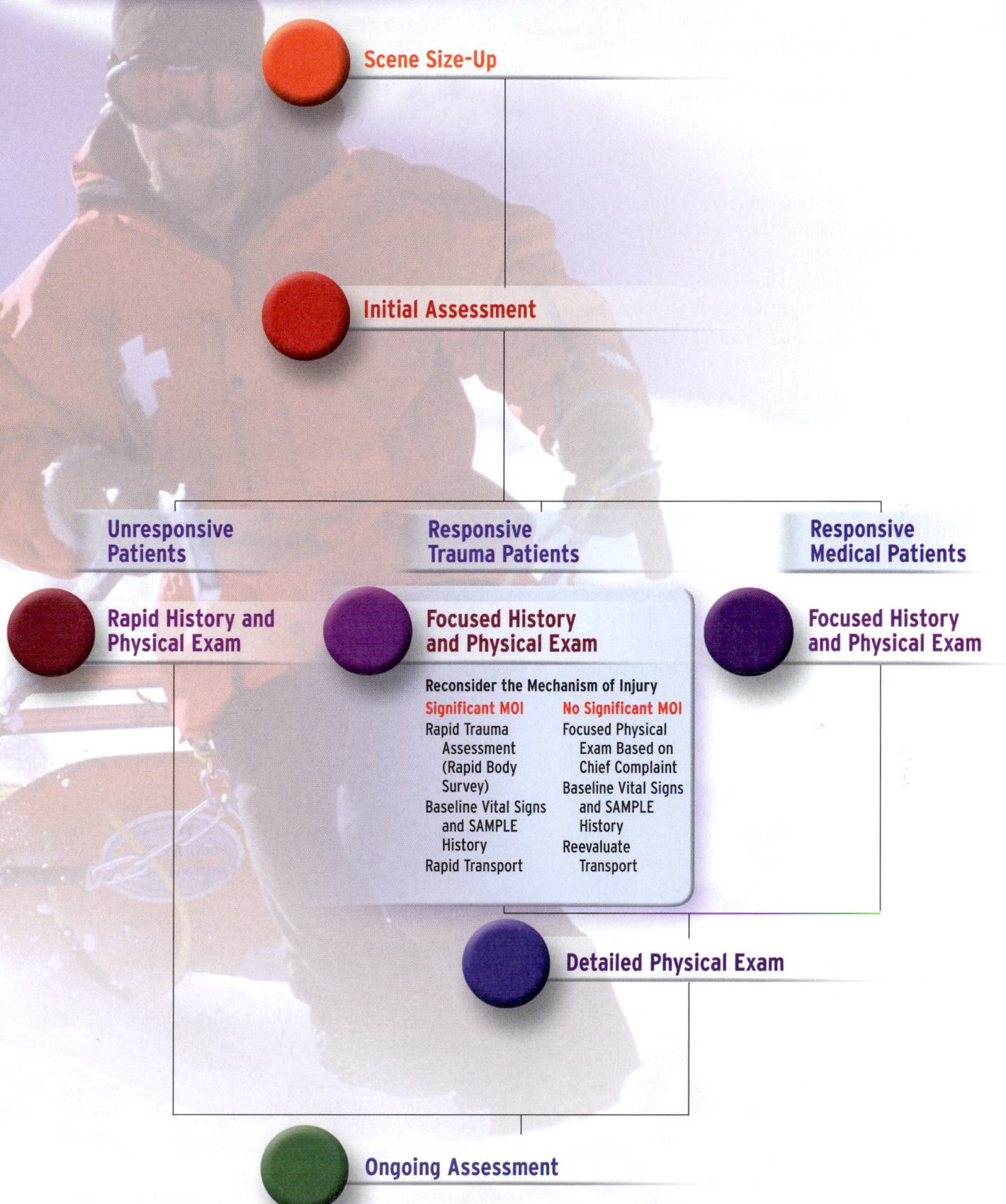

Scene Size-Up

Initial Assessment

Unresponsive Patients

Rapid History and Physical Exam

Responsive Trauma Patients

Focused History and Physical Exam

Reconsider the Mechanism of Injury

Significant MOI
Rapid Trauma Assessment (Rapid Body Survey)
Baseline Vital Signs and SAMPLE History
Rapid Transport

No Significant MOI
Focused Physical Exam Based on Chief Complaint
Baseline Vital Signs and SAMPLE History
Reevaluate Transport

Responsive Medical Patients

Focused History and Physical Exam

Detailed Physical Exam

Ongoing Assessment

As part of this physical exam, you should perform the following steps at the same time you are asking the patient questions:

- **Palpate** the patient's wrist and assess the rate, rhythm, and strength of the radial pulse.
- Note the wrist skin temperature, color, and moisture.
- Note whether the breathing rate is normal or abnormal and whether the patient has a cough or labored breathing.
- Note any difficulty in talking, such as shortness of breath that interferes with finishing a sentence.
- Listen for any abnormal sounds connected with breathing.
- Inspect the patient's face for expression, skin color, and obvious moisture.
- Note the patient's vocal inflections and emotional state.
- Assess the **capillary refill** time (not useful in a cold environment).

A patient who is experiencing pain will wear an expression of anxiety or discomfort. A patient with severe pain or a significant illness usually will be pale, cool to the touch, and sweaty. A normal pulse and breathing rate will help differentiate the patient with a less significant injury or illness from the patient with a severe, painful, or life-threatening condition. By this time, you probably will have established whether or not the patient has an adequate airway, breathing, circulation, and level of responsiveness and whether there is any obvious bleeding.

You should continue to observe the patient's face for unusual expression, color changes, and perspiration. Also, be sure to protect the patient from exposure to inclement weather.

If you determine that the patient has been injured, the first questions you should ask the patient are "Do you hurt anywhere?" or "Where do you hurt?" During the trauma **focused history and physical exam**, ask the patient to give you a detailed description of what happened so you can use this information, the mechanism of injury, to help you predict possible injuries.

Make sure you identify all painful and possibly injured areas. After discussing the initial signs and symptoms related by the patient, be sure to ask, "Did you hit your head, neck, or back?" and "Does your head, neck, or back hurt?" If the patient hit his or her head, always ask, "Were you knocked out?" Frequently,

the patient is not sure of the answers to these questions. If this is the case, companions or witnesses may be able to tell you whether the patient lost responsiveness. Finally, ask, "Did you get hurt anywhere else?"

Listen carefully to what the patient tells you and avoid asking leading questions. At the same time, note abnormal sounds, particularly in the respiratory system, and any abnormalities of speech.

Depending on the area injured, there are several important things you should ask injured patients about besides pain, as follows:

1. General
   - Weakness, lightheadedness, or excessive fatigue
   - Any bleeding

2. Head injury
   - Headache
   - Dizziness
   - Loss of responsiveness, even if momentary
   - Double vision or inability to see normally

3. Neck or back injury
   - Numbness, tingling, weakness, or inability to move
   - Difficulty breathing

4. Chest injury
   - Difficulty breathing
   - Cough
   - Blood in the sputum
   - Pain aggravated by breathing or coughing

5. Abdominal injury
   - Nausea, vomiting
   - Abdominal cramps
   - Blood in the feces or urine
   - Abdominal swelling
   - Time of last bowel movement
   - Pregnancy

6. Pelvic injury
   - Trouble urinating
   - Blood in the urine
   - Blood coming from the urethra, vagina, or rectum
   - Pregnancy

7. Extremity injury
   - Pain on motion
   - Numbness, tingling, weakness, or inability to move or use the extremity
   - Inability to bear weight on the lower extremity

Encourage patients not to respond to questions by nodding or shaking their head "yes" or "no." If you suspect a head, neck, or back injury based on the chief complaint, it is especially important that you assess the patient's head and neck, status of the pupils, and ability to move the extremities. In addition, you should assess the patient's ability to feel touch and pain both initially and during the ongoing assessment. If you suspect a neck or back injury and the patient is in a stable position, instruct the patient not to move while you continue your assessment. If the patient is uncooperative or in an unstable position, you may have to stop at that point and stabilize the patient's head and neck manually until more help arrives.

Next, perform a focused physical exam by assessing the major problem site(s) that the patient has identified ▶ Skill Drill 7-2 . Assess each site in question as described previously in the discussion on the rapid body survey. In particular, look for bleeding wounds. Then, provide appropriate care for any injuries you find, as detailed in the subsequent chapters of this textbook.

1. **Ensure scene safety, patient responsiveness, and recheck ABCs.** Continue to be alert for any changes in status and responsiveness since the initial assessment **(Step 1)**.

2. **Obtain consent from the patient** to continue your assessment. Take all the necessary BSI precautions **(Step 2)**.

3. **Move to the patient's specific injury site,** and assess the chief complaint. Make the patient comfortable by addressing him or her by name and at eye level **(Step 3)**.

4. **Assess the patient's pulse, skin temperature, breathing rate,** and examine any noticeable abnormalities. Avoid being distracted by conditions that are not limb- or life-threatening **(Step 4)**.

5. **Obtain a SAMPLE** history, if possible **(Step 5)**.

6. **Assess the injured site.** Ask the patient about important things other than pain. A responsive patient will be able to respond to your requests such as squeezing your hands **(Step 6)**.

7. **Inspect and expose** only what is necessary to determine the necessary emergency care **(Step 7)**.

8. **Splint and/or provide appropriate care** for any injuries using supplies in your aid pack and other emergency equipment at your disposal **(Step 8)**.

Baseline Vital Signs

Baseline vital signs provide useful information about the overall functions of the patient's heart and lungs. Remember, if the patient's condition is stable, you should reassess the vital signs every 15 minutes until you reach definitive care. If the patient is unstable, you should reassess at a minimum of every 5 minutes, or as often as the situation permits. Also obtain a SAMPLE history if possible.

Transport Decision

Following the focused history and physical exam, transport the patient to the aid room if injuries are minor, responsiveness is normal, and the patient can clearly indicate that no additional problems exist. It is best to quickly transport a patient who falls and sprains a knee to a warm aid room to prevent the risk of hypothermia that can occur when you conduct an assessment on the hill.

However, if the patient appears to be seriously injured, there is a significant mechanism of injury, the pulse or respirations are abnormal, or the patient presents a poor general impression, *immediately arrange for rapid transport to medical care.*

If you are in the aid room or another shelter, proceed to the detailed physical exam while awaiting transport to definitive care or transfer to family, etc. Give urgent interventions as indicated by your findings. Before you finish questioning the patient, always ask, "Is there anything else wrong with you?"

Again, assess every body area that the patient indicates or that you suspect is a site of pain or other abnormality.

SkillDrill 7-2 Performing a Focused History and Physical Exam–
Responsive Trauma Patient

1

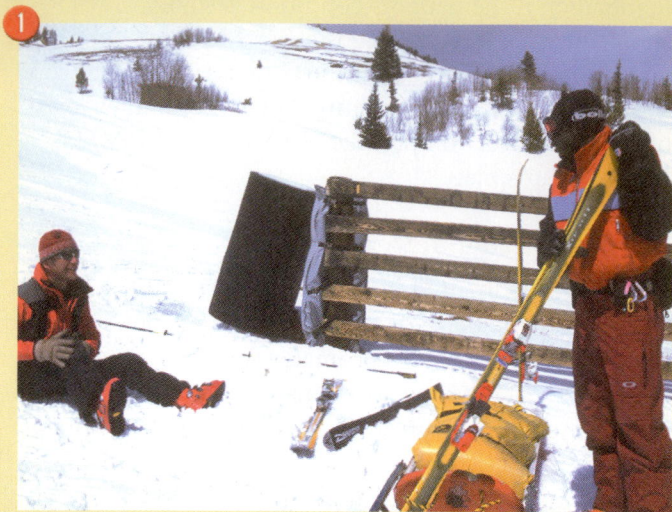

Ensure scene safety and patient responsiveness. Recheck ABCs.

2

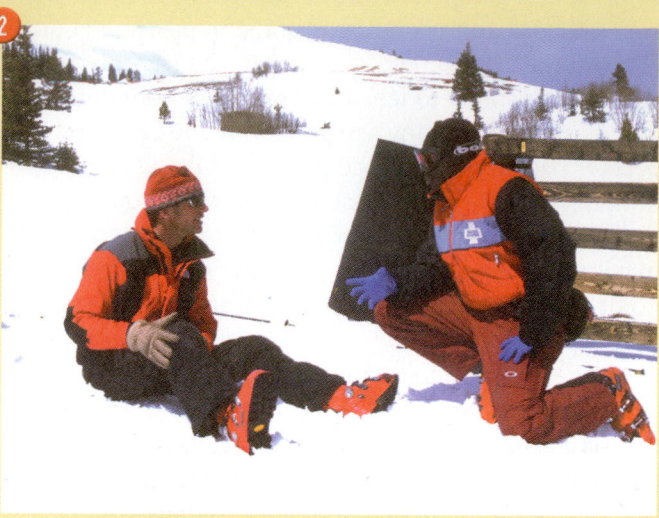

Institute BSI precautions and obtain the patient's consent for treatment.

3

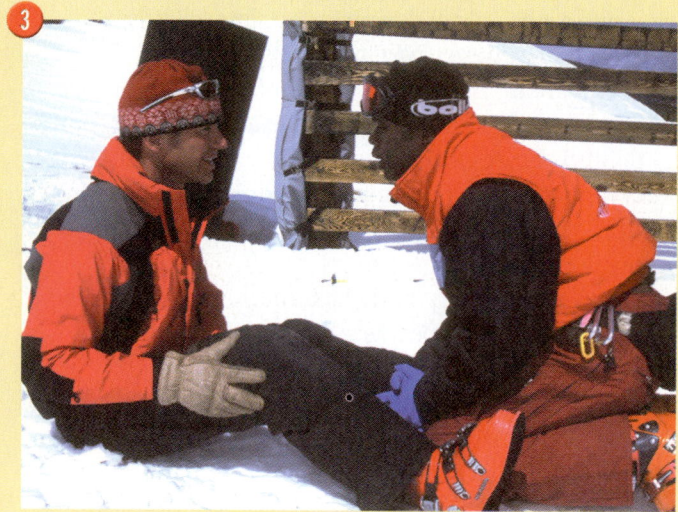

Determine the patient's chief complaint.

4

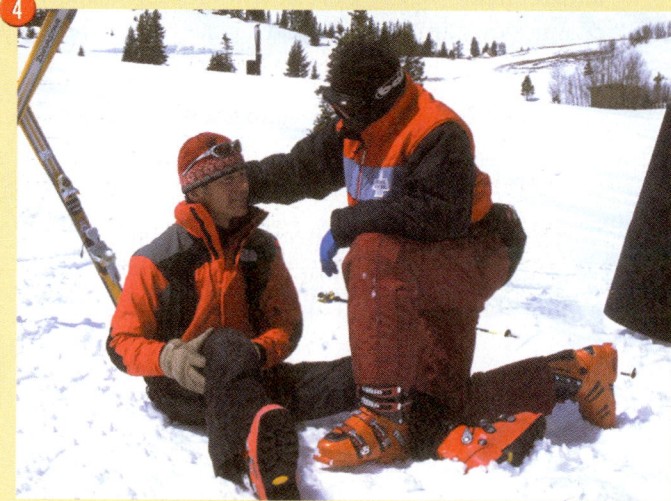

Assess the patient's head, neck, and back if a loss of responsiveness or spine or head injury is suspected.

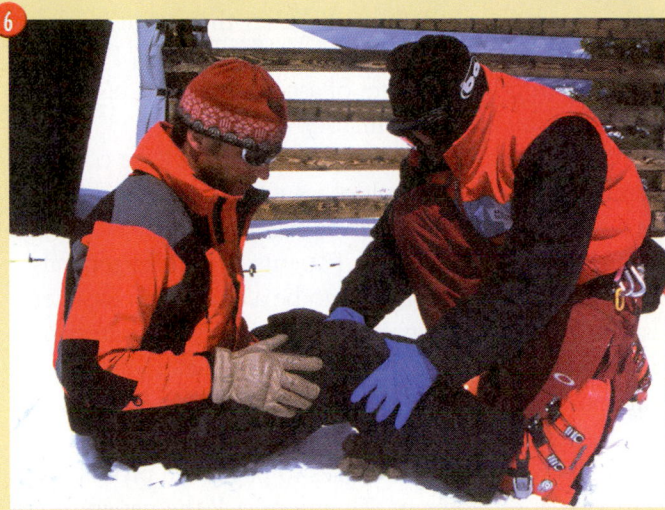

5 Obtain a SAMPLE history.

6 Perform a focused assessment of the injured site (chief complaint).

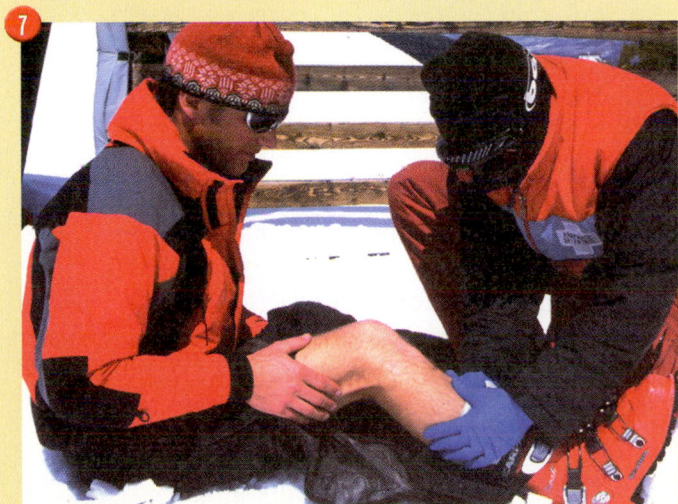

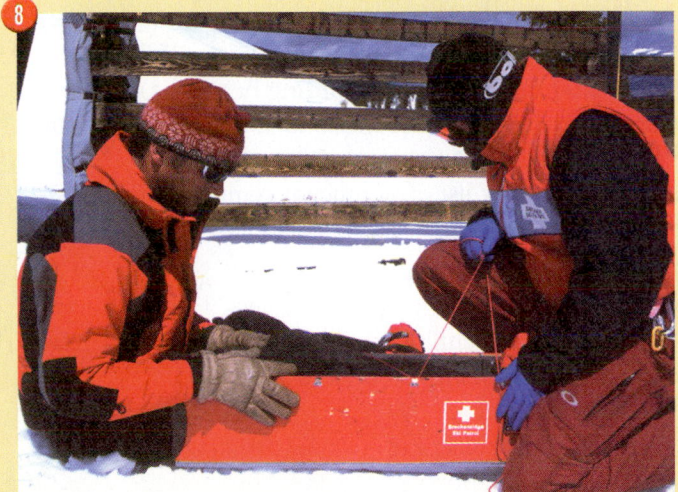

7 Expose only what is necessary to determine the essential emergency care.

8 Splint and/or provide appropriate care of injuries.

Assessment of Responsive Medical Patients

If the patient appears to be ill rather than injured, the approach is somewhat different ▶ **Table 7-13** . Probably the most important aspect of assessing a patient who is ill is to obtain a good history.

When dealing with an ill patient, one whose condition is not entirely a result of trauma, the focused history and physical exam can be the most important aspects of your assessment. Patients who have generalized and diffuse symptoms can be a challenge. Rescuers usually are unable to provide anything more than supportive care and arrange appropriate evacuation or transport. Determining the chronology of events and establishing past medical history provides definitive care providers with important clues to begin the process of diagnosis and treatment. Therefore, ask the patient how long it has been since he or she felt entirely well and try to reconstruct in chronologic order the events leading up to the patient's current status.

History of Illness

The most important signs and symptoms of illness are fever, pain in some area (including headache), and variations from the normal functions of one or more of the body systems.

Following is a list of significant symptoms that arise from these variations:

1. Nonspecific Symptoms
   - Tiredness or fatigue, weakness, lack of energy
   - Fever or chills (usually described as the sensation of being hot or cold)
   - Stiff neck
   - Trouble sleeping
   - Loss of appetite
   - Weight loss
   - Depression or other alteration of the emotional state
2. Respiratory System
   - Sore throat
   - Runny or stuffy nose
   - Postnasal discharge
   - Earache
   - Cough
   - Chest pain
   - Chest pain aggravated by a cough or deep breath
   - Difficulty breathing
   - Wheezing

Table 7-13 Responsive Medical Patient
Responsive Patient
• History of Illness
• SAMPLE History
• Focused Physical Exam: Based on Chief Complaint
• Baseline Vital Signs
• Reevaluate Transport

   - Pus in the sputum or nasal secretions
   - Hoarseness
3. Circulatory System
   - Palpitations
   - Chest pain
   - Difficulty breathing
   - Swelling of the ankles or legs
4. Digestive System
   - Painful or difficult swallowing
   - Heartburn
   - Sour stomach
   - Nausea
   - Vomiting
   - Vomiting blood
   - Diarrhea, constipation, or other changes in bowel habits
   - Excessive gas or bloating
   - Blood in bowel movements (black tarry stools)
   - Abdominal pain or cramps
5. Genitourinary system
   - Difficulty urinating
   - Burning sensation while urinating
   - Blood in the urine
   - Discharge from the vagina or penis
   - Change in menstrual periods
   - Pain in the lower abdomen, pelvis, genitals, or one side of the lower back (Note: With abdominal or pelvic pain in a woman of childbearing age, ask the patient when she had her last menstrual period, whether it was normal, and whether she might be pregnant.)
6. Musculoskeletal and Nervous System
   - Soreness, aching, or pain when moving a body part
   - Weakness, clumsiness, or paralysis of a body part

Patient Assessment

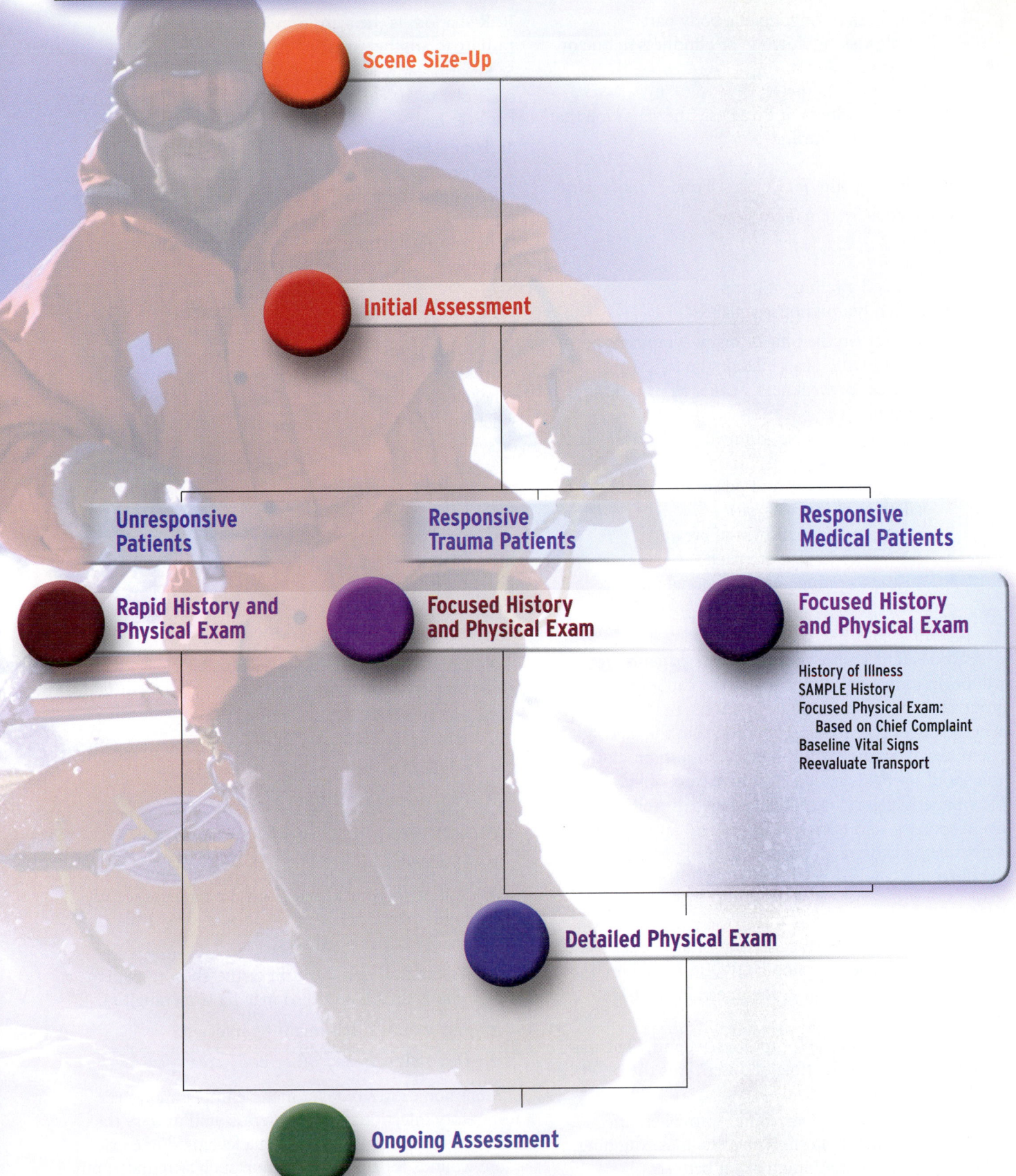

Scene Size-Up

Initial Assessment

Unresponsive Patients

Responsive Trauma Patients

Responsive Medical Patients

Rapid History and Physical Exam

Focused History and Physical Exam

Focused History and Physical Exam

History of Illness
SAMPLE History
Focused Physical Exam:
    Based on Chief Complaint
Baseline Vital Signs
Reevaluate Transport

Detailed Physical Exam

Ongoing Assessment

- Numbness or tingling of a body part
- Double vision, blurring, or blindness in one or both eyes
- Headache
- Lightheadedness or dizziness (the sensation that the room is whirling)
- Backache
- Stiffness, pain, or swelling of one or more joints

7. Cutaneous System (skin)
   - Itching
   - Rash
   - Localized swelling or lump
   - Swollen lymph nodes ("glands")

Depending on the illness, many symptoms occur in groups, which can include the following:
- Tiredness or weakness, aching all over, fever and chills
- Sore throat, earache, runny or stuffy nose, and cough
- Chest pain, cough, and pus in the sputum (yellow or green material)
- Chest pain and shortness of breath
- Heartburn and sour stomach
- Nausea, vomiting, and abdominal pain or cramps
- Diarrhea and cramps

As you interact with more and more patients, you will begin to recognize that symptoms can appear in groups and indicate specific conditions. Be wary, however, of diagnosing medical conditions in the field. Often, rescuers miss or misinterpret important clues. You should provide good supportive care, obtain a complete patient history including negative as well as positive responses, and transport the patient appropriately. A complete history is the cornerstone of good care for the ill patient.

OPQRST

Ask the patient to describe the pain or any other specific symptom. The mnemonic OPQRST is commonly used to help you remember the questions to ask about pain or other symptoms.

O: Onset. When did the symptom start and what was the patient doing at the time of onset? Was the onset sudden or gradual?

P: Provocation. What, if anything, "provokes" the symptom, ie, what makes it worse (such as coughing, eating, etc.)? Does anything make it better?

Q: Quality. What is the symptom like? For example, if the patient has pain, what is it like (dull, sharp, aching, throbbing, constant, intermittent, etc.)?

R: Radiation. Is the symptom localized or does it radiate to another area?

S: Severity. How bad is it? For example, rate it on a scale of 1 to 10, where 10 is the worst pain the patient has ever had.

T: Time. How long has it lasted? Is it getting better, worse, or staying the same over time? Is it changing in quality? Has the patient ever experienced anything like it in the past? Could it be part of a longstanding condition? Was there some change in the condition that made the patient seek help at this particular time?

If the patient has a fever or you suspect an acute infection, it is important that you find out what part of the body is involved. In addition to fever, other general symptoms of infection include chills, headache, backache, weakness, and aching all over. Ask the patient whether he or she has had any of the following signs or symptoms:

- Shaking (teeth chattering) chills, which, if present, is a sign of a significant infection.
- A cold, sore throat, or earache. If so, did the patient notice any yellow or green discharge from the nose?
- Coughing. If so, is the patient coughing anything up? What color is the discharge?
- Chest pain. If so, exactly where is it located? Is the pain worse when the patient coughs or takes a deep breath?
- Nausea, vomiting, or diarrhea; abdominal pain, tenderness, or cramps.
- Pain during urination.
- Backache, pain in the joints, or aching all over.
- Headache.
- Stiff or sore neck. If so, did the patient recently injure his or her neck or does he or she have a history of neck arthritis?
- Ability to touch the chin to the chest (a patient who is unable to do so may have meningitis).
- Any wounds that might be infected.
- Discomfort in any other body area.

Common causes of fever include upper and lower respiratory infections, gastroenteritis, and urinary tract infections. Inspect a patient with a fever and one or more wounds for signs of infection such as redness, pus discharge, swelling, and red streaks running proximally (toward the patient's trunk) from the wound.

Variations from the Normal Functions of Body Systems

DIFFICULTY BREATHING. If the patient has difficulty breathing, ask about a recent chest injury, cough, stuffy nose, sputum production, coughing up blood, fever, chills, wheezing, ankle swelling, palpitations, chest pain, and a history of heart disease, emphysema, or asthma.

Recent onset of shortness of breath in a previously healthy person should make you suspect acute conditions such as asthma, pneumonia, high-altitude pulmonary edema, or a spontaneous lung collapse (pneumothorax). You should suspect heart failure in a patient with known heart or lung disease in whom shortness of breath develops more gradually, especially if there is swelling of the ankles. In a patient with emphysema, you should suspect further deterioration of lung function resulting from a lung infection. A patient with a history of asthma may be having an asthma attack, usually indicated by audible wheezing. Find out whether the patient has recently had an upper respiratory infection (URI) or the flu, and ask if the pain is a new or recurring problem.

ABDOMINAL PAIN. If the patient has abdominal pain, ask about the time of onset, location of the pain at onset, the type of pain (dull, crampy, sharp, etc.), whether it has moved or changed in type or intensity, and whether it is related to eating, passing gas, or bowel movements.

Inquire about the presence of nausea, vomiting, constipation, or diarrhea; how long it has been since the patient had a bowel movement; and any activity that makes the pain better or worse. Ask about a history of ulcer, gallbladder disease, or colitis, and whether the patient's appendix has been removed. Ask when the patient last ate and, in the case of vomiting, when the patient was last able to keep food or liquids down. Ask whether it's possible that the patient recently consumed contaminated food or water.

Common abdominal pain syndromes include:

- The acute onset of upper abdominal pain, fever, nausea, vomiting, or diarrhea as part of a nonspecific viral infection; food poisoning; or a specific stomach or intestinal infection by a virus or bacterium
- Upper abdominal pain, sour stomach, and heartburn following a large or spicy meal
- Right lower quadrant pain caused by appendicitis
- Severe epigastric pain, caused by an ulcer or inflammation of the stomach, that improves with antacids or milk

- Right upper quadrant pain that is due to gallbladder disease
- A chronic left lower quadrant ache that is due to chronic constipation or colitis
- Right or left posterior flank pain due to kidney problem

If the patient has nausea or vomiting, ask about the duration, frequency, characteristics of the vomit, and the presence of blood or "coffee grounds" material (partly digested blood) in the vomit. Also ask if the patient has abdominal pain and, if so, whether the nausea and vomiting are related to the pain, particularly if the pain changes before or after the patient vomits. Ask if the patient has recently had a URI or the flu. To determine the status of the patient's hydration and nutrition, ask how long it has been since he or she has been able to keep anything down.

Most instances of nausea and vomiting are due to a viral stomach infection, but they also can accompany an ulcer, acute mountain sickness, severe headache, or overindulgence in food or alcohol. In addition, nausea and vomiting can be associated with almost any severe injury or illness.

DIARRHEA. If the patient has diarrhea, ask about the duration, the presence of chills and fever, the number and type of bowel movements, whether they contain pus or blood, and whether there is accompanying pain. Ask whether the patient has recently had a URI or flu. Most diarrhea that lasts longer than a few hours is caused by a specific bowel infection.

CHEST PAIN. If the patient has chest pain, ask him or her to describe the pain, specifically the type (sharp, squeezing, dull, pressure); location (beneath the sternum, over the lower ribs, over the heart); characteristics of onset; duration; whether the pain worsens with coughing or deep breathing or is brought on by exertion; and whether it radiates to the neck, jaw, back, shoulder, or arm, particularly the left shoulder and left arm. Find out if the pain is made worse if the patient uses the arms or twists the trunk.

Ask the patient whether he or she has symptoms of an infection such as cough and fever, whether similar pain has occurred before, and whether there is a history of angina, heart disease (particularly coronary artery disease), or lung disease.

WEAKNESS. If the patient complains about weakness, ask him or her to explain what is meant by weakness. Ask the patient if he or she can differentiate between tiredness and weakness, whether the weakness is chronic or of recent onset, and whether it is general or confined to an arm, a leg, or one side of the body. It is important to know whether the patient is capable of performing normal activities or if the weakness prevents sitting, standing, or walking.

Ask if the patient's sleeping habits have been normal or have recently changed and whether the onset of the weakness coincided with the onset of an illness such as a URI or the flu, another disease, an injury, an operation, or missing one or more meals.

Sudden weakness that involves one or more extremities usually is caused by injury or illness affecting the nerves that supply the weakened parts. Weakness affecting one side of the body may indicate a stroke. General body weakness can accompany many illnesses and injuries and be due to overwork and lack of sleep, or, if chronic, psychoneurosis. However, general weakness also can be caused by a subtle medical condition such as anemia, newly developing diabetes, chronic kidney disease, hidden malignant disease, or a low thyroid state.

DIFFICULTY VOIDING. If the patient complains about having difficulty voiding, ask him or her to elaborate. Elderly men with enlargement of the prostate gland have difficulty starting and stopping the urinary stream and have to get up frequently at night to void.

Women who have borne several children may have trouble with urine leaking involuntarily when they cough or laugh. Pain during urination and frequent voiding of small amounts usually indicates the presence of an infection.

A change in voiding habits also may be important. Urinating large amounts may be a sign of diabetes, especially if it is accompanied by increased thirst.

After thoroughly discussing the patient's chief complaint, obtain a SAMPLE history and assess the patient's body depending on his or her symptoms (▶ **Figure 7-9**). If you suspect a febrile illness, hypothermia, or hyperthermia and have a thermometer with you, take the patient's temperature; otherwise, wait until the detailed physical exam.

The SAMPLE History

Once you have obtained a clearer picture of the patient's chief complaint and have explored it using OPQRST questions, you should obtain a SAMPLE history. Remember that the purpose of this history is to gather information about the patient's past medical experiences. The elements of the SAMPLE history are repeated below for your review.

- **S**igns and symptoms of the episode
- **A**llergies, particularly to medications

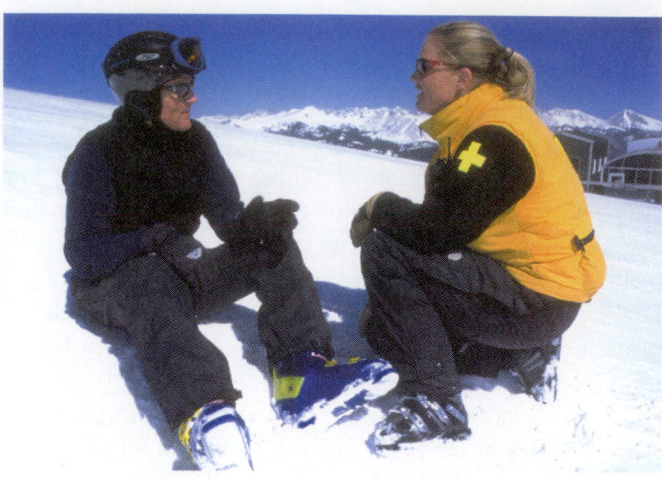

Figure 7-9 After discussing the chief complaint, obtain a SAMPLE history and assess the patient's body depending on his or her symptoms.

- **M**edications, including prescription, over-the-counter, and recreational (illicit) drugs
- **P**ast medical history, particularly involving similar episodes in the past
- **L**ast oral intake, including food and/or drinks. This is particularly important if the patient may need surgery
- **E**vents leading up to the episode

Be sure to ask whether the patient has any other problems that you should know about. This question is useful in that it provides the patient with an opportunity to tell you something about apparently unrelated previous medical problems. In most cases, this will serve as useful background information.

Medical Focused Physical Exam

Perform a medical focused physical exam by assessing the areas of chief complaint. Follow the assessment steps shown in (▶ **Skill Drill 7-3**):

1. **Ensure scene safety, reassess the patient's responsiveness, and recheck ABCs.** Continue to be alert for any changes in status and responsiveness since the initial assessment **(Step 1)**.

2. **Obtain consent from the patient** to continue your assessment. Take all the necessary BSI precautions **(Step 2)**.

3. **Obtain a clear picture of the patient's chief complaint.** Make the patient comfortable by addressing him or her by name and at eye level **(Step 3)**.

4. **Use OPQRST** to help clarify the history of the patient's illness **(Step 4)**.

5. **Take a SAMPLE history.** This information will help you reevaluate the chief complaint in light of potential new information **(Step 5)**.

6. **Assess the patient's body,** depending on his or her symptoms **(Step 6)**.

7. **Get baseline vital signs** to give you information about the overall functions of the patient's heart and lungs **(Step 7)**.

8. **Provide appropriate interventions and reevaluate transport decisions** made during the initial assessment to transferring the patient from the outdoor environment **(Step 8)**.

Perform your assessment of a responsive medical patient in a systematic and logical manner. Along with significant symptoms derived from questioning the patient, use the appropriate key points for assessing the various body parts as you focus on the chief complaint.

The Head

Assess the patient's pupils and note any color change in the whites of the eyes. Using a flashlight and tongue blade or spoon handle, check the patient's throat and tonsils by pressing down on the tongue and asking the patient to say "ah."

The Neck

Feel the patient's upper neck and under both sides of the jaw for tender or enlarged lymph nodes. Ask the patient to touch his or her chest with the chin. Inability to do this may indicate that the neck is abnormally stiff, which in a patient with fever could be a sign of meningitis. Listen for hoarseness or **stridor**.

The Chest

Note any rattles, crackling, wheezes, or bubbly sounds. These noises may be clearly audible, but you can hear them better with a stethoscope or by placing your ear against the patient's chest. If the patient is coughing up material from the lungs or blowing it out of the nose, inspect it for color (clear, yellow, green, or bloody [red, pink, or rust-colored]).

The Abdomen and Pelvis

Assess the patient's abdomen for distention, tenderness, rigidity, masses, and scars from previous operations or injuries. If the patient indicates a certain area as the site of pain or tenderness, assess this area last; if you hurt the patient by pressing on a tender area, he or she may resist further examination.

Listen for the loud gurgles of gastroenteritis or bowel obstruction.

The Skin and Extremities

Inspect any wounds for swelling, redness, tenderness, discharge, or red streaks leading away from the wound (in an extremity, these streaks usually will run toward the trunk). Inspect the patient's ankles for swelling, especially "pitting" edema (pressing a finger into the skin leaves a depression or "pit").

If the patient reports that an extremity is weak, compare its strength with that of the opposite, normal extremity by having the patient squeeze both of your hands or push his or her feet down and pull them back up against your hands.

The Back

Frequently patients with a urinary infection will exhibit tenderness of the kidneys. If the patient reports backache, assess for tenderness and tight muscles over each flank at the indicated area.

As with the injured patient, *if the patient looks seriously ill, has an abnormal pulse or respirations, or the patient presents a poor general impression, arrange for immediate transport to medical care.* While awaiting transport, expand your medical focused physical exam into a complete rapid body survey or, if the patient is sheltered, into a detailed physical exam. Provide care based on your findings.

When finished, always remember to ask the patient, "Is there anything else wrong with you that we should know about?"

Baseline Vital Signs

Baseline vital signs should be obtained after this exam to provide information for assessing trends in patient conditions. Remember, if the patient's condition is stable, you should reassess the vital signs every 15 minutes as soon as the patient has reached shelter. If the patient is unstable, you should reassess at a minimum of every 5 minutes, or as often as the situation permits.

Reevaluate the Transport Decision

Your next step is to provide the necessary emergency medical care in the field, addressing the chief complaint. Once the patient is transported to the shelter, aid room, or a warm environment, reevaluate the need for further definitive care and/or transport to a clinic or emergency department.

Skill Drill 7-3

Performing a Focused Physical Exam—Responsive Medical Patient

1

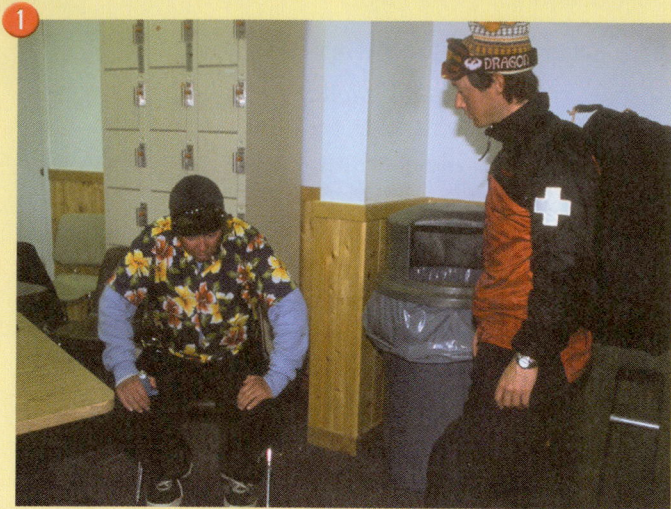

Inspect the scene for clues to the nature of illness such as medication vials, medic altert tags, or asthma inhalers.

2

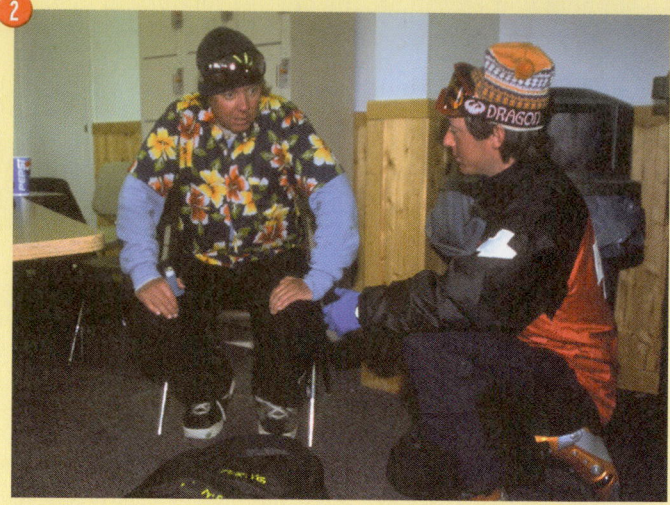

Institute BSI precautions and obtain the patient's consent for treatment.

3

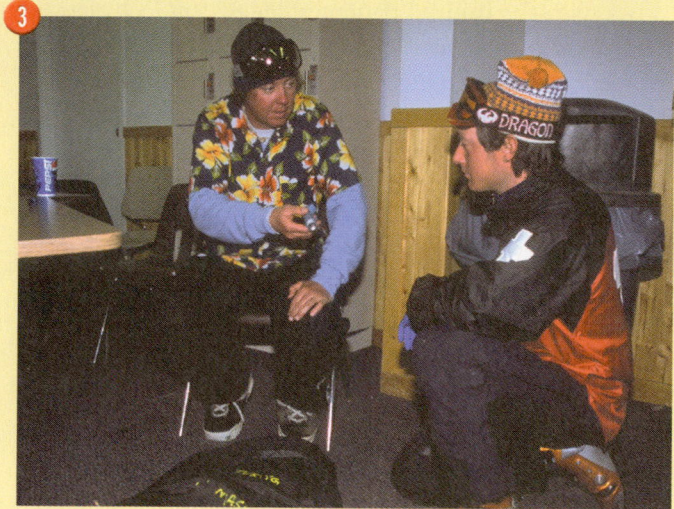

Determine the patient's chief complaint.

4

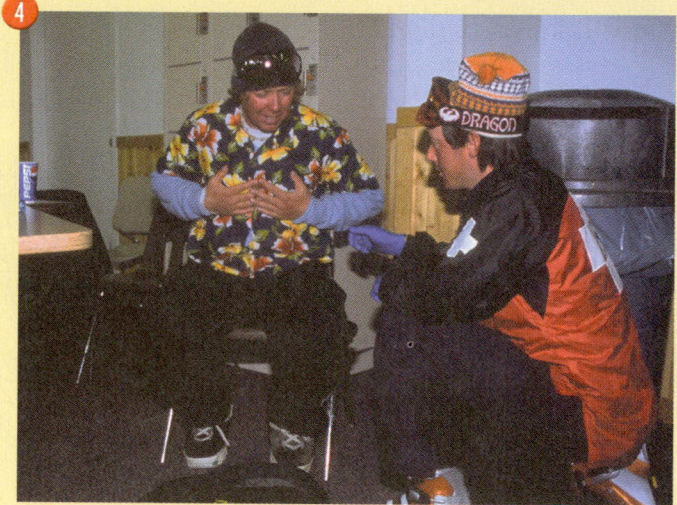

Use OPQRST to clarify the patient's illness.

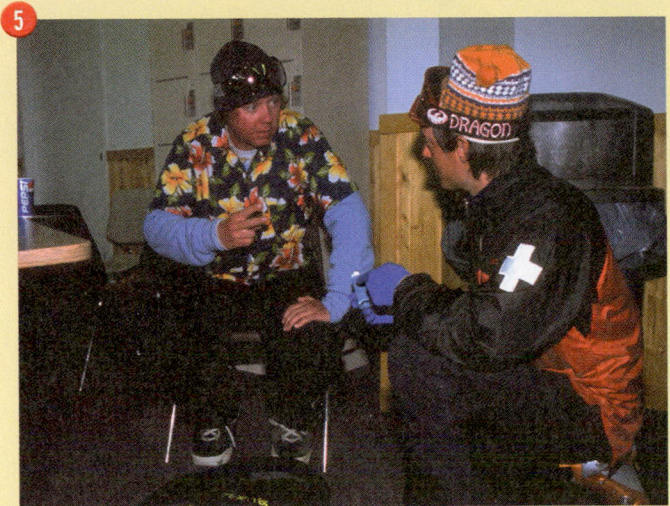

Take a SAMPLE history.

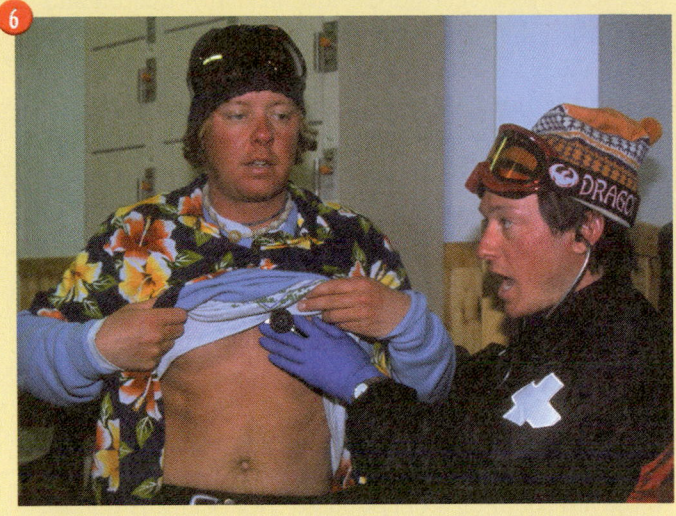

Perform a focused assessment of the body depending on the patient's chief complaint.

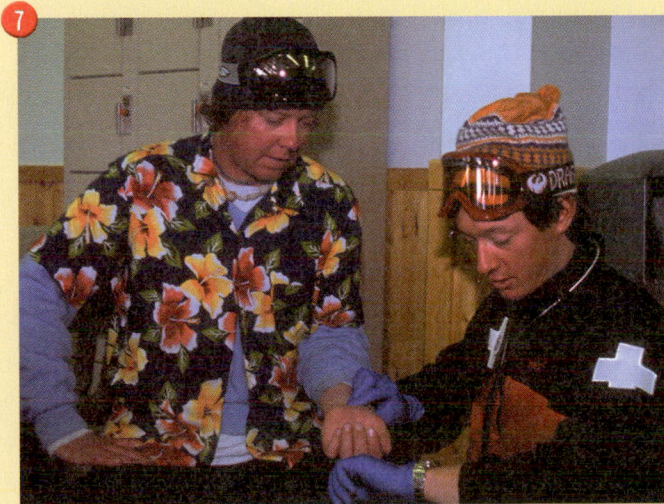

Obtain a baseline set of vital signs.

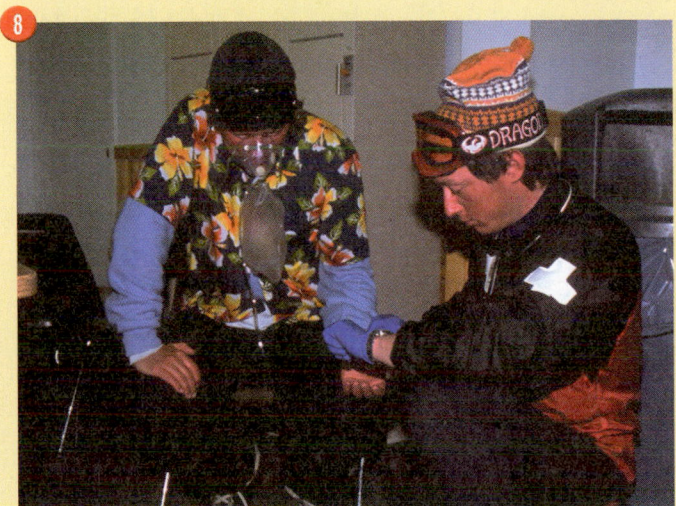

Provide needed treatments and reevaluate transport decisions and the patient's status.

Detailed Physical Exam

Recall that the assessment process began with anticipation when you received the dispatch information and performed the scene size-up. After that, you performed the initial assessment in which you identified and treated life-threatening conditions. If trauma was a factor in your patient's situation, you also initiated spinal immobilization. When indicated for an unresponsive or trauma patient with a significant MOI, you followed up on the initial assessment by performing a rapid history and physical exam. You also provided transport if your patient had an obvious life-threatening condition. On the basis of what you learned from the history, you assessed selected areas of the patient's body. You also have taken at least one set of vital signs.

In most instances, you have transported your patient to the aid room or other suitable shelter at this point (▼ **Figure 7-10**). If you are still on the scene, it is because the patient does not have any life-threatening conditions and you have not found the cause for the patient's complaints.

The extent of the **detailed physical exam** (► **Table 7-14**) depends partly on the nature of the primary injury or illness. Ideally, you should perform the head-to-toe steps as completely as possible when the patient has altered responsiveness, has sustained multiple or serious injuries, or appears to be seriously ill, unreliable, or mentally impaired. However, the detailed physical exam *should not delay* transport or EMS interface, especially if the patient's condition is critical (see Table 7-1).

You should understand that it usually is inappropriate to conduct an elaborate assessment on a seriously injured or ill patient in very cold weather in the same manner as you would in a warm aid room. Transporting

Table 7-14 Detailed Physical Exam
Head-to-toe Steps
Systematic Exam Using DCAP-BTLS
Baseline Vital Signs

the patient to shelter, where he or she will be more comfortable, other rescuers can assist, and the individual is that much closer to the next level of medical care, makes far more sense, as well as being better for the patient, than taking extra time to perform important but noncritical steps in the field.

You can abbreviate or omit the detailed physical exam if injuries are minor and the patient can clearly indicate that no additional problems exist. Because it is important to maintain spinal stabilization, do not unstrap a patient from a backboard during the detailed physical exam.

In both the rapid body survey and the detailed physical exam, you should try to obtain as much critical information about the patient's well-being as you can. However, this may be difficult because of conflicting requirements and environmental conditions. You must be as thorough as possible so you won't miss anything important, but you also must work with all possible speed to reduce the patient's exposure to the elements and avoid delaying transport.

If you don't suspect a spinal injury, the patient should be sitting up (if he or she is able) for assessment of the head, neck, chest, and back, and supine for assessment of the abdomen, pelvis, and extremities. If you do suspect a spinal injury, the entire assessment should be conducted with the patient supine.

If unexpected findings during the detailed physical exam indicate that the patient is seriously injured or ill, you should interrupt the exam to make arrangements for immediate transport to definitive medical care. Do not delay transport solely to complete the detailed physical exam, which can be performed en route as necessary.

Perform the detailed physical exam by looking (inspection), feeling (palpation), listening (auscultation), and smelling. Although these techniques are described separately, they are usually performed simultaneously. For example, as you palpate a suspected injured area, be sure to watch the patient's face for a grimace, which indicates that the area is tender or the manipulation is painful.

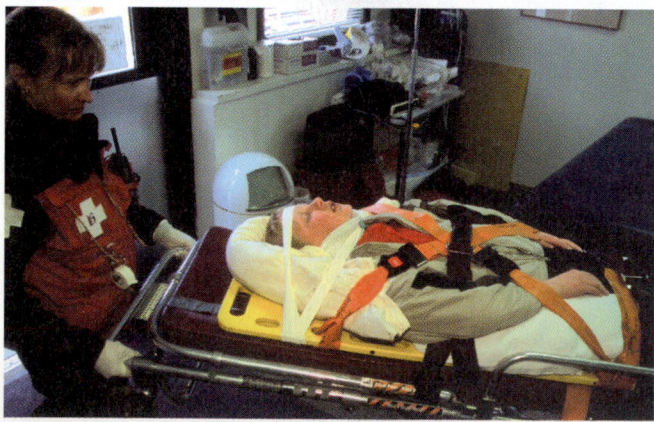

Figure 7-10   The detailed physical exam is best conducted in a comfortable environment.

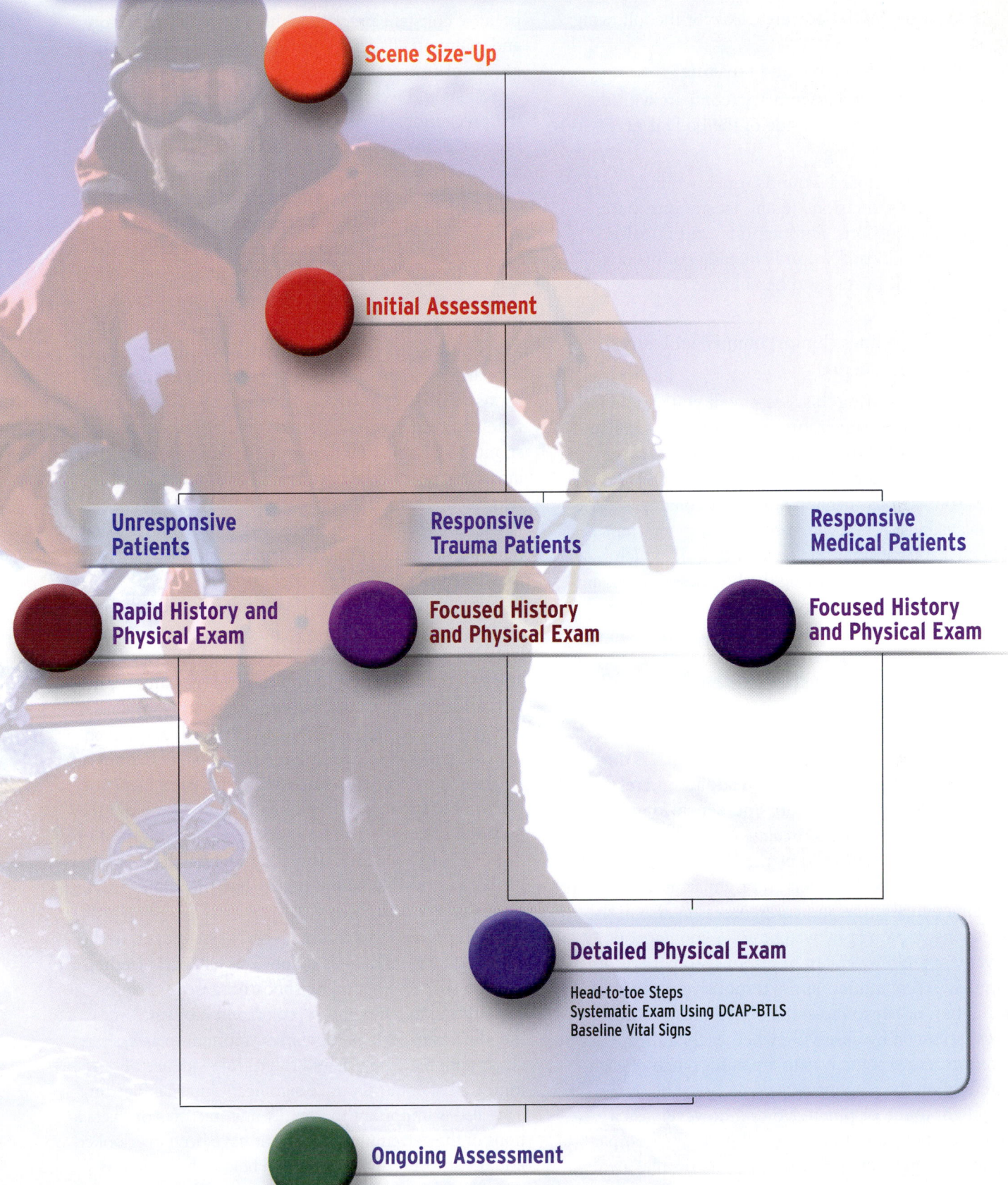

Scene Size-Up

Initial Assessment

Unresponsive Patients

Responsive Trauma Patients

Responsive Medical Patients

Rapid History and Physical Exam

Focused History and Physical Exam

Focused History and Physical Exam

Detailed Physical Exam

Head-to-toe Steps
Systematic Exam Using DCAP-BTLS
Baseline Vital Signs

Ongoing Assessment

As you assess each body area, *look* for the following signs:

- abnormal skin color and moisture
- deformities and asymmetry (compare with the uninjured, opposite side of the body if necessary)
- obvious bleeding
- open and closed wounds (open wounds include abrasions, incisions [cuts], lacerations, punctures, avulsions, amputations, and impaled objects; closed wounds include contusions [bruises], burns, and hematomas)
- scars
- small swellings (lumps, bumps) and large swellings (edema)

In addition, during this assessment you should feel the patient's skin temperature and moisture, small and large swellings (edema), and tenderness.

If you suspect a neck injury, stabilize the neck manually as soon as possible and apply a C-collar as soon as one is available. The collar, however, does not replace manual stabilization of the head and neck, which should be maintained during the body assessment and until the patient is fully immobilized on a backboard. Apply the collar with the least possible movement of the patient's head and neck, which usually means waiting until the individual is supine in the neutral position. However, always assess the neck (including the back of the neck) before applying the collar.

Continue to use the mnemonic DCAP-BTLS during your systematic physical exam. In addition, remember to check **circulation, motion, and sensation (CMS)** in the extremities. Assess *circulation* first by checking the carotid pulse, followed by the extremity pulses and noting whether both the left and right arms and legs are the same temperature and color. Assess *motion* in the unresponsive patient by watching for spontaneous movement and movement in response to pain or other stimulus; assess motion in the responsive patient by asking him or her to move the extremities in turn. Assess *sensation* by observing whether the unresponsive patient reacts in some way to a painful pinch of each extremity; in the responsive patient, ask if he or she can feel a light touch or pinch. Do not, however, ask a patient to move an injured part. If in doubt, compare any area in question with the opposite, normal area.

Head-to-Toe Steps

Despite these guidelines, you should take every opportunity to perform a thorough detailed physical exam,

because constant practice is the only way to develop and maintain efficient, thorough, and accurate techniques of assessment.

You should wear protective gloves and institute other BSI precautions during the detailed physical exam because of the likelihood of contact with the patient's moist body fluids. The first steps of the exam are to reassess responsiveness and assess and record the pulse rate, breathing rate, blood pressure, body temperature, and—in infants and young children—the skin perfusion as measured by the capillary refill test.

Grade the patient's level of responsiveness on the AVPU scale, and observe the facial skin for abnormal temperature, color, and moisture. While doing this, note any noises or movements, especially in the unresponsive patient, in which it is particularly important to note and record whether all four extremities move spontaneously. If all four extremities do not move spontaneously, note and record which ones move spontaneously and which do not.

Blood pressure can be recorded at this time if you have the apparatus available. If no blood pressure apparatus is available, estimate the blood pressure by locating the major pulses. If you can feel the radial pulse, the adult patient's systolic blood pressure is at least 80 mm Hg; if you can feel the femoral pulse, it is at least 70 mm Hg; and if you can feel the carotid pulse, it is at least 60 mm Hg. If a thermometer is available and you suspect hypothermia, hyperthermia, or fever, take the patient's temperature. Ask the patient about any new developments since the initial assessment was performed. If you have not already done so, obtain the SAMPLE history. In the unresponsive patient, repeat the SAMPLE history if anyone has arrived who is more likely to know the patient better than the witnesses you have already questioned.

Next, proceed to a thorough body assessment. In the injured patient, if there is no obvious external bleeding but you suspect impending shock because of changes in the pulse; skin temperature, color, and moisture; or blood pressure, it is particularly important to assess the chest, abdomen, pelvis, and thighs for evidence of injuries that could produce significant internal bleeding.

It also is important to identify any fractures or dislocations of the extremities that might have been overlooked initially so you can care for them before the patient is transported further. Although you should try to shield the patient from the eyes of curious bystanders, misguided concern for the patient's modesty is no excuse for missing a significant injury or illness.

If a patient has suffered a chemical burn to the eyes, you should remove their contact lenses. Be aware that hard contact lenses are difficult to remove without a special suction cup made for this purpose. Most individuals who need this equipment carry it with them. If you cannot remove a hard lens, you may be able to slide it from the clear part of the eye (cornea) onto the white of the eye, which will reduce the danger of corneal damage. Place the removed lenses in a lens container, which the patient probably will have, or in a clean, closed bottle containing a small amount of physiologic saline solution.

Some types of soft contact lenses are designed to be left in place for weeks and are unlikely to injure the eye as long as they remain moist. To prevent drying, tape the eyelids shut: pull each eyelid closed, lay a gauze pad firmly but gently over the eye, and tape over the gauze. Avoid applying tape directly to the eyelid, eyelashes, or eyebrow.

If it is necessary to remove soft contact lenses, you can usually lift them off by pinching them gently between your thumb and index finger. Rescuers who wear contact lenses are accustomed to doing this and can help.

The goals of the detailed physical exam are to further explore problems that were identified during the focused history and physical exam and to possibly identify the cause of complaints that were not identified earlier.

Here, organized by body region, are some additional assessments that you might want to perform during the detailed physical exam. As you evaluate each region, visualize and palpate to find evidence of signs of injury, again using the mnemonic DCAP-BTLS. Follow the steps in ▶ **Skill Drill 7-4** .

1. **Look at the patient's face** for obvious lacerations, bruises, or deformities **(Step 1)**.

2. **Inspect the area around the eyes and eyelids (Step 2)**.

3. **Examine the eyes** for redness and for contact lenses. Assess the pupils using a penlight **(Step 3)**.

4. **Pull the patient's ear forward** to assess for bruising (Battle's sign) **(Step 4)**.

5. **Use the penlight to look for drainage** or blood in the ears **(Step 5)**.

6. **Look for bruising and lacerations about the head.** Palpate for tenderness, depressions of the skull, and deformities **(Step 6)**.

7. **Palpate the zygomas and maxillae** for tenderness or instability **(Step 7)**.

8. **Palpate the mandible (Step 8)**.

9. **Assess the mouth for obstructions,** foreign bodies (including loose teeth or dentures), bleeding, lacerations, or deformities and cyanosis **(Step 9)**. **Check for unusual odors** on the patient's breath.

10. **Look at the neck** for obvious lacerations, bruises, and deformities **(Step 10)**.

11. **Palpate the front and the back of the neck** for tenderness and deformity **(Step 11)**.

12. **Look for distended jugular veins.** Note that distended neck veins are not necessarily significant in a patient who is lying down **(Step 12)**.

13. **Look at the chest** for obvious signs of injury before you begin palpation. Be sure to watch for movement of the chest with respirations **(Step 13)**.

14. **Gently palpate over the ribs** to elicit tenderness. Avoid pressing over obvious bruises or suspected rib fractures **(Step 14)**.

15. **Listen for breath sounds** over the midaxillary and midclavicular lines **(Step 15)**.

16. **Listen also at the bases and apices of the lungs (Step 16)**.

17. **Look at the abdomen and pelvis** for obvious lacerations, bruises, and deformities **(Step 17)**.

18. **Gently palpate the abdomen** for tenderness. If the abdomen is unusually tense, you should describe the abdomen as rigid **(Step 18)**.

19. **Gently compress the pelvis** from the sides to assess for tenderness **(Step 19)**.

20. **Gently press the iliac crests** to elicit instability, tenderness, or crepitus **(Step 20)**.

21. **Assess the lower extremities** for DCAP-BTLS, and medical alert anklets **(Step 21)**.

22. **Assess distal pulses and motor and sensory function** in the lower extremities **(Step 22)**.

23. **Assess the upper extremities.** Watch for medical alert bracelets **(Step 23)**.

24. **Assess distal pulses and motor and sensory function** in the upper extremities **(Step 24)**.

25. **Assess the back for tenderness or deformities.** Remember, if you suspect a spinal cord injury, use spinal precautions as you log roll the patient **(Step 25)**.

SkillDrill 7-4   Performing the Detailed Physical Exam

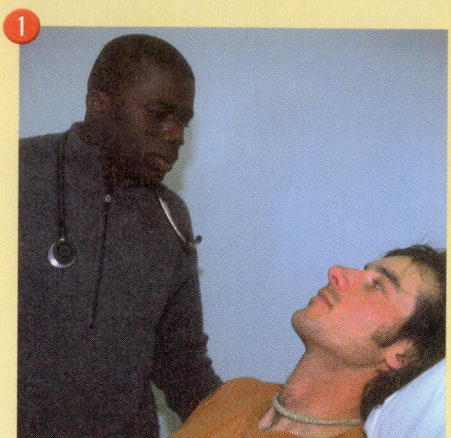
Observe the patient's face.

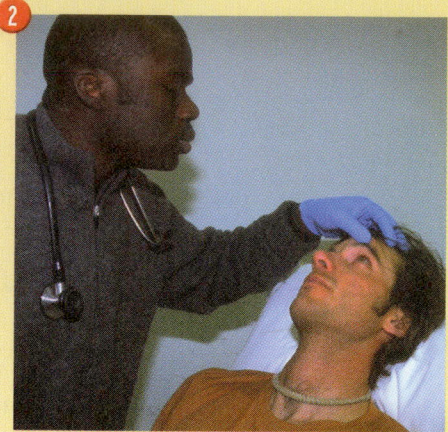
Inspect the eyelids and the area around the eyes.

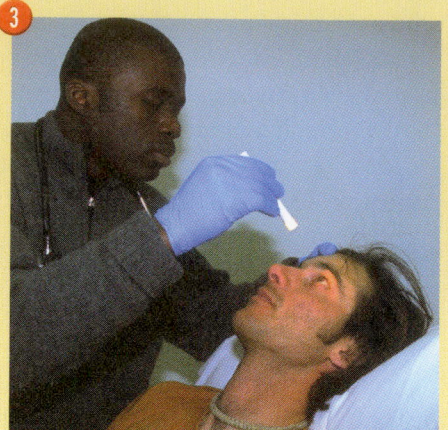
Examine the eyes for redness, contact lenses. Check pupil function.

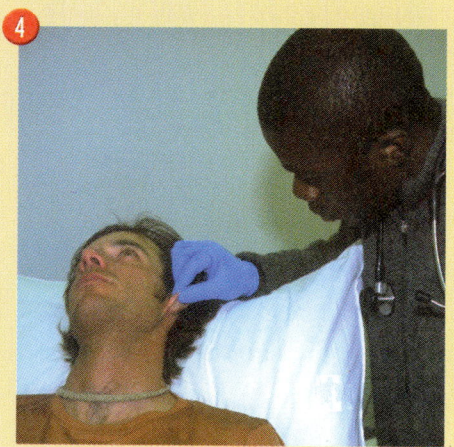
Look behind the ear for Battle's sign.

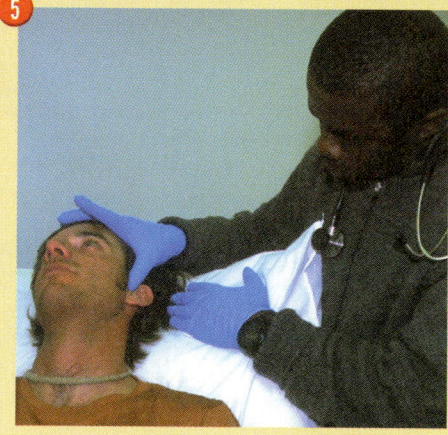
Check the ears for drainage or blood.

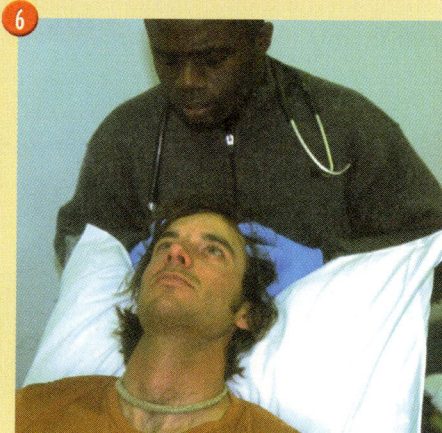
Observe and palpate the head.

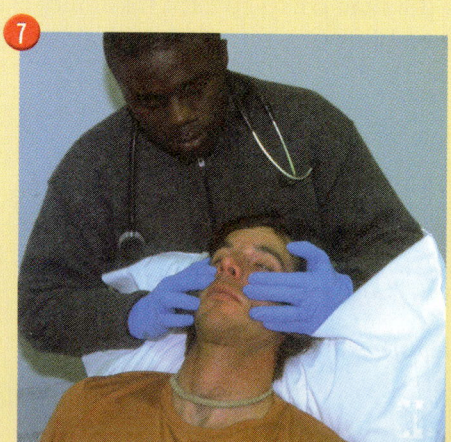
Palpate the zygomas and maxillae.

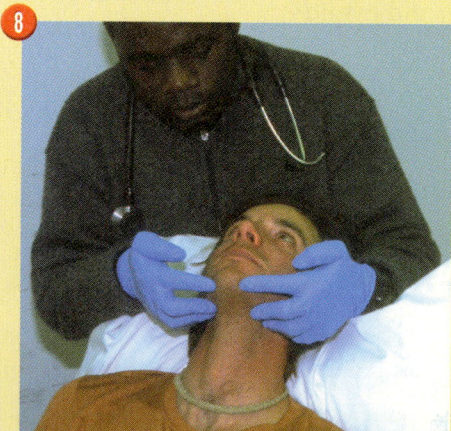
Palpate the mandible.

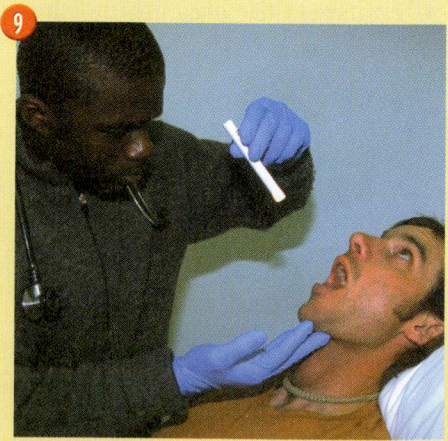
Assess the mouth.

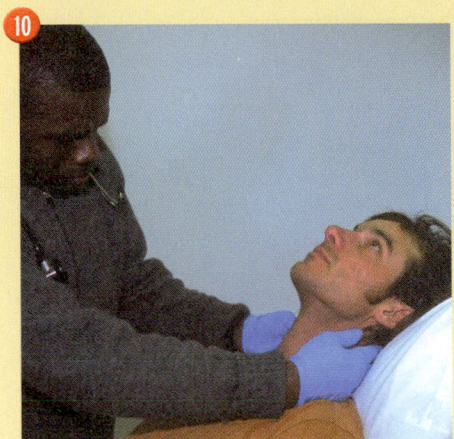

Inspect the neck.

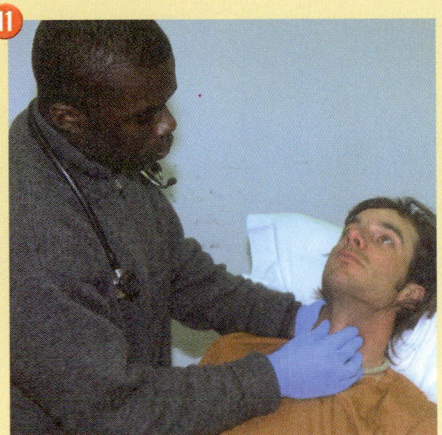

Palpate the neck, front and back.

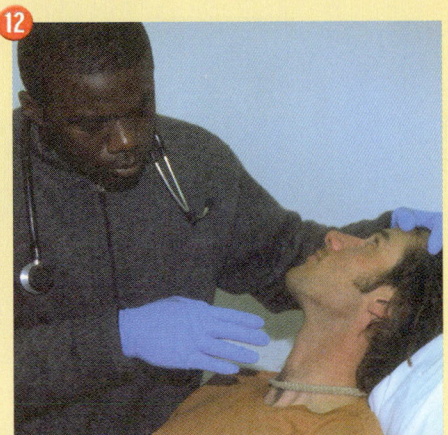

Observe for jugular vein distention.

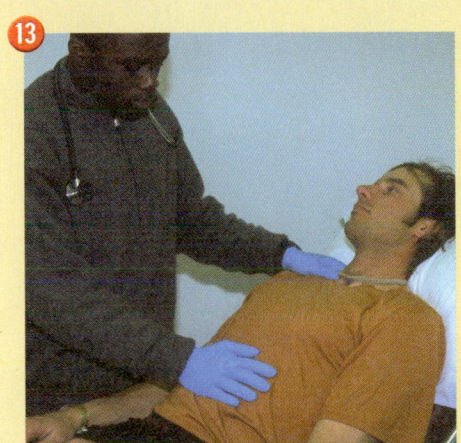

Inspect the chest and observe breathing motion.

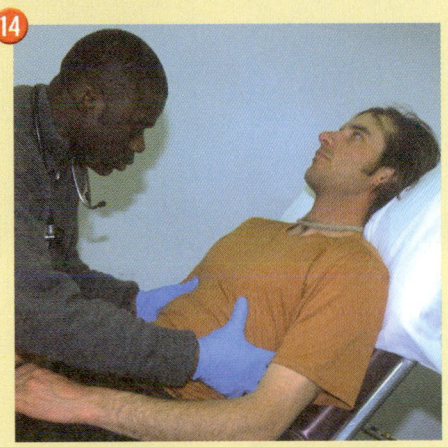

Gently palpate the ribs.

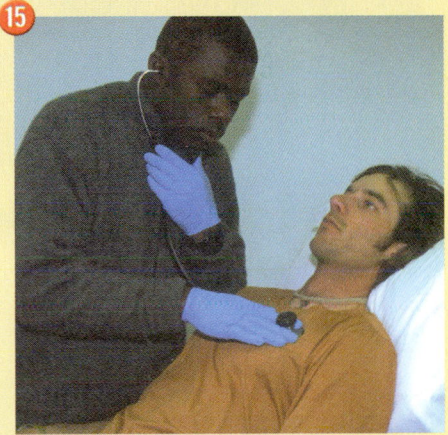

Listen to anterior breath sounds (midaxillary, midclavicular).

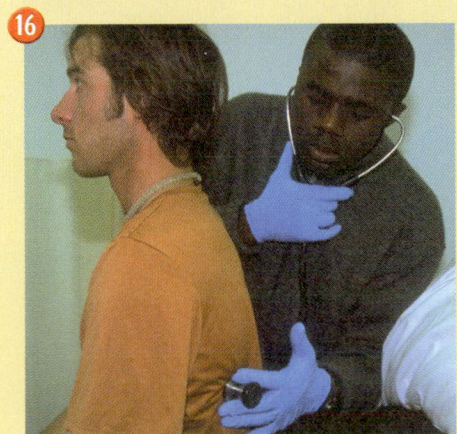

Listen to posterior breath sounds (bases, apices).

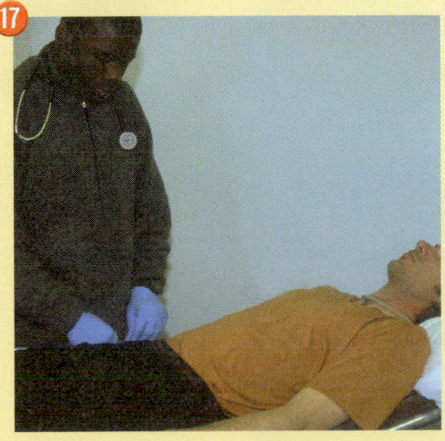

Observe the abdomen and pelvis.

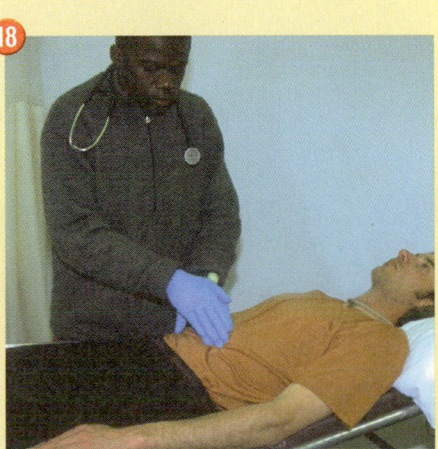

Gently palpate the abdomen.

Continued.

Skill Drill 7-4   Performing the Detailed Physical Exam–continued.

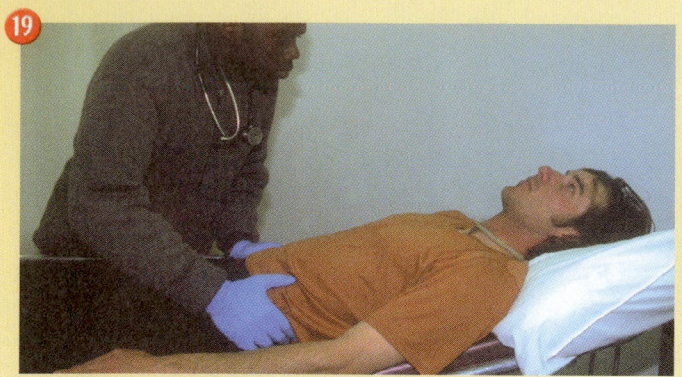

Gently compress the pelvis from the sides.

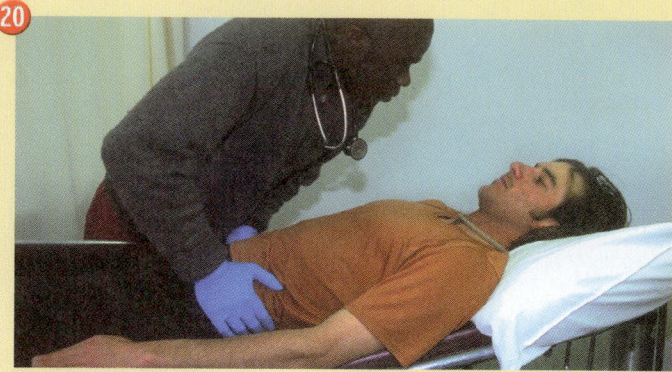

Gently press the iliac crests.

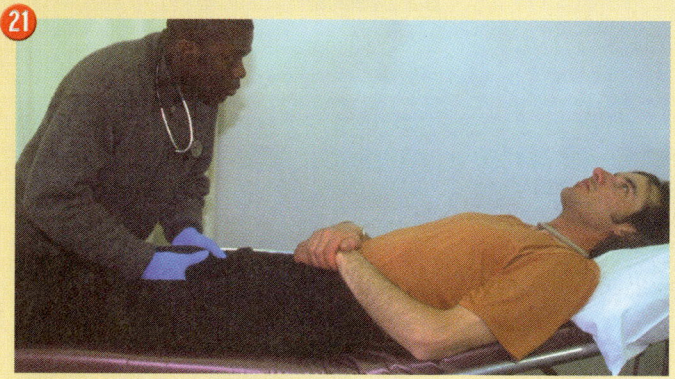

Assess the lower extremities.

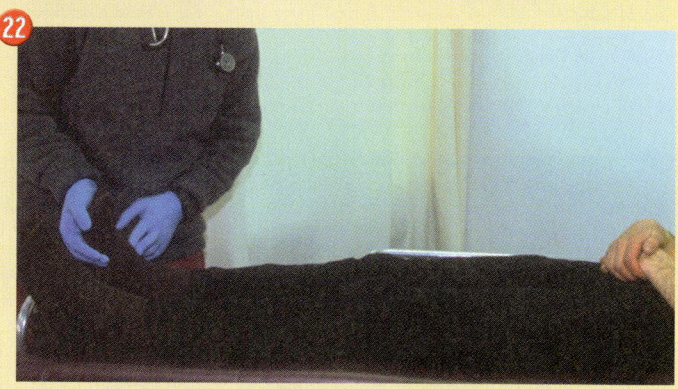

Assess distal circulation, motor, and sensory functions in the lower extremities.

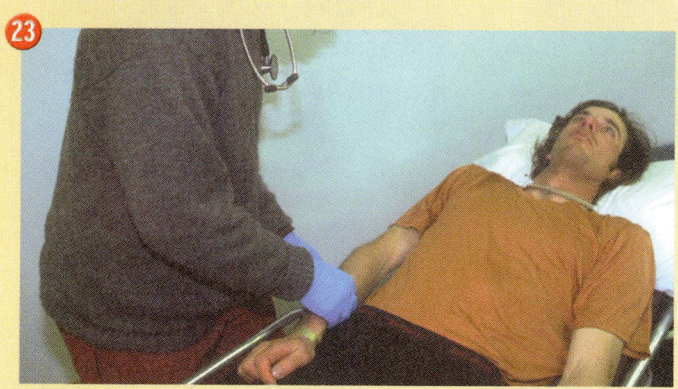

Assess the upper extremities.

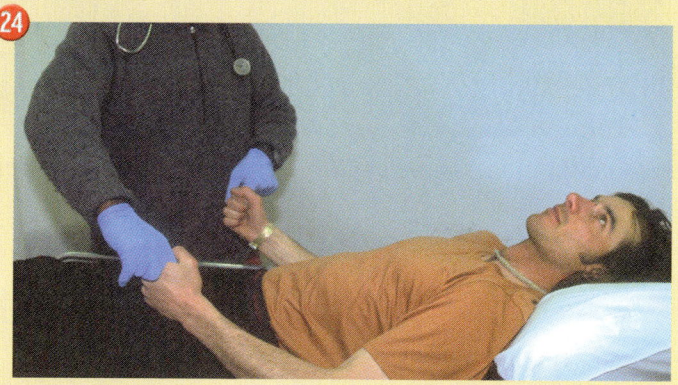

Assess distal circulation, motor, and sensory functions in the upper extremities.

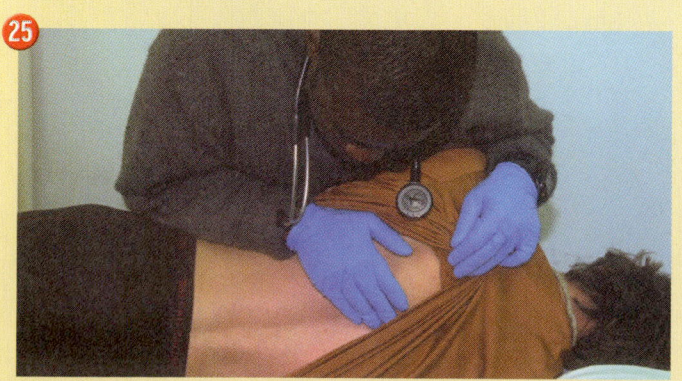

Log roll the patient. Inspect and palpate the back.

TABLE 7-15 Assessing the Skin

Color	Possible Cause	Temperature/Moisture	Possible Cause
Pink	• Normal color	Warm	• Normal condition
Ashen/Pale Face and/or Skin on Extremities	• Hypovolemia • Hypoxia	Hot	• Significant fever • Sunburn • Hyperthermia • Heavy exercise/sweating
Gray-Blue (cyanotic)	• Insufficient air exchange • Low blood oxygen levels (Hypoxia)	Cool	• Early shock • Heat exhaustion
Flushed	• High blood pressure • Carbon monoxide poisoning • Significant fever • Heatstroke • Sunburn • Allergic reaction	Cold	• Profound shock • Hypothermia • Frostbite
		Dry	• Normal condition
Jaundice	• Liver disease or dysfunction	Clammy, Damp, or Moist	• Shock • Heart attack

The Head

Starting at the top of the patient's head and proceeding downward, *look* at the scalp, face, and jaw for abnormal skin color, moisture (▲ Table 7-15), obvious bleeding, and open and closed wounds. Also look for burns—including singed hair, eyebrows, or eyelashes—scars, swelling, depressions, and asymmetry.

Inspect the patient's eyes for unequal prominence of the eyeballs, the pupils for size, equality, and response to light, the **conjunctivae** for discoloration or bleeding, and the areas around the eyes for bruising and swelling. In the responsive patient, ask if he or she is having trouble seeing. Note whether the patient is wearing contact lenses, which you should leave in place, at least until the detailed physical exam is completed.

In the unresponsive patient, it generally is safe to leave contact lenses in place as long as the eyes are kept closed, by taping if necessary, and the patient can be transported to a hospital within 2 to 3 hours. Alert hospital personnel by writing "contact lenses" on a piece of tape and sticking it to the patient's forehead.

Never remove a contact lens if the patient has sustained a direct injury to the eye. However, in facial injuries, consider removing contact lenses before the eyes swell shut, and always remove them in the case of a chemical or physical burn.

Using a flashlight, inspect the patient's ears and nose for bleeding or a clear, colorless or pink discharge, which may represent cerebrospinal fluid leaking from a skull fracture. If you are uncertain whether spinal fluid is present, allow a few drops of the discharge to fall on a white cloth during the detailed physical exam. A bulls-eye pattern with a red center and a pink rim indicates blood mixed with spinal fluid. Make sure you know whether blood in the ear is coming from the ear canal and is not merely blood trickling down from a scalp injury.

With a flashlight and a tongue blade or spoon handle, inspect the patient's mouth for dentures, foreign objects, broken teeth, bleeding, and wounds. Inspect the teeth for obvious injury and abnormal alignment. In the event the patient has sustained a facial injury, note whether the lower jaw is properly aligned under the upper jaw when the patient's mouth is closed; in the responsive patient, ask whether he or she can open and close the mouth normally.

Starting at the top of the patient's head and proceeding downward, *feel* the scalp, face, and jaw for lumps, tenderness, swelling, and the type of spongy, soft dent that may indicate a depressed skull fracture. If blood has matted the hair, palpate against the direction that the hair is matted, which will be more effective. Feel the temperature of the forehead skin, and feel as well as look for moisture.

Listen for abnormal noises in the patient's nose and throat, such as gurgles, wheezes, and crowing sounds. Also, smell the patient's breath for unusual odors such as alcohol; the fruity, acetone smell of diabetic acidosis; the urinous smell associated with kidney failure; or the fecal odor associated with bowel obstruction.

The Neck

Expose the patient's neck temporarily by unzipping a high jacket and pulling down a turtleneck or other shirt with a high collar. Starting just below the patient's jaw and moving downward, *look* for abnormal skin color and moisture, obvious bleeding, open and closed wounds, burns, scars, swelling, bumps, engorged neck veins, asymmetry, abnormal position, and deformity. Also look for a medical-alert tag on a chain.

Starting below the patient's jaw and moving downward, *feel* the front, sides, and back of the neck for tenderness, bumps, swellings, and **subcutaneous emphysema**, which should alert you to a significant airway injury and the possibility of an accompanying cervical spine injury.

If you find a large, open neck wound, cover it immediately with an occlusive dressing, taped on all four sides, to prevent the introduction of air into a vein, which can be fatal.

Check just above the sternal notch to see whether the trachea is in the midline. Do this by pushing your index finger inward medial to each sternomastoid muscle just above its attachment to the sternoclavicular joint. Resistance should be the same on each side. If resistance is less on one side than the other, for example, the space between the sternomastoid and the trachea is wider, the trachea may be deviated, or pushed or pulled to the opposite side because of a collapsed lung or tension pneumothorax.

In addition, *listen* for noises coming from the larynx, such as hoarseness and stridor (a high-pitched crowing noise on inhalation).

The Chest

During the initial assessment you should avoid exposing the patient's chest completely, however, you can assess it to some extent through the clothing or, if necessary, by pulling clothing partially up or down.

Characteristics of the pulse and breathing were noted during the first part of the initial assessment. The second time you assess them you should count and record the pulse and breathing rates and note any abnormal characteristics such as an irregular pulse or an abnormal breathing pattern.

Starting at the patient's clavicles and proceeding downward, assess for abnormal skin color, temperature, and moisture; deformities, obvious bleeding including blood-soaked clothing, open and closed wounds, scars, bumps, swelling, and asymmetry. Note the effort required for breathing, whether both sides of the chest move symmetrically with breathing, and whether there is any obvious pain produced by breathing or coughing.

Again, starting at the clavicles and proceeding downward, *feel* both clavicles, the sternum, and all the ribs in turn to detect swelling, bumps, tenderness (especially over the ribs), and subcutaneous emphysema. If you detect subcutaneous emphysema, the lung or other parts of the lower airway have been injured.

Assess both sides of the patient's chest together—preferably without clothing in place—so you can compare them. Place one hand on each side of the lower, anterior chest to determine whether both sides expand and contract equally during breathing. Feel whether a section of the chest moves paradoxically in and out on exhalation. This condition is referred to as a "flail chest."

Listen for audible wheezes, rattles, squeaks, bubbly sounds, and any other abnormal sounds. If the patient coughs up any material, examine it for color (clear, yellow, green, or bloody [red, pink, or rust-colored]).

Immediately seal any open wounds (see Chapter 19 for further details).

The Abdomen and Pelvis

Acquire the habit of always examining the abdomen from the same side each time you assess a patient. If you are right-handed, assess from the patient's right side because it is easier to detect enlargement or tenderness of the spleen, liver, or gallbladder with the hand nearest the patient's feet. If you are left-handed, assess from the patient's left side.

For the patient's comfort, try to warm your hands before this part of the assessment. You should not need to expose the abdomen completely during the initial assessment because you can do most of this with the patient's clothing in place. To quickly look for abnormalities, especially wounds and bleeding, you can pull the patient's clothing up or down to expose one part of the abdomen at a time. During the detailed physical

> **Remember**
>
> Establishing a baseline set of vital signs is important when assessing a patient's condition. Vital signs should be charted and repeated at regular intervals to identify trends in patient status. As a general rule, reassess the vital signs every 15 minutes in a stable patient and every 5 minutes in the unstable patient.

examination, the patient's abdomen should be completely exposed.

With as much of the patient's abdomen exposed as is practical, start at the **costal arches** and move downward, *looking* for abnormal skin color and moisture; deformities and asymmetry, obvious bleeding, open and closed wounds, scars, local swelling, and general abdominal swelling (distention).

Using the pads of your fingertips, assess the four quadrants of the abdomen in a clockwise manner, beginning with the quadrant farthest from any painful area indicated by the patient. Gently *feel* the abdominal wall to check for tenderness, rigidity, local swelling, masses, and tightening of the abdominal muscles overlying a tender area ("guarding"). In the detailed physical exam, assess for skin temperature and moisture as well.

In the event of trauma, unless the patient reports pelvic pain, has a pelvic deformity, or you already strongly suspect a pelvic fracture, you should gently press the sides of the pelvis toward the midline with a rotary motion to see if this maneuver causes pain or **crepitus**. Crepitus is the grating sensation caused by the grinding of fractured bone ends, which indicates that the pelvis probably is fractured. Position the patient's hands over the pelvic bones and then place your hands on top of the patient's. If the patient doesn't indicate any discomfort during this maneuver, gently push each side of the pelvis backward to see if this maneuver causes pain or crepitus.

Listen for audible gurgling noises and *smell* for abnormal odors, such as the smell of urine or feces, which indicates incontinence. A normal sign is the presence of bowel sounds; an abnormal sign is the absence of bowel sounds.

After shelter is reached, look for evidence of vaginal bleeding in a female patient and for **priapism** or bleeding from the penis in a male patient. Be sure that a witness of the same sex as the patient is present while you are doing this.

The Lower Extremities

It's important to compare the two lower extremities during assessment. Although tights and pants can be pulled down at the waist and pulled up at the ankles, it is difficult to expose a patient's thighs and legs adequately, even in a warm aid room, if the patient is wearing several layers of clothing. Therefore, in the initial assessment, start by *looking* for blood on the clothing, *asking* about pain or tenderness, and *feeling* for swelling, tenderness, and deformity through the clothing.

Note any difference in the length of the extremities and whether or not one foot is turned in or out more than the other, which may mean a fracture or dislocation. If you find any abnormality and suspect a significant injury, use trauma shears or a seam ripper to expose the area completely.

During the initial assessment, while the patient is still wearing boots, ask if he or she can feel the toes and wiggle them. You also can tap the sole and ask if the patient can feel the vibration. However, do not ask a patient to move the injured part of an extremity.

During the detailed physical exam, remove the patient's shoes or boots and socks to assess the feet and ankles (a detailed discussion of ski boot removal is included in Chapter 25). With the patient's extremities exposed as much as possible, start at the groin and move downward, *looking* at the thighs, knees, legs, ankles, and feet for abnormal skin color and moisture, deformities and asymmetry (including abnormal shortening and unusual positions), obvious bleeding, open and closed wounds, scars, and swelling. If in doubt, carefully compare the injured extremity with the opposite, normal one.

In the same order, *feel* the patient's skin and muscles for skin temperature and moisture, tender areas, swelling, and crepitus. Check CMS, and locate and palpate the dorsalis pedis and posterior tibial pulses. Watch for spontaneous motion in the unresponsive patient, and ask the responsive patient to move the hips, knees, and ankles, wiggle the toes, and push and pull the foot against your hand, unless extremity injuries are obvious.

To check the sensation in both thighs and legs in the unresponsive patient, pinch the skin or toenail moderately hard and see whether the patient moves or otherwise reacts. In the responsive patient, check whether the patient can feel you gently pinch him or her or scrape the skin with your fingernail. Ask if the legs or feet feel numb or tingly.

Always compare the reactions of the two extremities. It is especially important to check CMS in the part of an extremity *distal* to a fracture or other serious injury. Note any differences in skin temperature, color, and moisture between the two extremities.

If you are wearing proper facial BSI protection such as a splash shield, *smell* any open wounds that are more than a day or two old to detect abnormal odors, which may indicate infection or gangrene.

The Upper Extremities

Also compare the two upper extremities during the assessment. As with the lower extremities, you can assess the upper extremities fairly well through the clothing during the initial assessment, although you can pull jackets and shirts off the shoulders and push sleeves up temporarily if necessary. In the case of bleeding or a possible open fracture, expose the area by cutting or ripping along a seam.

Starting at the shoulders and moving distally, *look* at the skin for abnormal color and moisture. Look at each shoulder, arm, elbow, forearm, wrist, and hand for deformities, including abnormal shortening and unusual position, asymmetry, obvious bleeding, open and closed wounds, scars, and swelling. Again, if in doubt, compare an injured extremity with the opposite, normal extremity. Look for a medical alert bracelet.

In the same order, starting at the shoulder and moving distally, *feel* the clavicle, shoulder, arm, elbow, forearm, wrist, and hand, checking for skin temperature and moisture, abnormal swellings, tender areas, and depressions. Assess the radial pulse at each wrist.

In the unresponsive patient, check CMS by assessing the patient's radial pulse, looking for spontaneous motion, and testing his or her reaction to a painful pinch of the skin or fingertip.

In the responsive patient, check CMS by asking the individual to move the shoulder, elbow, wrist, and fingers and to tell you whether the arm, forearm, hand, and fingers feel numb or tingly. Ask the patient to squeeze both your hands simultaneously so you can test his or her strength and compare the grip of one hand with the other. To test the motor function of the three nerves that supply each hand, ask the patient to make a fist and then unclench the fist and spread the fingers apart. Record what the patient can and cannot do. Again, do not ask the patient to move the injured part of an extremity.

Check sensation by determining whether the patient can feel a gentle fingernail scrape on the skin of the arms, forearms, and hands and a gentle pinch on the skin of the wrists. Compare the reactions of both extremities. It is especially important to check CMS in the area of the extremity distal to a fracture or other serious injury.

Note any crepitus at the site of an injury, which indicates a fracture. Compare the two extremities for differences in skin color and temperature. Remove all jewelry from an injured extremity as soon as possible, documenting what you removed and what you did with it. Make sure that you have a witness for this step.

As with the lower extremities and if you are wearing proper facial BSI protection such as a splash shield, *smell* any open wounds that are more than a day or two old to detect abnormal odors that may indicate infection or gangrene.

The Back

In this section, the back includes the posterior part of the neck. To adequately assess the back, it must be accessible; that is, the patient can be prone, semiprone, or sitting up. Ideally you can remove or pull clothing out of the way as needed, but this may not be practical during the initial assessment. In fact, during this survey you usually can assess the back adequately through the clothing unless the patient has an open injury or is bleeding severely.

If you suspect a neck or back injury, do not log roll the supine patient to the side to repeat the back assessment during the detailed physical exam unless the movement is necessary to control bleeding or for other urgent reasons. Likewise, do not unstrap a patient already immobilized on a long backboard to assess the back.

If the patient is found in a prone or semiprone position, the rescuer should assess the patient's back and posterior neck before the individual is turned or log rolled to a supine position. If the signs (and symptoms in a responsive patient), mechanism of injury, or abnormalities you find while assessing the back make you suspect a back or neck injury, *unless it is absolutely necessary,* do not turn the patient into the supine position or otherwise move the person until enough help is available to use safe techniques.

If an unresponsive patient is found in a supine position, log roll the patient onto the side using spinal precautions to assess the back. Also log roll any patient in whom the mechanism of injury, location of pain, or abnormalities detected during assessment lead you to

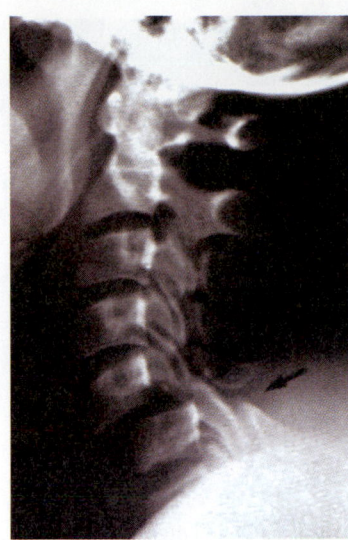

Figure 7-11 Step-off deformity.

suspect a neck or back injury. To avoid unnecessary movement, assess the patient's back when the patient is log rolled for placement on a long backboard.

While waiting for the backboard to arrive, you may begin assessing the back with the patient still supine. Caution the patient not to move. Wearing protective gloves, slide your hand under the neck and back, feeling each spinous process in turn from above and downward for swelling, tenderness, and deformity—especially an abnormal prominence or the step-off type of deformity that may mean a fracture or dislocation of the spine ▲ **Figure 7-11**. At times, you can detect bleeding this way as well.

After the patient is on his or her side, start at the neck and move downward. *Look* for any evidence of blood on the patient's clothing. If you are in a shelter, pull the patient's clothing up or down so you can look at the skin of the neck, back, and buttocks for abnormal skin color and moisture, deformities, asymmetry, open and closed wounds, scars, and swelling.

Next, beginning with the neck, *feel* the neck, back, buttocks, and especially the spinous processes for swelling, tenderness, deformities such as a step-off, unusual prominence, or unusual position. Assess both scapulae. Palpate each flank to assess for tenderness.

Baseline Vital Signs

If you have not assessed the vital signs, now is the time to do so.

Ongoing Assessment

The <u>ongoing assessment</u> (▶ Table 7-16) helps you to monitor changes in the patient's condition. If the changes are improvements, simply continue whatever treatment you are providing, However, in some instances, the patient's condition will deteriorate. When this happens, you should be prepared to modify treatment as appropriate and then begin new treatment on the basis of the problem identified.

All patients should be monitored regularly from the time the initial assessment is completed until they are turned over to a higher level of care. This means they should be reassessed to determine whether they are the same, better, or worse, any new developments have occurred, and any interventions performed have been effective.

Repeat the Initial Assessment and Vital Signs

Monitoring should take only a minute or two. If the patient's vital signs and responsiveness are normal and unchanging and there is no significant mechanism of injury or nature of illness, the patient is considered <u>stable</u>. Conversely, if the patient's vital signs or responsiveness are abnormal or changing, there is a significant mechanism of injury or nature of illness, or the individual's condition appears serious, the patient is considered <u>unstable</u>. Stable patients should be monitored about every 15 minutes and unstable patients every 5 minutes.

Be sure to reassess and record the following components of the assessment:

- Responsiveness (AVPU scale). If responsiveness is altered, also reassess the state of the pupils and the patient's ability to move the extremities on both sides of the body. In a patient with a head injury, this will help you detect the triad of decreasing level of responsiveness, progressive enlargement of one pupil, and decreasing ability to move on one side, which indicates increased bleeding into or swelling of part of the brain—a neurosurgical emergency.
- The airway, to make sure it remains open. This is especially important in the patient who has an altered responsiveness or a severe injury of the face or anterior neck.

Table 7-16 Ongoing Assessment
Repeat the Initial Assessment (ABCs)
Reassess Vital Signs
Repeat Focused Assessment
Check Interventions

Documentation Tips

Always document your findings during the ongoing assessment. Include pulse, blood pressure, respirations, responsiveness, and any other important findings along with the appropriate timelines. Make sure this information as well as earlier documentation accompanies the patient when transferred to EMS services or medical care.

- Breathing, for rate and effectiveness.
- Pulse, for rate, regularity, and quality.
- Blood pressure, recorded or estimated.
- Skin temperature, color, and moisture.

Repeat Focused Assessment

Question the responsive patient again regarding any new signs and symptoms or changes in previous ones. Always assume that something may have been overlooked.

Check Interventions

Recheck the adequacy of any interventions you started. Take a moment to make certain that the oxygen is still flowing, the backboard straps are still tight, bleeding has been controlled, and the airway is still open. Because changes often occur in the uncontrolled prehospital environment, this is a good time to be sure that your emergency care is still "working" the way you expect it to. Care for any changes or other problems immediately.

Patient Assessment

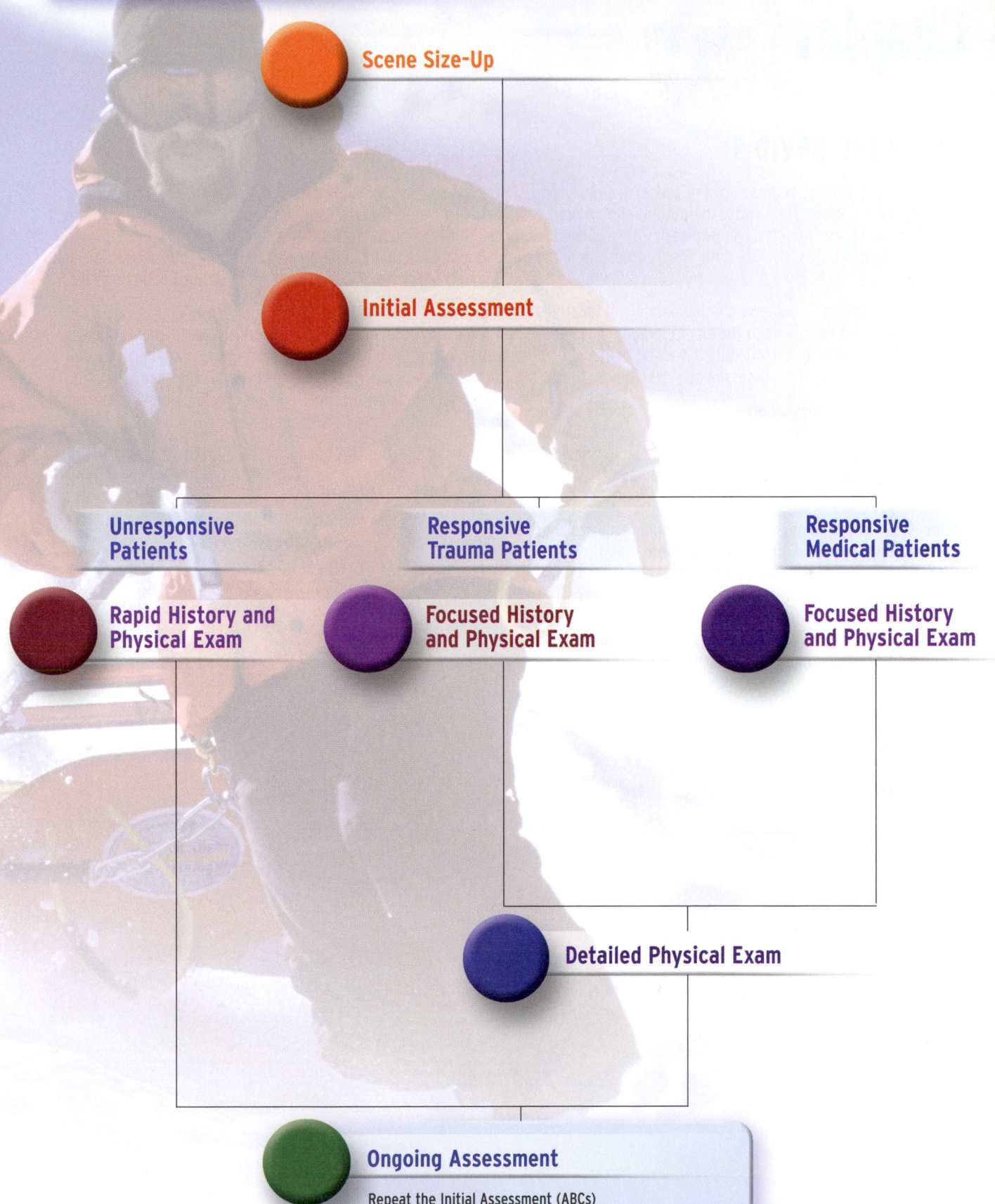

Scene Size-Up

Initial Assessment

Unresponsive Patients

Rapid History and Physical Exam

Responsive Trauma Patients

Focused History and Physical Exam

Responsive Medical Patients

Focused History and Physical Exam

Detailed Physical Exam

Ongoing Assessment

Repeat the Initial Assessment (ABCs)
Reassess Vital Signs
Repeat Focused Assessment
Check Interventions

Chapter *Sweep*

Ready for Review

The assessment process begins with the scene size-up, which identifies real or potential hazards. The patient should not be approached until these hazards have been dealt with in a way that eliminates or minimizes risk to both the rescuers and the patient(s).

The initial assessment is performed on all patients. It identifies any life-threatening conditions to the airway, breathing, and circulation (ABCs). Any life threats identified must be treated before moving to the next step of the assessment.

The rapid history and physical exam is performed quickly on any patient who is unresponsive or unable to articulate the nature of the problem to identify injuries or illnesses. When injuries and conditions are found, they should be prioritized and treated as appropriate.

The focused history and physical exam, trauma and medical, are performed on all patients once their ABCs are stabilized. The focused history and physical exam identify potentially life-threatening conditions and help you to identify and explore the patient's chief complaint. In most cases, the focused history and physical exam, trauma and medical, will provide adequate information to enable you to initiate treatment.

The detailed physical exam is performed on a select group of patients. It helps you to further understand problems that were identified during the focused exam and may also be used to evaluate problems that cannot be identified using the focused exam. The detailed physical exam should be performed in a controlled, warm environment, preferably indoors.

The ongoing assessment is also performed on all patients. It gives you an opportunity to reevaluate problems that are being treated and to recheck treatments to be sure that they are still being delivered correctly. Information from the ongoing assessment may be used to change treatment plans.

As you can see, the assessment process is both systematic and dynamic. All patients will be evaluated by using these same steps. However, because of the ability of the focused history and physical exam to center your actions on the major problems, each of your assessments—unresponsive or responsive, trauma or medical—will be slightly different, depending on the needs of the patient. The result will be a process that will enable you to quickly identify and treat the needs of all patients, both medical and traumatic, in a way that meets their unique needs.

Vital Vocabulary

AVPU A mnemonic for assessing a patient's level of responsiveness by determining whether a patient is Awake and alert, responsive to Verbal stimulus or Pain, or Unresponsive; used principally in the initial assessment.

body substance isolation (BSI) An infection control concept and practice that assumes that all body fluids are potentially infectious.

capillary refill A test that evaluates distal circulatory system function by squeezing (blanching) blood from an area such as a nail bed and watching the speed of its return after releasing the pressure.

chief complaint The reason a patient called for help; also, the patient's response to general questions such as "What's wrong?" or "What happened?"

circulation, motion, sensation (CMS) An abbreviation for what to check in an injured extremity.

conjunctiva The delicate membrane that lines the eyelids and covers the exposed surface of the eye.

costal arches The arch formed by the cartilage that connects the sixth through tenth ribs to each other and to the base of the sternum.

crepitus A grating or grinding sensation caused by fractured bone ends or joints rubbing together.

DCAP-BTLS A mnemonic for assessment in which each area of the body is evaluated for Deformities, Contusions, Abrasions, Punctures/Penetrations, Burns, Tenderness, Lacerations, and Swelling.

detailed physical exam The part of the assessment process in which a detailed area-by-area exam is performed on patients whose problems cannot be readily identified or when more specific information is needed about problems identified in the focused history and physical exam.

focused history and physical exam The part of the assessment process, either trauma or medical, in which the patient's major complaints or any problems that are immediately evident are further and more specifically evaluated.

Golden Hour The time from injury to definitive care, during which treatment of shock or traumatic injuries should occur because survival potential is the best.

hemorrhage Profuse bleeding.

hypothermia A condition in which the internal body temperature falls below 95°F (35°C) after exposure to a cold environment.

initial assessment The part of the assessment process that helps you to identify any immediately or potentially life-threatening conditions so that you can initiate lifesaving care.

intervention An urgent measure that interrupts assessment in order to care for a condition that threatens life or limb and requires immediate care.

mechanism of injury (MOI) The way in which traumatic injuries occur; the forces that act on the body to cause damage.

nature of illness (NOI) Effort to determine the general type of illness.

ongoing assessment The part of the assessment process in which problems are reevaluated and responses to treatment are assessed.

OPQRST The six pain questions: Onset, Provoking factors, Quality, Radiation, Severity, Time.

palpate Examine by touch.

priapism Painful persistent erection caused by spinal injury.

radiation A continuation of an area of pain or discomfort; gives the sensation that the pain is moving (radiating) away from the origin.

rapid body survey A quick, hands-on, clothes-on examination of the entire body during the initial assessment; designed to be performed on site before reaching shelter.

rapid history and physical exam A part of the assessment process for an unresponsive or a responsive trauma patient with a significant mechanism of injury with a goal of evacuating the patient to definitive care as quickly as possible.

recovery position The preferred body position for an unconscious patient with no suspected spine injury. The patient lies on his or her side with the opposite knee flexed and the head cushioned on the hand. Also called the semiprone, rescue, stable side, or NATO position.

responsiveness The way in which a patient responds to external stimuli, including verbal stimuli (sound), tactile stimuli (touch), and painful stimuli.

SAMPLE history A key brief history of a patient's condition to determine Signs/Symptoms, Allergies, Medications, Pertinent past history, Last oral intake, and Events leading to the illness/injury.

scene size-up A quick assessment of the scene and the surroundings made to provide information about its safety and the mechanism of injury or nature of illness, before you enter and begin patient care.

stable A patient whose vital signs and mental status are normal and unchanging, and there is no significant MOI or NOI.

stridor A harsh, high-pitched inspiratory sound that is often heard in acute laryngeal (upper airway) obstruction; may sound like crowing and be audible without a stethoscope.

subcutaneous emphysema A characteristic crackling sensation on palpation, caused by the presence of air in soft tissues.

supine Lying face up.

triage The process of establishing treatment and transportation priorities according to severity of injury and medical need.

unresponsive A patient who is less than alert, ie, less than A on the AVPU scale.

unstable A patient whose vital signs or mental status are abnormal or changing, or in whom there is a significant MOI or NOI.

www.OECzone.com

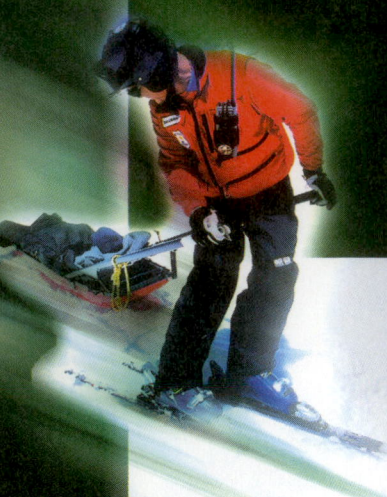

Assessment in Action

You respond to a call in the cafeteria where there has been a fire. A frying pan full of grease caught fire, spreading up the walls to the cupboards. The patient is a woman in her early 20s and is lying on the floor of the kitchen. She responds only by moaning when you pinch her fingers. Her pupils are dilated and barely reactive. Her face is pale with soot present. Her skin feels warm and moist but her lips are gray. You note burns on her hands and lower arms but no other wounds. Vital signs include a regular pulse of 130 beats/min, respirations of 26 breaths/min, and a blood pressure of 104/66 mm Hg.

1. Appropriate BSI precautions for this situation would include:
   A. gloves and goggles.
   B. gloves and mask.
   C. gloves.
   D. mask and goggles.

2. Which of the following terms would best describe the patient's current level of consciousness?
   A. Alert and oriented
   B. Responsive to pain
   C. Semiconscious
   D. Unresponsive

3. Which of the following characteristics of the patient's skin would suggest that the patient is not getting adequate oxygen?
   A. Pale
   B. Gray lips
   C. Warm
   D. Moist

4. Your general assessment suggests that your immediate action should be to:
   A. call for additional help.
   B. apply oxygen.
   C. dress her burns.
   D. apply spinal immobilization.

5. Part of your rapid trauma assessment includes listening for breath sounds. The best place to listen for accurate breath sounds is:
   A. from the back, over the shirt.
   B. from the front, over the shirt.
   C. from the back, under the shirt.
   D. from the front, under the shirt.

6. A SAMPLE history for this patient would include:
   A. finding her unconscious, in the room where a fire started.
   B. documenting that she has burns.
   C. any medications found with her.
   D. the suspicion that she was getting ready to eat.

7. In this patient, it is especially important to check which of the following?
   A. Back
   B. Abdomen
   C. Mouth
   D. Burns

Challenging Questions

8. From the little information you have, what is most likely causing her unconsciousness?

9. Immediate treatment is included during the initial and ongoing assessment. What immediate treatment is necessary for this patient?

10. During your assessment you note wheezing in all lobes. What is the most likely cause of her wheezing?

Points to Ponder

You are called to a mountain bike trail where an unresponsive woman is lying face down, bleeding from a facial laceration with some trail debris on her face as well. When you shake her gently, she moans but does not awaken. You reach under her head to see if you can feel her breathing and find that she has vomited. How would this situation affect your patient assessment? Would you be as thorough? What does your general assessment suggest you should do?

Issues BSI Precautions, Thorough and Consistent Patient Assessment; Airway Management, Transport Decisions

Online Outlook

During the initial assessment (ABCs), life-threatening conditions are identified and their management is begun. You can learn more about the initial assessment by following the Trauma Assessment link at www.OECzone.

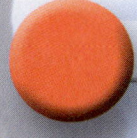

Scene Size-Up

Body Substance Isolation
Scene Safety
Determine Mechanism of Injury/Nature of Illness
Determine Number of Patients
Request Additional Assistance
Consider C-Spine Immobilization

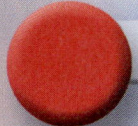

Initial Assessment

Form General Impression of the Patient
Assess Responsiveness
Assess the Airway, Breathing, and Circulation (ABCs)
Stabilize ABCs
Identify Priority Patients
Initiate Transport Decision

**Unresponsive
Patients**

**Responsive
Trauma Patients**

**Responsive
Medical Patients**

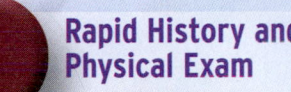

Rapid History and Physical Exam

Rapid Body Survey
Baseline Vital Signs
SAMPLE History
    (from friends, family,
    or bystanders)
Rapid Transport

Focused History and Physical Exam

Reconsider the Mechanism of Injury

Significant MOI	**No Significant MOI**
Rapid Trauma Assessment (Rapid Body Survey)	Focused Physical Exam Based on Chief Complaint
Baseline Vital Signs and SAMPLE History	Baseline Vital Signs and SAMPLE History
Rapid Transport	Reevaluate Transport

Focused History and Physical Exam

History of Illness
SAMPLE History
Focused Physical Exam:
    Based on Chief Complaint
Baseline Vital Signs
Reevaluate Transport

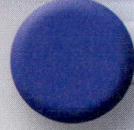

Detailed Physical Exam

Head-to-toe Steps
Systematic Exam Using DCAP-BTLS
Baseline Vital Signs

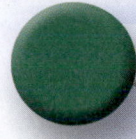

Ongoing Assessment

Repeat the Initial Assessment (ABCs)
Reassess Vital Signs
Repeat Focused Assessment
Check Interventions

Bleeding

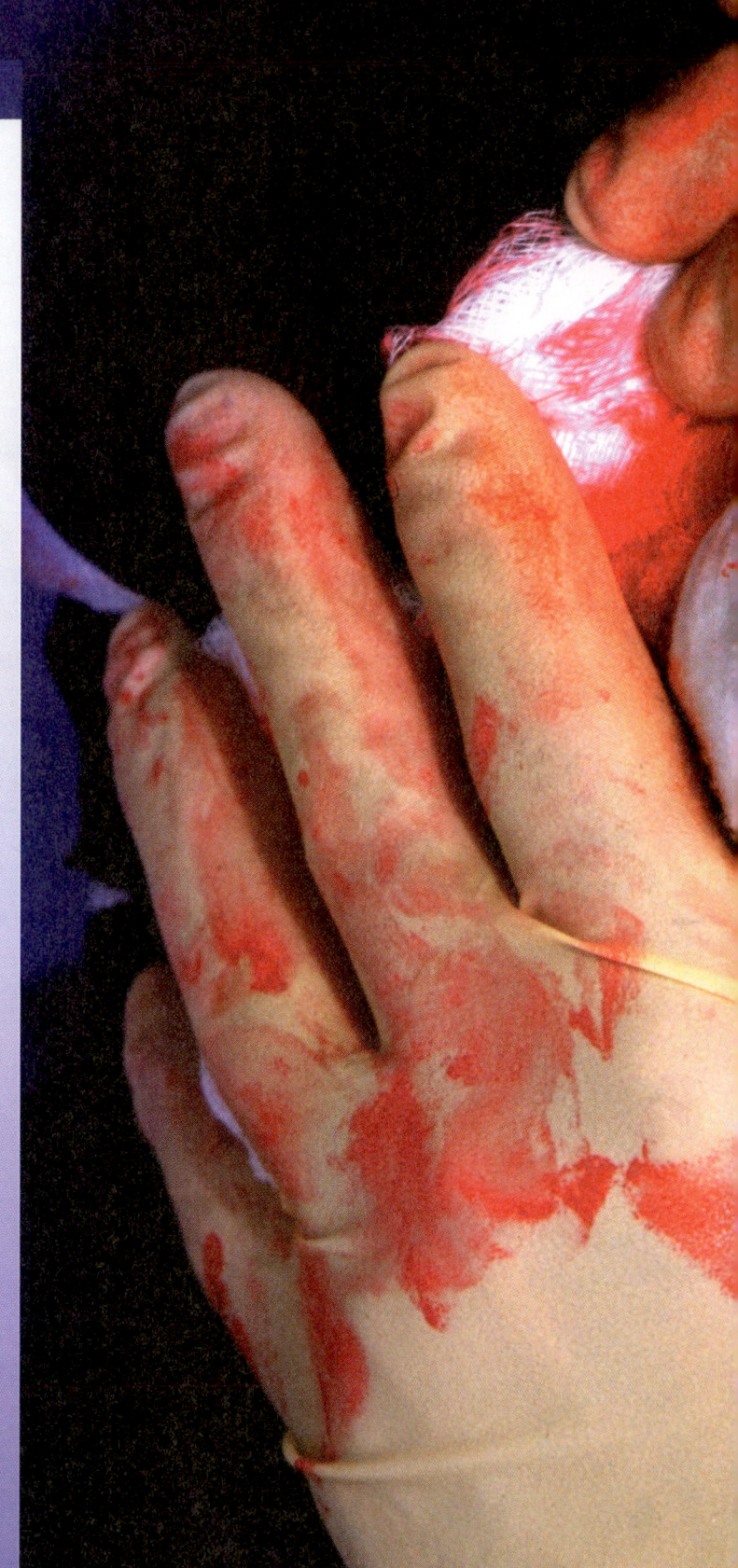

🌲 These are core concepts in initial patrol training.

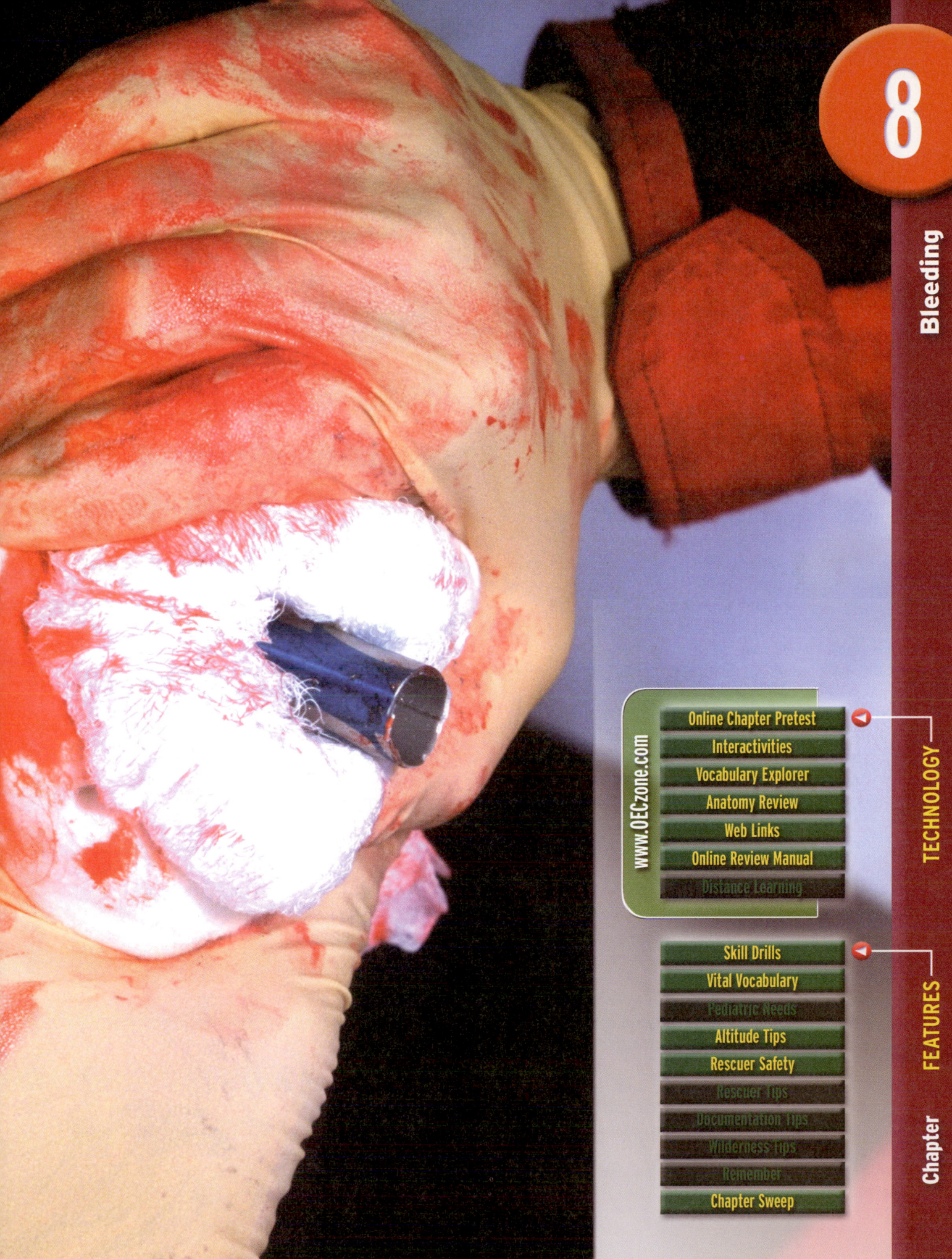

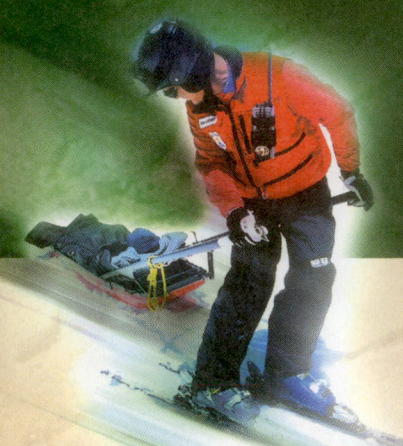

While skiing a mogul run, you and your partner come upon a guest who has fallen against a large rock. The skier's lower arm and wrist are already showing signs of swelling and a hematoma, as well as some surface bleeding.

Blunt trauma can produce injuries ranging from minor soft-tissue wounds to fatalities, either of which can present with little visible outward signs indicating the severity of the injury. This chapter will provide information on the methods recommended to control bleeding along with helping you answer the following questions:

1. Why does internal bleeding often go unnoticed until the patient "crashes"?

2. Under what circumstances might the rarely used tourniquet be the best choice for bleeding control?

Bleeding

After managing the airway, recognizing bleeding and understanding how it affects the body are perhaps the most important skills you will learn as a rescuer. Bleeding can be external and obvious or internal and hidden. Either way, it is potentially dangerous, causing first weakness and, if left uncontrolled, eventually shock and death. The most common cause of shock after trauma is bleeding.

The purpose of this chapter is to help you understand how the cardiovascular system reacts to blood loss. The chapter begins with a brief review of the anatomy and function of the cardiovascular system. It then describes the signs, symptoms, and emergency medical care of both external and internal bleeding. The chapter concludes with a discussion on the relationship between bleeding and hypovolemic shock.

Anatomy and Physiology of the Cardiovascular System

The cardiovascular system circulates blood to all of the body's cells and tissues, delivering oxygen and nutrients and carrying away metabolic waste products ▶ Figure 8-1 . Certain parts of the body, such as the brain, spinal cord, and heart, require a constant flow of blood to live. The cells in these organs cannot tolerate a lack of blood for more than a few minutes. Other organs, such as the lungs and kidneys, can survive for short periods of time without adequate blood flow. After that, their cells begin to die. This can lead to a permanent loss of function or, if enough cells die, death.

The cardiovascular system, the main system responsible for supplying and maintaining adequate blood flow, consists of three parts:

- The pump (the heart)
- A container (the blood vessels that reach every cell in the body)
- The fluid (blood and body fluids)

The Heart

The heart is a hollow muscular organ about the size of a clenched fist. It is an involuntary muscle that is under the control of the autonomic nervous system, but it has its own regulatory system. Thus, it can function even if the nervous system shuts down.

The heart is always working; all other organs depend on it to provide a rich blood supply. For this reason, it has a number of special features that other muscles do not. First, because the heart can tolerate a serious interruption of its blood supply for only a few seconds, its blood supply is as rich and well distributed as possible. Second, the heart works as two paired pumps ▶ Figure 8-2 . Each side of the heart has an upper chamber (atrium) and a lower chamber (ventricle), both of which pump blood. Blood leaves each chamber of a normal heart through a one-way valve, which keeps the blood moving in the proper direction by preventing a backflow.

The right side of the heart receives oxygen-poor (deoxygenated) blood from the veins of the body. Blood enters into the right atrium from the vena cava, then fills the right ventricle. After the right ventricle contracts, blood flows into the pulmonary artery and the pulmonary circulation. The now oxygen-rich (oxygenated) blood returns to the left side of the heart from the lungs through the pulmonary veins. Blood enters the left

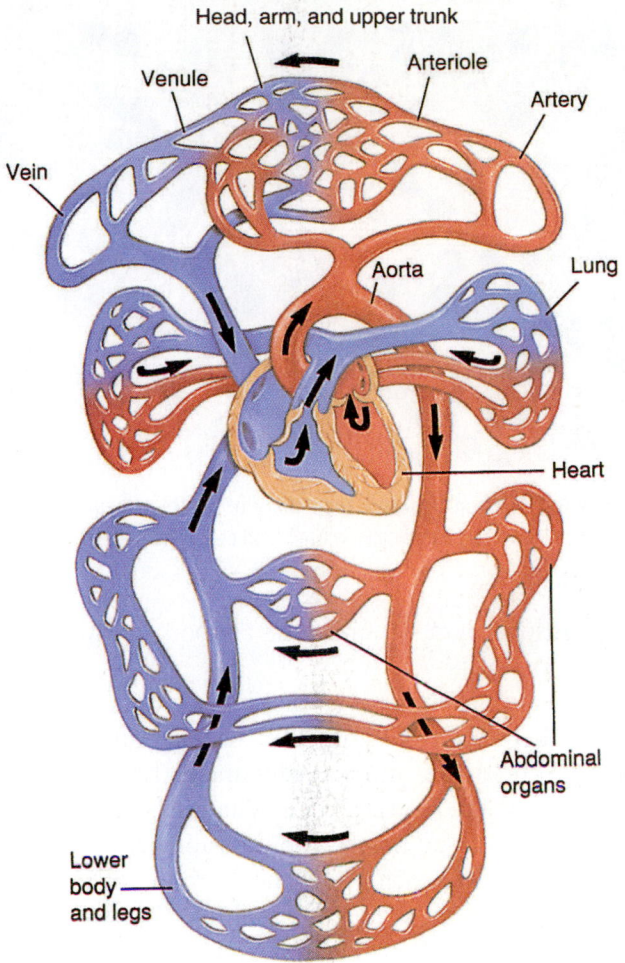

Figure 8-1   The cardiovascular system includes the heart, arteries, veins, and interconnecting capillaries. The exchange of nutrients and waste products that occurs in the capillaries is shown.

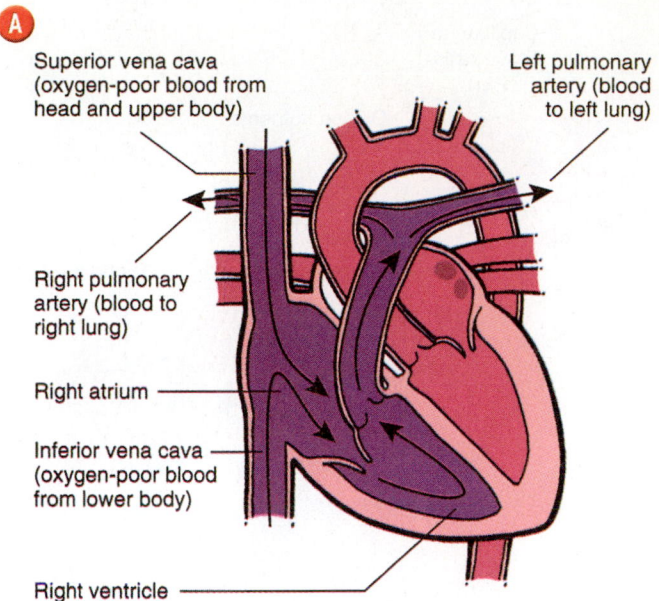

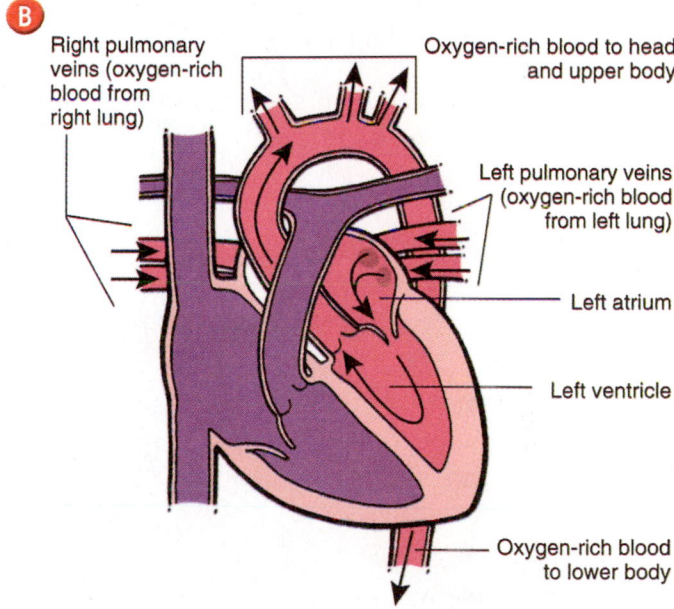

Figure 8-2   **A.** The left side of the heart circulates oxygen-rich blood to all parts of the body. It is the more muscular of the two pumps, as it must pump blood into the aorta and into the arteries. **B.** The right side of the heart circulates blood from the body to the lungs.

atrium, then passes into the left ventricle. This side of the heart is more muscular than the other because it must pump blood into the aorta and on to the arteries throughout the body.

Blood Vessels and Blood

There are five types of blood vessels:

- Arteries
- Arterioles
- Capillaries
- Venules
- Veins

As blood flows out of the heart, it passes into the **aorta**, the largest **artery** in the body. The arteries become smaller as they move away from the heart. The smaller vessels that connect the arteries and capillaries are called **arterioles**. **Capillaries** are small tubes, with the diameter of a single red blood cell, that pass among all the cells in the body, linking the arterioles and the venules. Blood leaving the distal side of the capillaries flows into the venules. These small, thin-walled vessels

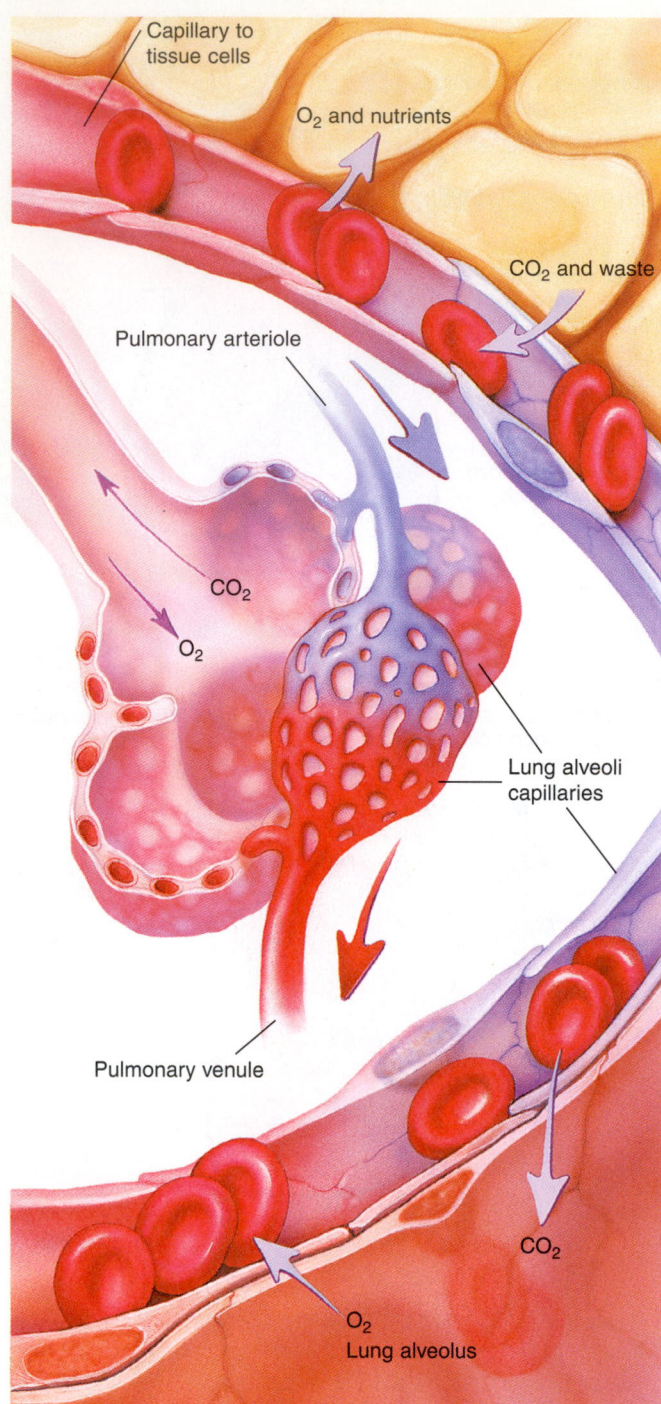

Figure 8-3   Oxygen and nutrients pass easily from the capillaries into the cells, and waste and carbon dioxide move out of the cells into the capillaries (top). Oxygen and carbon dioxide pass freely between the lungs and the capillaries (bottom).

empty into the **veins**, which return the blood to the heart. Oxygen and nutrients easily pass from the capillaries into the cells, and waste and carbon dioxide move out of the cells and into the capillaries (▲ **Figure 8-3**).

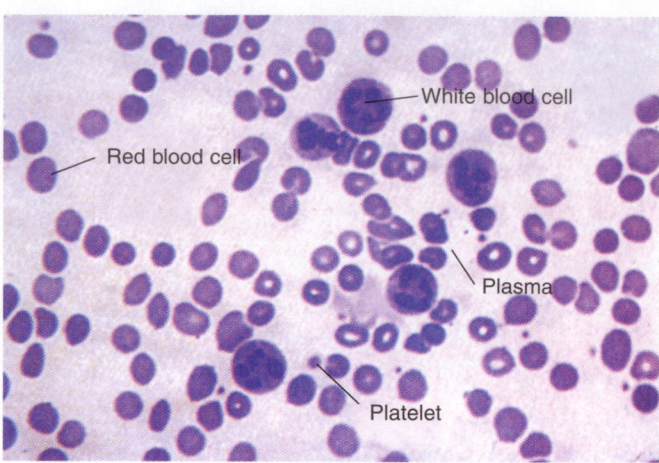

Figure 8-4   The microscopic appearance of the three major elements in blood: red blood cells, white blood cells, and platelets.

This transportation system allows the body to rid itself of waste products.

At the arterial ends of the capillaries and in the arteries themselves are circular muscular walls, which constrict and dilate automatically under the control of the autonomic nervous system. When these muscles open (dilate), blood passes into the capillaries into close proximity to each cell of the surrounding tissue; when the muscles are closed (constricted), there is no capillary blood flow. The muscles dilate and constrict in response to conditions such as fright, heat, cold, a specific need for oxygen, and the need to dispose of metabolic waste. In a healthy individual, all the vessels are never fully dilated or fully constricted at the same time.

The last part of the cardiovascular system is the contents of the container, or the blood. Blood contains red cells, white cells, platelets, and a liquid called plasma (▲ **Figure 8-4**).

Physiology and Perfusion

Perfusion is the circulation of blood within an organ or tissue in adequate amounts to meet the cells' current needs for oxygen, nutrients, and waste removal. Blood enters an organ or tissue first through the arteries, then the arterioles, and finally the capillary beds (▶ **Figure 8-5**). While passing through the capillaries, the blood delivers nutrients and oxygen to the surrounding cells and picks up the wastes they have generated. Then the blood leaves the capillary beds through the venules and finally reaches the veins, which take the blood back to the heart.

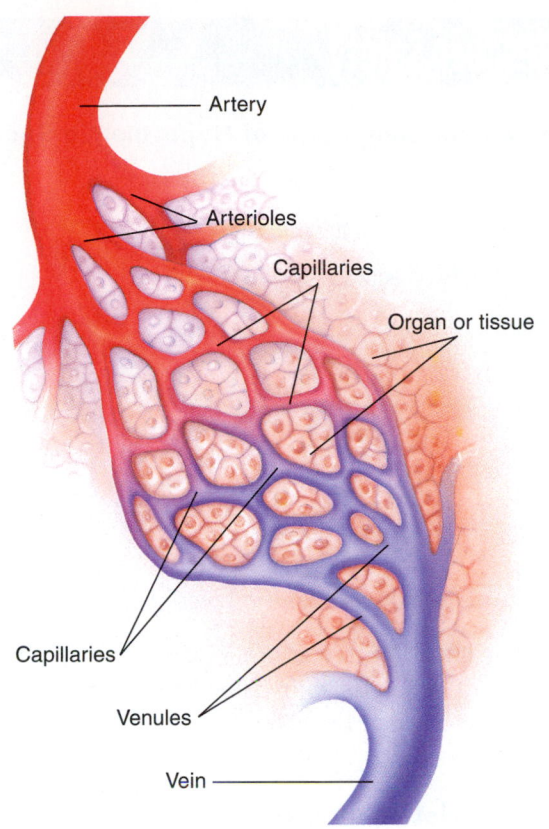

Rescuer Safety

Remember that a bleeding patient may expose you to potentially infectious body fluids; therefore, you must always follow BSI precautions in treating patients with external bleeding. Wear gloves and eye protection in all situations. Avoid direct contact with body fluids if possible. Take special care if you have an open sore, cut, scratch, or ulcer. Also remember that frequent, thorough handwashing between patients and after every run is a simple yet important protective measure. If there is a risk of blood splatter, wear a mask with eye protection and a disposable, fluid-resistant gown in the aid room. On the hill, a parka and wind pants preferably made of fluid-resistant material will be suitable, but you should also wear your ski goggles.

Figure 8-5 Perfusion occurs when blood circulates through tissues or an organ to provide the necessary oxygen and nutrients and remove waste products.

Oxygen and carbon dioxide exchange takes place in the lungs.

Blood must pass through the cardiovascular system at a speed that is fast enough to maintain adequate circulation throughout the body and slow enough to allow each cell time to exchange oxygen and nutrients for carbon dioxide and other waste products. While some tissues, such as the lungs and kidneys, never rest and require a constant blood supply, most require circulating blood only intermittently, especially when active. Muscles are a good example. When you sleep, they are at rest and require a minimal blood supply. However, during exercise, they need a very large blood supply. The gastrointestinal tract requires a high flow of blood after a meal. After digestion is completed, it can do quite well with a small fraction of that flow.

The autonomic nervous system monitors the body's needs from moment to moment and adjusts the blood flow as required. During emergencies, the autonomic nervous system automatically redirects blood away from other organs to the heart, brain, lungs, and kidneys.

Thus, the cardiovascular system is dynamic, constantly adapting to changing conditions. At times, the system fails to provide sufficient circulation for every body part to perform its function. This condition is called hypoperfusion, or **shock**.

Knowing which organs need adequate perfusion is the foundation on which your treatment of patients is based. Emergency medical care is designed to support the following systems:

- The heart (cardiovascular system)
- The brain (central nervous system)
- The lungs (respiratory system)
- The kidneys (renal system)

The heart requires constant perfusion, or it will not function properly. The brain and spinal cord cannot go for more than 4 to 6 minutes without perfusion, or the nerve cells will be permanently damaged. It is important to remember that cells of the central nervous system do not have the capacity to regenerate. The kidneys will be permanently damaged after 45 minutes of inadequate perfusion. Skeletal muscles cannot tolerate more than 2 hours of inadequate perfusion. The gastrointestinal tract can exist with limited (but not absent) perfusion for several hours. These times are based on a normal body temperature (98.6°F [37.0°C]).

External Bleeding

Hemorrhage means "bleeding." External bleeding is a visible hemorrhage. Examples include nosebleeds and bleeding from open wounds. As a rescuer, you must understand how to control external bleeding.

The Significance of Bleeding

Acute blood loss of greater than 20% of blood volume in an adult can be life threatening (▼ **Figure 8-6**). The typical adult has approximately 70 mL of blood per kilogram of body weight, or 6 L (10 to 12 pints) in a body weighing 80 kg (175 lb). If the typical adult loses more than 1 L of blood (about 2 pints), significant changes in vital signs will occur, including increasing heart and respiratory rates and decreasing blood pressure. Because infants and children have less blood volume to begin with, the same effect is seen with smaller amounts of blood loss. For example, a 1-year-old infant has a total blood volume of about 800 mL. Significant symptoms of blood loss will occur after only 100 to 200 mL of blood loss. To put this in perspective, a soft drink can holds roughly 345 mL of liquid.

How well people compensate for blood loss is related to how rapidly they bleed. A normal, healthy adult can comfortably donate 1 unit (500 mL) of blood over a period of 15 to 20 minutes, adapting well to this decrease in blood volume. However, if a similar blood loss occurs in a much shorter period of time, **hypovolemic shock**, a condition in which low blood volume results in inadequate perfusion and even death, may rapidly develop. The body simply cannot compensate for such a rapid blood loss.

You should consider bleeding to be serious if the following conditions are present:

- It is associated with a significant mechanism of injury.
- The patient has a poor general appearance.
- Assessment reveals signs and symptoms of shock (hypoperfusion).

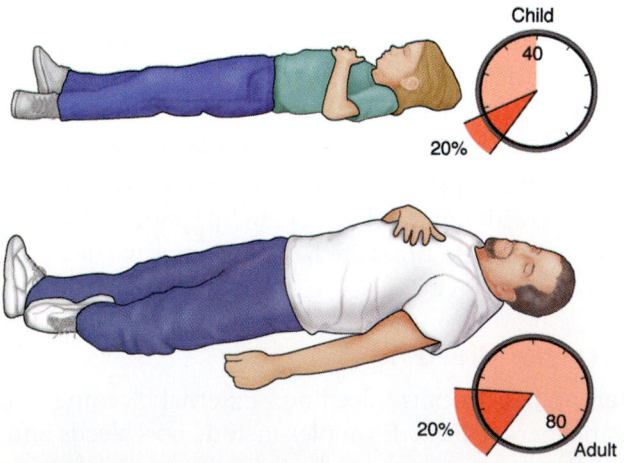

Figure 8-6 Loss of approximately 1 L of blood will cause significant changes in an adult; a much smaller blood loss will result in shock in a child or infant.

Signs and Symptoms of Hypovolemic Shock

Rapid, weak pulse

Low blood pressure (late sign)

Mental status changes

Cool, clammy skin

Cyanosis (lips, under nails)

- You note a significant amount of blood loss.
- The blood loss is rapid.
- You cannot control the bleeding.

In any situation, blood loss is an extremely serious problem. It demands your immediate attention as soon as you have cleared the airway and managed the patient's breathing.

Characteristics of Bleeding

Injuries and some illnesses can disrupt blood vessels and cause bleeding. Typically, bleeding from an open artery is bright red (high in oxygen) and spurts in time with the pulse. The pressure that causes the blood to spurt also makes this type of bleeding difficult to control. As the amount of blood circulating in the body drops, so does the patient's blood pressure and, eventually, the arterial spurting.

Blood from an open vein is much darker (low in oxygen) and flows steadily. Because it is under less pressure, most venous blood does not spurt and is easier to manage. Bleeding from damaged capillary vessels is dark red and oozes from a wound steadily but slowly. It may clot spontaneously (▶ **Figure 8-7**).

On its own, bleeding tends to stop rather quickly, within about 10 minutes, in response to internal mechanisms and exposure to air. When we are cut, blood flows rapidly from the open vessel. Soon afterward, the cut ends of the vessel begin to constrict, reducing the amount of bleeding. Then a clot forms, plugging the hole and sealing the injured portions of the vessel. This process is called **coagulation**. Small arteries may spasm and stop bleeding only to spontaneously start again if a solid clot has not formed. Direct contact with body tissues and fluids or the external environment commonly triggers the blood's clotting factors.

Despite the efficiency of this system, it may fail in certain situations. A number of medications, including aspirin, interfere with normal clotting. With a severe injury, the damage to the vessel may be so large that a clot cannot completely block the hole. Sometimes, only part of the vessel wall is cut, preventing it from constricting. In these cases, bleeding will continue unless it is stopped by external means. Occasionally, blood loss occurs very rapidly. In these instances, the patient might die before the body's defenses, such as clotting, could help.

A very small portion of the population lacks one or more of the blood's clotting factors. One such condition is called <u>hemophilia</u>. There are several forms of hemophilia, most of which are hereditary and some of which are severe. Sometimes, bleeding may occur spontaneously in hemophilia. Because the patient's blood does not clot, all injuries, no matter how trivial, are potentially serious. A bleeding patient with hemophilia should be transported immediately to the hospital. If external bleeding is present, continuous pressure on the source must be maintained.

Emergency Medical Care

As you begin to care for a patient with obvious external bleeding, remember to follow BSI precautions. As with all patient care, make sure that the patient has an open airway and is breathing adequately. Provide oxygen if it is needed. You may then concentrate on controlling the bleeding.

Several methods are available to control external bleeding. Starting with the most commonly used, these include the following:

- Direct pressure and elevation
- Pressure dressings
- Pressure points (for upper and lower extremities)
- Splints
- Air splints
- Pneumatic antishock garment
- Tourniquets (last resort)

BASIC METHODS. It will often be useful to combine these methods. ▶ Skill Drill 8-1 illustrates the basic techniques that do not require special equipment:

1. Almost all instances of external bleeding can be controlled simply by **applying direct local pressure to the bleeding site.** This method is by far the most effective way to control external bleeding. Pressure stops the flow of blood and permits normal coagulation to occur. You may apply pressure with your gloved fingertip or hand, over the top of a sterile dressing if one is immediately available.

2. **Elevating a bleeding extremity** by as little as 6" often stops venous bleeding. Whenever possible, use both techniques: direct pressure and elevation. In most cases, this will stop the bleeding. However, if it does not, you still have several options **(Step 1)**.

3. **Once you have applied a dressing and controlled the bleeding,** you can create a pressure dressing to maintain the pressure by firmly wrapping a sterile, self-adhering roller bandage around the entire wound. Use 4" × 4" or 4" × 8" sterile gauze pads for small wounds, and sterile universal dressings for larger wounds. If sterile gauze pads are not immediately available, use a clean handkerchief,

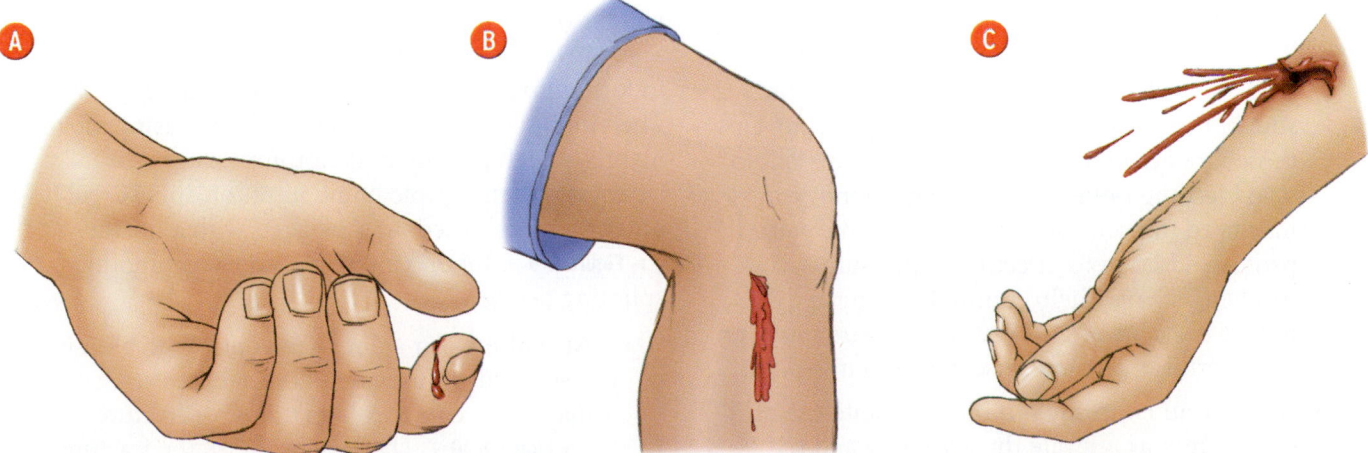

Figure 8-7 **A.** Bleeding from capillary vessels is dark red and oozes from the wound slowly but steadily. **B.** Venous bleeding is darker than arterial bleeding and flows steadily. **C.** Arterial bleeding is characteristically bright red and spurts in time with the pulse.

Skill Drill 8-1   Controlling External Bleeding

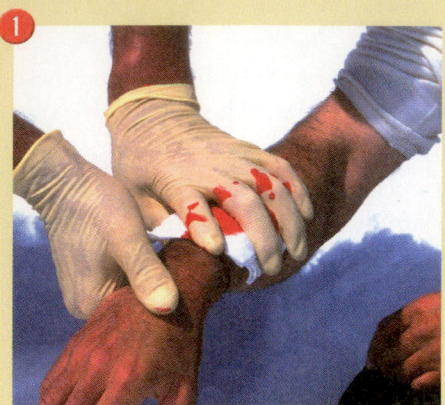
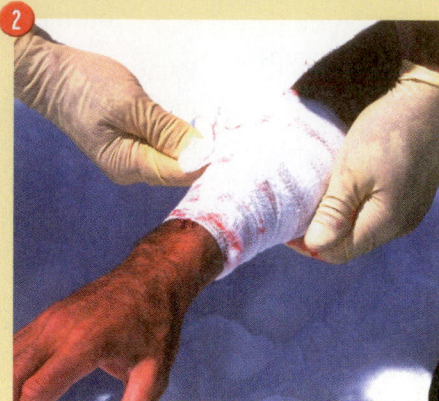
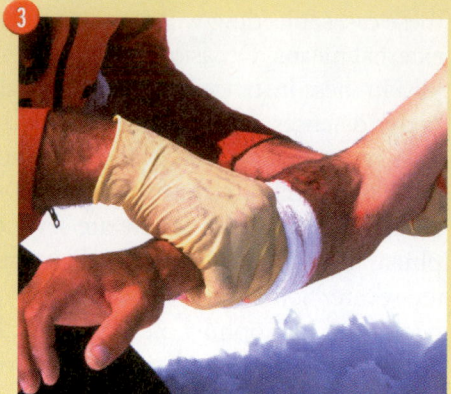

1 Apply direct pressure over the wound. Elevate the injury above the level of the heart if no fracture is suspected.

2 Apply a pressure dressing.

3 Apply pressure at the appropriate pressure point while continuing to hold direct pressure and elevation.

---

sanitary napkin, or clean cloth. If no material is available, use your gloved hand to continue to provide the necessary pressure.

Cover the entire dressing, above and below the wound. Stretch the bandage tight enough to control bleeding but not so tight as to decrease blood flow to the extremity. You should still be able to palpate a distal pulse on the injured extremity after applying the pressure dressing. If bleeding continues, the dressing is probably not tight enough. Do not remove a dressing until a physician has evaluated the patient. Instead, apply additional manual pressure through the dressing. Then add more gauze pads over the first dressing, and secure them both with a second, tighter, roller bandage.

Bleeding will almost always stop when the pressure of the dressing exceeds arterial pressure. On those rare occasions when direct pressure fails to stop bleeding from a large gaping wound, you may need to pack the wound with sterile gauze pads, in addition to direct hand pressure. Applying ice may help control bleeding and reduce the pain **(Step 2)**. Beware, an extremity with poor perfusion is more susceptible to frostbite.

4. **If a wound continues to bleed** despite use of direct pressure, elevate the extremity and try placing additional pressure over a proximal **pressure point**, or pulse point. A pressure point is a spot where a blood vessel lies near a bone. This

technique is also useful if you have no material on hand to use for a dressing. Because a wound usually draws blood from more than one major artery, proximal compression of a major artery rarely stops bleeding completely, but it helps to slow the loss of blood. You must be thoroughly familiar with the location of the pulse points for this to work ▶ **Figure 8-8** **(Step 3)**.

SPECIAL TECHNIQUES. Much of the bleeding associated with broken bones occurs because the sharp ends of the bones cut muscles and other tissues. Also, the marrow inside the bone will bleed at the fracture site. As long as a fracture remains unstable, the bone ends will move and continue to injure partially clotted vessels. Movement at the fracture site does not allow a clot to form into a solid mass that stops bleeding. Therefore, stabilizing a fracture and decreasing movement is a high priority in the prompt control of bleeding. Often, simple immobilization splints will quickly control bleeding associated with a fracture ▶ **Figure 8-9** . If not, you may need to use another splinting device.

- **Air splints.** Air splints can control the bleeding associated with severe soft-tissue injuries, such as massive or complex lacerations, or fractures ▶ **Figure 8-10** . They also stabilize the fracture itself. An air splint acts like a pressure dressing applied to an entire extremity rather than to a small, local area. Once you have applied an air

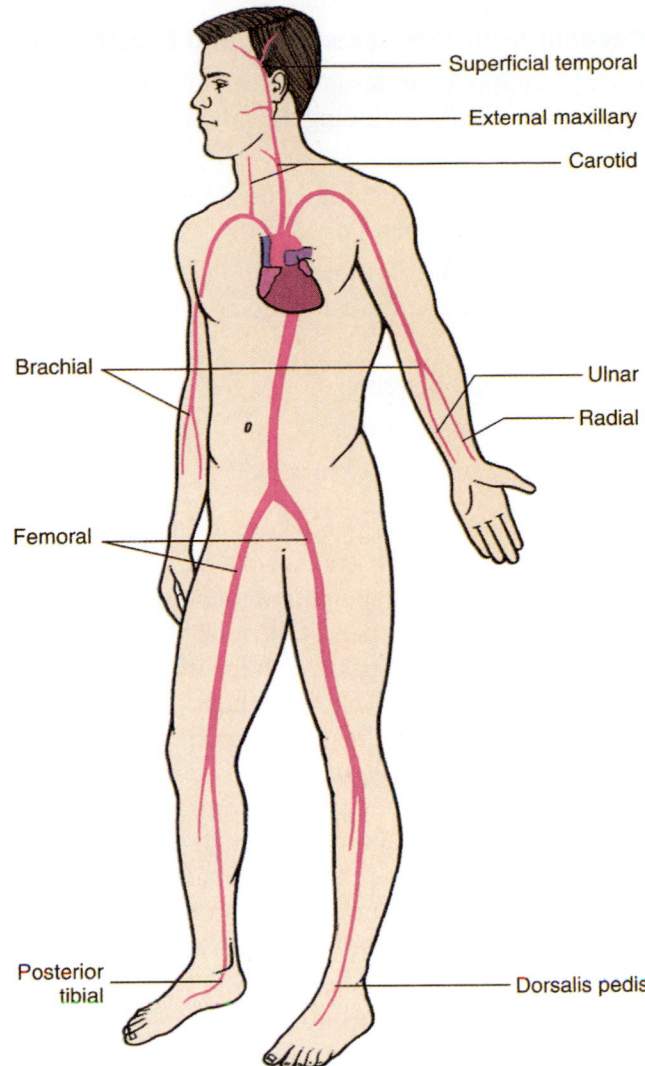

- Superficial temporal
- External maxillary
- Carotid
- Brachial
- Ulnar
- Radial
- Femoral
- Posterior tibial
- Dorsalis pedis

Figure 8-8 You should be familiar with the locations of arterial pressure points.

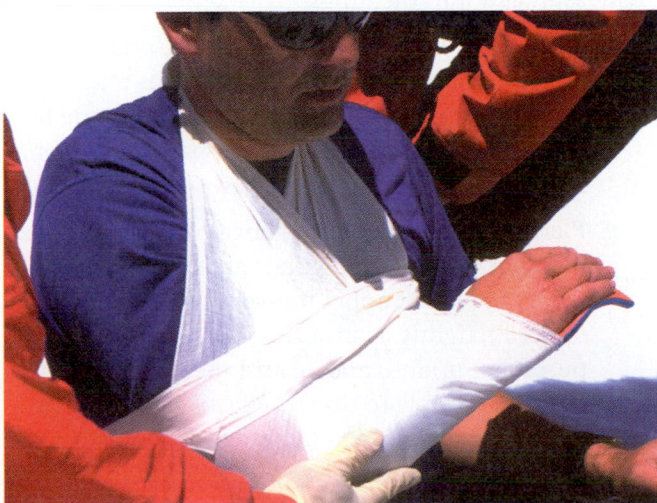

Figure 8-9 Use of a simple splint will often quickly control bleeding associated with a fracture. As long as a fracture is not immobilized, the bone ends are free to move and may continue to injure partially clotted vessels.

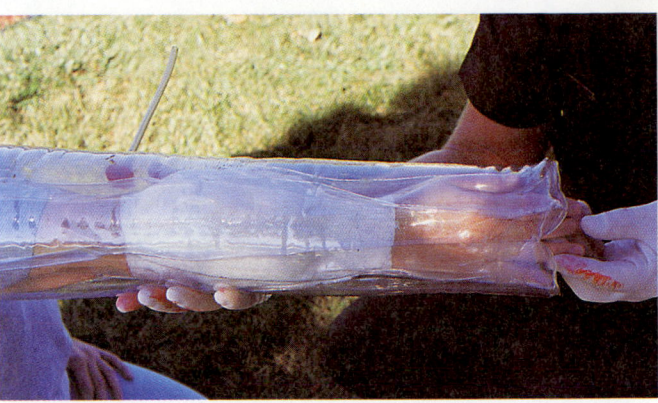

Figure 8-10 Air splints can also be used to control bleeding as they act as a pressure bandage for the entire extremity.

splint, be sure to monitor circulation in the distal extremity. Use only BSI-approved, clean, or disposable valve stems when orally inflating air splints.

- **Pneumatic antishock garments. Pneumatic antishock garment (PASG)** is a splinting device sometimes used in the EMS environment, but this remains a controversial therapy. Due to special training and medical control requirements, this is not a device used by outdoor rescuers.

- **Tourniquets.** A **tourniquet** is rarely needed to control bleeding. When your efforts to control life-threatening bleeding have failed and there is no reasonable alternative, apply a tourniquet. A tourniquet often creates, rather than solves, problems. Application of a tourniquet can cause permanent damage to nerves, muscles, and blood vessels, resulting in the loss of an extremity. In addition, tourniquets are often improperly applied.

If you cannot control bleeding from the major vessel in an extremity *in any other way,* a properly applied tourniquet may save a patient's life. Specifically, the tourniquet is useful if a patient is bleeding severely from a partial or complete amputation.

Follow these steps to apply a tourniquet
▶ **Skill Drill 8-2**):

1. **Fold a triangular bandage** until it is 4″ wide and six to eight layers thick.

2. **Wrap the bandage** around the extremity twice. Choose an area only slightly proximal to the bleeding, to reduce the amount of tissue damage to the extremity **(Step 1)**.

3. **Tie one knot** in the bandage. Then place a stick or rod on top of the knot, and tie the ends of the bandage over the stick in a square knot **(Step 2)**.

Altitude Tips

With changing elevation, the relative pressure in air and vacuum splints does not remain constant. When going from high to low elevation, the air splint can become soft and ineffective. A vacuum splint can become soft when subject to increased elevation during air evacuation. Therefore, the rescuer must monitor and make adjustments to these devices as needed.

4. **Use the stick as a handle,** and twist it to tighten the tourniquet until the bleeding has stopped; then stop twisting **(Step 3)**.

5. **Secure the stick in place,** and make the wrapping neat and smooth.

6. **Write "TK"** and the exact time (hour and minute) that you applied the tourniquet on a piece of adhesive tape. Use the phrase "time applied." Securely fasten the tape to the patient's forehead. Notify hospital personnel on your arrival that your patient has a tourniquet in place. Record this same information on the ambulance run report form **(Step 4)**.

7. **As an alternative method,** you can use a blood pressure cuff as an effective tourniquet. Position the cuff proximal to the bleeding point, and inflate it just enough to stop the bleeding. Leave the cuff inflated. If you use a blood pressure cuff, monitor the gauge continuously to make sure that the pressure is not gradually dropping. You may have to clamp the tube with a hemostat leading from the cuff to the inflating bulb to prevent loss of pressure **(Step 5)**.

Whenever you apply a tourniquet, make sure you observe the following precautions:

- Do not apply a tourniquet directly over any joint. Keep it as close to the injury as possible.

- Use the widest bandage possible. Make sure that it is tightened securely.

- Never use wire, rope, a belt, or any other narrow material. It could cut into the skin.

- Use wide padding under the tourniquet if possible. This will protect the tissues and help with arterial compression.

- Never cover a tourniquet with a bandage. Leave it open and in full view.

- Do not loosen the tourniquet after you have applied it. Hospital personnel will loosen it once they are prepared to manage the bleeding.

Bleeding from the Nose, Ears, and Mouth

Several conditions can result in bleeding from the nose, ears, and/or mouth, including the following:

- Skull fracture

- Facial injuries, including those caused by a direct blow to the nose

- Sinusitis, infections, nose drop use and abuse, dried or cracked nasal mucosa, or other abnormalities

- High blood pressure

- Coagulation disorders

- Digital trauma (nose picking)

Epistaxis, or nosebleed, is a common emergency. Occasionally, it can cause enough of a blood loss to send a patient into shock. Keep in mind that the blood you see may be only a small part of the total blood loss. Much of the blood may pass down the throat into the stomach as the patient swallows. A person who swallows a large amount of blood may become nauseated and start vomiting the blood, which is sometimes confused with internal bleeding. Most nontraumatic nosebleeds occur from sites in the septum, the tissue dividing the nostrils. You can usually handle this type of bleeding effectively by pinching the nostrils together.

Follow these steps to treat a patient with epistaxis ▶ Skill Drill 8-3 :

1. **Follow BSI precautions.**

2. **Help the patient to sit,** leaning forward, with the head tilted forward. This position stops the blood from trickling down the throat or being aspirated into the lungs.

3. **Apply direct pressure** for at least 15 minutes by pinching the fleshy part of the nostrils together. This is the preferred method. This technique may also be self-administered by the patient if he or she is capable and bleeding is severe **(Step 1)**.

4. **Placing a rolled 4" × 4" gauze bandage** between the upper lip and the gum is another option. Have the patient apply pressure by stretching the upper lip tightly against the rolled bandage and pushing it up into and against the nose. If the patient is unable to do this effectively, use your gloved fingers to press the gauze against the gum.

5. **Keep the patient calm and quiet,** especially if he or she has high blood pressure or is anxious. Anxiety tends to increase blood pressure, which could worsen the nosebleed **(Step 2)**.

6. **Apply ice over the nose.**

Skill Drill 8-2 Applying a Tourniquet

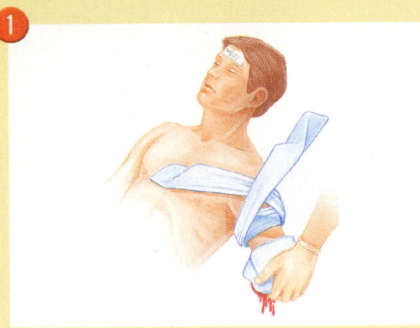
1 Create a 4"-wide, multilayered bandage. Wrap the bandage twice around the extremity, just above the bleeding site.

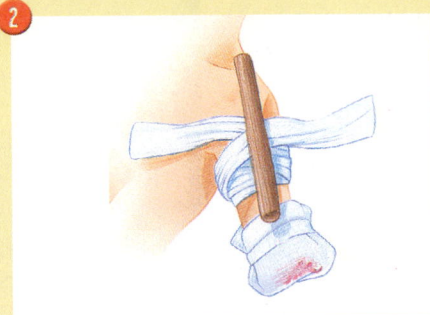
2 Tie a single knot, and place a stick on the top of it.

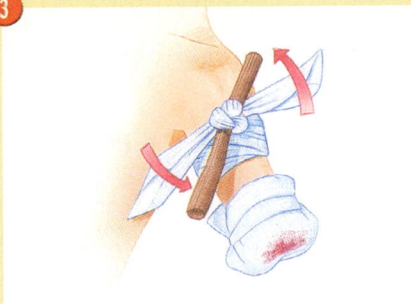
3 Tie a square knot over the stick, and then twist the stick until the bleeding stops.

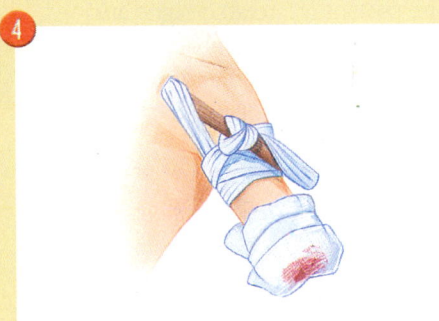
4 Secure the stick so that it will not unwind.

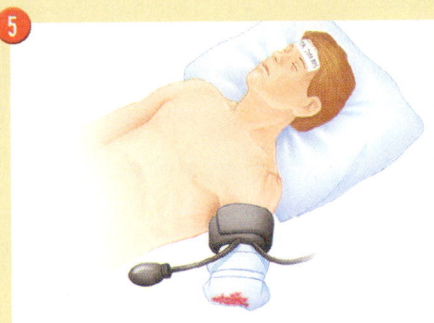
5 Write "TK" and the exact time you applied the tourniquet on a piece of adhesive tape, fasten the tape to the patient's forehead, and notify hospital personnel on arrival. You can also use a blood pressure cuff as an effective tourniquet.

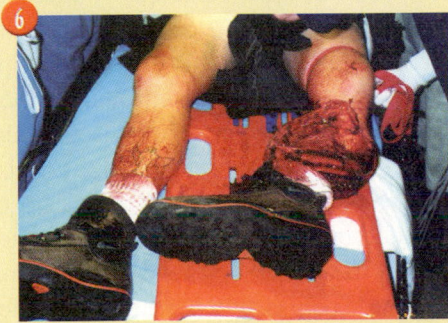
6 Tourniquets are rarely used to control bleeding, but they may be useful if a patient is bleeding severely from an amputation.

Skill Drill 8-3 Controlling Epistaxis

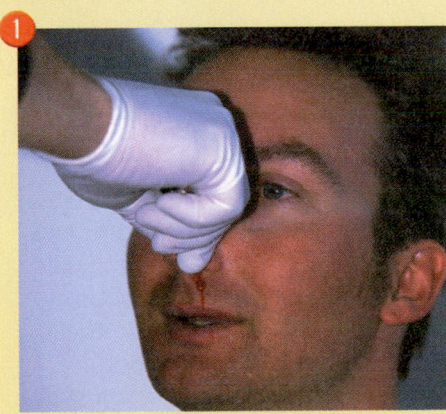
1 Use BSI precautions. Position the patient: sitting, leaning forward. Apply direct pressure, pinching the fleshy part of the nostrils.

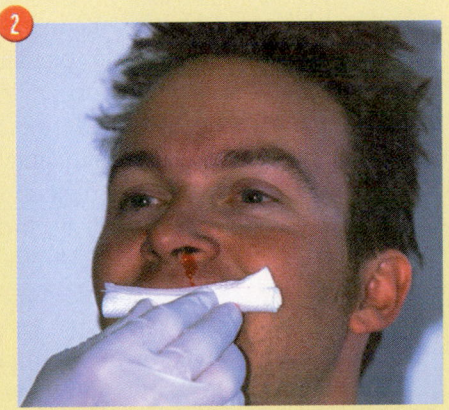
2 Alternate method: Use pressure with a rolled gauze bandage between the upper lip and gum. Calm the patient.

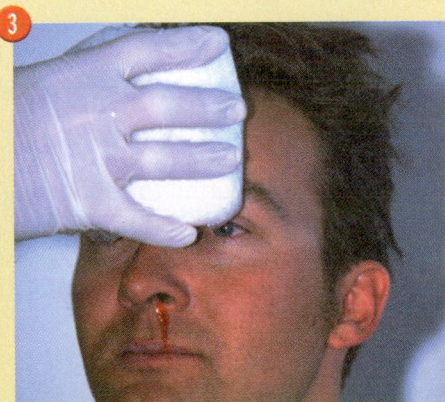
3 Apply ice over the nose. Maintain pressure until bleeding is controlled. Provide prompt transport after bleeding stops. Transport immediately if indicated. Assess and treat for shock, including oxygen, as needed.

7. **Maintain the pressure** until the bleeding is completely controlled, usually no more than 15 minutes (assuming that this is the patient's only problem). Most often, failure to stop a nosebleed is the result of releasing the pressure too soon.

8. **Provide prompt transport** once the bleeding has stopped.

9. **If you cannot control the bleeding,** if the patient has a history of frequent nosebleeds, or if there is a significant amount of blood loss, transport the patient immediately. Assess the patient for signs and symptoms of shock. Treat appropriately for shock and administer oxygen via mask, if necessary **(Step 3)**.

Bleeding from the nose or ears following a head injury may indicate a skull fracture. In these instances, you should not attempt to stop the blood flow. This bleeding may be difficult to control. Second, applying excessive pressure to the injury may force the blood leaking through the ear or nose to collect within the head. This could increase the pressure on the brain and possibly cause permanent damage. If you suspect a skull fracture, loosely cover the bleeding site with a sterile gauze pad to collect the blood and help keep contaminants away from the site. There is always a risk of infection to the brain. Apply light compression by wrapping the dressing loosely around the head ▶ **Figure 8-11** . If blood or drainage contains cerebrospinal fluid, a characteristic staining of the dressing, much like a target, will occur.

Internal Bleeding

Internal bleeding can be very serious, especially because you might not be aware that it is happening. Injury or damage to internal organs commonly results in extensive internal bleeding, which can cause hypovolemic shock before you realize the extent of blood loss. A person with a bleeding stomach ulcer may lose a large amount of blood very quickly. Similarly, a person who has a lacerated liver or a ruptured spleen may lose a considerable amount of blood within the abdomen. Yet the patient has no obvious shock and no outward signs of bleeding.

Broken bones also may cause serious internal blood loss. With rib fractures and associated internal soft-tissue lacerations from the sharp bone ends, this bleeding extends into the chest cavity and the soft tissues of the chest wall. A broken femur can easily result in the loss of 1 L or more of blood into the soft tissues of the thigh. Often, the only signs of such bleeding are local swelling and bruising due to the accumulation of blood around the ends of the broken bone. Severe pelvic fractures may result in life-threatening hemorrhage.

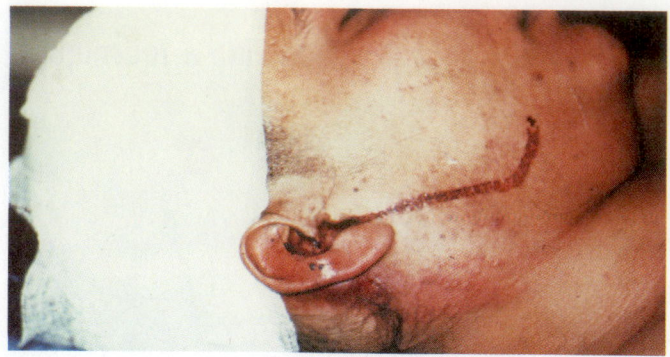

Figure 8-11   Bleeding from the ear after a head injury may indicate a skull fracture. Loosely cover the bleeding site with a sterile gauze pad, and apply light compression by wrapping the dressing loosely around the head.

You must always be alert to the possibility of internal bleeding and assess the patient for related signs and symptoms, particularly if the mechanism of injury is severe. If you suspect that a patient is bleeding internally, you should promptly transport him or her to the hospital.

Mechanism of Injury

Internal bleeding is possible whenever the mechanism of injury suggests that severe forces affected the abdomen and/or the chest. These forces include blunt and penetrating trauma. Internal bleeding commonly occurs as a result of falls, hitting fixed objects such as lift towers, snowmobile or motorcycle crashes, and mountain bike crashes.

As you assess a patient, look for signs of injury over the chest or abdomen, including contusions, abrasions, lacerations, or other signs of injury or deformity. You should always suspect internal bleeding in a patient who has penetrating injury or blunt trauma.

Nature of Illness

Nontraumatic internal bleeding can lead to shock just as easily as bleeding caused by injury. Usually, internal bleeding occurs in the abdomen as a result of irritable bowel syndrome, an aneurysm, an ulcer, a ruptured ectopic pregnancy, or another condition. Abdominal pain and distention are frequent in these situations but are not always present. In older patients, dizziness, faintness, or weakness may be the first sign of nontraumatic internal bleeding. Ulcers or other gastrointestinal problems may cause vomiting of blood or black tarry stools.

It is not as important for you to know the specific organ involved as it is to recognize that the patient is in shock and *respond appropriately*.

Signs and Symptoms

The most common symptom of internal abdominal bleeding is acute abdominal pain. Another common sign is bruising around the abdomen. This can occur with or without trauma. Bruising is also called **contusion**, or **ecchymosis**. A **hematoma**, a mass of blood in the soft tissues beneath the skin, indicates bleeding into soft tissues and may be the result of either a minor or a severe injury. Bruising or ecchymosis may not be present initially; the only sign of severe pelvic or abdominal trauma may be redness or skin abrasions acutely.

Bleeding, however slight, from any body opening is serious. It usually indicates internal bleeding that is not easy to see or control. Bright red bleeding from the mouth or rectum (hematochezia) or blood in the urine (hematuria) may suggest serious internal injury or disease. Nonmenstrual vaginal bleeding is always significant.

Other signs and symptoms of internal bleeding in both trauma and medical patients include the following:

- **Hematemesis.** This is vomited blood. It may be bright red or dark red, or if the blood has been partially digested, it may look like coffee ground vomitus.

- **Melena.** This is a black, foul-smelling, tarry stool that contains digested blood.

- **Hemoptysis.** This is bright red blood that is coughed up by the patient, coming from the pulmonary system.

- **Pain, tenderness, bruising, guarding, or swelling.** These signs and symptoms may mean that a closed fracture is bleeding.

- **Broken ribs, bruises over the lower chest, or a rigid, distended abdomen.** These signs and symptoms may indicate a lacerated spleen or liver. Patients with an injury to either organ may have referred pain in the right shoulder (liver) or left shoulder (Kerr's sign; spleen). You should suspect internal abdominal bleeding in a patient with referred pain.

The first sign of hypovolemic shock (hypoperfusion) is a change in mental status, such as anxiety, restlessness, or combativeness. In nontrauma patients, weakness, faintness, or dizziness on standing is another early sign. Changes in skin color, or pallor, are seen often in both trauma and medical patients. Later signs of hypoperfusion suggesting internal bleeding include the following:

- Tachycardia
- Weakness, fainting, or dizziness at rest
- Thirst
- Nausea and vomiting

- Cold, moist (clammy) skin
- Shallow, rapid breathing
- Dull eyes
- Slightly dilated pupils that are slow to respond to light
- Capillary refill in infants and children of more than 2 seconds
- Weak, rapid (thready) pulse
- Decreasing blood pressure
- Altered level of consciousness

Patients with these signs and symptoms are at risk. Some may be in danger. Even if their bleeding stops, it could begin again at any moment. Therefore, prompt transport is necessary.

Emergency Medical Care

Controlling internal bleeding or bleeding from major organs usually requires surgery or other procedures that must be done in the hospital. Your role as a rescuer in these cases is to keep the patient still to promote clot formation and to provide high-flow oxygen and prompt transport. However, you can usually control internal bleeding into the extremities quite well in the field simply by splinting the extremity.

Follow these steps to care for patients with possible internal bleeding:

1. **Follow BSI precautions.**

2. **Maintain the airway** with cervical spine immobilization if the mechanism of injury suggests the possibility of spinal injury.

3. **Administer high-flow oxygen** and provide artificial ventilation as necessary.

4. **Control all obvious external bleeding.**

5. **Treat suspected internal bleeding** in an extremity by applying a splint.

6. **Monitor and record the vital signs** at least every 5 minutes.

7. **Give the patient nothing** (not even small sips of water) by mouth.

8. **Elevate the patient's legs 6″ to 12″** to help the blood return to the vital organs.

9. **Keep the patient warm.**

10. **Provide immediate transport** for all patients with signs and symptoms of shock (hypoperfusion). Report any changes in the patient's condition to EMS and/or emergency department personnel.

Chapter *Sweep*

Ready for Review

Perfusion is the circulation of blood in adequate amounts to meet each cell's current needs for oxygen, nutrients, and waste removal. Hypoperfusion, or shock, occurs when the cardiovascular system fails to provide adequate perfusion. Both internal and external bleeding can cause shock. You must know how to recognize and control both.

The six methods for controlling external bleeding are direct local pressure, elevation, pressure dressings, pressure points, splinting, and as a last resort, using a tourniquet. Do not remove a dressing until a physician has evaluated the patient; instead, apply additional dressings as needed. Stabilizing a serious fracture has a high priority in the control of bleeding.

Bleeding from the nose, ears, and/or mouth may result from skull fracture, facial injuries, sinusitis, high blood pressure, and coagulation disorders. To treat epistaxis, apply direct pressure for at least 15 minutes by pinching the nostrils together or using gauze between the upper lip and gum. If you suspect a skull fracture, cover the bleeding site (usually the nose or ear) loosely with a sterile gauze pad.

You should assess and promptly transport any patient who may have internal bleeding, particularly if the mechanism of injury is severe and has affected the abdomen and/or the chest. The most common sign of internal abdominal bleeding is acute abdominal pain. Bleeding from any body opening is serious. Signs of internal bleeding include hematemesis, melena, hemoptysis, broken ribs, bruised chest, distended abdomen, and referred pain. Signs of shock that suggest internal bleeding include change in mental status, pallor, weakness and dizziness, tachycardia, thirst, nausea and vomiting, and shallow, rapid breathing. If you suspect that a patient is bleeding internally, maintain the airway, administer high-flow oxygen, keep the patient still, apply a splint to any affected extremity, monitor vital signs at least every 5 minutes, and, in nontrauma patients, elevate the legs.

Vital Vocabulary

aorta The main artery, which receives blood from the left ventricle and delivers it to all the other arteries that carry blood to the tissues of the body.

arterioles The smallest branch of an artery leading to the vast network of capillaries.

artery A blood vessel, consisting of three layers of tissue and smooth muscle that carries blood away from the heart.

capillary Any one of the small blood vessels that connect arteriole and venule and through whose walls various substances pass into and out of the interstitial tissues and then on to the cells.

coagulation Formation of clots to plug openings in injured blood vessels and stop blood flow.

contusion Bruising, or ecchymosis.

ecchymosis Discoloration of the skin associated with a closed wound; bruising.

epistaxis Nosebleed.

hematoma Mass of blood in the soft tissues beneath the skin.

hemophilia A congenital condition in which the patient lacks one or more of the blood's normal clotting factors.

hemorrhage Bleeding.

hypovolemic shock A condition in which low blood volume, due to either massive internal or external bleeding or extensive loss of body water, results in inadequate perfusion.

perfusion Circulation of blood within an organ or tissue in adequate amounts to meet the cells' current needs.

pneumatic antishock garment (PASG) An inflatable device that covers the legs and abdomen; used to splint the lower extremities or pelvis, or to control bleeding in the lower extremities, pelvis, or abdominal cavity.

pressure point A point where a blood vessel lies near a bone; useful when direct pressure and elevation do not control bleeding.

shock A condition in which the circulatory system fails to provide sufficient circulation so that every body part can perform its function; also called hypoperfusion.

tourniquet The bleeding control method of last resort that occludes arterial flow; used only when all other methods have failed and the patient's life is in danger.

vein Any blood vessel that carries blood from the tissues to the heart.

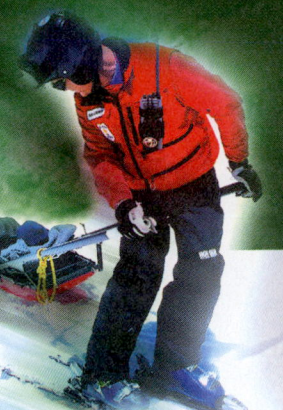

Assessment in Action

You are dispatched to lift five, tower six, where one of the maintenance crew had gotten his arm caught between the cable and the shim. He has already been extricated and brought to the ground. He is conscious and answering questions, although he appears somewhat disoriented.

Given what he has just been through, you consider that his mental status may be normal. A coworker is kneeling in a puddle of blood as he holds a piece of torn cloth around the man's injured upper arm. You look quickly under the cloth and see a 5" laceration from which bright red blood immediately spurts. The patient appears pale, but you find no other injuries on your exam.

1. Your first priority on this call is to:
   A. determine whether the patient is showing signs of shock.
   B. notify area management regarding the potential liability from the injury.
   C. check for avalanche danger.
   D. call for a helicopter.

2. In this case, the patient's bright red blood spurting from his laceration is most likely from a/an:
   A. vein.
   B. capillary.
   C. arteriole.
   D. artery.

3. Why does blood continue to spurt from the laceration on his arm?
   A. Profuse bleeding is common when the patient is young.
   B. Muscle spasms in the arm are forcing the blood out.
   C. There is a surge in arterial pressure with each heart contraction.
   D. Any injury in which the patient goes into shock causes bleeding.

4. Which artery in the patient's arm may have been lacerated?
   A. Jugular
   B. Carotid
   C. Brachial
   D. Femoral

5. When obtaining a blood pressure on this patient, you are measuring the pressure that the circulating blood is exerting on the walls of the:
   A. veins when the right atrium contracts.
   B. veins when the right ventricle contracts.
   C. arteries when the left ventricle contracts.
   D. arteries when the left atrium contracts.

6. If the patient's blood pressure is low, due to blood loss, other signs that should be apparent include pale, cold, clammy skin and:
   A. tachycardia.
   B. bradycardia.
   C. slower breathing.
   D. bounding pulse.

7. Immediate treatment for this type of bleeding includes:
   A. a tourniquet.
   B. a compression dressing.
   C. elevation.
   D. direct pressure.

8. Further assessment of this patient reveals continued disorientation. What might his disorientation be indicating?
   A. Head injury
   B. Shock
   C. Intoxication
   D. Psychological impact of what happened

Challenging Questions

9. Why does direct pressure work?

10. Of the signs of shock, which will occur first?

Points to Ponder

You are sent from the patrol aid room to a gift store at the area's shopping mall in response to a patient who slipped and fell. You are led to the rear of the store, where you find that the patient not only fell, but fell through a display case and is bleeding severely. You immediately recognize the need for much more BSI protection, yet your patrol belt is minutes away in the aid room.

Would you leave this severely bleeding patient to get more protection for yourself? If so, why? If you did leave and the patient died, would you be liable?

Issues BSI Precautions, HIV Testing, HIV Risks, Exposure Reporting, Workers' Compensation.

Online Outlook

Six ways to control external bleeding are presented in this chapter. Test your ability to choose the appropriate way to control bleeding for different situations by completing Exercise 8 at www.OECzone.com.

www.OECzone.com

Shock

Objectives

Cognitive

♣ 1. List signs and symptoms of shock (p 267).

♣ 2. State the steps in the emergency medical care of the patient with signs and symptoms of shock (p 271).

Affective

♣ 3. Explain the sense of urgency to transport patients who are bleeding and show signs of shock (p 266).

Psychomotor

♣ 4. Demonstrate the care of the patient exhibiting signs and symptoms of shock (p 271).

5. Demonstrate completing an incident report for the patient with bleeding and/or shock (p 77-78).

♣ These are core concepts in initial patrol training.

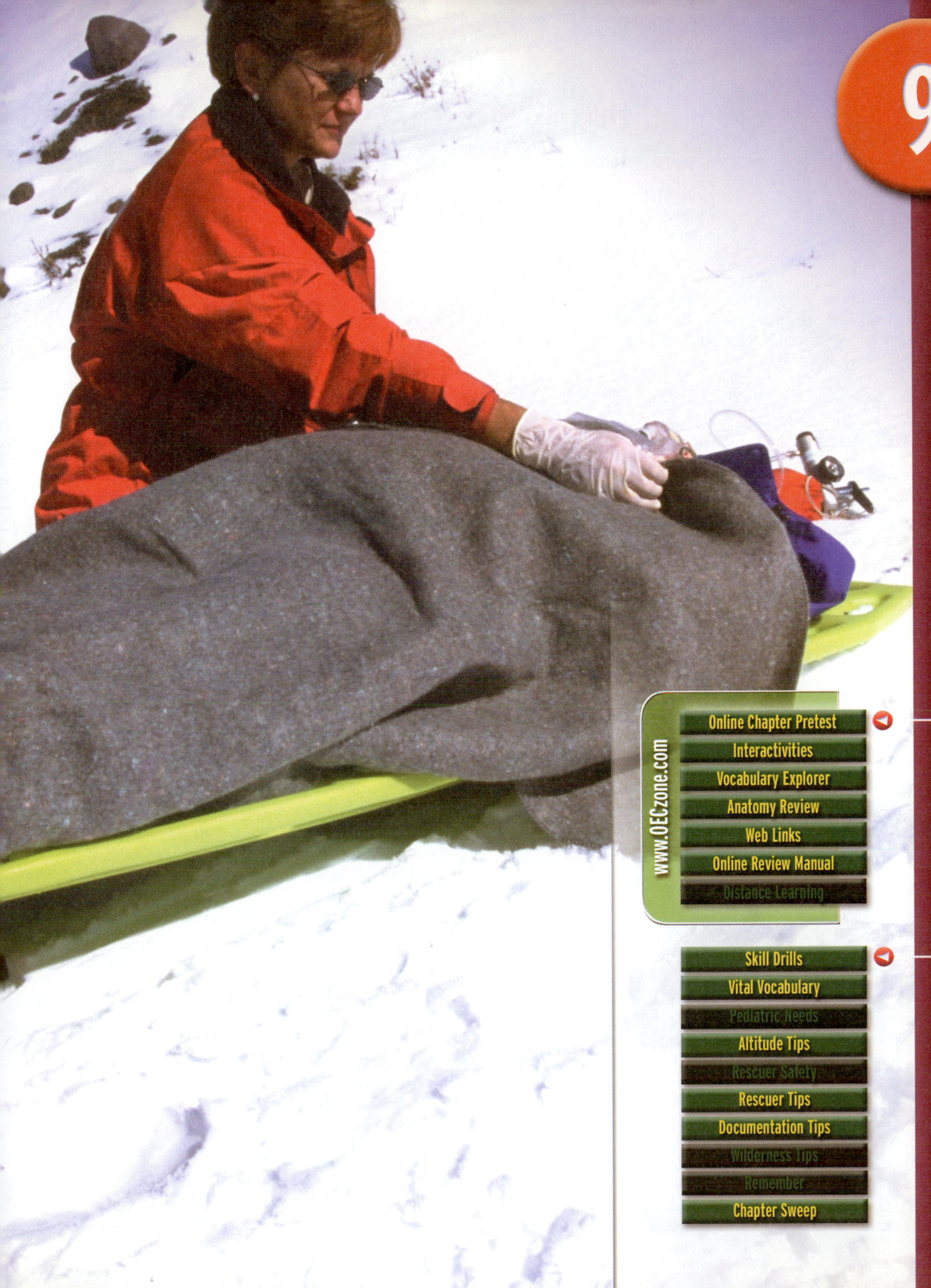

www.OECzone.com

Online Chapter Pretest
Interactivities
Vocabulary Explorer
Anatomy Review
Web Links
Online Review Manual
Distance Learning

Skill Drills
Vital Vocabulary
Pediatric Needs
Altitude Tips
Rescuer Safety
Rescuer Tips
Documentation Tips
Wilderness Tips
Remember
Chapter Sweep

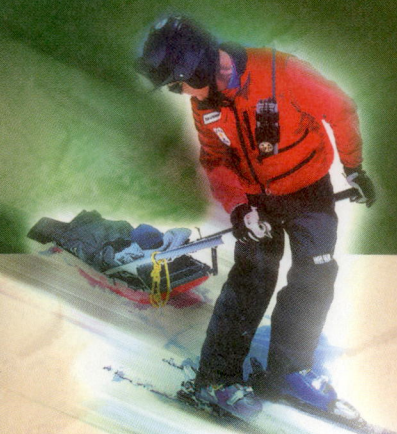

You are the rescuer

Rescuer 21 at mountain bike aid station #3 responds to a racer down on the sidewinder turn. On arrival, you find a 38-year-old man with abdominal bleeding from an impaled tree branch.

A critical part of the rescuer's job is having an understanding of shock and shock management. This chapter will present valuable information on the topic of shock in addition to helping you answer the following questions.

1. How does compensated shock differ from decompensated shock? Does your care differ as well?

2. Is there a difference in how children and adults compensate for severe traumatic injuries?

Shock

Shock has a number of meanings. For example, we often say that a person who has received a fright or a piece of bad news is in shock. An electric current passing through the body delivers a shock. In this chapter, shock describes a state of collapse and failure of the cardiovascular system in which blood circulation slows and eventually ceases. If not treated promptly, shock can be fatal.

Shock often accompanies the events, such as trauma, or medical problems such as heart attacks. Therefore, you should always be able to anticipate, recognize, and treat shock in order to manage patients effectively.

This chapter begins with a close-up look at perfusion, the function that fails in shock. Next it looks at the physiologic causes of shock, describing each of its major forms. Finally, it discusses the emergency treatment of shock in general and of each kind of shock in particular.

Perfusion

Shock, or hypoperfusion, refers to a state of collapse and failure of the cardiovascular system that leads to inadequate circulation. Shock cannot be seen. It is not a specific disease or injury. However, it is a dangerous condition that results in the inadequate flow of blood to the body's cells and failure to rid cells of metabolic wastes. As the cells begin to die, the body attempts to compensate by redirecting blood flow from nonessential organs (skin and intestines) to essential organs (heart, lungs, and brain). If the conditions causing shock are not promptly addressed, the patient will soon die.

As we have seen, the cardiovascular system consists of three parts: a pump (heart), a container (vessels), and the container's contents (blood) ▶ Figure 9-1). Blood is the vehicle for carrying oxygen and nutrients through the vessels to the capillary beds, where these supplies are exchanged for waste products. The blood keeps moving as a result of pressure that is generated by the contractions of the heart and affected by the dilating and constricting of the vessels. This pressure, which we call blood pressure, is usually carefully controlled by the body so that there is always sufficient circulation, or perfusion, in the various tissues and organs. Blood pressure is, in fact, a rough measure of perfusion. It tells us how well the body's oxygen, nutrient, and waste removal needs are being met.

Remember that blood pressure is really the pressure of blood within the vessels at any one time. The systolic pressure is the arterial pressure, or pressure generated every time the heart contracts; the diastolic pressure is the pressure maintained within the system.

Blood flow through the capillary beds is regulated by the capillary sphincters, circular muscular walls that constrict and dilate. These sphincters are under the control of the autonomic nervous system, which regulates involuntary functions such as sweating and digestion. Capillary sphincters also respond to other stimuli such as heat, cold, the need for oxygen, and the need for waste removal. Keep in mind that, under normal circumstances, not all cells have the same needs at the same time. For example, the stomach and intestines have a high need for blood flow during and shortly after eating, when digestion is at a peak. Between meals, blood flow is lessened, and blood is diverted to other areas. The brain, by contrast, needs a constant and consistent supply of blood to function.

Thus, regulation of blood flow is determined by cellular need and is accomplished by vessel constriction or dilation, together with sphincter constriction or dilation. Maintenance of blood flow, or perfusion, is accomplished by the heart, blood vessels, and blood, working together.

Perfusion requires more than just having a working cardiovascular system, however. It also requires adequate oxygen exchange in the lungs, adequate nutrients in the form of glucose in the blood, and adequate carbon dioxide removal, primarily through the lungs. Therefore, the respiratory system is also a major contributor to maintaining adequate perfusion.

In addition, the body also has mechanisms in place to help support the respiratory and cardiovascular systems when the need for perfusion of vital organs is increased. These mechanisms, including the autonomic nervous system and certain chemicals called hormones, are triggered when the body senses that the pressure in the system is falling. The action of the hormones stimulates an increase in heart rate and in the strength of cardiac contractions and vasoconstriction in nonessential areas, primarily in the skin and gastrointestinal tract (peripheral vasoconstriction). Together, these actions are designed to maintain pressure in the system and, as a result, perfusion of all vital organs.

Eventually, there is also a shifting of body fluids to help maintain pressure within the system. However, the response of the autonomic nervous system and

Altitude Tips

The hormonal response to decreased circulating blood volume resulting from cold and high altitude, "hohendiorese," causes an urge to urinate.

hormones comes within seconds. It is this response that causes all the signs and symptoms of a patient in shock.

Causes of Shock

Shock can result from many different conditions, including respiratory failure, acute allergic reactions, and overwhelming infection. In all cases, however, the damage occurs because of insufficient perfusion of organs and tissues. As soon as perfusion stops or becomes impaired, tissues start to die, affecting all local body processes. If the conditions causing shock are not promptly arrested and reversed, death soon follows.

Understanding the basic physiologic causes of shock will better prepare you to treat it (▼ **Figure 9-2**).

A **CARDIOGENIC SHOCK**
Poor pump function
Causes: Heart attack, trauma to heart

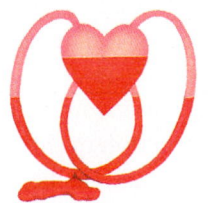
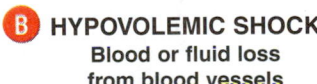

B **HYPOVOLEMIC SHOCK**
Blood or fluid loss
from blood vessels
Causes: Trauma to vessels or tissues, fluid loss from gastrointestinal tract (vomiting/diarrhea can also lower the fluid component of blood)

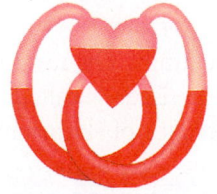
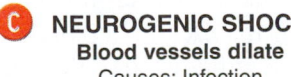

C **NEUROGENIC SHOCK**
Blood vessels dilate
Causes: Infection

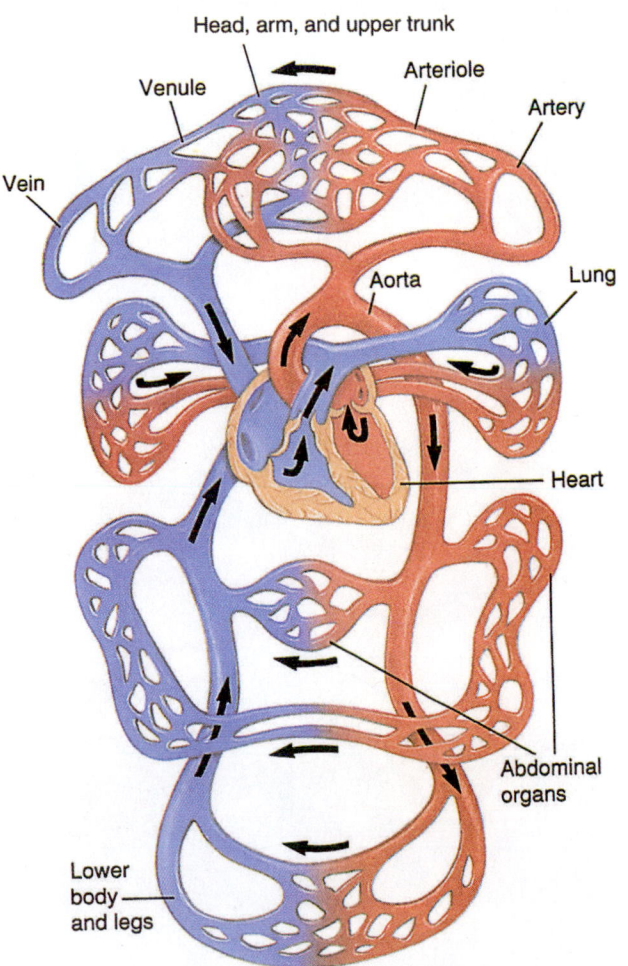

Figure 9-1 The cardiovascular system consists of three parts: the pump (heart), the container (vessels), and the contents (blood). The blood carries oxygen and nutrients through the vessels to the capillary beds, where they are exchanged for waste products.

Figure 9-2 There are three basic causes of shock and impaired tissue perfusion. **A.** Pump failure occurs when the heart is damaged by disease or injury. The heart does not generate enough energy to move the blood through the system. **B.** Decreased blood volume, usually a result of bleeding, results in inadequate perfusion. **C.** The blood vessels can dilate enough that the blood within them, even though it is of normal volume, is inadequate to fill the system and provide efficient perfusion.

There are both cardiovascular and noncardiovascular causes of shock. The three major cardiovascular causes of shock are as follows:

- **Poor pump function.** The heart, if damaged by muscular disease or injury, may fail to perform properly as a pump. That is, it does not generate sufficient energy to move blood through the system.

- **Blood or fluid loss from blood vessels.** If enough blood or plasma is lost, the volume of fluid contained within the vascular system is insufficient to perfuse all tissues and organs.

- **Poor vessel function.** If all the blood vessels dilate at once, the normal volume of blood will be insufficient to fill the system and provide efficient perfusion.

Cardiovascular Causes of Shock

PUMP FAILURE. Cardiogenic shock is caused by inadequate function of the heart, or pump failure. Circulation of blood throughout the vascular system requires the constant pumping action of a normal and vigorous heart muscle. Many diseases can cause destruction or inflammation of this muscle. Within certain limits, the heart can adapt to these problems. If too much muscular damage occurs, however, as sometimes happens after a heart attack, the heart no longer functions well. A major effect is the backup of blood into the lungs. The resulting buildup of fluid within the pulmonary tissue is called pulmonary edema. **Edema** is the presence of abnormally large amounts of fluid between cells in body tissues, causing swelling of the affected area ▶ **Figure 9-3** . Pulmonary edema leads to impaired ventilation, which may be manifested by an increased respiratory rate and abnormal lung sounds.

The muscular contraction of the heart moves blood through the vessels at distinct pressures. For blood to circulate efficiently throughout the entire system, there must be both the right amount of pressure and an adequate number of heartbeats. For this reason, the heart has its own electrical system that initiates and regulates its beating. Disease or injury can damage or destroy this system, causing irregular and uncoordinated beats, beats that are too slow (fewer than 60/min), or beats that are too fast (greater than 150/min).

Cardiogenic shock develops when the heart muscle can no longer generate enough pressure to circulate the blood to all organs or when the regularity of the heartbeat is so disrupted that the volume of blood within the system can no longer be handled efficiently. In either case, direct pump failure is the cause of shock.

CONTENT FAILURE. Following injury, shock is often a result of fluid or blood loss. This type of shock is called **hypovolemic** (low-volume) **shock** or, when caused by blood loss, hemorrhagic shock. The loss may be due to external bleeding, which is common in patients who have suffered severe lacerations or fractures. Or it may be due to internal bleeding, which follows a variety of

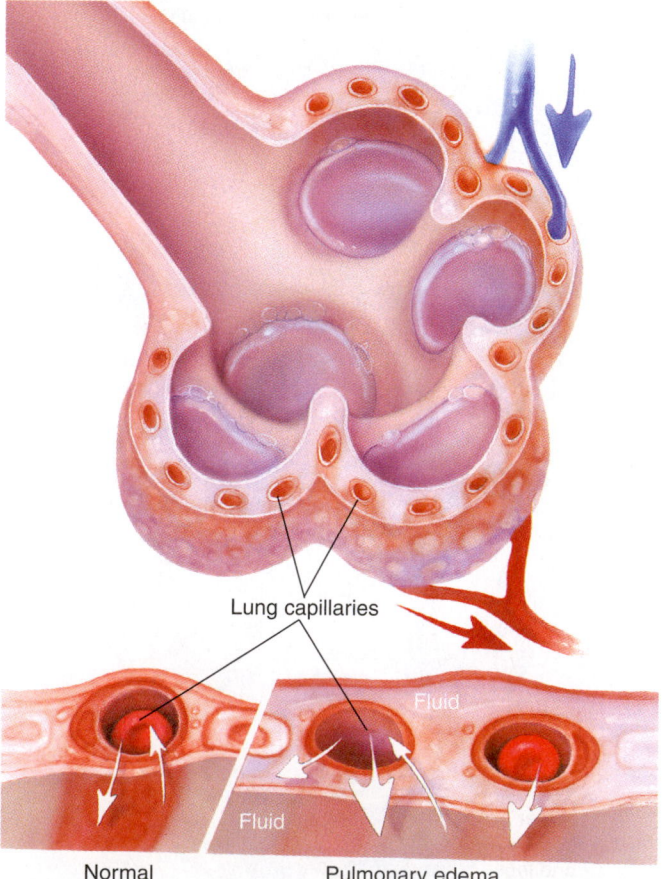

Lung capillaries

Fluid

Fluid

Normal   Pulmonary edema

Figure 9-3 Pulmonary edema develops as a result of fluid buildup within the pulmonary tissue. The edema causes swelling and leads to impaired ventilation.

injuries or diseases, such as rupture of the liver or the spleen, lacerations of the great vessels within the abdomen or the chest, bleeding peptic ulcers, and tumors, among others.

Hypovolemic shock also occurs with severe thermal burns. In this case, it is intravascular plasma (the colorless part of the blood) that is lost, leaking from the circulatory system into the burned tissues that lie adjacent to the injury. Likewise, crushing injuries may result in the loss of blood and plasma from damaged vessels into injured tissues. <u>Dehydration</u>, the loss of water from body tissues, excessive secreting, diarrhea, or vomiting aggravates shock.

In these circumstances, the common factor is an insufficient volume of blood within the vascular system to provide adequate circulation to the organs of the body.

POOR VESSEL FUNCTION. Damage to the spinal cord, particularly at the upper cervical levels, may cause significant injury to the part of the nervous system that controls the size and muscular tone of the blood vessels. <u>Neurogenic shock</u> is usually the result. Although not as common, there are medical causes as well. These include brain conditions, tumors, pressure on the spinal cord, or spina bifida. In this condition, the muscles in the walls of the blood vessels are cut off from the nerve impulses that cause them to contract. There-fore, all the vessels below the level of the spinal injury dilate widely, increasing the size and capacity of the vascular system (▼ **Figure 9-4**), and causing blood to pool. The available 6 L of blood in the body can no longer fill the enlarged vascular system. Even though no blood or fluid has been lost, perfusion of organs and tissues becomes inadequate, and shock occurs. In this condition, a radical change in the size of the vascular system has caused shock. A characteristic sign of this type of shock is the absence of sweating below the level of injury.

With this type of injury, many other functions that are under the control of the same part of the nervous system are also lost. The most important of them, in an acute injury setting, is the ability to control body temperature. Body temperature in the patient with neurogenic shock can rapidly fall to match that of the environment. In many situations, significant hypothermia occurs, severely complicating the situation. <u>Hypothermia</u> is a condition in which the internal body temperature falls below 95°F (35°C), usually after prolonged exposure to cool or freezing temperatures. Maintenance of body temperature is always an important element of treatment for a patient in shock. It is important to emphasize that neurogenic shock is an unusual form of shock. In the acute setting with evidence of spinal cord damage, *always* assume shock to be due to hypovolemia, ie, internal or external bleeding.

COMBINED VESSEL AND CONTENT FAILURE. In some patients who have severe bacterial infections, toxins (poisons) generated by the bacteria or by infected body tissues produce a condition called <u>septic shock</u>. In this condition, the toxins damage the vessel walls, causing them to become leaky and unable to contract well. Widespread dilation of vessels, in combination with plasma loss through the injured vessel walls, results in shock.

Septic shock is a complex problem. First, there is an insufficient volume of fluid in the container, because much of the blood has leaked out of the vascular system (hypovolemia). Second, the fluid that has leaked out often collects in the respiratory system, interfering with ventilation. Third, there is a larger-than-normal vascular bed to contain the smaller-than-normal volume of intravascular fluid.

Septic shock is almost always a complication of some very serious illness, injury, or surgery.

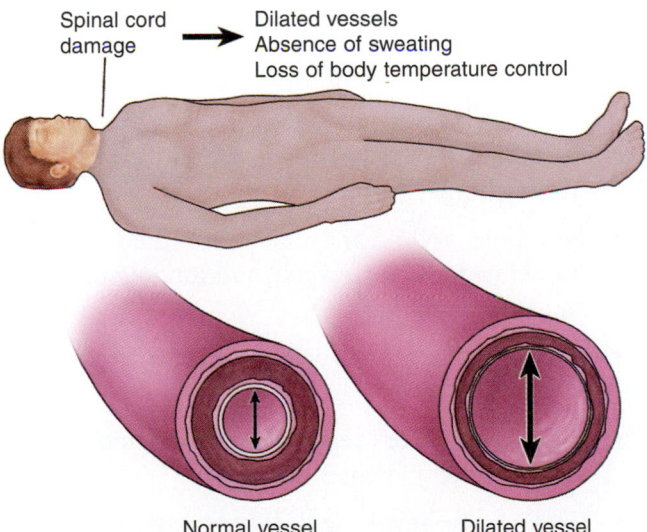

Figure 9-4 Damage to the spinal cord can cause significant injury to the part of the nervous system that controls the size and muscle tone of blood vessels. If the muscles in the blood vessels are cut off from their impulses to contract, then the vessels dilate widely, increasing the size and capacity of the vascular system. The blood in the body can no longer fill the enlarged vessels, resulting in inadequate perfusion.

Noncardiovascular Causes of Shock

There are two causes of shock that do not result from disturbances of the cardiovascular system: respiratory insufficiency and anaphylaxis.

RESPIRATORY INSUFFICIENCY. A patient with a severe chest injury or obstruction of the airway may be unable to breathe in an adequate amount of oxygen. An insufficient concentration of oxygen in the blood can produce shock as rapidly as vascular causes, even if the volume of blood, the volume of the vessels, and the action of the heart are all normal. Without oxygen, the organs in the body cannot survive, and their cells promptly start to deteriorate.

This is why the first two steps in resuscitation are always securing an airway and restoring respirations. Circulation of nonoxygenated blood will not benefit the patient.

ANAPHYLACTIC SHOCK. **Anaphylaxis**, an exaggerated allergic reaction, or **anaphylactic shock**, occurs when a person reacts violently to a substance to which he or she has been sensitized. **Sensitization** means becoming sensitive to a substance that did not initially cause a reaction. Do not be misled by a patient who reports no history of allergic reaction to a substance on first or second exposure.

Instances that cause severe allergic reactions commonly fall into the following four categories:

- Injections (tetanus antitoxin, penicillin)
- Stings (honeybee, wasp, yellow jacket, hornet)
- Ingestion (shellfish, nuts, oral penicillin)
- Inhalation (dusts, pollens, latex glove powder)

Anaphylactic reactions can develop in minutes or even seconds after contact with the substance to which the patient is allergic. The signs of such allergic reactions are very distinct and not seen with other forms of shock. (▶ Table 9-1) shows the signs of anaphylactic shock in the order in which they typically occur.

In anaphylactic shock, there is no loss of blood, no vascular damage, and only a slight possibility of direct cardiac muscular injury. Instead, there is widespread vascular dilation. The combination of poor oxygenation and poor perfusion in anaphylactic shock may easily prove fatal.

PSYCHOGENIC SHOCK. A patient in **psychogenic shock** has had a sudden reaction of the nervous system that produces a temporary, generalized vascular dilation, resulting in fainting or **syncope**. Blood pools in the dilated vessels, reducing the blood supply to the brain; as a result, the brain ceases to function normally, and the patient faints. Causes of syncope range from fear, bad news, or unpleasant sights (often the sight of blood) to life-threatening cardiac arrhythmia or **aneurysm**, a

TABLE 9-1 Signs of Anaphylactic Shock

Skin
- Flushing, itching, or burning, especially over the face and upper chest
- Urticaria (hives), which may spread over large areas of the body
- Edema, especially of the face, tongue, and lips
- Cyanosis (a bluish cast to the skin resulting from poor oxygenation of circulating blood) about the lips

Circulatory System
- Dilation of peripheral blood vessels
- A drop in blood pressure
- A weak, barely palpable pulse
- Pallor
- Dizziness
- Fainting and coma

Respiratory System
- Sneezing or itching in the nasal passages
- Tightness in the chest, with a persistent dry cough
- Wheezing and **dyspnea**, or difficulty in breathing
- Secretions of fluid and mucus into the bronchial passages, alveoli, and lung tissue, causing coughing
- Constriction of the bronchi; difficulty drawing air into the lungs
- Forced expiration, requiring exertion and accompanied by wheezing
- Cessation of breathing

weakening of the artery wall that results in swelling or enlargement of the artery.

The Progression of Shock

Although you cannot see shock, you can see its signs and symptoms ▶ Table 9-2 . The early stage of shock, while the body can still compensate for blood loss, is called **compensated shock**. The late stage, when blood pressure is falling, is called **decompensated shock**. The last stage, when shock has progressed to a terminal stage, is called **irreversible shock**. A transfusion of any type at this point will not save the patient's life.

Remember that blood pressure may be the last measurable factor to change in shock. As we have seen, the body has several automatic mechanisms to compensate for initial blood loss and to help maintain blood pressure. Thus, by the time you detect a drop in blood pressure, shock is well developed. This is particularly true of infants and children, who can maintain their blood pressure until they have lost more than half their blood volume. By the time blood pressure drops in infants and children who are in shock, they are close to death.

You should expect shock in many emergency medical situations. For example, you would expect shock to accompany massive external or internal bleeding. You should also expect shock if a patient has any one of the following conditions:

- Multiple severe fractures
- Abdominal or chest injury
- Trauma
- A severe infection
- A major heart attack
- Anaphylaxis

Emergency Medical Care

You must begin immediate treatment for shock as soon as you realize that the condition may exist. Follow the steps in ▶ Skill Drill 9-1 :

1. As with any type of patient care, you should **begin by following BSI precautions,** making sure the patient has an open airway, and checking breathing and pulse. In general, keep the patient in a supine position. Patients who have had a severe heart attack or who have lung disease may find it easier to breathe in a sitting or semisitting position (Step 1).

Documentation Tips

Just as they make for thorough written reporting, taking and recording frequent vital signs—and observing perfusion indicators such as skin condition and mental status—will give you a window into the progression of shock. Use your documentation to remind you to suspect shock early and treat it aggressively.

TABLE 9-2 Progression of Shock

Compensated Shock

Agitation

Anxiety

Restlessness

Feeling of impending doom

Altered mental status

Weak, rapid (thready), or absent pulse

Clammy (pale, cool, moist) skin

Pallor, with cyanosis about the lips

Shallow, rapid breathing

Air hunger (shortness of breath), especially if there is a chest injury

Nausea or vomiting

Capillary refill in infants and children of longer than 2 seconds in warm environment

Marked thirst

Decompensated Shock

Falling blood pressure (systolic blood pressure of 90 mm Hg or lower in an adult)

Labored or irregular breathing

Ashen, mottled, or cyanotic skin

Thready or absent peripheral pulses

Dull eyes, dilated pupils

Poor urinary output

Skill Drill 9-1 Treating Shock

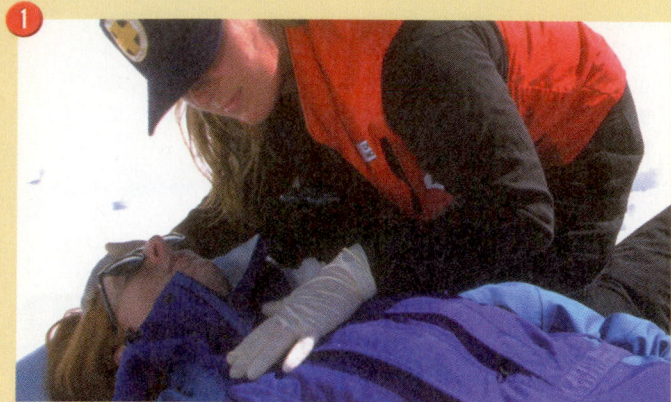

Keep the patient supine, open the airway, and check breathing and pulse.

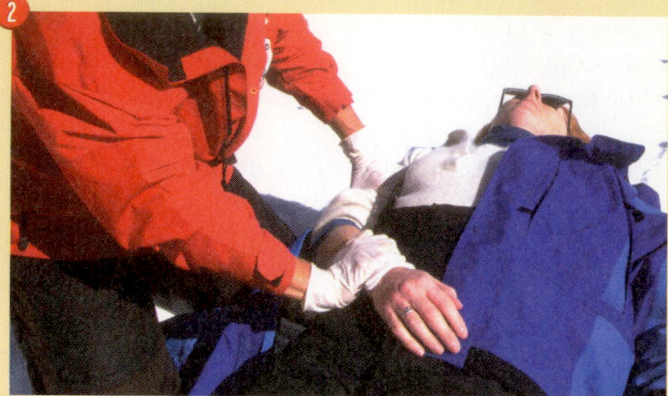

Control obvious external bleeding.

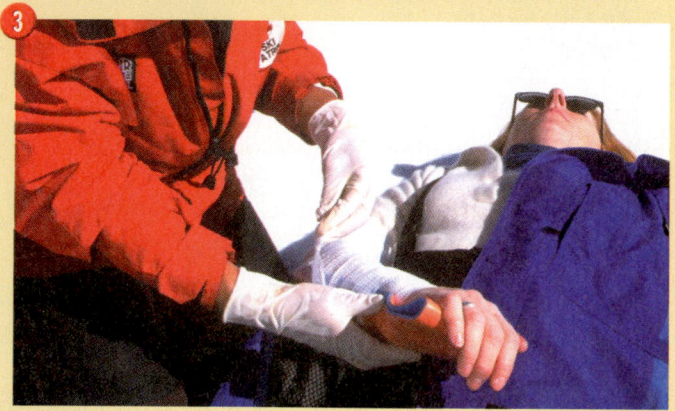

Splint any broken bones or joint injuries.

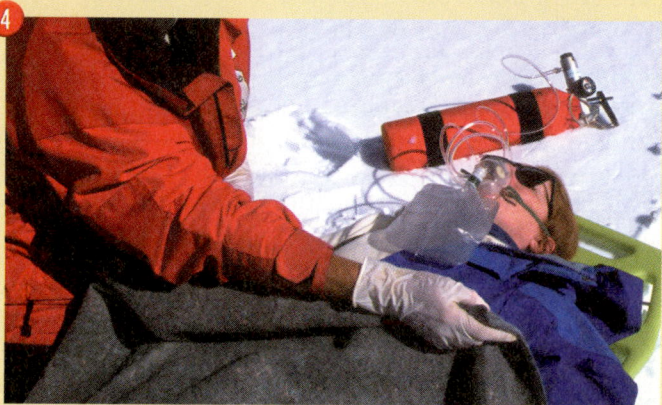

Give high-flow oxygen if you have not already done so, and place blankets under and over the patient.

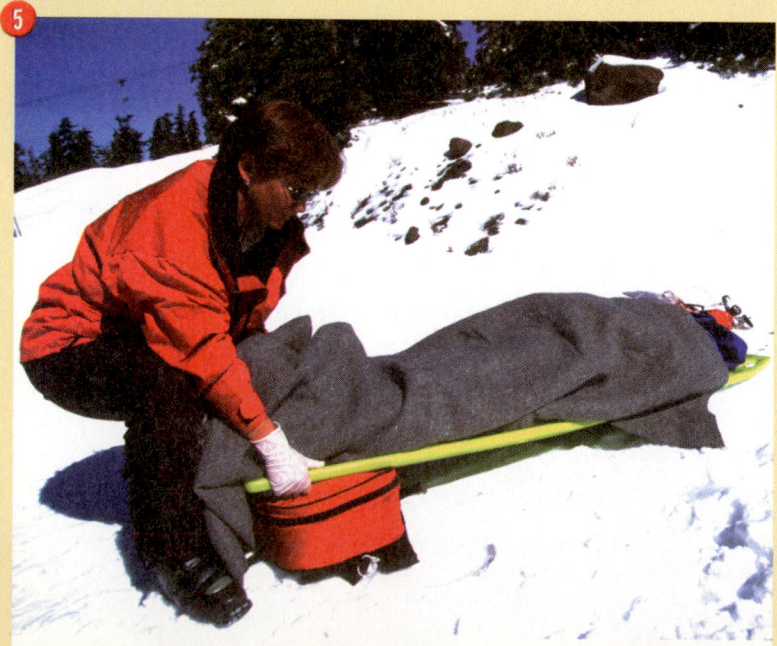

If no fractures are suspected, elevate the legs 6" to 12".

2. **Next, control all obvious external bleeding.** Place dry, sterile dressings over the bleeding sites, and secure with bandages **(Step 2)**.

3. **Splint any bone or joint injuries.** This minimizes pain, bleeding, and discomfort, all of which can aggravate shock. It also prevents the broken bone ends from further damaging adjacent soft tissue. In general, splinting also makes it easier to move the patient. Handle the patient gently and no more than is necessary **(Step 3)**.

4. **Remember that inadequate ventilation** may be the primary cause of shock or a major factor in its development. Always provide oxygen, assist with ventilations as needed, and continue to monitor the patient's breathing. To prevent the loss of body heat, place blankets under and over the patient. Remember to cover the head. Remove wet clothes and place a vapor barrier, such as a garbage bag, over the patient. It may be better for the patient to be slightly cool rather than too hot **(Step 4)**.

5. **If there are no broken bones,** elevate the lower extremities 6″ to 12″ with attention to the spine if the mechanism suggests possible spinal injury. This not only stops venous bleeding in an extremity, it allows blood in the legs to return to the heart more rapidly **(Step 5)**.

In some cases, a shock patient may also have lung congestion from heart failure, lung disease, or lung injury, and may need to sit up because of the inability to breathe when lying flat. In this situation, use the Rothberg position, in which the patient's upper body is raised at a 45° angle, the abdomen is flat, and the lower extremities are elevated by flexing the hips at about 15° or bending the knees.

Do not give the patient anything by mouth, no matter how urgently you are asked. To relieve the intense thirst that often accompanies shock, give the patient a moistened piece of gauze to chew or suck. Never give a patient in shock an alcoholic drink or other depressant. A stimulant, such as coffee, also has little value in treating shock.

Accurately record the patient's vital signs approximately every 5 minutes throughout treatment and transport. It is essential to transport the trauma patient to the hospital as rapidly as possible for definitive treatment. The Golden Hour refers to the first 60 minutes after injury, which is felt to be a critically important period for the early resuscitation and treatment of severely injured trauma patients.

> **Early resuscitation and definitive treatment of a patient in shock or with severe injuries is critically important during the Golden Hour immediately after injury.**

This concept underscores the importance of rapid evaluation, stabilization, and transport. The goal of prehospital care rescuers is to limit on-scene time (time on-scene until transport to the hospital is started). Remember to speak calmly and reassuringly to a conscious patient throughout assessment, care, and transport.

▶ **Table 9-3** lists the general supportive measures for the major types of shock. Not every measure is used for every type of shock.

Treating Cardiogenic Shock

The patient who is in shock as a result of a heart attack does not require a transfusion of blood, IV fluids, or elevation of the legs. There is already a greater volume of blood in circulation than the heart can handle. The damaged heart muscle simply cannot generate the necessary power to pump blood throughout the circulatory system.

Keep in mind that chronic lung disease will aggravate cardiogenic shock. If the patient has chronic obstructive pulmonary disease, as well as heart disease, oxygenation of the blood passing through the lungs is impaired. Because fluid is collecting in the lungs, this patient is often able to breathe better in a sitting or semisitting position and may tell you so.

Usually, patients with cardiogenic shock do not have any injury, but they may be having chest pain. Such a patient may have taken nitroglycerin before your arrival and may want to take more. Before helping the patient self-administer nitroglycerin, if possible, consult with medical control for instructions. You will also need to perform an accurate assessment and to ensure that the patient's blood pressure meets the criteria for this medication. If the blood pressure is too low, nitroglycerin may increase the problem. Remember that patients in cardiogenic shock usually have a low blood pressure. Other signs include a weak, irregular pulse, cyanosis about the lips and underneath the fingernails, anxiety, and nausea.

Treatment of cardiogenic shock should begin by placing the patient in the position in which breathing is easiest as you give high-flow oxygen. Be ready to assist

TABLE 9-3 Types of Shock

Types of Shock	Examples of Potential Causes	Signs/Symptoms
Anaphylactic	Allergic reaction	Can develop within seconds Mild itching/rash Burning skin Vascular dilation Generalized edema Profound coma Rapid death
Cardiogenic	Inadequate heart function Disease of muscle tissue Impaired electrical system Disease or injury	Chest pains Irregular pulse Weak pulse Low blood pressure Cyanosis (lips, under nails) Anxiety
Hypovolemic	Loss of blood or fluid	Rapid, weak pulse Low blood pressure Change in mental status Cyanosis (lips, under nails) Cool, clammy skin Increased respiratory rate
Respiratory Insufficiency	Severe chest injury, airway obstruction	Rapid, weak pulse Low blood pressure Change in mental status Cyanosis (lips, under nails) Cool, clammy skin Increased respiratory rate
Neurogenic	Damaged cervical spine, which causes widespread blood vessel dilation	Bradycardia (slow pulse) Low blood pressure Signs of neck injury
Psychogenic (fainting)	Temporary, generalized vascular dilation Anxiety, bad news, sight of injury/blood, prospect of medical treatment, severe pain, illness, fatigue	Rapid pulse Normal or low blood pressure
Septic	Severe bacterial infection	Warm skin Tachycardia (rapid pulse) Low blood pressure

ventilations as necessary, and have suction nearby in case the patient vomits. Arrange for prompt transport to the hospital. Remember also to approach a patient who has had a suspected heart attack with calm reassurance.

Treating Neurogenic Shock

Shock that accompanies spinal cord injury is best treated by a combination of all the known supportive measures. The patient who has sustained this kind of injury usually will require hospitalization for a long time. Emergency treatment must be directed at obtaining and maintaining a proper airway, providing spinal immobilization, assisting inadequate breathing as needed, conserving body heat, and providing the most effective circulation possible.

This patient is not losing blood. However, the capacity of his or her blood vessels has become significantly larger than the volume of blood they contain. Supplemental oxygen will boost the concentration of oxygen in the blood. If respirations are weak or inadequate, provide assisted ventilations. Keep the patient as warm as possible with blankets, because the injury may have disabled the body's normal temperature controls. Arrange for prompt transport.

Treating Hypovolemic Shock

The emergency treatment of hypovolemic or hemorrhagic shock includes the control of all obvious external bleeding. To prevent continued bleeding, you must apply sufficient pressure to control obvious external bleeding, splint any bone and joint injuries, and ensure that you use great care to handle the patient gently. If there are no fractured extremities, you should raise the legs 6″ to 12″, keeping the torso in a horizontal position. This will increase blood flow to the heart from the lower body and keep unwanted pressure off the diaphragm. This method combats shock by using the patient's own blood to its best advantage.

Although you cannot control internal bleeding in the field, you must recognize its existence and provide aggressive general support. Secure and maintain an airway, and provide respiratory support, including supplemental oxygen and, if needed, assisted ventilations. Start the oxygen as soon as you suspect shock, and continue it during transport; with too little circulating blood, additional oxygen may be lifesaving. Be sure the patient does not aspirate blood or vomitus. Most important, you must transport the patient as rapidly as possible to the ambulance for transport directly to the hospital.

Treatment

Manage the airway
Assist ventilations
Administer high-flow oxygen
Determine cause
Assist with administration of epinephrine
Transport promptly

Position comfortably
Administer oxygen
Assist ventilations
Transport promptly

Secure airway
Assist ventilations
Administer high-flow oxygen
Control external bleeding
Elevate legs
Keep warm
Transport promptly

Secure airway
Clear air passages
Assist ventilations
Administer high-flow oxygen
Transport promptly

Secure airway
Spinal immobilization
Assist ventilations
Administer high-flow oxygen
Transport promptly

Determine duration of unconsciousness
Record initial vital signs and mental status
Suspect head injury if patient is confused or slow to regain consciousness
Transport promptly

Transport promptly
Administer oxygen en route
Provide full ventilatory support
Elevate legs
Keep patient warm

> Although you cannot
> control internal bleeding in the field,
> you must recognize its existence and
> provide aggressive support.

Treating Septic Shock

The proper treatment of septic shock requires complex hospital management. If you suspect that a patient has septic shock, you must transport him or her as promptly as possible. Use high-flow oxygen during transport. Ventilatory support may be necessary to maintain adequate tidal volume in this patient. Use blankets to conserve body heat.

Treating Respiratory Insufficiency

In treating the patient who is in shock as a result of inadequate respiration, you must immediately secure and maintain the airway. Clear the mouth and throat of anything obstructing the air passages, including mucus, vomitus, and foreign material. If necessary, provide ventilations with a bag-valve-mask device. Give supplemental oxygen, and transport the patient promptly.

Treating Anaphylactic Shock

The only really effective treatment for a severe, acute allergic reaction is to administer epinephrine by way of subcutaneous, intramuscular, or intravenous injection. For more information on the emergency care for allergic reactions, see Chapter 13. A patient who is aware of having a specific sensitivity may carry a bee sting kit containing epinephrine (▶ Figure 9-5).

If he or she is unable to inject the medication, you may have to do so if you are allowed by local protocol. If the patient's signs and symptoms recur or deteriorate, you should repeat the injection after consulting with medical control.

Promptly transport the patient to the ambulance or other transport, then directly to the hospital while providing all possible support, primarily supplemental oxygen and ventilatory assistance. You should also try to find out what agent caused the reaction (eg, a drug, an insect bite or sting, a food item) and how it was received (eg, by mouth, by inhalation, or by injection). The severity of allergic reactions can vary greatly, with

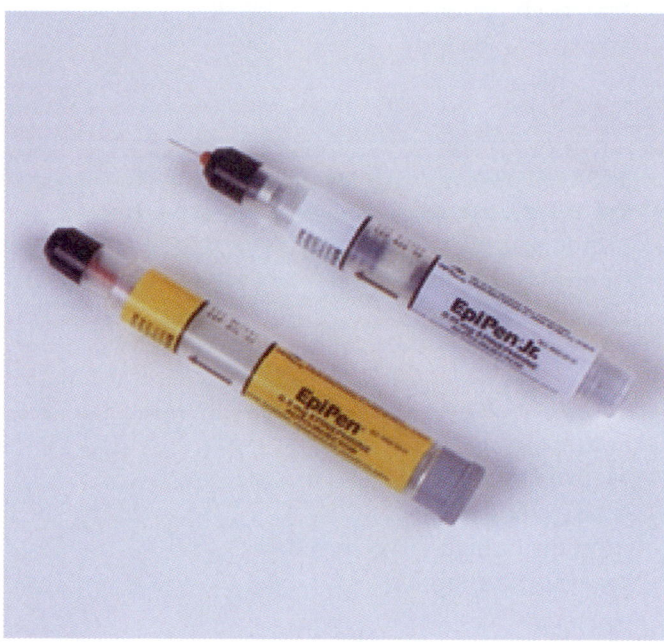

Figure 9-5 Patients who are allergic to bee stings often carry commercial bee sting kits, such as an intramuscular (IM) injector or autoinjector, containing epinephrine.

symptoms ranging from mild itching to profound coma and rapid death. Keep in mind that a mild reaction may worsen suddenly or over time. Consider requesting advanced life support backup, if available.

Treating Psychogenic Shock

In an uncomplicated case of fainting, once the patient collapses and becomes supine, circulation to the brain is usually restored, and with it a normal state of functioning. If the attack has caused the patient to fall, you must check for injuries, especially in older patients. However, you should also assess the patient thoroughly for any other abnormality. If, after regaining consciousness, the patient is unable to walk without weakness, dizziness, or pain, you should suspect another problem, such as head injury. You should transport this patient promptly.

Be sure to record your initial observations of vital signs and level of consciousness. In addition, try to learn from bystanders whether the patient complained of anything before fainting and how long he or she had been unconscious.

Rescuer Tips

When concerned about hemorrhage, remember that the body of an average 150-lb (67-kg) adult man contains about 6 quarts (5.7 L) of blood. The loss of 1.1 pints (500 mL) of blood is almost always well tolerated by a normal, healthy adult; however, the loss of 1.1 quarts (1 L) may cause *mild shock*. This type of shock is marked by a fast pulse and decreased pulse pressure, with low blood pressure when the patient sits up or attempts to stand, although the blood pressure may be normal or near-normal when the individual is lying down. A 1.6 to 2.1 quart (1.5 to 2 L) loss of blood causes *clinical shock*, marked by a fast pulse, low blood pressure, and altered mental status when the patient is lying down. A loss of more than 2.1 quarts (2 L) causes severe shock with unresponsiveness.

Chapter *Sweep*

Ready for Review

Shock (hypoperfusion) is the collapse and failure of the cardio-vascular system, in which blood circulation slows and eventually ceases. Perfusion requires a cardiovascular system with all three parts (the pump, container, and contents) working, but it also requires a functioning respiratory system. The signs and symp-toms of shock are caused by the actions of the autonomic nervous system and of hormones responding to the need for addi-tional perfusion.

The cardiovascular causes of shock include poor pump function (cardiogenic shock), blood or fluid loss from blood vessels (hypo-volemic shock), and/or poor vessel function (neurogenic shock), as when all vessels dilate at once. Septic shock is a combination of vessel and content failure; it is the result of a serious infection.

Signs of compensated shock include agitation or anxiety, a weak, rapid pulse, clammy skin, air hunger, nausea or vomiting, slow capillary refill in children and infants, and marked thirst. Signs of decompensated shock include labored or irregular breathing, ashen or cyanotic skin, thready or absent peripheral pulses, dilated pupils, poor urinary output, and, finally, falling blood pres-sure. By the time you detect a drop in blood pressure, shock is well developed. Expect shock in cases of massive internal or external bleeding, multiple severe fractures, abdominal or chest injury, spinal injury, severe infection, a major heart attack, and anaphylaxis.

Treat patients with shock by (1) opening and maintaining the airway; (2) providing oxygen and, if necessary, assisting ventila-tions; (3) controlling all obvious external bleeding; (4) conserving body heat with blankets; and (5) transporting promptly. Use high-flow oxygen for all patients in shock.

Vital Vocabulary

anaphylactic shock Severe shock caused by allergic reactions.

anaphylaxis An unusual or exaggerated allergic reaction to foreign protein or other substances.

aneurysms A swelling or enlargement of a part of an artery, resulting from weakening of the arterial wall.

autonomic nervous system The part of the nervous system that regulates involuntary functions, such as digestion and sweating.

cardiogenic shock Shock caused by inadequate function of the heart, or pump failure.

compensated shock The early stage of shock, in which the body can still compensate for blood loss.

cyanosis Bluish color of the skin resulting from poor oxygenation of the circulating blood.

decompensated shock The late stage of shock, when blood pressure is falling.

dehydration Loss of water from the tissues of the body.

dyspnea Difficulty in breathing.

edema The presence of abnormally large amounts of fluid between cells in body tissues, causing swelling of the affected area.

hypothermia A condition in which the internal body temperature falls below 95°F (35°C), usually as a result of prolonged exposure to cool or freezing temperatures.

hypovolemic shock Shock caused by fluid or blood loss.

irreversible shock The final stage of shock, resulting in death.

neurogenic shock Circulatory failure caused by paralysis of the nerves that control the size of the blood vessels, leading to widespread dilation; seen in spinal cord injuries.

perfusion Circulation of blood within an organ or tissue in adequate amounts to meet the cells' current needs.

psychogenic shock Shock caused by a sudden, temporary reduction in blood supply to the brain that causes fainting (syncope).

sensitization Developing a sensitivity to a substance that initially caused no allergic reaction.

septic shock Shock caused by severe bacterial infection.

shock A condition in which the circulatory system fails to provide sufficient circulation to enable every body part to perform its function; also called hypoperfusion.

sphincters Circular muscles that encircle and, by contracting, constrict a duct, tube, or opening.

syncope Fainting.

Assessment in Action

You are on patrol for the ski area's "Extreme Cliff Competition." You feel your heart sink as you watch the current competitor catch an edge and tumble over a rock band into a steep and rocky chute. He emerges at the bottom "ragdolling" for an additional 200'.

As you ski toward him, you expect the worst. You and three other patrollers are the first to arrive at the victim. He is unconscious but breathing. He appears pale but you can feel a carotid pulse and you estimate a rate of about 140 beats/min. Your quick size-up reveals chest wall trauma; the patient reacts with apparent pain to palpation of his left upper abdomen. His pelvis moves when you compress it and he has obvious deformity of both femurs, one of which protrudes through his ski pants.

1. Which of the following would be most appropriate for this patient?
   A. Provide c-spine stabilization on a backboard, splint the legs, apply oxygen, and notify the aid room to expect you in 15 minutes.
   B. Call for immediate Medevac and have the receiving hospital placed on alert, apply oxygen, provide c-spine stabilization on a backboard, splint the legs, and apply a dressing to the open wound. Move the patient rapidly to the landing zone.
   C. Apply oxygen, move the patient to the aid room without further intervention due to the seriousness of the injuries.

2. With serious trauma leading to shock from internal bleeding, what is the most important determinant of survival?
   A. Placing oxygen on the patient within the first 5 minutes of the trauma
   B. Meticulous wound care at the scene
   C. Rapid transport to a facility that can perform emergency surgery
   D. A full-coverage medical health plan

3. On the basis of the patient's signs and symptoms, you suspect:
   A. neurogenic shock due to a probable c-spine fracture.
   B. hypovolemic shock due to internal bleeding.
   C. psychogenic shock due to the fear of the fall.
   D. anaphylactic shock due to regurgitation of stomach contents.

4. Based on the vital signs, you would expect the capillary refill to be:
   A. almost instantaneous.
   B. less than 2 seconds.
   C. greater than 2 seconds.
   D. virtually nonexistent.

5. If the patient's ventilatory rate increases to about 40 breaths/min and becomes more shallow, you should:
   A. apply oxygen by nasal cannula at 2 L/min.
   B. try a jaw-thrust or head tilt-chin lift maneuver to open the airway.
   C. begin rescue breathing.
   D. try a brisk sternal rub.

6. The greatest threat to this patient's life at this point is:
   A. head injury.
   B. internal bleeding.
   C. hypothermia.
   D. delay in transport.

7. If the patient cannot be immediately transported off the hill and you have to take him to the aid room, what measures can you provide that might help decrease internal bleeding?
   A. Pelvic swathe, traction splints to the femurs
   B. Direct pressure to the femoral wound
   C. Direct pressure to the abdomen
   D. High-flow oxygen

Challenging Question

8. This patient may have a serious head injury in addition to internal bleeding. How does that change your management of the shock state?

Points to Ponder

You are asked to assist in the first aid room for an injured biker. Upon observation, you notice that the patient is pale, flushed, anxious, and restless. The only injury the patient has sustained is a tibia/fibula fracture. The fellow rescuer notices that the patient's mental status seems to be deteriorating. How would this situation affect your patient assessment? What interventions need to be initiated, if any?

Issues BSI Precautions, Long-Term Effects of Infectious Disease, Reporting Requirements, Reasonable Risk, Responsibility to Patients and Employers.

Online Outlook

The signs and symptoms of shock are presented in this chapter. Test your ability to recognize shock by completing Exercise 9 at www.OECzone.com.

www.OECzone.com

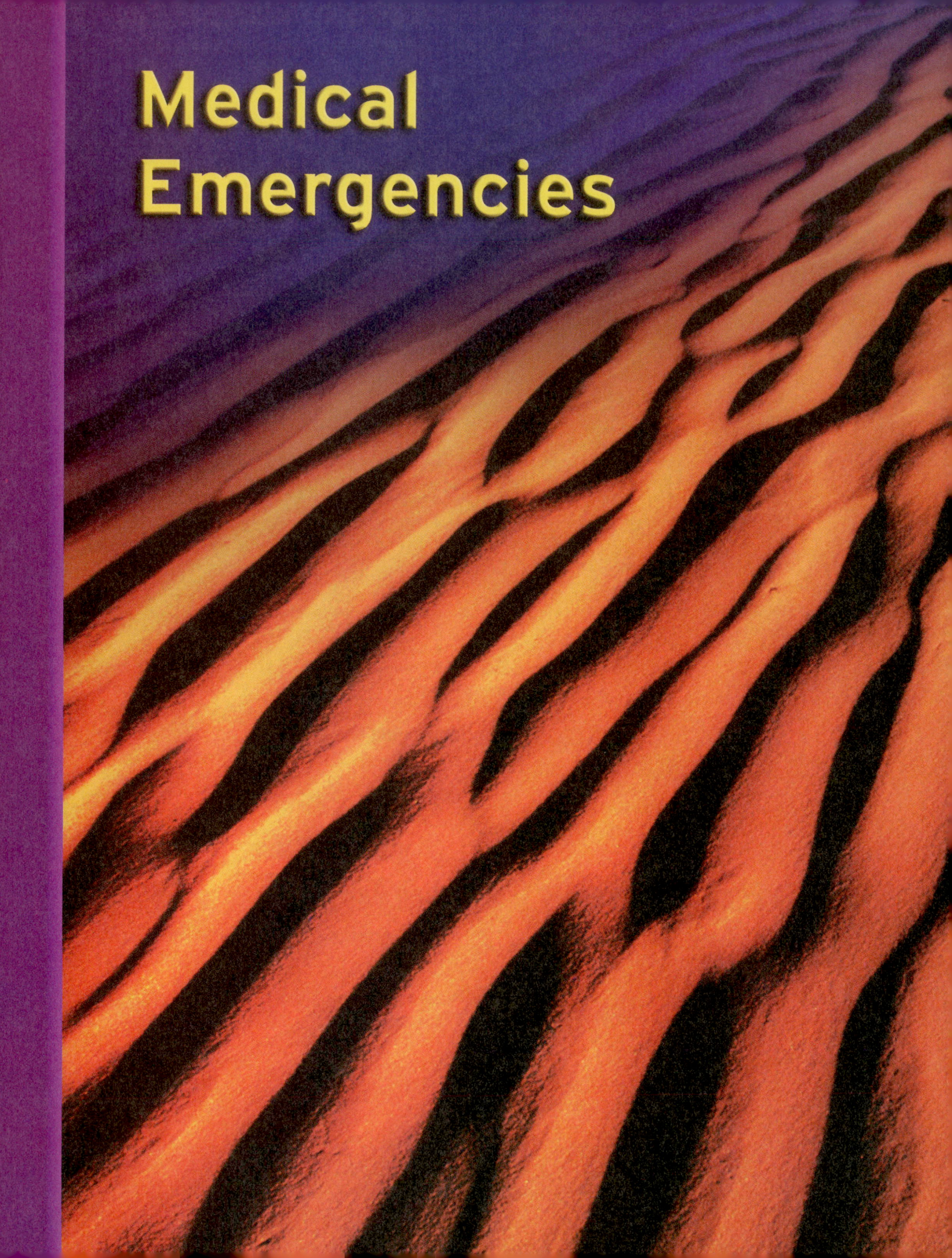

Medical Emergencies

Section

4

Respiratory Emergencies

Objectives

Cognitive

🌲 **1.** List the structure and function of the respiratory system (p 285).

🌲 **2.** State the signs and symptoms of a patient with breathing difficulty (p 286).

🌲 **3.** Describe the emergency medical care of the patient with breathing difficulty (p 295).

4. Recognize the need for medical direction to assist in the emergency medical care of the patient with breathing difficulty (p 295).

5. Describe the emergency medical care of the patient with breathing distress (p 295).

6. Establish the relationship between airway management and the patient with breathing difficulty (p 295).

7. List signs of adequate air exchange (p 286).

8. State the generic name, medication forms, dose, administration, action, indications, and contraindications for the prescribed inhaler (p 296).

🌲 **9.** Distinguish between the emergency medical care of the infant, child, and adult patient with breathing difficulty (p 298).

10. Differentiate between upper airway obstruction and lower airway disease in the infant and child patient (p 299).

🌲 **11.** Describe the special considerations due to high altitude (p 290).

Affective

🌲 **12.** Defend OEC treatment regimens for various respiratory emergencies (p 295).

13. Explain the rationale for administering an inhaler (p 296).

Psychomotor

🌲 **14.** Demonstrate the emergency medical care for breathing difficulty (p 295).

15. Perform the steps in facilitating the use of an inhaler (p 297).

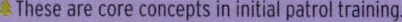 These are core concepts in initial patrol training.

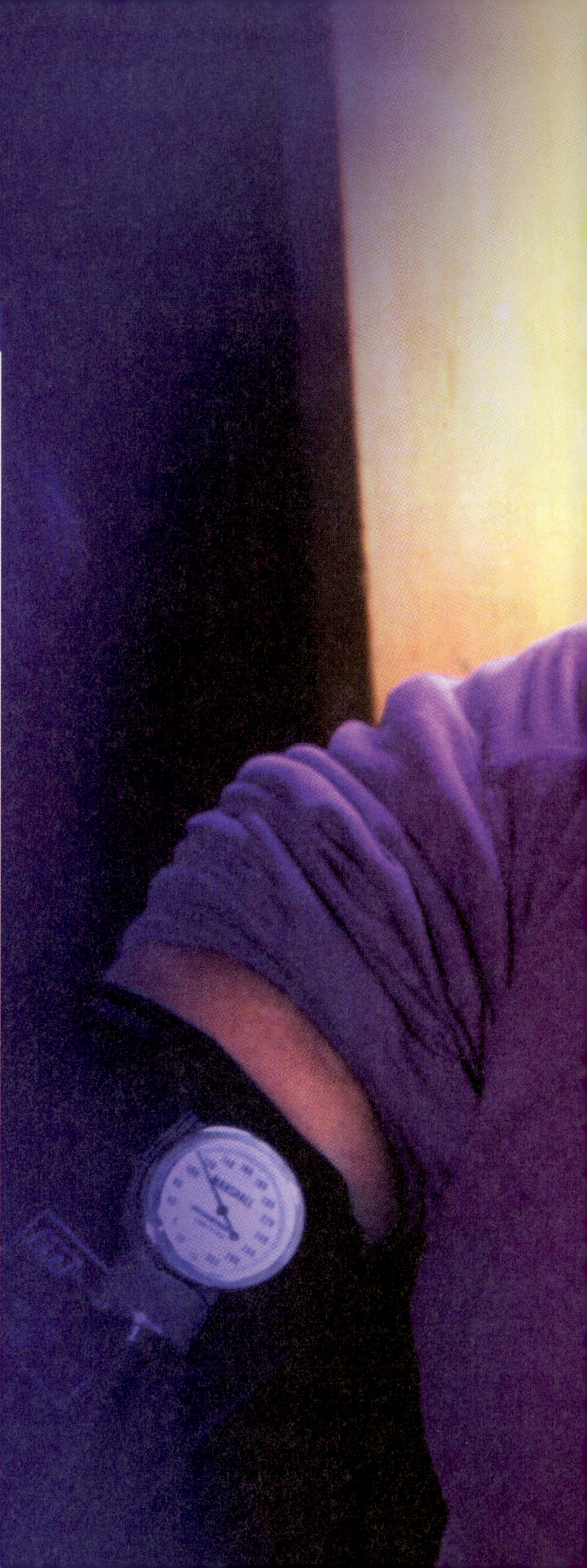

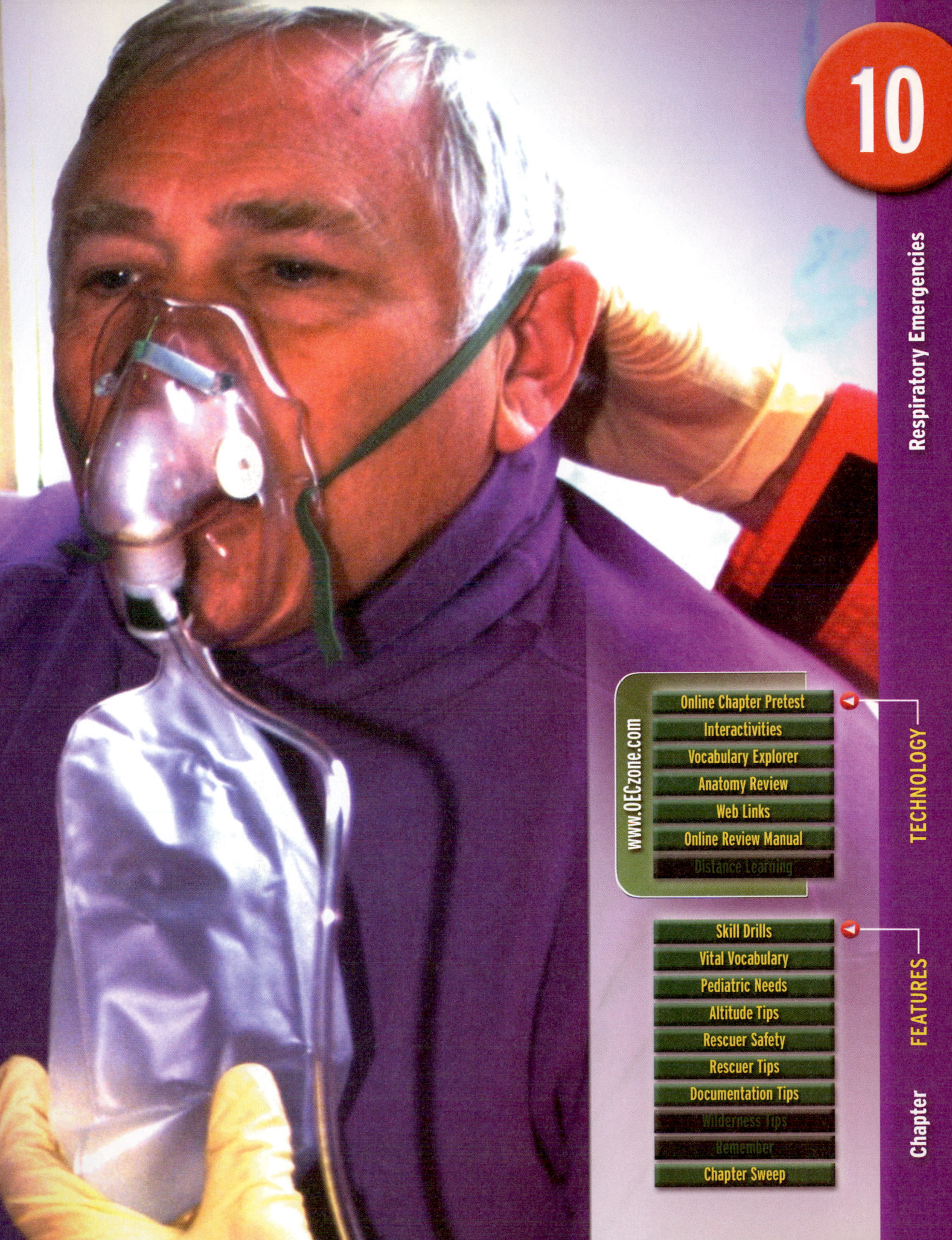

Chapter

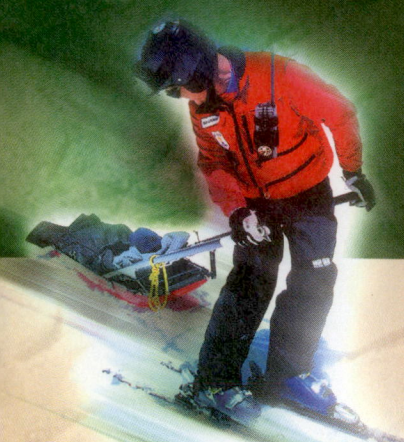

Your team is dispatched to a midmountain restaurant for a "sick skier." You arrive to find a 31-year-old woman complaining that she "just can't breathe" and "has a sharp pain in the chest."

Given the frequency with which emergency calls are related to breathing, it is paramount that a rescuer be prepared to handle them. This chapter will prepare you to do just that as well as to answer the following questions:

1. What are the most common signs and symptoms of patients with breathing difficulties?

2. What is the relationship between airway management and breathing difficulty?

Respiratory Emergencies

Dyspnea, the feeling of being short of breath, is a complaint that you will encounter often. It is a symptom of many different conditions, from the common cold and asthma to heart failure and pulmonary embolism. Some degree of dyspnea is normal at high altitudes (more than 8,000′). You may or may not be able to determine what is causing dyspnea in a particular patient; this can be difficult even for physicians in a hospital setting. Also, several different problems may contribute to a patient's dyspnea at the same time, including some that are serious or life threatening. Even without a definitive diagnosis, however, you may still be able to save a life.

This chapter begins with a basic explanation of how the lungs function. It then looks at common medical problems that can impede normal functioning and cause dyspnea, including acute pulmonary edema, chronic obstructive pulmonary disease, and asthma. You will learn the signs and symptoms of each condition. You should keep all these possible medical problems in mind as you take the patient's history and perform a physical assessment, a process that the chapter describes in detail. The information that you collect will help you to decide on the proper treatment, which differs according to the probable cause of the dyspnea.

Remember, the sensation of not getting enough air can be terrifying, regardless of its cause. As a rescuer, you should be prepared to treat not just the symptom and the underlying problem, but also the anxiety that it produces.

Anatomy and Function of the Lungs

The respiratory system consists of all the structures of the body that contribute to the breathing process. Important anatomic features include the upper and lower airways, the lungs, and the diaphragm (▶ Figure 10-1). Air enters the trachea and moves along the bronchial tubes to the air spaces, called alveoli, where oxygen and carbon dioxide are exchanged.

The principal function of the lungs is respiration, which is the exchange of oxygen and carbon dioxide. The two processes that occur during respiration are inspiration, the act of breathing in or inhaling, and expiration, the act of breathing out or exhaling. During respiration, oxygen is provided to the blood, and carbon dioxide is removed from it. This exchange of gases takes place rapidly in normal lungs at the level of the alveoli. Alveoli are microscopic, thin-walled air sacs that lie against the pulmonary capillary vessels. Oxygen and carbon dioxide must be able to pass freely between the alveoli and the capillaries (▶ Figure 10-2). Oxygen entering the alveoli from inhalation passes through tiny passages in the alveolar wall into the capillaries, which carry the oxygen-rich blood to the heart. The heart pumps the oxygen around the body. Carbon dioxide produced by the body's cells (▶ Figure 10-3A) returns to the lungs in the blood that circulates through and around the alveolar air spaces. The carbon dioxide diffuses back into the alveoli and travels back up the bronchial tree and out the upper airways during exhalation (▶ Figure 10-3B). Again, carbon dioxide is "exchanged" for oxygen, which travels in exactly the opposite direction (during inhalation).

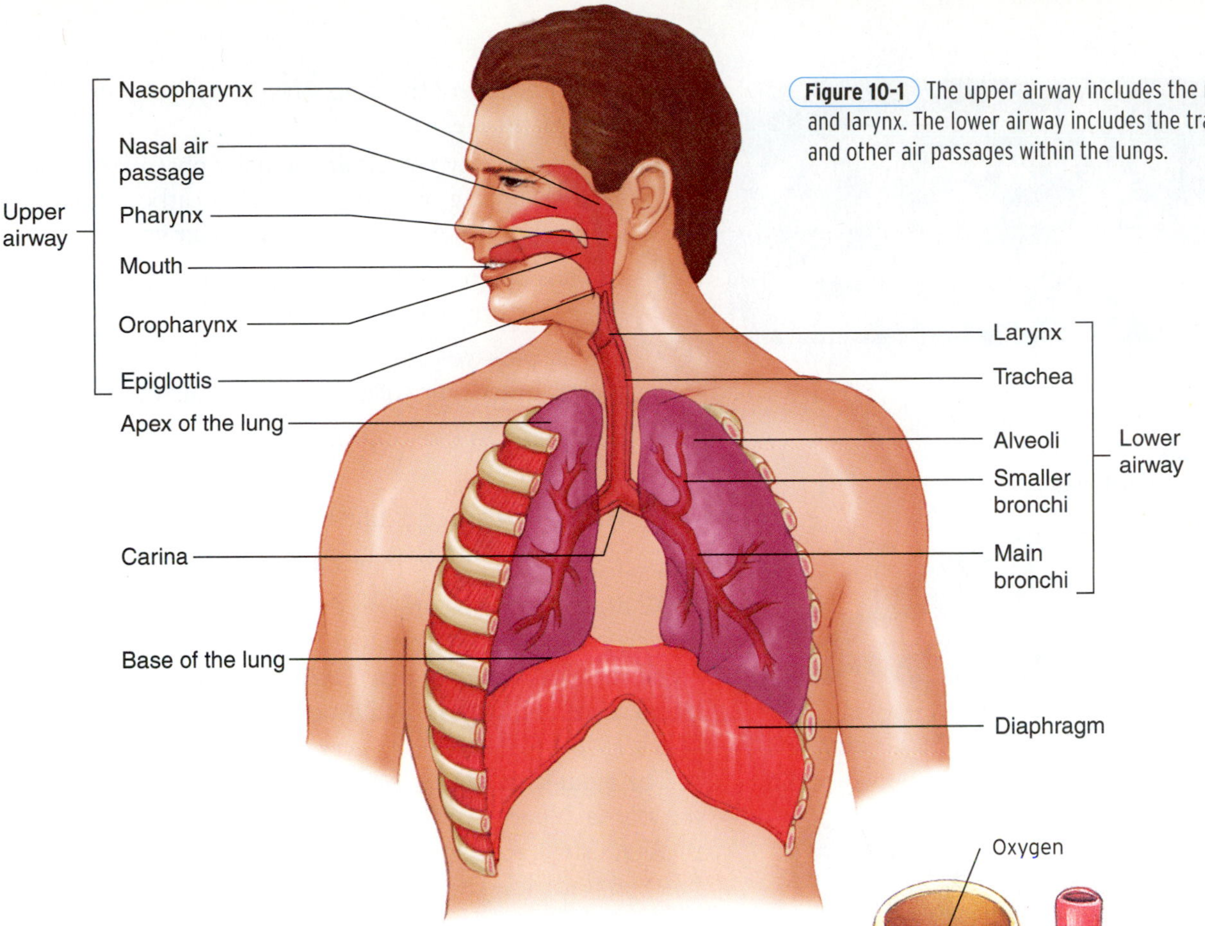

Upper airway
Nasopharynx
Nasal air passage
Pharynx
Mouth
Oropharynx
Epiglottis
Apex of the lung
Carina
Base of the lung

Larynx
Trachea
Alveoli
Smaller bronchi
Main bronchi
Diaphragm

Lower airway

Figure 10-1 The upper airway includes the mouth, nose, pharynx, and larynx. The lower airway includes the trachea, major bronchi, and other air passages within the lungs.

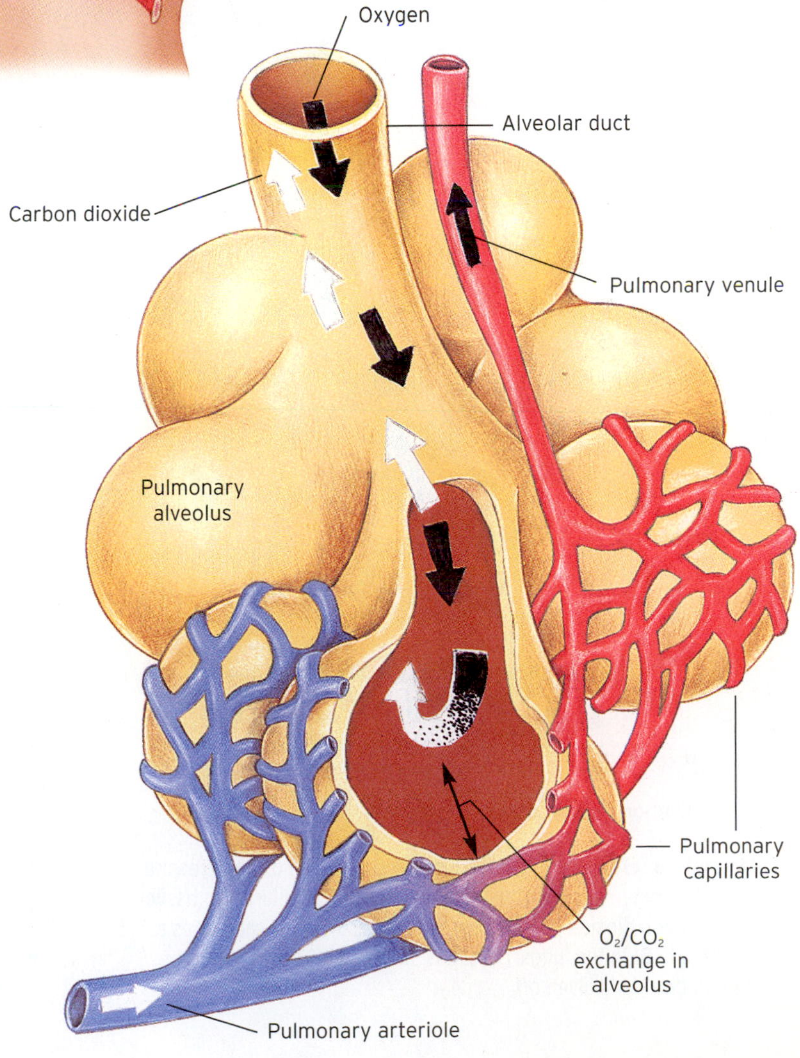

Oxygen
Alveolar duct
Carbon dioxide
Pulmonary venule
Pulmonary alveolus
Pulmonary capillaries
O₂/CO₂ exchange in alveolus
Pulmonary arteriole

Figure 10-2 An enlarged view of a single alveolus (air sac) showing where the exchange of oxygen and carbon dioxide between air in the sac and blood in the pulmonary capillaries takes place.

Pulmonary edema occurs when the undamaged right side of the heart continues to pump blood *into* the lungs but the damaged left side is too weak to handle even a normal volume of blood coming *from* the lungs.

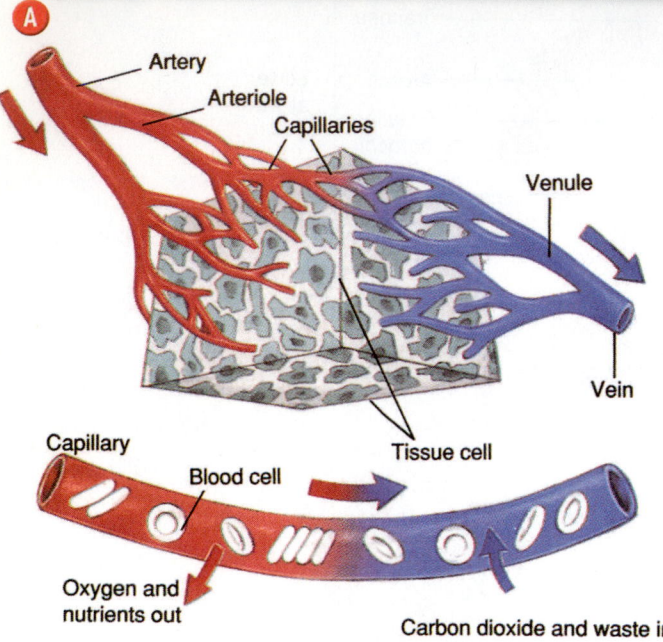

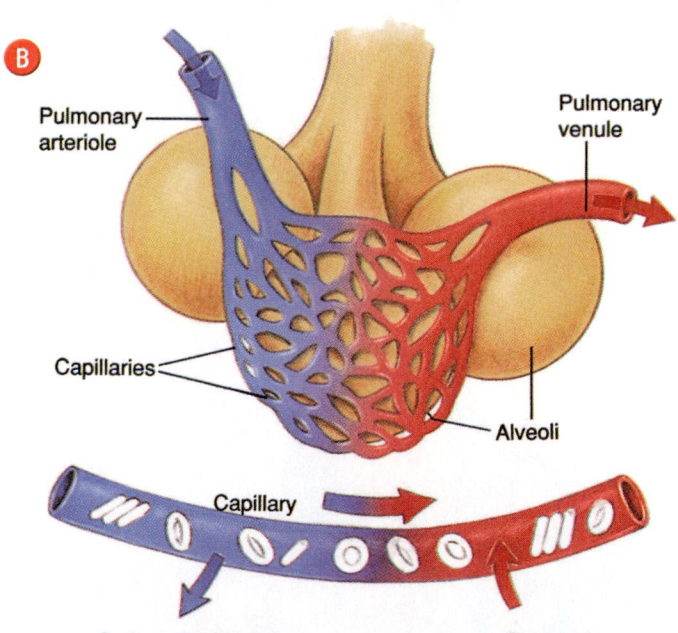

Figure 10-3 The exchange of oxygen and carbon dioxide in respiration. **A.** Oxygen passes from the blood through capillaries to tissue cells. Carbon dioxide passes from tissue cells through capillaries to the blood. **B.** In the lungs, oxygen is picked up by the blood and carbon dioxide is given off.

In most disorders of the lung, one or more of the following situations exists:

- The pulmonary vessels are actually obstructed from absorbing oxygen or releasing carbon dioxide by fluid, infection, or collapsed air spaces.
- The alveoli are damaged and cannot transport gases properly across their own walls.
- The air passages are obstructed by muscle spasm, mucus, or weakened floppy airway walls.
- Blood flow to the lungs is obstructed by blood clots.
- The pleural space is filled with air or excess fluid, so the lungs cannot properly expand.

All these conditions prevent the proper exchange of oxygen and carbon dioxide. In addition, the pulmonary blood vessels themselves may have abnormalities that interfere with blood flow and thus with the transfer of gases.

The brain stem senses the level of carbon dioxide in the arterial blood. The level of carbon dioxide bathing the brain stem is what stimulates a healthy person to breathe. If the level drops too low, the person automatically breathes at a slower rate and less deeply. As a result, less carbon dioxide is expired, allowing carbon dioxide levels in the blood to return to normal. If the level of carbon dioxide in the arterial blood rises above normal, the patient breathes more rapidly and more deeply. When more fresh air (containing no carbon dioxide) is brought into the alveoli, more carbon dioxide diffuses out of the bloodstream, thereby lowering the level. During acclimatization to high altitude, the brain stem resets the level of carbon dioxide to a lower level, thereby increasing breathing and raising the oxygen level. At high altitude, low oxygen also stimulates breathing.

The following are the characteristics of adequate breathing:

- A normal rate and depth
- A regular pattern of inhalation and exhalation
- Good audible breath sounds on both sides of the chest
- A regular rise and fall movement on both sides of the chest
- Pink, warm, dry skin

The following are signs of inadequate breathing:

- A rate of breathing that is slower than 8 breaths/min or faster than 24 breaths/min

- Muscle retractions above the clavicles, between the ribs, and below the rib cage, especially in children
- Pale or cyanotic skin
- Cool, damp (clammy) skin
- Shallow or irregular respirations
- Pursed lips
- Nasal flaring
- Drowsiness or depressed consciousness

The level of carbon dioxide in the arterial blood can rise for a number of reasons. The exhalation process may be impaired by various types of lung disease. The body may also produce too much carbon dioxide, either temporarily or chronically, depending on the disease or abnormality.

If, over a period of years, arterial carbon dioxide levels rise slowly to an abnormally high level and remain there, the respiratory center in the brain, which senses carbon dioxide levels and controls breathing, may work less efficiently. The failure of this center to respond normally to a rise in arterial levels of carbon dioxide is called chronic **carbon dioxide retention**. If the condition is severe, respiration will stop unless there is a secondary drive, called the **hypoxic drive**, to stimulate the respiratory center. Fortunately, a second stimulus does develop in patients with chronically high blood carbon dioxide levels, namely, a low level of oxygen in the blood. Low blood oxygen causes the respiratory center to respond and stimulate respiration. If the arterial level of oxygen is then raised, as happens when the patient is given additional oxygen, there is no longer any stimulus to breathe; both the high carbon dioxide and low oxygen drives are lost. Patients with chronic lung diseases frequently have a chronically high level of blood carbon dioxide. Therefore, giving too much oxygen to these patients may actually depress, or completely stop, the respirations. Individuals older than 65 years are especially prone to problems with respiration, either from occult (not obvious) stroke, lung disease, cardiovascular disease, liver disease, or certain medications.

Causes of Dyspnea

Dyspnea is shortness of breath or difficulty breathing. Many different medical problems may cause dyspnea. Be aware that if the problem is severe and the brain is deprived of oxygen, the patient may not be alert enough to complain of shortness of breath. More commonly, altered mental status is a sign of hypoxia of the brain.

Breathing difficulty or hypoxia often develops in patients with the following medical conditions:

- Upper or lower airway infection
- Acute pulmonary edema
- Chronic obstructive pulmonary disease (COPD)
- Spontaneous pneumothorax
- Asthma or allergic reactions
- Pleural effusion
- Prolonged seizures
- Obstruction of the airway
- Hypothermia
- Pulmonary embolism
- Hyperventilation
- Severe pain, particularly chest pain
- High altitude illness

Upper or Lower Airway Infection

Infectious diseases causing dyspnea may affect all parts of the airway. Some cause mild discomfort. Others obstruct the airway to the point that patients require a full range of respiratory support. In general, the problem is always some form of obstruction, either to the flow of air in the major passages (colds, diphtheria, epiglottitis, and croup) or to the exchange of gases between the alveoli and the capillaries (pneumonia). ▶ Table 10-1 shows infectious diseases that are associated with some degree of dyspnea.

Acute Pulmonary Edema

Sometimes, the heart muscle is so injured after an acute myocardial infarction or other illness that it cannot circulate blood properly. In these cases, the left side of the heart cannot remove blood from the lung as fast as the right side delivers it. As a result, fluid builds up within the alveoli as well as in the lung tissue between the alveoli and the pulmonary capillaries. This accumulation of fluid, called **pulmonary edema**, can develop

TABLE 10-1 Infectious Diseases Associated with Dyspnea

Disease	Characteristics	Disease	Characteristics
Common Cold	• A viral infection usually associated with swollen nasal mucous membranes and the production of fluid from the sinuses and nose. • Dyspnea is not severe; patients complain of "stuffiness" or difficulty breathing through the nose.	Epiglottitis	• A bacterial infection of the epiglottis that can produce severe swelling of the flap over the larynx. • In preschool and school-aged children especially, the epiglottis can swell to two to three times its normal size (▼ Figure 10-4A). • The airway may become almost completely obstructed, sometimes quite suddenly (▼ Figure 10-4B).
Diphtheria	• Although well controlled in the past decade, it is still highly contagious and serious when it occurs. • The disease causes the formation of a diphtheritic membrane lining the pharynx that is composed of debris, inflammatory cells, and mucus. This membrane can rapidly and severely obstruct the passage of air into the larynx.		
Pneumonia	• An acute bacterial or viral infection of the lung that damages lung tissue, usually associated with fever, cough, and production of sputum. • Fluid also accumulates in the surrounding normal lung tissue, separating the alveoli from their capillaries. (Sometimes, fluid also accumulates in the pleural space.) • The lung's ability to exchange oxygen and carbon dioxide is impaired. • The breathing pattern in pneumonia does not indicate major airway obstruction, but the patient may experience tachypnea, an increase in the breathing rate, which is an attempt to compensate for the reduced amount of normal lung tissue and for the buildup of fluid.		

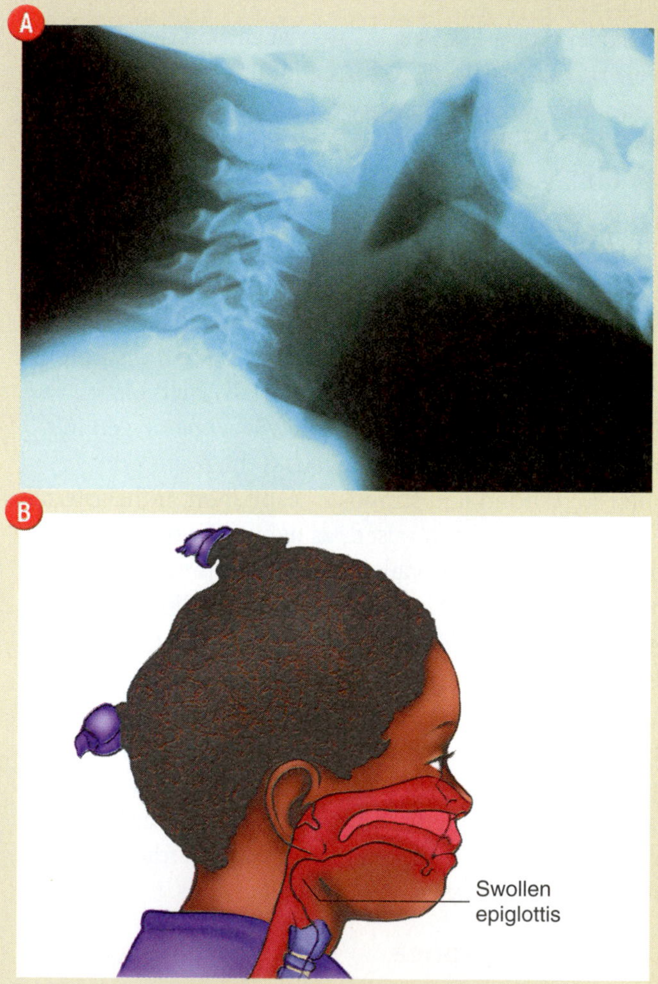

Figure 10-4 Acute epiglottitis. **A.** Epiglottitis is caused by a bacterial infection resulting in severe swelling of the epiglottis. **B.** The epiglottis is massively swollen and almost fully obstructs the airway.

Disease	Characteristics
Epiglottitis continued	• **Stridor** (harsh, high-pitched, rough barking inspiratory sounds) may be heard late in the development of airway obstruction. • Acute epiglottitis in the adult is characterized by a severe sore throat. • The disease is now much less common than it was 20 years ago because of a vaccine that can help to prevent most cases.
Croup	• An inflammation and swelling of the lining of the larynx, the narrowest point of the airway, typically seen in children between ages 6 months and 3 years ▼ **Figure 10-5** . • The common signs of croup are stridor and a seal-bark cough, which signal a significant narrowing of the air passage of the larynx that may progress to significant obstruction. • Croup often responds well to the administration of humidified oxygen.

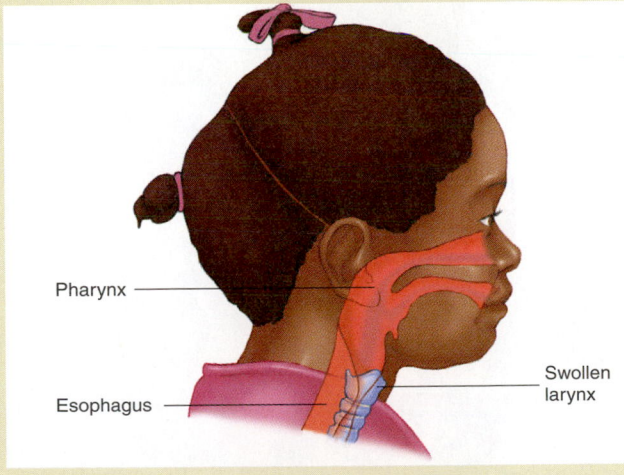

Pharynx

Esophagus

Swollen larynx

Figure 10-5 Croup swells the lining of the larynx, which is the narrowest point in a child's airway.

quickly after a major heart attack. By physically separating alveoli from pulmonary capillary vessels, the edema interferes with the exchange of carbon dioxide and oxygen. There is not enough room left in the lung for slow, deep breaths. The patient usually experiences dyspnea with rapid, shallow respirations. In the most severe instances, you will see a frothy pink sputum at the nose and mouth.

In most cases, patients have a longstanding history of chronic congestive heart failure that can be kept under control with medication. However, an acute onset may occur if the patient stops taking the medication, eats food that is too salty, or has a stressful illness, a new heart attack, or an abnormal heart rhythm. Pulmonary edema is one of the most common causes of hospital admission in the United States ▼ **Figure 10-6** . It is not uncommon for a patient to have repeated bouts.

Some patients who have pulmonary edema do not have heart disease. Inhaling large amounts of smoke or toxic chemical fumes can produce pulmonary edema, as can traumatic injuries of the chest. In these cases, fluid

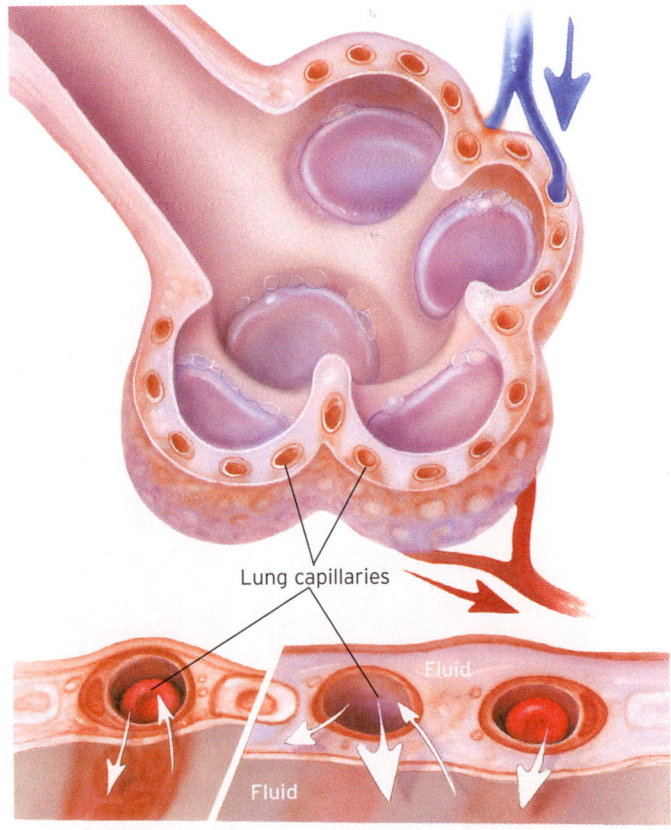

Lung capillaries

Fluid

Fluid

Normal

Pulmonary edema

Figure 10-6 In pulmonary edema, fluid fills the alveoli and separates the capillaries from the alveolar wall, interfering with the exchange of oxygen and carbon dioxide.

collects in alveoli and lung tissue in response to damage to the tissues of the lung or the bronchi. High altitude can cause pulmonary edema in perfectly healthy people by increasing capillary pressure in the lungs.

Chronic Obstructive Pulmonary Disease

<u>Chronic obstructive pulmonary disease (COPD)</u> is a common lung condition, affecting some 10% to 20% of the entire adult population in the United States. It is the end of a slow process, which over several years results in disruption of the airways, the alveoli, and the pulmonary blood vessels. The process itself may be a result of direct lung and airway damage from repeated infections or inhalation of toxic agents such as industrial gases, but most often, it results from cigarette smoking. Although it is well known that cigarettes are a direct cause of lung cancer, their role in the development of COPD is far more significant and less well publicized.

Tobacco smoke is itself a bronchial irritant and can create a <u>chronic bronchitis</u>, an ongoing irritation of the trachea and bronchi.

With bronchitis, excess mucus is constantly produced, obstructing small airways and alveoli. Protective cells and lung mechanisms that remove foreign particles are destroyed, further weakening the airways. Chronic oxygenation problems can also lead to right heart failure and fluid retention, such as edema in the leg.

Pneumonia develops easily when the passages are persistently obstructed. Ultimately, repeated episodes of irritation and pneumonia cause scarring in the lung and some dilation of the obstructed alveoli, leading to COPD (▼ Figure 10-7).

Another type of COPD is called <u>emphysema</u>. Emphysema is a loss of the elastic material around the air spaces as a result of chronic stretching of the alveoli when bronchitic airways obstruct easy expulsion of gases. Smoking can also directly destroy the elasticity of the lung tissue. Normally, lungs act like a spongy balloon that is inflated; once they are inflated, they will naturally recoil because of their elastic nature, expelling gas rapidly. However, when they are constantly obstructed or when the "balloon's" elasticity is

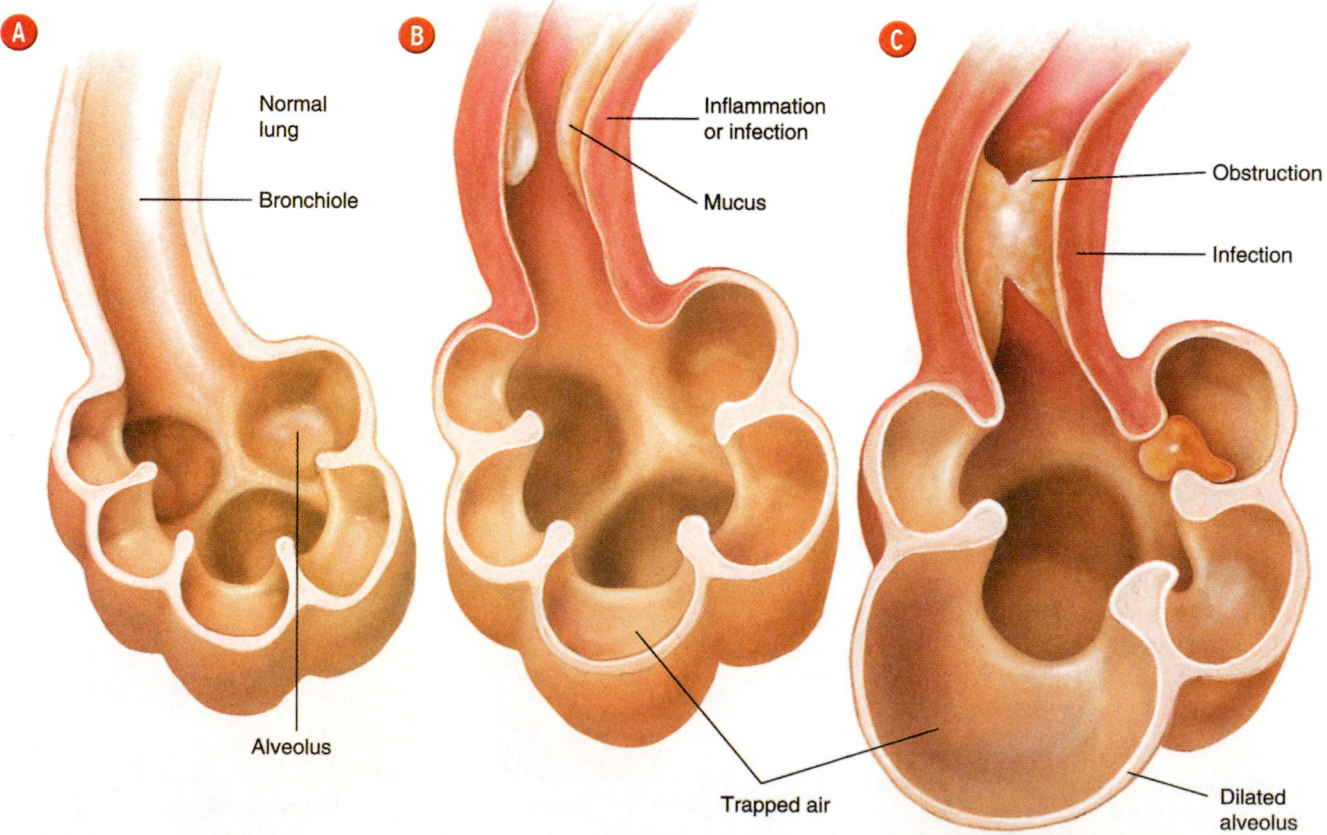

Normal lung

Bronchiole

Alveolus

Inflammation or infection

Mucus

Trapped air

Obstruction

Infection

Dilated alveolus

Figure 10-7 Repeated episodes of irritation and inflammation in the alveoli result in the obstruction, scarring, and some dilation of the alveolar sac characteristic of COPD. **A.** Normal alveolus. **B.** Infection produces mucus and swelling. **C.** A mucous plug creates an obstruction and further dilation of the alveolus.

diminished, air is no longer expelled rapidly, and the walls of the alveoli eventually fall apart, leaving large "holes" in the lung that resemble a large air pocket or cavity. This condition is called emphysema.

Most patients with COPD have elements of both chronic bronchitis and emphysema. Some patients will have more elements of one condition than the other; few patients will have only emphysema or bronchitis. Therefore, most patients with COPD will chronically produce sputum, have a chronic cough, and have difficulty expelling air from their lungs, with long expiration phases and wheezing.

Patients with COPD cannot handle pulmonary infections well, because the existing airway damage makes them unable to cough up the mucus or sputum produced by the infection. The chronic airway obstruction makes it difficult to breathe deeply enough to clear the lungs. Gradually, the arterial oxygen level falls, and the carbon dioxide level rises. If a new infection of the lung occurs in a patient with COPD, the arterial oxygen level may fall rapidly. In a few patients, the carbon dioxide level may rise high enough to cause sleepiness. These patients require respiratory support and careful administration of oxygen.

Patients with COPD usually are older than 50 years. They will always have a history of recurring lung problems and are almost always long-term cigarette smokers. Patients with COPD may complain of tightness in the chest and constant fatigue. Because air has been gradually and continuously trapped in their lungs in increasing amounts, their chests often have a barrel-like appearance ▶ **Figure 10-8** . If you listen to the chest with a stethoscope, you will hear abnormal breath sounds. These may include **rales**, which are crackling, rattling sounds that are usually associated with fluid in the lungs but here are related to chronic scarring of small airways. **Rhonchi**, which are coarse, gravelly sounds caused by mucus in the airways, and high-pitched, whistling **wheezes**, which are expiratory sounds common to patients with asthma, may be heard as well. Because of large emphysematous air pockets and diminished airflow, sounds of breathing are frequently hard to hear and may be detected only high up on the posterior chest.

The patient with COPD usually presents with a long history of dyspnea with a sudden increase in shortness of breath. There is rarely a history of chest pain. More often, the patient will remember having had a recent "chest cold" with fever and either inability to cough up mucus or a sudden increase in sputum. If the patient is able to cough up sputum, it will be thick and is often green or yellow, denoting a concurrent pulmonary infection. The blood pressure of patients with COPD is normal; however, the pulse is rapid and occasionally irregular. Pay particular attention to the respirations. They may be rapid, or they may be very slow.

Spontaneous Pneumothorax

Normally, the "vacuum" pressure in the pleural space keeps the lung inflated. When the surface of the lung is disrupted, however, air escapes into the pleural cavity, and the negative vacuum pressure is lost; the natural elasticity of the lung tissue causes the lung to collapse. The accumulation of air in the pleural space, which may be partial or complete, is called a **pneumothorax** ▶ **Figure 10-9** . Pneumothorax is most often caused by trauma, but it can also be caused by some medical conditions without any injury. In these patients, the condition is called a "spontaneous" pneumothorax.

Spontaneous pneumothorax may occur in patients with certain chronic lung infections or in young people born with weak areas of the lung. Patients with emphysema and asthma are at high risk for spontaneous pneumothorax when a weakened portion of lung ruptures,

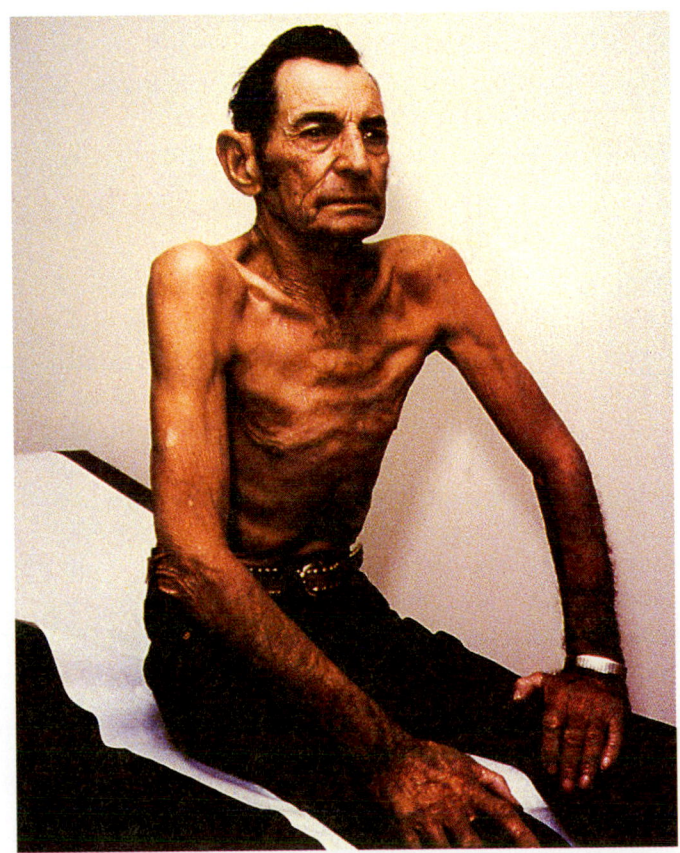

Figure 10-8 Typically, a patient with COPD uses accessory muscles and pursed lips for breathing. Notice, also, that the patient is sitting in the tripod position.

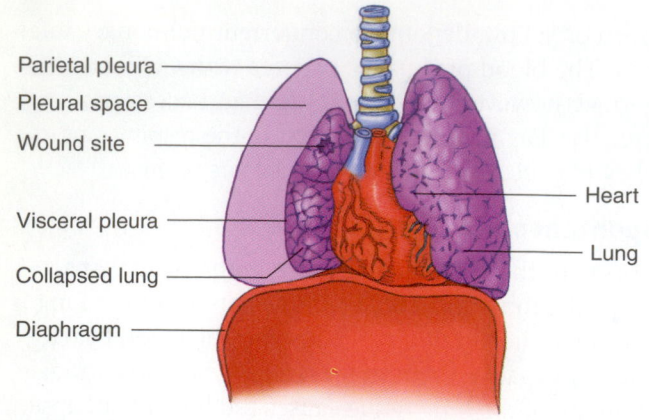

Parietal pleura
Pleural space
Wound site
Visceral pleura
Collapsed lung
Diaphragm
Heart
Lung

Figure 10-9 A pneumothorax occurs when air leaks into the pleural space from an opening in the chest wall or the surface of the lung. The lung collapses as air fills the pleural space and the two pleural surfaces are no longer in contact.

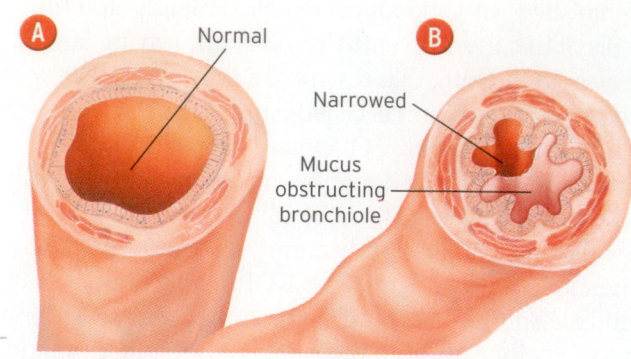

A   Normal   B
Narrowed
Mucus obstructing bronchiole

Figure 10-10 Asthma is an acute spasm of the bronchioles. **A.** Cross-section of a normal bronchiole. **B.** The bronchiole in spasm; a mucous plug has formed and partially obstructed the bronchiole.

often during coughing. A patient with a spontaneous pneumothorax becomes dyspneic (short of breath) and can complain of **pleuritic chest pain**, a sharp, stabbing pain on one side that is worse during breathing or with certain movement of the chest wall. By listening to the chest with the stethoscope, you can sometimes tell that breath sounds are absent or decreased on the affected side. However, altered breath sounds are very difficult to detect in a patient with severe emphysema. Spontaneous pneumothorax may be the cause of sudden dyspnea in a patient with underlying emphysema.

Asthma and Allergic Reactions

Asthma is an acute spasm of the smaller air passages called bronchioles, associated with excessive mucus production and sometimes with spasm of the bronchiolar muscles (▶ **Figure 10-10**). It is a common but serious disease, affecting about 6 million Americans and killing some 4,000 to 5,000 Americans each year. Asthma produces a characteristic wheezing as patients attempt to exhale through partially obstructed air passages. These same air passages open easily during inspiration. In other words, when patients inhale, breathing appears relatively normal; the wheezing is heard only when they exhale. This wheezing may be so loud that you can hear it without a stethoscope. In other cases, the airways are so blocked that no air movement is heard. In severe cases, the actual work of exhaling is very tiring, and cyanosis and/or respiratory arrest may quickly develop, even within minutes.

Asthma affects patients of all ages and is usually the result of an allergic reaction to an inhaled, ingested, or injected substance. Note that the substance itself is not the cause of the allergic reaction; rather, it is an exagger-

ated response of the body's immune system to that substance that causes the reaction. In some cases, however, there is no identifiable substance, or **allergen**, that triggers the body's immune system. Almost anything can be considered an allergen. An allergic response to certain foods or some other allergen may produce an acute asthma attack. Between attacks, patients may breathe normally. In its most severe form, an allergic reaction can produce anaphylaxis and even anaphylactic shock. This, in turn, may cause respiratory distress that is severe enough to result in coma and death. Asthma attacks may also be caused by severe emotional stress, being exposed to a cold environment, exercise, or respiratory infections.

Most patients with asthma are familiar with their symptoms and know when an attack is imminent. Typically, they will have appropriate medication either with them or at home. You should listen carefully to what these patients tell you; they often know exactly what they need.

ASTHMA AND ANAPHYLACTIC REACTIONS. Patients who do not have asthma may still have severe allergic reactions. The same allergens that may cause asthma attacks may cause anaphylaxis, a reaction characterized by airway swelling and dilation of blood vessels all over the body, which may lower blood pressure significantly. Anaphylaxis may be associated with widespread itching and an asthmalike condition. The airway may swell so much that breathing problems can progress from extreme difficulty in breathing to total airway obstruction in a matter of a few minutes. Most anaphylactic reactions occur within 30 minutes of exposure to the allergen, which can be anything from eating certain nuts to receiving a penicillin injection. For some patients, this may be the first time they had such a reaction to the substance. Therefore, they may not know what caused the swelling and allergic reaction. In other cases, the patient may know of the allergen but not be aware of exposure. In severe cases, epinephrine is the treatment of choice. Oxygen and antihistamines are also useful. As always, medical direction should guide appropriate therapy.

HAY FEVER. A much milder and more common allergy problem is hay fever. This is caused by an allergic reaction to pollen. In some areas of the country where pollen is present in the air throughout the year, hay fever is almost a universal illness. Generally, it does not produce major emergency problems. It does produce a number of difficulties in the upper respiratory tract, such as a stuffy or runny nose and sneezing.

Pleural Effusions

A **pleural effusion** is a collection of fluid outside the lung on one or both sides of the chest; in compressing the lung or lungs, it causes dyspnea (▼ **Figure 10-11**). This fluid may collect in large volumes in response to any irritation, infection, or cancer. Though it can build up gradually, over days or even weeks, patients often

report that their dyspnea came on suddenly. Pleural effusions should be considered as a contributing diagnosis in any patient with lung cancer and shortness of breath.

When you listen with a stethoscope to the chest of a patient with dyspnea resulting from pleural effusions, you will hear decreased breath sounds over the region of the chest where fluid has moved the lung away from the chest wall. These patients frequently feel better if they are sitting upright. Nothing will really relieve their symptoms, however, except removal of the fluid, which must be done by a physician.

Mechanical Obstruction of the Airway

As a rescuer, you should always be aware of the possibility that a patient with dyspnea may have a mechanical obstruction of the airway and be prepared to treat it quickly. In semiconscious and unconscious individuals, the obstruction may be the result of aspiration of vomitus or a foreign object (▼ **Figure 10-12A**), or of a position of the head that causes obstruction by the tongue (▼ **Figure 10-12B**). Opening the airway with the head tilt-chin lift maneuver may solve the problem. You should perform this maneuver only after you have

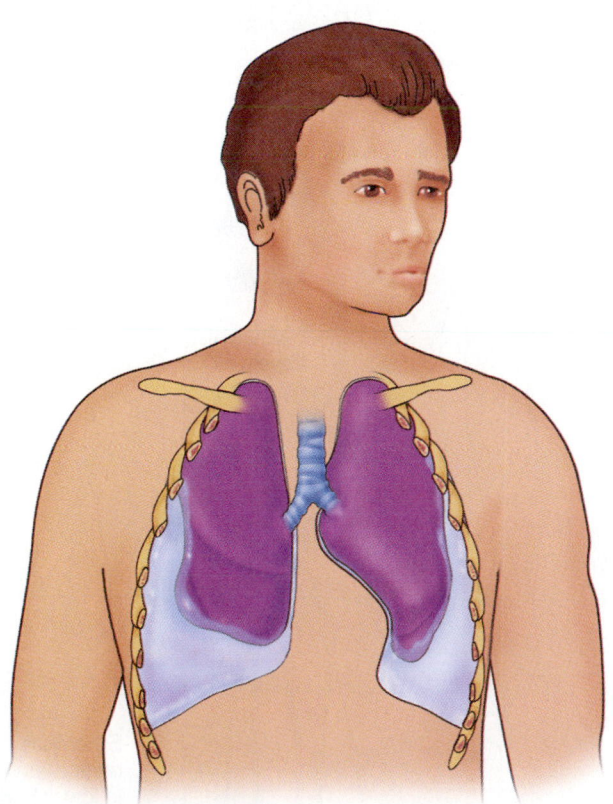

Figure 10-11 With a pleural effusion, fluid may accumulate in large volumes on one or both sides, compressing the lungs and causing dyspnea.

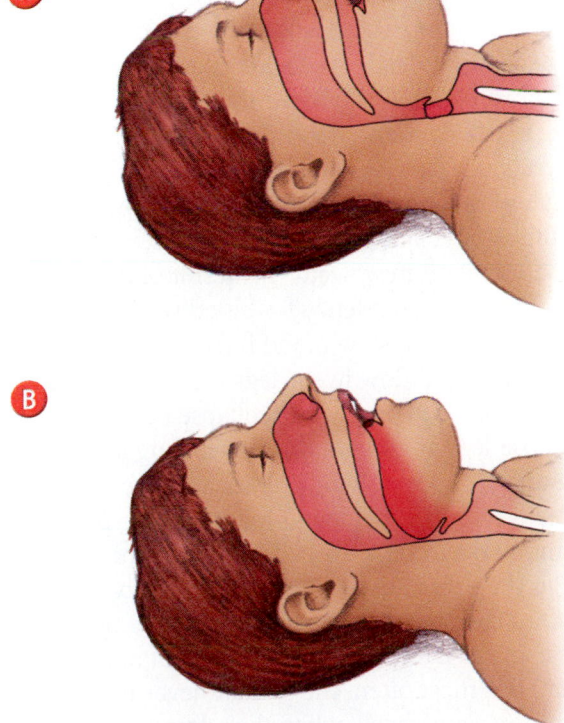

Figure 10-12 A. Foreign body obstruction occurs when an object, such as food, is lodged in the airway. B. Mechanical obstruction also occurs when the head is not properly positioned, causing the tongue to fall back into the throat.

ruled out a head or neck injury. If simply opening the airway does not correct the breathing problem, you will have to assess the upper airway for the obstruction.

Always consider upper airway obstruction from a foreign body first in patients who were eating just before becoming short of breath. The same is true of young children, especially crawling babies, who might have swallowed and choked on a small object.

Pulmonary Embolism

An **embolus** is anything in the circulatory system that moves from its point of origin to a distant site and lodges there, obstructing subsequent blood flow in that area. Beyond the point of obstruction, circulation can be completely cut off or at least markedly decreased, which can result in a serious, life-threatening condition. Emboli can be fragments of blood clots in an artery or vein that break off and travel through the bloodstream. They also can be foreign bodies that enter the circulation, such as a bullet or a bubble of air.

A **pulmonary embolism** is the passage of a blood clot formed in a vein, usually in the legs or pelvis, that breaks off and circulates through the venous system. The large clot moves through the right side of the heart and into the pulmonary artery or one of its arterial branches, where it becomes lodged, significantly decreasing or blocking blood flow (▶ Figure 10-13). Even though the lung is actively involved in inhalation and exhalation of air, no exchange of oxygen or carbon dioxide takes place in the areas of blocked blood flow because there is no effective circulation. In this circumstance, the level of arterial carbon dioxide usually rises, and the oxygen level may drop enough to cause cyanosis. More importantly, blood clots can inhibit circulation and cause significant dyspnea.

Pulmonary emboli may occur as a result of damage to the lining of vessels, a tendency for blood to clot unusually fast, or, most often, slow blood flow in a lower extremity. Slow blood flow in the legs is usually caused by bed rest, which can lead to the collapse of veins. Patients whose legs are immobilized following a fracture or recent surgery are at risk for pulmonary emboli for days or weeks after the incident. Only rarely do pulmonary emboli occur in active, healthy individuals.

Although they are fairly common, pulmonary emboli are difficult to diagnose. They occur about 650,000 times a year in the United States. Ten percent are immediately fatal, but most often, the patient never notices them. Symptoms and signs, when they do occur, include the following:

- Dyspnea
- Acute pleuritic chest pain
- Hemoptysis (coughing up blood)
- Cyanosis
- Tachypnea
- Varying degrees of hypoxia

With a large enough embolus, complete, sudden obstruction of the right heart's output of blood flow can result in sudden death.

Hyperventilation Syndrome

When dyspnea occurs in a patient with no lung abnormalities, it is called hyperventilation syndrome. **Hyperventilation** is defined as overbreathing to the point that the level of arterial carbon dioxide falls below normal. This is normal at high altitude but may be an indicator of major, life-threatening illness. For example, a patient with diabetes who has very high

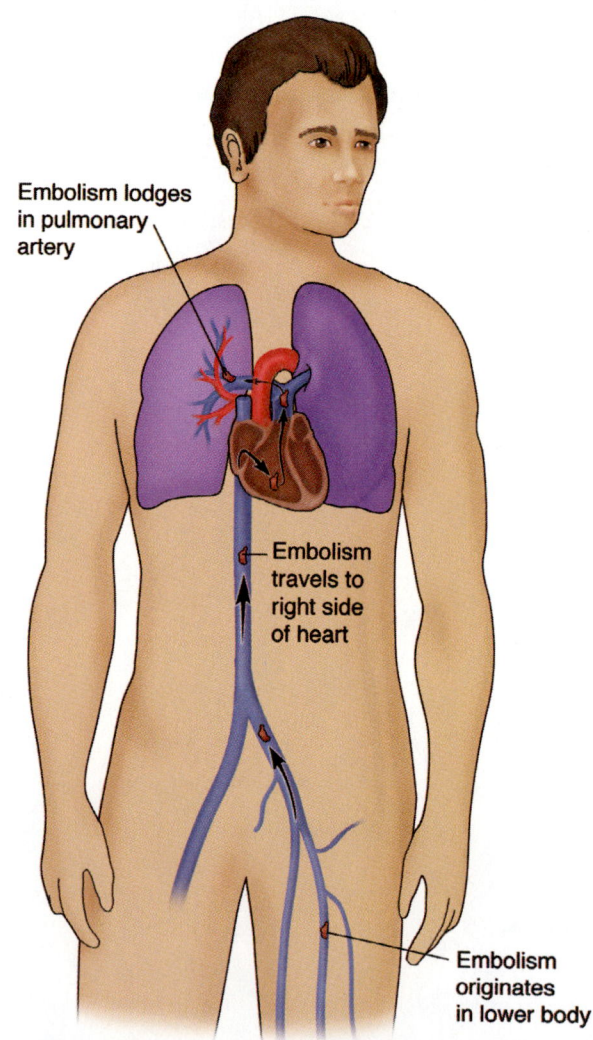

Embolism lodges in pulmonary artery

Embolism travels to right side of heart

Embolism originates in lower body

Figure 10-13 A pulmonary embolus is a blood clot from the vein that breaks off, circulates through the venous system, and moves through the right side of the heart into the pulmonary artery. Here, it can become lodged and significantly obstruct blood flow.

blood glucose levels, a patient who has overdosed with aspirin, or a patient with a severe infection is likely to hyperventilate. In these patients, rapid, deep breathing is the body's attempt to stay alive. The body is trying to compensate for *acidosis*, the buildup of excess acid in the blood or body tissues, resulting from the primary illness. Because carbon dioxide, mixed with water in the bloodstream, can add to the blood's acidity, lowering the level of carbon dioxide helps to compensate for the other acids.

Similarly, in an otherwise healthy person, blood acidity can be diminished by excessive breathing during a panic attack, because it "blows off" too much carbon dioxide. The result is a relative lack of acids. The resulting condition, *alkalosis*, is the buildup of excess base (lack of acids), in the body fluids.

Alkalosis is the cause of many of the symptoms associated with *hyperventilation syndrome*, including anxiety, dizziness, numbness, tingling of the hands and feet, and even a sense of dyspnea despite the rapid breathing. Although hyperventilation can be the response to illness and a buildup of acids, hyperventilation syndrome is not the same thing. Instead, this syndrome occurs in the absence of other physical problems. However, it is very common during psychological stress, affecting some 10% of the population at one time or another. The respirations of an individual who is experiencing hyperventilation syndrome may be as high as more than 40 shallow breaths/min or as low as only 20 very deep breaths/min.

The decision whether hyperventilation is being caused by a life-threatening illness or a panic attack should not be made outside the hospital. All patients who are hyperventilating should be given supplemental oxygen and transported to the hospital, where physicians will make that medical decision.

Emergency Care of Respiratory Emergencies

When taking the initial vital signs of a person with dyspnea, you should pay particular attention to respirations. Always speak with assurance and assume a concerned, professional approach to reassure the patient, who is probably very frightened. You will usually administer oxygen. Take great care in monitoring the respirations as you do so. Reevaluate the respirations and the patient's response to oxygen repeatedly, at least every 5 minutes, until you reach the emergency department. In a person with a chronically high carbon dioxide level (eg, certain patients with COPD), this is critical, because the supplemental oxygen may cause a rapid rise in the arterial oxygen level. This, in turn, may abolish the secondary respiratory oxygen drive and cause respiratory arrest.

Altitude Tips

The most dangerous of the common types of altitude illness is pulmonary edema. As low as 8,000' (2,400 m), but normally above 9,000' (2,700 m), high-pressure shunts and hypoxia cause both increased capillary pressure and capillary wall damage. Regardless of what causes the pulmonary edema, the result is that the lung stiffens and can no longer take in oxygen. Bubbly sounds, wheezes, and rattles are often audible with an unaided ear. The patient is short of breath, coughs frequently, may be cyanotic, and finds it easier to breathe in a sitting position.

Do *not* withhold oxygen for fear of depressing or stopping breathing in a patient with COPD who needs oxygen. Slowing of respirations after administration of oxygen does not necessarily mean that the patient no longer needs the oxygen; he or she may need it even more. If respirations slow and the patient becomes unconscious, you should assist breathing with a BVM device.

Approach to the Patient in Respiratory Distress

Your first questions are always the same: Is the patient conscious? Is he or she breathing? If not, you must take action. Assess the airway and give two ventilations. As you ventilate, you need to ask another series of questions, as follows:

1. **Is air going into the lungs?** Look for clues in the rise and fall of the chest, the respirations, and the heart rate.

2. **When you squeeze the BVM device, does the chest wall expand?**

3. **When you release the bag, does the chest fall?** If not, something is wrong. Try to reposition the patient and insert an oral airway to keep the tongue from blocking the airway. Reposition the head. Reassess your hand position and face mask seal.

Next, assess the rate at which you are assisting the patient's ventilations. You need to give breaths at roughly the same rate as the patient would if he or she were breathing spontaneously (eg, 12 to 20/min). Rescuers often get excited and ventilate the patient too quickly. Breathing for the patient too rapidly can cause harm. With rapid squeezing of the bag, higher pressures force the air rapidly into the lungs. Higher pressures can fill the stomach, as well as the lungs, with air. If the air and fluid in the stomach come back up the esophagus, vomit may enter the lungs, which can cause a serious form of pneumonia. Adults should be given one breath every 5 seconds. School-aged children need a smaller breath every 3 seconds. Infants need a small breath every 3 seconds. Use an appropriately sized BVM device for each.

Finally, assess the pulse. If the patient has a pulse, continue to support respirations. Measure the pulse rate; if it is normal, chances are that the patient is receiving enough oxygen to support life. If the pulse rate is too fast (more than 100/min) or too slow (less than 60/min), the patient may not be getting enough oxygen. Recheck everything. Is the oxygen bottle hooked up to the mask? Is the oxygen turned on? Is the flow rate adequate (10 to 15 L/min)? Is there a good face mask seal? Is the chest rising and falling with each breath? Is the airway blocked with vomit or the tongue?

SIGNS AND SYMPTOMS. If the patient is breathing, you need to decide whether the breathing is adequate. ▶ Table 10-2 lists the clues that will help you to decide if there is a breathing difficulty.

FOCUSED HISTORY AND PHYSICAL EXAMINATION. After you form your general impression and have completed the initial assessment, ask the patient to describe the problem. Begin by asking an open-ended question: "What can you tell me about your breathing?" Pay close attention to OPQRST: when the problem began (onset), what makes the breathing difficulty worse (provocation), how the breathing feels (quality), and whether the discomfort moves (radiation). How much of a problem is the patient having (severity)? Is the problem continuous or intermittent (time)? If it is intermittent, how long does it last? Does the patient smoke?

Find out what the patient has already done for the breathing problem. Does the patient use a prescribed inhaler? If so, when was it used last? How many doses have been taken? Does the patient use more than one inhaler? Find out whether the patient has any allergies or history of medication reactions.

INTERVENTIONS. If the patient complains of breathing difficulty, you should administer supplemental oxygen. In general, you do not need to worry about giving too much oxygen. Put a nonrebreathing face mask on the patient and supply oxygen at a rate of 10 to 15 L/min (enough to maintain the reservoir bag) in a patient with severe difficulty breathing. Then continue your assessment. Obtain a set of vital signs and document them.

As was stated previously, there is some concern about suppression of the "hypoxic" drive to breathe in some patients with COPD. Unless these patients are unresponsive, a more conservative approach is suggested. In patients who have longstanding COPD and probable carbon dioxide retention, administration of low-flow oxygen (2 L/min) is a good place to start, with adjustments to 3 L/min, then 4 L/min, and so on until symp-

toms have improved (for example, the patient has less dyspnea or a better mental status). When in doubt, err on the side of more oxygen, and monitor the patient closely.

Patients who call for help because of breathing difficulty are likely to have had the same trouble before. They probably have prescribed medications to use that are delivered by inhaler. If so, you may be able to help them use it. Remember to report what the medication is, when the patient last took a puff, how many puffs were used at that time, and what the label states regarding dosage. Be certain that the inhaler belongs to the patient, it contains the correct medication, the expiration date has not passed, and the correct dose is being administered. Help the patient repeat doses of the medication if the maximum dose has not been exceeded and the patient is still experiencing shortness of breath.

If the patient does not have a prescribed inhaler, continue with the focused history and physical exam. Even patients who use their inhaler may continue to get worse. You need to reassess breathing frequently and be prepared to assist ventilations in severe cases. If you must assist ventilation in a patient who is having an asthma attack, use slow, gentle breaths. Remember, the problem in asthma is getting the air out of the lungs, not into them. Resist the temptation to squeeze the bag hard and fast. Always assist with ventilations as a last resort, and then provide only about 10 to 12 shallow breaths/min.

Prescribed Inhalers

Some of the most common medications used for shortness of breath are called inhaled beta-agonists, which dilate breathing passages. Typical trade names are Proventil, Ventolin, Alupent, Serevent, and Brethine. The generic name for Proventil and Ventolin is albuterol; for Alupent, it is metaproterenol; for Serevent, it is salmeterol; and for Brethine, it is terbutaline. The action of most of these medications is to relax the muscles that surround the bronchioles in the lungs, leading to enlargement (dilation) of the airways and easier passage of air. Common side effects of inhalers used for acute shortness of breath include increased pulse rate, nervousness, and muscle tremors.

If the patient has a prescribed metered-dose inhaler, read the label carefully to make sure that the medication is to be used for shortness of breath and that it has, in fact, been prescribed by a physician ▶ Figure 10-14 . When in doubt, consult medical control.

Before helping a patient to self-administer any metered-dose inhaler medication, make sure that the medication is indicated, that is, the patient has signs and symptoms of shortness of breath. Finally, check that there are no contraindications for its use, such as the following:

TABLE 10-2 Signs and Symptoms of Inadequate Breathing

- **The patient complains of difficulty breathing.**
- **The patient appears anxious or restless.** This can happen if the brain is not getting enough oxygen for its needs. Check the vital signs.
- **The patient's respiratory rate is too slow** (respirations are less than 8 breaths/min), you may need to assist ventilations with a BVM device.
- **The patient's skin is blue (cyanotic).** The tongue, nailbeds, and inside the lips are good places to look for cyanosis. These all have a large collection of blood vessels and thin skin, making bluish blood easy to see.
- **The patient is wheezing, gurgling, snoring, or crowing.** Common causes of stridor include a foreign body obstruction and infection.
- **The patient cannot speak more than a few words between breaths.** Ask the patient something such as "How are you doing?" If the patient cannot speak at all, he or she probably has a respiratory emergency that will need immediate attention.
- **The patient is using the accessory muscles in the neck to assist breathing.** If the patient is using only the diaphragm to breathe, suspect damage to the nerves that carry breathing commands to the chest muscles; the diaphragm may be getting the command to breathe, but because of spinal cord injury, the chest muscles may not.
- **The patient has an altered mental status associated with shallow or slow breathing.**

- **The patient is coughing excessively,** which might mean that the patient has anything from a mild upper respiratory infection or hay fever to pneumonia, asthma, or pulmonary edema.
- **The patient's breathing rhythm is irregular.** Because the brain controls breathing, an irregular breathing rhythm may indicate a head injury. In this case, the patient will probably be unresponsive.
- **The patient is sitting up, leaning forward** with palms flat on the table or the arms of the chair. This is called the tripod position, because the back and two arms are working together to support the upper body. This position allows the diaphragm the most room to function and helps the patient to use accessory muscles to assist breathing. It is usually a good idea to let the patient stay in the most comfortable position.
- **The chest has a barrel shape.** In certain chronic lung diseases, because air has been gradually and continuously trapped within the lung in increasing amounts, the distance from front to back gets longer, nearly equaling the side-to-side distance. A barrel chest may indicate a long history of breathing problems.
- **The conjunctivae are pale.** Perhaps the patient is short of breath because there are not enough red blood cells to carry oxygen to the tissues.
- **The patient has an increased pulse and respirations** (heart rate more than 100 beats/min or respirations more than 24 breaths/min).

- The patient is unable to help coordinate inhalation with depression of the trigger, perhaps because the patient is too confused.
- The inhaler is not prescribed for this patient.
- Your local protocol prohibits assisting patients to self-administer medications.
- The patient had already met the maximum prescribed dose before your arrival.

ADMINISTRATION OF METERED-DOSE INHALER MEDICATION. To help a patient self-administer medication from an inhaler, follow these steps (▶ **Skill Drill 10-1**):

1. **Obtain the patient's permission** to help with self-administration.
2. **Check that you have** the right medication, the right patient, and the right route **(Step 1)**.

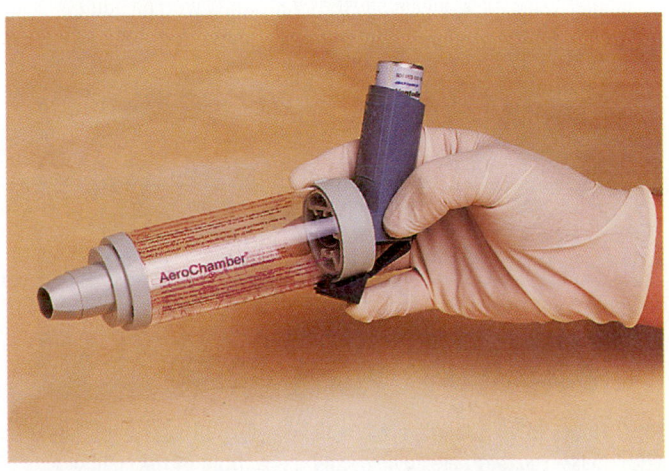

Figure 10-14 Make sure the inhaler has been prescribed by a physician.

3. **Make sure that the patient is alert** enough to use the inhaler.

4. **Check the expiration date** of the inhaler.

5. **Check to see whether the patient** has already taken any doses.

6. **Make sure the inhaler** is at room temperature or warmer.

Rescuer Tips

While one rescuer is getting oxygen ready, the second rescuer should try to coach the patient with asthma or COPD to use "pursed-lip" breathing. The increase in back pressure will help air flow through narrowed bronchioles.

Pediatric Needs

Asthma is a common childhood illness. When assessing a pediatric patient, look for retraction of the skin above the sternum and between the ribs. Retractions are typically easier to see in children than in adults. Cyanosis is a late finding in children. Keep in mind that a cough may not be a symptom of a cold; it could signal pneumonia or asthma. Even if you do not hear much wheezing, the presence of a cough can indicate that some degree of reactive airway disease, or an acute asthma attack may be taking place.

The emergency care of a child with shortness of breath is the same as it is for an adult, including the use of supplemental oxygen. However, many small children will not tolerate (or may refuse to wear) a face mask. Rather than fighting with the child, hold the oxygen mask in front of the child's face or ask the parent to hold the mask (▼ **Figure 10-15**). Many children with asthma also will have prescribed hand-held metered-dose inhalers. Use these inhalers just as you would with an adult.

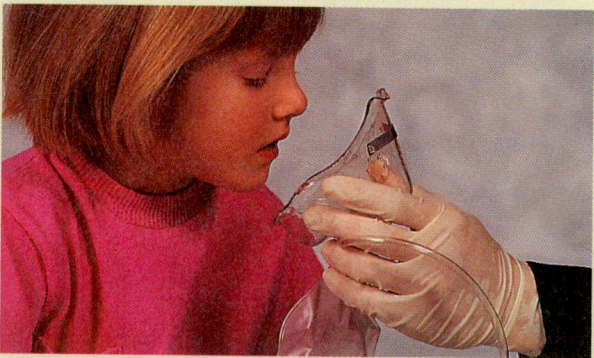

Figure 10-15 Because children may refuse to wear an oxygen mask, you may have to hold the mask in front of the child's face. If the child still refuses, enlist the parents' help.

7. **Shake the inhaler** vigorously several times.

8. **Stop administering** supplemental oxygen and remove any mask from the patient's face.

9. **Ask the patient** to exhale deeply and, before inhaling, to put his or her lips around the opening of the inhaler.

10. **If the patient has a spacer,** use it to allow more effective use of the medication **(Step 2)**.

11. **Have the patient** depress the hand-held inhaler as he or she begins to inhale deeply.

12. **Instruct the patient** to hold his or her breath for as long as is comfortable to help the body absorb the medication **(Step 3)**.

13. **Continue to administer** supplemental oxygen.

14. **Allow the patient** to breathe a few times, then repeat with a second dose if indicated by instructions on the inhaler **(Step 4)**.

REASSESSMENT. You need to carefully watch patients with shortness of breath. About 5 minutes after the patient uses an inhaler, obtain the vital signs again and perform a focused reassessment. Ask the patient whether the treatment made any difference. Look at the patient's chest to see whether the patient is still using accessory muscles to breathe. Listen to the patient's speech pattern. Keep in mind that the patient may get worse instead of better, and be prepared to assist ventilations with a BVM device.

After helping the patient with the inhaler treatment, transport the patient to the emergency department. While en route, continue to assess the patient's breathing. Try talking to calm and reassure the patient and continue to give supplemental oxygen.

Treatment of Specific Conditions

INFECTION OF THE UPPER OR LOWER AIRWAY. Dyspnea associated with acute infections is quite common. Except for the patient with pneumonia, acute bronchitis, or epiglottitis, it is rarely serious. The acute congestion and stuffiness of a common cold hardly ever require emergency care. Indeed, most people with colds treat themselves with over-the-counter medications. However, individuals with a common cold who have underlying problems such as asthma or heart failure may experience a worsening of their condition as a result of the additional stress of the infection. In addition, cold medications may also have stressful side effects, such as agitation, increased heart rate, and increased blood pressure.

For patients with upper airway infections and dyspnea, administer humidified oxygen (if available). Do not attempt to suction the airway or place an oropharyngeal airway in a patient with suspected epiglot-

Skill Drill 10-1   Assisting a Patient with a Metered-Dose Inhaler

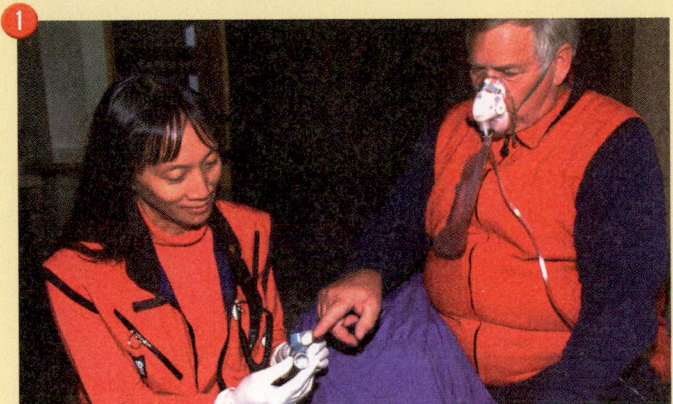

Check that you have the right medication, the right patient, and the right route.

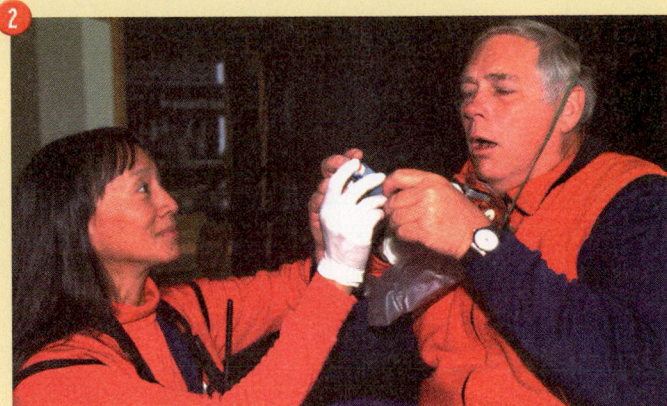

Remove oxygen mask.
Hand inhaler to the patient. Instruct the patient about breathing and lip seal.
Use a spacer if the patient has one.

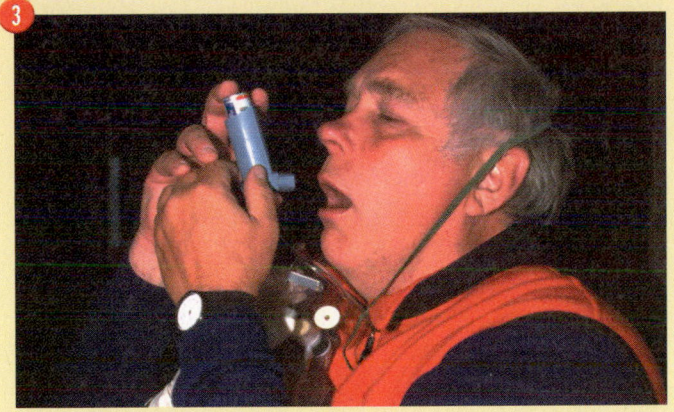

Instruct the patient to press the inhaler and inhale.
Instruct the patient about breath holding.

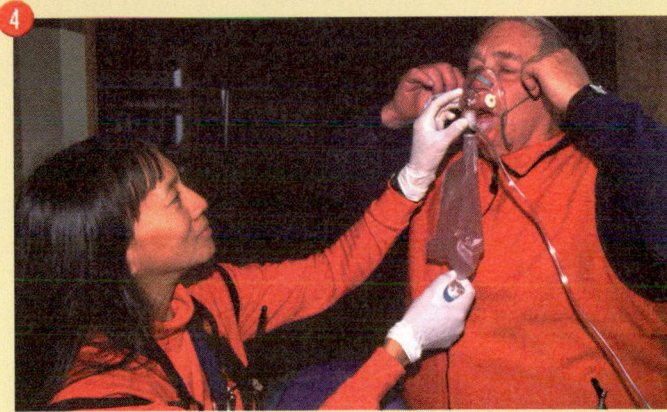

Reapply oxygen.
After a few breaths, have the patient repeat the dose if order/protocol allows.

titis. These maneuvers may cause a spasm and complete airway obstruction. Transport the patient promptly to the hospital. Allow the patient to sit in the position that is most comfortable. For someone with epiglottitis, this is usually sitting upright and leaning forward, the "sniffing position" ▶ **Figure 10-16** . To force a patient with epiglottitis to lie supine may cause upper airway obstruction that could result in death.

The dyspnea of pneumonia is caused not by upper airway obstruction but by the loss of effective lung volume and a need for more rapid air exchange. Here again, the problem will not be helped by the use of artificial airways but may improve with the administration of oxygen.

ACUTE PULMONARY EDEMA. Dyspnea caused by acute pulmonary edema may be associated with cardiac dis-

ease, direct lung damage, or high altitude. Administer 100% oxygen, and, if necessary, carefully suction any secretions from the airway. Provide prompt transport to the emergency department. The best position for a con-

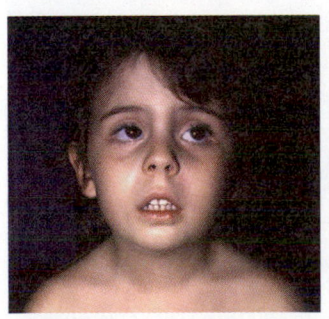
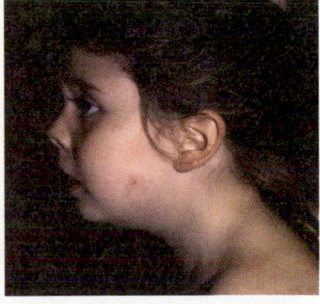

Figure 10-16 A child with respiratory edema may be more comfortable sitting up and leaning forward.

scious patient who has pulmonary edema is the one in which it is easiest to breathe. Usually, this is sitting up. Rarely will you need to use an artificial airway, because no upper airway obstruction problem exists. However, an unconscious patient with acute pulmonary edema may require full ventilatory support, including airway, positive pressure ventilation with oxygen, and suctioning.

CHRONIC OBSTRUCTIVE PULMONARY DISEASE. Patients with COPD may be semiconscious or unconscious from hypoxia, a condition in which the body's cells and tissues do not get enough oxygen, or from carbon dioxide retention. They may appear to be in respiratory distress and/or be cyanotic. They may have pursed lips and may be using accessory muscles to breathe, including those in the neck and shoulders.

Assist with the patient's prescribed inhaler if they have one. Transport patients with COPD as promptly as possible to the emergency department, allowing them to sit upright if this is most comfortable ▼ Figure 10-17 . Patients with COPD often find breathing difficult when lying down.

SPONTANEOUS PNEUMOTHORAX. Patients with spontaneous pneumothorax may have severe respiratory distress, or they may have no distress at all and complain only of pleuritic chest pain. Provide supplemental oxygen, and provide prompt transport to the hospital. Like most dyspneic patients, those with spontaneous pneumothorax are usually more comfortable sitting up. Monitor the patient carefully, watching for any sudden deterioration in the respiratory status. Be ready to support the airway, assist respirations, and give full cardiopulmonary support if it becomes necessary.

ASTHMA OR ALLERGIC REACTIONS. Many lung problems are incorrectly labeled "asthma"; therefore, your assessment of the patient is critical. A patient who truly has asthma will have a history of repeated episodes of sudden shortness of breath, in which he or she had difficulty exhaling. Confirm whether the patient is able to breathe normally at other times. If possible, ask family members to describe the patient's asthma. Even if they only identify wheezing as a problem, be aware that some forms of heart failure, foreign body aspiration, or high-altitude pulmonary edema may cause wheezing.

As you assess the patient's vital signs, note that the pulse rate will be normal or elevated, the blood pressure may be slightly elevated, and respirations will be increased. Assist with the patient's prescribed inhaler if he or she has one. Administer oxygen, and allow the patient to sit in an upright position, which makes breathing easier. Be reassuring; tension and anxiety make asthma attacks worse.

Ask questions about how and when the symptoms began, because reactions that follow a bee or wasp sting may progress rapidly to anaphylactic shock. A patient in anaphylactic shock may quickly become unconscious and require assisted ventilations and supplemental oxygen. If the patient is already unconscious upon your arrival, look for a medical identification tag that may provide a clue ▼ Figure 10-18 . Unconscious patients require prompt transport to the emergency department.

As you care for the patient, be prepared to suction large amounts of mucus from the mouth and to administer oxygen. If you do suction, do not withhold oxygen for more than 15 seconds for an adult patient, 10 seconds for a child, and 5 seconds for an infant. Allow some time for oxygenation between suction attempts. If the patient is unconscious, you may have to provide airway management.

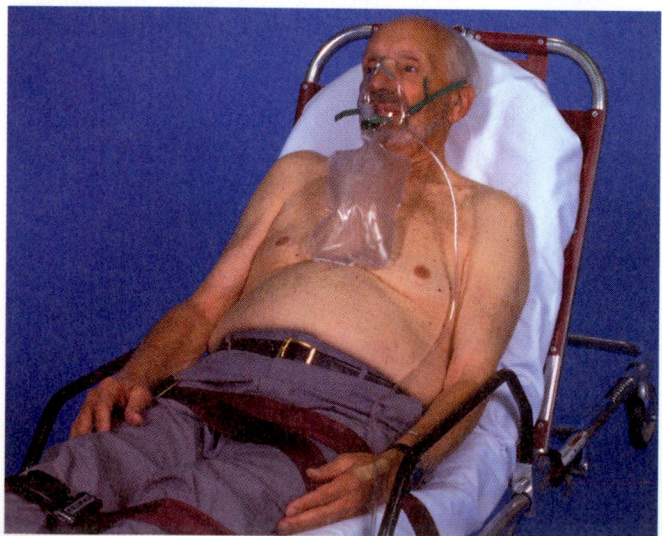

Figure 10-17 Transport a patient with COPD in an upright position if it is most comfortable. Ensure that you continue to monitor the patient.

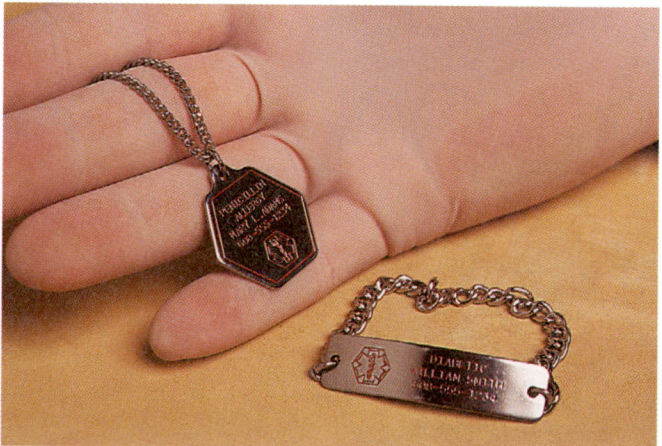

Figure 10-18 Some patients who are known to be severely allergic to bee stings, certain medications, or other substances often wear a medical identification tag.

If the patient carries medication, such as an epinephrine auto-injector, for an asthma attack or allergic reaction, you may help with its administration, as directed by local protocol. Keep in mind that epinephrine is a very potent agent with a number of significant side effects. Do not give it unless you are certain that the patient is having a severe asthma attack or severe allergic reaction and you know the history of the episode. Patients who experience an acute asthma or allergic attack and improve with administration of epinephrine should still be administered oxygen and transported to the hospital.

A prolonged asthma attack that is unrelieved by epinephrine may progress into a condition known as *status asthmaticus*. The patient is likely to be frightened, frantically trying to breathe, while using all the accessory muscles. Status asthmaticus is a true emergency, and the patient must be given oxygen and transported immediately to the emergency department.

The effort to breathe during an asthma attack is very tiring, and the patient may be exhausted by the time you arrive. An exhausted patient may have stopped feeling anxious or even struggling to breathe. This patient is not recovering; he or she is at a very critical stage and is likely to stop breathing. Aggressive airway management, oxygen administration, and prompt transport are essential in this situation. Tiering with ALS should be considered. Follow local protocol.

PLEURAL EFFUSIONS. Treatment of pleural effusions consists of removal of fluid collected outside the lung, which must be done by a physician in a hospital setting. However, you should provide oxygen and other routine support measures to these patients.

OBSTRUCTION OF THE UPPER AIRWAY. If the patient is a small child or someone who was eating just before dyspnea developed, you may assume that the problem is an inhaled or aspirated foreign body. If the patient is old enough to talk but cannot make any noise, upper airway obstruction is the likely cause. Generally, the patient will clutch his or her throat, try to speak, but be unable to do so.

The first thing to do is clear the upper airway. Using the Heimlich maneuver with abdominal thrusts for an adult or backblows for an infant can be lifesaving.

If you are successful in dislodging a foreign object, breathing should return to normal. If you are unsuccessful, or if breathing does not return to normal, administer supplemental oxygen and transport the patient promptly to the emergency department.

PULMONARY EMBOLISM. Because a considerable amount of lung tissue may not be functioning, supplemental oxygen is mandatory in a patient with a pulmonary embolism. Place the patient in a comfortable position, usually sitting, and assist breathing as necessary. Hemoptysis, if present, is usually not severe, but any blood that has been coughed up should be cleared from the airway. The patient may have an unusually rapid and possibly irregular heartbeat. Transport the patient to the emergency department promptly. Be aware that pulmonary emboli may cause cardiac arrest.

The following conditions require that the patient be transported rapidly to a hospital:

- Respiratory distress accompanied by one or more of these signs and symptoms: stridor, cyanosis, inability to speak, extreme or worsening fatigue or exhaustion, fever or shaking chills, signs and symptoms of shock, or a pulse rate of more than 130 beats/min.

- Suspected pneumonia, severe bronchitis, or pulmonary embolus.

- Evidence of heart disease, such as a positive medical history; an abnormal heart rate or rhythm; suspicious pain in the chest, neck, shoulder, or arm; or swelling of the ankles.

- An asthma attack that does not improve within 20 minutes of the patient taking his or her medication.

- Severe respiratory distress due to any cause, or respiratory distress of uncertain cause that does not improve with rest, reassurance, and a short period of high-flow oxygen.

HYPERVENTILATION. When you respond to a patient who is hyperventilating, complete an initial assessment and history of the event. Is the patient having chest pain? Is there a history of cardiac problems or diabetes? You must always assume a serious underlying problem even if you suspect that the underlying problem is stress. Do not have the patient breathe into a paper bag, even though it is thought to be the traditional technique for managing hyperventilation syndrome. In theory, breathing into a paper bag causes the patient to rebreathe exhaled carbon dioxide, allowing the level of carbon dioxide in the blood to return to normal. In fact, if the patient is hyperventilating because of a serious medical problem, this maneuver could make things worse. A patient with underlying pulmonary disease who breathes into a bag may become severely hypoxic. Treatment should instead consist of reassuring the patient in a calm, professional manner; supplying supplemental oxygen; and providing prompt transport to the emergency department. Patients who hyperventilate need to be evaluated in the hospital setting.

Chapter Sweep

Ready for Review

Dyspnea is a common complaint that may be caused by numerous medical problems, including infections of the upper or lower airway, acute pulmonary edema, chronic obstructive pulmonary disease, spontaneous pneumothorax, asthma or allergic reactions, pleural effusions, mechanical obstruction of the airway, pulmonary embolism, and hyperventilation. Each of these lung disorders interferes in one way or another with the exchange of oxygen and carbon dioxide that takes place during respiration. This interference may be in the form of damage to the alveoli, separation of the alveoli from the pulmonary vessels by fluid or infection, obstruction of the air passages, or air or excess fluid in the pleural space. Patients with longstanding lung diseases often have chronically high levels of blood carbon dioxide; in some cases, giving too much oxygen to these patients may depress or stop respirations. However, judicious use of oxygen is always an important priority in patients with dyspnea.

Signs and symptoms of breathing difficulty include abnormal respiratory rates, unusual breath sounds, including wheezing, stridor, rales, and rhonchi; nasal flaring; pursed lip breathing; cyanosis; inability to talk; use of accessory muscles to breathe; and sitting in the tripod position, which allows the diaphragm the most room to function.

In treating dyspnea, it is important to reassure the patient and provide supplemental oxygen. Remember to maintain the patient in a position that is comfortable for breathing, usually sitting upright. If the patient is not breathing, use a BVM device with oxygen to assist breathing. If the patient is breathing inadequately, apply oxygen through a nonrebreathing face mask with the oxygen flow set at 10 to 15 L/min. Next, perform a focused history and physical exam, including vital signs. If the patient has a prescribed inhaler or epinephrine auto-injector, the rescuer may assist with its use as directed by local protocol. Then transport the patient to the hospital, monitoring his or her condition on the way. Talking with the patient is a good way to monitor a breathing problem.

Remember, a patient who is breathing rapidly may be getting insufficient oxygen as a result of respiratory distress from a variety of problems, including high-altitude pulmonary edema, pneumonia, or a pulmonary embolism; trying to "blow off" more carbon dioxide to compensate for acidosis caused by a poison, a severe infection, or a high level of blood glucose; or having a stress reaction. In every case, prompt recognition of the problem, giving oxygen, and prompt transport are essential.

Vital Vocabulary

allergen A substance that causes an allergic reaction.

asthma A disease of the lungs in which muscle spasm in the small air passageways and the production of large amounts of mucus result in airway obstruction.

carbon dioxide retention A condition characterized by a chronically high blood level of carbon dioxide in which the respiratory center no longer responds to high blood levels of carbon dioxide.

chronic bronchitis Irritation of the major lung passageways, from either infectious disease or irritants such as smoke.

chronic obstructive pulmonary disease (COPD) A slow process of dilation and disruption of the airways and alveoli, caused by chronic bronchial obstruction.

common cold A viral infection usually associated with swollen nasal mucous membranes and the production of fluid from the sinuses and nose.

croup An infectious disease of the upper respiratory system that may cause partial airway obstruction and is characterized by a barking cough; usually seen in children.

diphtheria An infectious disease in which a membrane lining the pharynx is formed that can severely obstruct passage of air into the larynx.

dyspnea Shortness of breath or difficulty breathing.

embolus A blood clot or other substance in the circulatory system that travels to a blood vessel where it causes blockage.

emphysema A disease of the lungs in which there is extreme dilation and eventual destruction of pulmonary alveoli with poor exchange of oxygen and carbon dioxide; it is one form of chronic obstructive pulmonary disease (COPD).

epiglottitis An infectious disease in which the epiglottis becomes inflamed and enlarged and may cause upper airway obstruction.

hyperventilation Rapid or deep breathing that lowers blood carbon dioxide levels below normal.

hypoxia A condition in which the body's cells and tissues do not have enough oxygen.

hypoxic drive Backup system to control respirations when oxygen levels fall.

pleural effusion A collection of fluid between the lung and chest wall that may compress the lung.

pleuritic chest pain Sharp, stabbing pain in the chest that is worsened by a deep breath or other chest wall movement; often caused by inflammation or irritation of the pleura.

pneumonia An infectious disease of the lung that damages lung tissue.

pneumothorax A partial or complete accumulation of air in the pleural space.

pulmonary edema A buildup of fluid in the lungs, usually as a result of congestive heart failure, also from high altitude.

pulmonary embolism A blood clot that breaks off from a large vein and travels to the blood vessels of the lung, causing obstruction of blood flow.

rales Crackling, rattling breath sounds signaling fluid in the air spaces of the lungs or chronic scarring of small airways in patients with COPD.

rhonchi Coarse breath sounds heard in patients with chronic mucus in the airways.

stridor A harsh, high-pitched, barking inspiratory sound often heard in acute laryngeal (upper airway) obstruction.

wheeze A high-pitched, whistling breath sound, characteristically heard on expiration in patients with asthma or COPD.

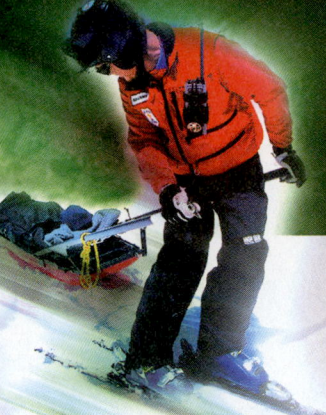

Assessment in Action

You receive a call for an adult with difficulty breathing at the warming hut. On arrival, you find a 38-year-old man sitting up, leaning forward, with his hands braced on his knees. You notice that his neck muscles are straining when he inhales and he appears pale. As you begin to ask him questions, he answers in short, three- to four-word phrases. He manages to tell you that he is allergic to cats, and two cats are in the hut.

The patient also tells you that he has a history of asthma and uses a Ventolin inhaler, but he left it in his car. The patient also tells you that he is allergic to dust, pollen, and penicillin. Your partner obtains baseline vital signs, which include a pulse of 122 beats/min and regular shallow respirations of 34 breaths/min; and a blood pressure of 152/90 mm Hg. His skin is cool and dry. Lung sounds disclose wheezes in both sides of his chest.

1. Which of the following assessment signs tell you that the patient has difficulty breathing?
   A. Vital signs and history
   B. Position and speech
   C. Vital signs and skin color
   D. History of allergies

2. The medical term for this patient's chief complaint is:
   A. apnea.
   B. dyspnea.
   C. anoxia.
   D. hyperventilation.

3. How do you know that this patient has accessory muscle use?
   A. His neck muscles are straining when he inhales.
   B. He is sitting in a hunched-over position.
   C. He is talking in three- to four-word phrases.
   D. His respiratory rate is 34 breaths/min.

4. This patient is sitting up, leaning forward with his hands braced on his knees. What is this position called?
   A. Hunched position
   B. COPD position
   C. Fowler's position
   D. Tripod position

5. A bystander offers to let the patient use her inhaler when the patient states that he left his inhaler in the car. The most appropriate course of action would be to:
   A. thank the bystander and state that the patient needs his own inhaler
   B. check the inhaler, then assist the patient with using the bystander's inhaler
   C. observe the patient as the bystander helps administer the inhaler
   D. obtain another set of vital signs, then assist the patient in using the inhaler

6. The patient finds an almost-empty inhaler in his briefcase and uses it. Which of the following would be considered a side effect of his Ventolin inhaler?
   A. Symptom relief and bradycardia
   B. Bradycardia and nervousness
   C. Nervousness and tachycardia
   D. Tachycardia and low blood pressure

7. This patient has asthma with wheezes in both sides of his chest. The sound of wheezes in a patient with asthma is caused by which of the following?
   A. Enlargement of the pulmonary blood vessels
   B. Excessive pleural effusions outside the lungs
   C. Excess fluid and scarring in the lungs
   D. Excess mucus and spasm of the bronchioles

Challenging Questions

8. En route to the hospital, this patient has a bout of coughing that resulted in a sudden onset of sharp, stabbing pain on one side of his chest wall that is worse during breathing and with certain movement of the chest wall. You listen with a stethoscope and can tell that breath sounds are decreased on that side. What has most likely happened to your patient, and why is your patient prone to this problem?

9. Patients with chronic lung diseases frequently have a chronically high level of blood carbon dioxide, which is the normal stimulus to breathe. When that happens, what takes over their stimulus to breathe?

10. If this patient exhibited a barrel chest, what would that tell you in terms of his respiratory problem?

Points to Ponder

You are returning from lunch when you hear the dispatch of another unit to a snow submersion about 6 minutes away from where you are. You "jump" the call and go to the scene. You arrive as rescuers hand out a 10-year-old boy. The child is cyanotic and unresponsive. You find a pulse but no breathing. Your partner has a child about that same age and is shaken by this call. Just before transport, the child "crashes," losing his pulse also. Even with the best care you could provide, the child dies. Now you are back out on duty, your partner is barely functioning, and when you close your eyes, you can see the child and the look on your partner's face as you took control of the scene. There are about 6 hours left

in your shift. Would you stay on duty? What would you do to help your partner? What would you do to help yourself?

Issues Incident Investigation, Risks of Being a Rescuer, Duty to Act, Signs of Irreversible Death, Critical Incident Stress Debriefing (CISD), Helping a Grieving Family

Online Outlook

The term COPD comprises emphysema and chronic bronchitis. The number of lives that are claimed by chronic lung disease has increased sharply over the past 20 years. To learn more about COPD, complete Exercise 10 at the www.OECzone.com.

www.OECzone.com

Cardiovascular Emergencies

Objectives

Cognitive

- ♠ 1. Describe the structure and function of the cardiovascular system (p 306).
- ♠ 2. Describe the emergency medical care of the patient experiencing chest pain/discomfort (p 313).
- ♠ 3. List the indications for automated external defibrillation (AED) (p 320).
- 4. List the contraindications for automated external defibrillation (p 320).
- ♠ 5. Define the role of rescuer in the emergency cardiac care system (p 306).
- 6. Explain the impact of age and weight on defibrillation (p 324).
- ♠ 7. Discuss the position of comfort for patients with various cardiac emergencies (p 312).
- ♠ 8. Establish the relationship between airway management and the patient with cardiovascular compromise (p 316).
- ♠ 9. Predict the relationship between the patient experiencing cardiovascular compromise and basic life support (p 315).
- ♠ 10. Discuss the fundamentals of early defibrillation (p 320).
- 11. Explain the rationale for early defibrillation (p 320).
- 12. Explain that not all chest pain patients result in cardiac arrest and do not need to be attached to an automated external defibrillator (p 320).
- ♠ 13. Explain the importance of prehospital ACLS intervention if it is available (p 324).
- ♠ 14. Explain the importance of urgent transport to a facility with Advanced Cardiac Life Support if it is not available in the prehospital setting (p 313).
- 15. Discuss the various types of automated external defibrillators (p 319).
- 16. Differentiate between the fully automated and the semiautomated defibrillator (p 319).
- ♠ 17. Discuss the procedures that must be taken into consideration for standard operations of the various types of automated external defibrillators (p 321).
- 18. State the reasons for assuring that the patient is pulseless and apneic when using the automated external defibrillator (p 320).
- 19. Discuss the circumstances which may result in inappropriate shocks (p 320).
- 20. Explain the considerations for interruption of CPR when using the automated external defibrillator (p 321).
- 21. Discuss the advantages and disadvantages of automated external defibrillators (p 319).
- 22. Summarize the speed of operation of automated external defibrillation (p 320).
- 23. Discuss the use of remote defibrillation through adhesive pads (p 320).
- 24. Discuss the special considerations for rhythm monitoring (p 320).
- 25. List the steps in the operation of the automated external defibrillator (p 321).
- 26. Discuss the standard of care that should be used to provide care to a patient with persistent ventricular fibrillation and no available ACLS (p 323).
- 27. Discuss the standard of care that should be used to provide care to a patient with recurrent ventricular fibrillation and no available ACLS (p 323).
- 28. Differentiate between the single rescuer and multi-rescuer care with an automated external defibrillator (p 323).
- 29. Explain the reason for pulses not being checked between shocks with an automated external defibrillator (p 321).
- ♠ 30. Discuss the importance of coordinating ACLS trained providers with personnel using automated external defibrillators (p 324).
- 31. Discuss the importance of postresuscitation care (p 323).
- 32. List the components of postresuscitation care (p 323).
- 33. Explain the importance of frequent practice with the automated external defibrillator (p 327).
- 34. Discuss the need to complete the Automated Defibrillator: Operator's Shift Checklist (p 326).
- 35. Discuss the role of the American Heart Association (AHA) in the use of automated external defibrillation (p 320).
- ♠ 36. Explain the role medical direction plays in the use of automated external defibrillation (p 327).
- 37. State the reasons why a case review should be completed following the use of the automated external defibrillator (p 327).
- 38. Discuss the components that should be included in a case review (p 327).
- 39. Discuss the goal of quality improvement in automated external defibrillation (p 327).
- ♠ 40. Recognize the need for medical direction of protocols to assist in the emergency medical care of the patient with chest pain (p 327).
- 41. Define the function of all controls on an automated external defibrillator, and describe event documentation and battery defibrillator maintenance (p 325).

Affective

- ♠ 42. Defend the reasons for obtaining initial training in automated external defibrillation and the importance of continuing education (p 319).
- 43. Defend the reason for maintenance of automated external defibrillators (p 325).

Psychomotor

- ♠ 44. Demonstrate the assessment and emergency medical care of a patient experiencing chest pain/discomfort (p 313).
- 45. Demonstrate the application and operation of the automated external defibrillator (p 321).
- 46. Demonstrate the maintenance of an automated external defibrillator (p 325).
- 47. Demonstrate the assessment and documentation of patient response to the automated external defibrillator (p 321).
- 48. Demonstrate the skills necessary to complete the Automated Defibrillator: Operator's Shift Checklist (p 327).
- ♠ 49. Practice completing a prehospital care report for patients with cardiac emergencies (p 312).

♠ These are core concepts in initial patrol training.

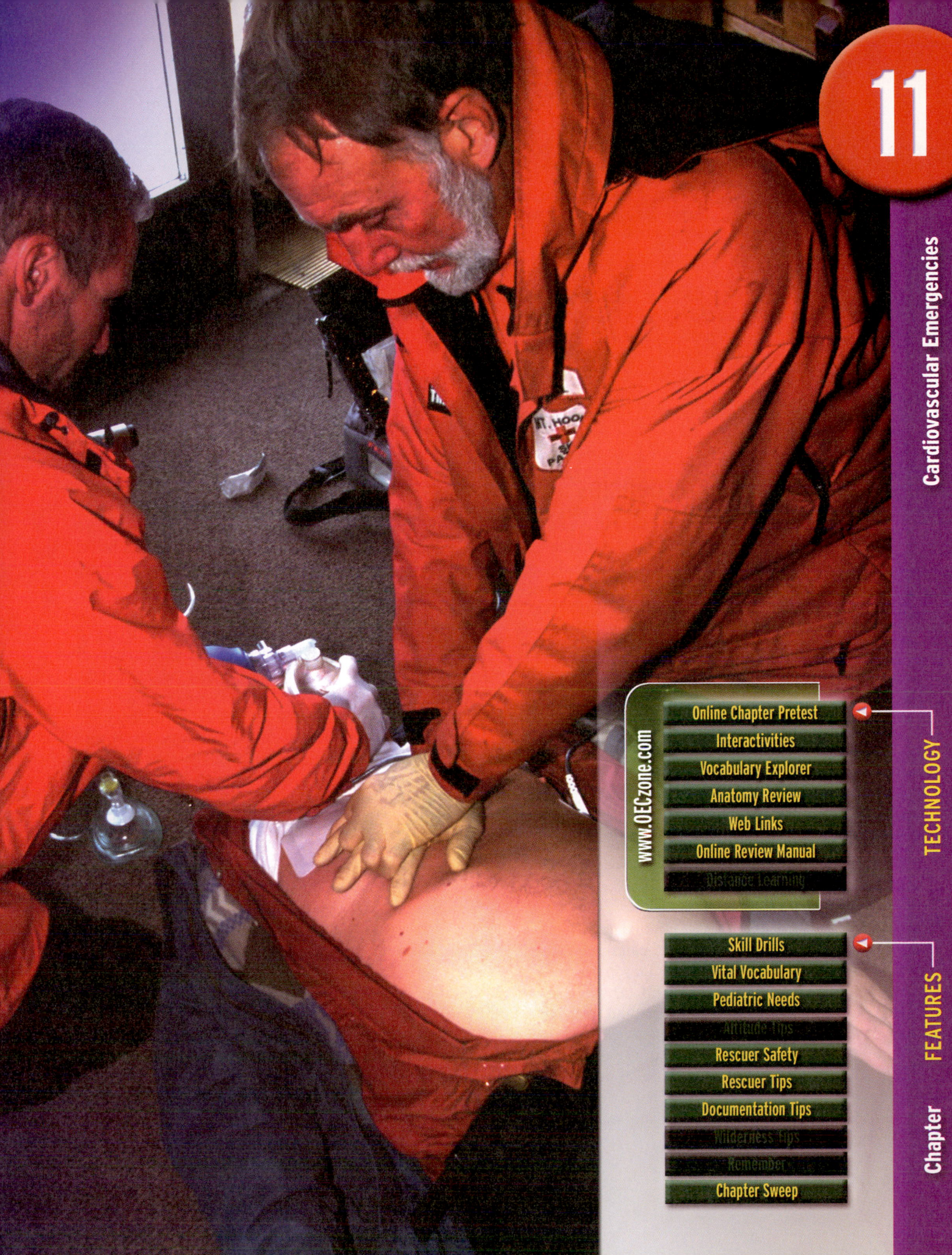

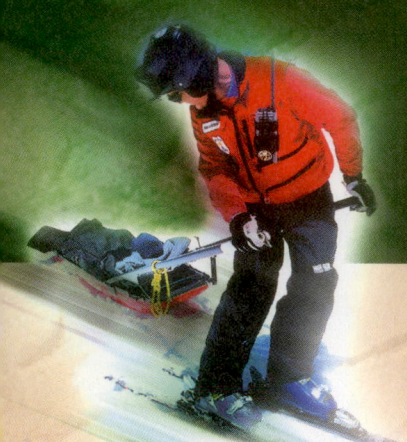

A 50-year-old man comes to the aid room asking for an antacid for "indigestion." Ten minutes later you are summoned to the day lodge because he has had a cardiac arrest.

Heart disease is very prevalent in the United States. Exercise, particularly at an elevated altitude, may precipitate an acute coronary event in individuals with diagnosed or undiagnosed coronary disease.

1. What is "cardiac denial," and why is it a factor in the mortality/morbidity of patients with cardiac emergencies?

2. Can you identify the most common presenting cardiac rhythm for patients who experience sudden cardiac death as well as the appropriate emergency intervention for it?

Cardiovascular Emergencies

The American Heart Association reports that cardiovascular disease (CVD) claimed 953,110 lives in the United States in 1997. This is 41.2% of all deaths, or 1 of every 2.4 deaths. CVD was about 60% of total mortality, which means that of the more than 2,000,000 deaths from all causes, CVD was listed as a primary or contributing cause on more than 1,406,000 death certificates. Heart disease has been the leading killer of Americans since 1900. This statistic is still true today. As a result, heart disease remains the leading cause of death. Thus, an OEC provider may be called upon to provide help for some type of cardiac emergency.

It is important for OEC providers to understand that many deaths caused by CVD occur from problems that may have been avoided by people living more prudent lifestyles and by access to improved medical technology. We can help to reduce these numbers of deaths with better public awareness, early access, increased numbers of laypeople trained in cardiopulmonary resuscitation (CPR), and with public access defibrillation.

This chapter begins with a brief description of the heart and how it works. It then discusses the relationship between chest pain and ischemic heart disease. It explains how to recognize and treat acute myocardial infarction (classic heart attack) and the complications of sudden death, cardiogenic shock, and congestive heart failure. The use of nitroglycerin is described. The last part of the chapter is devoted to the use and maintenance of the automated external defibrillator (AED).

Cardiac Structure and Function

The heart is a relatively simple organ with a simple job. It has to pump blood to supply oxygen-enriched red blood cells to the tissues of the body. The heart is divided down the middle into two sides (left and right) by a wall called the septum. Each side of the heart has an **atrium**, or upper chamber, and a **ventricle**, or lower chamber ▶ Figure 11-1 . Blood leaves each of the four chambers of the heart through a one-way valve. These valves keep the blood moving through the circulatory system in the proper direction. The largest valve is the **aortic valve**, lying between the left ventricle and the aorta. The **aorta**, the body's main artery, receives the blood ejected from the left ventricle and delivers it to all the other arteries so that they can carry blood to the tissues of the body.

The right side of the heart receives oxygen-poor (deoxygenated) blood from the veins of the body ▶ Figure 11-2A . Blood enters into the right atrium from the vena cava, which then fills the right ventricle. After contraction of the right ventricle, blood flows into the pulmonary artery and the pulmonary circulation, where the blood is oxygenated. The left side of the heart receives oxygen-rich (oxygenated) blood from the lungs through the pulmonary veins ▶ Figure 11-2B . Blood enters into the atrium, then passes into the left ventricle. This side of the heart is more muscular than the other because it must pump blood into the aorta and all the other arteries of the body.

The heart contains more than muscle tissue. The heart's electrical system, which is distributed throughout the entire heart, controls heart rate and enables the atria

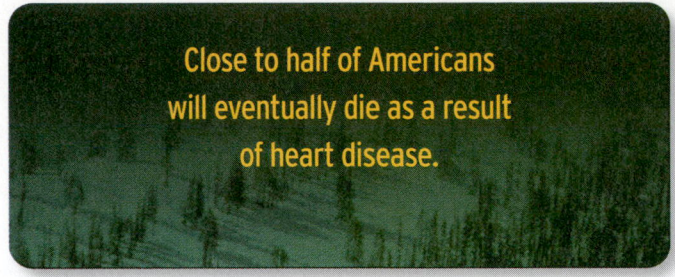

Close to half of Americans will eventually die as a result of heart disease.

and ventricles to work together (▶ Figure 11-3). Normal electrical impulses begin in the sinus node, just above the atria. The impulses travel across both atria, causing them to contract. Between the atria and the ventricles, the impulses cross over a bridge of special electrical tissue called the atrioventricular (AV) node. Here the signal is slowed down for about one tenth to two tenths of a second to allow blood time to pass from the atria to the ventricles. Then the impulses exit the AV node and spread throughout both ventricles, causing the ventricular muscle cells to contract.

Circulation

To carry out its function of pumping blood, the myocardium, or heart muscle, must have a continuous supply of oxygen and nutrients. During periods of physical exertion or stress, the myocardium requires more oxygen, so the heart must increase its output of bloodflow. In the normal heart, the increased need for blood is easily supplied by dilation, or widening, of the coronary arteries, which increases blood flow. The coronary arteries are the blood vessels that supply blood to the heart muscle. They start at the first part of the aorta, just above the aortic valve. The right coronary artery supplies blood to the right ventricle and, in most people, the bottom part, or inferior wall, of the left ventricle. The left coronary artery divides into two major branches, both of which supply the left ventricle (▶ Figure 11-4).

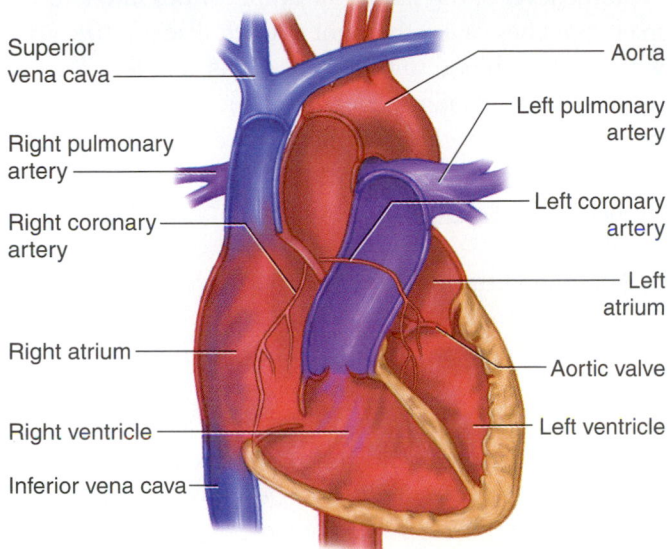

Figure 11-1 The heart is a four-chambered muscle that pumps blood to all parts of the body.

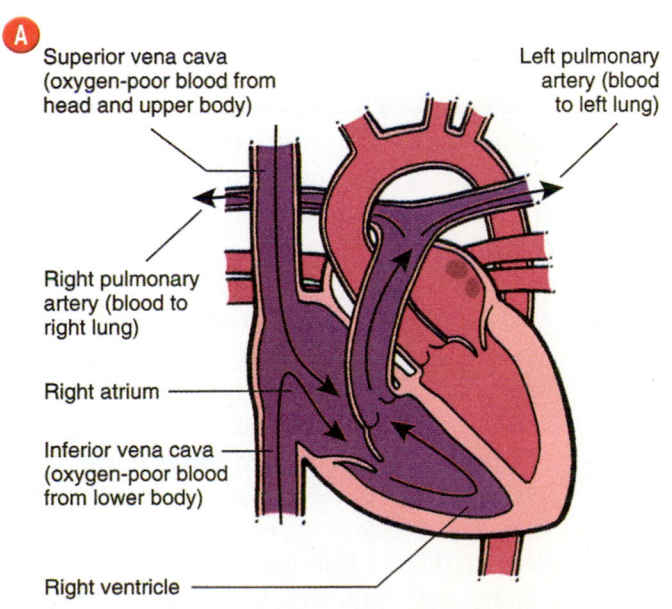

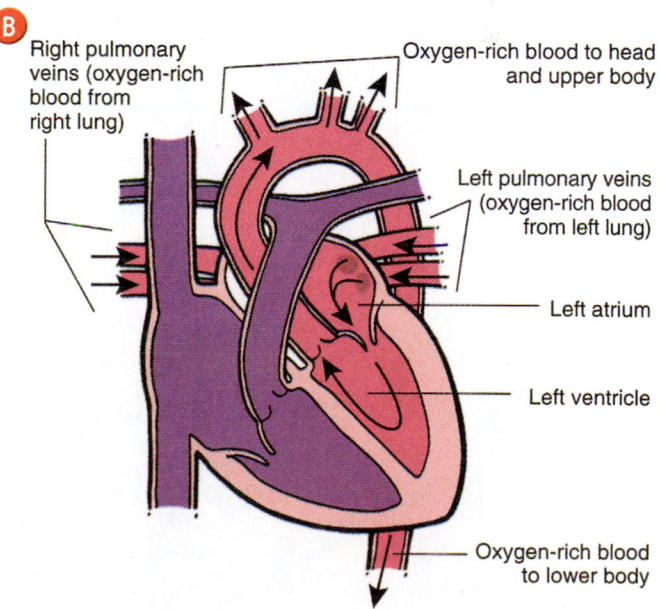

Figure 11-2 **A.** The right side of the heart receives oxygen-poor blood from the veins. **B.** The left side of the heart receives oxygen-rich blood from the lungs through the pulmonary veins.

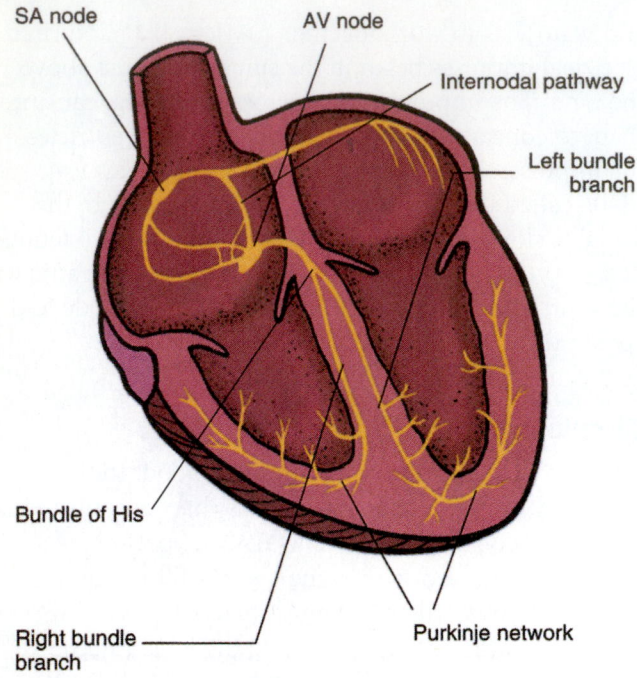

SA node   **AV node**   **Internodal pathway**   **Left bundle branch**   **Bundle of His**   **Right bundle branch**   **Purkinje network**

Figure 11-3 The electrical conduction system of the heart controls most aspects of heart rate and enables the four chambers to work together.

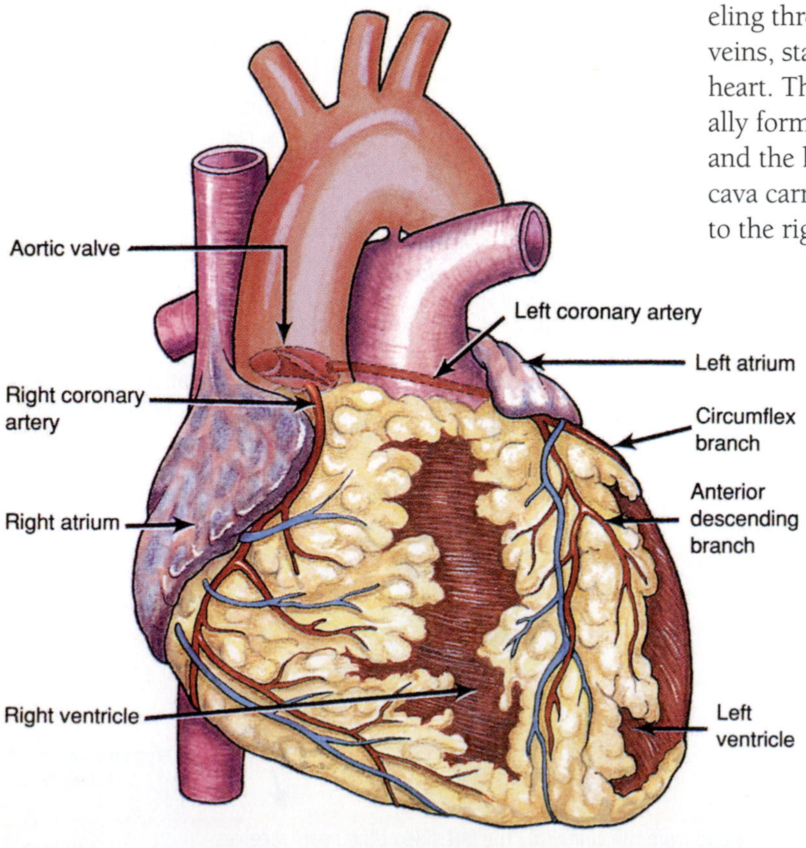

Aortic valve   **Right coronary artery**   **Right atrium**   **Right ventricle**   **Left coronary artery**   **Left atrium**   **Circumflex branch**   **Anterior descending branch**   **Left ventricle**

Figure 11-4 The coronary arteries carry the blood supply to the heart.

Two major arteries branching from the upper aorta supply blood to the head and arms. The right and left carotid arteries supply the head and brain with blood. The subclavian arteries (under the clavicles) supply blood to the upper extremities. As the subclavian artery enters each arm, it becomes the brachial artery, the major vessel that supplies blood to each arm. Just below the elbow, the brachial artery divides into two major branches: the radial and ulnar arteries (▶ **Figure 11-5**).

At the level of the navel, the aorta divides into two main branches called the right and left iliac arteries, which supply blood to the groin, pelvis, and legs. As the iliac arteries enter the legs through the groin, they become the right and left femoral arteries. At the level of the knee, the femoral artery divides into the **anterior** (front) and **posterior** (back) tibial artery and the peroneal artery.

After blood travels through the arteries, it enters smaller and smaller vessels, called arterioles and capillaries. The capillaries are tiny blood vessels about one cell thick that connect arterioles to venules. Capillaries, which are found in all parts of the body, allow the exchange of nutrients and waste at the cellular level.

Venules are the smallest branches of veins. After traveling through the capillaries, blood enters the system of veins, starting with the venules, on its way back to the heart. The veins become larger and larger and eventually form the two large venae cavae: the upper vena cava and the lower vena cava. The **superior** (upper) vena cava carries blood from the head, arms, and chest back to the right atrium. The **inferior** (lower) vena cava carries blood from the abdomen, kidneys, and legs back to the right atrium. The superior and inferior venae cavae join at the right atrium of the heart, where blood is eventually returned into the pulmonary circulation for oxygenation (▶ **Figure 11-6**).

Blood consists of several types of cells and fluid (▶ **Figure 11-7**). *Red blood cells* are the most numerous and give the blood its color. Red blood cells carry oxygen to the body's tissues and then remove carbon dioxide. Larger *white blood cells* help to fight infection. *Platelets*, which help the blood to clot, are much smaller than either red or white blood cells. *Plasma* is the fluid that the cells float in. It is a mixture of water, salts, nutrients, and proteins.

Blood pressure is the pressure of circulating blood against the walls of the arteries. Systolic blood pressure is the maximum

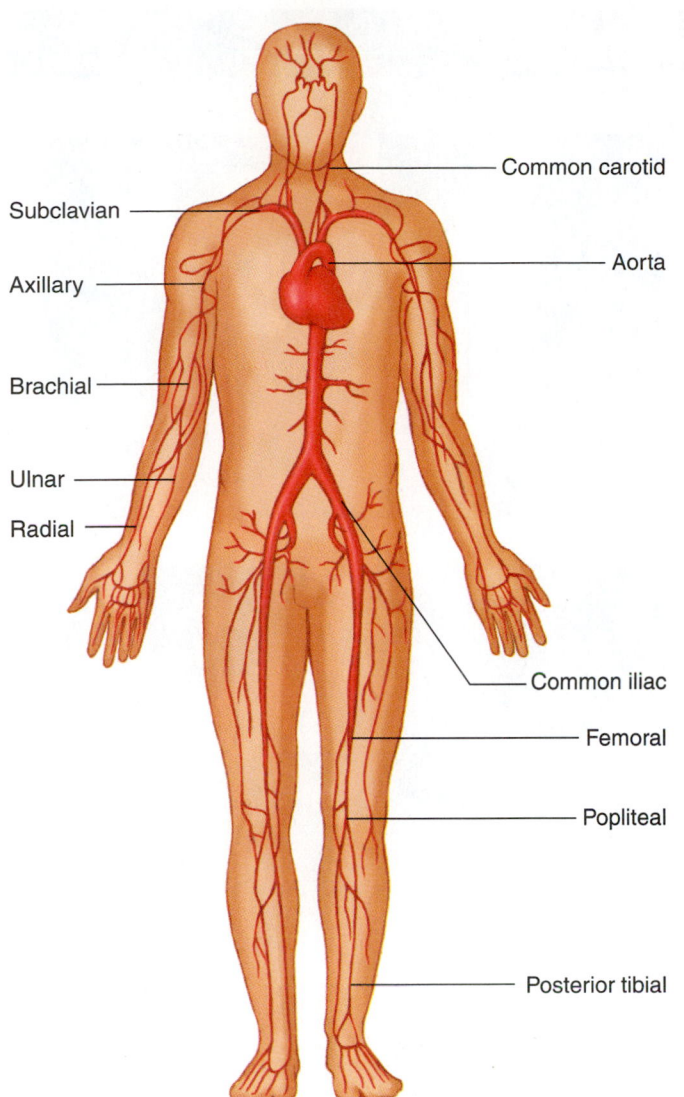

Common carotid

Subclavian

Axillary

Aorta

Brachial

Ulnar

Radial

Common iliac

Femoral

Popliteal

Posterior tibial

Figure 11-5 The major arteries of the body carry oxygen-rich blood to all parts of the body.

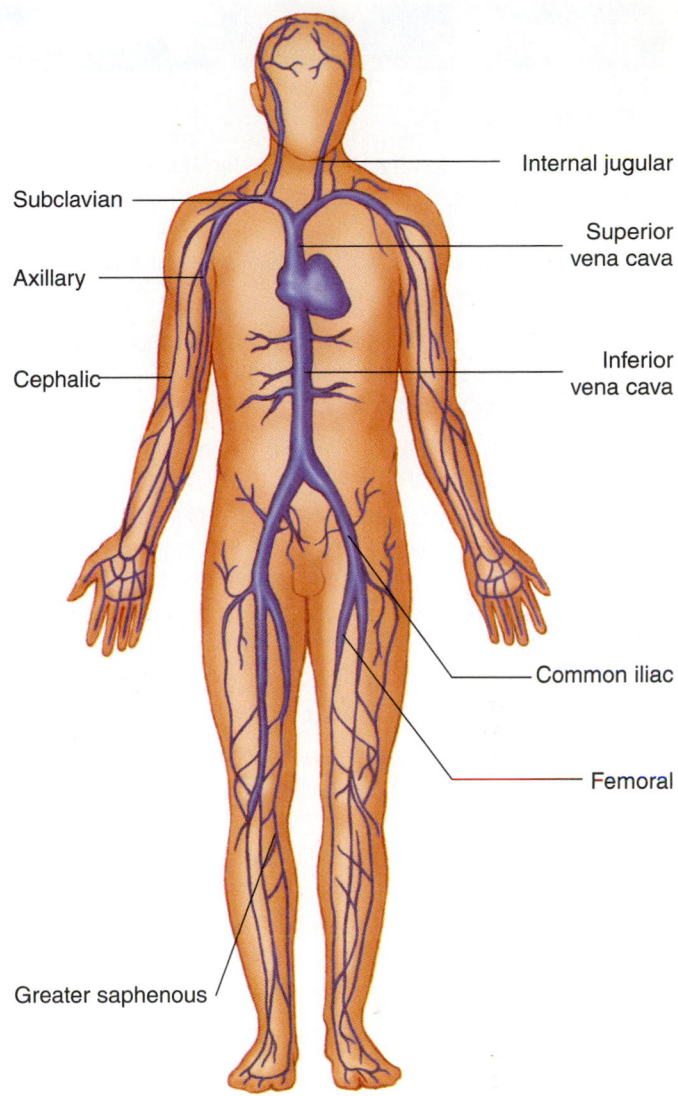

Internal jugular

Subclavian

Superior vena cava

Axillary

Cephalic

Inferior vena cava

Common iliac

Femoral

Greater saphenous

Figure 11-6 The veins carry blood from the body back to the heart, which pumps it through the lungs for oxygenation.

pressure exerted by the left ventricle as it contracts. As the left ventricle relaxes, the arterial pressure falls. When the aortic valve closes, blood flow stops. The diastolic blood pressure is the pressure exerted against the walls of the arteries while the left ventricle is at rest. Remember that the top number in a blood pressure reading is the systolic pressure, and the bottom number is the diastolic or resting pressure.

Cardiac Compromise

Chest pain or discomfort that is related to the heart usually stems from a condition called **ischemia**, or insufficient oxygen. Because of a partial or complete blockage of blood flow through the coronary arteries, heart tissue fails to get enough oxygen and nutrients.

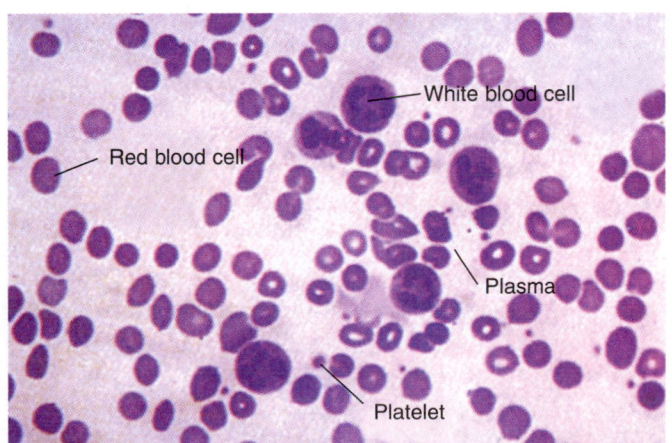

White blood cell

Red blood cell

Plasma

Platelet

Figure 11-7 Blood consists of several types of cells and fluids, including red blood cells, white blood cells, and platelets. The cells float in a fluid called plasma.

Rescuer Tips

Pulsation

As the left ventricle contracts, it ejects a forceful wave of blood through the arteries. You can feel that wave in areas where the artery lies over a bone and is near the surface of the skin. This wave is called the pulse. Common places to feel for a pulse include the following (▶ **Figure 11-8**):

- The *carotid pulse* can be felt in the neck, two fingerbreadths on either side of the Adam's apple (thyroid cartilage), and should be taken on side closest to the rescuer.

- The *femoral pulse* can be felt in the groin, right at the crease dividing the lower abdomen from the leg.

- The *brachial pulse* can be felt on the medial aspect of the elbow, right at the level of the crease. Pulsations also can be palpated on the inside of the arm between the elbow and armpit. This is the pulse that you listen to when you take blood pressure.

- The *radial pulse* can be felt on the thumb side of the wrist, about one finger width above the wrist crease.

- The *posterior tibial pulse* can be felt on the inside of the ankle, just posterior to the medial malleolus. The medial malleolus is the bony bump at the end of the tibia.

- The *dorsalis pedis pulse* can be felt at the top of the foot. This artery is not in the exact same place in all people. To find its pulse, place your hand across the top of the foot just below the ankle crease. Once you feel something that might be a pulse, use your fingertips to confirm that finding.

Practice feeling for these pulses on yourself and on friends and family members.

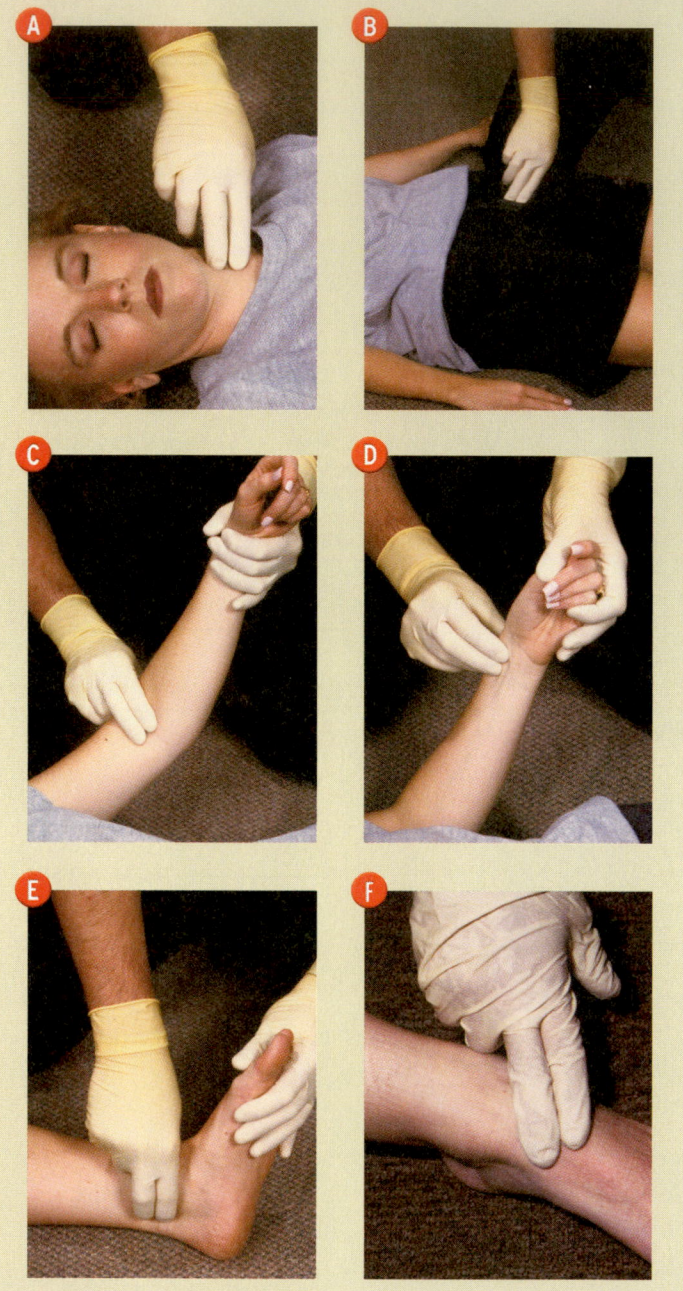

Figure 11-8   Common pulse points.
A. The carotid pulse is taken at the neck.
B. The femoral pulse is felt in the groin area.
C. The brachial pulse can be felt on the inside of the upper arm.
D. The radial pulse can be felt on the thumb side of the wrist.
E. The posterior tibial pulse can be felt on the inside of the ankle.
F. The dorsalis pedis pulse can be felt at the top of the foot.

The tissue soon begins to starve and, if blood flow is not restored, eventually dies. Ischemic heart disease, then, is disease involving a decrease in blood flow to one or more portions of the heart muscle.

Atherosclerosis

Most often, the low blood flow to heart tissue is caused by coronary artery atherosclerosis. **Atherosclerosis** is a disorder in which calcium and a fatty material called cholesterol build up and form a plaque inside the walls of blood vessels, obstructing flow and interfering with their ability to dilate or contract (▶ **Figure 11-9**). Eventually, atherosclerosis can even cause complete **occlusion**, or blockage, of a coronary artery. Atherosclerosis usually involves other arteries of the body, as well.

The problem begins when the first deposit of cholesterol is laid down on the inside of an artery. This may happen during the teenage years. As a person ages, more of this fatty material is deposited; the **lumen**, or the inside diameter of the artery, narrows. As the cholesterol deposits grow, calcium deposits can form as well. The inner wall of the artery, which is normally smooth and elastic, becomes rough and brittle with these atherosclerotic plaques. Damage to the coronary arteries may become so extensive that they cannot accommodate increased blood flow at times of maximum need.

For reasons that are still not completely understood, a brittle plaque will sometimes develop a crack, exposing the inside of the atherosclerotic wall. Acting like a torn blood vessel, the ragged edge of the crack activates the blood-clotting system, just as it does when an injury has caused bleeding. In this situation, however, the resulting blood clot will partially or completely

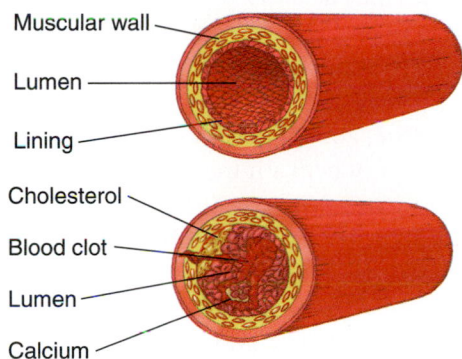

Figure 11-9   In atherosclerosis, calcium and cholesterol build up inside the walls of the blood vessels, causing an obstruction in blood flow to the heart.

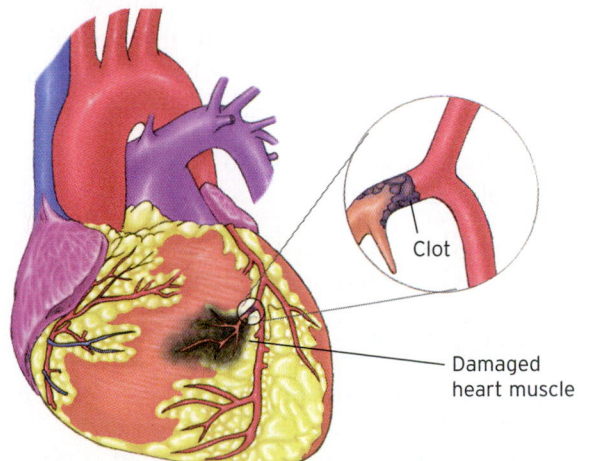

Figure 11-10   An acute myocardial infarction occurs when a blood clot prevents blood flow to an area of the heart muscle. If left untreated, this can result in death of heart tissue.

block the lumen of the artery. Tissues downstream from the blood clot will suffer from lack of oxygen (ischemia). If blood flow is resumed in a short time, the ischemic tissues will recover. However, if too much time goes by before blood flow is resumed, the tissues will die. This sequence of events is known as an **acute myocardial infarction (AMI)**, a classic heart attack **▼ Figure 11-10**. **Infarction** means the death of tissue. The same sequence may also cause the death of cells in other organs, such as the brain. The death of heart muscle can lead to severe diminishment of the heart's ability to pump, or **cardiac arrest**.

In the United States, coronary artery disease is the number one cause of death for both men and women. The peak incidence of heart disease occurs between ages 40 and 70 years, but it can also strike teens or individuals in their 90s. You must be alert to the possibility that, although less likely, a 26-year-old person with chest pain could actually be having a heart attack, especially if he or she has a higher than usual risk.

Factors that place a person at higher risk for a myocardial infarction are called risk factors. The major controllable factors are cigarette smoking, high blood pressure, elevated cholesterol levels, elevated blood sugar levels (diabetes), lack of exercise, and stress. The major risk factors that cannot be controlled are older age, family history of atherosclerotic coronary artery disease, and male gender.

Angina Pectoris

Chest pain does not always mean that a person is having an AMI. When, for a brief period of time, heart tissues are not getting enough oxygen, the pain is called **angina pectoris**, or angina. Although it can result from a spasm of the artery, angina is most often a symptom of atherosclerotic coronary artery disease. Angina occurs when the heart's need for oxygen exceeds its supply, usually during periods of physical or emotional stress when the heart is working hard. A large meal or sudden fear may also trigger an attack. When the increased oxygen demand goes away (eg, the person stops exercising), the pain typically goes away.

Angina pain is typically described as crushing, squeezing, or "like somebody standing on my chest." It is usually felt in the midchest, under the sternum. However, it can radiate to the jaw, the arms (frequently the left arm), the midback, or the epigastrium (the upper-middle region of the abdomen). The pain usually lasts from 3 to 8 minutes, rarely longer than 15 minutes. It may be associated with shortness of breath, nausea, or sweating. It disappears promptly with rest, supplemental oxygen, or nitroglycerin, all of which increase the supply of oxygen to the heart. Although angina pectoris is frightening, it does not mean that heart cells are dying, nor does it usually lead to death or permanent heart damage. It is, however, a warning that you and the patient should both take seriously. Even with angina, because oxygen supply to the heart is diminished, the electrical system can be compromised and the person is at risk for significant cardiac rhythm problems.

Keep in mind that it can be very difficult even for doctors in hospitals to distinguish between the pain of angina and the pain of a myocardial infarction.

Heart Attack

Most heart attacks are caused by an acute myocardial infarction, which means acute death (infarction) of part of the myocardium. The left side of the heart is most commonly involved because it is stressed more than the right side, as in cases of high blood pressure. Infarction usually occurs when a blood clot or some other process blocks or narrows a diseased coronary artery in a patient with coronary artery disease. If a blood clot is responsible, in many cases it can be dissolved with special intravenous drugs if the patient can get to medical care within 12 hours of the onset of symptoms.

In this section, although the term "heart attack" will be used for any sudden episode caused by malfunction of the heart, please note that the signs and symptoms, assessment, and emergency care described are for an acute myocardial infarction. Other types of heart attacks, which can be caused by the sudden onset of a rapid or irregular heartbeat or by sudden failure of the heart muscle in patients with diseased heart valves, are difficult to distinguish from a myocardial infarction in the field and are cared for in the same way.

Because increasing numbers of middle-aged and elderly persons are participating in skiing, snowboarding, and other outdoor activities, the incidence of heart attacks at ski areas and other outdoor locations will continue to increase.

Signs and Symptoms of Acute Myocardial Infarction

The signs and symptoms of AMI are caused by the heart muscle's sudden lack of oxygen. This oxygen depletion usually causes pain, which triggers anxiety and an autonomic nervous system response. Depending on the size and location of the involved

Documentation Tips

Documenting exactly how a patient describes chest discomfort, in the patient's own words, is a valuable source of information for hospital staff. Remember—OPQRST.

area, an AMI can interfere with the normal rhythm and rate of the heartbeat and/or diminish the strength of the heart's contractions. Involvement of a large area of myocardium may lead to **cardiogenic shock**. Sudden death due to cardiac arrest may be the first sign of an AMI. In less severe cases, a patient having an AMI usually wants to sit up, but occasionally will want to lie down or even walk around. The full range of signs and symptoms of AMI are as follows (▶ Table 11-1):

1. Pain, *which may be the only symptom of an AMI,* is similar to that of angina pectoris, but is usually more severe and longer lasting. It is described as heavy, squeezing, crushing, vise-like, burning, or a severe ache; almost never as sharp or sticking. It is commonly beneath the sternum (substernal), but may occur in the pit of the stomach (epigastrium), throat, or in the back between the shoulder blades. The pain frequently radiates from the chest to the neck, teeth, jaw, left shoulder and left arm, and occasionally the right shoulder and arm or both shoulders and arms. It is usually unrelated to exertion and is *not* relieved by rest or nitroglycerin.

   The patient may have had a previous AMI or previous episodes of angina. Occasionally, an AMI will occur without pain ("silent" myocardial infarction), but its detection is beyond the realm of the care provider trained at the OEC level.

2. The patient's pulse and blood pressure may be normal or abnormal.

3. Changes due to pain, anxiety, and autonomic nervous system response include the following signs and symptoms (some of which are also seen in cardiogenic shock):
   - Fear of impending doom
   - Cold, clammy, pale skin
   - Respiratory distress
   - Fast or very slow heart rate
   - High blood pressure

4. Changes due to heart muscle damage include the following:
   - Low blood pressure
   - Weak pulse
   - Irregular pulse
   - Generalized weakness
   - Cyanosis
   - Signs and symptoms of cardiogenic shock or pulmonary edema

Complications of Myocardial Infarction

The following complications increase the risk of death in a patient with a myocardial infarction.

Cardiac arrest

The risk of cardiac arrest is greatest in the first few hours or days after a myocardial infarction. Cardiac arrest occurs when the heart ceases to pump blood because of a sudden, irregular, and ineffective quivering of the ventricular myocardium (**ventricular fibrillation**), a heartbeat that is too fast and weak to pump enough blood (**ventricular tachycardia**), or complete cessation of heart contractions (**asystole**). The most common of these is ventricular fibrillation.

Cardiogenic shock

Damage to the myocardium may reduce the heart's output of blood to the point where the blood pressure can no longer be maintained. The signs and symptoms of cardiogenic shock are those of shock (see Chapter 9) that stem from the myocardial damage caused by a heart attack.

Pulmonary edema

Pulmonary edema occurs when the undamaged right side of the heart continues to pump blood *into* the lungs but the damaged left side is too weak to handle even a normal volume of blood coming *from* the lungs. Blood accumulates in the lungs, increasing the hydrostatic pressure in their capillaries. This forces the fluid part of the blood out into the alveoli. The signs and symptoms of pulmonary edema are discussed in Chapter 10.

The assessment of a patient with a heart attack is summarized in ▶ **Table 11-2** . Be aware that conditions that may be hard to distinguish from a heart attack include pulmonary embolus, spontaneous pneumothorax, pericarditis (inflammation of the sac around the heart), a perforated peptic ulcer, disease of the pancreas or gallbladder, hyperventilation, certain types of indigestion, esophageal spasm, and inflammation of the muscles or joints of the chest wall. Differentiating these conditions from a heart attack may require the expertise of a physician and the facilities of a hospital, so treat all such cases as potential heart attacks.

Emergency Care of a Patient with a Heart Attack

Many people have died of myocardial infarctions and other types of heart attacks when, with proper and timely treatment, they could have lived normal lives for many years. Therefore, *the most important emergency care for a patient with a heart attack is rapid access to an advanced life support (ALS) team* that is equipped with a heart monitor, defibrillator, intravenous fluids, intubation equipment, and appropriate medications, and in contact by radio with a hospital emergency department.

The ALS team will rapidly transport the patient by ambulance or helicopter to a hospital with an intensive care unit. Therefore, as soon as assessment indicates the suspicion of a heart attack, the ALS team and/or rescuers with **defibrillation** capability *must be summoned immediately.*

Table 11-1 Summary of Signs and Symptoms of AMI

1. Pain, usually but not always, is typical in type and location. It is similar to, but worse than, that of angina pectoris. In some cases, pain may be absent. Pain is not relieved by rest or nitroglycerin.
2. Anxiety and a feeling of impending doom.
3. Possible respiratory distress.
4. Pale, cold, and occasionally cyanotic skin.
5. Profuse sweating.
6. Pulse may be normal, slow, fast, irregular, strong, or weak.
7. Normal or abnormal blood pressure.
8. Patient usually prefers to sit up.
9. Possible complications:
   - Cardiac arrest
   - Cardiogenic shock
   - Pulmonary edema

Rescuer Tips

More about shock

Signs and symptoms

- One of the first signs of shock is *anxiety* or *restlessness* as the brain becomes relatively starved for oxygen. The patient may complain of *"air hunger."* Think of the possibility of shock when the patient is yelling, "I can't breathe." Obviously, the patient can breathe, because he or she can talk. However, the patient's brain is sensing that it is not getting enough oxygen.

- As the shock continues, the body tries to send blood to the most important organs, such as the brain and heart, and away from less important organs, such as the skin. Therefore, you may see *pale, clammy skin* in patients with shock.

- As the shock gets worse, the body will attempt to compensate by increasing the amount of blood pumped through the heart. Therefore, the *pulse rate will be higher than normal*. In severe shock the heart rate will usually, but not always, be greater than 120 beats/min.

- Shock can also be characterized by rapid and shallow breathing, nausea and vomiting, and a decrease in body temperature.

- Finally, as the heart and other organs begin to malfunction, the *blood pressure will fall below normal*. A systolic blood pressure of less than 90 mm Hg is easy to recognize, but it is a late finding that indicates decompensated shock. Do not assume that shock is not present just because the blood pressure is normal (compensated shock).

Treatment of patients with cardiogenic shock. Take the following steps when treating patients with signs and symptoms of shock:

1. Position the patient comfortably. Most patients with heart failure will be more comfortable in semi-Fowler's position; however, those with low blood pressure may not tolerate a semi-upright position. These patients may be more comfortable and be more alert in a supine position.

2. Administer high-flow oxygen.

3. Assist ventilations as necessary.

4. Provide prompt transport to the emergency department.

More about congestive heart failure

Signs and symptoms

Watch for the following signs and symptoms in a patient you suspect has **congestive heart failure (CHF)**:

- The patient finds it easier to breathe when sitting up. When the patient is lying down, more blood is returned to the right ventricle and lungs, causing further pulmonary congestion.

- Often, the patient is mildly or severely agitated.

- Chest pain may or may not be present.

- The patient often has distended neck veins that do not collapse even when the patient is sitting.

- The patient may have swollen ankles from **pedal edema** (backup of fluid).

- The patient generally will have a high blood pressure, rapid heart rate, and rapid respirations.

- The patient will usually be using accessory breathing muscles of the neck and ribs, reflecting the additional hard work of breathing.

- The fluid surrounding small airways may produce rales, best heard by listening to either side of the patient's chest, about midway down the back. In CHF, these soft sounds can be heard even at the top of the lung.

Once CHF develops, it can be treated but not cured. Regular use of medications may alleviate the symptoms. However, these patients often become ill again and are frequently hospitalized. Approximately half will be dead within 5 years of the onset of symptoms.

Treatment. Treat the patient with CHF the same way as the patient with chest pain:

1. Take the vital signs, monitor heart rhythm, and give oxygen by nonrebreathing face mask with an oxygen flow of 10 to 15 L/min.

2. Allow the patient to remain sitting in an upright position with the legs down.

3. Be reassuring; many patients with CHF are quite anxious because they cannot breathe.

4. Patients who have had problems with CHF before will usually have specific medications for its treatment. Gather these medications and take them along to the hospital.

5. Nitroglycerin may be of value if the patient's systolic blood pressure is greater than 100 mm Hg. If the patient has prescribed nitroglycerin, you may assist the patient to use it sublingually or by spray. Be sure to follow local protocol.

6. Prompt transport to the emergency department is essential.

Table 11-2 Summary of Assessment of a Patient With a Heart Attack

1. Scene size-up: the patient appears to have an illness rather than an injury. Institute BSI precautions.

2. Introduce yourself. Ask, "Can I help you?" and "What seems to be the problem?"

3. Begin the initial assessment, assessing the airway, breathing, and, especially, the pulse. Check skin for temperature, color, and moisture. Does the patient look critically ill?

4. Have the patient describe his or her symptoms in detail, especially pain.

5. Obtain a SAMPLE history, specifically asking whether the patient has a history of chest pain and heart disease. Measure the patient's blood pressure, if possible.

6. Assess the neck, chest, and abdomen or, in the case of a critical patient or one with abnormal pulse and respirations, perform a focused history and physical examination.

7. Arrange for rapid transport to a hospital.

8. Perform the detailed physical examination as appropriate.

9. Perform the ongoing assessment en route to the hospital or while awaiting emergency transport.

Table 11-3 Survival Rates for Patients with Cardiac Arrest

Emergency Care	Timeframe for Delivery of Care (min)					Survival Rate
	2	4	6	8	10	
No CPR, delayed defibrillation					Defibrillation	0% to 2%
Early CPR, delayed defibrillation	CPR				Defibrillation	2% to 8%
Early CPR, early defibrillation	CPR		Defibrillation			20%
Early CPR, very early defibrillation, early ALS	CPR		Defibrillation	ALS		30%

Modified with permission from *Basic Life Support for Healthcare Providers*, American Heart Association, 1997, p. 9-2.

Should cardiac arrest occur before the ALS team arrives, the patient's best chance of survival is to be given CPR within 2 minutes and defibrillation within 4 minutes, with ALS available within 8 minutes ▲ Table 11-3 . If an ALS team is not available, EMT-Bs or other emergency care providers who have access to automated external defibrillators (AEDs) and are trained in their use may be able to help. Ski patrols should identify, in advance, the location and contact information for the nearest ALS team and AED-equipped rescuers. Keep in mind, however, that these resources may not be readily available in every outdoor situation and may be totally unavailable in the backcountry or wilderness.

The AED is a recent development that shows promise in decreasing the death rate from cardiac arrest. This battery-operated device is equipped to identify "shockable rhythms" (ventricular fibrillation and ventricular tachycardia) immediately using two electrodes attached to the patient's chest, and to advise the rescuer when electric shocks should be given. The AED would appear to be a very useful piece of equipment to have on hand where large numbers of people are congregated in remote areas, such as ski resorts and national parks. Many larger ski areas have AEDs available. Although the device is easy to use, special training, certification, and licensing are required.

After summoning an ALS team, first responders should perform the following emergency care measures for any patient suspected of having had a heart attack ▼ Table 11-4 :

1. Keep the patient still and in the most comfortable position, which usually will be sitting up, especially if he or she is short of breath. Prevent the patient from becoming chilled or overheated.

2. Administer high-flow oxygen.

3. Take steps to minimize noise and distractions around the patient, and shield him or her from bystanders. Calm and reassure the patient.

4. Watch for complications:
   - If shock develops, the patient's accompanying shortness of breath may require that you place him or her in the Rothberg position by raising the person's head and chest and bending his or her knees ▶ Figure 11-11 .
   - If the patient's breathing becomes ineffective, support it with rescue breathing and supplemental oxygen administered via mouth-to-pocket mask or a bag-valve-mask (BVM) device.
   - If cardiac arrest occurs, administer CPR.
   - Treat pulmonary edema by propping the patient up in a seated position and administering high-flow oxygen.

CPR on the Ski Hill

The following technique for administering CPR on the ski hill is recommended by the Medical Committee of the National Ski Patrol. With this technique as a foundation, each ski patrol should develop its own CPR protocol with the input of the patrol medical advisor

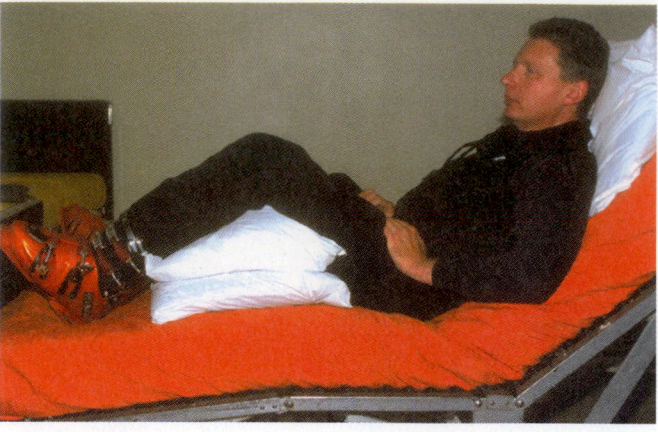

Figure 11-11 The Rothberg position is used in the emergency care of a heart-attack patient.

and area management.

1. Start CPR on the spot as soon as possible.

2. Administer high-flow oxygen as soon as it is available.

3. If an AED is available, use it as soon as it arrives. The rescuer may use the AED on snow or in rain as long as routine precautions are observed.

4. Transfer the patient to a toboggan and continue CPR during transport to the aid room or a waiting helicopter or ambulance.

Administering CPR in a moving toboggan is difficult on all but the most flat and smooth snow—and evidence of its effectiveness is lacking. Therefore, the "leap frog" technique is recommended when providing CPR during transport by toboggan over uneven or steep terrain, unless the patient is very close to the aid room. This approach, which entails alternating between periods of

---

Table 11-4 Summary of Emergency Care of a Heart Attack Patient

1. Perform the initial assessment and deal with urgent problems. Provide airway management, ventilation, or CPR, if needed.

2. Contact an ALS team without delay.

3. Summon a rescuer with defibrillator capability, if possible.

4. Keep the patient in the most comfortable position.

5. Give high-flow oxygen.

6. Calm and reassure the patient.

7. Shield the patient from bystanders.

8. Watch for complications and care for them if they occur:
   - Cardiac arrest
   - Cardiogenic shock
   - Pulmonary edema

9. Continue to monitor and record vital signs since they may change during the course of assessment and care.

10. Rapidly transport the patient to a hospital.

CPR and periods of transport as described below, is similar to the American Heart Association's recommended technique for moving a patient in cardiac arrest down several flights of stairs.

Use a standard toboggan to transport the patient and necessary equipment. Do not delay toboggan transport while waiting for oxygen or the AED to arrive. Stop CPR only long enough to lift the patient into the toboggan, continuing it until actual transport begins. As soon as the patient is loaded and ready to go, stop CPR and run the toboggan for about 30 seconds. At the end of this time, stop the toboggan, park it across the fall line in a suitable place so that the patient's body is as level as possible, and administer a minute of CPR. Use either the one- or two-rescuer technique with the rescuer(s) stationed at the downhill side of the toboggan. Then, run the toboggan for another 30 seconds. Repeat this sequence until you reach the bottom of the hill or the terrain is so flat that CPR can be given while the toboggan is moving.

If an AED arrives while the patient is being transported, use it as soon as you reach the next stopping site. Be careful to avoid contact with the patient or any metal objects the patient might be touching. The same applies to oxygen.

Two teams of two patrollers each are recommended in addition to the toboggan handler(s). The second team members ski (or snowboard) ahead to the next stopping site while the first team is giving 1 minute of CPR and are ready to start CPR as soon as the toboggan arrives at their site.

In some instances, the patient can be transported directly from the site to a hospital by helicopter. It is also possible to give effective CPR in the bed of a large, slow-moving over-snow vehicle. When transporting a patient who has had a heart attack from the aid room to the hospital, a vehicle other than an ambulance or helicopter should only be used as a last resort. In these cases, a station wagon or van is preferable. At a minimum, oxygen, airways, a BVM device, and suction equipment should be taken along, and two or more patrollers should accompany the patient and driver.

Because a patient with a massive AMI may die even in the best-equipped hospital intensive care unit, rescuers should be realistic about their ability to resuscitate such patients. Under nonurban conditions, the fatality rate depends on development of complications and can be as high as 100% for patients in whom cardiac arrest develops.

Heart Operations and Pacemakers

Over the last 20 years, hundreds of thousands of open heart operations were performed to bypass damaged

Altitude Tips

The level of exercise an individual can maintain at high elevations is limited by the oxygen supply to the tissues, not by cardiac output. At higher altitudes, there is a smaller amount of oxygen in the atmosphere, which results in the heart not being pushed to work at a maximum level.

segments of coronary arteries in the heart. In the coronary artery bypass graft (CABG) operation, a blood vessel from the chest or leg is sewn directly from the aorta to a coronary artery beyond the point of the obstruction. Other patients may have had a procedure called percutaneous transluminal coronary angioplasty (PTCA), which aims to dilate, rather than bypass, the coronary artery. In this procedure, usually called an angioplasty or balloon angioplasty, a tiny balloon is attached to the end of a long, thin tube. The tube is introduced through the skin into a large vein, usually in the groin, and then threaded into the narrowed coronary artery, with radiographs serving as a guide. Once the balloon is in position inside the coronary artery, it is inflated. The balloon is then deflated, and the tube is removed from the body. Sometimes, a metal mesh called a stent is placed inside the artery either instead of or after the balloon. The stent is left in place permanently to help keep the artery from narrowing again.

You may see a patient with previous AMI or angina who has had one of these procedures. Patients who have had a bypass graft will have a long surgical scar on their chest from the operation ▼ **Figure 11-12** . Patients who have had an angioplasty or coronary

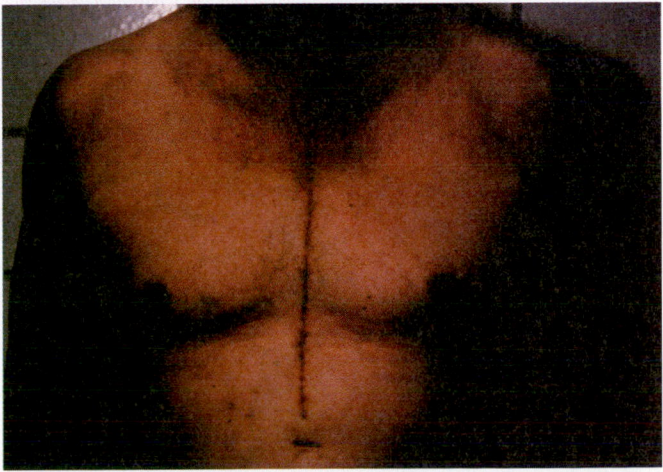

Figure 11-12 The surgical scar on the patient's chest implies a previous coronary artery bypass graft (CABG) surgery.

artery stent usually will not. However, newer "keyhole" surgical techniques may not produce a large scar. You should not assume that a patient who has a small scar has not had bypass surgery. Chest pain in a patient who has had any of these procedures should be treated the same as chest pain in patients who have not had any heart surgery. In any event, chest pain in a patient who has undergone either procedure is treated exactly the same as chest pain in a patient who has not. Carry out all the described tasks, and transport the patient promptly to the emergency department. If CPR is required, perform it in the usual way, regardless of the scar on the patient's chest. Likewise, if indicated, an AED should be used as well.

Many people with heart disease in the United States have cardiac pacemakers to maintain a regular cardiac rhythm and rate. Pacemakers are inserted when the electrical control system of the heart is so damaged that it cannot function properly. These battery-powered devices deliver an electrical impulse through wires that are in direct contact with the myocardium. The generating unit is generally placed under a heavy muscle or a fold of skin; it typically resembles a small silver dollar under the skin in the left upper chest (▼ Figure 11-13).

Normally, you do not need to be concerned about problems with pacemakers. Thanks to modern technology, an implanted unit will not require replacement or a battery charge for years. Wires are well protected and rarely broken. In the past, pacemakers sometimes malfunctioned when a patient got too close to an elec-

trical radiation source, such as a microwave oven, but this is no longer the case. Every patient with a pacemaker still should be aware of the precautions, if any, that must be taken to maintain its proper functioning.

If a pacemaker does not function properly, as when the battery wears out, the patient may experience syncope, dizziness, or weakness because of an excessively slow heart rate. The pulse ordinarily will be less than 60 beats/min because the heart is beating without the stimulus of the pacemaker and without the regulation of its own electrical system, which may be damaged. In these circumstances, the heart tends to assume a fixed slow rate that is not fast enough to allow the patient to function normally. A patient with a malfunctioning pacemaker should be promptly transported to the emergency department; repair of the problem may require an operation. When an AED is used, the patches should not be placed directly over the pacemaker. This will ensure a better flow of electricity through the patient's body.

Automatic Implantable Cardiac Defibrillators

More and more patients who survive ventricular fibrillation cardiac arrests have a small automatic implantable cardiac defibrillator (AICD) implanted. Some patients who are at particularly high risk for a cardiac arrest have them as well. These devices are attached directly to the heart and can prolong the lives of certain patients. They continuously monitor the heart rhythm, delivering shocks as needed (▼ Figure 11-14). Regardless of whether a patient having an AMI has an AICD, he or

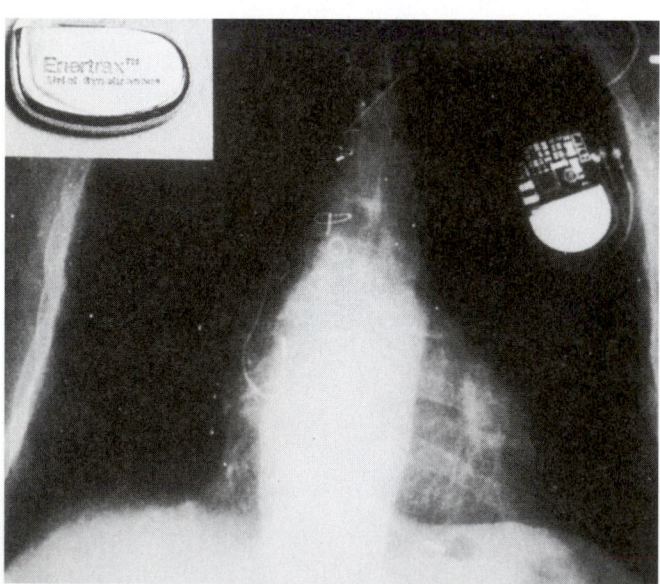

Figure 11-13 A pacemaker, which is typically inserted under the skin in the left upper chest, delivers an electrical impulse to regulate heartbeat.

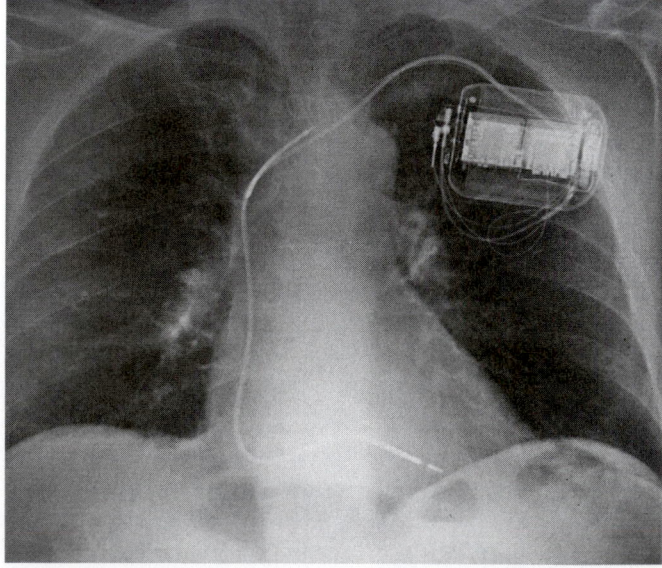

Figure 11-14 An AICD is attached directly to the heart and continuously monitors heart rhythm, delivering shocks as needed. The electricity from the AICD is so low that it has no effect on rescuers.

she should be treated like all other AMI patients; treatment should include performing CPR and using an AED if the patient goes into cardiac arrest. Generally, the electricity from an AICD is so low that it will have no effect on rescuers and therefore should not be of concern to you.

Automated External Defibrillation

In the late 1970s and early 1980s, scientists developed a small computer that could analyze electrical signals from the heart and determine when ventricular fibrillation was taking place. This development, along with improved battery technology, made possible the automated portable defibrillator, which can automatically administer an electrical shock to the heart when needed.

AED machines come in models with different features (▶ **Figure 11-15**). All of them require a certain degree of operator interaction, beginning with applying the pads and turning the machine on. The operator also has to push a button to deliver an electrical shock, regardless of the model. Many AEDs use a computer voice synthesizer to advise the rescuer which steps to take on the basis of the AED's analysis. Some have a button that tells the computer to analyze the heart's electrical rhythm; other models start doing this as soon as they are turned on. In the United States, most of the AEDs are semiauto-

mated. Even though most defibrillators are now semi-automated, we are using the term *automated external defibrillators* (AED) as the general term to describe all of these machines. There are very few actual AEDs left; all manufacturers are only producing semiautomated external defibrillators.

AEDs also come equipped to give a monophasic shock or a biphasic shock. Monophasic means to send the energy in one direction, from negative to positive and biphasic means to send the energy in two directions simultaneously. The advantage of biphasic shock is that it produces a more efficient defibrillation and may require a lower energy setting. The energy setting for ventricular fibrillation on a monophasic machine is generally 200 joules to start then moves to 200 or 300 joules, and then to 360 joules. With the biphasic technology, the energy can be set at 120 joules for all three shocks and all subsequest shocks after that.

The computer inside the AED is specially programmed to recognize rhythms that require defibrillation to correct, most commonly ventricular fibrillation. The current programs are extremely accurate. It would be extremely rare for them to recommend a shock when a shock would not be called for, and they rarely fail to recommend one when it would be helpful. Therefore, if the AED recommends a shock, you can believe that it is indicated.

When an error does occur, it is usually the operator's fault. The most common error is not having a charged battery. To avoid this problem, many defibrillator companies have built smarter machines that will warn the operator that the battery is unlikely to work. However, some of the older models do not have this feature. You should check the AED regularly and exercise the battery as often as the manufacturer recommends.

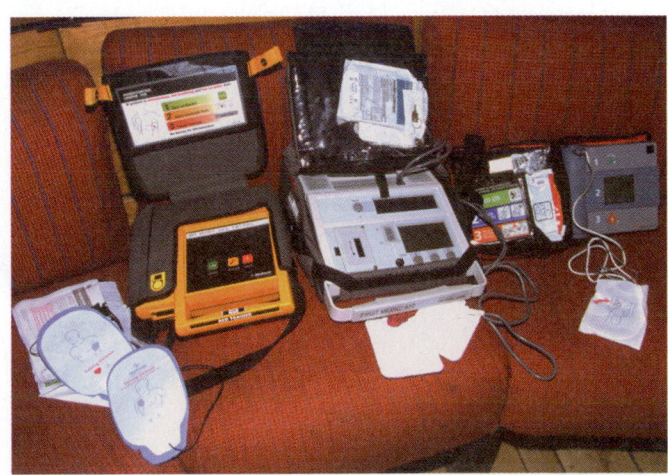

Figure 11-15 AEDs vary in their design, features, and operation.

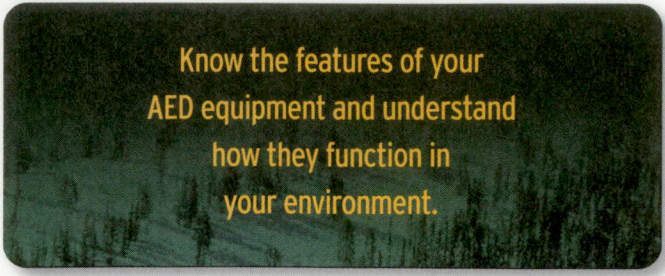

Know the features of your AED equipment and understand how they function in your environment.

Another error with some AED machines occurs when the AED is applied to a patient who is moving. The computer may be unable to tell the difference between electrical signals from the heart and electrical signals from the arms and chest muscles that are moving. The way to avoid this error is to apply the AED only to pulseless, unresponsive patients and to stay clear of the patient (do not touch the patient) during analysis and shocking.

A third error can occur when the AED is applied to a responsive patient with a rapid heart rate. Most computers identify a regular rhythm faster than 150 or 180 beats/min as ventricular tachycardia, which should be shocked. Sometimes, though, a patient has another heart rhythm that should not be shocked but that is fast enough to confuse the computer. Again, to avoid this problem, you should apply the AED only to unresponsive patients with no pulse.

Automated external defibrillation offers the rescuer a number of advantages. First, it delivers the most important treatment for the patient in ventricular fibrillation: an electrical shock. It can be delivered within 1 minute of the rescuer's arrival at the patient's side. Second, you will find that using an AED is easier than

performing CPR. ALS providers do not have to be on the scene to provide this definitive care.

Current AEDs offer two other advantages. The shock can be given through remote, adhesive defibrillator pads, which are safer for you than paddles. Usually, there are pictures on the pads to remind you where they go on the patient's chest.

Not all patients in cardiac arrest require an electrical shock. Although all patients in cardiac arrest should be analyzed with an AED, some do not have shockable rhythms (eg, pulseless electrical activity or asystole). Asystole (flatline) indicates that no electrical activity remains. Pulseless electrical activity usually refers to a state of cardiac arrest with disorganized ventricular fibrillation or ventricular tachycardia despite an electrical activity without a medical response. In both cases, CPR should be initiated as soon as possible.

Rationale for Early Defibrillation

Few patients who experience sudden cardiac arrest survive unless a rapid sequence of events takes place. The chain of survival is a way of describing the ideal sequence of events that can take place when such an arrest occurs.

The four links in the chain of survival are as follows ▼ **Figure 11-16**):

- Recognition of early warning signs and immediate activation of EMS
- Immediate bystander CPR
- Early defibrillation
- Early advanced cardiac life support

If any one of the links in the chain is absent or delayed, the patient is more likely to die. For example,

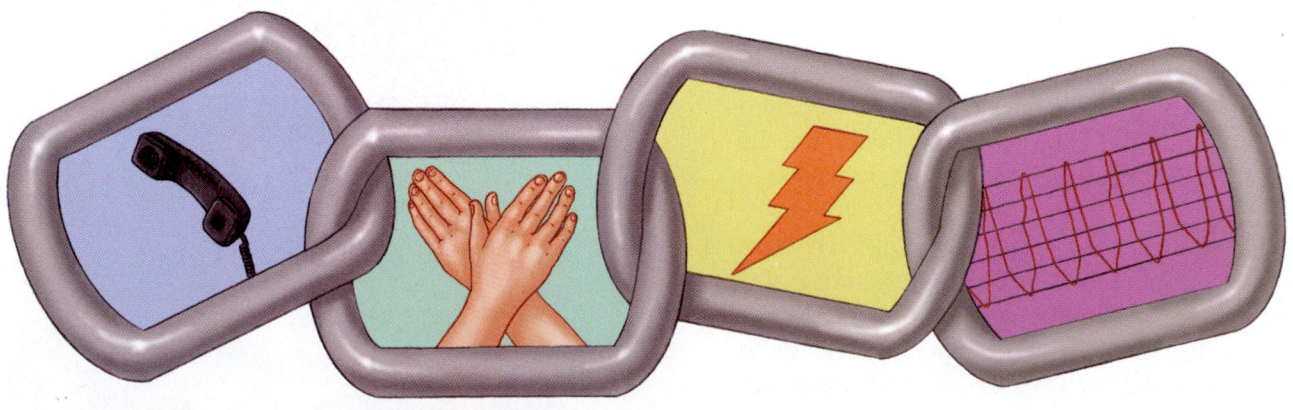

Early access   Early CPR   Early defibrillation   Early advanced care

Figure 11-16 The four links of the chain of survival.
Source: American Heart Association

there is a rapid decrease in patient survival rate (7% to 10% per minute) if early defibrillation is not implemented. Perform CPR in the first 2 to 3 minutes if the AED is not available to defibrillate. If all links in the chain are strong, the patient has the best possible chance of survival. The link with the most determinant for survival is the third link—early defibrillation.

CPR helps patients in cardiac arrest because it prolongs the period of time during which defibrillation can be effective. Rapid defibrillation has successfully resuscitated many patients with cardiac arrest from ventricular fibrillation. However, defibrillation works best if it takes place within 2 minutes of the onset of the cardiac arrest. To try to achieve better survival rates among cardiac arrest victims, many ski areas are supplying AEDs following state public access regulations. Area management must also approve AED usage. Remember, seconds really do matter when the patient is in cardiac arrest.

Integrating the AED and CPR

Since most cardiac arrests occur in the home, a bystander at the scene may already have started CPR before you arrive. For this reason, you must know how to work the AED into the CPR sequence. Remember, depending on internal technology, that some AEDs may not be able to distinguish other movements from ventricular fibrillation. Therefore, do not touch the patient while the AED is analyzing the heart rhythm and delivering shocks. Stop CPR, and let the AED do its job. CPR may be stopped for up to 90 seconds if three shocks are necessary. This is entirely proper; defibrillation is more important than CPR when ventricular fibrillation is present.

Upon arrival at the scene, make sure that the scene is safe to enter and that you use BSI techniques. Ask any bystanders or first responders who are performing CPR to stop so that you can apply the AED and defibrillate the patient. Take the following steps if allowed by your local protocols (▶ **Skill Drill 11-1**):

1. **Arrive on scene and perform your initial assessment.** Assess responsiveness. If the patient is responsive, do not apply the AED.
2. **Stop CPR** if it is in progress.
3. **Verify pulselessness and apnea.** Check for breathing and a pulse even if the patient appears to be breathing. Absent a pulse check step, lay rescuers are required to assess signs of circulation by assessing signs of normal breathing, coughing, or movement in response to two rescue breaths. *AHA Guidelines 2000 for Cardiopulmonary*

Rescuer Safety

When clearing the patient before an AED shock, ensure that no one is touching the patient and that no object is touching the patient, including the stretcher or other furniture if the patient is not on the floor or ground.

Resuscitation and Emergency Cardiovascular Care, p. I-37+, I-3; and *BLS for Healthcare Providers* text, p. 75–76.

4. If the patient is unresponsive and not breathing or is breathing agonally (slow, gasping breaths), **give two ventilations** using a BVM device or a pocket mask **(Step 1)**.
5. **Have your partner start or resume CPR.**
6. If an AED is on the scene, **prepare the AED pads.**
7. **Turn on the machine (Step 2).** Remove excess chest hair or wipe chest if wet, or pads will not adhere properly.
8. **Remove clothing from the patient's chest area.** Apply the pads to the chest: one just to the right of the breastbone (sternum) just below the collarbone (clavicle), the other on the left chest with the top of the pad 2″ to 3″ below the armpit. Ensure that the pads are attached to the patient cables (and that they are attached to the AED in some models).
9. **Stop CPR (Step 3).**
10. **State aloud, "Clear the patient,"** and ensure that no one is touching the patient.
11. **Push the analyze button,** if there is one.
12. **Wait for the computer** in the AED to determine whether a shockable rhythm is present.
13. If a shock is not needed, go to step 18 (CPR only). If a shock is advised, make sure that no one is touching the patient. When the area is clear, **push the shock button.**
14. **After the shock is delivered,** most AEDs will automatically reanalyze the rhythm; if not, push the analyze button again.
15. **If the machine advises a shock, deliver a second shock.**

Skill Drill 11-1   Integrating the AED and CPR

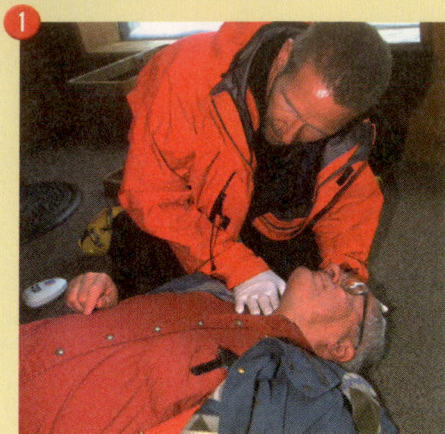

Stop CPR if in progress.
Assess responsiveness.
Check breathing and pulse.
If unresponsive and not breathing adequately, give two slow ventilations.

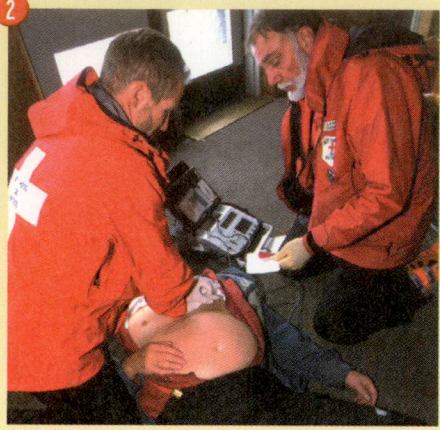

If pulseless, begin CPR.
Prepare the AED pads.
Turn on the AED; begin narrative if needed.

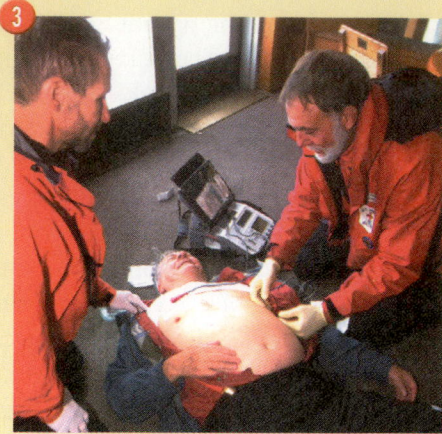

Apply AED pads.
Stop CPR.

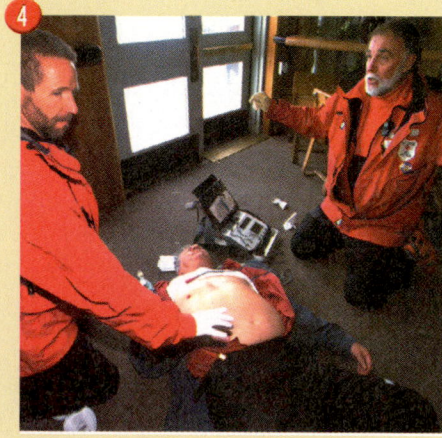

Verbally and visually clear the patient.
Push the analyze button if there is one.
Wait for the AED to analyze rhythm.
If no shock advised, perform CPR for 1 minute.
If shock advised, recheck that all are clear and push the shock button.
Push the analyze button, if needed, to analyze rhythm again.
Press the shock button if advised (second shock).
Push the analyze button, if needed, to analyze rhythm again.
Press the shock button if advised (third shock).

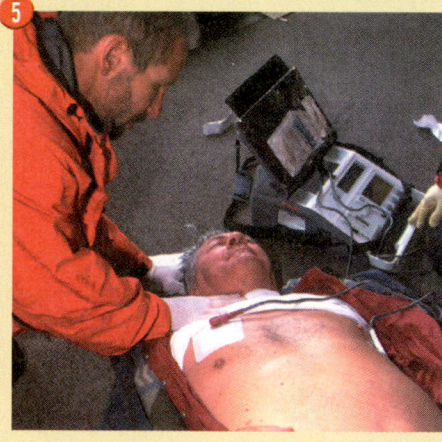

Check pulse.
If pulse is present, check breathing.

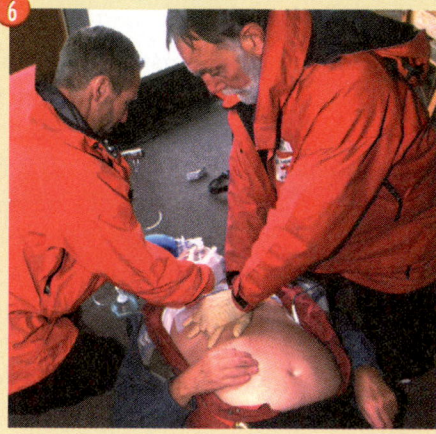

If breathing adequately, give oxygen and transport. If not, open airway, ventilate, and transport.
If no pulse, perform CPR for 1 minute.
Clear the patient and analyze again.
If necessary, repeat one cycle of up to three shocks.
Transport and call medical control.
Continue to support breathing or perform CPR, as needed.

16. **Reanalyze the rhythm.**

17. **If the machine advises a shock, deliver a third shock (Step 4).**

18. **Check for a pulse.**

19. **If the patient has a pulse,** check the patient's breathing **(Step 5)**.

20. **If the patient is breathing adequately,** give the patient oxygen via nonrebreathing mask and transport. If the patient is not breathing adequately, use necessary airway adjuncts and proper positioning of the head and jaw to ensure an open airway. Provide artificial ventilations with high-concentration oxygen and transport.

21. **If the patient has no pulse,** perform 1 minute of CPR.

22. **After 1 minute of CPR,** make sure no one is touching the patient. Push the analyze button again (as applicable).

23. **If necessary, repeat one cycle of up to three stacked shocks.**

24. **Transport and check with medical control.**

25. **Continue to support the patient** as needed: ventilate until the patient begins to breathe normally, and continue CPR if needed **(Step 6)**.

If, after any rhythm analysis, the AED advises no shock, check the patient's pulse. If the patient has a pulse, check the patient's breathing. If the patient is breathing adequately, give high-concentration oxygen via nonrebreathing mask and transport. If the patient is not breathing adequately, provide artificial ventilations with high-concentration oxygen via a BVM device and transport. Ensure that appropriate airway techniques are used at all times.

If the patient has no pulse, resume CPR for 1 minute, then have the AED reanalyze the heart rhythm. If the AED advises shock, deliver up to two sets of three stacked shocks. Separate each set of three shocks with 1 minute of CPR.

If the AED advises no shock and the patient has no pulse, resume CPR for 1 minute, then stop and reanalyze the heart rhythm for a third time. If the AED advises shock, deliver up to two sets of three stacked shocks with 1 minute of CPR between the two sets. If the AED still advises no shock, check with medical control, resume CPR, and transport.

If you are the only rescuer at the scene and you have an AED, take the following steps:

1. Perform an initial assessment. Assess responsiveness. If the patient is responsive, do not apply the AED.

2. Verify that the patient has no pulse and is not breathing (or is breathing with inadequate gasping breaths).

3. If the patient is not breathing or is gasping, give two slow breaths using a BVM device or pocket mask.

4. Expose the patient's chest. Apply one pad just to the right of the breastbone (sternum), just below the collarbone (clavicle), and the other on the left side of the chest with the top of the pad 2" to 3" below the armpit.

5. Turn on the AED.

6. Push the analyze button, if there is one.

7. Deliver up to three shocks, if indicated.

8. Follow your local protocol. If the AED indicates no need for shocks, provide CPR.

If another person is available who knows CPR, ask for help. You will perform the steps in the same order. The only difference is that the other person can continue CPR while you are getting the AED out and applied to the patient.

After AED Shocks

The care of the patient after the AED delivers its shock depends on your location, facilities, and resources; therefore, you should follow your local protocols. After the AED protocol is completed, the patient is likely to have had one of the following occur:

- Regained a pulse

- No pulse, and the AED indicates that no shock is advised

- No pulse, and the AED indicates that a shock is advised

If you got to the patient quickly and the patient started breathing on his or her own, administer oxygen by nonrebreathing face mask with the oxygen flow set to 10 to 15 L/min. Check the patient's pulse. If the patient has a pulse but is not breathing adequately, assist ventilations, using a BVM device with high-flow oxygen. Prepare for transport, keeping

Rescuer Tips

AED operational tips

- One rescuer operates the defibrillator while another does CPR.
- Defibrillation comes first. Do not apply oxygen or do anything else that delays analysis of rhythm or defibrillation.
- Be familiar with the AED device used by your area.
- Avoid all contact with the patient during analysis of the rhythm.
- State, "Clear the patient" before shocking. Another popular phrase is "I'm clear, you're clear, we're all clear" before delivering shocks.
- In applicable models of AEDs, check the batteries at the beginning of your shift; carry an extra charged battery with your AED.
- Do not use an AED for cardiac arrest in children younger than age 8 years or who weigh less than 55 lb (25 kg) unless you have access to pediatric pads.
- Unless indicated otherwise by local protocol, you do not need to perform pulse checks during rhythm analysis; typically, there will be no pulse check between stacked shocks 1 and 2 and stacked shocks 2 and 3.
- Continued airway maintenance and artificial ventilation are of prime importance.

the AED attached to the patient. Recheck the pulse frequently, at least every 30 seconds. In applicable devices, push the analyze button on the AED if the pulse is lost. Commonly, patients who are successfully defibrillated by AED will develop a normal heart rhythm for a while. However, since the heart still is not receiving optimal amounts of oxygen, ventricular fibrillation will often recur. Be sure you know your patrol's procedures for managing patients in this situation ▶ **Figure 11-17** .

Cardiac Arrest During Transport

If you are transporting a patient while performing CPR or using an AED, you need to a plan for managing the patient on the toboggan.

If you are transporting an unconscious patient in a toboggan, check the pulse at least every 30 seconds. If a pulse is not present, take the following steps:

1. Have the toboggan stopped and held secure by other patrollers. Have the patrollers stay in the handles for quick transport. Rescuers need to be cautious not to touch or let the patient touch any metal parts of the toboggan.

2. If the AED is not immediately ready, perform CPR until the unit is available. Have the toboggan held secure and do a full minute of CPR, then transport the patient for 30 seconds, stop, do a full minute of CPR, transport for 30 seconds, and so on until the AED is available or transport complete.

3. If the AED becomes available, have the toboggan stopped and held secure. Analyze the rhythm.

4. Deliver shocks, if indicated.

5. Continue resuscitation using the "leapfrog" technique of CPR if indicated and according to your local protocol.

If you are transporting a conscious adult patient who is having chest pain and becomes unconscious in a toboggan, take the following steps:

1. Check for a pulse.

2. Have the toboggan stopped and secured. Have the patrollers ready for immediate transport.

3. If the AED is not immediately available, perform a full minute of CPR, transport for 30 seconds, stop, do a full minute of CPR, transport, and so on until the AED is available or until toboggan transport is complete.

4. When the AED is available, analyze the rhythm.

5. Deliver shocks, if indicated.

6. Continue resuscitation according to your local protocol. If a "no shock" message is given and no pulse is present, you should use the "leapfrog" technique of CPR until toboggan transport is complete.

Coordination with ALS

The time to defibrillation is critical to survival after cardiac arrest. As a rescuer equipped with an AED, you have the one tool that the dying patient in ventricular fibrillation needs most. Furthermore, it is very hard to hurt someone with an AED. Therefore, if you have an AED available, do not wait for the more highly trained medical personnel to arrive to administer a shock. Waiting might seem like a good idea. It is not. It is throwing away the patient's best chance for survival.

If the patient is unresponsive and does not have a pulse, apply the AED and push the analyze button (if there is one) as quickly as you can. Notify the ALS per-

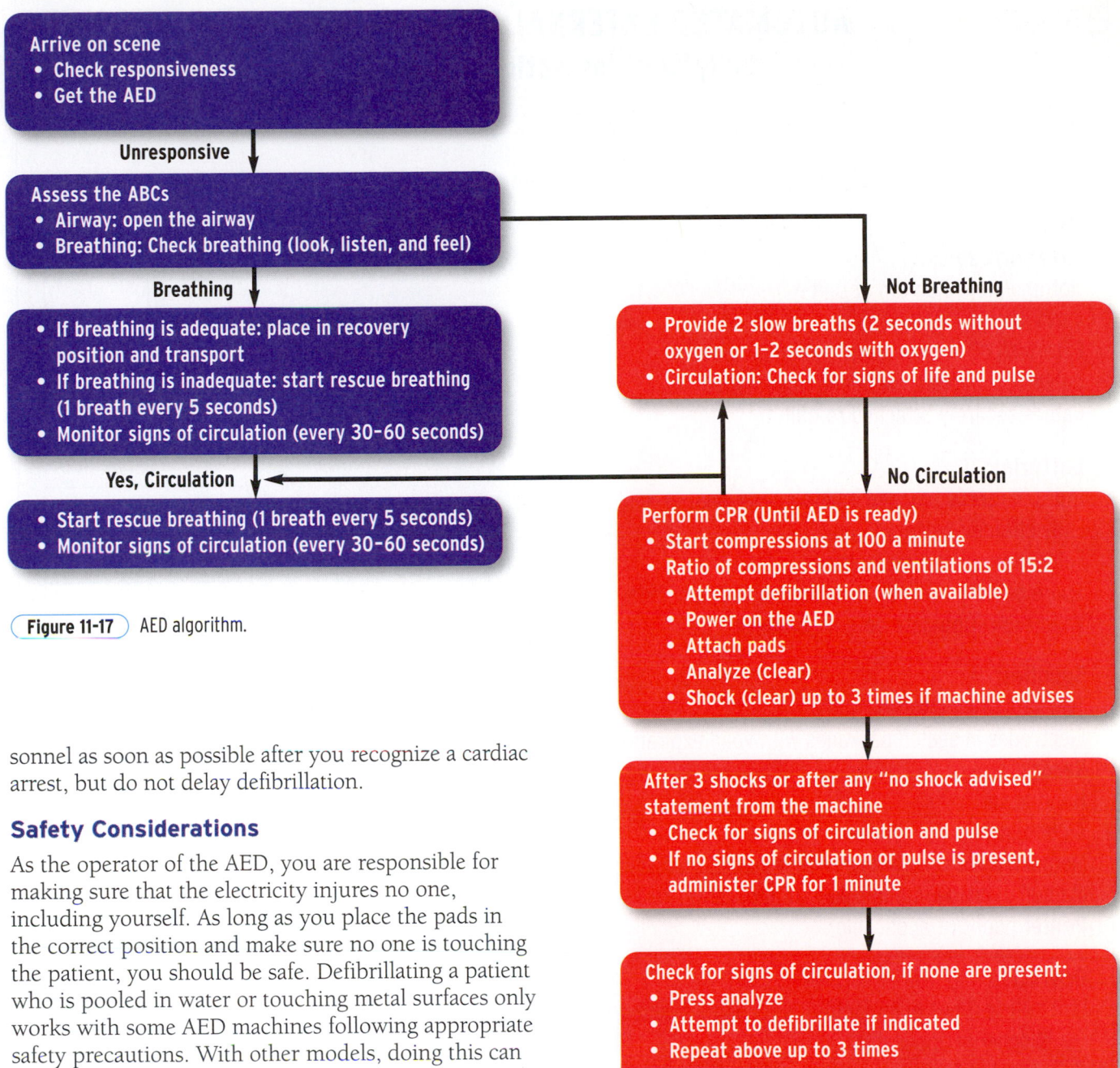

Arrive on scene
• Check responsiveness
• Get the AED

Unresponsive

Assess the ABCs
• Airway: open the airway
• Breathing: Check breathing (look, listen, and feel)

Breathing

• If breathing is adequate: place in recovery position and transport
• If breathing is inadequate: start rescue breathing (1 breath every 5 seconds)
• Monitor signs of circulation (every 30-60 seconds)

Yes, Circulation

• Start rescue breathing (1 breath every 5 seconds)
• Monitor signs of circulation (every 30-60 seconds)

Not Breathing

• Provide 2 slow breaths (2 seconds without oxygen or 1-2 seconds with oxygen)
• Circulation: Check for signs of life and pulse

No Circulation

Perform CPR (Until AED is ready)
• Start compressions at 100 a minute
• Ratio of compressions and ventilations of 15:2
   • Attempt defibrillation (when available)
   • Power on the AED
   • Attach pads
   • Analyze (clear)
   • Shock (clear) up to 3 times if machine advises

After 3 shocks or after any "no shock advised" statement from the machine
• Check for signs of circulation and pulse
• If no signs of circulation or pulse is present, administer CPR for 1 minute

Check for signs of circulation, if none are present:
• Press analyze
• Attempt to defibrillate if indicated
• Repeat above up to 3 times
Note: additional shock sequences are by local protocol.

Figure 11-17 AED algorithm.

sonnel as soon as possible after you recognize a cardiac arrest, but do not delay defibrillation.

Safety Considerations

As the operator of the AED, you are responsible for making sure that the electricity injures no one, including yourself. As long as you place the pads in the correct position and make sure no one is touching the patient, you should be safe. Defibrillating a patient who is pooled in water or touching metal surfaces only works with some AED machines following appropriate safety precautions. With other models, doing this can be a danger to you and your patient. Again, know the features of the AED you are using. Check your unit for safe use on snow. There is another problem. Electricity follows the path of least resistance; instead of traveling between the pads and through the patient's heart, it will diffuse into the water. Therefore, the heart will not receive enough electricity to cause defibrillation. You can defibrillate a soaking wet patient, but try first to dry the patient's chest. Do not defibrillate someone who is touching metal that others are touching, and carefully remove a nitroglycerin patch from a patient's chest and wipe the area with a dry towel before defibrillation to prevent ignition of the patch.

AED Maintenance

One of your primary missions as a rescuer is to deliver an electrical shock to a patient in ventricular fibrillation. To accomplish this mission, you need to have a functioning AED. You must become familiar with the maintenance procedures required for the brand of AED your service uses. Read the operator's manual. If your defibrillator does not work on the scene, someone will want to know what went wrong. That

AUTOMATED EXTERNAL DEFIBRILLATOR
Daily/Shift Inspection Checklist

Serial # _____   Date _____   Time _____

Model # _____   Inspected by _____

Item	Pass	Fail
Exterior/Cables:		
Nothing stored on top of unit		
Carry case intact and clean		
Exterior/LCD screen clean and undamaged		
Cables/connectors clean and undamaged		
Cables securely attached to unit		
Batteries:		
Unit charger is plugged in and operational (if applicable)		
Fully charged battery in unit		
Fully charged spare battery		
Spare battery charger plugged in and operational (if applicable)		
Valid expiration date on both batteries		
Supplies:		
Two sets of electrodes		
Electrodes in sealed packages with valid expiration dates		
Razor		
Hand towel		
Alcohol wipes		
Memory/voice recording device–module, card, microcassette		
Manual override–module, key (if applicable)		
Printer paper (if applicable)		
Operation:		
Unit self-test per manufacturer's recommendation/instructions:		
Display (if applicable)		
Visual indicators		
Verbal prompts		
Printer (if applicable)		
Attach AED to simulator/tester:		
Recognizes shockable rhythm		
Charges to correct energy level within manufacturer's specifications		
Delivers charge		
Recognizes nonshockable rhythm		
Manual override system in working order (if applicable)		

Signature:

Figure 11-18 A sample daily checklist for the AED.

person may be your system's administrator, your medical director, the local newspaper reporter, or the family's attorney. You will be asked to show proof that you maintained the defibrillator properly and attended any mandatory in-services.

The main legal risk in using the AED is failing to deliver a shock when one was needed. The most common reason for this failure is that the battery did not work, usually because it was not properly maintained. Another problem is operator error. This means not pushing the analyze or shock buttons when the machine advises you to do so or failing to apply the AED to a patient in cardiac arrest. Of course, the AED is like any other manufactured item. It can fail, although this is rare. Ideally, you will encounter any such failure while doing routine maintenance, not while caring for a patient in cardiac arrest. Check your equipment, including your AED, at the beginning of each shift. Ask the manufacturer for a checklist (◄ **Figure 11-18**) of items that should be checked daily, weekly, or less often.

If you do have an AED failure while caring for a patient, you must report that problem to the manufacturer and the US Food and Drug Administration. Be sure to follow the appropriate area procedures for notifying these organizations.

Medical Direction

Defibrillation of the heart is a medical procedure. While AEDs have made the process of delivering electricity much simpler, there is still a benefit in having a physician's involvement. The medical advisor of your resort should help to teach you how to use the AED. At the very least, he or she should approve the written protocol that you will follow in caring for patients in cardiac arrest. If a medical advisor is not part of your operations, a local emergency department physician may be willing to provide medical direction.

There should be a review of each incident in which the AED is used. Sit down with the rest of the team and go over what happened. This discussion will help all members of the team to learn from the incident. Review such events by using the written report, any voice-ECG tape recorder, and the device's solid-state memory modules and magnetic tape recordings, if applicable.

Mandatory continuing education with skill competency review is generally required for AED providers, with a continuing competency skill review periodically.

Chapter *Sweep*

Ready for Review

The heart is divided down the middle into two sides, right and left, each with an upper chamber called the atrium and a lower chamber called the ventricle. The largest of the four heart valves that keep blood moving through the circulatory system in the proper direction is the aortic valve, which lies between the left ventricle and the aorta, the body's main artery. The heart's electrical system controls heart rate and helps to keep or maintain that the atria and ventricles work together.

During periods of exertion or stress, the myocardium requires more oxygen. This is supplied by dilation of the coronary arteries, which increases blood flow.

Common places to feel for a pulse include the carotid, femoral, brachial, radial, ulnar, posterior tibial, and dorsalis pedis arteries.

Low blood flow to the heart is usually caused by coronary artery atherosclerosis, a disease in which cholesterol plaques build up inside blood vessels, eventually occluding them. Occasionally, a brittle plaque will crack, causing a blood clot to form. Heart tissue downstream suffers from a lack of oxygen and, within 30 minutes, will begin to die. This is called an acute myocardial infarction (AMI), or heart attack. Heart tissues that are not getting enough oxygen but are not yet dying can cause pain called angina. The pain of AMI is different from the pain of angina in that it can come at any time, not just with exertion; it lasts up to several hours, rather than just a few moments; and it is not relieved by rest or nitroglycerin. In addition to crushing chest pain, signs of AMI include sudden onset of weakness, nausea, and sweating; sudden arrhythmia; pulmonary edema; and even sudden death.

Heart attacks can have three serious consequences. One is sudden death, usually the result of cardiac arrest caused by abnormal heart rhythms called arrhythmias. These include tachycardia, bradycardia, ventricular tachycardia, and, most commonly, ventricular fibrillation. The second consequence is cardiogenic shock. Symptoms include restlessness; anxiety; pale, clammy skin; pulse rate higher than normal; and blood pressure lower than normal. Patients with these symptoms should receive oxygen, assisted ventilations as needed, and immediate transport.

The third consequence of AMI is congestive heart failure, in which damaged heart muscle can no longer contract effectively enough to pump blood through the system. The lungs become congested with fluid, breathing becomes difficult, the heart rate increases, and the left ventricle enlarges. Signs include swollen ankles from pedal edema, high blood pressure, rapid heart rate and respirations, rales, and sometimes the pink sputum and dyspnea of pulmonary edema. Treat a patient with CHF as you would a patient with chest pain. Monitor the patient's heart rhythm, give the patient oxygen via nonrebreathing face mask, allow the patient to remain sitting up.

In treating patients with chest pain, obtain a SAMPLE history, following the OPQRST mnemonic to assess the pain; measure and record vital signs; put the patient in a comfortable position, usually sitting up; administer prescribed nitroglycerin and oxygen; and transport the patient, reporting to medical control as you do. If a patient is not responsive and is 8 years or older and weighs at least 55 lb, you must decide whether to use the automated external defibrillator (AED). If the patient weighs less than 55 lb, begin CPR.

The AED requires the operator to apply the pads, power on the unit, analyze the rhythm, and press the shock button. The computer inside the AED recognizes rhythms that require shocking and will not mislead you. The three most common errors in using certain AEDs are failure to keep a charged battery in the machine, applying the AED to a patient who is moving, and applying the AED to a responsive patient with a rapid heart rate. Do not touch the patient while the AED is analyzing the heart rhythm or delivering shocks. In integrating use of the AED and CPR, you should perform CPR only after giving up to three shocks, if these are all needed. If you still cannot get a pulse, perform CPR for 1 minute.

The chain of survival, which is the sequence of events that must occur for a patient with cardiac arrest to have the best chance of survival, includes recognition of early warning signs and immediate activation of EMS, immediate CPR by bystanders, early defibrillation, and early advanced care. Seconds count at every stage.

Vital Vocabulary

acute myocardial infarction (AMI)   Heart attack; death of heart muscle following obstruction of blood flow to it. Acute in this context means "new" or "happening right now."

angina pectoris   Transient (short-lived) chest discomfort caused by partial or temporary blockage of blood flow to the heart muscle.

anterior   The front surface of the body; the side facing you in the standard anatomic position.

aorta   The main artery, which receives blood from the left ventricle and delivers it to all the other arteries that carry blood to the tissues of the body.

aortic valve   The one-way valve that lies between the left ventricle and the aorta. It keeps blood from flowing back into the left ventricle after the left ventricle ejects its blood into the aorta. One of four heart valves.

asystole   Complete absence of heart electrical activity.

atherosclerosis   A disorder in which cholesterol and calcium build up inside the walls of blood vessels, eventually leading to partial or complete blockage of blood flow.

atrium   One of two (right and left) upper chambers of the heart. The right atrium receives blood from the vena cava and delivers it to the right ventricle. The left atrium receives blood from pulmonary veins and delivers it to the left ventricle.

cardiac arrest   A state in which the heart fails to generate an effective and detectable blood flow; pulses are not palpable in cardiac arrest, even if muscular and electrical activity continues in the heart.

cardiogenic shock   A state in which not enough oxygen is delivered to the tissues of the body, caused by low output of blood from the heart. It can be a severe complication of a large acute myocardial infarction, as well as other conditions.

congestive heart failure (CHF)   A disorder in which the heart loses part of its ability to effectively pump blood, usually as a result of damage to the heart muscle and usually resulting in a backup of fluid into the lungs.

coronary artery   A blood vessel that carries blood and nutrients to the heart muscle.

defibrillation   To shock a fibrillating (chaotically beating) heart with specialized electrical current in an attempt to restore a normal rhythmic beat.

dilation   Widening of a tubular structure such as a coronary artery.

infarction   Death of a body tissue, usually caused by interruption of its blood supply.

inferior   The part of the body, or any body part, nearer to the feet.

ischemia   A lack of oxygen that deprives tissues of necessary nutrients, resulting from partial or complete blockage of blood flow; potentially reversible since permanent injury has not yet occurred.

lumen   The inside diameter of an artery or other hollow structure.

myocardium   Heart muscle.

occlusion   Blockage, usually of a tubular structure such as a blood vessel.

pedal edema   Swelling of the feet and ankles caused by collection of fluid in the tissues; a possible sign of congestive heart failure (CHF).

posterior   The back surface of the body; the side away from you in the standard anatomic position.

superior   The part of the body, or any body part, nearer to the head.

ventricle   One of two (right and left) lower chambers of the heart. The left ventricle receives blood from the left atrium (upper chamber) and delivers blood to the aorta. The right ventricle receives blood from the right atrium and pumps it into the pulmonary artery.

ventricular fibrillation   Disorganized, ineffective twitching of the ventricles, resulting in no blood flow and a state of cardiac arrest.

ventricular tachycardia   Rapid heart rhythm in which the electrical impulse begins in the ventricle (instead of the atrium), which may result in inadequate blood flow and eventually deteriorate into cardiac arrest.

www.OECzone.com

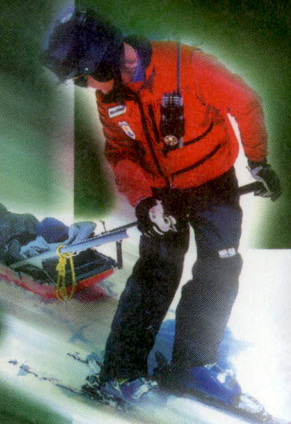

Assessment in Action

You are dispatched to the aid room at the top of Lift Eight for a "man with chest pain." The patient's wife meets you at the door. She tells you he has had indigestion for the last hour but as they got off the chair lift he started complaining of severe chest pressure, so they skied to the aid room.

As the wife begins introducing her husband, you note that he is very pale, his lips are gray, and sweat is beading up on his forehead. He is clutching his chest and looks at you with frightened eyes. His vital signs include a pulse of 110 beats/min and regular, shallow respirations of 20 breaths/min, and a blood pressure of 98/56 mm Hg. His skin is cold and clammy. He is alert and oriented with a history of gastric reflux disease, hypertension, and angina. He is on nitroglycerin for angina pectoris, Tinormen for hypertension, and Prilosec for gastric reflux. He has no allergies.

1. Chest pain that is cardiac in origin is usually caused by:
   A. too much oxygen to the lungs.
   B. insufficient oxygen to the heart.
   C. excess oxygen to the heart.
   D. trauma to the chest wall.

2. Which of the following signs or symptoms that this patient is exhibiting indicates a high suspicion for cardiac involvement? Chest pain, clutching his chest, and:
   A. pale, cold, clammy skin and blood pressure.
   B. his pulse, blood pressure, and respiratory rate.
   C. a history of indigestion and now chest pain.
   D. the frightened look in his eyes and mental status.

3. The most likely reason this patient has ashen gray skin is because:
   A. his skin is normally that color.
   B. he has poor cardiac output.
   C. his blood pressure is abnormally high.
   D. he is getting ready to vomit.

4. Treatment should include high-flow oxygen and:
   A. lying him flat with his feet elevated.
   B. keeping him in an upright position.
   C. placing him in the recovery position.
   D. applying the AED.

5. This patient has his own nitroglycerin that is current. Your protocols will allow you to use nitroglycerin, so your partner gets ready to administer it. Appropriate actions include:
   A. rechecking his blood pressure and assisting with administration.
   B. ensuring that his mouth is moist prior to administration.
   C. reminding your partner that his blood pressure is too low.
   D. listening to breath sounds and assisting with administration.

6. When you listen to breath sounds, you hear crackles. This suggests that which of the following is present?
   A. Sudden death
   B. Spontaneous pneumothorax
   C. Pulmonary edema
   D. Pulmonary emboli

7. You notice that this patient's neck veins are becoming distended, his color is getting worse, and he is becoming confused. Vital signs are now: pulse 120 and irregular, respirations 28 and labored, blood pressure 90/64. What is happening?
   A. Congestive heart failure
   B. A cerebrovascular accident
   C. An unrelated pulmonary problem
   D. Cardiogenic shock

Challenging Questions

8. This patient cannot lie down. Why?

9. This patient is going into cardiac arrest. Why shouldn't the AED be applied?

10. Why should you encourage patients to lie down after they are given nitroglycerin?

Points to Ponder

You are the first person to respond to a report of chest pain. The patient is on the upper floor of the ski lodge. Being first on the scene, you are the designated care provider for this situation. When you walk into the ski lodge you immediately recognize the patient as a man who is inappropriately suing your father and asking for a large financial settlement. It has been an ugly case with very hard feelings on both sides of the lawsuit. The patient is in obvious respiratory distress and has significant chest pain. He immediately recognizes you but does not say anything. How would you deal with this situation? Do you need to document this interaction any differently? Should it be reported and, if so, to whom?

Issues Conflict of Interest, Best Patient Care, Reporting Non-medical Issues.

Online Outlook

In an average lifetime, the heart beats more than two and a half billion times, without ever pausing to rest. Like a pumping machine, the heart provides the power that is needed for life. To learn more about the heart and cardiovascular system, complete Exercise 11 at www.OECzone.com.

Neurologic Emergencies

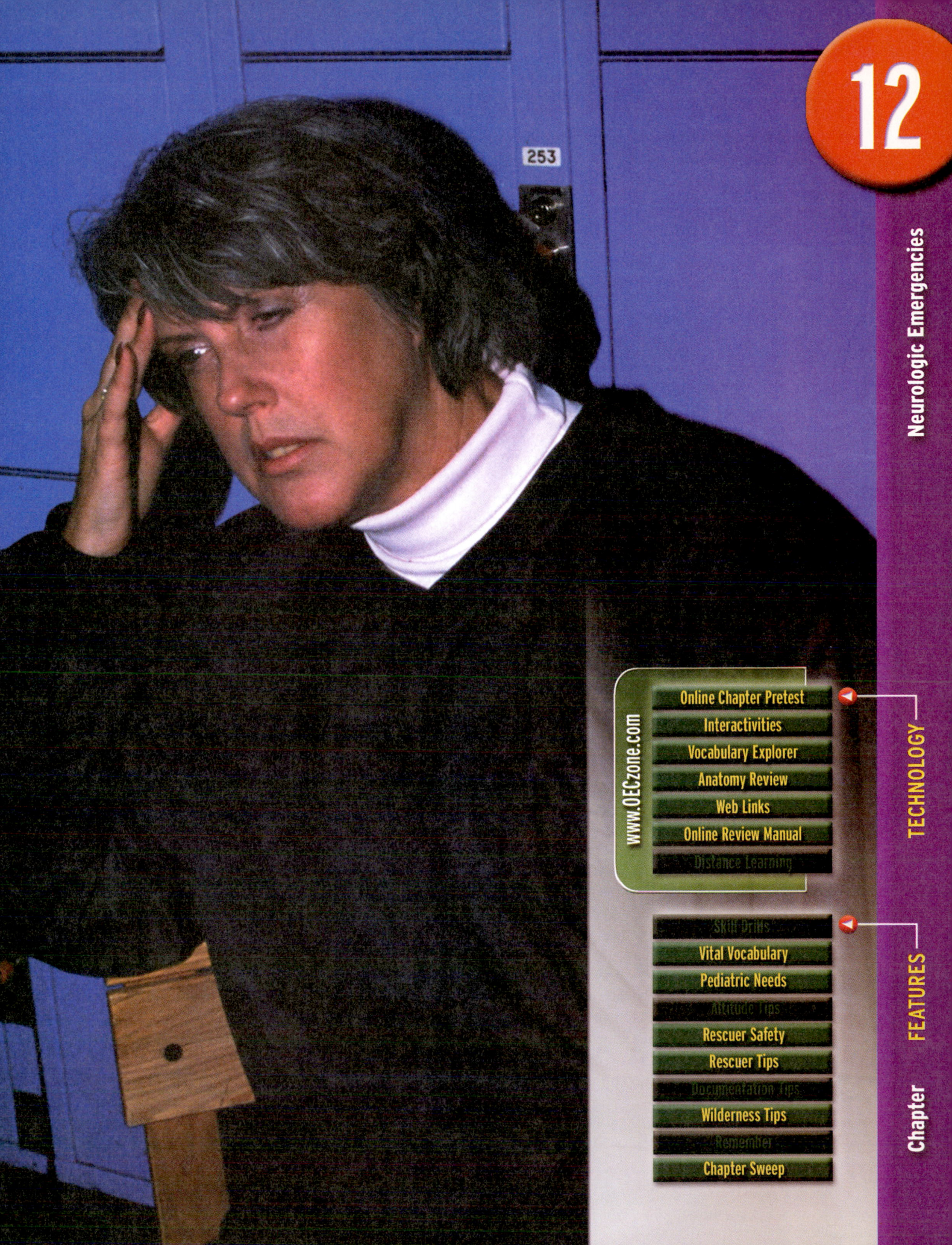

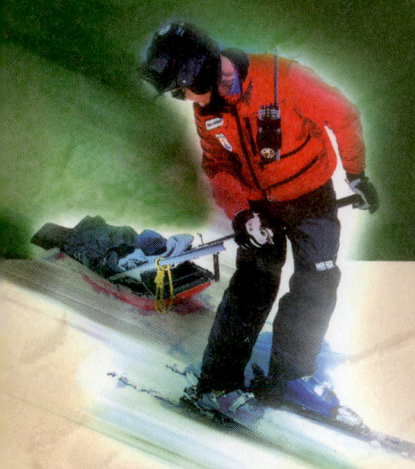

"609 Randy, this is Lunch Rock Dispatch."

"Lunch Rock Dispatch, 609, go ahead."

"Randy, 10-50 CODE RED on Derailer, skier versus tree, halfway down the run in the trees on the left. Party is unresponsive. When out, use Com 3, time out 13.28."

"I'm en route, Derailer on the left, 609 clear."

This chapter will lay the foundation of knowledge necessary for you to provide quality care for patients with traumatic brain injuries or neurologic dysfunction and will also help you answer the following questions:

1. Why does a person become unresponsive soon after blood flow to the brain ceases?

2. What are the key components for an abbreviated trauma neurologic exam in the field and the importance of early interventions and rapid transport?

Neurologic Emergencies

Stroke, seizures, and altered responsiveness are neurologic emergencies commonly seen by emergency care providers. In fact, stroke is the third most common cause of death in the United States, after heart disease and cancer. In the past few years, there has been a revolution in the treatment of stroke. For the most part, emergency treatment had not previously been available for patients with stroke, who typically faced years of painful rehabilitation or lifelong paralysis. Now, prehospital care providers, emergency physicians, neurologists, and neurosurgeons can help some patients with acute stroke to avoid the most devastating consequences of this condition, assuming that they get to the hospital in time.

Seizures and altered responsiveness also occur when there is a disorder in the brain. Seizures may occur as a result of a recent or old brain injury, a brain tumor, a metabolic problem, or simply a genetic predisposition. Your ability to recognize when a seizure has occurred or is occurring is critical for the patient, as it helps to direct appropriate treatment.

Altered responsiveness is a common presentation in patients with a wide variety of medical problems. Though it is tempting, you should not make assumptions about the cause of altered mental status. Causes range from alcohol intoxication to stroke. Obviously, treatment varies widely as well. Patients with altered responsiveness present a particular challenge in that they may be difficult to handle and frustrating to treat at times. Your professionalism and compassion are paramount in these situations.

The chapter opens with a description of the structure and function of the brain and what goes wrong in the most common causes of brain disorder, including stroke, seizure, and altered mental status. It then discusses the signs and symptoms of each condition. You will learn how to approach and assess a patient with a brain disorder and why prompt transport (usually load and go on the ski slope) to an appropriate medical facility is so important. The chapter then describes key assessment strategies for stroke, seizure, and altered awareness. Appropriate management of each is then discussed.

Brain Structure and Function

The brain is like the body's computer. It controls breathing, speech, and all other body functions. All your thoughts, memories, wants, needs, and desires reside in the brain. Different parts of the brain perform different functions. For example, some receive input from the senses, including sight, hearing, taste, smell, and touch; others control the muscles and integrated movement, while others interpret language and control speech.

The brain is divided into three major parts: the brain stem, the cerebellum, and the largest part, the cerebrum ▶ Figure 12-1). The brain stem controls the most basic automatic functions of the body, such as breathing, blood pressure, swallowing, and pupil constriction. Next to the brain stem, the cerebellum controls integrated muscle and body coordination. It is responsible for smooth coordination of muscle movement such as standing on one foot without falling, walking, picking up a coin, or skiing the bumps.

The cerebrum, located above the cerebellum and brain stem, is divided down the middle into the right and left cerebral hemispheres. Each hemisphere controls activities on the opposite side of the body. The frontal lobe of the cerebrum controls emotion and thought, and

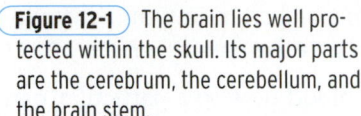 **Figure 12-1** The brain lies well protected within the skull. Its major parts are the cerebrum, the cerebellum, and the brain stem.

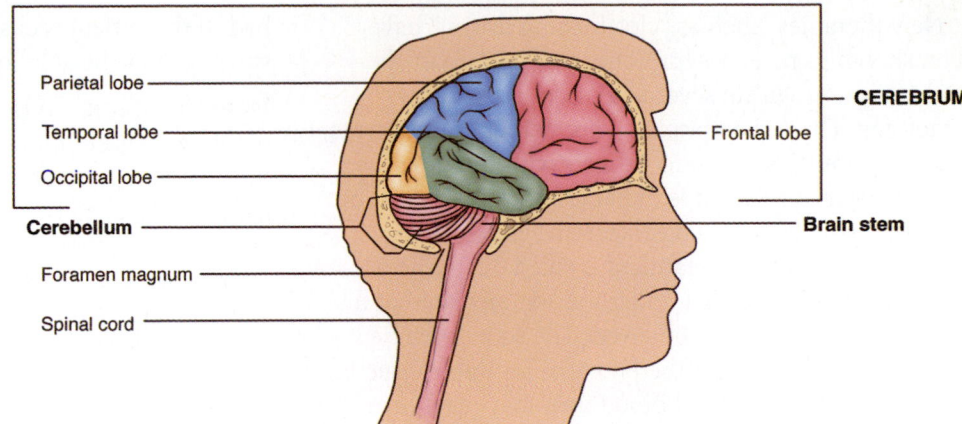

the parietal lobe interprets sensation and controls movement. The occipital lobe of the cerebrum processes sight. In most people, speech is controlled by the left side of the brain near the temporal lobe.

All the messages traveling to and from the brain travel along nerves. Twelve cranial nerves run directly from the brain to various parts of the head, such as the eyes, ears, nose, and face. All the rest of the nerves join in the spinal cord and exit the cranium through a large hole in the base of the skull called the foramen magnum ► **Figure 12-2** . At each vertebra in the neck and back, two nerves (left and right), called spinal nerves, branch out from the spinal cord and carry signals to and from the body.

Common Causes of Nontraumatic Brain Injury

Stroke is a common cause of brain disorder that is potentially treatable. Other brain disorders include hemorrhage, infection, and tumor. Although these specific problems are not covered here, the seizures or altered mental status that often accompany them are discussed. The information in this section will help you better understand, communicate with, and care for patients who have experienced some type of brain injury.

Stroke

A <u>cerebrovascular accident (CVA)</u> is an interruption of blood flow to the brain that results in the loss of brain function. <u>Stroke</u> is the loss of brain function that results from a CVA and occurs when part of the blood flow to the brain is suddenly cut off. Lacking oxygen and the main nutrient glucose, brain cells stop working and begin to die; these dead cells are called <u>infarcted cells</u>. Once these cells are dead, they no longer control body function. However, it may take

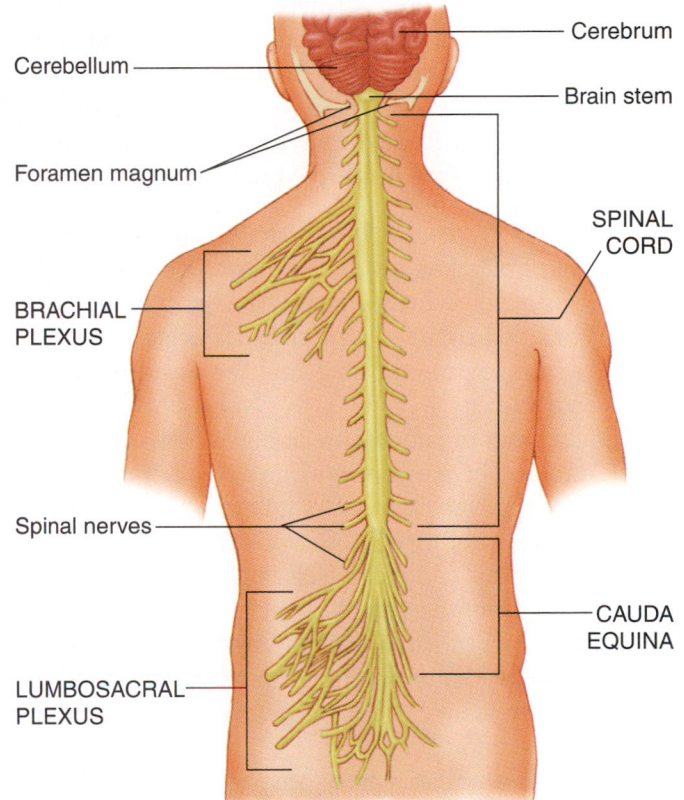

Figure 12-2 The spinal cord is the continuation of the brain stem. It exits the skull at the foramen magnum and extends down to the level of the second lumbar vertebra.

several hours or more for cell death to occur, even when it appears that severe disability has occurred. Also, in some cases, a trickle of blood may still be getting through to the affected area of the brain. This blood may supply enough oxygen to keep alive a group of brain cells, called <u>ischemic cells</u>, although they may not work properly and perform their given jobs.

New therapies, such as "clot-busting drugs," have been shown to reverse symptoms and thus abort the stroke, if given within several hours of the start of symptoms. These therapies may not work for all patients, and they cannot be given to patients with bleeding-type (hemorrhagic) strokes. It is imperative that a CT scan be obtained as soon as possible. Nevertheless, until the potential for definitive treatment is ruled out at the hospital, you should proceed under the assumption that the area of the brain can still be saved. The sooner the treatment is begun, the better the potential for improvement.

Interruption of cerebral blood flow may result from **thrombosis**, clotting of the cerebral arteries; **arterial rupture**, rupture of a cerebral artery; or **cerebral embolism**, obstruction of a cerebral artery caused by a clot that was formed elsewhere and traveled to the brain.

There are two main types of stroke: hemorrhagic (usually from arterial rupture) and ischemic (from embolism or thrombosis). Their symptoms are the same, although the events taking place inside the brain are different.

HEMORRHAGIC STROKE. A **hemorrhagic stroke** occurs as a result of bleeding inside the brain. The free blood then forms a clot, which squeezes the brain tissue next to it. When that tissue is compressed, oxygenated blood cannot get into the area, and the surrounding cells begin to die.

Certain types of patients are at higher risk of hemorrhagic stroke. The patients who are at highest risk are those who have very high or long-term elevated blood pressure that is not treated. After many years of high blood pressure, the blood vessels in the brain weaken. Eventually, one of the vessels may rupture, and blood will spurt out of the hole and into the brain, increasing the pressure inside the cranium. Proper treatment of high blood pressure can help to prevent this long-term damage to the blood vessels.

Some individuals may have been born with weaknesses, called *aneurysms*, in the blood vessels of the brain. An aneurysm is a swelling or enlargement of part of an artery, resulting from weakening of the arterial wall. Many of these individuals complain of a sudden onset of a "bad headache." When a hemorrhagic stroke occurs in an otherwise healthy young person, the likely cause is often a weakness in a blood vessel called a *berry aneurysm*. This type of aneurysm resembles a tiny balloon (or berry) that juts out from the artery. When the aneurysm is overstretched and ruptures, blood spurts into an area around the coverings of the brain called the subarachnoid space. Therefore, these types of strokes are called subarachnoid hemorrhages. Again, patients with this type of stroke experience a sudden severe headache, typically described as the worst headache they have ever

had. If the patient seeks medical attention immediately, surgeons may be able to repair the aneurysm.

ISCHEMIC STROKE. When blood flow to a particular part of the brain is cut off by a blockage inside a blood vessel, the result is a nonhemorrhagic or bland stroke called an **ischemic stroke**. This can be from a thrombosis or an embolism that blocks blood flow. As with coronary artery disease, atherosclerosis in the blood vessels is usually the cause. **Atherosclerosis** is a disorder in which calcium and cholesterol build up, forming a plaque inside the walls of blood vessels. This plaque obstructs blood flow, interfering with the vessel's ability to dilate. Eventually, atherosclerosis can cause complete occlusion (blockage) of an artery (▼ **Figure 12-3**). In other cases, an atherosclerotic plaque in the carotid artery in the neck ruptures. A blood clot forms over the crack in the plaque, sometimes growing big enough to completely block all blood flow through that artery. This is consistent with thrombosis of the carotid artery. Deprived of oxygen, parts of the brain supplied by the artery will stop working. Patients with such ischemic strokes will have dramatic symptoms, including loss of movement on the opposite side of the body.

Even if the blockage in the carotid artery is not complete, smaller pieces of the clot may embolize (break off and be carried by the blood flow) deep into the brain. This is called a cerebral embolism. There, a piece of clot

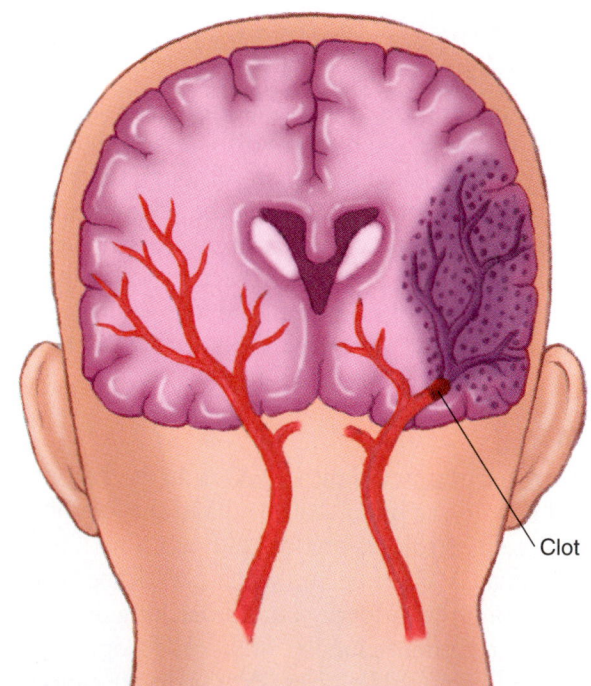

Figure 12-3 Atherosclerosis can damage the wall of a cerebral artery, producing narrowing and a clot. When the vessel is narrowed or completely blocked, blood flow to that part of the brain may be blocked, and the cells begin to die.

will lodge in a branch blood vessel. This cerebral embolism then blocks blood flow (▼ **Figure 12-4**). Depending on the location of the lodged clot, the patient may experience anything from no symptoms to a complete loss of body functions or unresponsiveness.

TRANSIENT ISCHEMIC ATTACK. In some patients, normal processes in the body will break up a blood clot in the brain. When that happens quickly, blood flow is restored to the affected area, and the patient will regain use of the affected body part. When stroke symptoms go away on their own in less than 24 hours, the event is called a **transient ischemic attack (TIA)**. Some patients call these mini-strokes.

Although most patients with TIAs do well, every TIA is an emergency. It may be a warning sign that a larger, permanent stroke is about to occur. For this reason, all patients with TIAs should be evaluated by a physician to determine whether preventive action can be taken.

Seizures

A **seizure**, or convulsion, is typically characterized by unresponsiveness and a generalized severe uncontrolled twitching of all of the body's muscles that lasts several minutes or longer. This type of seizure is often called a **generalized seizure** or *grand mal seizure*. In other

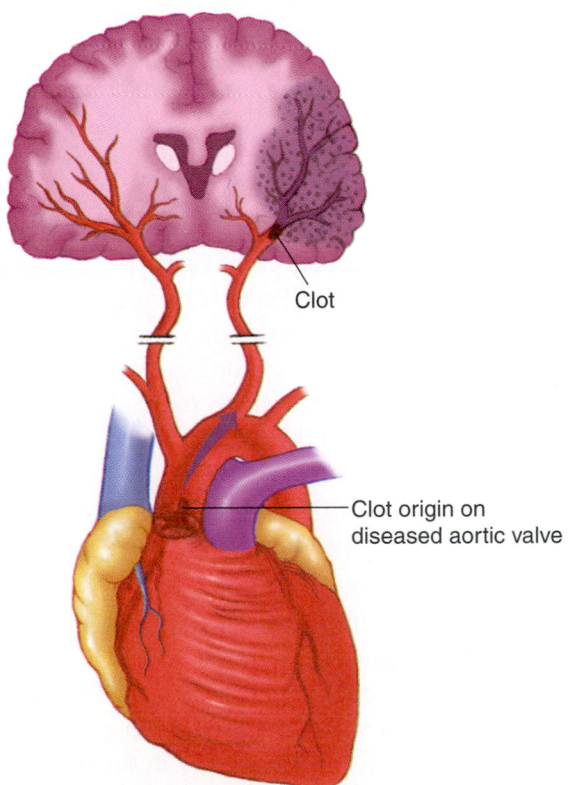

Clot

Clot origin on
diseased aortic valve

(**Figure 12-4**)   An embolus, a blood clot usually formed on a diseased heart valve, can travel through the body's vascular system, lodge in a cerebral artery, and cause a stroke.

cases, the seizure may simply be characterized by a brief lapse of attention in which the patient seems to just stare and does not seem to respond to anyone. This type of seizure, called an **absence seizure** or *petit mal seizure*, typically occurs in young children.

CHARACTERISTICS OF SEIZURES. Some seizures occur on only one side of the body. These are classified as partial seizures. Others begin on one side and gradually progress to a generalized seizure that affects the entire body. Most individuals with lifelong or chronic seizures tolerate these events reasonably well without complications, but in some situations, seizures may signal life-threatening conditions.

Most seizures last 3 to 5 minutes and are followed by a lengthy period (5 to 30 minutes or more) of what is called a **postictal state**, in which the patient remains calm yet unresponsive. Gradually, in most cases, the patient will begin to recover and become responsive. In contrast, a petit mal seizure can last for just a fraction of minute, after which the patient fully recovers immediately with only a brief lapse of memory of the event.

Seizures that continue for longer than 20 minutes are referred to as **status epilepticus**. For obvious reasons, recurring seizures should be considered potentially life-threatening situations in which patients need immediate emergency medical care.

CAUSES OF SEIZURES. Some seizure disorders are congenital, which means that the patient was born with the condition. Patients with recurrent seizures that require long-term or permanent medication to control them are considered to have a medical condition called epilepsy. Other types of seizures may be due to high fevers, microscopic abnormalities in the brain, or metabolic or chemical problems in the body (▶ **Table 12-1**). Seizures can usually be controlled with medications such as phenytoin (Dilantin), phenobarbital, or carbamazepine (Tegretol). Patients with epilepsy will often have seizures if they stop taking their medications or if they do not take an adequate dose. Excesses in exercise, altitude, alcohol, or minor medical conditions such as respiratory infections or trauma can precipitate a seizure in patients with epilepsy.

Seizures may also be caused by an area of abnormality in the brain, such as a benign or cancerous tumor, an infection (brain abscess), or a scar from some type of prior injury. These seizures are said to have a *structural* cause; in other cases, the seizures are *metabolic*. Seizures from a metabolic cause can be caused by abnormal levels of certain blood chemicals (eg, extremely low sodium levels), hypoglycemia (low blood glucose levels), poisons, drug overdoses, or sudden withdrawal from

TABLE 12-1 Common Causes of Seizures

Type	Cause
Epileptic	Congenital in origin
Structural	Tumor (benign or cancerous)
	Infection (brain abscess)
	Scar from injury
Metabolic	Abnormal blood chemistry
	Hypoglycemia
	Poisoning
	Drug overdose
	Sudden withdrawal from alcohol, medications
Febrile	Sudden high fever

Rescuer Safety

Patients may behave violently during the postictal phase. Though most seizure patients pose no threat to responders, signs of alcohol or drug abuse should heighten your awareness of the potential for dangerous behavior.

Documentation Tips

Physician evaluation of a patient who has had a seizure depends heavily on reports of the seizure pattern and changes in that pattern. Record all pertinent information about the seizure in terms of duration, areas of body movement, and possible triggering factors. This requires effective interviewing of available witnesses, family members, or caregivers.

routine and heavy alcohol or sedative drug usage or even from prescribed medications. Dilantin, a drug that is used to control seizures, can cause seizures itself if the person takes too much.

Seizures can also result from sudden high fevers, particularly in children. Such convulsions, known as **febrile seizures**, are usually very unnerving for parents to observe but are generally well tolerated by the child. Nevertheless, you should arrange for transport of a child who has had a febrile seizure, as this condition needs to be evaluated by a physician. The fact that a second seizure may occur is worrisome, and if it occurs, the patient requires hospital evaluation to identify possible causes, such as serious infection within the brain or tissues covering the brain.

THE IMPORTANCE OF RECOGNIZING SEIZURES. Regardless of the type of seizure, it is extremely important for you to recognize when a seizure is occurring or whether one has already occurred. You must also determine whether this episode differs from any previous ones. For example, if the previous seizure occurred on only one side of the body and this seizure occurs over the entire body, some additional or new problem may be involved. In addition to recognizing that seizure activity has occurred and/or that something different may now be occurring, you must also recognize the postictal state as well as the complications of seizures.

Because most seizures involve a vigorous twitching of the muscles, they use a lot of oxygen. This excessive demand consumes oxygen that was being delivered by

the circulation to the vital functions of the body. It is similar to a situation in which you exercise vigorously without giving your body a chance to rest. As a result, there is a buildup of acids in the bloodstream. With lack of adequate oxygenation, the patient may turn cyanotic (bluish lips, tongue, and skin). Often, the seizures prevent the patient from breathing normally, making the problem worse.

Recognizing seizure activity also means looking at other problems associated with the seizure. For example, the patient may have fallen during the seizure episode and injured some part of the body; brain injury is the most serious possibility. Patients having a generalized seizure may become **incontinent**, meaning that they may lose bowel and bladder control. Therefore, one clue that unresponsive or disoriented patients may have had a seizure is to find that they urinated into their clothing. Although incontinence is possible with other medical conditions, sudden incontinence is very likely a sign that a seizure has occurred.

THE POSTICTAL STATE. Once a seizure has stopped, the patient's muscles relax, becoming almost flaccid, or floppy, and the breathing becomes labored (fast and deep) in an attempt to compensate for the buildup of acids in the bloodstream. By breathing faster and more deeply, the body can balance the acidity in the bloodstream. With a normal circulation and liver function, the acids clear away within minutes, and the patient will begin to breathe more normally. Intuitively, the longer and harder the convulsions are, the longer it will

> Besides recognizing that a seizure has occurred, it is important to document whether this is the first seizure or if the patient has a history of seizures. Most patients with recurrent seizures will be on medication. Ask what medication the patient is taking.

take for this imbalance to correct itself. Likewise, longer and more severe seizures will result in longer postictal unresponsiveness and confusion.

In some situations, the postictal state may be characterized by **hemiparesis**, or weakness on one side of the body, resembling a stroke. Unlike the typical stroke, hypoxic hemiparesis soon resolves itself. Most commonly, the postictal state is characterized by disorientation (for example to person, place, and date) and altered responsiveness. The patient may be combative and appear angry. You must be prepared for these circumstances, both in your approach to scene control and in your treatment of the patient's symptoms. If the patient's condition does not improve over several minutes, you should consider other possible underlying problems, including hypoglycemia or infection.

Altered Responsiveness

Aside from stroke and seizures, another neurologic emergency is disorientation and altered responsiveness. Simply put, the patient is not appropriately interacting with his or her immediate environment. In some instances, patients will be unresponsive (▼ Figure 12-5); in others, they may be alert but confused. The range of problems is wide, and the causes are many, including common problems such as **hypoglycemia** (low blood glucose levels), hypoxemia, intoxication, drug over-

dose, unrecognized head injury, brain infection, body temperature abnormalities, and uncommon conditions such as brain tumors, glandular abnormalities, and overdoses/poisonings.

HYPOGLYCEMIA. The clinical picture of patients with altered mental status due to hypoglycemia is very complex. Patients can have signs and symptoms that mimic stroke and seizures. Because both oxygen and glucose are needed for brain function, hypoglycemia can mimic conditions in the brain such as those associated with stroke. In these instances, the patient may have hemiparesis, similar to what occurs as a result of a stroke. The principal difference, however, is that a patient who has had a stroke may be alert and attempting to communicate normally, whereas a patient with hypoglycemia almost always has an altered or decreased level of consciousness (▼ Figure 12-6).

Patients with hypoglycemia commonly, but not always, take medications that lower blood glucose levels. They may have taken medication to lower the body's glucose levels, yet haven't consumed enough nutrients to prevent dangerously low glucose levels. Thus, if the patient appears to have signs and symptoms of stroke and an altered awareness or disorientation, obtain the best history you can from relatives, friends, or bystanders and report your findings to EMS or medical personnel. Check for and report medications, but remember that not all patients who have diabetes take insulin or other medications to lower their blood glucose levels. Remember also that patients with a decreased level of responsiveness should not be given anything by mouth. Again, local protocols should guide your actions.

Patients with hypoglycemia can also experience seizures, and you may arrive at the scene to find a patient in a postictal state: confused and disoriented or unresponsive. The mental status of a patient who has

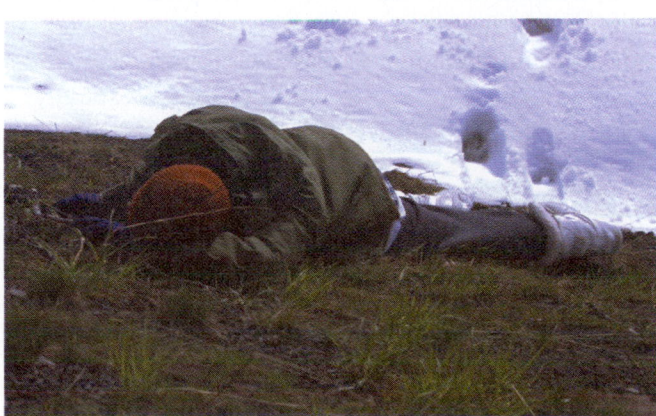

Figure 12-5 A patient with altered mental status can be unconscious in some instances; in others, the patient may be alert but confused.

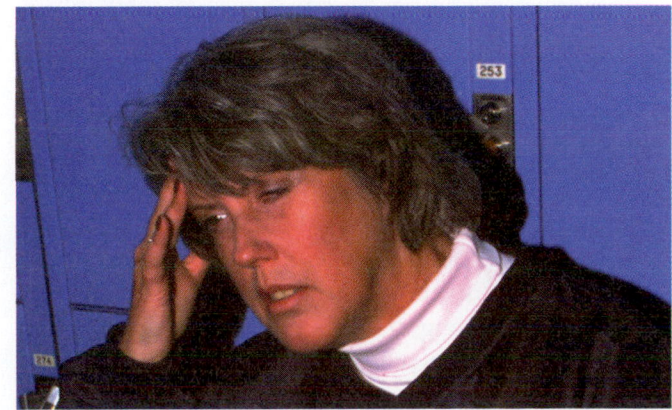

Figure 12-6 During your assessment of a patient with an altered or decreased level of consciousness, consider the possibility of hypoglycemia.

had a typical seizure is likely to improve; however, in a patient with hypoglycemia, the mental status is not likely to improve, even after several minutes. Therefore, you should consider the possibility of hypoglycemia in a patient who has had a seizure, especially if the blood glucose tested below normal.

Likewise, you should consider hypoglycemia in a patient who is disoriented and unresponsive after an injury such as a motor vehicle crash, even when there is the possibility of an accompanying head injury. As with any other patient, you should look for medical identification bracelets or medications that might confirm your suspicions.

OTHER CAUSES OF ALTERED RESPONSIVENESS. Altered responsiveness can occur as a result of hypoglycemia, but there are many other possibilities as well, including unrecognized brain injury, a body temperature that is too high or too low, or severe alcohol intoxication. Your consideration of other possibilities becomes important because a patient who is disoriented may be combative and refuse treatment and transport. You should be prepared for difficult patient encounters and follow local protocols for dealing with these situations, recognizing the potential for serious underlying problems.

In most cases, a patient who appears intoxicated most likely is just that; however, you must consider other problems as well. Individuals with chronic alcoholism can have abnormalities in liver function and in their blood-clotting and immune systems, which can predispose them to intracranial bleeding, brain and bloodstream infections, and hypoglycemia.

Psychological problems and complications from medications are also possible causes of altered responsiveness. A person who appears to have a psychological problem may also have an underlying medical condition.

Infections are another possible cause, particularly those involving the brain or bloodstream. Infections in these areas are obviously life threatening and need immediate attention. Patients may not demonstrate typical signs of infection, such as fever, particularly if they are very young or very old or have impaired immune systems; however, minor changes in the body's temperature result in brain dysfunction.

Altered responsiveness can also be caused by drug overdose or poisonings; therefore, you should monitor patients closely for accompanying cardiac and breathing problems.

Thus, the presentation of altered mental status varies widely from simple confusion to coma and may be the result of multiple factors. No matter what the cause, you should consider disorientation or altered responsiveness to be an emergency that requires immediate attention even when it appears that the culprit may simply be alcohol intoxication or a minor car crash or fall.

Signs and Symptoms of Brain Disorder

Many different conditions can cause brain or other neurologic symptoms, which can affect level of responsiveness, speech, and voluntary muscle control. As a general rule, if the brain problem is caused primarily by disorders in the heart and lungs, the entire brain will be affected. For example, without any blood flow (cardiac arrest), the patient will go into a coma and can have permanent brain damage within minutes, even if CPR is performed immediately. However, if the primary problem is in the brain, such as an inadequate supply to the parietal lobe of the left cerebral hemisphere, the patient may not be able to move some parts of the right side of the body. This might be the right arm, the right leg, or the facial muscles. Low oxygen levels in the bloodstream, due to lung disease, for example, will affect the entire brain, causing disorientation.

Stroke

LEFT HEMISPHERE PROBLEMS. If the left cerebral hemisphere has been affected, the patient may have a speech disorder called <u>aphasia</u>, an inability to produce or understand speech. Speech problems can vary widely. Patients may have trouble understanding speech but can speak clearly. This condition is called receptive aphasia. You can detect this problem by asking the patient a question such as "What day is today?" In response, the patient with aphasia may say, "Green," in other words, the patient may give an inappropriate response with clear pronunciation. The speech is clear, but it does not make sense. Other patients will be able to understand the question but cannot produce the right sounds in order to answer. Usually, the patient appears to understand and may even follow commands but will not be able to form words or sentences. Only grunts or other incomprehensible sounds emerge. These patients have expressive aphasia.

RIGHT HEMISPHERE PROBLEMS. If the right cerebral hemisphere of the brain is not getting enough blood, patients will have trouble moving the muscles on the left side of the body. Usually, they will understand language and be able to speak, but their words may be slurred and hard to understand. This problem is called <u>dysarthria</u>.

Interestingly, patients with right hemisphere strokes may be completely oblivious to their problem. If you ask these patients to lift their left arm and they cannot, they will lift their right arm instead. They seem to have forgotten that the left arm even exists. This symptom is called neglect. Patients with a problem affecting the occipital lobe of the cerebrum may neglect certain parts of their vision. Generally, this is hard to detect, but you should be aware of the possibility. Try to sit or stand on the patient's good side, since he or she may be unable to see objects in the affected visual field.

The problem of neglect causes many patients who have had large strokes to delay seeking help. Strokes are not painful. Therefore, a patient may be unaware that there is a problem until a family member or friend points out that some part of the patient's body is not working correctly. Occasionally, patients may have a fixed gaze with their eyes to the left or right. The direction of the gaze is important to note and document as it can represent a destructive lesion in one hemisphere (stroke) or an irritative lesion in the other (seizure).

BLEEDING IN THE BRAIN. Patients who have bleeding in their brain from a weakness of a blood vessel typically present with a severe headache (the worst headache of their lives) and altered responsiveness. They may have very high blood pressure. Sometimes, this is the cause of the bleeding, but many times it is a response to the bleeding: the brain is raising the blood pressure in an attempt to force more oxygen into its injured parts. High blood pressure in stroke patients should not be treated in the field. Quite often, blood pressure in stroke patients will return to normal on its own.

Other Conditions

The following three conditions may simulate stroke:
- Hypoglycemia
- A postictal state
- Subdural or epidural bleeding (a blood clot near the skull that presses on the brain)

Because both oxygen and glucose are needed for brain metabolism, a patient with hypoglycemia may look like a patient who is having a stroke. You should find out whether the patient has diabetes and takes insulin or a glucose-lowering medication.

A patient in the postictal state may look like a patient who is having a stroke. However, in most cases, a patient having a seizure will recover rapidly, within the next few minutes.

Subdural and epidural bleeding usually occur as a result of trauma. The dura is a leathery covering over the brain, next to the skull. A fracture near the temples may cause an artery to bleed on top of the dura and the resulting clot presses on the brain (▼ **Figure 12-7A**). Onset of this *epidural* bleeding is usually very rapid after injury. In other cases, the veins just below the dura may be torn and bleed, a *subdural* bleed (▼ **Figure 12-7B**). Onset occurs more slowly, sometimes over a period of several days.

The onset of stroke-like signs and symptoms may be subtle; the original injury may not even be remembered.

Assessing the Patient

Stroke

When you are called to assist a patient with a possible stroke, you should first determine whether the patient is responsive and breathing. Friends and family members frequently mistake other medical conditions, such as cardiac arrest, for strokes or seizures. It is very important that you consider all reports of a stroke or seizure as an emergency until you are able to assess the patient yourself.

INITIAL ASSESSMENT. Upon arrival, you should check and care for immediate problems with the patient's ABCs. If the patient is responsive and breathing, obtain a history. Also try to speak with relatives or friends who may have seen what happened (▼ **Figure 12-8**).

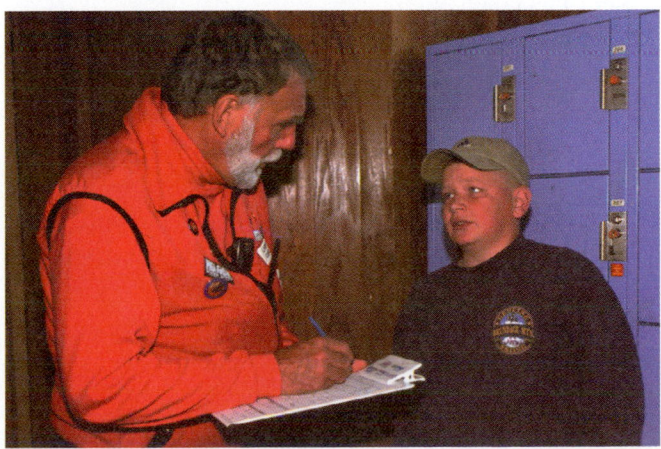

Figure 12-8 Obtain a history from family members or bystanders who may have seen what happened. They may also be able to tell you when the patient last appeared "normal."

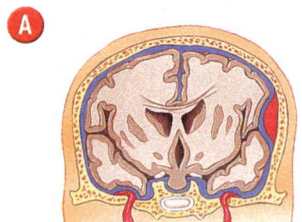 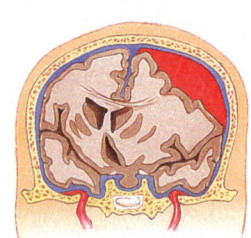

Figure 12-7 Trauma to the head can result in intracranial bleeding.
A. Bleeding outside the dura and under the skull is epidural.
B. Bleeding beneath the dura but outside the brain is subdural.

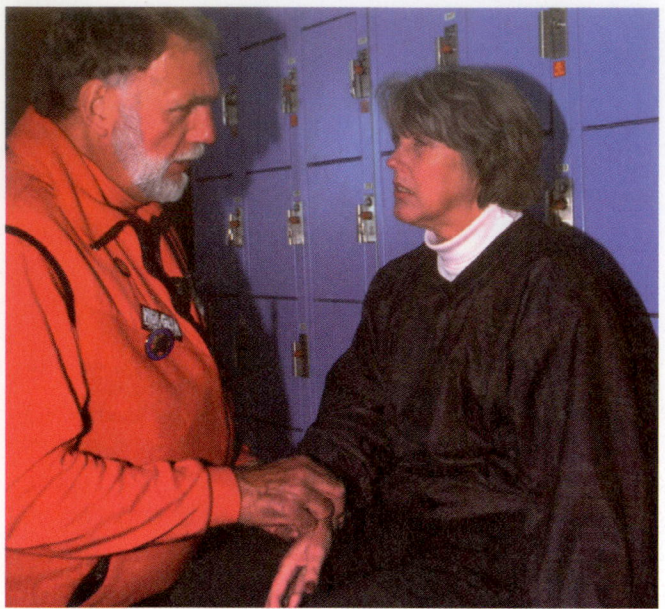

Figure 12-9   Make a special effort to establish communication with a patient who may have had a stroke. Look for indications that the patient understands you, such as a glance, gaze, squeeze of the hand, efforts to speak, or nodding of the head.

Rescuer Tips

An abbreviated neurologic exam should assess three things: the patient's level of responsiveness (alert), pupillary status (pupils 4mm, reactive to light on both sides), and quality of motor response (follows commands on both sides). Together, these components help the rescuer quickly assess brain function and localize an injury. The more severe the brain injury as indicated by the exam, the more important early intervention on the scene with supplemental oxygen and rapid transport are in preventing secondary injury and a bad outcome.

Make a special effort to determine when the patient last appeared to be normal. This will tell physicians in the emergency department whether it is safe to begin certain treatments that must be given in the first hours after onset. Since you may be the only person on the rescue team with the opportunity to speak with bystanders, you may be the only one who can make this critical determination. Many times, you will be able to find out only that the patient was normal when he or she went to sleep the night before. Note that in such cases, the time the patient was last seen to be normal should be recorded. Collect or list all medications the patient has taken.

Although a stroke patient may appear to be unresponsive and unable to speak, the patient may still be able to hear and understand what is taking place. Be careful what you say, avoiding all unnecessary or inappropriate remarks. Try to communicate with the patient by looking for indications that the patient can understand you, such as a glance, gaze, motion or pressure of the hand, efforts to speak, or nodding the head. Establishing effective communication can help you to calm the patient and lessen the fear that accompanies an inability to communicate ▲ Figure 12-9.

As you perform the initial assessment, administer supplemental oxygen. Then begin your focused assessment, including vital signs. If necessary, provide assisted ventilation, protect the airway, and suction to prevent aspiration. Remember to check for any history of diabetes, seizure, or recent head injury.

FOCUSED HISTORY AND PHYSICAL EXAM. As soon as possible, perform a neurologic exam as part of your focused physical exam. The neurologic exam should consist of the level of responsiveness, the pupillary exam, and a motor test of strength. In addition, you should perform at least three key physical tests on patients you suspect of having had a stroke: tests of speech, facial movement, and arm movement. If any one of the three is positive (abnormal), the patient may be having a stroke.

The rescuer should use the Cincinnati Stroke Scale, which tests speech, facial droop, and arm drift. The examination is identified in ▶ Table 12-2.

To test speech, simply ask the patient to repeat a simple phrase such as "The sky is blue in Cincinnati." If the patient does this correctly, you know that he or she both understands and can produce speech. If the patient cannot repeat the phrase, the problem may be with either function: understanding speech or producing it.

To test facial movement, ask the patient to show his or her teeth (or gums, if there are no teeth). Watch to see that both sides of the face around the mouth move equally. If only one side is moving well, then you know that something is wrong with the control of the muscles on the other side.

To test arm movement, ask the patient to hold both arms in front of his or her body, palms up toward the sky, with eyes closed and without moving. Over 20 seconds, watch the patient's hands. If you see one side drift down toward the ground, then you know that side is weak. If both arms stay up and do not move, then you know that both sides of the brain are working.

If both arms fall to the patient's side, you have not really learned anything. Perhaps the patient did not

TABLE 12-2 Cincinnati Stroke Scale

Test	Normal	Abnormal
Facial Droop (Ask patient to show teeth or smile.)	Both sides of face move equally well.	One side of face does not move as well as the other.
Arm Drift (Ask patient to close eyes and hold both arms out with palms up.)	Both arms move the same, or both arms do not move.	One arm does not move, or one arm drifts down compared with the other side.
Speech (Ask patient to say, "The sky is blue in Cincinnati.")	Patient uses correct words with no slurring.	Patient slurs words, uses inappropriate words, or is unable to speak.

TABLE 12-3 Glasgow Coma Scale

Eye Opening		Best Verbal Response		Best Motor Response	
Spontaneous	4	Oriented conversation	5	Obeys commands	6
In response to speech	3	Confused conversation	4	Localizes pain	5
In response to pain	2	Inappropriate words	3	Withdraws to pain	4
None	1	Incomprehensible sounds	2	Abnormal flexion	3
		None	1	Abnormal extension	2
				None	1

Score: 14-15 Mild dysfunction
Score: 11-13 Moderate to severe dysfunction
Score: 10 or less is severe dysfunction

understand your instructions. Try the arm test again, but this time move the patient's arms into position yourself. Another possibility to consider is that the patient is having a problem other than stroke. This is likely to be the answer if both sides of the brain are working improperly.

Although not a triage tool, if it is part of your medical protocol, patients with a possible stroke should also have a Glasgow Coma Scale performed, which can be seen in ▲ Table 12-3 .

TRANSPORT CONSIDERATIONS. After you have performed the neurologic exam, prepare the patient for transport as soon as possible. You want to spend as little time on the scene as possible. Remember, stroke is an emergency. There may be treatment available for the patient at the hospital. Place the patient in a comfortable posi-

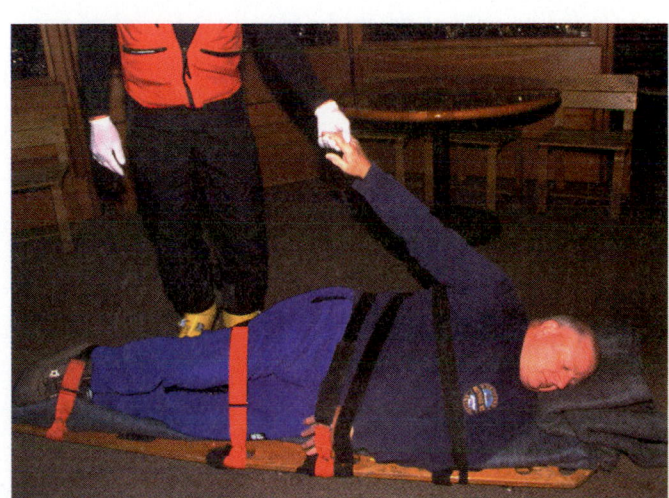

Figure 12-10 A patient who has had a stroke should be positioned with the paralyzed side down and well protected with padding. Elevate the head about 6".

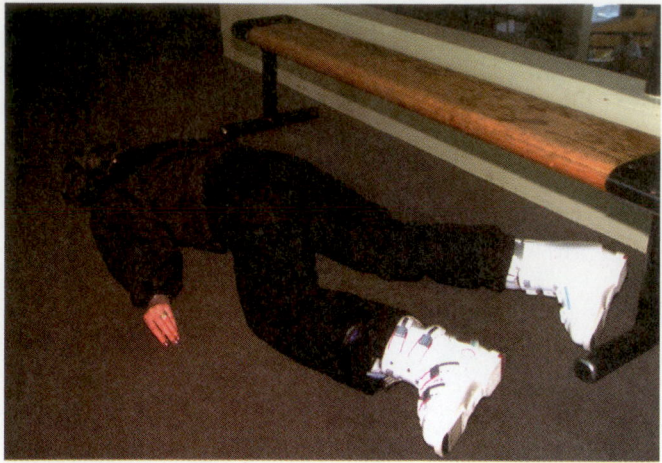

Figure 12-11 A patient who has had a seizure may be found in the postictal state when you arrive. If this is the case, be sure to ask family members or bystanders to verify that a seizure has occurred and how the seizure developed.

tion, usually supine ◀ **Figure 12-10** . The patient's head should be elevated about 6″. Continue giving oxygen while transporting the patient. Watch for airway compromise and be prepared to suction both saliva, which the patient may not be able to swallow, or vomitus.

You should always relay the information you have learned to the receiving EMS service. Be sure to include the time that the patient was last seen to be normal and the findings of your neurologic examination. This information will help EMS and the emergency department.

Seizures

You are typically called to care for a patient who has had a seizure because someone actually witnessed the seizure. However, you may also be called to see an unresponsive patient when the patient is found in a postictal state ▲ **Figure 12-11** . In other situations, you may be called to care for a patient who is having seizures and find that the patient actually has some other medical problem, such as cardiac arrest or some psychological problem. Therefore, thorough assessment is key because the information gathered at the scene may be extremely important to the hospital staff who must soon care for the patient.

In most instances, you will arrive sometime after the seizure has occurred, as it only lasts a few minutes. By the time someone recognizes the problem, calls for help, and receives a response, the patient is usually in a postictal state. Thus, you must gather as much information from family or bystanders as possible to verify that a seizure has occurred and to obtain a description of the way the seizure developed.

Rescuer Tips

As part of your emergency care for seizures, allow the patient to rest in the recovery position until he or she is fully responsive and functional. Rapidly transport the patient to medical care if:

- The cause of seizure is unknown or uncertain.
- The seizure accompanies injury or illness.
- Recovery is delayed.
- Significant injuries result from a fall.
- Status epilepticus occurs.

Advise the patient to see a physician if there is no history of seizures.

Wilderness Tips

If a patient having a seizure is in an exposed or dangerous location such as in water or on a cliff, he or she should be removed immediately or secured in some way if possible. Remember that cold and reduced atmospheric oxygen at higher altitudes also can add to the patient's stress of this condition. As soon as possible, prompt evacuation and transport to definitive medical care is essential.

INITIAL ASSESSMENT. As with any other situation, you should focus on the ABCs upon arrival. The patient may have been eating or chewing gum at the time of the seizure, and so there may be a foreign body obstruction. Bystanders may have tried to put objects in a patient's mouth "to help them breathe better," even though this practice is ill advised. Breathing and circulation should be confirmed as normal or treated as necessary. Again, in the immediate postictal state following a major seizure, you should anticipate rapid, deep respirations and an accompanying fast heart rate due to the stress of the severe convulsions. However, both respirations and heart rate should begin to slow to normal rates after several minutes. If not, you might suspect problems beyond the seizure alone.

FOCUSED HISTORY AND PHYSICAL EXAM. You should obtain a SAMPLE history, including whether the patient has a history of seizures. If so, it is important to find out how the patient's seizures typically occur and whether this episode differs in some way from previous episodes. You should also ask what medications the patient has been taking. If the patient takes phenytoin (Dilantin®) or phenobarbital, he or she most likely has chronic problems. You might find that the patient ran out of medication or stopped taking medication for a while.

If the patient has no history of convulsions and now has a sudden focal (not generalized) seizure, a serious condition, such as brain tumor, intracranial bleeding, or serious infection should be suspected. Document whether the patient takes medications that lower blood glucose, such as insulin or oral hypoglycemic agents. You may want to inquire about drug use or exposure to poisons.

As you document the physical signs of seizure, observe for recurrent seizures. If they occur, note whether the seizure starts at a focal part of the body (eg, one arm or one leg) and then progresses to the rest of the body. Most important, evaluate the patient's level of responsiveness and orientation and monitor it every several minutes to verify progressive improvement. The patient should be checked for other injuries that may have occurred as a result of the seizure, including head lacerations, shoulder dislocations, tongue lacerations, and occasional extremity fractures. Also assess for weakness or loss of sensation on one side of the body, and reassess for improvement in such findings.

Altered Responsiveness

Altered responsiveness is a sign of an underlying problem with brain function. It may range from alcohol intoxication to stroke. Use the AVPU scale to assess responsiveness.

During your assessment, consider other underlying medical conditions; the most important are those that are easily reversible. Therefore, you should consider hypoxemia and hypoglycemia as possible causes. Continually reassess these patients closely for depressed respirations; assist ventilations if needed. Likewise, a patient with a decreased level of responsiveness may not be able to protect the airway. Therefore, you should make sure that basic airway maneuvers are followed and suctioning is available ▼ Figure 12-12 . Prompt transport is necessary, with close monitoring of vital signs en route.

Coordination with ALS

If paramedics are available, you should request their assistance if the patient is unresponsive, has abnormal vital signs, or has any signs of airway compromise, particularly if the patient has a history of diabetes.

Emergency Medical Care

Stroke

After assessment, continue high-flow oxygen; place the patient supine and transport as soon as possible. In most patients with suspected stroke, physicians in the emergency department need to determine whether there is bleeding in the brain. If there is no bleeding, the patient may be a candidate for medication to help break up the blood clot or to help brain cells survive the reduced amount of oxygen. The only reliable way to tell whether there is bleeding is with a special type of X-ray test called computed tomography (CT). Blood is usually easy to see on the CT scan ▼ Figure 12-13 .

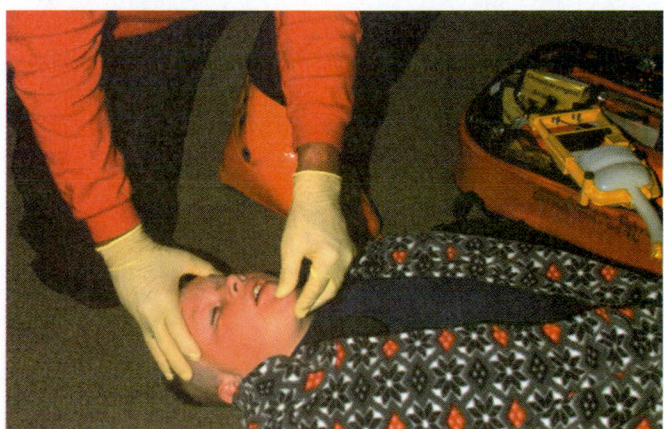

Figure 12-12 Securing and maintaining the airway in a patient who is unresponsive is critical; also be sure to have suction readily available in the event that the patient vomits.

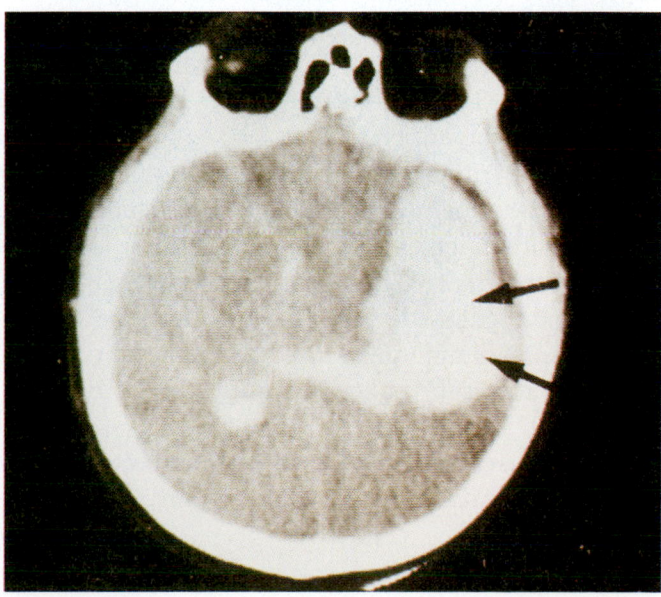

Figure 12-13 A CT scan of a ruptured cerebral aneurysm. The light area represents hemorrhage into the brain tissue (arrows).

Keep in mind that most treatments for stroke must be started as soon as possible after the onset of the event (▶ Table 12-4). Few, if any, current treatments do any good if they are started more than 3 to 6 hours after the stroke or stroke symptoms begin. Even if 3 hours have passed, prompt action on your part is essential.

Seizures

In most situations, patients who have had a seizure require quick transport and definitive evaluation and treatment in the hospital. Protect the patient from further injury during the active muscular twitching phase of seizing. Maintain an airway and administer high-flow oxygen. Do not put your fingers in the patient's mouth during a seizure—however, insert an oral airway if the gag response is low and the patient is unresponsive. Use a suction device if the patient is gurgling or has vomited. Even a patient who has a history of chronic epilepsy that is controlled with medications may have an occasional seizure, commonly referred to as a breakthrough seizure. These patients should also be taken to the hospital for observation. At the hospital, blood levels of seizure medications are checked to ensure that patients are receiving the correct dose. Clearly, patients who have just had their first seizure or those with chronic seizures who have had an episode that is "different" require immediate examination to rule out life-threatening conditions. Unless the patient has a well-established history of seizures and is completely alert and oriented, supplemental oxygen is strongly advised, not only to provide extra oxygen but also to prevent the possibility of a recurrent seizure if there is a hypoxic component to the source of the convulsion.

Depending on local protocols, you should assess and treat the patient for possible hypoglycemia (patient with diabetes with disorientation or altered responsiveness who takes insulin or oral agents that lower blood glucose levels). If trauma is suspected, provide spinal immobilization. With recurrent seizures, protect the patient from further injury and manage the airway once the seizure ceases.

If you are treating a child whom you suspect is having a febrile seizure, you should attempt to lower

---

TABLE 12-4 Tips on Patient Care

- Patients who experience a TIA may have most of the same signs and symptoms as patients with a stroke. These signs and symptoms can last from minutes up to 24 hours. Therefore, the signs of stroke that you note on arrival may gradually disappear. Patients who appear to have had a TIA should be transported for further evaluation.

- Place the patient's affected or paralyzed extremity in a secure and safe position during patient movement and transport.

- Some patients who have had a stroke may be unable to communicate, but they can often understand what is being said around them. Be aware of this possibility.

- New therapies for stroke must be used shortly after the start of symptoms. Minimize time on the scene and notify the receiving hospital as soon as possible.

---

the child's temperature by loosening or removing his or her clothing and cooling the child with tepid water, particularly about the head and neck, and then fanning the moistened areas. Be careful not to make the patient shiver, which will increase body temperature.

If the patient has been exposed to a toxin or poison, you should safely remove the source if possible. Suction should be readily available in case a patient with a decreased level of responsiveness begins to vomit.

In all instances, you should be patient and tolerant with these individuals, as many of them are likely to be confused and occasionally frightened. Many patients who experience seizures are frustrated with their condition and may refuse transport. Kindness and professional behavior are required to help convince the patient that transport is necessary for definitive care.

Pediatric Needs

Children can have altered responsiveness caused by strokes, seizures, and other brain emergencies. However, children who have subarachnoid hemorrhages may not have a berry aneurysm; instead, they may have a congenital problem with the blood vessels in the brain. Children who have sickle cell anemia are at particularly high risk for ischemic stroke. Treat stroke in children the same way that you do in adults.

As was mentioned earlier in this chapter, seizures can result from sudden high fevers, particularly in children. Remember that although febrile seizures are generally well tolerated by children, you must transport these patients to the hospital. The possibility of a second seizure makes transport mandatory so that if other problems develop, the child is in the hospital and can receive immediate definitive care.

If you suspect that a patient with disorientation has hypoglycemia and you have the ability to test for it, you should do so and treat the patient according to local protocols. Also, these patients require close monitoring, particularly of the airway, en route to the hospital.

Chapter Sweep

Ready for Review

The cerebrum, the largest part of the brain, is divided into right and left hemispheres, each controlling the opposite side of the body. Different parts of the brain control different functions: the front part of the cerebrum controls emotion and thought; the middle controls touch and movement; the back part of the cerebrum is involved with vision. In most people, speech is controlled on the left side of the brain, near the temporal lobe of the cerebrum.

Many different disorders can cause brain or other neurologic symptoms. As a general rule, if the problem is primarily in the brain, only part of the brain will be affected. If the problem is in the heart or lungs, the whole brain will be affected. Stroke is a significant brain disorder because it is common and potentially treatable. Seizures and altered responsiveness are also common, and you must learn to recognize the signs and symptoms of each. Other causes of neurologic dysfunction include hemorrhage, infections, and tumors.

Strokes occur when part of the blood flow to the brain is suddenly cut off; within minutes, brain cells begin to die. Signs and symptoms of stroke include receptive or expressive aphasia, dysarthria, muscle weakness or numbness on one side, facial droop, and sometimes high blood pressure. You should always do three additional neurologic tests on patients you suspect of having a stroke: testing speech, facial movement, and arm movement. In a transient ischemic attack (TIA), normal body processes break up the blood clot, restoring blood flow and ending symptoms in less than 24 hours. However, patients with TIAs are at high risk for a permanent stroke. Because current treatments must be administered within 3 to 6 hours of the onset of symptoms to be most effective, you should provide prompt transport.

Seizures are characterized by unconsciousness and generalized twitching of all or part of the body. Most seizures last between 3 and 5 minutes and are followed by a postictal state in which the patient may be unresponsive, have labored breathing, hemiparesis, and urinary incontinence. Continually monitor airway assessment and control during transport. It is important for you to recognize the signs and symptoms of seizures so that you can provide EMS or emergency department staff with information as the patient is transported.

Altered responsiveness is also a common neurologic problem that you will encounter as a rescuer. Signs and symptoms vary widely, as do the causes for this condition. Among the most common causes are hypoglycemia, intoxication, drug overdose, and poisoning. As you assess the patient with altered responsiveness, do not always assume intoxication; hypoglycemia is just as likely a cause. Prompt transport with close monitoring of vital signs en route is indicated.

Vital Vocabulary

absence seizure Seizure that may be characterized by a brief lapse of attention in which the patient may stare and does not respond. Also known as petit mal seizure.

aphasia The inability to understand or produce speech.

arterial rupture Rupture of a cerebral artery that may contribute to interruption of cerebral blood flow.

atherosclerosis A disorder in which cholesterol and calcium build up inside the walls of blood vessels, forming plaque, which eventually leads to partial or complete blockage of blood flow. An atherosclerotic plaque can also become a site where blood clots can form, break off, and embolize elsewhere in the circulation.

cerebral embolism Obstruction of a cerebral artery caused by a clot that was formed elsewhere in the body and traveled to the brain.

cerebrovascular accident (CVA) An interruption of blood flow to the brain that results in the loss of brain function.

dysarthria The inability to pronounce speech clearly, often a result of loss of blood flow to the right hemisphere of the brain.

febrile seizures Convulsions that result from sudden high fevers, particularly in children.

generalized seizure Seizure characterized by severe twitching of all the body's muscles that may last several minutes or more; also known as a grand mal seizure.

hemiparesis Weakness on one side of the body.

hemorrhagic stroke One of the two main types of stroke; occurs as a result of bleeding inside the brain.

hypoglycemia A condition characterized by low blood glucose levels.

incontinent Loss of bowel and bladder control due to a generalized seizure.

infarcted cells Cells in the brain that die as a result of loss of blood flow to the brain.

ischemic cells Cells in the brain that receive enough blood after a cerebrovascular accident to stay alive but not to function properly.

ischemic stroke One of the two main types of stroke; occurs when blood flow to a particular part of the brain is cut off by a blockage (eg, a clot) inside a blood vessel.

postictal state Period following a seizure that lasts between 5 and 30 minutes, characterized by labored respirations and some degree of altered mental status.

seizure Generalized, uncoordinated muscular activity associated with loss of responsiveness; a convulsion.

status epilepticus A condition in which seizures last more than 20 minutes.

stroke A loss of brain function in certain brain cells that do not get enough oxygen. Usually caused by obstruction of the blood vessels in the brain that feed oxygen to those brain cells.

thrombosis Clotting of the cerebral arteries that may result in the interruption of cerebral blood flow and subsequent stroke.

transient ischemic attack (TIA) A disorder of the brain in which brain cells temporarily stop working because of insufficient oxygen, causing stroke-like symptoms that resolve completely within 24 hours of onset.

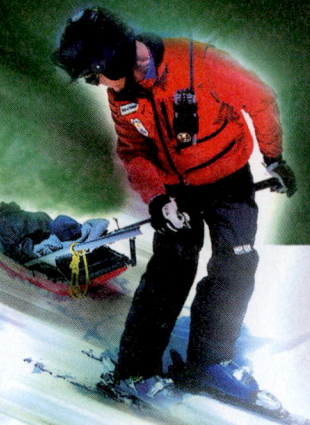

Assessment in Action

You are dispatched to a woman who has fallen. On arrival, you find a 57-year-old woman propped against an espresso stand in a resort lodge. She appears alert and focuses on you as you approach. Her friend tells you that they were walking by the vendor when your patient seemed to stumble. She was caught by a passerby and eased to the ground. There is no trauma involved.

The patient attempts to answer your questions but her speech is garbled. As you observe her, you note that the right side of her face appears to droop. Her skin is pale, cool, and dry. As you continue with your assessment your partner determines that her vital signs include a pulse of 88 beats/min and irregular, respirations of 16 breaths/min, and a blood pressure of 156/96 mm Hg.

1. The first step in caring for this patient should be to:
   A. ask the patient to try and stand on her own.
   B. obtain a history of her medications.
   C. contact a family member to obtain permission to treat.
   D. ensure that her airway is open and clear.

2. What potentially life-threatening problem is associated with the patient's facial droop?
   A. Serious depression
   B. Impending heart attack
   C. Possible airway compromise
   D. Increasing hyperventilation

3. For any patient with a neurologic problem, additional neurologic assessment should include assessing:
   A. breath sounds, chest rise, and skin color.
   B. speech, facial movement, and arm movement.
   C. skin color, blood pressure, and capillary return.
   D. skin moisture and degree of dehydration.

4. Which of the following is vitally important to determine with this patient?
   A. A history of physical activity prior to the incident
   B. A history of diabetes, seizures, or a brain injury
   C. A family history of cardiovascular disease
   D. When she last saw her physician

5. Transport considerations for this patient include which of the following?
   A. Protecting the paralyzed extremities
   B. Elevating her feet and keeping her warm
   C. Placing her in the recovery position
   D. Placing her in a head down position

6. On the way to the hospital, her speech becomes clear and distinct and she moves all her extremities to command. At the emergency department, she has no complaints and wants to go home. A return of function in this patient suggests that:
   A. she has suffered a very short stroke.
   B. what happened was not a neurologic event.
   C. the patient was faking her signs and symptoms.
   D. she most likely had a transient ischemic attack.

7. This patient has signs and symptoms that suggest a stroke. Stroke patients are also at risk for developing which of the following?
   A. Vomiting
   B. Allergic reactions
   C. Seizures
   D. Diabetic reactions

Challenging Questions

8. Because this patient is having trouble speaking, which part of her body may also be affected?

9. If this patient were taking medication such as Tegretol or Dilantin, what other condition might you suspect?

10. There is a difference between a patient who has had an ischemic stroke and a patient who has stroke-like symptoms due to a hypoglycemic reaction. What is the difference?

Points to Ponder

You are dispatched to the cafeteria for an "unconscious person." When you arrive, a man in his mid-20s approaches you. It quickly becomes noticeable that the man is mentally impaired. He leads you to his elderly mother whom you determine may have experienced a stroke. The man is very scared and agitated. He wants to know if his mother is all right. He has no other family. The mother seems stable but unresponsive. How would you calm the son? How much time would you spend on scene with the son? Would you transport the son with the mother?

Issues Special Populations, Personal Biases, Care for Non-Patients at the Scene.

Online Outlook

Different parts of the brain do different things. For example, some parts receive input from the senses, including sight, hearing, taste, smell, and touch; others control the muscles and movement; and still others control the formation of speech. To see many pictures of the brain and learn more about its function centers, complete Exercise 12 at www.OECzone.com.

www.OECzone.com

Common Medical Emergencies

♣ These are core concepts in initial patrol training.

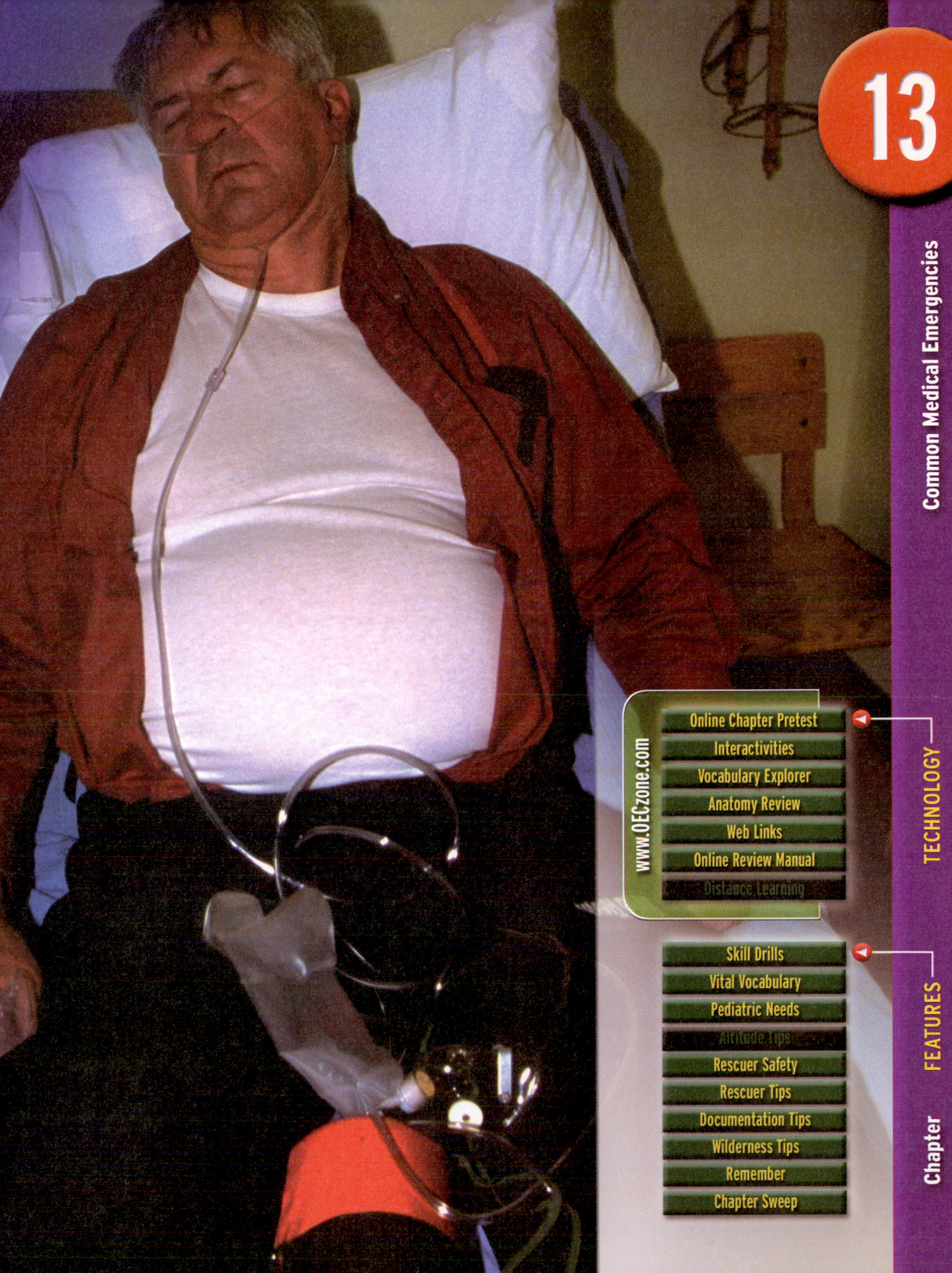

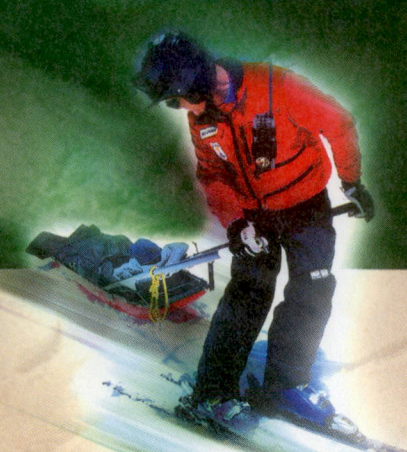

A brief stop for coffee in the lodge cafeteria turns into work when a 25-year-old woman just in front of you in the line collapses. You help ease the woman to the floor. She is complaining of "terrible stomach pain."

An acute abdomen is one kind of common medical emergency. It can be the result of something as minor as indigestion or as life threatening as a ruptured appendix. This chapter will prepare you to care properly for patients with an acute abdomen, diabetic emergencies, allergic reactions, envenomations, and emergencies resulting from substance abuse and poisoning, as well as help you answer the following questions:

1. Why would a patient with a serious abdominal problem complain of pain elsewhere, such as the shoulder?

2. How is it possible to go into shock from an "acute abdomen?" Give at least two examples.

Common Medical Emergencies
The Acute Abdomen

Abdominal pain is a common complaint, but the cause is often difficult to identify, even for a physician. As a rescuer, you do not need to determine the exact cause of acute abdominal pain. You simply need to be able to recognize a life-threatening problem and act swiftly in response. Remember, the patient is in pain and is probably anxious, requiring all your skills of rapid assessment and emotional support.

This section begins by explaining the physiology of the abdomen. It then describes the signs and symptoms of the acute abdomen and explains how to examine the abdomen. Next, it discusses the different causes of the acute abdomen and appropriate emergency medical care.

The Physiology of the Abdomen

Acute abdomen is a medical term referring to the sudden onset of abdominal pain that indicates an irritation of the peritoneum, the thin membrane that lines the entire abdominal cavity. This condition, called peritonitis, can be caused by an infection, a penetrating abdominal wound, a blunt injury severe enough to damage abdominal organs, and many diseases. In all cases, the major symptom is the same: severe pain. The major clinical signs are abdominal tenderness and distention.

Anatomically, the peritoneum is not one membrane, but two. The *parietal peritoneum* lines the walls of the abdominal cavity; the *visceral peritoneum* covers the surface of each of the organs in the abdominal cavity.

Two different types of nerves supply these two areas of the peritoneum. The parietal peritoneum is supplied by the same nerves from the spinal cord that supply the skin of the abdomen; it can therefore perceive much the same sensations: pain, touch, pressure, heat, and cold. These sensory nerves can easily identify and localize a point of irritation. In contrast, the visceral peritoneum is supplied by the autonomic nervous system. These nerves are far less able to localize sensation. The visceral peritoneum is stimulated when distention or contraction of the hollow abdominal organs activates the stretch receptors. This sensation is usually interpreted as colic, a severe, intermittent cramping pain. Other painful sensations that occur because of an irritated visceral peritoneum may be perceived at a distant point on the surface of the body, such as the back or shoulder. This phenomenon is called referred pain.

Referred pain is the result of connections between the body's two separate nervous systems. The spinal cord supplies sensory nerves to the skin and muscles; these nerves are called the somatic nervous system. The autonomic nervous system controls the abdominal organs and the blood vessels. The nerves connecting these two systems cause the stimulation of the autonomic nerves to be perceived as stimulation of the spinal sensory nerves. For example, *acute cholecystitis* (inflammation of the gallbladder) may cause pain in the right shoulder, because the autonomic nerves serving the gallbladder lie near the spinal cord at the same anatomic level as the spinal sensory nerves that supply the skin of the shoulder ▶ Figure 13-1 .

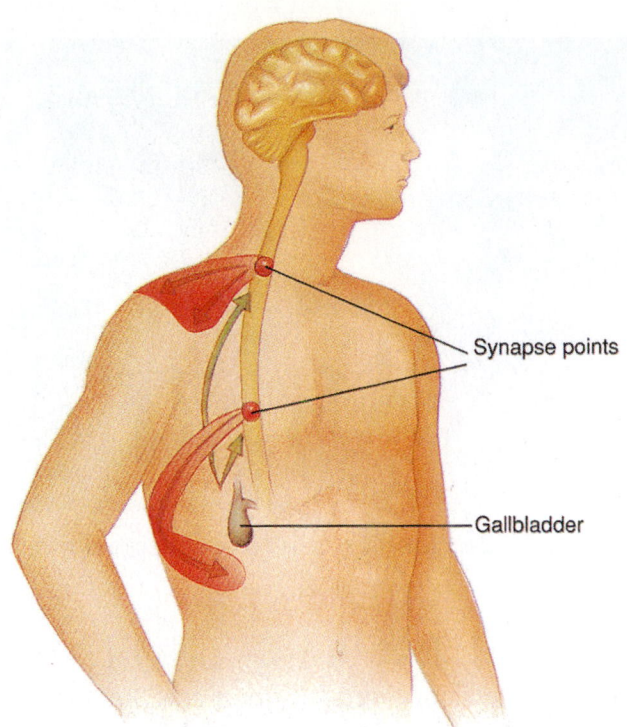

Figure 13-1 Acute cholecystitis causes referred pain in the shoulder as well as abdominal pain.

Synapse points

Gallbladder

Documentation Tips

An acute abdomen usually indicates peritonitis, in which generalized signs can make it challenging to determine exactly where the problem lies, even for physicians. Knowing abdominal assessment steps well, and recording your findings in detail, are important early factors in the process that leads to diagnosis.

Signs and Symptoms of Acute Abdomen

Peritonitis typically causes **ileus**, or paralysis of the muscular contractions that normally propel material through the intestine. The retained gas and feces, in turn, cause abdominal distention. In the presence of such paralysis, nothing that is eaten can pass normally out of the stomach or through the bowel. The only way the stomach can empty itself, then, is by **emesis**, or vomiting. For this reason, peritonitis is almost always associated with nausea and vomiting, usually in that order. These complaints do not point to a particular cause, since they can accompany almost every type of gastrointestinal disease or injury.

Similarly, **anorexia**, loss of hunger or appetite, is a nonspecific symptom. It, too, is an almost universal complaint in gastrointestinal and abdominal disease or injury. In fact, if a patient does not have anorexia, the situation may not be as serious as it otherwise appears.

Peritonitis is associated with a loss of body fluid into the abdominal cavity. The loss of fluid usually results from abnormal shifts of fluid from the bloodstream into body tissues. This decreases the volume of circulating blood and may eventually cause *hypovolemic shock*. This problem can be compounded by massive internal or external bleeding, resulting in severely inadequate perfusion. The patient may have

normal vital signs or, if the peritonitis has progressed farther, may have tachycardia and hypotension. When peritonitis is accompanied by hemorrhage, the signs of shock are much more apparent.

As we have seen, an acute abdomen is characterized by abdominal pain and tenderness. The pain may be sharply localized or diffuse and will vary in its severity. Localized pain gives a clue to the problem organ or area causing it. Tenderness may be minimal or so great that the patient will not allow you to touch the abdomen.

Another sign of the acute abdomen is tenseness of the abdominal muscles over the irritated area. In some instances, the muscles of the abdominal wall become rigid in an involuntary effort to protect the abdomen from further irritation. This board-like muscle spasm, called **guarding**, can be seen with major problems such as a perforated peptic ulcer or **pancreatitis**. In some situations, patients are comfortable only when lying in one particular position, which tends to relax muscles adjacent to the inflamed organ and thus lessen the pain. Therefore, the position of the patient may provide an important clue. For example, a patient with appendicitis may draw up the right knee. A patient with pancreatitis may lie curled up on one side.

Remember, the patient with peritonitis usually has abdominal pain, even when lying quietly. The patient can be quiet but have difficulty breathing and may take rapid, shallow breaths because of the pain. Usually, you will find tenderness on palpation of the abdomen or when the patient moves. The degree of pain and tenderness is usually related directly to the severity of peritoneal inflammation.

The following is a checklist of common signs and symptoms of irritation or inflammation of the peritoneum that you can use to determine whether a patient has an acute abdomen:

- Local or diffuse abdominal pain and/or tenderness

- A quiet patient who is guarding the abdomen (in shock)
- Loss of bowel sounds
- Rapid and shallow breathing
- Referred (distant) pain in the shoulder or back
- Anorexia, nausea, vomiting
- Tense, often distended, abdomen
- Sudden constipation or bloody diarrhea
- Tachycardia
- Hypotension
- Fever
- Rebound tenderness (hurts less when direct pressure is applied, but very painful when pressure is released)

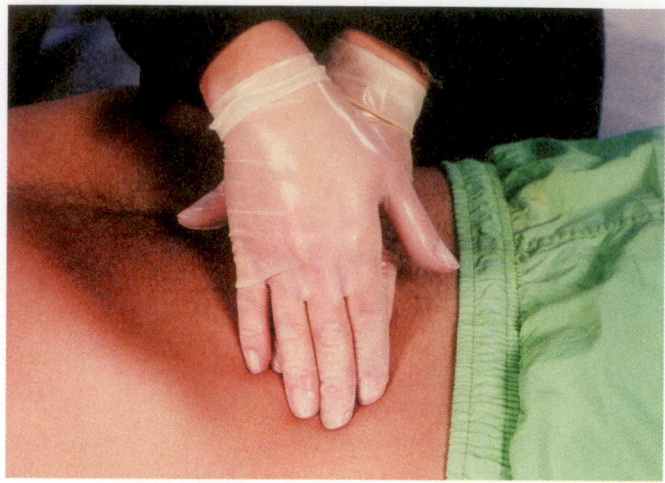

Figure 13-2 Check tenderness or rigidity by gently palpating the abdomen.

Use the following steps to assess the abdomen:

1. Explain to the patient what you are about to do.

2. Place the patient in a supine position with the legs drawn up and flexed at the knees to relax the abdominal muscles, unless there is any trauma, in which case the patient will remain supine and immobilized.

3. Determine whether the patient is restless or quiet; whether motion causes pain; or whether any characteristic position, distention, or obvious abnormality is present. Ask the patient to point with one finger to where the most pain is located.

4. Palpate the four quadrants of the abdomen gently to determine whether it is tense (guarded) or soft ▶ **Figure 13-2** . Leave the suspect quadrant for last.

5. Determine whether the patient can relax the abdominal wall on command.

6. Determine whether the abdomen is tender when palpated.

Although such an examination will yield much information, it should not be prolonged. The physician will do a much more detailed examination in the hospital. Remember to be very gentle when palpating the abdomen. Occasionally, an organ within the abdomen will be enlarged and very fragile, and rough palpation could cause further damage.

Causes of Abdominal Pain

Gastrointestinal and Urinary Tract

The abdominal cavity contains the solid and hollow organs that make up the gastrointestinal, genital, and urinary systems ▶ **Figure 13-3** . Many of these organs, such as the bowel, are covered by visceral peritoneum;

parietal peritoneum covers the inside aspect of the abdominal wall that forms the abdominal cavity. The entire abdominal cavity normally contains a very small amount of peritoneal fluid to bathe the organs. Any condition that allows pus, blood, feces, urine, gastric juice, intestinal contents, bile, pancreatic juice, amniotic fluid, or other foreign material to lie within or adjacent to this cavity can cause an acute abdomen. Technically, organs such as kidneys, ovaries, and other genitourinary structures are *retroperitoneal* (behind the peritoneum) ▶ **Figure 13-4** . However, because they lie next to the peritoneum, problems in these organs can lead to an acute abdomen. Therefore, nearly every kind of abdominal problem can cause an acute abdomen.

INDIGESTION. Indigestion is a sign that the upper part of the gastrointestinal tract, particularly the stomach, is not functioning normally. Symptoms include pain (including heartburn), nausea, and vomiting.

The symptoms of indigestion are caused by a mild to severe inflammation of the stomach, duodenum, or lower esophagus and are frequently associated with excessive acid production. Symptoms may be brought on by stress, a viral infection, excessive alcohol intake, or a meal that is too large, too rich, or too spicy. Indigestion can also be an early symptom of an ulcer or stomach cancer. Persistent indigestion should be evaluated by a physician.

The pain associated with indigestion can be a burning pain, dull discomfort, cramping, or a feeling of fullness or pressure. It is usually felt in the epigastric area and is often accompanied by epigastric tenderness.

Heartburn is a burning feeling in the epigastric area that radiates to the substernal region and throat. It is

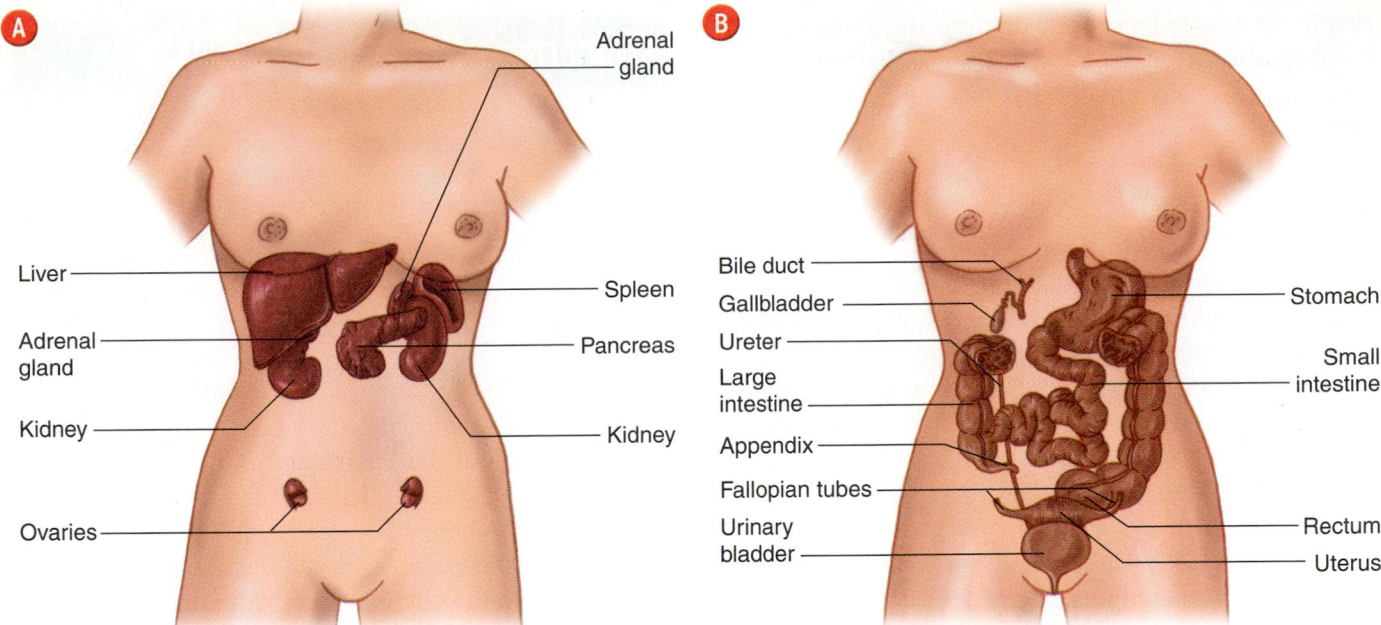

Figure 13-3 The solid and hollow organs of the abdomen. **A.** Solid organs include the liver, spleen, pancreas, kidneys, adrenal gland, and ovaries (in women). **B.** Among the hollow organs are the gallbladder, stomach, small and large intestine, and bladder.

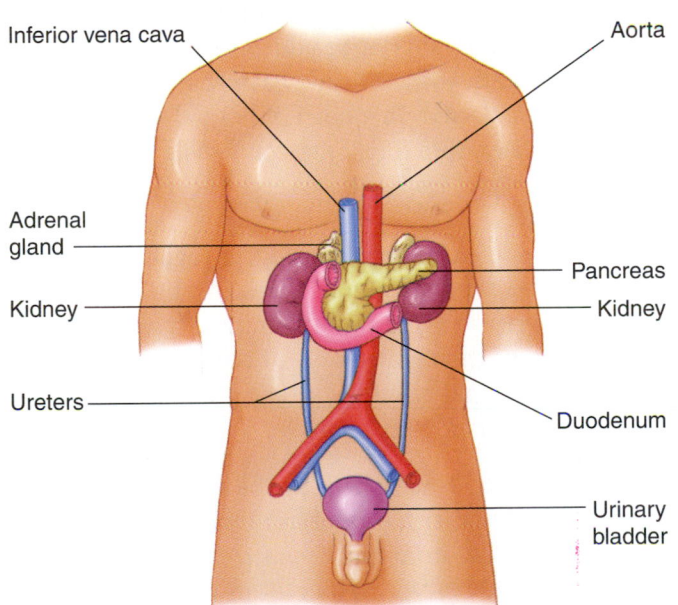

Figure 13-4 The major organs of the retroperitoneal space include the kidneys, ovaries, and other genitourinary structures.

caused by the regurgitation of acid stomach contents into the lower esophagus. This can mimic cardiac pain.

Nausea is the unpleasant feeling that you are going to vomit, and **vomiting** is the actual process of contracting the stomach muscles and ejecting the stomach contents through the mouth.

These two common symptoms reflect the stomach's tendency to react to noxious stimuli by emptying its contents. Stimuli that act directly on the stomach include infection, food poisoning, potentially irritating drugs or chemicals such as aspirin or ibuprofen, alcohol, abdominal trauma, ulcers, and tumors of the stomach. Stimuli that act indirectly on the stomach through nerve impulses include effects of high altitude, severe headache, motion sickness, stress ("nervous stomach"), psychosomatic illness, or a severe injury or illness of any type.

Nausea and vomiting may be mild or severe, acute or chronic. Severe, prolonged nausea limits a person's ability to eat and drink. The major serious effects of vomiting are as follows:

1. A loss of fluids and electrolytes and an inability to eat, leading to starvation, dehydration, metabolic abnormalities, and occasionally even shock.

2. Aspiration of vomit, causing airway obstruction and severe lung infection.

3. Bleeding due to tears in the stomach or esophagus.

In the outdoor setting, vomiting is usually caused by gastroenteritis, food poisoning, or the effects of altitude, and it eventually subsides. However, if vomiting is prolonged or recurrent, the patient must be rapidly transported to medical care.

Vomiting of blood almost always indicates a serious condition. Although it can result from swallowing blood during a nosebleed, it is usually caused by bleeding associated with disease of the stomach or esophagus. The most common causes are inflammation of the stomach, a stomach or duodenal ulcer, a tear in the esophagus caused by severe vomiting, or rupture of esophageal varices (large, fragile veins in the lower esophagus that accompany cirrhosis and other chronic liver diseases).

Vomited blood can be bright red or, if partly digested, resemble coffee grounds. A patient who is vomiting blood requires rapid transport to a hospital.

DIARRHEA. Diarrhea is the passage of soft or liquid stools with abnormally high frequency. In severe cases, there may be pus or blood in the stools. Prolonged, severe diarrhea can lead to dehydration, starvation, and occasionally even shock because a considerable amount of food and fluid may be lost through the frequent passage of stools. Diarrhea may be accompanied by nausea and vomiting.

Since diarrheal diseases usually stem from contaminated food or water, the causes and incidence of diarrhea differ in different parts of the world due to variables such as climate and quality of sanitation. In the urban areas of developed countries, the most common cause of moderate to severe diarrhea is a bowel infection caused by a virus (usually a rotavirus or adenovirus) or the bacterium *Campylobacter*. Serious bacterial infections, such as cholera and bacillary dysentery, are rare. Another significant cause of diarrhea is *Staphylococcus*, or "staph." These bacteria—a common cause of minor skin infections—grow easily in bland, creamy foods left unrefrigerated. They produce a toxin that causes violent vomiting, diarrhea, and cramps. This toxin is not destroyed by reheating the contaminated food.

A protozoan, *Giardia lamblia*, carried by beaver and many other wild animals, is a common cause of diarrhea in persons who drink untreated surface water in the backcountry. Another protozoan, *Cryptosporidium*, is an increasingly frequent cause of diarrhea attributed to contaminated water, both in urban and rural—even backcountry—areas. Chronic, mild diarrhea may also be caused by chronic emotional stress.

Severe diarrhea is common in underdeveloped countries, especially affecting travelers from developed countries, giving rise to the name "traveler's diarrhea." It is usually caused by microorganisms introduced into food by flies or dirty hands or into ground water through contamination by human feces. The most common cause is a particularly toxic form of the common colon bacillus *Escherichia coli* (often called *E. coli*). Varieties of this organism have also caused epidemics of severe, occasionally fatal, diarrhea in industrialized countries, traced to contaminated

Wilderness Tips

Persons who drink untreated surface water in the backcountry commonly experience diarrhea caused by a protozoan carried by beaver and other wild animals.

commercial food products. Other bacteria, such as *Campylobacter, Salmonella,* and *Shigella*, and amoebae can also cause traveler's diarrhea.

Traveler's diarrhea can be prevented through scrupulous attention to personal cleanliness, by washing hands before eating and preparing food, by protecting food from spoilage and contamination by flies, and by proper treatment of drinking water. In underdeveloped countries, avoid raw or partly cooked meat or seafood, salads, cooked food that has cooled before being served, and raw fruit or vegetables (unless they can be peeled). Bottled drinks are usually safe, but ice, which can be contaminated, should not be added to them. Do not brush your teeth with or drink water that has not been boiled or disinfected. In a hotel, if bottled water is not available, water from the hot tap (as hot as possible) is "safer" than water from the cold tap, but it should still be disinfected.

When diarrhea and vomiting occur together, vomiting prevents the fluid and minerals lost by diarrhea from being replaced orally. Dehydration, starvation, and shock are thus even more likely to occur than with diarrhea alone. Hospitalization with intravenous fluid therapy is frequently necessary.

BLOOD IN THE STOOLS. Bright red blood in the stools usually means either bleeding from the rectum or lower colon or bleeding from higher in the gastrointestinal tract with rapid passage of blood through the bowel.

The most common cause of blood in stools is bleeding from hemorrhoids or a fissure (crack or small ulcer) of the anus. The color of blood in the stools depends on how long it has been in the bowel. Maroon or reddish-black blood (frequently called "tarry stools") usually comes from the upper part of the gastrointestinal tract. It most commonly comes from a bleeding ulcer of the stomach or duodenum, but at times from a bleeding polyp or cancer of the colon. The darker color is caused by partial digestion of the blood. Bismuth preparations (such as Pepto-Bismol) and vitamin-mineral supplements that contain iron can turn the stool black. Eating large amounts of beets can turn the stool (and urine) red. Inflammatory bowel disease due to infection or other causes may produce either bright red or dark blood in the stools.

Dark or reddish-black blood in the stool almost always signifies a serious condition; the patient should see a physician as soon as possible. Bright red blood accompanied by pain in the anal area after a bowel movement is almost always caused by bleeding from hemorrhoids, a fissure, or an abrasion from a hard stool. A patient repeatedly passing more than minimal amounts of bright red blood should be transported rapidly to a hospital.

COLIC. Colic is intermittent, severe abdominal pain caused by obstruction of a hollow, tubular organ such as the gallbladder, bowel, or ureter. The pain is caused by the strong contractions of the muscles of the organ as they try to force the organ contents past the obstruction. Pain resembling colic also can occur with severe gastroenteritis because the irritation causes spasm of the bowel muscles.

Common causes of colic or colic-like pain are stones in the gallbladder or bile ducts, severe gastroenteritis, stones in the ureter, and intestinal obstruction caused by adhesions, a twisted bowel, or a tumor. Gallbladder or bile duct colic is usually felt in the right upper abdominal quadrant and in the back near the lower angle of the right scapula; ureteral colic is felt in the flank; and intestinal colic around the navel.

Colic is frequently a symptom of serious disease and, in any case, is so painful that rapid medical assistance is required.

CONSTIPATION. Constipation is the passage of hard, dry stools at less-than-normal intervals. It can be caused by insufficient physical activity, dehydration, chronic anxiety, or lack of bulk in the diet.

Constipation must be distinguished from the infrequent passage of stools of normal consistency, a situation that is normal in many people. Excessive bowel consciousness is a common human preoccupation, encouraged by laxative peddlers. The elderly, who may be inactive and subsist on a bulk-poor diet, are more likely to be afflicted with constipation than younger, more active people.

Persistent constipation or other changes in bowel habits without apparent cause should be investigated because they may be early symptoms of bowel cancer. In some cases of constipation, hard stool accumulates in the rectum, cannot be passed normally, and must be dug out of the rectum with a lubricated, gloved finger.

This condition, called "fecal impaction," may cause intestinal obstruction if not cared for promptly.

DIFFICULTY IN SWALLOWING. Coordinated contractions of the esophageal muscles usually move food and liquids easily from the mouth and pharynx into the stomach, so that normal swallowing is painless and free of effort. Difficulty in swallowing (**dysphagia**) may be caused either by abnormal function of the esophageal muscles (as in stroke) or by obstruction of the esophagus by scar tissue, tumor, or a swallowed foreign body.

Dysphagia may be acute, chronic, or intermittent. The most common cause is a temporary spasm of the esophageal muscles, which occasionally is severe enough to cause pain suggesting a heart attack. The most serious cause is cancer of the esophagus, which usually causes slowly progressive dysphagia characterized at first by difficulty swallowing solids, followed by difficulty swallowing both solids and liquids. All patients with dysphagia should be examined by a physician.

JAUNDICE. Jaundice is yellow discoloration of the skin, mucous membranes, and the whites of the eyes caused by an abnormal accumulation of **bilirubin** in the blood. It may be accompanied by brown urine or pale stools. Bilirubin, which is a yellow compound that is a byproduct of the normal breakdown of red blood cells, is metabolized by the liver, and the leftover products of its metabolism are excreted through the bile into the intestines, then in the urine and stools. It will accumulate if red-cell breakdown rises above normal or if the normal metabolism or excretion pathways are diseased or blocked.

The most common causes of jaundice are liver disease (such as hepatitis) and obstruction of the bile ducts by a gallstone or tumor. Since jaundice is always a sign of a serious condition, the patient should see a physician promptly.

Uterus and Ovaries

Gynecologic problems are a common cause of acute abdominal pain. Always consider that a woman with lower abdominal pain and tenderness may have a problem related to her ovaries, fallopian tubes, or uterus.

Abdominal pains may also be related to the normal menstrual cycle. A common lower abdominal pain, often confused with appendicitis but fairly short lived, is called *mittelschmerz*. It is associated with the release of an egg from the ovary, characteristically occurring in the middle of the menstrual cycle, between menstrual periods. Mittelschmerz may also be associated with lower abdominal tenderness. Some women experience painful cramps at the time of their menstrual periods.

Between 1% and 2% of all pregnancies are ectopic. The term *ectopic pregnancy* means that a fertilized egg has come to lie in an area outside the uterus, usually in a fallopian tube. A fallopian tube is simply not large enough to support the growth of a fetus and placenta for more than about 6 to 8 weeks. When the tube ruptures, it produces massive internal hemorrhage and abrupt abdominal pain. In this situation, the acute abdomen may be associated with the onset of hypovolemic shock. This combination mandates immediate transport to the hospital.

Other Organ Systems

The aorta lies immediately behind the peritoneum on the spinal column. In older individuals, the wall of the aorta sometimes develops weak areas that swell to form an **aneurysm**. The development of an aneurysm is rarely associated with symptoms because it occurs slowly, but if the aneurysm ruptures, massive hemorrhage may occur and, with it, the signs of acute peritoneal irritation. The patient may also experience severe back pain, because the peritoneum can, at times, be rapidly stripped away from the wall of the main abdominal cavity by the hemorrhage. Pain can also be associated with the pressure of blood on the back itself. In such instances, bleeding usually leads to profound shock. Again, the association of acute abdominal signs and symptoms with shock requires prompt transportation. Because this is a fragile situation with a large, leaking artery, avoid unnecessary or vigorous palpation of the abdomen. Remember to handle the patient gently during transport.

Pneumonia, especially in the lower parts of the lung, may cause both ileus pain and abdominal pain. In this instance, the problem lies in an adjacent body cavity, but the intense inflammatory response can affect the abdomen. Treat and transport this patient as you would any patient with abdominal pain.

A **hernia** is a protrusion of an organ or tissue through a hole in the body wall covering its normal site. Virtually every organ or tissue in the body will herniate through its covering membranes in certain circumstances. Hernias can occur as a result of the following:

- A congenital defect, as around the umbilicus
- A surgical wound that has failed to heal properly
- Some natural weakness in an area such as in the groin

Hernias always produce a mass or lump that the patient will be aware of. At times, the mass will disappear back into the body cavity in which it belongs. In this case, the hernia is said to be *reducible*. If the mass cannot be pushed back within the body, it is said to be *incarcerated*.

Reducible hernias pose little risk to the patient; some individuals live with them for years. When a hernia is incarcerated, however, its contents may become seriously compressed by the surrounding tissue, eventually compromising the blood supply. This situation, called **strangulation**, is a serious medical emergency. Immediate surgery is required to remove any dead tissue and repair the hernia.

The following signs and symptoms indicate a serious hernia problem:

- The existence of the hernia itself
- A clear statement that a mass that was reducible can no longer be pushed back inside the body
- Pain at the hernia site
- Tenderness when the hernia is palpated
- Red or blue skin discoloration over the hernia

Any of these signs and symptoms, other than the hernia itself, is cause for prompt transport to the emergency department.

Emergency Medical Care

The signs and symptoms of an acute abdomen signal a serious medical or surgical emergency. Ensure that you provide prompt, gentle transport for the patient; do not delay transport. Carry out the following steps as quickly as possible before transport.

1. **Assess the abdomen as previously described** to determine whether the patient has an acute abdomen.

2. **Clear and maintain the airway.**

3. **Anticipate vomiting.**

4. **Administer high-flow oxygen.**

5. **Do not give the patient anything by mouth.** The presence of food in the stomach will make any emergency surgery more dangerous.

6. **Document all pertinent information:** Onset, Provocation, Quality, Radiation, Severity, Time and treatment (OPQRST). Note the presence of abdominal tenderness, distention, or guarding.

7. **Anticipate the development of hypovolemic shock.** Treat the patient for shock when it is evident.

8. **Make the patient as comfortable** as possible for transport. Conserve body heat with blankets, as needed.

9. **Monitor vital signs**; these may change quickly.

Diabetic Emergencies

Diabetes is a very common disease, affecting about 6% of the population. It is a metabolic disorder in which the hormone that is needed to regulate blood glucose levels is missing or ineffective. Without treatment, blood glucose levels become too high and can cause coma and death. If properly treated, most people with diabetes can live a relatively normal life. However, diabetes can have many severe complications that affect the length and quality of life, including blindness, cardiovascular disease, and kidney failure. Also, treatment to lower high blood glucose levels can overshoot and cause a life-threatening state of hypoglycemia (low blood glucose). Therefore, as a rescuer, you need to know the signs and symptoms of a blood glucose level that is either too high or too low so that you can provide the proper lifesaving treatment.

This section explains two types of diabetes and how they are controlled, including the role of glucose and insulin. You will learn how to distinguish between diabetic coma and insulin shock, which often resemble each other. The section discusses how to identify and treat diabetic emergencies in the prehospital setting. Complications, such as seizures, altered mental status, and heart attack are also briefly discussed, as are the emergency medical care for each.

Diabetes

Defining Diabetes

The term diabetes refers to a metabolic disorder in which the body's ability to metabolize simple carbohydrates (blood glucose) is impaired. It is characterized by the passage of large quantities of urine containing glucose, significant thirst, and deterioration of body functions. **Glucose**, or dextrose, is one of the basic sugars in the body and, along with oxygen, is the primary fuel for cellular metabolism.

The central problem in diabetes is the lack or ineffective action of **insulin**, a hormone that is normally produced by the pancreas that enables glucose to enter the cells. A **hormone** is a chemical substance produced by

a gland that has special regulatory effects on other body organs and tissues. Without insulin, cells begin to "starve" because insulin is needed, like a key, to let glucose into the cells.

Left untreated, diabetes leads to a wasting of body tissues and death. Even with medical care, some patients with particularly aggressive forms of diabetes will die relatively young from one or more complications of the disease. Most patients with diabetes, however, can live out a normal life span. But they must be willing to adjust their lives to the demands of the disease, especially their eating habits and activities.

Types of Diabetes

Diabetes mellitus is a disease with two distinct onset patterns. It may become evident when the patient is a child, or it may develop in later life, usually when the patient is middle-aged.

In **type I diabetes**, most patients do not produce insulin at all; they have insulin-dependent diabetes mellitus (IDDM). They need daily injections of supplemental, synthetic insulin throughout their lives to control blood glucose. Since this is the type of diabetes that strikes children, it used to be called "juvenile diabetes." However, it can, in some cases, develop in later life as well. Patients with type I diabetes are more likely to have metabolic problems and organ damage, such as blindness, heart disease, kidney failure, and nerve disorders.

In **type II diabetes**, which usually appears later in life, patients produce inadequate amounts of insulin. In other cases, they may produce a fairly normal amount but the insulin does not function effectively. Although some patients with noninsulin-dependent diabetes (NIDD) may require some supplemental insulin, most can be treated with diet and non-insulin-type oral medications. These medications work by stimulating the pancreas to produce more insulin or by allowing the patient's own normal insulin to work better and thus lower blood glucose. In some cases, these medications can lead to hypoglycemia, particularly when patient activity and exercise levels are too vigorous or excessive. Patients with **hypoglycemia** have an abnormally low level of blood glucose. Noninsulin-dependent diabetes used to be called adult (maturity)-onset diabetes. Again, some patients with noninsulin-dependent diabetes may, in fact, be dependent on insulin.

The two types of diabetes are equally serious, although noninsulin-dependent diabetes is easier to regulate. Both can affect many tissues and functions other than the glucose-regulating mechanism. Both require lifelong medical management. Diabetes is considered to be an autoimmune problem, in which the body becomes allergic to its own tissues and literally destroys them. The severity of diabetes relates to the amount of insulin-producing tissue that is damaged or destroyed, as well as the time of life when the process started.

The Role of Glucose and Insulin

Glucose is the major source of energy for the body, and all cells need it to function properly. Some cells will not function at all without glucose. A constant supply of glucose is as important as oxygen to the brain. Without glucose, or with very low levels, brain cells rapidly suffer permanent damage. With the exception of the brain, insulin is needed to allow glucose to enter individual body cells to fuel their functioning. For this reason, insulin is said to be a "cellular key" ▶ **Figure 13-5**.

Without insulin, glucose from food remains in the blood and gradually rises to extremely high levels. This condition is called **hyperglycemia**. Once the blood glucose levels reach 200 mg/dL or more, or twice the usual amount (normally 80 to 120 mg/dL), excess glucose is excreted by the kidney. This process requires a large amount of water. The loss of water in such large amounts causes the classic symptoms of uncontrolled diabetes, the "3 Ps":

- **Polyuria**: frequent and plentiful urination

- **Polydipsia**: frequent drinking of liquid to satisfy continuous thirst (secondary to the loss of so much body water)

- **Polyphagia**: excessive eating as a result of cellular "hunger"; seen only occasionally

Without glucose to supply energy for cells, the body must turn to other fuel sources. The most abundant is fat. Unfortunately, when fat is used as an immediate energy source, chemicals called *ketones* and *fatty acids* are formed as waste products and are hard for the body to excrete. As they accumulate in blood and tissue, certain ketones can produce a dangerous condition called **acidosis**. The form of acidosis seen in uncontrolled diabetes is called **diabetic ketoacidosis (DKA)**, in which an accumulation of certain acids occurs when insulin is not available in the body. Signs and symptoms of diabetic ketoacidosis include a sweet, fruity odor on the

breath, vomiting, abdominal pain, and a type of deep, rapid breathing called **Kussmaul respirations**. When the acid levels in the body become too high, individual cells will cease to function. If the patient is not given proper fluid and insulin to reverse fat metabolism and restore use of glucose as a source of energy, ketoacidosis will progress to unconsciousness, diabetic coma, and eventually death.

As we have seen, diabetes mellitus is treatable; however, treatment must be tailored for the individual patient. The trick is to balance constantly the patient's need for glucose with the available supply of insulin by testing either the blood or the urine. Most patients measure the level of glucose in the blood instead, using a *blood glucose self-monitoring unit*. This is a simple and accurate procedure: A drop of blood from the fingertip is placed on a thin strip of chemically treated paper. The paper turns color and is compared with a color chart, which matches colors with approximate blood glucose readings. A more elaborate unit that automatically ana-

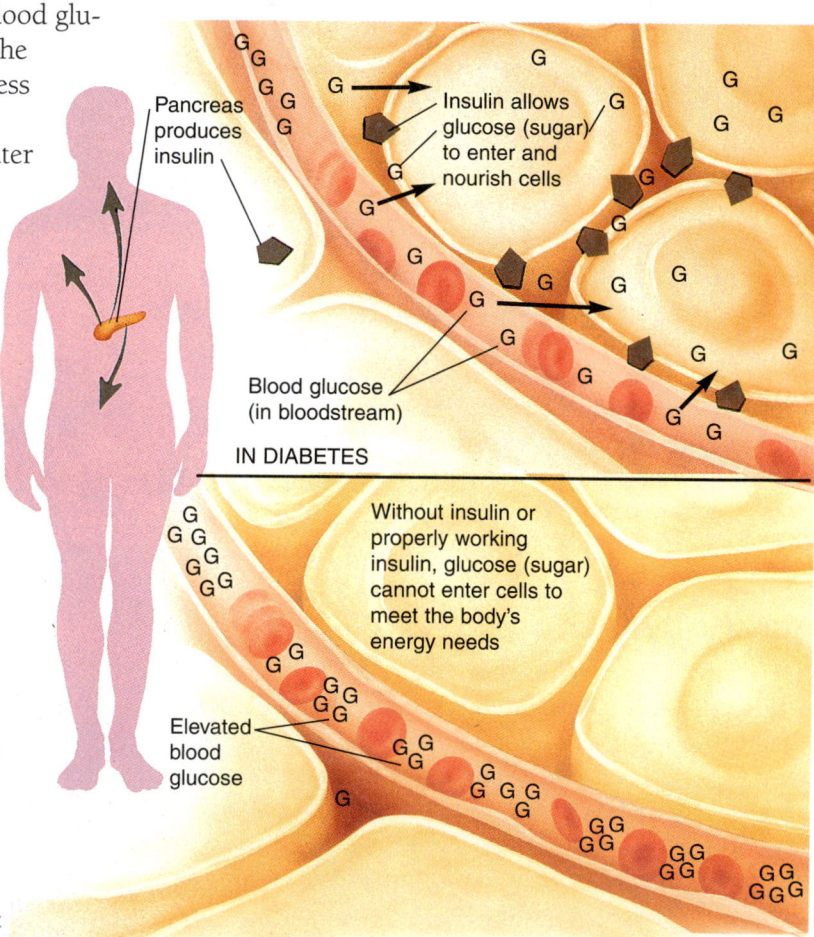

Pancreas produces insulin

Insulin allows glucose (sugar) to enter and nourish cells

Blood glucose (in bloodstream)

IN DIABETES

Elevated blood glucose

Without insulin or properly working insulin, glucose (sugar) cannot enter cells to meet the body's energy needs

Figure 13-5 Diabetes is defined as a lack of or ineffective action of insulin. Without insulin, cells begin to "starve" because insulin is needed to allow glucose to enter and nourish the cells.

lyzes the test strip and provides a digital readout of the blood glucose level is known as a glucometer.

Diabetic Coma and Insulin Shock

Two different conditions can lead to a diabetic emergency: diabetic coma (high blood glucose, or extreme hyperglycemia) or insulin shock (low blood glucose, or hypoglycemia) ▶ Figure 13-6 . The signs and symptoms of the two conditions can be quite similar ▶ Table 13-1 . For example, staggering and an intoxicated appearance or complete unresponsiveness are signs and symptoms of both. Note that your assessment of these potential emergencies should not prevent you from providing prompt care and transport as detailed in this chapter. However, in such urgent emergencies, the earlier clues are gathered, the better for the patient. With specific information about the type of emergency, you can help the hospital to prepare prompt, definitive care for the patient.

DIABETIC COMA. **Diabetic coma** is a state of unconsciousness resulting from several problems, including ketoacidosis, dehydration because of excessive urination, and hyperglycemia. Too much blood glucose by itself does not always cause diabetic coma, but on some occasions, it can lead to it.

Diabetic coma may occur in the patient who is not under medical treatment, who takes insufficient insulin, who markedly overeats, or who is undergoing some sort of stress, such as an infection, illness, overexertion, fatigue, or drinking alcohol. Usually, ketoacidosis develops over a period of time lasting from hours to days. The patient may ultimately be found comatose with the following physical signs:

- Dehydration, as indicated by dry, warm skin and sunken eyes
- A sweet or fruity (acetone) odor on the breath, caused by the unusual waste products in the blood (ketones)
- A rapid, weak ("thready") pulse
- A normal or slightly low blood pressure
- Varying degrees of unresponsiveness
- Kussmaul respirations

INSULIN SHOCK. In **insulin shock**, the problem is hypoglycemia, insufficient glucose in the blood. When insulin levels remain high, glucose is rapidly taken out of the blood to fuel the cells. If glucose levels get too low, there may be an insufficient amount to supply the brain. If blood glucose remains low, unconsciousness and permanent brain damage can quickly follow.

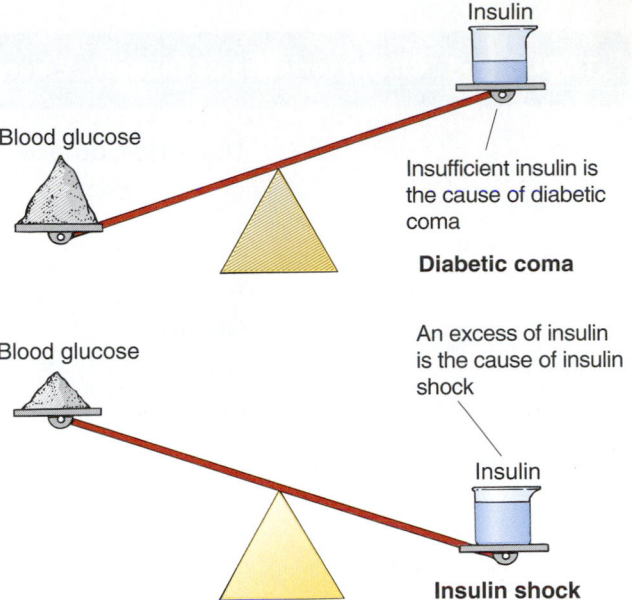

Figure 13-6 The two most common diabetic emergencies, diabetic coma and insulin shock, develop when the patient has either too much or too little glucose in the blood, respectively.

Insulin shock occurs when the patient has done one of the following:

- Taken too much insulin
- Taken a regular dose of insulin but has not eaten enough food
- Had an unusual amount of activity or vigorous exercise and used up all available glucose
- Has been ill, vomiting, and cannot eat
- Taken an overdose of oral hypoglycemic medication

Insulin shock may also occur after the patient vomits a meal on a day he or she took a regular dose of medication for diabetes. At times, insulin shock may occur with no identifiable predisposing factor.

Children who have diabetes may pose a particular management problem. First, their high levels of activity mean that they can use up circulating glucose more quickly than adults do, even after a normal insulin injection. Second, they do not always eat correctly and on schedule. As a result, insulin shock can develop more often and more severely in children than in adult patients.

Insulin shock develops much more quickly than diabetic coma. In some instances, it can occur in a matter of minutes. Hypoglycemia can be associated with the following signs and symptoms:

- Normal or rapid respirations
- Pale, moist (clammy) skin

TABLE 13-1 Characteristics of Diabetic Emergencies

	Diabetic Coma	Insulin Shock
History		
Food intake	Excessive	Insufficient
Insulin dosage	Insufficient	Excessive
Onset	Gradual	Rapid, within minutes
Skin	Warm and dry	Pale and moist
Infection	Common	Uncommon
Gastrointestinal Tract		
Thirst	Intense	Absent
Hunger	Absent	Intense
Vomiting	Common	Uncommon
Respiratory System		
Breathing	Rapid, deep (Kussmaul respirations)	Normal or rapid
Odor of breath	Sweet, fruity	Normal
Cardiovascular System		
Blood pressure	Normal to low	Low
Pulse	Normal or rapid and full	Rapid, weak
Nervous System		
Consciousness	Restless merging to coma	Irritability, confusion, seizure, or coma
Urine		
Sugar	Present	Absent
Acetone	Present	Absent
Treatment		
Response	Gradual, within 6 to 12 hours following medication and fluid	Immediately after administration of glucose

- Diaphoresis (sweating)
- Dizziness, headache
- Rapid pulse
- Normal to low blood pressure
- Altered mental status, aggressive, confused, lethargic, or unusual behavior
- Anxious or combative behavior
- Hunger
- Seizure, fainting, or coma
- Weakness on one side of the body (may mimic stroke)

Both diabetic coma and insulin shock produce unconsciousness and, in some instances, death. But they call for very different treatment. Diabetic coma is a complex metabolic condition that usually develops over time and involves all the tissues of the body. Correcting this condition may take many hours in a well-controlled hospital setting. Insulin shock, however, is an acute condition that can develop rapidly. A patient with diabetes who has taken his or her standard insulin dose and missed lunch may be in insulin shock before dinner. The condition is just as quickly reversed by giving the patient glucose. Without that glucose, however, the patient will suffer permanent brain damage. Minutes count.

Most individuals with diabetes understand and manage their disease well. Still, emergencies occur. In addition to diabetic coma and insulin shock, patients with diabetes may have "silent," or painless, heart attacks, a possibility that you should always consider. Their only symptom may be "not feeling so well."

Emergency Medical Care

You should ask the following questions of any ill patient who you know has diabetes:

- Do you take insulin or any pills that lower your blood sugar?
- Have you taken your usual dose of insulin (or pills) today?
- Have you eaten normally today?
- Have you had any illness, unusual amount of activity, or stress today?

If the patient has eaten but has not taken insulin, it is more likely that diabetic ketoacidosis is developing. If the patient has taken insulin but has not eaten, the problem is more likely to be insulin shock. A patient with diabetes will often know what is wrong. If the patient is not thinking or speaking clearly (or is unconscious), ask a family member or bystander the same questions.

The first step is to perform an initial assessment to verify that the airway is open. If the patient is not breathing or is having difficulty breathing, open the airway, give oxygen, and assist ventilations. Continue to monitor the airway as you provide care. Perform the focused history and physical exam while another rescuer obtains the baseline vital signs and SAMPLE history.

When you are assessing a patient whom you suspect might have diabetes, check to see whether he or she has an emergency medical identification symbol: a wallet card, necklace, or bracelet. Or ask the patient or family if the patient has diabetes. Remember, however, that just because a person has diabetes does not mean that the diabetes is causing the current problem. He or she might be having a heart attack, stroke, or other medical emergency. For this reason, you must always do a full, careful assessment, paying attention to the ABCs. Ask the patient or family about the patient's last meal and insulin dose.

In the outdoor environment, when unable to check the patient's blood sugar, always give glucose to a conscious patient who can swallow and who is in a diabetic emergency. Avoid hard candy, as the patient could aspirate the candy. Glucose given to a person with insulin shock can be lifesaving, while the amount of glucose given to someone with diabetic coma will not change

the eventual outcome. After oral glucose, the patient with insulin shock will usually become more responsive, while the one with diabetic coma will continue to deteriorate.

In the past, rescuers were often advised to place oral glucose gel or glucose tablets under the tongue or in the mouth of the unconscious patient. Very little sugar is actually absorbed in this manner. The risk of choking or aspirating liquid into the lungs probably outweighs the benefits of providing such small amounts of glucose. Therefore, although glucose is very important to give to patients with diabetes with altered mental status, *you should not attempt to give anything by mouth to an unconscious patient,* even if you suspect insulin shock. These patients need IV glucose, which you are not authorized to give. Your responsibility is to provide prompt transport to ALS caregivers who can give proper care.

Keep in mind that any unconscious patient may have undiagnosed diabetes. In patients with an altered mental status, you may not be able to determine this in the field. Treat this patient as you would any other unconscious individual. Provide emergency medical care, particularly airway management, and prompt transport. At the emergency department, the diabetes and its complication can quickly be diagnosed.

Giving Oral Glucose

Oral glucose is a commercially available gel that dissolves when placed in the mouth (▼ Figure 13-7). One toothpaste-type tube of gel equals one dose. Trade names for the gel include Glutose and Insta-Glucose. Glucose gel, which acts to increase blood glucose levels, should be given to any patient with a decreased level of consciousness who has a history of diabetes. The only contraindications to glucose are an inability to swallow or unconsciousness, since aspiration (inhalation of the substance) can occur. Oral glucose itself has no side

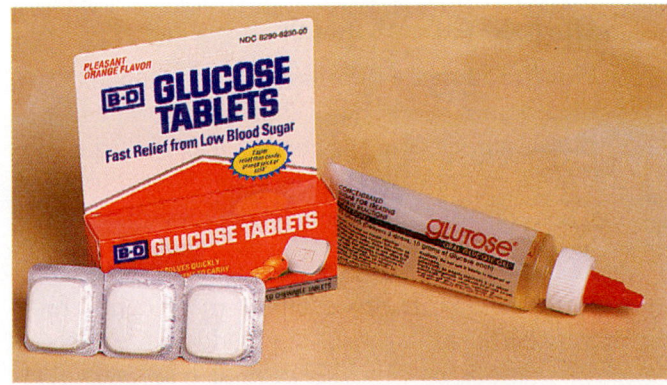

Figure 13-7 Oral glucose is commercially available in gel and tablet form. One tube of gel equals one dose.

SkillDrill 13-1   Administering Glucose

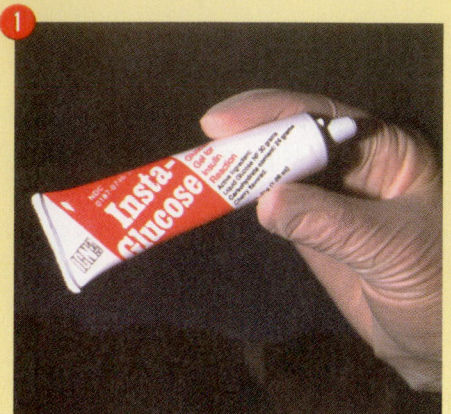

Make sure that the tube of glucose is intact and has not expired.

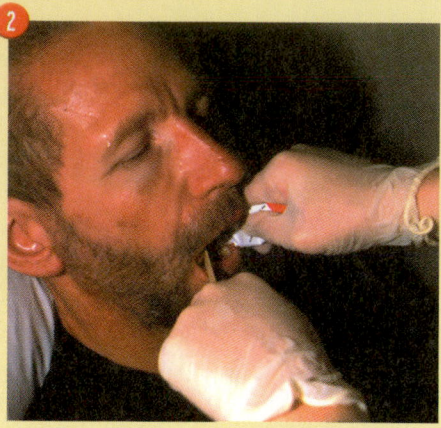

Squeeze the entire tube of oral glucose onto the bottom third of a bite stick or tongue depressor.

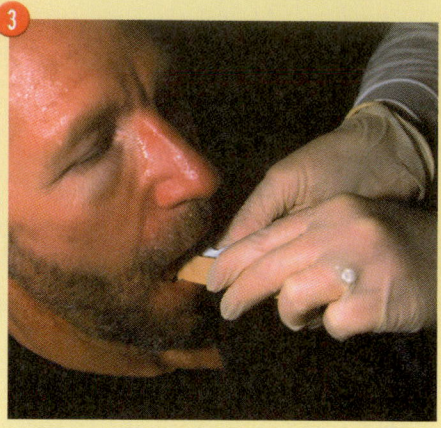

Open the patient's mouth.
Place the tongue depressor on the mucous membranes between the cheek and the gum with the gel side next to the cheek.

effects if it is administered properly; however, the risk of aspiration in a patient who does not have a gag reflex can be dangerous. A conscious patient (even if confused) who does not really need glucose will not be harmed by it. Therefore, do not hesitate to give it under these circumstances.

As always, be sure to wear gloves before placing anything into a patient's mouth. After you have confirmed that the patient is conscious and able to swallow, follow these steps to administer oral glucose (▲ Skill Drill 13-1):

1. **Examine the tube** to ensure that it is not open or broken. Check the expiration date **(Step 1)**.

2. **Squeeze the entire tube** onto the bottom third of a bite stick or tongue depressor **(Step 2)**.

3. **Open the patient's mouth.**

4. **Place the tongue depressor** on the mucous membranes between the cheek and gum, with the gel side next to the cheek. Once the gel is dissolved, or if the patient loses consciousness or has a seizure, remove the tongue depressor **(Step 3)**.

Reassess the patient regularly after giving glucose, even if you see rapid improvement in the patient's condition. Watch for airway problems, sudden loss of consciousness, or seizures. Provide prompt evacuation to definitive care; do not delay transport just to give additional oral glucose.

Rescuer Safety

Patients with well-regulated diabetes are able to lead almost normal lives and can participate in skiing, snowboarding, hiking, climbing, and other outdoor sports. Patients with diabetes who require emergency care for the disease are usually suffering from either hypoglycemia (low blood sugar) or ketoacidosis (acidosis formed by incomplete fat metabolism in uncontrolled diabetes).

Pediatric Needs

Signs and symptoms of hypoglycemia can be nonspecific.

A patient in insulin shock (rapid onset of altered mental status—hypoglycemia) needs sugar immediately, and a patient in diabetic coma (acidosis, dehydration, hyperglycemia) needs insulin and IV fluid therapy. These patients need prompt evacuation to a hospital or clinic for appropriate medical care.

For the conscious patient in insulin shock, protocols usually recommend oral glucose. These will usually reverse the reaction within several minutes. Do not be afraid to give too much sugar. The problem often will not be solved with just a sip of juice. An entire candy bar or a full glass of sweetened juice is often needed. Do not give sugar-free drinks that are sweetened with saccharin or other synthetic sweetening compounds, as they will have little or no effect. Remember that even if the patient responds after receiving glucose, he or she may still need additional treatment. Therefore, you must evacuate the patient to a hospital or clinic as soon as possible.

Complications of Diabetes

Diabetes is a systemic disease affecting all tissues of the body, especially the kidneys, eyes, small arteries, and peripheral nerves. Therefore, you are likely to be called to treat patients with a variety of complications of diabetes, such as heart disease, visual disturbances, renal failure, stroke, and ulcers or infections of the feet or toes. With the exception of heart attack and stroke, most of these will not be acute emergencies. Considering that diabetes is a major risk factor for cardiovascular disease, individuals with diabetes should always be suspected of having a potential for heart attack, particularly older patients, even when they do not present with classic symptoms such as chest pain.

Seizures

Although seizures are rarely life threatening, you should consider them very serious, even in patients with a history of chronic seizures, Seizures, which may be brief or prolonged, are caused by fever, infections, poisoning, hypoglycemia, trauma, or decreased levels of oxygen. They can also be idiopathic (of unknown cause) in children. Although brief seizures are not harmful, they may indicate a more dangerous and potentially life-threatening underlying condition. Because seizures can be caused by head injury, consider trauma as a cause. In the patient with diabetes, you should also consider hypoglycemia.

Emergency medical care of seizures includes ensuring that the airway is clear and placing the patient on his or her side if there is no possibility of cervical spine trauma. Do not attempt to place anything in the patient's mouth (eg, a bite stick or oral airway). Be sure to have suctioning equipment ready in case the patient vomits. Provide artificial ventilation if the patient is cyanotic or appears to be breathing inadequately, and provide prompt transport.

Altered Mental Status

Although altered mental status is often caused by complications of diabetes, it may also be caused by a variety of conditions, including poisoning, part of the post-seizure state, infection, head injury, and decreased levels of oxygen.

Begin emergency medical care of altered mental status by ensuring that the airway is clear. Be prepared to provide artificial ventilation and suctioning in case the patient vomits, and provide prompt transport.

Relationship to Airway Management

Patients with altered mental status, particularly those who are difficult to awaken, are at risk for losing their gag reflex. When the gag reflex is not working, patients cannot reject foreign materials in their mouth (including vomit), and their tongues will often relax and obstruct the airway. Therefore, you must carefully monitor the airway in patients with hypoglycemia, diabetic coma, or a diabetic complication such as stroke or seizure. Place the patient in a lateral recumbent position, and make sure suction is readily available.

Allergic Reactions and Envenomations

Every year, at least 1,000 Americans die of acute allergic reactions. In dealing with allergy-related emergencies, you must be aware of the possibility of acute airway obstruction and cardiovascular collapse and be prepared to treat these life-threatening complications. You must also be able to distinguish between the body's usual response to a sting or bite and an allergic reaction, which may require epinephrine. Your ability to recognize and manage the many signs and symptoms of allergic reactions may be the only thing standing between a patient and imminent death.

This section begins by describing the five categories of stimuli that may provoke allergic reactions. It then goes into considerable detail about insect stings and the typical reactions to them that occur among people who are, and those who are not, allergic to bees, wasps, yellow jackets, and hornets. You will learn what to look for in assessing patients who may be having an allergic reaction and how to care for them, including helping with the administration of epinephrine. The chapter then describes specific bites from poisonous spiders and snakes, ticks, dogs, humans, and marine animals.

Allergic Reactions

Contrary to what many people think, an **allergic reaction**, an exaggerated immune response to any substance, is not caused directly by an outside stimulus, such as a bite or sting. Rather, it is a reaction by the body's immune system, which releases chemicals to combat the stimulus. Among these chemicals are **histamines** and **leukotrienes**.

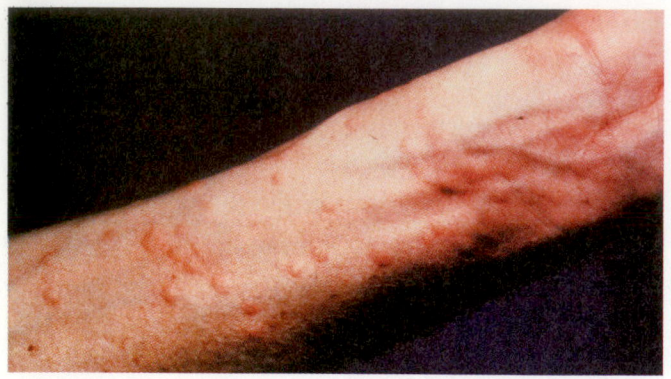

Figure 13-8 Urticaria, or hives, may appear following a sting and is characterized by multiple, small, raised areas on the skin. Urticaria may be one of the warning signs of impending anaphylactic reaction.

> Anaphylaxis is a severe reaction that may be life threatening and typically involves multiple organ systems.

Remember

Environmental stimuli for hives formation and spontaneous anaphylaxis include cold exposure, exercise, and sun exposure.

An allergic reaction may be mild and local, involving hives, itching, or tenderness, or it may be severe and systemic, resulting in shock and respiratory failure.

Anaphylaxis is an extreme allergic reaction that is not always life threatening, but it typically involves multiple organ systems. In severe cases, anaphylaxis can rapidly result in death. Two of the most common signs of anaphylaxis are wheezing, a high-pitched, whistling breath sound usually resulting from bronchospasm and typically heard on expiration, and widespread urticaria, or hives. Urticaria consists of small areas of generalized itching or burning that appear as multiple, small, raised areas on the skin (▲ Figure 13-8).

Given the right person and the right circumstances, almost any substance can trigger the body's immune system and cause an allergic reaction: animal bites, food, latex gloves, or even semen can be an allergen. The most common allergens, however, fall into the following five general categories:

- **Insect bites and stings.** When an insect bites you and injects the bite with its venom, the act is called envenomation or, more commonly, a sting. The sting of a honeybee, wasp, ant, yellow jacket, or hornet may cause a severe reaction with the swiftness of an injected medication. The reaction may be local, causing swelling and itchiness in the surrounding tissue, or it may be systemic, involving the entire body. Such a total body reaction would be considered an anaphylactic reaction.

- **Medications.** Injection of medications such as penicillin may cause an immediate (within 30 minutes) and severe allergic reaction. However, reactions to oral medications, such as oral penicillin, may be slower in onset (more than 30 minutes) but equally severe. The fact that a person has taken a medication once without experiencing an allergic reaction is no guarantee that he or she will not have an allergic reaction to it the next time around.

- **Plants.** Individuals who inhale dusts, pollens, or other plant materials to which they are sensitive may experience a rapid and severe allergic reaction.

- **Food.** Eating certain foods, such as shellfish or nuts, may result in a relatively slow (more than 30 minutes) reaction that still can be quite severe. The person may be unaware of the exposure or inciting agent.

- **Chemicals.** Certain chemicals, makeup, soap, latex, and various other substances can cause severe allergic reactions.

Insect Stings

There are more than 100,000 species of bees, wasps, and hornets. Deaths from anaphylactic reactions to stinging insects far outnumber deaths from snake bites. The stinging organ of most bees, wasps, yellow jackets, and hornets is a small hollow spine projecting from the abdomen. Venom can be injected through this spine directly into the skin. The stinger of the honeybee is barbed, so the bee cannot withdraw it (▶ Figure 13-9A). Therefore, the bee leaves a part of its abdomen embedded with the stinger and dies shortly after flying away. Wasps and hornets have no such handicap; they can sting repeatedly (▶ Figure 13-9B). Since these insects usually fly away after stinging,

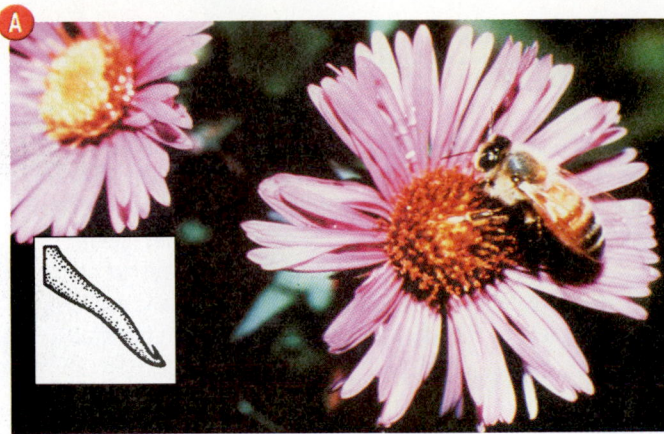

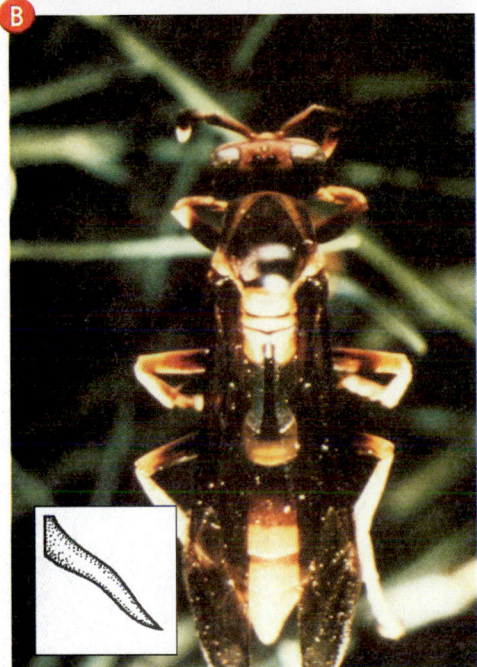

Figure 13-9   Most stinging insects inject venom through a small, hollow spine that projects from the abdomen. **A.** The stinger of the honeybee is barbed and cannot be withdrawn once the bee has stung someone. **B.** The wasp's stinger is unbarbed, meaning that it can inflict multiple stings.

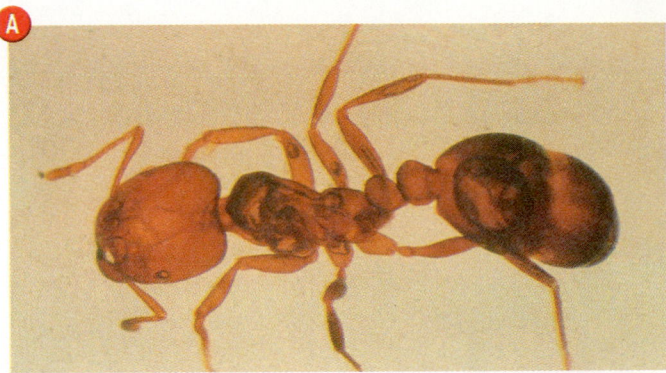

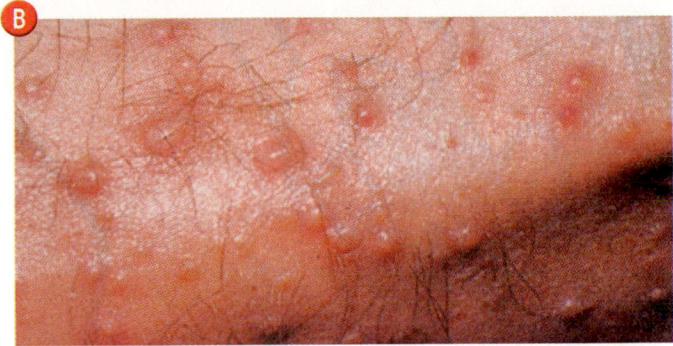

Figure 13-10   **A.** The fire ant. **B.** Fire ants inject an irritating toxin at multiple sites. Bites are generally found on the feet and the legs and appear as multiple small raised pustules.

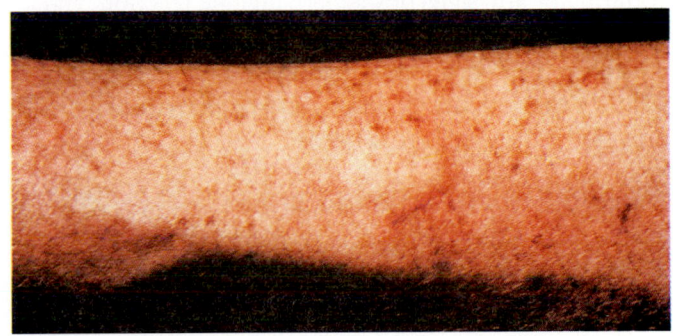

Figure 13-11   A wheal is a whitish, firm elevation of the skin that occurs after an insect sting or bite.

it is often impossible to identify which species was responsible for the injury.

Some ants, especially the fire ant (Formicoidea, ▶ **Figure 13-10A**), also strike repeatedly, often injecting a particularly irritating **toxin**, or poison, at the bite sites. It is not uncommon for a patient to sustain multiple ant bites, usually on the feet and legs, within a very short period of time ▶ **Figure 13-10A** .

Signs and symptoms of insect stings or bites include sudden pain, swelling, localized heat, and redness in light-skinned individuals, usually at the site of injury. There may be itching and sometimes a **wheal**, which

is a raised, swollen, well-defined area on the skin ▲ **Figure 13-11** . There is no specific treatment for these injuries, although applying ice sometimes makes them less irritating. The swelling associated with an insect bite may be dramatic and sometimes frightening to patients. However, these local manifestations are usually not serious.

Because the stinger of the honeybee remains in the wound, it can continue to inject venom for up to 20 minutes after the bee has flown away. In caring for a patient who has been stung by a honeybee, you should gently attempt to remove the stinger and attached muscle by

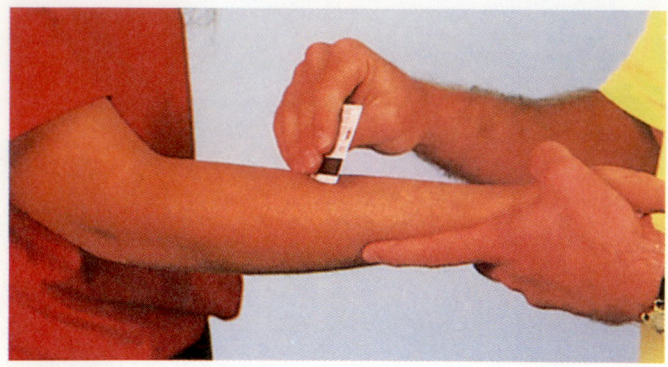

Figure 13-12 To remove the stinger of a honeybee, gently scrape the skin with the edge of a sharp, stiff object such as a credit card.

scraping the skin with the edge of a sharp, stiff object such as a credit card (▲ **Figure 13-12**). Generally, you should not use tweezers or forceps, as squeezing may cause the stinger to inject still more venom into the wound. Gently wash the area with soap and water or a mild antiseptic. Try to remove any jewelry from the area before swelling begins. Position the injection site slightly below the level of the heart and apply ice or cold packs to the area, but not directly on the skin, to help relieve pain and slow the absorption of the toxin. Be alert for vomiting or any signs of shock or allergic reaction, and do not give the patient anything by mouth. Place the patient in the shock position and give oxygen if needed. Monitor the patient's vital signs and be prepared to provide further support as needed.

Anaphylactic Reaction to Stings

Approximately 5% of all people are allergic to the venom of the bee, hornet, yellow jacket, or wasp. This type of allergy, which accounts for about 200 deaths per year, can cause very severe reactions, including anaphylaxis. Patients may experience generalized itching and burning, widespread urticaria, wheals, swelling about the lips and tongue, bronchospasm and wheezing, chest tightness and coughing, dyspnea, anxiety, abdominal cramps, and hypotension. Occasionally, respiratory failure occurs.

If untreated, such an anaphylactic reaction can proceed rapidly to death. In fact, more than two thirds of patients who die of anaphylaxis do so within the first half hour, so speed on your part is essential.

Patient Assessment

Begin by performing a scene size-up, which in some cases of envenomation can lead you to possible

Rescuer Tips

The appropriate emergency care for a victim of poisoning varies depending on how the poison has been introduced into the body. When a rescuer encounters a patient with an allergic reaction, frequently monitor the patient's airway, breathing, and level of responsiveness. Provide suction, rescue or assisted breathing, CPR, and treatment for shock and convulsions as needed. Rapidly transport the patient to a hospital.

answers. Second, perform your initial assessment. A patient may have bite or sting marks that, with other signs and symptoms, may identify an allergic reation. Assess baseline vital signs and get a SAMPLE history. Then collect a focused history and perform a physical examination. Allergic symptoms are almost as varied as allergens themselves. Your assessment of the patient experiencing an allergic reaction should include evaluations of the respiratory system, circulatory system, mental status, and the skin (▶ **Table 13-2**).

Wheezing occurs because excessive fluid and mucus are secreted into the bronchial passages, and muscles around these passages tighten in reaction to the allergen. Exhalation, normally the passive, relaxed part of breathing, becomes harder as the patient tries to cough up the secretions or move air past the constricted airways. The fluid in the air passages and the constricted bronchi together produce the wheezing sound. Breathing rapidly becomes more difficult, and the patient may even stop breathing. Prolonged respiratory difficulty can cause a rapid heartbeat (tachycardia), shock, and even death. **Stridor**, a harsh, high-pitched inspiratory sound, occurs when swelling in the upper airway (near the vocal cords and throat) closes off the airway and can eventually lead to total obstruction.

Remember, the presence of hypoperfusion (shock) or respiratory distress indicates that the patient is having a severe enough allergic reaction to lead to death.

Emergency Medical Care

If the patient seems to be having an allergic reaction, you should give 100% oxygen by nonrebreathing mask as you complete the initial assessment. Perform a focused history and physical examination. Find out whether the patient has a history of allergies, what the patient was exposed to, and how the patient was exposed. Determine what the effects of the exposure have been and how they have progressed. Find out what interventions have been

TABLE 13-2   Common Signs and Symptoms of Allergic Reaction

Respiratory System

- Sneezing or an itchy, runny nose (initially)
- Tightness in the chest or throat
- Irritating, persistent dry cough
- Hoarseness
- Respirations that become rapid, labored, or noisy
- Wheezing and/or stridor

Circulatory System

- Decrease in blood pressure as the blood vessels dilate
- Increase in pulse rate (initially)
- Pale skin and dizziness, as the vascular system fails
- Loss of consciousness and coma

Skin

- Flushing, itching, or burning skin; especially common over the face and upper chest
- Urticaria over large areas of the body, both internally and externally
- Swelling, especially of the face, neck, hands, feet, and/or tongue
- Swelling and cyanosis or pallor around the lips
- Warm, tingling feeling in the face, mouth, chest, feet, and hands

Other Findings

- Anxiety, a sense of impending doom
- Abdominal cramps
- Headache
- Itchy, watery eyes
- Decreasing mental status

---

completed. Inform dispatch about the patient's condition to arrange for ALS, then find out whether the patient has any prescribed, preloaded medications for allergic reactions. If necessary, be prepared to use standard airway procedures and to assist ventilations if necessary.

If the patient appears to be having a severe allergic (or anaphylactic) reaction, you should administer BLS at once and provide prompt evacuation to a hospital or clinic. In addition to providing oxygen, you should be prepared to maintain an airway or give CPR. Placing ice over the injury site has been thought to slow absorption of the toxin and diminish swelling, but ice packs placed directly on the skin may freeze it and cause more damage. Like any other attempt to reduce swelling with ice, you should be careful not to overdo the icing. Anaphylactic reactions are usually treated with injectable adrenaline, **epinephrine**. This drug works rapidly to raise the pulse rate and blood pressure by constricting the blood vessels. More importantly, it inhibits the allergic reaction and dilates the bronchioles, making breathing easier. Bee sting kits or "pens" contain a prepared syringe of epinephrine, ready for subcutaneous injection, along with instructions for use. If the patient has had a previous serious anaphylactic reaction, he or she will usually have one of these. The rescuer should help the patient self-

administer the epinephrine. The most common device is an EpiPen, which delivers 0.3 mg of epinephrine to an adult, and 0.15 mg to the child (▶ Figure 13-13).

If the patient is able to use the auto-injector on his or her own, your role is limited to helping. To use, or help the patient use, the auto-injector, you should first receive training and a direct order from your medical director or follow local protocols or standing orders. Follow BSI precautions, and make sure the medication has been prescribed specifically for that patient. If it has not, do not give the medication: inform the responding EMS unit, and provide immediate evacuation. Finally, make sure the medication is not discolored or expired.

Once you have done these things, follow the steps in (▶ Skill Drill 13-2) to use an auto-injector.

1. **Remove the safety cap** from the auto-injector and, if possible, wipe the patient's thigh with alcohol or some other antiseptic. However, do not delay administration of the drug **(Step 1)**.

2. **Place the tip of the auto-injector** against the lateral part of the patient's thigh, midway between the waist and the knee **(Step 2)**.

3. **Push the injector firmly** against the thigh until the injector activates, about 5 to 10 seconds. This action will help prevent the kick that the

SkillDrill 13-2   Using an Auto-Injector

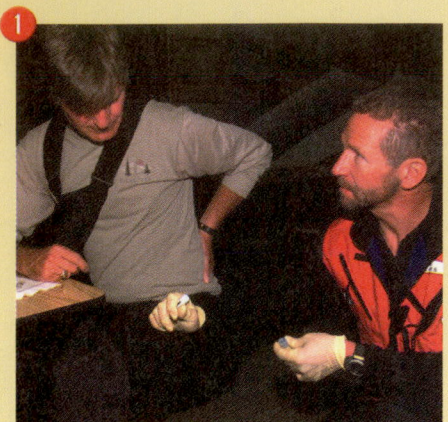

1 Remove the auto-injector's safety cap.

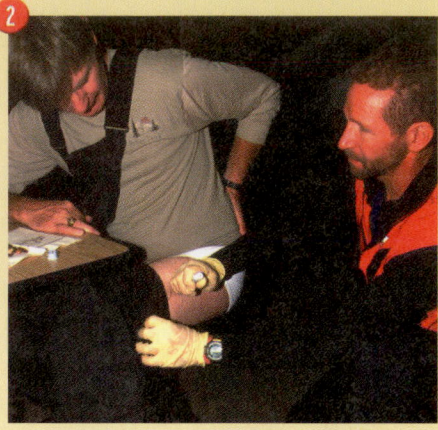

2 Place the tip of the auto-injector against the lateral thigh.

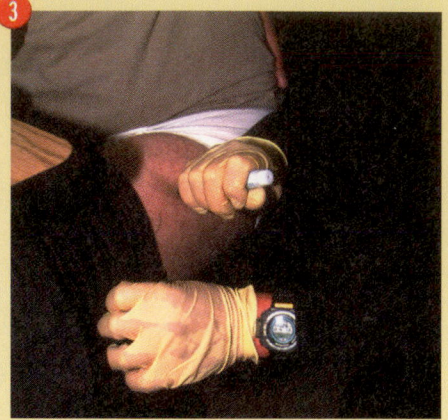

3 Help the patient push the auto-injector firmly against the thigh and hold it in place until all the medication is injected.

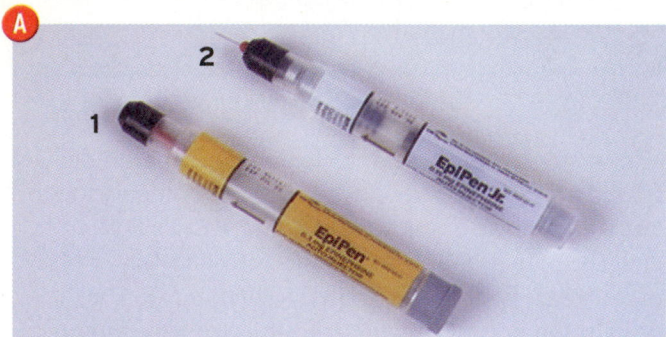

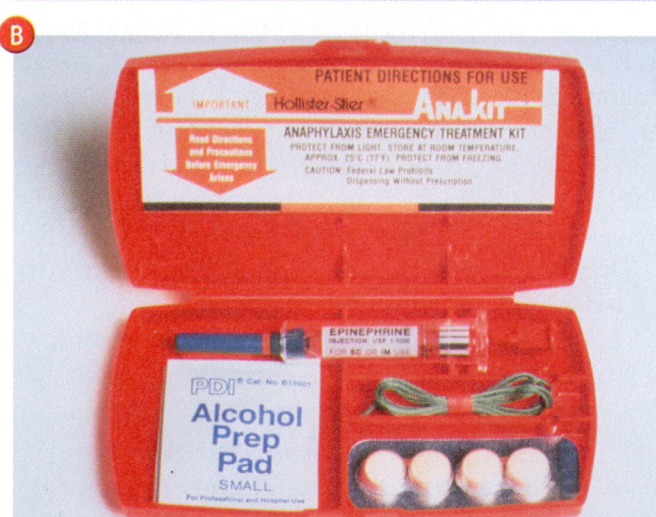

Figure 13-13 Patients who experience severe allergic reactions often carry their own epinephrine, which comes predosed in an auto-injector or a standard syringe. **A.** EpiPen auto-injectors (1–unfired adult model, 2–fired junior model). **B.** AnaKit with epinephrine syringe.

Rescuer Tips

If your local protocols allow it, and your patient has an inhaler as well as an epinephrine auto-injector, one rescuer can help administer the inhaler while the other helps administer the epinephrine. Then transport them quickly to definitive care. Basic life support may be required.

spring-loaded syringe can cause when the needle is pulled from the injection site too soon. Hold the injector in place until the medication is injected (10 seconds). **(Step 3)**.

4. **Remove the injector** from the patient's thigh and dispose of it in the proper biohazard container.

5. **Record the time and dose** of the injection.

6. **Reassess and record** the patient's vital signs after using the auto-injector.

If the patient is known to be allergic, he or she might carry a commercial bee sting kit (AnaKit) that contains a standard syringe of epinephrine for intramuscular injection (◄ **Figure 13-13**). If you help the patient administer this epinephrine, make the same general preparations you make for an auto-injector. Take BSI precautions, and ensure that the medicine is the patient's and is not discolored or expired.

Whether or not your emergency treatment includes epinephrine, you should always provide prompt evacuation for any patient who may be having an allergic reaction or has experienced a poisonous envenomation or bite. Continue to reassess the patient's vital signs en route; remember that signs and symptoms may change rapidly. As with any patient you are transporting, be prepared to treat for shock, begin BLS measures, or use the AED if necessary.

If the patient's condition improves, provide supportive care, including giving the patient oxygen during transport.

Specific Bites and Envenomations

Spider Bites

Spiders are both numerous and widespread in the United States. Many species of spiders bite. However, only two, the female black widow spider and the brown recluse spider, are able to deliver serious, even life-threatening bites. When you care for a patient who has had some type of bite, be alert to the possibility that the spider may still be in the area, although it is not likely. Remember that your safety is of paramount importance.

BLACK WIDOW SPIDER. The female black widow spider (*Latrodectus*) is fairly large as far as spiders go, measuring approximately 2″ long with its legs extended. It is usually black and has a distinctive, bright red-orange marking in the shape of an hourglass on its abdomen (▶ **Figure 13-14**). The female is larger and more toxic than the male. Black widow spiders are found in every state except Alaska. They prefer dry, dim places around buildings, in woodpiles, and among debris.

The bite of the black widow spider is sometimes overlooked. If the site becomes numb right away, the patient may not even recall being bit. However, most black widow spider bites cause localized pain and symptoms, including agonizing muscle spasms. In some cases, a bite on the abdomen causes muscle spasms so severe that the patient may be thought to have an acute abdomen, possibly peritonitis. The main danger with this type of bite, however, comes from the fact that the black widow's venom is poisonous to nerve tissues (neurotoxic). Other systemic symptoms include dizziness, sweating, nausea, vomiting, and rashes. Tightness in the chest and difficulty breathing develop within 24 hours, as well as severe cramps, with board-like rigidity of the abdominal muscles. Generally, these signs and symptoms subside over 48 hours.

In general, emergency treatment of a black widow spider bite consists of BLS for the patient in respiratory distress. Much more often, the patient will merely require relief from pain. Evacuate the patient to the emergency department as soon as possible for treatment of both pain and muscle rigidity. If possible, bring the spider along.

BROWN RECLUSE SPIDER. The brown recluse spider (*Loxosceles*) is dull brown and, at 1″, somewhat smaller than the black widow (▼ **Figure 13-15**). The short-haired body has a violin-shaped mark, brown to yellow in color, on its back. Although it lives mostly in the southern and central parts of the country, the brown recluse may be found throughout the continental United States. The spider takes its name from the fact that it tends to live in dark areas: in corners of old, unused buildings, under rocks, and in woodpiles. In cooler areas, it moves indoors to closets, drawers, cellars, and old piles of clothing.

In contrast to the venom of the black widow spider, the venom of the brown recluse spider is not neurotoxic but cytotoxic; that is, it causes severe local tissue damage. Typically, the bite is not painful at first but becomes so within hours. The area becomes swollen and tender, developing a pale, mottled, cyanotic center and possibly a small blister (▼ **Figure 13-16**). Over the next several days, a scab of dead skin, fat, and debris will form and dig down into the skin, producing a large ulcer that may not heal unless treated promptly. Evacuate patients with such symptoms as soon as possible.

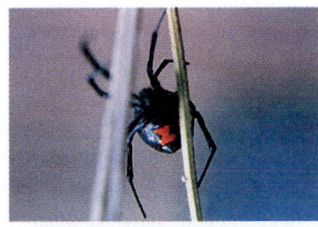

Figure 13-14 Black widow spiders are distinguished by their glossy black color and bright orange hourglass marking on the abdomen.

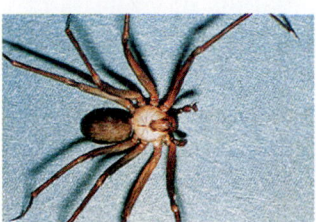

Figure 13-15 Brown recluse spiders are dull brown and have a dark, violin-shaped mark on the back.

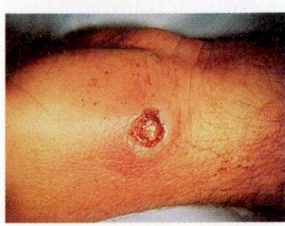

Figure 13-16 The bite of a brown recluse spider is characterized by swelling, tenderness, and a pale, mottled cyanotic center. There may also be a small blister on the bite.

Brown recluse spider bites rarely cause systemic symptoms and signs. When they do, the initial treatment is BLS and evacuation to an emergency department. Again, it is helpful if you can identify the spider and bring it to the hospital along with the patient.

Snake Bites

Snake bites are a worldwide problem of some significance. More than 300,000 injuries from snake bites occur annually, including 30,000 to 40,000 deaths. The greatest number of the fatalities occur in Southeast Asia and India (25,000 to 30,000) and in South America (3,000 to 4,000). In the United States, 40,000 to 50,000 snake bites are reported annually; about 7,000 of them are caused by poisonous snakes. However, snake bite fatalities in the United States are extremely rare, about 15 a year for the entire country.

Of the approximately 115 different species of snakes in the United States, only 19 are venomous. These include the rattlesnake (*Crotalus*), the copperhead (*Agkistrodon contortrix*), the cottonmouth, or water moccasin (*Agkistrodon piscivorus*), and the coral snakes (*Micrurus* and *Micruroides*) ▶ **Figure 13-17** . At least one of these poisonous species is found in every state except Alaska, Hawaii, and Maine. As a general rule, these creatures are timid. They usually do not bite unless provoked, angered, or accidentally injured, as when they are stepped on. There are a few exceptions to these rules. Cottonmouths are often rather aggressive, and very little provocation is needed to annoy a rattlesnake. Coral snakes, by contrast, are very shy and usually bite only when they are being handled.

Most snake bites occur between April and October, when the animals are active. Remember, almost any time you are caring for a patient with a snake bite, another snake could come along and create a second victim: you. Therefore, use extreme caution and be sure to wear the proper protective equipment for the area.

With the exception of the coral snake, poisonous snakes native to the United States all have hollow fangs in the roof of the mouth that inject the poison from two sacs at the back of the head. The classic appearance of the poisonous snake bite, therefore, is two small puncture wounds, usually about 1/2" apart, with discoloration, swelling, and pain surrounding them ▶ **Figure 13-18** . Nonpoisonous snakes can also bite, usually leaving a horseshoe of tooth marks. However, some poisonous snakes have teeth as well as fangs, making it impossible to say which kind is responsible for a given set of tooth marks. On the other hand, fang marks are a clear indication of a poisonous snake bite.

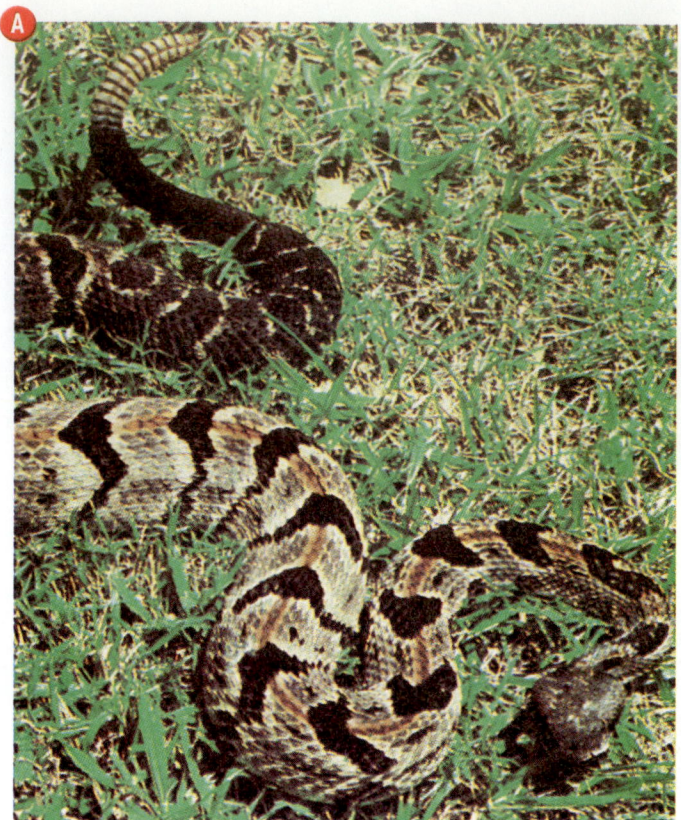

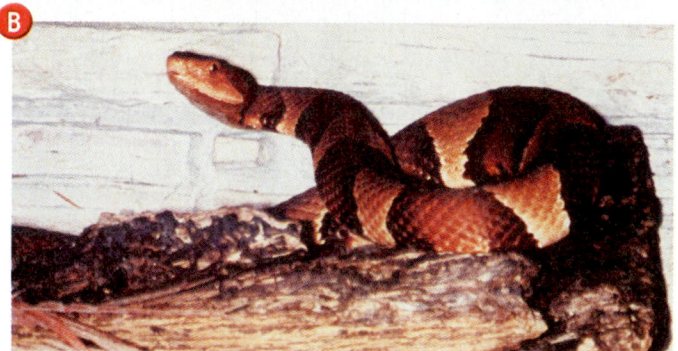

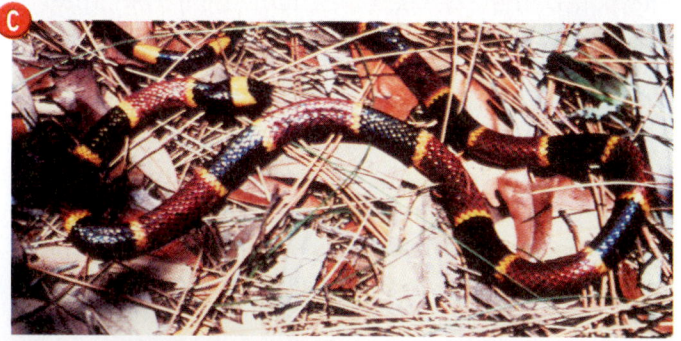

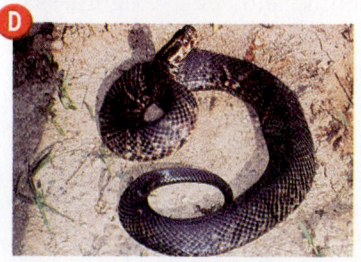

Figure 13-17
A. Rattlesnake.
B. Copperhead.
C. Coral snake.
D. Cottonmouth.

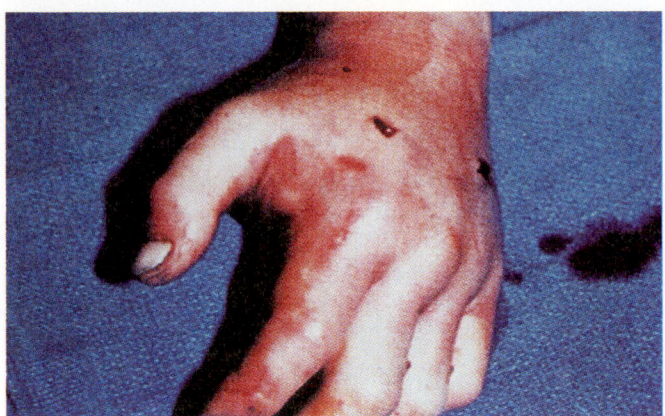

Figure 13-18   A snake bite wound from a poisonous snake has characteristic markings: two small puncture wounds about $\frac{1}{2}$" apart, discoloration, and swelling.

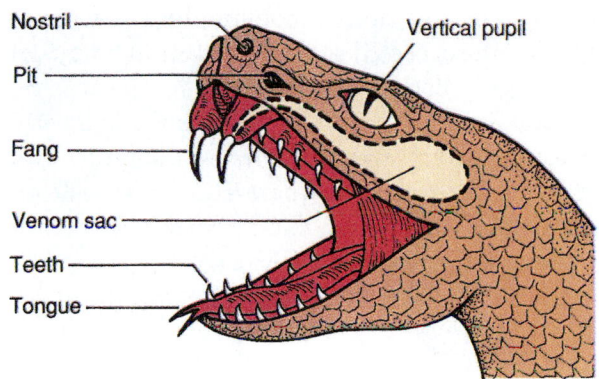

Figure 13-19   Pit vipers have small, heat-sensing organs (pits) located in front of their eyes that allow them to strike at warm targets, even in the dark.

Wilderness Tips

Of all animals, venomous snakes are the most dangerous to humans. If you are in a remote area where transport to definitive medical care cannot be reached for hours, suggestions for emergency care include:

- Some experts recommend using a single constricting band to slow absorption of the venom in extremity bites. Tie a snug cloth or cravat around the extremity, directly over the bite, so there is pressure on the wound. This reduces blood flow to the area, decreasing systemic release of the venom. The pressure should not be so tight that peripheral pulses are absent.
- Use a commercial negative pressure device, which should be part of the emergency care kit carried in snake country. Use it immediately after the bite occurs.
- Send a member of the party for help.
- Clean the bite with soap and water and cover it with a sterile compress.
- Splint a bitten extremity.
- Give the patient electrolyte-containing fluids to replace fluid lost from the blood into the bitten area.

Set up camp and have the patient rest until help arrives. If the group is large enough and a litter can be improvised, carry the patient out. During tick season (spring and early summer), outdoor recreationists should inspect each other for ticks nightly. It is important to inspect all hidden and hairy areas carefully, particularly the scalp, armpits, and perianal and genital areas.

PIT VIPERS. Rattlesnakes, copperheads, and cottonmouths are all pit vipers, with triangular-shaped, flat heads (▲ **Figure 13-19**). They take their name from the small pits located just behind each nostril and in front of each eye. The pit is a heat-sensing organ that allows the snake to strike accurately at any warm target, especially in the dark when it cannot see through its vertical, slit-like pupils.

The fangs of the pit viper normally lie flat against the roof of the mouth and are hinged to swing back and forth as the mouth opens. When the snake is striking, the mouth opens wide and the fangs extend; in this way, the fangs penetrate whatever the mouth strikes. The fangs are actually special hollow teeth that act much like hypodermic needles. They are connected to a sac containing a reservoir of venom, which in turn is attached to a poison gland. The gland itself is a specially adapted salivary gland, which produces powerful enzymes that digest and destroy tissue. The primary purpose of the venom is to kill small animals and to start the digestive process prior to their being eaten.

The most common form of pit viper is the rattlesnake. Several different species of rattlesnake can be identified by the rattle on the tail. The rattle is actually numerous layers of dried skin that were shed but failed to fall off, coming to rest against a small knob on the end of the tail. Rattlesnakes have many patterns of color, often in a diamond shape. They can grow to 6' or more.

Copperheads are smaller than rattlesnakes, usually 2' to 3' long, with a reddish coppery color crossed with brown or red bands. These snakes typically inhabit woodpiles and abandoned dwellings, often close to areas of habitation. Although they account for most of the venomous snake bites in the eastern United States, copperhead bites are almost never fatal; however, note that the venom can destroy extremities.

Cottonmouths grow to about 4' in length. Also called water moccasins, these snakes are olive or brown, with black cross-bands and a yellow undersurface. They are water snakes, with a particularly aggressive pattern of behavior. Although fatalities from these snake bites are rare, tissue destruction from the venom may be severe.

The signs of envenomation by a pit viper are severe burning pain at the site of the injury, followed by swelling and a bluish discoloration (ecchymosis) in light-skinned individuals that signals bleeding under the skin. These signs are evident within 5 to 10 minutes after the bite has occurred and spread over the next 36 hours. In addition to destroying tissues locally, the venom of the pit viper can also interfere with the body's clotting mechanism and cause bleeding at various distant sites. Other systemic signs, which may or may not occur, include weakness, sweating, fainting, and shock. If the patient has no local signs an hour after being bitten, it is safe to assume that envenomation did not take place. If swelling has occurred, you should mark its edges on the skin with an ink pen. This will allow physicians to assess what has happened, and when it happened, with greater accuracy.

Occasionally, a patient bitten by a snake will faint from fright. The patient will usually regain consciousness promptly when placed in a supine position. Do not confuse a fainting spell with shock. If shock occurs, it will happen much later.

In treating a snake bite from a pit viper, follow these steps to get the patient to the hospital in a timely fashion:

1. Calm the patient; assure him or her that poisonous snake bites are rarely fatal. Keep the patient supine, and explain that staying quiet will slow the spread of any venom through the system. Remove rings, watches, bracelets, or any article that might constrict circulation.

2. Locate the bite area; clean it gently with soap and water or a mild antiseptic. **Do not apply ice to the area.**

3. If the bite occurred on an arm or leg, splint the extremity to decrease movement.

4. Be alert for vomiting, which may be a sign of anxiety rather than the toxin itself.

5. Do not give anything by mouth.

6. If, as rarely happens, the patient was bitten on the trunk, keep him or her supine and quiet and evacuate the patient as quickly as possible.

7. Monitor the patient's vital signs and mark the skin with a pen over the area that is swollen, proximal to the swelling, to note whether swelling is spreading.

8. If there are any signs of shock, place the patient in the shock position and give oxygen.

9. If the snake has been killed, as is often the case, be sure to bring it with you so that physicians can identify it and administer the proper antivenin.

10. Notify the hospital that you are bringing in a snake bite patient; if possible, describe the snake.

11. Evacuate the patient promptly to the hospital.

If the patient shows no sign of envenomation, provide BLS as needed, place a sterile dressing over the suspected bite area, and immobilize the injury site. All patients with suspected snake bites should be taken to the emergency department, whether they show signs of envenomation or not. Treat the wound as you would any deep puncture wound to prevent infection.

If you work in an area where poisonous snakes are known to live, you should know the local protocol for handling snake bites. You should also know the address of the nearest facility where antivenin is available.

CORAL SNAKES. The coral snake is a small reptile with a series of bright red, yellow, and black bands completely encircling the body. Many harmless snakes have similar coloring, but only the coral snake has red and yellow bands next to one another, as this helpful rhyme suggests: "Red on yellow will kill a fellow; red on black, venom will lack."

A rare creature that lives primarily in Florida and in the desert Southwest, the coral snake is a relative of the cobra. It has tiny fangs and injects the venom with its teeth by a chewing motion, leaving behind one or more puncture or scratch-like wounds. Because of its small mouth and teeth and limited jaw expansion, the coral snake usually bites its victims on a small part of the body, such as a finger or toe.

Coral snake venom is a powerful toxin that causes paralysis of the nervous system. Within a few hours of being bitten, a patient will exhibit bizarre behavior, followed by progressive paralysis of eye movements and respiration. Often, there are limited or no local symptoms.

Successful treatment, either emergency or long term, depends on positive identification of the snake and support of respiration. Antivenin is available, but most hospitals do not stock it. Therefore, you should notify the hospital of the need for it as soon as possible. The steps for emergency care of a coral snake bite are as follows:

1. Immediately quiet and reassure the patient.

2. Flush the area of the bite with 1 to 2 quarts of warm, soapy water to wash away any poison left on the surface of the skin. **Do not apply ice to the region.**

3. Splint the extremity to minimize movement and the spread of venom at the site.

4. Check the patient's vital signs and continue to monitor them.

5. Keep the patient warm and elevate the lower extremities to help prevent shock.

6. Give supplemental oxygen if needed.

7. Evacuate the patient promptly to the emergency department, giving advance notice that the patient has been bitten by a coral snake.

8. Give the patient nothing by mouth.

Scorpion Stings

Scorpions are eight-legged arachnids from the biological group Arachnida with a venom gland and a stinger at the end of their tail (▼ **Figure 13-20**). Scorpions are rare; they live primarily in the southwestern United States and in deserts. With one exception, a scorpion's sting is usually very painful but not dangerous, causing localized swelling and discoloration. The exception is the *Centruroides sculpturatus*. Although it is found naturally in Arizona and New Mexico, as well as parts of Texas, California, and Nevada, it may be kept as a pet by anyone. The venom of this particular species may produce a severe systemic reaction that brings about circulatory collapse, severe muscle contractions, excessive salivation, hypertension, convulsions, and cardiac failure. Antivenin is available but must be administered by a physician. If you are called to care for a patient with a suspected sting from *sculpturatus*, you should notify medical control as soon as possible. Administer all the elements of BLS and evacuate the patient to the emergency department as rapidly as possible.

Tick Bites

Found most often on brush, shrubs, trees, sand dunes, or other animals, ticks usually attach themselves directly to the skin (▼ **Figure 13-21**). Only a fraction of an inch long, they can easily be mistaken for a freckle, especially since their bite is not painful. Indeed, the danger with a tick bite is not from the bite itself, but from the infecting organisms that the tick carries. Ticks commonly carry two infectious diseases: Rocky Mountain spotted fever and Lyme disease. Both are spread through the tick's saliva, which is injected into the skin when the tick attaches itself.

Rocky Mountain spotted fever, which is not limited to the Rocky Mountains, occurs within 7 to 10 days after a bite by an infected tick. Its symptoms include nausea, vomiting, headache, weakness, paralysis, and possibly cardiorespiratory collapse.

Lyme disease, spread by deer ticks, has received extensive publicity. It is, after AIDS, the second most rapidly growing infectious disease in the United States. Originally seen only in Connecticut, Lyme disease has now been reported in 35 states. It occurs most commonly in the Northeast, the Great Lake States, and the Pacific Northwest; New York State reports the largest number of cases. The first symptom, a rash that may spread to several parts of the body, begins about 3 days after the bite of an infected tick. The rash may eventually resemble a target bull's-eye pattern in one third of patients (▼ **Figure 13-22**). After a few more days or weeks, painful swelling of the joints, particularly the knees, occurs. Lyme disease may be confused with rheumatoid arthritis and, like that disease, may result in permanent disability. However, if it is recognized and treated promptly with antibiotics, the patient may recover completely.

Tick bites occur most commonly during the summer months, when people are out in the woods wearing little protective clothing. Transmission of the infection from

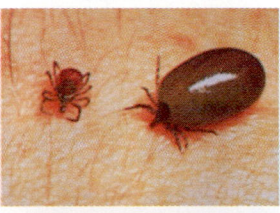

Figure 13-21 Ticks typically attach themselves directly to the skin and eventually become engorged with blood, as shown on the right.

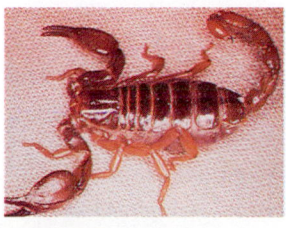

Figure 13-20 The sting of a scorpion is usually more painful than it is dangerous, causing localized swelling and discoloration.

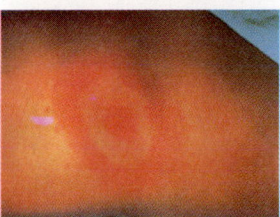

Figure 13-22 The rash associated with Lyme disease has a characteristic "bull's-eye" pattern.

Wilderness Tips

During tick season (spring and early summer), outdoor recreationists should inspect each other for ticks nightly. It is important to inspect all hidden and hairy areas carefully, particularly the scalp, armpits, and perianal and genital areas. Embedded ticks should be removed with forceps rather than with the fingers. Lift the tick's body so that it is perpendicular to the skin. To avoid leaving the tick's mouth-parts in the wound, remove a small area of the surrounding skin along with the front end of the tick, using a sturdy pair of splinter forceps and cleaning them afterward with alcohol or by flaming them with a match.

Rescuer Safety

In snake country, never put a hand, foot, or other body part in a place that isn't in your full view. Always use caution when reaching overhead to grasp a rocky ledge or when stepping over a log, and carry a sturdy walking stick to poke logs and rocks before stepping over them.

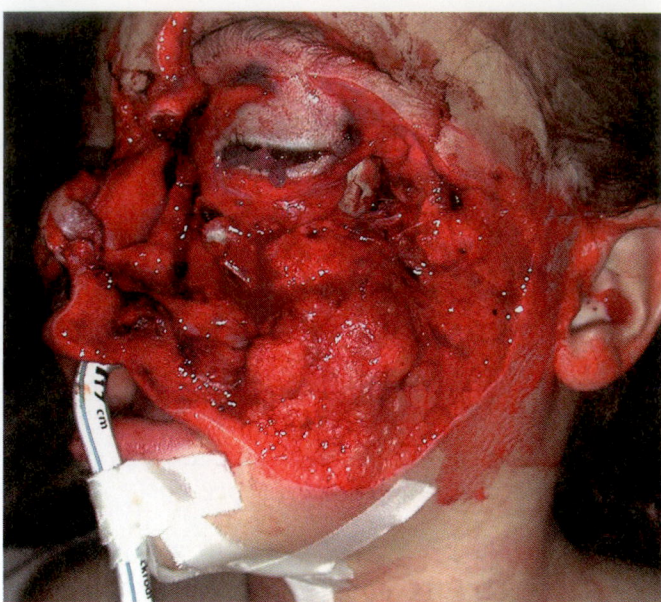

Figure 13-23 Dog bite wounds should be examined at the hospital, as these wounds are heavily contaminated with virulent bacteria.

tick to person takes at least 12 hours, so if you are called on to remove a tick, you should proceed carefully and slowly. Do not attempt to suffocate the tick with gasoline or Vaseline or burn it with a lighted match; you will only burn the patient. Instead, using fine tweezers, grasp the tick by the body and pull it straight out of the skin. This method will usually remove the whole tick. Even if part of the tick is left embedded in the skin, the part containing the infecting organisms has been removed. Cleanse the area with disinfectant and save the tick in a glass jar or other container so that it can be identified. Do not handle the tick with your fingers. Provide any necessary supportive emergency care, and transport the patient to a hospital or clinic if necessary.

Dog Bites and Rabies

Most people who are bitten by dogs do not report the incident to a physician, believing that dog bites are not serious. They can be very serious, however. A dog's mouth is heavily contaminated with virulent bacteria. You should consider all dog bites as contaminated and potentially infected wounds that may require antibiotics, tetanus prophylaxis, and suturing (▶ **Figure 13-23**). Occasionally, dog bites result in mangled, complex wounds that require surgical repair. For these reasons, all dog bites should be treated by a physician. Place a dry, sterile dressing over the wound, and promptly

evacuate the patient to the emergency department. If an arm or leg was injured, splint that extremity. Often, the patient will be extremely upset and frightened, a situation that calls for calm reassurance on your part.

A major concern with dog bites is the spread of *rabies*, an acute, fatal viral infection of the central nervous system that can affect all warm-blooded animals. Although rabies is extremely rare today, particularly with widespread inoculation of pets, it still exists. Stray dogs that have not been inoculated can be carriers of the disease, as can squirrels, bats, foxes, skunks, and raccoons. The virus is in the saliva of a **rabid**, or infected, animal and is transmitted through biting or licking an open wound. Infection can be prevented in a person who has been bitten by such an animal only by a series of special vaccine injections, a painful procedure that must be begun soon after the bite. Since animals that have rabies do not always show it immediately in their behavior, a person's only chance to avoid the vaccine is to find the animal and turn it over to the health department for observation and/or testing. Refer to your local animal control procedures.

Human Bites

The human mouth, more so than even the dog's, contains an exceptionally wide range of virulent bacteria and viruses. For this reason, you should regard any human bite that has penetrated the skin as a very serious injury. Similarly, any laceration caused by a human tooth can result in a serious, spreading infection (▶ **Figure 13-24**). Remember this if you have occasion to treat someone

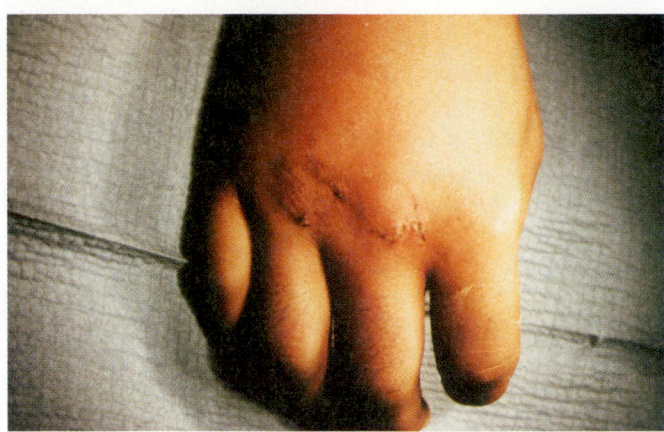

Figure 13-24 Human bites can result in serious, spreading infection. Thus, patients must be evaluated at the hospital.

who has been punched in the mouth: The person who delivered the punch may also need treatment.

The emergency treatment of human bites consists of the following steps:

1. Wash the area with soap and water.

2. Apply a dry, sterile dressing.

3. Promptly immobilize the area with a splint or bandage.

4. Provide transport to the emergency department for surgical cleansing of the wound and antibiotic therapy.

Injuries from Marine Animals

Coelenterates, including the fire coral, Portuguese man-of-war, sea wasp, sea nettles, true jellyfish, sea anemones, true coral, and soft coral, are responsible for more envenomations than any other marine animals ▶ **Figure 13-25** . The stinging cells of the coelenterate are called nematocysts, and large animals may discharge hundreds of thousands of them. Envenomation causes very painful, reddish lesions in light-skinned individuals, extending in a line from the site of the sting. Systemic symptoms include headache, dizziness, muscle cramps, and fainting.

To treat a sting from the tentacles of a jellyfish, a Portuguese man-of-war, various anemones, corals, or hydras, remove the patient from the water and pour any type of alcohol on the affected area. Unlike fresh water, alcohol will inactivate the nematocysts. Do not try to manipulate the remaining tentacles; this will only cause further discharge of the nematocysts. Remove the tentacles by scraping them off with the edge of a sharp, stiff object such as a credit card. Persistent pain may respond to immersion of the area in hot water (110° to 115°F, 43° to 46°C) for 30 minutes. On very rare occasions, a

TABLE 13-3 Common Marine Envenomations

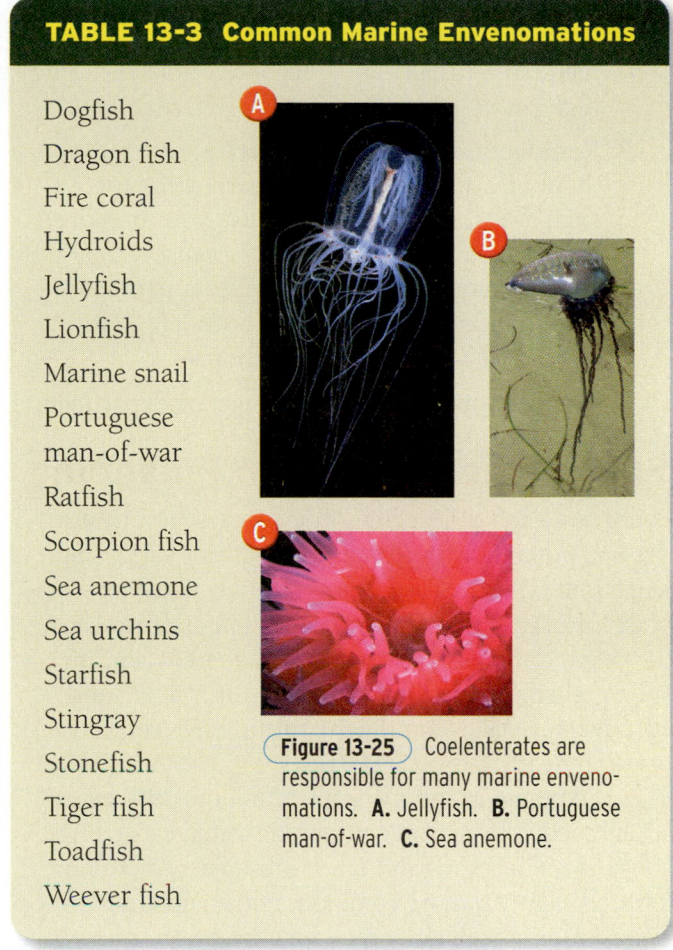

Dogfish
Dragon fish
Fire coral
Hydroids
Jellyfish
Lionfish
Marine snail
Portuguese man-of-war
Ratfish
Scorpion fish
Sea anemone
Sea urchins
Starfish
Stingray
Stonefish
Tiger fish
Toadfish
Weever fish

Figure 13-25 Coelenterates are responsible for many marine envenomations. **A.** Jellyfish. **B.** Portuguese man-of-war. **C.** Sea anemone.

patient may have a systemic allergic reaction to the sting of one of these animals. Treat such a patient for anaphylactic shock. Give BLS, and provide immediate transport to the hospital.

Toxins from the spines of urchins, stingrays, and certain spiny fish such as the lionfish, scorpion fish, or stonefish are heat sensitive ▲ **Table 13-3** . Therefore, the best treatment for such injuries is to immobilize the affected area and soak it in hot water for 30 minutes. This will often provide dramatic relief from local pain. However, the patient still needs to be transported to the emergency department, since an allergic reaction or infection, including tetanus, could develop.

If you work near the ocean, you should be familiar with the marine life in your area. The emergency treatment of common coelenterate envenomations consists of the following steps:

1. **Limit further discharge** of nematocysts by avoiding fresh water, wet sand, showers, or careless manipulation of the tentacles. Keep the patient calm, and reduce motion of the affected extremity.

2. **Inactivate the nematocysts** by applying alcohol. (Although isopropyl or rubbing alcohol is recommended, virtually any type of alcohol, including high proof liquor or cologne, is effective.)

3. **Remove the remaining tentacles** by scraping them off with the edge of a sharp, stiff object such as a credit card. Do not use your ungloved hand to remove the tentacles, because self-envenomation will occur. Persistent pain may respond to immersion in hot water (110° to 115°F, 43° to 46°C) for 30 minutes.

4. **Provide transport** to the emergency department.

Substance Abuse and Poisoning

Every day, each of us comes into contact with things that are potentially poisonous. This is not surprising when you consider that almost any substance may be a poison in certain circumstances. Different doses can turn even a remedy into a poison. Consider aspirin. When taken in recommended doses, it is a safe and effective analgesic. Too much aspirin, however, can result in death.

Acute poisoning affects some 5 million children and adults each year. Chronic poisoning, often caused by abuse of medications and other substances, including tobacco, is much more common. Fortunately, deaths from poisoning are fairly rare. Rates of death from poisoning for children have decreased steadily since the 1960s, when safety caps were introduced for drug bottles and containers. Deaths from poisoning in adults, though, have been rising, the majority the result of drug abuse or overdose.

In this section, the term "poisoned" includes both acute and chronic poisonings. As a rescuer, you must recognize that patients with either type of problem may have a variety of injuries. Although you cannot stop a chronic substance abuse problem, you may be able to prevent death from the acute effects of the poison.

This section discusses how to identify the patient who has been poisoned and how to gather clues about the poison. It describes the different ways in which poison is introduced into the body. It then discusses the signs, symptoms, and treatment of specific poisons, including sedatives and **opioids** (medicines with actions similar to morphine). Food poisoning and plant poisoning are also discussed.

Identifying the Patient and the Poison

A **poison** is any substance whose chemical action can damage body structures or impair body function. A poison can be introduced into the body through a

Rescuer Tips

Poison Control Centers

There are several hundred poison control centers in the United States. The phone number of a local poison control center is typically found on the inside cover of a local phone book. Staff at every center have access to information about virtually all of the commonly used medications, chemicals, and substances that could possibly be poisonous. They know the appropriate emergency treatment for each, including the antidote, if there is one. An **antidote** is a substance that will counteract the effects of a particular poison.

If you believe that a patient has been poisoned, you should immediately provide medical control with all relevant information: when the poisoning occurred; a description of the suspected poison, including the amount involved; and the patient's size, weight, and age.

variety of means. Poisons act by changing the normal metabolism of cells or by actually destroying them. Poisons may act acutely, as in an overdose of heroin, or chronically, as in years of alcohol or other substance abuse. **Substance abuse** is the knowing misuse of any substance to produce a desired effect (eg, cocaine intoxication).

Your primary responsibility to the patient who has been poisoned is to recognize that a poisoning has occurred. Keep in mind that very small amounts of some poisons can cause considerable damage or death. If you have even the slightest suspicion that a patient has taken a poisonous substance, you should call for transport and begin emergency treatment at once.

Symptoms and signs of poisoning vary according to the specific agent, as shown in (▶ **Table 13-4**). These groups of signs and symptoms are known as toxidromes. Some poisons cause the pulse to speed up, while others cause it to slow down; some cause the pupils to dilate, while others cause the pupils to constrict. If respiration is depressed or difficult, cyanosis may occur. Some chemical compounds will irritate or burn the skin or mucous membranes, resulting in burning or blistering. The presence of such injuries at the mouth strongly suggests the **ingestion** (swallowing) of a poison, such as lye. If possible, consider asking the patient the following questions:

- What substance did you take?
- When did you take it (or become exposed to it)?
- How much did you ingest?
- What actions have been taken?
- How much do you weigh?

TABLE 13-4 Toxidromes: Typical Signs and Symptoms of Specific Drug Overdose

Opioid (eg, codeine)	Hypoventilation/ respiratory arrest Pinpoint pupils (miosis) Sedation/coma Hypotension	**Anticholinergics** (eg, jimson weed)	Tachycardia Hyperthermia Hypertension Dilated pupils (mydriasis) Dry skin and mucous membranes Sedation/agitation/seizures/ coma/delirium Decreased bowel sounds
Sympathomimetics (eg, amphetamines)	Hypertension Tachycardia Dilated pupils (mydriasis) Agitation/seizures Hyperthermia	**Cholinergics** (eg, insecticides, mushrooms)	Excess defecation/urination Muscle fasciculations Pinpoint pupils (miosis) Excess lacrimation/ salivation Airway compromise Nausea/vomiting
Sedative-Hypnotics (eg, valium)	Slurred speech Sedation/coma Hypoventilation Hypotension		

Try to determine the nature of the poison. Objects at the scene may provide clues: an overturned bottle, a needle or syringe, scattered pills, chemicals, even an overturned or damaged plant. The remains of any nearby food or drink may also be important. Place any suspicious material in a plastic bag, and take it to the hospital, along with any containers you find.

Containers can provide critical information. In addition to the name and concentration of the drug, a pill bottle label may list specific ingredients, the number of pills that were originally in the bottle, the name of the manufacturer, and the dose that was prescribed. This information can help emergency department physicians to determine how much has been ingested and what specific treatment may be required. For certain food poisonings, a food container that lists the name and location of the maker or the vendor may be of equal importance in saving the life of the patient and possibly other people.

If the patient vomits, collect the material, called **vomitus**, in a separate plastic bag so that it can be analyzed at the hospital. After providing emergency care, collecting and bagging suspicious materials and vomitus may be the most important thing you can do for the patient.

How Poisons Get Into the Body

Emergency care for the patient who has been poisoned may include a range of actions from reassuring an anxious parent to instituting CPR. Most often, it will not include administering a specific antidote, because most poisons do not have one. Therefore, in general,

the most important treatment for poisoning is diluting and/or physically removing the poisonous agent. How you do this depends on how the poison gets into the patient's body in the first place. Essentially, the four avenues to consider are as follows (▶ Figure 13-26):

- Ingestion
- Inhalation
- Injection
- Absorption (surface contact)

Injection often can be the most worrisome avenue of poisoning. You can administer oxygen to a patient who has inhaled a poison, and you can give activated charcoal to one who has ingested a poison. You can flood the skin with water and wash out the eyes of one who has contacted a poison. However, it is difficult to remove or dilute injected poisons, a fact that makes these cases especially urgent. On the other hand, all routes of poisoning can be deadly, and each should be thought of as being equally serious.

Ingested Poisons

Approximately 80% of all poisoning is by mouth (ingestion). Ingested poisons include liquids, household cleaners, contaminated food, plants, and, in most cases, drugs. Ingested poisoning is usually accidental in children and, except for contaminated food, deliberate in adults. Plant poisonings are common among children, who like to explore and often bite the leaves of various bushes or shrubs.

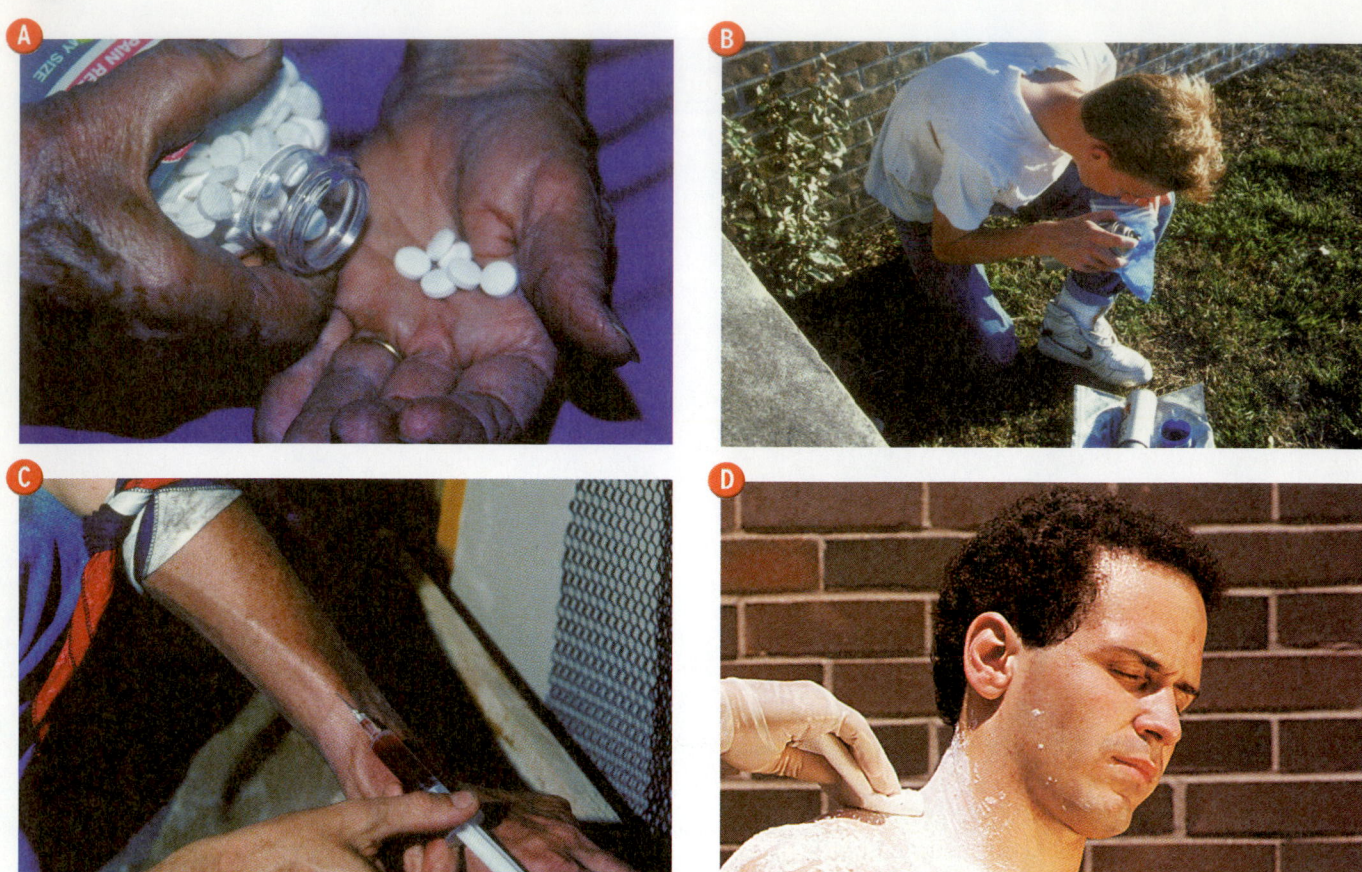

Figure 13-26   There are four routes by which a poison can enter the body. **A.** Ingestion. **B.** Inhalation. **C.** Injection.
D. Absorption (surface contact).

Your goal as a rescuer is to rapidly remove as much of the poison as possible from the gastrointestinal tract. For most poisoning victims, this emergency treatment is sufficient. Call your local poison control center for appropriate information.

In the past, syrup of ipecac was used to cause vomiting, but today it is recommended in only a few situations in which the risk of losing consciousness is clearly ruled out. Because syrup of ipecac induces vomiting, individuals who have ingested substances that may cause diminished alertness over time might vomit and inhale the vomit into the lungs as they lose consciousness. Activated charcoal comes as a suspension that binds to the poison in the stomach and carries it out of the system. Therefore, it is both more effective and safer than syrup of ipecac. Because activated charcoal is an inky, messy fluid, you may have to do some coaxing to get the patient to drink it; try to give it in a covered cup with a straw ▶ **Figure 13-27** . Remember, you should never force this (or any other) liquid into a patient's mouth.

Although every poison will result in a specific set of symptoms and signs, you should always assess the airway, breathing, and circulation of every patient who has been poisoned. Many patients have died as a result of problems with the ABCs that might have been managed easily. Be prepared to provide aggressive ventilatory support and CPR to a patient who has ingested an opiate, sedative, or barbiturate, each of which can cause depression of the central nervous system (CNS) and slow breathing. Whenever poisoning is involved, you should provide prompt evacuation to the emergency department. The patient may need IV support and other treatments that can be given only in a hospital or clinic.

Inhaled Poisons

Patients who have inhaled poison, including natural gas, certain pesticides, carbon monoxide, chlorine, or other gases, should be moved into fresh air immediately ▶ **Figure 13-28** . Depending on how long they were exposed, they may require supplemental oxygen. Remember that once patients are removed from the toxic environment, they are not toxic to you. However, make certain that only trained rescuers remove the patient from the poisonous environment.

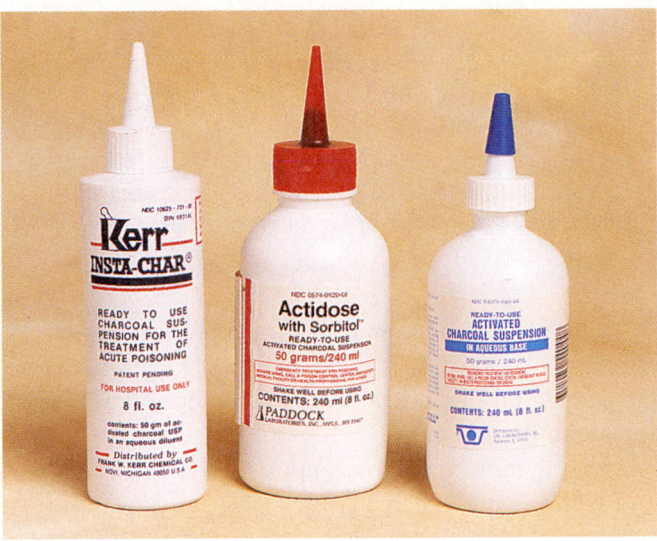

Figure 13-27 Activated charcoal comes as a premixed suspension that you should give, if local protocol allows, in a covered cup with a straw.

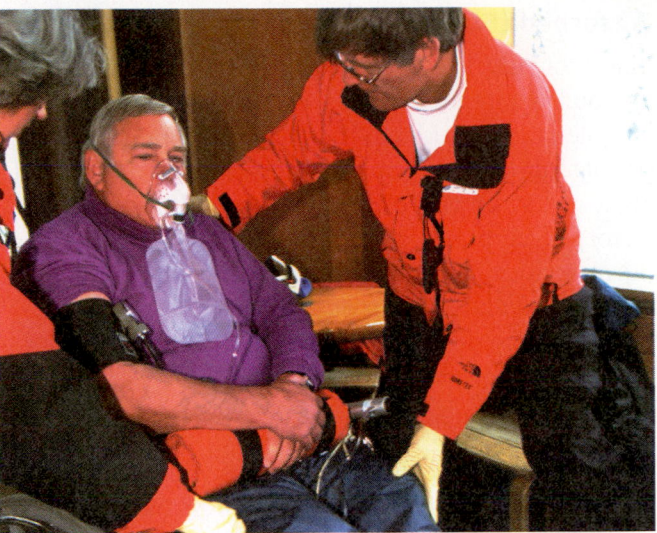

Figure 13-28 Patients who have inhaled poisons need supplemental oxygen and prompt evacuation to an emergency department or clinic.

Some inhaled poisons, such as carbon monoxide and powder from latex gloves, are odorless and produce severe hypoxia without damaging or even irritating the lungs. Others, such as chlorine, are very irritating and cause airway obstruction and pulmonary edema. The patient may report the following signs and symptoms: burning eyes, sore throat, cough, chest pain, hoarseness, wheezing, respiratory distress, dizziness, confusion, headache, or stridor in severe cases. The patient may also have seizures or an altered mental status. Some inhaled agents cause progressive lung damage, even after the patient is removed from direct exposure; the damage may not be evident for a few hours. Meanwhile, it may take 2 or 3 days or more of intensive care to reestablish normal lung function. For this reason, all patients who have inhaled poison require immediate transport to an emergency department. Be prepared to use supplemental oxygen via nonrebreathing mask and/or ventilatory support with a bag-valve-mask device, if necessary. Make sure a suctioning unit is available in case the patient vomits. As with other poisonings, it is helpful to have containers, bottles, and labels accompany the patient to the hospital.

Injected Poisons

Poisoning by injection is almost always the result of a deliberate drug overdose, such as heroin or cocaine ▶ **Figure 13-29** . Contrary to the thinking of television detectives, the only other parties who are likely to have injected a patient with poison are insects and animals.

Signs and symptoms of poisoning by injection can

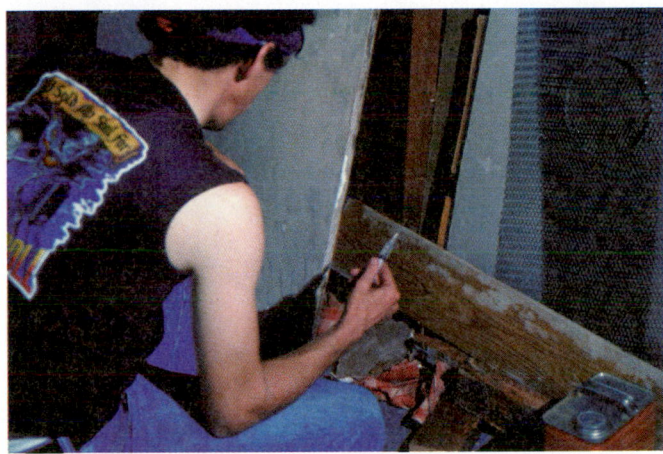

Figure 13-29 Injected poisons are impossible to dilute or remove from the body; therefore, prompt transport to the emergency department is critical.

have a multitude of presentations, including weakness, dizziness, fever, chills, easy excitability, or unresponsiveness.

In general, injected poisons are impossible to dilute or remove, as they are usually absorbed quickly into the body or cause intense local tissue destruction. If you suspect that rapid absorption has occurred, monitor the patient's airway, provide high-flow oxygen, and be alert for nausea and vomiting. Remove rings, watches, and bracelets from areas around the injection site if swelling occurs. Prompt transport to the emergency department is essential. Bring all containers, bottles, syringes, and labels with the patient to the hospital.

Absorbed (Surface Contact) Poisons

Many corrosive substances will damage the skin, mucous membranes, or eyes, causing chemical burns, tell-tale rashes, or lesions. Acids, alkalis, and some petroleum (hydrocarbon) products are very destructive. Signs and symptoms of absorbed poisoning include a history of exposure, liquid or powder on a patient's skin, burns, itching, irritation, redness of the skin in light-skinned individuals, or typical odors of the substance.

Emergency treatment of a typical contact poisoning includes the following two steps:

1. Avoid contaminating yourself or others.

2. Remove the irritating or corrosive substance from the patient as rapidly as possible.

Remove all clothing that has been contaminated with poisons or irritating substances, thoroughly brush off any dry chemicals, flush the skin with running water, then wash the skin with soap and water. When a large amount of material has been spilled on a patient, flooding the affected part for at least 20 minutes may be the fastest and most effective treatment. If the patient has a chemical agent in the eyes, you should irrigate them quickly and thoroughly, at least 5 to 10 minutes for acid substances and 15 to 20 minutes for alkali substances. *As you irrigate the eyes, make sure that the fluid runs from the bridge of the nose outward* (▼ **Figure 13-30**).

Many chemical burns occur in industrial settings, where showers and specific protocols for handling surface burns are available. If you are called to such a scene, trained people usually will be there to assist you.

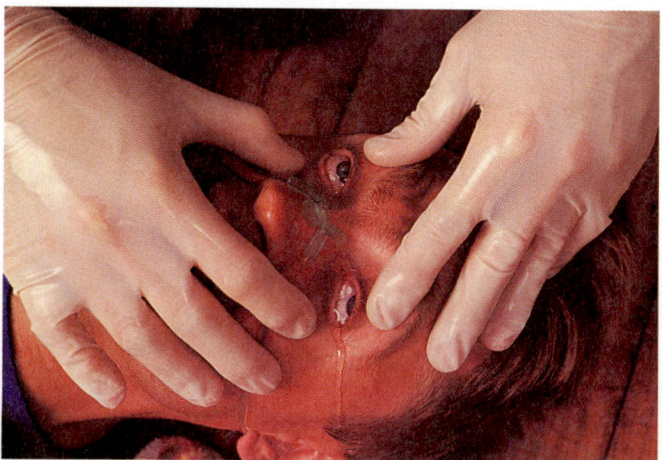

Figure 13-30 If chemical agents are in the patient's eyes, irrigate the eyes quickly and thoroughly, ensuring that the irrigation fluid runs from the bridge of the nose outward. (Use of a nasal cannula is pictured.)

Do not spend time trying to neutralize substances on the skin with additional chemicals. This may actually be more harmful. Instead, wash the substance off immediately with lots of water.

The only time you should not irrigate the contact area with water is when a poison reacts violently with water, such as contamination with phosphorus or elemental sodium. These substances ignite when they come into contact with water. Instead, brush the chemical off the patient, remove contaminated clothing, and apply a dry dressing to the burn area. Be sure to wear gloves and the proper protective clothing.

Provide prompt transport to the emergency department for definitive care. En route, continue irrigation and provide oxygen if possible.

Emergency Medical Care

External decontamination is important. Remove tablets or fragments from the patient's mouth, wash or brush poison from the patient's skin, and monitor the patient's breathing. Treatment focuses on support: assessing and maintaining the patient's ABCs.

Specific Poisons

Over time, a person who routinely misuses a substance needs increasing amounts of it to achieve the same result. This is called developing a **tolerance** to the substance. Increasing tolerance can lead to addiction. A person with an **addiction** has an overwhelming desire or need to continue using the agent, at whatever cost, with a tendency to increase the dosage. This does not happen only with the classic drugs of abuse, such as cocaine. Almost any substance can be abused, including laxatives, nasal decongestants, diet pills, vitamins, and food.

The importance of BSI precautions in caring for victims of drug abuse cannot be stressed enough. Known drug abusers have a fairly high incidence of serious and undiagnosed infections, including HIV and hepatitis. These patients may bite, spit, hit, or otherwise injure you, causing you to come into contact with their blood and other body fluids. Always be sure to wear appropriate protective equipment. A calm, professional approach can defuse frightening situations, but keep your safety and that of your team uppermost in mind. Expect the unexpected and remember: The drug user, not the drug, can pose the greatest threat.

Alcohol

The most commonly abused drug in the United States is alcohol (▼ Figure 13-31). It affects people from all walks of life and kills more than 200,000 of them each year. More than 50% of all traffic fatalities or injuries, 67% of murders, and 33% of suicides are related to alcohol, which impairs the capacity to think and function rationally. Alcoholism is one of the greatest national health problems, along with heart disease, cancer, and stroke.

Alcohol is a powerful central nervous system (CNS) depressant. It is both a **sedative**, a substance that decreases activity and excitement, and a **hypnotic**, meaning that it induces sleep. In general, alcohol dulls the sense of awareness, slows reflexes, and reduces reaction time. It may also cause aggressive and inappropriate behavior and lack of coordination. However, a person who appears intoxicated may have other medical problems as well. Look for signs of head trauma, toxic reactions, or uncontrolled diabetes. Severe acute alcohol ingestion may cause hypoglycemia, which may contribute to the symptoms. At the very least, you should assume that all intoxicated patients are experiencing a drug overdose and may require thorough examination by a physician. In most states, such patients cannot legally refuse treatment.

If a patient exhibits signs of serious CNS depression, you must provide respiratory support. This may be difficult, however, because depression of the respiratory system can also cause emesis, or vomiting. The vomiting may be very forceful or even bloody (**hematemesis**), since large amounts of alcohol irritate the stomach. Internal bleeding should also be considered if the patient appears to be in shock (hypoperfusion), as blood might not clot effectively in a patient who has a prolonged history of alcohol abuse.

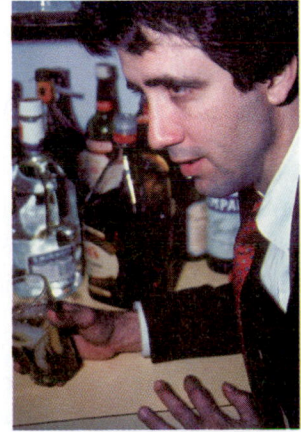

Figure 13-31 Alcohol intoxication causes altered mental status, slowed reflexes, and impaired reaction time.

A patient in alcohol withdrawal may experience frightening hallucinations or **delirium tremens (DTs)**, a syndrome characterized by restlessness, fever, sweating, disorientation, agitation, and even convulsions. These conditions may develop if patients no longer have their daily source of alcohol. Alcoholic hallucinations come and go. A patient with an otherwise fairly clear mental state may see fantastic shapes or figures or hear odd voices. Such auditory and visual hallucinations often precede DTs, which are a much more severe complication.

DTs may develop 1 to 7 days after a person stops drinking or when consumption levels are decreased suddenly. Again, patients may experience one or more of the following signs and symptoms:

- Agitation and restlessness
- Fever
- Sweating
- Confusion and/or disorientation
- Delusions and/or hallucinations
- Seizures

Provide prompt transport for these patients after you have completed your assessment and given necessary care. A person who is experiencing hallucinations or DTs is extremely ill. Should seizures develop, treat them as you would any other seizure. The patient should not be restrained, although you must protect him or her from self-injury. Give the patient oxygen and watch carefully for vomiting. Hypovolemia may develop from sweating, fluid loss, insufficient fluid intake, or vomiting associated with DTs. If you see signs of hypovolemic shock, elevate the patient's feet slightly, clear the airway, and turn the head to one side to minimize the chance of aspiration during transport. These patients may not respond appropriately to suggestions or conversation; they are often confused and frightened. Therefore, your approach should be calm and relaxed. Reassure the patient and provide emotional support.

Opioids

The pain relievers called opioid analgesics are named for the opium in poppy seeds, the origin of heroin, codeine, and morphine. On the list of frequently abused drugs, they have been joined by a number of synthetic opioids, with origins in the laboratory. These include meperidine (Demerol), hydromorphone (Dilaudid), propoxyphene (Darvon), oxycodone (Percocet, Tylox), hydrocodone (Vicodin), and methadone. New narcotic tablets (OxyContin) also have a high abuse potential ▶ Table 13-5 . Most of these drugs have legitimate medical uses. With the exception of heroin, which is illegal in the United States, many addicts may have started using any of the opioids with an appropriate medical prescription.

These agents are CNS depressants and can cause severe respiratory depression. When administered intravenously, however, they produce a characteristic "high" or "kick." Tolerance develops rapidly, so some users may require massive doses to experience the same high. In general, emergency medical problems related to opioids are caused by respiratory depression, including a decreased volume of inspired air and decreased respirations. Patients typically appear sedated and cyanotic and have pinpoint pupils.

Treatment includes supporting the airway and breathing. You may try to arouse patients by talking loudly to them or shaking them gently. Always give supplemental oxygen and be prepared for vomiting. Many home remedies are believed to reverse the respiratory depression associated with heroin overdose, including applying ice to the groin or forcing milk into the mouth. *None of these work, and they frequently complicate the clinical picture.* Nevertheless, you should be aware that a patient's friends may have attempted inappropriate methods of resuscitation. The only effective antidote to reverse the symptoms and signs of opioid overdose are certain narcotic antagonists such as naloxone (Narcan). Patients will respond within 2 minutes to naloxone

TABLE 13-5 Common Opioid Drugs

Butorphanol (Stadol)

Codeine

Fentanyl derivatives ("China White")

Heroin

Hydrocodone (Hycodan)

Hydromorphone (Dilaudid)

Meperidine (Demerol)

Methadone (Dolophine)

Morphine

Oxycodone (Percodan, Tylox, OxyContin)

Pentazocine (Talwin)

Propoxyphene (Darvon)

when it is given intravenously. Naloxone is usually administered by paramedics or by physicians at the emergency department.

Sedative-Hypnotic Drugs

Barbiturates and benzodiazepines have been a part of legitimate medications for a long time. They are easy to obtain and relatively cheap. People sometimes solicit prescriptions from several physicians for the same hypnotics or a variety of sedative-hypnotics. These drugs are CNS depressants and alter level of consciousness, with effects similar to those of alcohol so that the patient may appear drowsy, peaceful, or intoxicated ▶ Table 13-6 . By themselves, these drugs do not relieve pain, nor do they produce a specific high, although users often take alcohol or an opioid at the same time to boost their effects.

In general, these agents are taken by mouth. Occasionally, however, contents of capsules are suspended or dissolved in water and injected to produce a rather sudden state of ease and contentment. Unfortunately, use of IV sedative-hypnotic drugs quickly induces tolerance, so an individual requires increasingly larger doses. As a result, you are less likely to be called upon to treat an acute overdose in someone who chronically abuses these drugs. However, you may be called to a scene of an attempted suicide in which the patient has taken large quantities of these drugs. In these situations,

TABLE 13-6 Examples of Sedative-Hypnotic Drugs

Barbiturates	Benzodiazepines	Others
Amobarbital	Alprazolam (Xanax)	Carisoprodol (Soma)
Butabarbital	Chlordiazepoxide (Librium)	Chloral hydrate ("Mickey Finn")
Pentobarbital	Diazepam (Valium)	Cyclobenzaprine (Flexeril)
Phenobarbital	Flunitrazepam (Rohypnol)	Ethchlorvynol (Placidyl)
Secobarbital	Lorazepam (Ativan)	Ethyl alcohol (drinking alcohol)
	Oxazepam (Serax)	Glutethimide (Doriden)
	Temazepam (Restoril)	Hydrocarbon inhalants
		Isopropyl alcohol (rubbing alcohol)
		Meprobamate (Equagesic)

patients will have marked respiratory depression and may even be in a coma.

Sedative-hypnotic drugs may also be given to unsuspecting people as a "knock-out" drink, or "Mickey Finn." More recently, drugs such as flunitrazepam (Rohypnol) have been abused as a "date rape drug," causing the unwary individual to become sedated and even unconscious. The individual later begins to awaken, confused and unable to remember what happened.

In general, your treatment of patients who have overdosed with sedative-hypnotics and have respiratory depression is to provide airway clearance, ventilatory assistance, and arrange for prompt transport. Give supplemental oxygen and be ready to assist ventilations. You may attempt to stimulate the person by speaking loudly or gently shaking him or her; remember to watch for vomiting.

As multidrug use becomes more common, you may find it increasingly difficult to determine what agents the patients have taken. Your best approach is to treat any obvious injuries or illnesses, keeping in mind that drug use may complicate the picture and make full life support necessary. Focus on the ABCs, especially the possibility of airway problems (relaxation of the tongue, causing obstruction), vomiting, respiratory depression, and, in severe cases, cardiac arrest.

Abused Inhalants

Many abused inhalants produce several of the same CNS effects as other sedative-hypnotics, but these agents are inhaled instead of ingested or injected.

Some of the more common agents include acetone, toluene, xylene, and hexane, which are found in glues, cleaning compounds, paint thinners, and lacquers. Similarly, gasoline and various halogenated hydrocarbons, such as Freon, used as propellants in aerosol sprays, and nitrous oxide in some plastic containers, are also abused as inhalants. None of these inhalants is a medication. Since these are products that can be bought in hardware stores, they are commonly abused by teenagers seeking an alcohol-like high.

Always use special care in dealing with a patient who may have used inhalants. Their effects range from mild drowsiness to coma, but unlike most other sedative-hypnotics, these agents may often cause seizures. Also, halogenated hydrocarbon solvents can make the heart supersensitive to the patient's own adrenaline, putting the patient at high risk for sudden cardiac death from ventricular fibrillation; even the action of walking may release enough adrenaline to cause a fatal ventricular arrhythmia. You must try to keep such patients from struggling with you or exerting themselves. Give supplemental oxygen and use a stretcher to move the patient. Prompt transport to the hospital is essential.

Sympathomimetics

Sympathomimetics are CNS stimulants that frequently cause hypertension, tachycardia, and dilated pupils. A **stimulant** is an agent that produces an excited state. Amphetamine and methamphetamine ("ice") are commonly taken by mouth. They are also injected by abusers in many cases. They typically are taken to make the user "feel good," improve task performance, suppress appetite, or prevent sleepiness. They may just as easily produce irritability, anxiety, lack of concentration, or seizures. Other common examples include phentermine and Benzedrine. Caffeine, theophylline, and phenylpropanolamine (a nasal decongestant) are all mild sympathomimetics. So-called "designer drugs," such as Ecstasy and Eve, are also frequently abused in certain areas of the country.

Sympathomimetic drugs are frequently called "uppers" (▼ Table 13-7). Someone using one of these agents may display disorganized behavior, restlessness, and sometimes anxiety or great fear. Paranoia and delusions are common with sympathomimetic abuse.

Cocaine, also called coke, crack, crystal, snow, freebase, rock, gold dust, blow, and lady, may be taken in a number of different ways. Classically, it is inhaled into the nose and absorbed through the nasal mucosa, damaging tissue, causing nosebleeds, and ultimately destroying the nasal septum. It can also be injected intravenously or subcutaneously (skin-popping). Cocaine can be absorbed through all mucous membranes and even across the skin. In any form, the immediate effects of a given dose last less than an hour.

Another method of abusing cocaine is by smoking it. Crack is pure cocaine. It melts at 93°F (34°C) and vaporizes at a slightly higher temperature. Therefore, crack is easily smoked. In this form, it reaches the capillary network of the lungs and can be absorbed into the body in seconds. The immediate outflow of blood from the heart speeds the drug to the brain, so its effect is felt at once. Smoked crack produces the most rapid means of absorption and therefore the most potent effect.

Cocaine is one of the most addicting substances known, more so than heroin or nicotine. Its immediate effects include excitement and euphoria. Acute cocaine overdose is a genuine emergency, as patients are at high

risk for seizures and cardiac arrhythmias. Chronic cocaine abuse may cause hallucinations; patients with "cocaine bugs" think that bugs are crawling out of their skin.

In caring for patients who have been poisoned with any of the sympathomimetics, be aware that their severe agitation can lead to tachycardia and hypertension. Patients may also be paranoid, putting you and other health care providers in danger.

All of these patients need to get to the emergency department promptly because of the risk of seizures, cardiac arrhythmias, and stroke. You may see blood pressures as high as 250/150 mm Hg. Give supplemental oxygen and be ready to provide suctioning. If the patient is already having a seizure, you must protect him or her against self-injury.

Marijuana

The flowering hemp plant *Cannabis sativa*, called marijuana, is abused throughout the world. It has been estimated that as many as 20 million people use marijuana daily in the United States. Inhaling marijuana smoke from a cigarette or pipe produces euphoria, relaxation, and drowsiness. It also impairs short-term memory and the capacity to do complex thinking and work, and decreases coordination and balance. In some people, the euphoria progresses to depression and confusion. An altered perception of time is common, and anxiety and panic can occur. With very high doses, patients experience hallucinations.

A person who has been using marijuana rarely needs transport to the hospital. Exceptions may include someone who is hallucinating, very anxious, or paranoid. However, you should be aware that marijuana is often used as a vehicle to get other drugs into the body. For example, it may be covered with crack or PCP.

Hallucinogens

Hallucinogens alter an individual's sensory perceptions (▶ Table 13-8). The classic hallucinogen is lysergic acid diethylamide (LSD). Abuse of another hallucinogen, phencyclidine (PCP, "angel dust") is relatively uncommon among young adults. PCP is a dissociative anesthetic that is easily synthesized and highly potent. Its effectiveness by oral, nasal, pulmonary, and IV routes makes it easy to add to other street drugs. PCP is dangerous, as it causes severe behavioral changes in which individuals often inflict injury to themselves.

All these agents cause visual hallucinations, intensify both vision and hearing, and generally separate the user from reality. The user, of course, expects that the altered

TABLE 13-7 Street Names for Amphetamines		
Adam	Fen-phen	Psychodrine
Bennies	Golden eagle	Speed
Crank	Ice	STP
DOM	MDA	Uppers
Ecstasy	Meth	
Eve		

sensory state will be pleasurable. Often, however, it can be terrifying. At some point, you may encounter patients who are having a "bad trip." They will usually be hypertensive, tachycardic, anxious, and probably paranoid.

Many of the hallucinogens have sympathomimetic properties. Indeed, your care for a patient who is having a bad reaction to a hallucinogenic agent is the same as that for a patient who has taken a sympathomimetic. Use a calm, professional manner, and provide emotional support. Do not use restraints unless you or the patient is in danger of injury and then always within the guidelines specified by local authorities. These patients may suddenly experience hallucinations or odd perceptions, so you must watch them carefully throughout transport. Never leave a patient who has taken a hallucinogen unattended and unmonitored.

Anticholinergic Agents

The classic picture of a person who has taken too much of an anticholinergic medication is "hot as a hare, blind as a bat, dry as a bone, red as a beet, and mad as a hatter." These are medications that have properties that, among other effects, block the parasympathetic nerves. Common drugs with a significant anticholinergic effect include atropine, diphenhydramine (Benadryl), jimson weed, and certain tricyclic antidepressants. With the exception of jimson weed, these medications usually are not abused drugs but may be taken as an intentional overdose. You will find that it is often difficult to distinguish between an anticholinergic overdose and a sympathomimetic overdose. In both groups of patients,

TABLE 13-8 Commonly Abused Hallucinogens

Bufotenine (toad skin)

Dimethyltryptamine (DMT)

Jimson weed

Lysergic acid diethylamide (LSD)

Marijuana

Mescaline

Morning glory

Nutmeg

Phencyclidine (PCP)

Psilocybin (mushroom)

patients may be agitated and tachycardic and have dilated pupils.

Cholinergic Agents

The "nerve gases" designed for chemical warfare are cholinergic agents. These agents overstimulate normal body functions that are controlled by parasympathetic nerves, resulting in increased salivation, mucous secretion, urination, crying, and heart rate. Obviously, you are unlikely to run across these. However, you may well be called to care for patients who have been exposed to one of the organophosphate insecticides or certain wild mushrooms, which are also cholinergic agents. The signs and symptoms of cholinergic drug poisoning are easy to remember because of the mnemonic DUMBELS:

- **D**efecation
- **U**rination
- **M**iosis (constriction of the pupils)
- **B**ronchorrhea (discharge of mucus from the lungs)
- **E**mesis
- **L**acrimation (tearing)
- **S**alivation

Alternatively, you can use the mnemonic SLUDGE:
- **S**alivation
- **L**acrimation
- **U**rination
- **D**efecation
- **G**I irritation
- **E**ye constriction/Emesis

In poisonings, patients will have excessive amounts of these normal functions and body secretions. In addition, patients may have either bradycardia or tachycardia.

The most important consideration in caring for a patient who has been exposed to an organophosphate insecticide or some other cholinergic agent is to avoid exposure yourself. Because such agents may cling to a patient's clothing and skin, decontamination may take priority over immediate transport to the emergency department. At the hospital, the anticholinergic drug atropine can be used to dry up the patient's secretions. In the meantime, your priority after decontamination is to decrease the secretions in the mouth and trachea that threaten to suffocate the patient, and provide airway support. Let your local EMS system know you are in a HazMat situation.

Weapons of Mass Destruction

Although the use of weapons of mass destruction (WMD) still remains more prevalent in wartime and more closely associated with the military, it has become a threat during peacetime and could involve OEC technicians practicing in civilian life. We have seen WMD used to produce tragedies such as the Oklahoma bombing of a federal building. We now protect ourselves against terrorist attacks at events such as the Olympic games. Protection involves military presence and in the event of an attack, we are equipped with military medical teams and civilian teams, which include the disaster medical assistance teams (DMATs). These DMATs are made up of experts that include physicians, nurses, respiratory therapists, EMT-Bs, paramedics, and clergy. During these events, DMATs are federalized and operate under the Department of Health and Human Services.

Biological, chemical, and nuclear warfare are used for mass destruction. Many different agents are used. Treatment after an attack is typically divided into three zones. The first zone is the red or hot zone, which is usually managed by the military or other highly trained individuals. In the hot zone, patients are triaged and go through early decontamination (called decon). In the next zone, the yellow or warm zone, extensive decontamination takes place by trained individuals. The last zone, the green zone or cold zone, is where EMS will transport the patient. Although OEC technicians and EMTs do not manage patients who are in a hot zone, they will have to manage patients after the decontamination team has completed and cleared the patients for transport. EMS providers do not enter the red or yellow area unless they are trained and are wearing the proper clothing. It is important to understand that you should never enter a situation that is potentially dangerous without proper training.

Miscellaneous Drugs

While not as common as it was 30 years ago, aspirin poisoning remains a potentially lethal condition. Ingesting too many aspirin tablets, either acutely or chronically, may result in nausea, vomiting, hyperventilation, and ringing in the ears. Patients with this problem are frequently anxious, confused, tachypneic, and in danger of having seizures. They should be transported quickly to the hospital.

Overdosing with *acetaminophen* is also very common, probably because acetaminophen is available in so many different preparations, such as Tylenol. The good news is that acetaminophen is generally not very toxic. A healthy patient could ingest 140 mg of acetaminophen for every kilogram of body weight without serious adverse effects. The bad news is that the symptoms of an overdose generally do not appear until it is too late. For example, massive liver failure may not be apparent for a full week. And patients may not provide the information necessary for a correct diagnosis. For this reason, gathering information at the scene is very important. By finding an empty acetaminophen bottle, you may save a patient's life. If given early enough

(before liver failure occurs), a specific antidote may prevent liver damage.

Be extremely careful in dealing with a child who has unintentionally ingested a poisonous substance. Although such incidents usually do not lead to death, family members may be distraught, and your professional attitude will help to ease the tension. Remember, however, that a single swallow of some substances can kill a child ▶ Table 13-9 .

Some alcohols, including methyl alcohol and ethylene glycol, are even more toxic than ethyl alcohol (drinking alcohol). Although they may be used as a substitute by the chronic alcoholic who is unable to obtain ethyl alcohol, they are more often taken by someone attempting suicide. In either case, immediate transport to the emergency department is essential. Methyl alcohol is found in dry gas products and Sterno; ethylene glycol is found in some antifreeze products. Both cause a "drunken" feeling. Left untreated, both will also cause severe tachypnea, blindness (methyl alcohol), renal failure (ethylene glycol), and eventually death. Even ethyl alcohol (typical drinking alcohol) can stop a patient's

TABLE 13-9 Fatal Ingested Poisons
Benzocaine
Calcium channel blockers (verapamil, nifedipine, diltiazem)
Camphor
Chloroquine
Hydrocarbon solvents
Lomotil
Methanol/ethylene glycol
Methylsalicylate (oil of wintergreen)
Phenothiazines (Thorazine)
Quinine
Theophylline
Tricyclic antidepressants (amitriptyline [Elavil], imipramine [Tofranil], nortriptyline [Pamelor])
Visine

breathing if taken in too high a dose or too fast, particularly in children.

Food Poisoning

The term "ptomaine poisoning" was coined in 1870 to indicate poisoning by a class of chemicals found in rotting food. It is still used today in many news accounts of food poisoning. This is unfortunate, because the term is misleading. Food poisoning is almost always caused by eating food that is contaminated by bacteria. The food may appear perfectly good, with little or no decay or odor to suggest danger.

There are two main types of food poisoning. In one, the organism itself causes disease; in the other, the organism produces toxins that cause disease. A toxin is a poison or harmful substance produced by bacteria, animals, or plants.

One organism that produces direct effects of food poisoning is the *Salmonella* bacterium. The condition called salmonellosis is characterized by severe gastrointestinal symptoms within 72 hours of ingestion, including nausea, vomiting, abdominal pain, and diarrhea. In addition, patients suffering from salmonellosis may be systemically ill with fever and generalized weakness. Some people are carriers of certain bacteria; although they may not become ill themselves, they may transmit diseases, particularly if they work in the food services industry. Usually, proper cooking kills bacteria, and proper cleanliness in the kitchen prevents the contamination of uncooked foods.

The more common cause of food poisoning is the ingestion of powerful toxins produced by bacteria, often in leftovers. The bacterium *Staphylococcus*, a common culprit, is quick to grow and produce toxins in foods that have been prepared in advance and kept too long, even in the refrigerator. Foods prepared with mayonnaise, when left unrefrigerated, are a common vehicle for the development of staphylococcal toxins. Usually, staphylococcal food poisoning results in sudden gastrointestinal symptoms, including nausea, vomiting, and diarrhea. Although time frames may vary from individual to individual, usually these symptoms may start within 2 to 3 hours after ingestion or as long as 8 to 12 hours after ingestion.

The most severe form of toxin ingestion is botulism. This often-fatal disease usually results from eating improperly canned food, in which the spores of *Clostridium* bacteria have grown and produced a toxin. The symptoms of botulism are neurologic: blurring of vision, weakness, and difficulty in speaking and breathing. Symptoms may develop as long as 4 days after ingestion or as early as the first 24 hours.

In general, you should not try to determine the specific cause of acute gastrointestinal problems. After all, severe vomiting may be a sign of a self-limiting food poisoning, a bowel obstruction requiring surgery, or another poison, such as copper, arsenic, zinc, cadmium, scombrotoxin (fish poison), or Clitocybe or Inocybe mushrooms. Instead, you should gather as much history as possible from the patient, and transport him or her promptly to the hospital. When two or more individuals in one group have the same illness, you should bring along some of the suspected food. In advanced cases of botulism, you may have to assist respirations and give basic life support.

Plant Poisoning

Several thousand cases of poisoning from plants occur each year, some severe. Many household plants are poisonous if ingested, as they may be by children who like

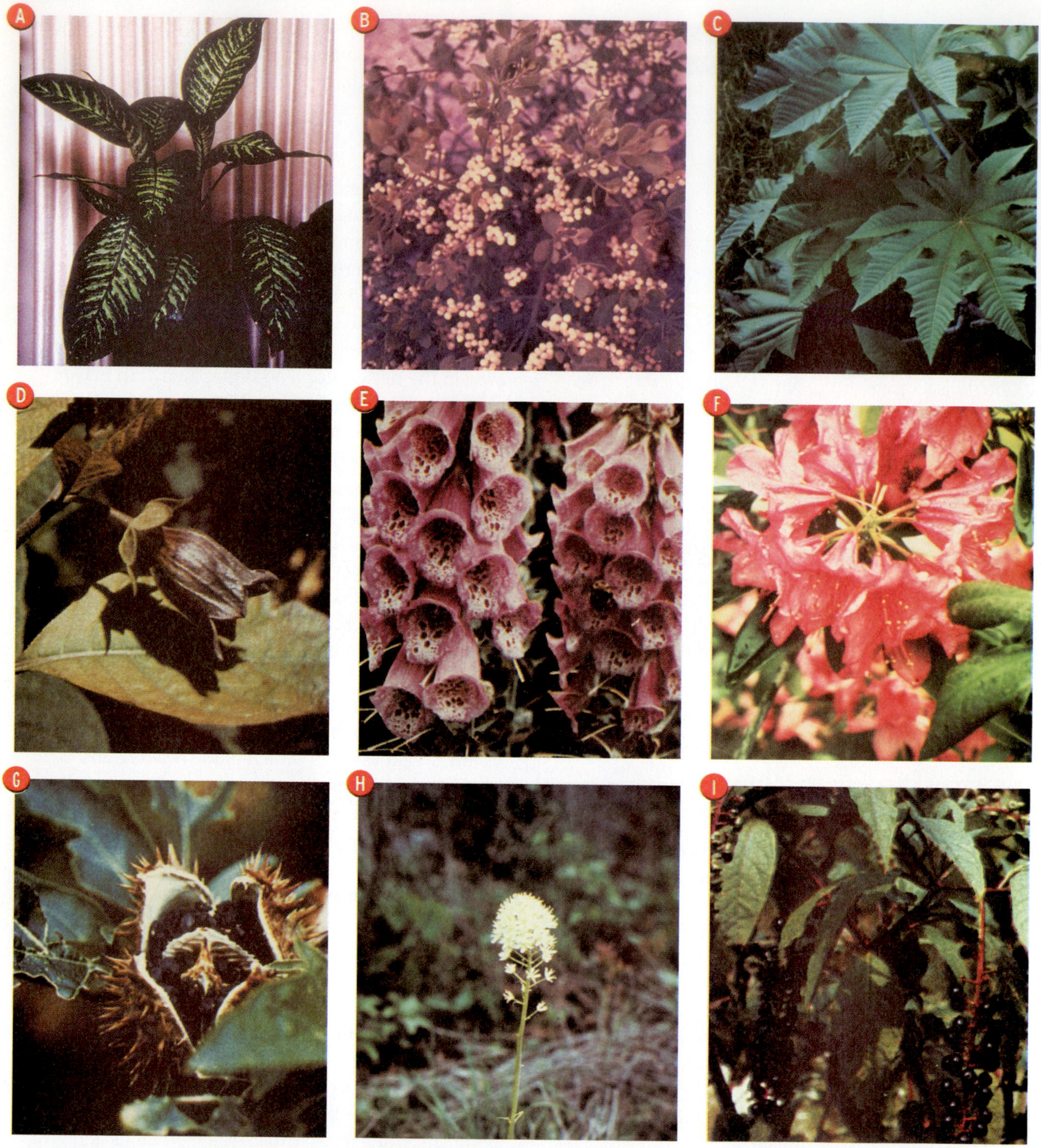

Figure 13-32 The toxins in these common poisonous plants are often ingested or absorbed through the skin. **A.** Dieffenbachia. **B.** Mistletoe. **C.** Castor bean. **D.** Nightshade. **E.** Foxglove. **F.** Rhododendron. **G.** Jimson weed. **H.** Death camus. **I.** Pokeweed. **J.** Rosary pea. **K.** Poison ivy. **L.** Poison oak. **M.** Poison sumac.

to nibble leaves (▼ **Table 13-10**). Some poisonous plants cause local irritation of the skin; others can affect the circulatory system, the gastrointestinal tract, or the central nervous system. It is impossible for you to memorize every plant and poison, let alone their effects (◄ **Figure 13-32**). You can and should do the following:

1. Assess the patient's airway and vital signs.
2. Notify the regional poison control center for assistance in identifying the plant.
3. Give the plant to the EMS service to take to the emergency department.
4. Arrange for prompt transport.

TABLE 13-10 Common Toxic Plants

Scientific Name	Common Name	Scientific Name	Common Name
Abrus precatorius	Jequirity bean/rosary pea	*Nerium oleander*	Oleander/rose laurel
Cicuta species	Water hemlock/wild carrot	*Nicotiana glauca*	Tree tobacco
Colchicum autumnale	Autumn crocus	*Phoradendron leucarpum*	Mistletoe
Conium maculatum	Poison hemlock	*Phytolacca americana*	Pokeweed
Convallaria majalis	Lily of the valley	*Rhododendron*	Rhododendron/azalea
Datura species	Jimson weed/stinkweed	*Ricinus communis*	Castor bean
Dieffenbachia	Dumbcane	*Solanum nigrum*	Nightshade
Digitalis purpurea	Foxglove	*Zigadenus* species	Death camus
Euphorbia pulcherrima	Poinsettia		

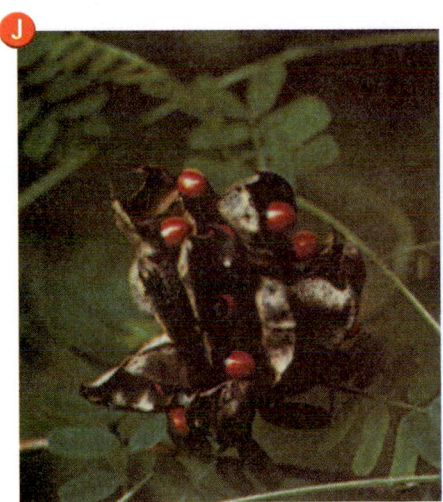

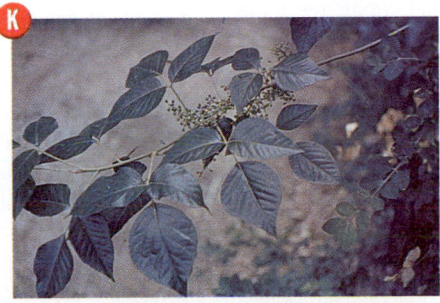

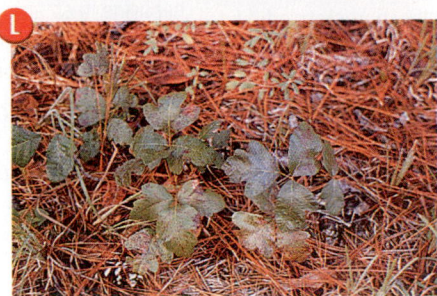

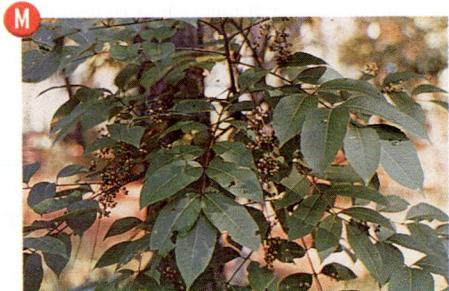

Chapter *Sweep*

Ready for Review

"Acute abdomen" is a collective term for a number of painful abdominal conditions.

Gastrointestinal-related maladies are perhaps some of the most common medical complaints. Whether the problem is caused by something as simple as what a person eats or as complex as an underlying disease, the discomfort can be great and, depending on the source of the affliction, death can result. Therefore, the care provider must pay close attention to the signs and symptoms of gastrointestinal complaints. Your first impression of a person with a gastrointestinal complaint will be that the patient appears to have an illness rather than an injury.

Your first priorities are to assess airway, breathing, and circulation and then apply oxygen. Next, obtain a pertinent medical history: When did the symptoms begin? How have they changed over time? Where exactly is the pain? What does it feel like? How long does it last and how intense is it? Has there been a loss of fluid volume as a result of vomiting or diarrhea? Take vital signs and gently palpate the abdomen. The presence of abdominal tenderness will confirm the need to transport the patient to the emergency department in an urgent manner.

There is no effective field treatment for the patient who is vomiting blood, has an abdominal injury, severe rectal bleeding, or a severe illness of any type with gastrointestinal symptoms. In the outdoor setting, any patient with persistent or severe abdominal pain should be evacuated promptly.

In the outdoor environment, consuming contaminated food containing such bacteria as *Staphylococcus* or *E. coli* and water carrying the protozoan *Giardia lamblia* can cause diarrhea and abdominal discomfort and often lead to more serious problems.

Diabetes mellitus is a metabolic disorder caused by the lack of insulin, a hormone that enables glucose to enter the cells, where it can be used for energy. Diabetes is typically characterized by excessive urination and resulting thirst, along with deterioration of body tissues. There are two types of diabetes. Type I diabetes, or insulin-dependent diabetes mellitus, usually starts in childhood and requires daily insulin to control blood glucose. Type II diabetes, or noninsulin-dependent diabetes, usually develops in middle age and often can be controlled with diet and oral medications. Both are serious systemic diseases, especially affecting the kidneys, eyes, small arteries, and peripheral nerves.

Patients with diabetes have chronic complications that place them at risk for other diseases such as heart attack, stroke, and infection. Most often, however, you will be called upon to treat the acute complications of blood glucose imbalance. These include hyperglycemia (excess blood glucose) and hypoglycemia (not enough blood glucose). Symptoms of hypoglycemia classically include confusion; rapid respirations; pale, moist skin; diaphoresis; dizziness; fainting; and even coma and seizures. This condition, called insulin shock, is rapidly reversible with the administration of glucose or sugar. Without treatment, however, permanent brain damage and death can occur. Hyperglycemia is usually associated with dehydration and ketoacidosis. It can result in diabetic coma, marked by rapid (often deep) respirations; warm, dry skin; a weak pulse; and a fruity breath odor. Hyper-glycemia must be treated in the hospital or clinic with insulin and IV fluids.

Since either too much or too little blood glucose can result in altered mental status, you must perform a thorough history and patient assessment. When you cannot determine the nature of the problem, it is best to treat the patient for hypoglycemia. Be prepared to give oral glucose to a conscious patient who is confused or has a slightly decreased level of consciousness; however, do not give oral glucose to a patient who is unconscious or otherwise unable to swallow properly or protect his or her own airway. Remember, in all cases, providing emergency medical care and prompt transport is your primary responsibility.

An allergic reaction is a response to chemicals the body releases in order to combat certain stimuli, called allergens. Allergic reactions occur most often in response to five categories of stimuli: insect bites and stings, medications, food, plants, and chemicals. The reaction may be mild and local, involving itching, redness, and tenderness; or severe and systemic, including shock and respiratory failure. Anaphylaxis is a life-threatening allergic reaction mounted by multiple organ systems, which must be treated with epinephrine. Wheezing and skin wheals can be signs of anaphylaxis. People who know that they are allergic to bee, hornet, yellow jacket, or wasp venom often carry a bee sting kit that contains epinephrine in an auto-injector. You may help to administer this medication in this form with authorization from medical control. All patients with suspected anaphylaxis require oxygen.

In assessing a person who may be having an allergic reaction, you should check for flushing, itching, and swelling skin; hives; wheezing and stridor; a persistent cough; a decrease in blood pressure; a weak pulse; dizziness; abdominal cramps; and headache.

Poisonous spiders include the black widow spider and the brown recluse spider. Poisonous snakes include pit vipers and coral snakes. A person who has been bitten by a pit viper needs prompt transport; clean the bite area and keep the patient quiet to slow the spread of venom. Notify the hospital as soon as possible if a patient has been bitten by a coral snake, as its venom can cause paralysis of the nervous system, and most hospitals do not have appropriate antivenin on hand.

Patients who have been bitten by ticks may be infected with Rocky Mountain spotted fever or Lyme disease and should see a doctor within a day or two. Remove the tick using tweezers, and save it for identification.

Dog and human bites can both lead to serious infection and must be treated by a physician. Dogs can carry rabies, a fatal viral infection present in their saliva. Painful vaccine treatment is necessary to prevent rabies in a person who has been bitten by a dog that cannot be captured or identified.

Remember that a hundred times more people die every year from allergic reactions to food, bee stings, or medications than from the bites of venomous snakes or marine animals. Many venomous snake bites may be treated with antivenin. Many marine envenomations may benefit from submersion in hot water to deactivate the heat-sensitive toxins.

Always provide prompt transport to the hospital for any patient who is having an allergic reaction or has been bitten by a poisonous insect or animal. Remember that signs and symptoms can deteriorate rapidly. Carefully monitor the patient's vital signs en route, especially for airway compromise.

Poisons act acutely or chronically to destroy or impair body cells. If you believe a patient may have taken a poisonous substance, you should notify medical control and begin emergency treatment at once. This may include administration of an antidote, usually at the hospital, if an antidote exists. It also entails collecting any evidence of the type of poison that was used and bringing it to the hospital; diluting and physically removing the poisonous agent; providing respiratory support; and transporting the patient promptly to the hospital.

A poison can be introduced into the body in one of four ways: ingestion, inhalation, injection, or surface contact (absorption). Approximately 80% of all poisoning is by ingestion, including plants, contaminated food, and most drugs. In general, activated charcoal should be used in these patients. In the case of surface contact poisons, be sure to avoid contaminating yourself. You should then remove all contaminated substances and clothing from the patient, and flood the affected part. Move patients who have inhaled poison into the fresh air; be prepared to use supplemental oxygen via nonrebreathing mask and/or ventilatory support via BVM device. Some patients may need BLS, especially those who have injected poison, which is almost always a deliberate act.

Two main types of food poisoning cause gastrointestinal symptoms. In one type, bacteria in the food directly cause disease, such as salmonellosis; in the other, bacteria such as *Staphylococcus* produce powerful toxins, often in leftover food. The most severe form of toxin ingestion is botulism, which can first produce neurologic symptoms as late as 4 days after ingestion. Plant poisoning can affect the circulatory system, the gastrointestinal system, or the central nervous system.

Vital Vocabulary

acidosis A pathologic condition resulting from the accumulation of acids in the body.

acute abdomen A condition of sudden onset of pain within the abdomen, usually indicating peritonitis; demands immediate medical or surgical treatment.

addiction A state of overwhelming obsession or physical need to continue the use of a drug or agent.

allergen A substance that causes an allergic reaction.

allergic reaction The body's exaggerated immune response to an internal or surface agent.

anaphylaxis An extreme, possibly life-threatening systemic allergic reaction that may include shock and respiratory failure.

aneurysm A swelling or enlargement of a part of an artery, resulting from weakening of the arterial wall.

anorexia Lack of appetite for food.

antidote A substance that is used to neutralize or counteract a poison.

bilirubin A yellow compound that is a byproduct of the normal breakdown of red blood cells. It is removed by the liver and excreted through the bile into the intestines.

colic Acute, intermittent cramping abdominal pain.

delirium tremens (DTs) A severe withdrawal syndrome seen in patients with alcohol withdrawal who are deprived of ethyl alcohol; characterized by restlessness, fever, sweating, disorientation, agitation, and convulsions.

diabetic coma Unconsciousness caused by dehydration, very high blood glucose, and acidosis in diabetes.

diabetic ketoacidosis (DKA) A form of acidosis in uncontrolled diabetes in which certain acids accumulate when insulin is not available.

dysphagia Difficulty in swallowing.

emesis Vomiting.

envenomation The act of injecting venom.

epinephrine A substance produced by the body (commonly called adrenaline), and a drug produced by pharmaceutical companies that increases pulse rate and blood pressure; the drug of choice for an anaphylactic reaction.

www.OECzone.com

Chapter Sweep

Vital Vocabulary

glucose One of the basic sugars; it is the primary fuel, along with oxygen, for cellular metabolism.

guarding Involuntary muscle contractions (spasm) of the abdominal wall, an effort to protect the inflamed abdomen.

hallucinogen An agent that produces false perceptions in any one of the five senses.

heartburn A type of indigestion characterized by a burning sensation in the epigastric area or beneath the sternum.

hematemesis Vomiting blood.

hernia The protrusion of an organ or tissue through an abnormal body opening.

histamine A substance released by the immune system in allergic reactions that is responsible for many of the symptoms of anaphylaxis.

hormone A chemical substance that regulates the activity of body organs and tissues; produced by a gland.

hyperglycemia Abnormally high glucose level in the blood.

hypnotic A sleep-inducing effect or agent.

hypoglycemia Abnormally low glucose level in the blood.

ileus Paralysis of the bowel, arising from any one of several causes; stops contractions that move material through the intestine.

ingestion Swallowing; taking a substance by mouth.

insulin A hormone produced by the pancreas that enables sugar in the blood to enter the cells of the body; used in synthetic form to treat and control diabetes mellitus.

insulin shock Unconsciousness or altered mental status in a patient with diabetes caused by significant hypoglycemia; usually the result of excessive exercise and activity or failure to eat after a routine dose of insulin.

Kussmaul respirations Deep, rapid breathing; usually the result of an accumulation of certain acids when insulin is not available in the body.

leukotrienes Chemical substances that contribute to anaphylaxis; released by the immune system in allergic reactions.

nausea An unpleasant sensation in the epigastrium that often leads to vomiting.

opioids Any drug or agent with actions similar to morphine.

pancreatitis Inflammation of the pancreas.

peritoneum The membrane lining the abdominal cavity (parietal peritoneum) and covering the abdominal organs (visceral peritoneum).

peritonitis Inflammation of the peritoneum.

poison A substance whose chemical action could damage structures or impair function when introduced into the body.

polydipsia Excessive thirst persisting for long periods of time despite reasonable fluid intake; often the result of excessive urination.

polyphagia Excessive eating; in diabetes, the inability to use glucose properly can cause a sense of hunger.

polyuria The passage of an unusually large volume of urine in a given period; in diabetes, this can result from wasting of glucose in the urine.

rabid Describes an animal that is infected with rabies.

referred pain Pain felt in an area of the body other than the area where the cause of pain is located.

sedative A substance that decreases activity and excitement.

stimulant An agent that produces an excited state.

strangulation Complete obstruction of blood circulation in a given organ as a result of compression or entrapment, an emergency situation causing death of tissue.

stridor A harsh, high-pitched respiratory sound, generally heard during inspiration, that is caused by partial blockage or narrowing of the upper airway.

substance abuse The knowing misuse of any substance to produce some desired effect.

tolerance The need for increasing amounts of a drug over time to obtain the same effect.

toxin A poison or harmful substance.

type I diabetes The type of diabetic disease that usually starts in childhood and requires insulin for proper treatment and control.

type II diabetes The type of diabetic disease that usually starts in later life and often can be controlled through diet and oral medications.

urticaria Small spots of generalized itching and/or burning that appear as multiple raised areas on the skin; hives.

vomit The verb form refers to ejection of stomach contents through the mouth due to the contraction of the muscles of the stomach.

vomitus Vomited material.

weapons of mass destruction Biological, chemical, and nuclear warfare mediums used for mass destruction, more prevalent in wartime and more closely associated with the military.

wheal A raised, swollen, well-defined area on the skin resulting from an insect bite or allergic reaction.

wheezing A high-pitched, whistling breath sound, usually caused by a partial airway blockage and typically heard on expiration.

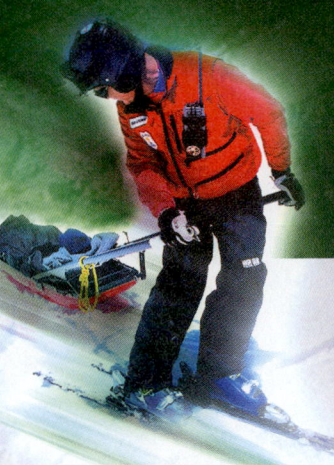

Assessment in Action

Two college students, John and Bob, have driven to your local ski area for Christmas break and are staying in an RV in the parking lot. John went in early for lunch, and Bob kept skiing, returning to the RV about an hour later. When he entered the RV, he found John lying on the bed, unconscious and unresponsive. He immediately ran to the patrol office for help. When you arrive, you find a 20-year-old man dressed in ski gear. The patient appears very pale, and is unresponsive to any stimuli. He is breathing quickly with no apparent airway problems.

As you check for a pulse, you notice that his skin is cool and clammy. According to Bob, John said he was not feeling well at breakfast, and promised to eat something later. He also tells you that the patient has no known allergies, and the only medication he takes is insulin. He also remembers to tell you that John started jogging and exercising every day a few weeks ago to try to get back into shape. His vital signs are a pulse of 128 beats/min, respirations of 28 breaths/min, and a blood pressure of 88/54 mm Hg.

1. The most important part of this patient's history that helps determine your treatment is a history of:
   A. unresponsiveness.   B. not feeling well.
   C. recent jogging.   D. diabetes.

2. Based on this patient's assessment findings and history, the best position for transport would be:
   A. supine.   B. Fowler's.
   C. lateral recumbent.   D. prone.

3. Which of the following indicates treatment with oral glucose?
   A. A history of diabetes with unconsciousness
   B. Altered mental status with a history of diabetes
   C. Altered mental status in any adult
   D. A history of diabetes in any patient with a problem

4. Proper administration of oral glucose in a patient with diabetes with an altered mental status includes confirming that the patient is conscious and able to swallow and:
   A. applying it as a topical ointment.
   B. placing it between the cheek and gum.
   C. placing it in an inhaler.
   D. injecting it in the lateral thigh.

5. In situations where oral glucose has been given, what complications should you watch for and be prepared to manage?
   A. Airway problems, sudden loss of consciousness, and seizures
   B. Sudden loss of consciousness, vomiting, and severe headache
   C. A drop in blood pressure, chest pain, and difficulty breathing
   D. A rise in blood pressure, severe headache, and chest pain

Challenging Questions

6. Altered mental status in the older patient with diabetes may mimic the signs and symptoms of what conditions?

7. Why is hypoglycemia (insulin shock) considered more of an immediate emergency than hyperglycemia (diabetic coma)?

Points to Ponder

You are enjoying a day off by going for a hike. You are about 2 hours from where you started when you come across a woman who asks if you can help her. You find out that her friend is a short distance off of the trail and is having trouble breathing. She tells you that he is "allergic to bee stings" and has been stung. When you find the friend, he is unresponsive, barely breathing and showing many signs of anaphylactic shock. You quickly check his pockets and find his "Epi kit." Would you administer the EpiPen? If you are off-duty, are you functioning as a rescuer? Could the woman give you permission to give the injection? Is administration of epinephrine covered under Good Samaritan laws?

Issues Provisions of Care, Consent, Local/State Regulations, Good Samaritan Laws, Invasive Procedures.

Online Outlook

There is a wealth of information about gastrointestinal complaints, diabetes, substances that trigger the body's immune system and cause an allergic reaction, and poisoning on the World Wide Web. Explore some of these Internet resources by completing Exercise 13 at www.OECzone.com.

www.OECzone.com

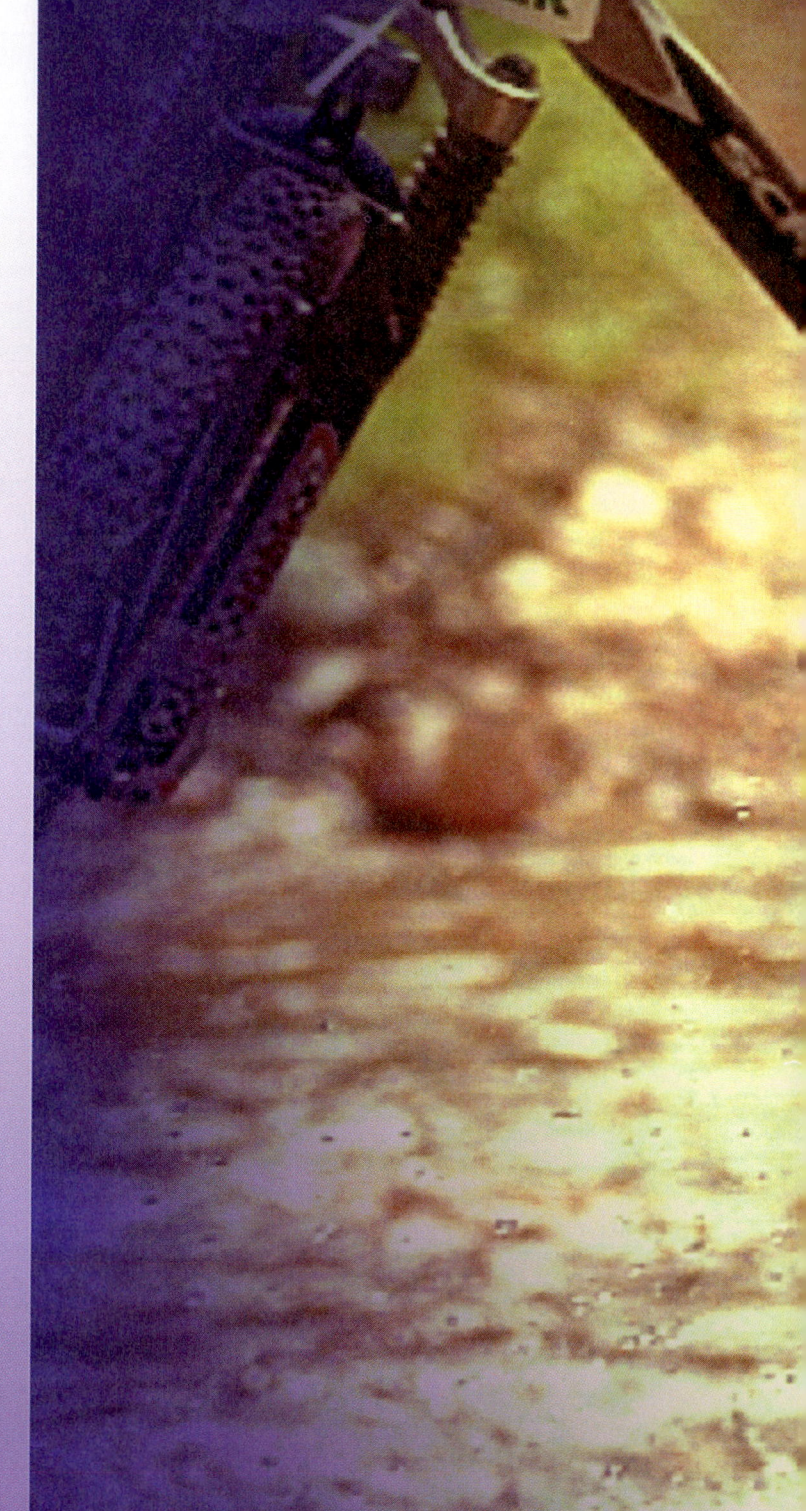

Snowsports and Mountain Biking Emergencies

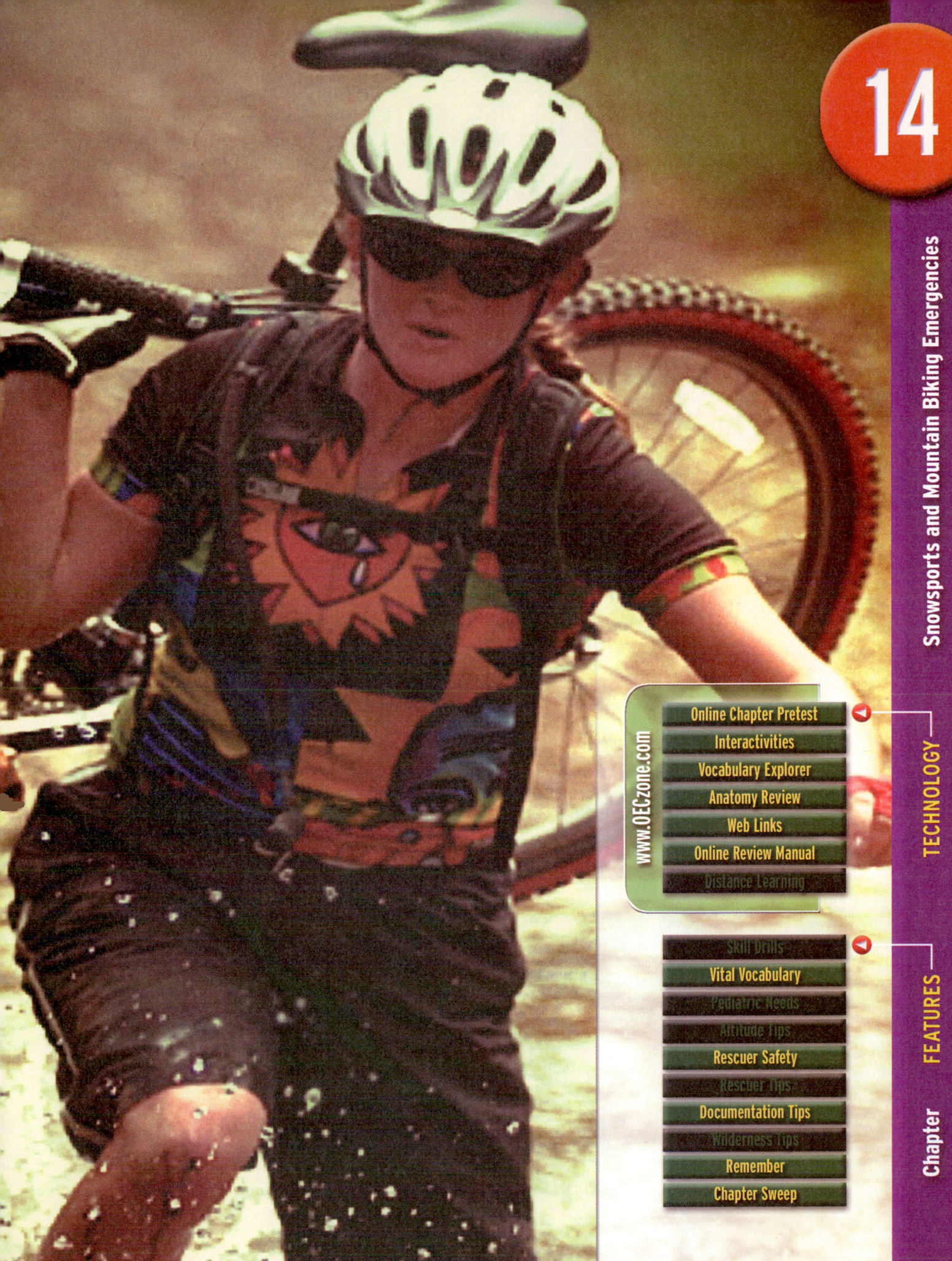

Chapter

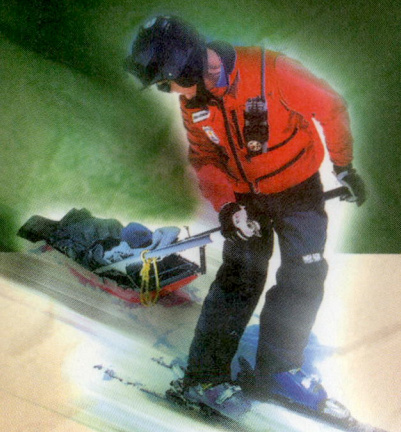

You are the rescuer

You are doing your morning trail check. You need to make sure that the grooming vehicles didn't hit anything or leave anything that might present a hazard. You also need to mark all the bare spots, particularly at the breakovers, or check for erosion and rocks that turn up.

A very important task while on patrol duty at any time of year is the morning trail check. The resort depends on its patrollers to scour the trails for anything that requires fixing or changing, post warning or information signs, and ensure that compliance-type signs are in proper placement. This chapter focuses on providing the rescuer with the knowledge and insights of the types of snowsports and mountain bike emergencies that can occur and raises the level of appreciation for safety and the prevention of accidents.

1. What are the common types of injuries resulting from various snowsports and what safety efforts can occur as part of a rescuer's responsibilities to help reduce these incidents?

2. What needs to be done to warn the guests of spring or summer conditions to make this a safe environment for everyone?

Snowsports and Mountain Biking Emergencies

Snowsports, mountain biking, climbing, rafting, and other outdoor sports provide tremendous opportunities for fun and exhilaration in a beautiful environment, but that does not mean that these activities are free of risk. Mishaps can result in a variety of injuries, some of which are described in this chapter.

Skier/snowboarder visits to ski areas have remained stable and even increased slightly during the first part of the new millennium. Mountain biking has shown an increase in popularity as have many other pastimes that occur out of doors. It is increasingly common to spend a weekend climbing, rafting or hiking, rather than staying indoors and watching TV. With the increase in popularity of outdoor activity comes a parallel increase in the potential for outdoor emergencies.

Skiing and snowboarding deaths are relatively rare. ◄ Table 14-1 shows the number of deaths per year in the United States for four types of accidents. A skier or snowboarder is six to eight times more likely to die in an automobile or commercial aircraft than on the slopes.

Snowsports Injuries

Skiing (fixed heel, free heel, and cross-country) and snowboarding have certain inherent risks considering that participants propel themselves down steep slopes, strapped to objects with sharp edges at moderate to high rates of speed with minimal protective gear.

During the last 30 years, the frequency and patterns of ski injuries have changed. Data vary depending on the source, location, and weather and snow conditions each year, but certain generalizations can be made. Ability and experience are probably the most important factors in determining a skier's likelihood of injury. The decline in the overall alpine injury rate during the last 40 years is likely due to increased numbers of older and more experienced skiers on the slopes, better teaching methods, better slope grooming, better bindings, better rental equipment, the use of ski brakes, and the availability of shorter skis. The incidence rate in men and women is essentially the same when controlled for ability level. There is a higher incidence of injuries during the late afternoon. This is due to a combination of higher skier density on the hill, fatigue, poor lighting, and deteriorating snow conditions. Skiing in large groups or when the slopes are crowded seems to increase the injury rate, which is lowest on weekdays. In alpine ski racing, almost half the injuries occur on the last third of the course, a sta-

Table 14-1 Deaths Per Year by Accident Type	
Accident Type	**Average Number of Deaths per Year in the United States**
Skiing and snowboarding accidents	34
Lightning strikes	89
Bathtub falls	300
Automobile collisions	42,000

tistic that probably reflects the importance of fatigue as a contributor to ski injuries.

Certain types of snow conditions are associated with higher injury rates. These include heavy, wet snow and deep powder, which increase knee sprains, tibial fractures, and other rotational injuries; icy conditions, which are associated with more head and upper body injuries due to hard falls; and breakable crust, which makes skis harder to control and increases the frequency of falls.

Modern alpine bindings are safer than the old cable and long-thong bindings, but the perfect binding has yet to be invented. Such a binding would have to be inexpensive, simple to install, and easy to adjust and maintain. It would have to release during a fall but not during a hard turn, release equally well during all types of falls, and be unaffected by dirt, snow, ice, or corrosion.

Alpine Skiing Injuries

The overall alpine injury rate has been steadily falling to its current level of about 2.5 accidents per 1,000 skier/snowboarder visits in the United States. Advances in ski equipment design have helped to decrease the overall rate of injury (▼ **Figure 14-1**). However, all the advances have been unable to significantly reduce injuries to the knee.

Despite the most sophisticated advances in ski boot and binding technology, skiing technique, and ski hill design, there will always be skiing accidents. Nonetheless, skiing is relatively safe when compared with other sports (► **Figure 14-2**).

Mechanisms and Patterns of Injury

There are two basic types of ski accidents: falls and collisions (▼ **Table 14-2**). Collisions occur in many different ways and can injure almost any part of the body.

Falls can be divided into two general types: **rotational** (twisting) and **nonrotational** (nontwisting). The specific

Table 14-2 Breakdown of Number of Accidents by Sport	
Sport	**Number of Accidents per 1,000 Participants**
Skiing/Snowboarding	2
Swimming	2
Tennis	2
Ice Skating	4
Snowmobiling	4
Soccer	13
Bicycle riding	14
Football	18
Basketball	20

Rates calculated from 1999 injury rates.

Sources: *National Safety Council Injury Facts 2001 Edition,* and Rochester Institute of Technology, Jasper Shealy, PhD.

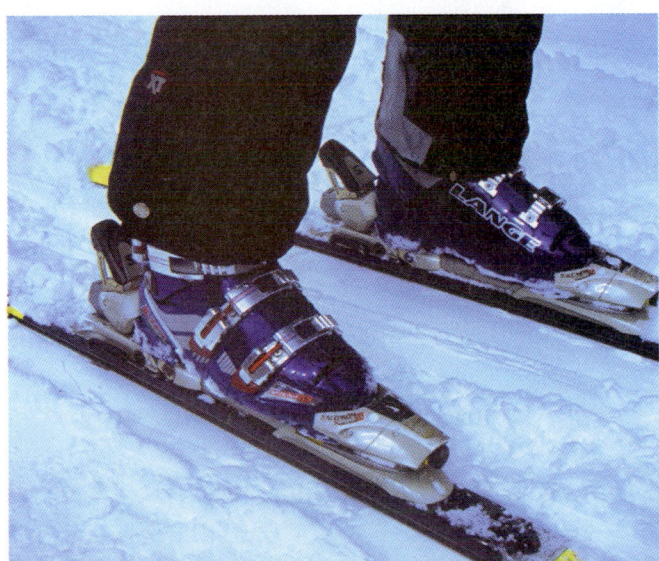

Figure 14-1 Advances in ski equipment design have helped decrease the overall rate of injury.

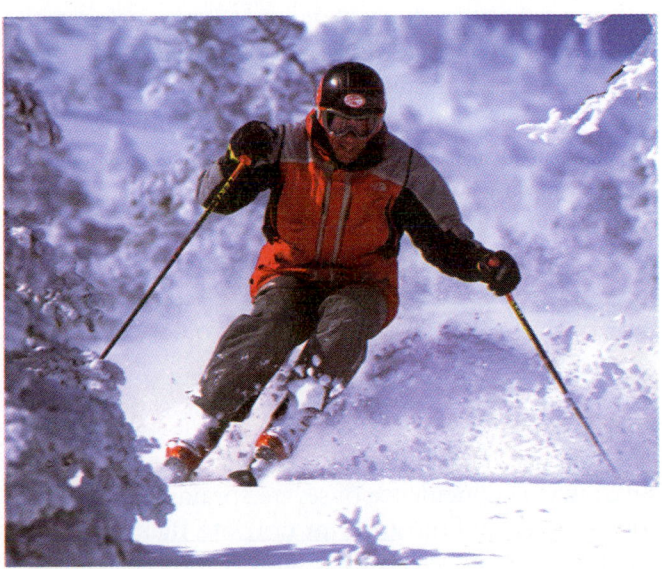

Figure 14-2 Skiing is a safe and enjoyable winter activity.

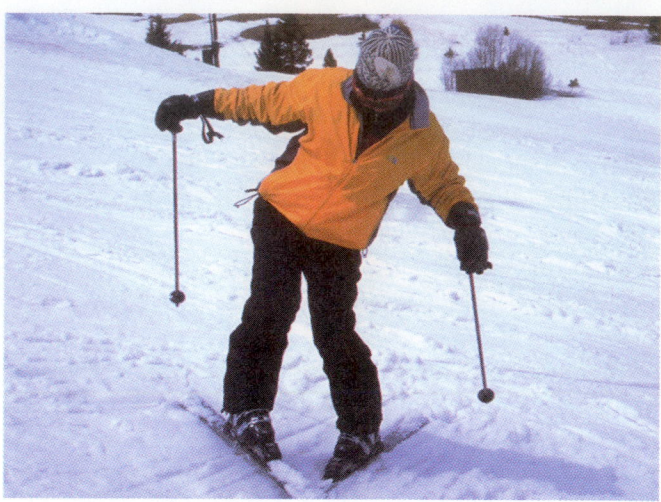

Figure 14-3 Rotational fall.

type and extent of any injury produced by a fall depend on the type, magnitude, and direction of the resulting forces and whether these forces are concentrated on one or more body parts in a manner that exceeds their threshold of injury. The type of equipment (ie, high, low, stiff, or soft boots; ski poles held with straps around the wrists), as well as the physical condition, flexibility, weight, and bone structure may influence the skier's chances of injury. Other important factors include whether the heel is free or fixed and whether the bindings release normally, prematurely, or not at all.

A rotational fall most commonly rotates the foot outward and forces the leg outward at the knee, eg, when a skier catches an inside edge while falling forward or to the side ▶ **Figure 14-3** . A nonrotational fall typically occurs when a skier falls forward over the ski tips, tending to bend the leg over the front edge of the boot ▶ **Figure 14-4** .

Ankle

Ankle sprains and fractures are relatively uncommon with new boot design but they still do occur. Lower leg fractures and knee injuries have become relatively more frequent, probably because higher, stiffer ski boots transmit forces to a different and more proximal area of the lower extremity. Leg fractures that occur near the top of the boot (boot-top fractures) continue to be common, but the incidence of spiral fractures of the tibia and fibula has decreased, apparently due to advances in lateral toe release technology and the reduction of friction between modern ski boots and bindings. However, there has been recent anecdotal evidence of an increase in spiral fractures of the tibia and fibula related to the popularity of snowboards or new short skis, which do not have releasable bindings.

Knee

Knee sprains continue to be the most common serious ski injury. The incidence of severe sprains, especially complete tears of the **anterior cruciate ligament (ACL)**, has more than tripled since 1980. These serious injuries, which pose a permanent threat to an active lifestyle, can occur without a fall. Wearing high, stiff boots seems to increase their incidence.

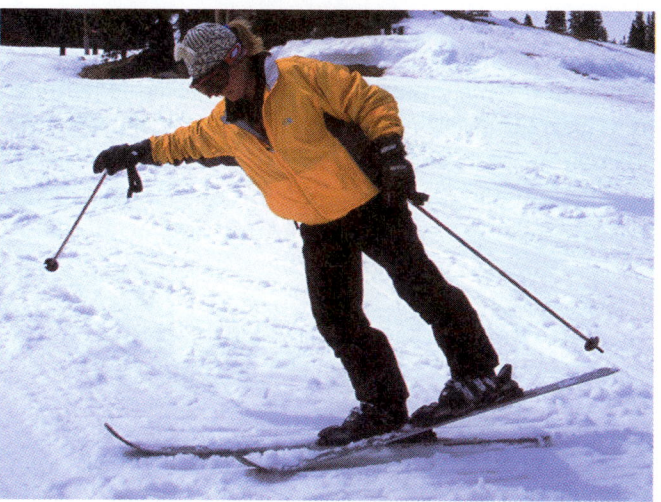

Figure 14-4 Nonrotational fall.

The ACL runs from the posterior femur to the anterior tibia and prevents the forward dislocation of the tibia. The mechanisms of many ACL injuries have recently been identified. They include the following:

- hyperextension of the knee
- external rotation and abduction of the lower leg on the thigh during a forward fall (often occurs when the skier catches an inside edge)
- the top of the skier's boot thrusts the tibia forward during a backward fall
- internal rotation of the thigh when the knee is hyperflexed (often occurs when the skier catches the inside edge of his or her ski tail while sitting back; known as "**phantom foot syndrome**." It typically happens when novices try to stop by sitting down.)

The four most common patterns of ligament injury to the knee are:

1. <u>Medial collateral ligament (MCL)</u> injury alone.
2. ACL with MCL injury.
3. Complete ACL injury.
4. ACL and/or MCL with tibial plateau fracture.

Knee (not patella) dislocations are rare but signify a potential limb-threatening situation because of possible arterial damage. Knee dislocations require expedient transport to the nearest medical facility.

Knee injuries constantly challenge equipment manufacturers to design a binding that will provide better knee protection and encourage ski instructors to perfect techniques that will help prevent knee injuries.

Thigh, Hip, and Pelvis

Injuries to the thigh, hip, and pelvis usually involve contusions and lacerations, but when enough force is involved, fractures of the femur, hip, and pelvis occur as well as hip dislocations.

Hand

Hand injuries can involve contusions, fractures, sprains, and dislocations. The most common hand injury is called "<u>skier's thumb</u>," which occurs when the thumb is bent backwards in the process of a fall. Skiers often do not seek medical attention for this injury. If the injury is left untreated, however, significant long-term disability of the hand, with loss of ability to pinch firmly, may occur.

Upper Extremity

Upper extremity injuries to the wrist, forearm, elbow, and upper arm are less common but can involve fractures and dislocations. Common shoulder injuries include dislocations, rotator cuff strains, <u>acromioclavicular separations</u>, and clavicle fractures. Some studies show that shoulder injuries account for up to 11% of alpine ski injuries.

Overuse of Body Parts

Overuse can cause lower back pain, patella pain, chronic lower extremity muscle strains, and ankle and foot pain caused by tight, rigid boots. These injuries are more common in nordic skiers than in alpine skiers.

Multiple Anatomic Parts

An ominous development has been the increase in serious injuries to multiple areas of the body, including combinations of injuries to the head, spine, chest, and abdomen that resemble injuries seen in motor vehicle crashes. This worrisome trend, noted in both North America and Europe, is probably a by-product of improvements in equipment, technique, and slope grooming, which have led to higher speeds involving greater kinetic energy. With the higher speeds have come more serious injuries due mainly to deceleration trauma. Another factor that has led to more frequent collisions is slope crowding. As a result, alpine ski areas now emphasize improved trail design, lift layout, and more effective skier/snowboarder education.

Head and Chest

Although skier and snowboarder deaths are relatively uncommon, they are largely due to head and chest injuries resulting from collisions with trees and other stationary objects.

Snowboarding Injuries

The sport of snowboarding has seen an exponential growth since its inception in the mid 1980s. In the last 4 years, there has been more than a fourfold increase in visits to ski areas by snowboarders. The early fears of the "reckless, dangerous, young, and foolish" prompted banning of the equipment and/or designated areas for use. Only recently have all but a few major resort areas opened the lift lines to boarders. In contrast to the early years, the snowsports industry has now embraced riding (the sport of snowboarding) to include major ski area modifications and engineering. With the growth of riding and its promotion by the ski industry, this alternative winter sport has evolved into a significant business sector of the ski resort industry ▼ Figure 14-5.

Mechanisms and Patterns of Injury

The combination of slope, gravity, and minimal friction creates the potential for injury when boarding. Though

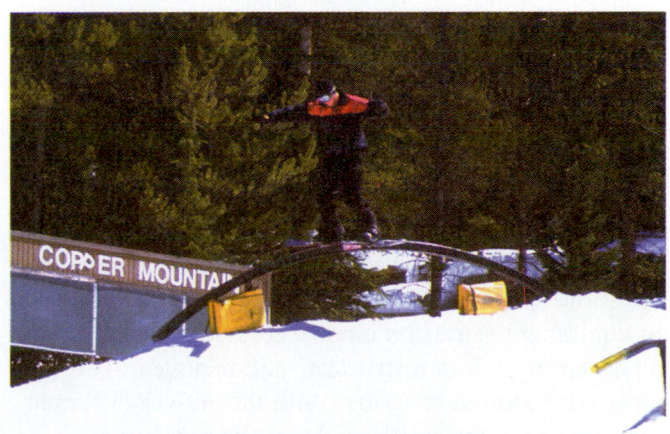

Figure 14-5 Snowboarding has evolved into a significant business sector of the ski resort industry.

Rescuer Safety

In early and late season, patrollers highlight bare spots on the slopes with markers, particularly at breakovers. Develop sign boards to warn guests of conditions ahead, such as "You will have to walk a little if you go this way!"

boarding has a short history when compared to skiing, many significant similarities and differences in injury patterns are emerging. In addition, the evolution of equipment design has resulted in changes in the injury pattern.

Injury risk for boarding is slightly higher than that for skiing. The typical injured boarder profile is the young, inexperienced man with no skiing background who has had no professional instruction. A New Hampshire study found injury rates between first time skiers and snowboarders to be the same for both groups (4%). Snowboarders, however, sustained a significantly greater number of emergent injuries requiring immediate intervention, such as concussion, fracture, dislocation, and dental avulsion.

Whereas skiers experience a predominance of lower extremity injuries, riders experience more injuries to the upper extremities. Head and lower limb (mostly ankle) injuries are common among riders as well. The risk of fracture in snowboarding is twice that of skiing—there is a 28% risk of fracture when snowboarding compared to a 14% risk of fracture when skiing. Also, men have a higher percentage of ankle and lower leg injuries, while women have a higher percentage of wrist and knee injuries.

There are specific injury mechanisms unique to snowboarding. The mechanics of snowboarding results in a different set of forces being applied to the rider than in skiing. With sudden deceleration of the board (catching a heel or toe edge), forward momentum is focused in the skeletal system and resulting injuries are generally due to impact. The more distant an object is from the center of rotation (specifically the outstretched arm or the head), the greater the force upon impact with the snow (or other surfaces). Unrelated to the actual fall or equipment is the combination of issues surrounding a new sport, lack of instruction, and relative unfamiliarity with mountain sports. With the growth of formal training programs, it is hoped that the number of injuries from this sport will decline.

Lower Extremity

On average, lower leg injuries among snowboarders are 60% fewer than those among skiers. This decreased frequency is attributed to the unique mechanical differences between the snowboard and the ski. The reduced length of many boards decreases rotational forces to the legs. This rotational force is halved, as the rider has both feet attached nearly parallel. Riding on one board (with two edges) as opposed to two skis (with four edges) also mitigates isolated lower extremity injuries. The most common cause of leg injury, therefore, is direct impact. Experienced riders tend to sustain more ACL injuries. This usually occurs after "catching air" when the knee flexes forcefully during the landing. Occasionally a rider will sustain a fracture of the tibial plateau when landing on a straight leg. As riders typically have a "lead leg," that extremity is at most risk for direct blow injury. Injury patterns include contusion, laceration, and fracture. When the board is attached to only the lead foot (lift lines and "scootering"—dragging the board with one foot still in the binding—on the flats), the knee is at increased risk of rotational, and therefore ligament, injury.

The rate of boarder ankle injury is more than twice that for the skier because of a combination of numerous mechanical factors: softer boots, nonreleasable bindings, and directional force application. The ankle frequently is injured as a result of **compression**, **inversion**, and **dorsiflexion** of the joint. Sprain and fracture are generally differentiated at the hospital. **Snowboarder's ankle**, or fracture of the **talus** (the support structure for both the tibia and fibula) is frequent and sometimes very difficult to identify even on x-ray. This fracture is important to recognize because of the long-term complications that result if treatment is not received. Any rider with persistent ankle pain that is not improving should be evaluated for this injury. Special x-rays at the hospital may be required.

Abdominal, Thoracic, and Back

Spinal injuries are of equal frequency for both boarders and skiers. These injuries generally involve high speed or sudden decelerations, for example, striking an immovable object. Injuries to the spleen are more common in severely injured riders and are potentially fatal due to intra-abdominal hemorrhage.

Blunt thoracic trauma is the second most common cause of snowboarding fatalities. When the thorax suddenly decelerates, the heart can forcefully swing and tear from its pendulum attachment to the aorta. Direct penetration of the chest can result in lung collapse.

Table 14-3 Breakdown of Upper Extremity Injuries in Snowboarding	
Type of Upper Extremity Injury	Percentage
Fractures	56
Sprains	27
Dislocations	10

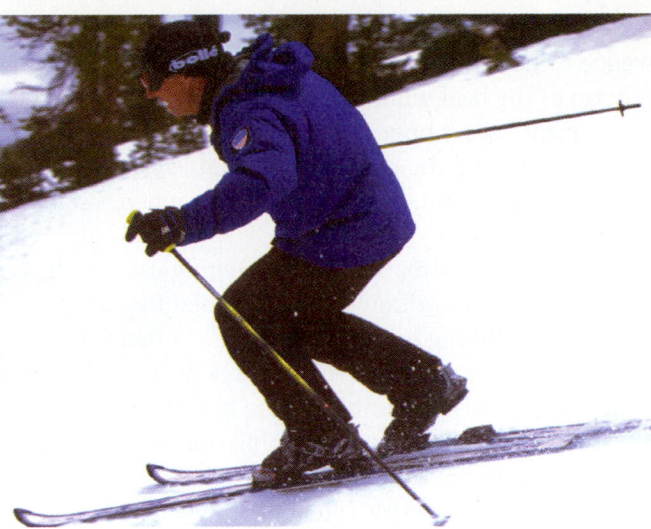

Figure 14-6 Telemark skiing is the third most popular winter sport at major ski areas in the US.

Rapid **tension pneumothorax**—an expanding collection of air outside the lung with resulting pressure on the heart and blood vessels—can result. This requires immediate recognition, treatment, and rapid evacuation as death can quickly occur.

Upper Extremity

More than 50% of all boarding injuries involve the upper extremities (▲ Table 14-3). Wrist injuries are most commonly seen in beginners, women, and the younger age groups. Intermediate and expert male boarders experience a higher frequency of hand, elbow, and shoulder injuries.

The upper extremity is at high risk of injury as the arm and hand are used to decelerate a fall. Commonly known as FOOSH (Fall Onto Outstretched Hand), this mechanism is the cause of most wrist injuries. The risk of a wrist injury is 13 to 15 times greater for a boarder than for a skier. Wrist fractures (distal radius and **scaphoid**) are commonly seen in the rider. Point tenderness over a bone surface in a child is most frequently due to fracture rather than sprain.

Other upper extremity injuries include those to the elbow and shoulder. The risk of fracture and/or dislocation of the elbow is greater for boarders than for skiers. Injury to the shoulder includes sprain, dislocation, and rotator cuff injury. A direct blow to the outside of the shoulder can result in damage to the ligaments supporting the **acromion** and the clavicle resulting in various degrees of **shoulder separation**, or acromioclavicular separation.

Head

There are fewer head injuries than other types of injuries; they comprise 3% to 15% of all skiing and boarding injuries. However, head injury is the leading cause of death and disability for both these groups. In head injuries from boarding, a high incidence of impact to the base of the skull, or occiput, is described. This injury typically occurs from falling backwards, when the boarder's head rapidly snaps back, extending the cervical spine. Collision and fall both contribute to head injury.

Telemark Ski Injuries

Telemark skiing at alpine areas is the third most popular winter sport at major ski areas in the United States (▲ Figure 14-6). With the introduction of ever increasing stiffer and higher telemark ski boots and higher performance skis (including parabolic telemark skis), the injury pattern is becoming similar to alpine ski injuries. It was once thought that because the heel was free, ACL and spiral tibia fractures would not occur. This has proven not to be true with the higher stiffer plastic telemark boots. In a similar fashion to the evolution of alpine equipment technology, telemark equipment manufacturers are developing safer gear. Releasable bindings with ski brakes are now available and are highly recommended for their injury prevention potential.

Nordic Skiing Injuries

Nordic skiing includes diagonal stride or classic ski racing, skate skiing, cross-country day tours at nordic centers or in nearby fields and forests, backcountry and wilderness skiing, multiday ski camping, ski mountaineering, and telemark skiing in alpine areas.

There are estimated to be more than 7 million nordic skiers in the United States. Unlike alpine skiing, the boot heel in nordic skiing is not permanently affixed to the ski. The traditional nordic binding is a light, three-pin, nonreleasable binding. A device such as a heel wedge or heel locator is frequently used to limit side motion of the heel while it is in contact with the ski. The typical nordic boot is either street-shoe height or ankle height, and the nordic ski is double **cambered** so that its midpoint touches the snow only when weighted ▼ **Figure 14-7** .

Backcountry telemark skiers frequently use higher, stiffer boots and bindings with heel cables that limit side-to-side shifting motion of the heel ▼ **Figure 14-8** . Ski mountaineers may use high, stiff boots resembling alpine boots and convertible release bindings that allow the heel to be free when going uphill but locked down for alpine-style descents (often referred to as randonne equipment) ▼ **Figure 14-9** . Telemarking and mountaineering skis are lighter than alpine skis, but they share some alpine features, including single camber and parabolic design, which permit easier turns ▼ **Figure 14-10** .

Although the types of nordic skiing are generally felt to be safer than alpine skiing, it is not a completely benign sport. The informal nature of nordic skiing makes data collection difficult, but the injury rates are estimated to be 0.5 or less per 1,000 skier visits. The development of faster, lighter-weight equipment, more frequent trail grooming at nordic skiing areas, and the increasing popularity of the skating technique are making it possible for skiers to move faster, and consequently, increasing the potential for injuries. Because nordic skiers often travel in places far removed from a heated lodge, cold injuries are more common in nordic skiers than alpine skiers. Although rare, deaths are most often due to avalanche burial.

In nordic skiing, most injuries result from falls that follow loss of balance on downhill terrain, where skiers on groomed trails can reach speeds of more than 35 mph (almost 16 m/sec). Upper body injuries occur about as often as lower body injuries. However, like alpine skiing, knee and thumb injuries occur the most

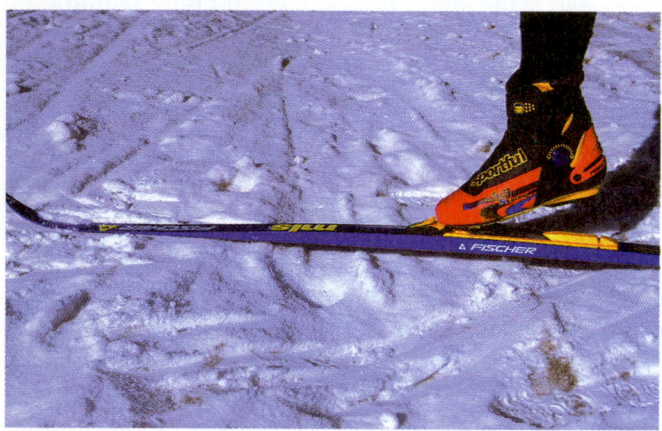

Figure 14-7 The nordic ski is double cambered so that its midpoint touches the snow only when weighted.

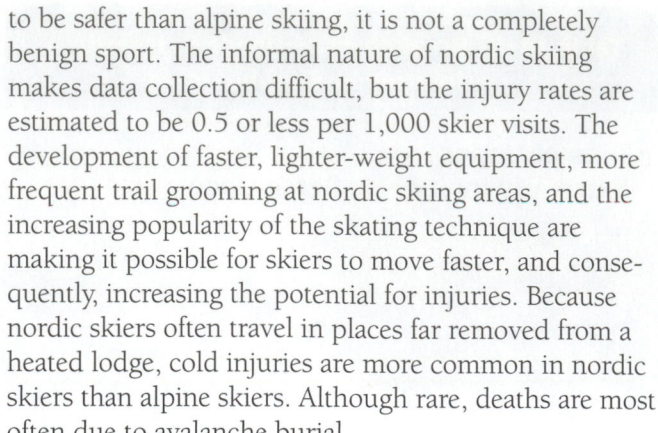

Figure 14-8 Backcountry telemarkers skiers frequently use higher, stiffer boots and bindings with heel cables that limit side-to-side shifting.

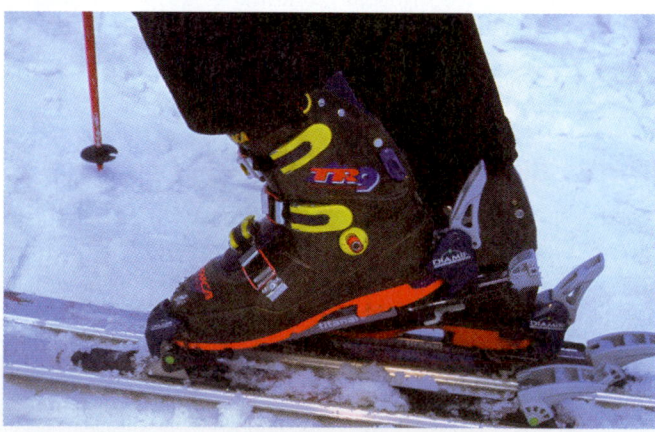

Figure 14-9 Randonne equipment may be used by mountaineers.

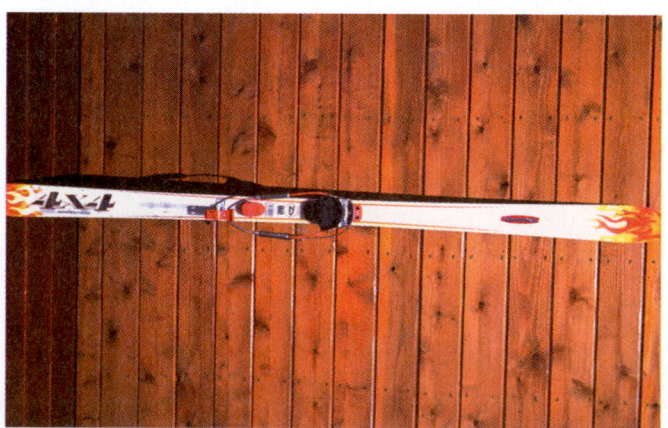

Figure 14-10 Telemarking and mountaineering skis include single camber and parabolic design.

frequently. Other common injuries include acromioclavicular (shoulder) separations, clavicle fractures, wrist fractures, rotator cuff tears, and ankle sprains. Ankle injuries occur more often in skiers who wear low boots. Fractures of the lower leg and femur and serious head and trunk injuries occur only occasionally.

In track skiing, devices that restrain lateral motion of the heel on the ski increase the lower extremity injury rate. Skate skiing, during which skiers can move up to 20 mph (9 m/sec)—compared with the 13 mph (6 m/sec) speeds of classic cross-country nordic skiers—increases the amount of kinetic energy involved but does not seem to alter injury patterns.

Severe eye injuries occur occasionally due to collisions with frozen branches, especially during night skiing. Freezing injuries of the cornea due to cold exposure and that require corneal transplant have also been reported.

Overuse injuries seen in nordic skiers include stress fractures, upper extremity tendinitis caused by poling, lower back pain, shin splints (anterior leg pain), and pain in the patella and anterolateral thigh. **Skier's toe**, characterized by pain in the big toe caused by repeated dorsiflexion, is another common complaint.

Snowblade Injuries

A recent trend in snowsports has been the widespread availability and use of very short skis (▼ **Figure 14-11**). While these have been around for many years, they were used primarily as a teaching tool and were simply cut down skis with alpine-style bindings. The new generation of these skis, known as ski boards, figls, and Snowblades are meant to provide the thrill of skiing without the lengthy period of learning. Adolescents are readily attracted to them and enjoy the ability to access terrain at a ski area almost immediately. More experi-

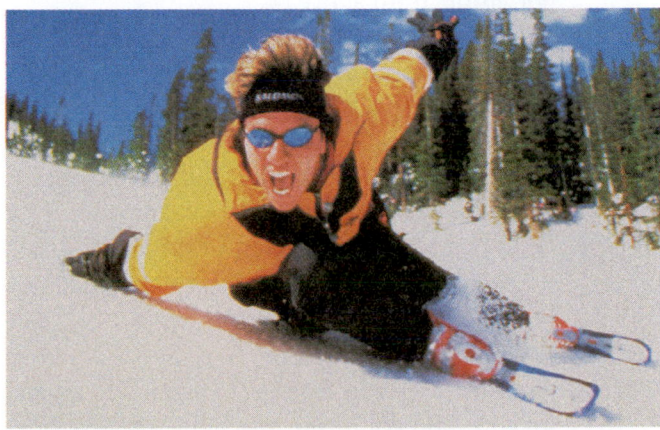

Figure 14-11 The snowsports industry continues to introduce new types of "sliding" equipment, like Snowblades.

> Stop where you obstruct
> a trail or are not visible from above.
> Failure to heed this can result in collision and
> the possibility of serious or fatal injuries.

enced users are becoming adept at performing aerial tricks in terrain parks and half pipes. Some ski area workers occasionally use them to move about the resort while wearing plastic mountaineering boots. Most are sold with nonreleasable plate bindings similar to the type used in snowboard racing. For the most part, injuries incurred when using this new generation of skis are consistent with those seen in both skiing and snowboard riding. Usually Snowblade users slide without poles, so upper extremity injuries that occur are consistent with snowboard riding. Anecdotal evidence suggests a connection between the nonreleasable bindings and a pattern of boot-top and spiral fractures of the tibia and fibula.

Tubing Injuries

Tubing, or riding downhill on an inner tube, is a popular sport in snowy, hilly areas. However, inner tubes accelerate rapidly, cannot be steered, and are difficult to stop. Soft-tissue injuries, head and spine injuries, and multiple fractures caused by collisions and rollovers are common.

Injury Prevention

Skiers and snowboarders can lessen their chances of injury by following a few basic steps.

1. Stay in good physical condition, preferably all-year long. Mountain biking, in-line skating, stair climbing, balance boards, and ski-simulation machines are particularly effective off-season exercises.

2. Purchase good equipment and keep it tuned and repaired. Buy the best bindings you can afford. Keep ski and snowboard edges sharpened and bases repaired and waxed.

3. Learn the mechanics of your bindings and keep them properly maintained, lubricated, and adjusted according to the manufacturer's specifications. Keep bindings clean and free of snow and ice when not in use.

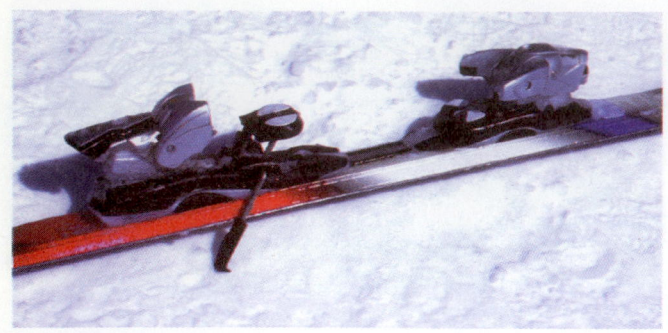

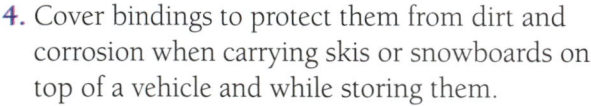

Figure 14-12 Ski brakes can decrease your likelihood of being hit by a windmilling ski during a fall.

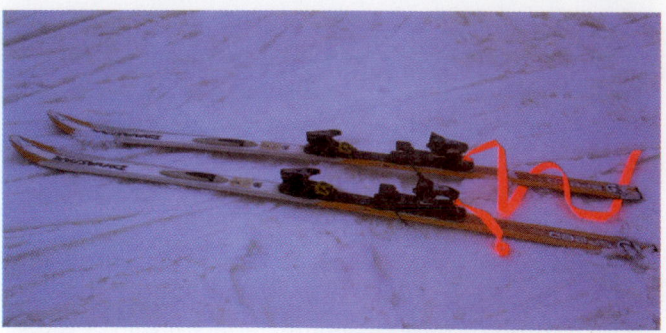

Figure 14-13 Powder cords help to locate buried skis.

4. Cover bindings to protect them from dirt and corrosion when carrying skis or snowboards on top of a vehicle and while storing them.

5. Use devices to avoid runaway and lost skis and snowboards. In alpine skiing, use ski brakes instead of safety straps to decrease your likelihood of being hit by a windmilling ski during a fall (▲ **Figure 14-12**). Snowboard riders and telemark skiers should use safety straps, but be aware of the potential risks involved with nonrelease bindings while accessing terrain with avalanche hazard. Powder skiers should use powder cords so that buried skis can be located more easily, and all skiers who use ski brakes should be careful not to unintentionally release a binding while riding on an aerial lift (▲ **Figure 14-13**).

6. Do not ski or ride on slopes or in snow conditions that you do not know how to handle.

7. Be aware of your surroundings. Ski and ride carefully at intersections and in slow speed and crowded areas. Do not stop unexpectedly.

8. Do not use alcohol, tranquilizers, sleeping pills, or any drugs (such as antihistamines) that interfere with alertness or coordination before or while skiing or riding.

9. Do not skip meals during skiing or other strenuous physical activities. High-carbohydrate meals and snacks are the best fuel for replenishing and maintaining muscle glycogen.

10. When you are tired or cold, go inside to warm up, rest, and have a snack.

11. Dress for a variety of conditions. Carry spare clothing in a backpack or in your vehicle. Carry emergency equipment when nordic or back-country skiing. At a minimum, always carry matches and a sturdy knife.

12. Be familiar with the area where you are skiing or snowboarding. Carry a map of the area, plus a compass if you are heading out of bounds. Backcountry skiers and riders should always carry a topographic map and compass, and if possible, a Global Positioning System (GPS) unit. If in avalanche-prone areas, avalanche transceivers are essential.

13. Do not ski or ride alone in isolated locations, even at an alpine ski area. If you must go alone (because it is part of your job or for any other reason), carry a radio.

14. Follow your responsibility code and urge others to do the same.
    a. Always stay in control, and be able to stop or avoid other people or objects.
    b. People ahead of you have the right of way. It is your responsibility to avoid them.
    c. Do not stop where you obstruct a trail or are not visible from above.
    d. When starting downhill or merging into a trail, look uphill and yield to others.
    e. Always use devices to help prevent runaway equipment.
    f. Observe all posted signs and warnings. Keep off closed trails and out of closed areas.
    g. Before using any lift, you must have the knowledge and ability to load, ride, and unload safely.

15. Other snowsports equipment:
    a. Goggles should be flexible, ventilated to avoid fogging, and equipped with light-sensitive or interchangeable yellow and dark lenses. The dark lenses should filter out 85% to 98% of the sun's ultraviolet rays.

b. Helmets are highly recommended and widely accepted in many sports involving significant kinetic energy and a high risk of deceleration trauma, such as motorcycling, bicycling, hockey, in-line skating, football, and horse-back riding. A significant cause of death and serious disability may be prevented by wearing helmets. Some experts recommend that all skiers and snowboarders wear helmets. In the United States, however, helmet use is widespread only in children and racers. Although helmet use is a matter of personal choice, make sure it fits properly, is comfortable, and offers the appropriate level of protection for your activity of choice.

(▼ **Table 14-4**) summarizes methods for preventing skiing and snowboarding emergencies.

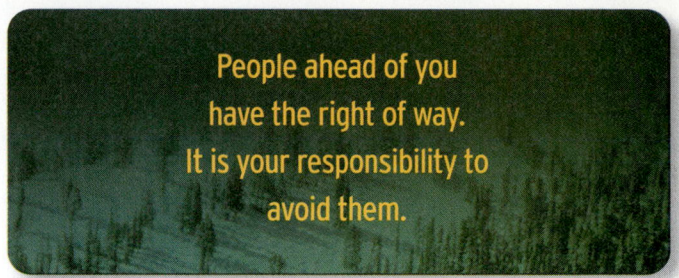

People ahead of you have the right of way. It is your responsibility to avoid them.

Snowmobiling Injuries

Snowmobiles are widely used for winter recreation and, during the snowy months, are an important means of travel in state and national forests, national parks, ski areas, and in the logging, trapping, mining, oil drilling, and farming industries. They are essential when secondary roads are unplowed or when off-road travel is required. Along with steadily increasing use, there are a

Table 14-4 Summary of Methods for Preventing Emergencies

1. Stay in good physical condition all year long.
2. Get good equipment and take care of it.
3. Know your bindings and test them regularly.
4. Cover bindings when carrying skis or snowboards on top of a vehicle or storing them.
5. Use devices to prevent runaway and buried skis and snowboards.
6. Avoid slopes and snow conditions that you cannot handle.
7. Be aware of your surroundings.
8. Avoid alcohol and drugs while skiing.
9. Stay well nourished while skiing.
10. Rest, warm up, and eat when tired and cold.
11. Dress for a variety of conditions. Have spare clothing handy.
12. Be familiar with the ski area.
13. Avoid skiing or snowboarding alone if possible.
14. Follow your responsibility code, and urge others to do the same.
15. Carry emergency survival equipment when skiing or snowboarding out of bounds.
16. Use high-quality eyewear and ski poles.
17. Whenever wearing a helmet, make sure it fits, is comfortable, and provides adequate protection.

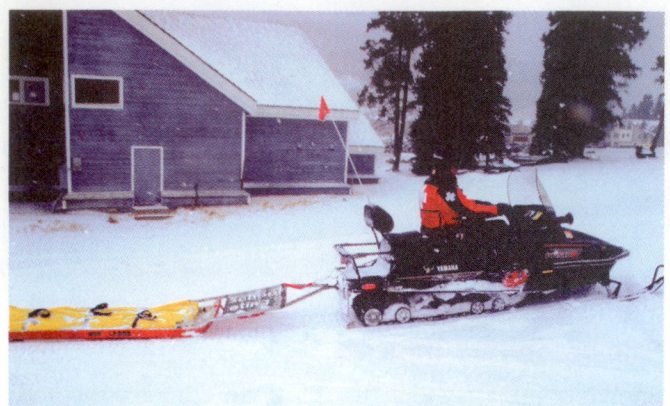

Figure 14-14 Rescue toboggans for patient transport should be used with a rigid hitch so they do not contact the moving snowmobile track.

growing number of accidents, most of which occur during recreational use.

Snowmobiles are rugged, and, during certain maneuvers and conditions, can be unstable. Modern models can travel faster than 100 mph (160 kph). Good judgment, a high level of skill, and a moderate amount of strength are required to drive these vehicles safely. Children often are not strong enough, experienced enough, or properly trained to handle them.

Acute snowmobiling injuries resemble motorcycle injuries. Risk factors include multiple riders, excessive speed, use of alcohol and drugs, lack of proper equipment such as helmets and high boots, riding at night, riding in unfamiliar terrain, riding in avalanche terrain or on bodies of water covered by unstable ice, and advertising that sometimes depicts snowmobiles jumping off embankments. In many cases, multiple risk factors are involved, such as the combination of excessive speed, alcohol use, and riding at night.

Most snowmobile injuries occur in teenagers and young adults. Extremities, especially the lower extremity, are the most commonly injured body areas. Fractures make up about half of all lower extremity injuries. Spine injuries due to compression trauma occur twice as often as they do in skiers, and multiple injuries are frequent.

Most snowmobile fatalities occur at dusk or at night and are due to head or neck trauma. About half the deaths are associated with alcohol use. Avalanche burial and drowning are somewhat common in risky locations. Occasionally, individuals who try to lift a stuck snowmobile suffer heart attacks.

Overuse injuries are frequent. They include hearing loss; vibration-induced vascular injury to the hands (**Raynaud's syndrome**); tendinitis of the hands, wrists,

and shoulders; and lower back pain. Many of these injuries are related to the poor ergonomics of snowmobile construction (unadjustable seat and handlebar positions, inadequate cushioning, strong vibration, loud engine noise), and improper driving habits (leaning forward at the hips, driving with one knee on the seat, wearing a backpack while riding).

Snowmobile rescue organizations have been formed in areas of high snowmobile use. Rescue sleds for patient transport, which are towed behind a snowmobile, should be used with a rigid hitch so they do not contact the moving snowmobile track ◄ **Figure 14-14** .

Off-Road Mountain Biking Injuries

Like snowboarding, mountain biking is another new Olympic sport. Off-road or mountain bikes now make up the majority of bicycles sold in the United States. They are 10- to 21-speed bicycles with rugged frames, horizontal handlebars, and wide tires designed to let the rider venture off paved roads—specifically onto dirt roads and hiking trails. During the warm months, many ski areas promote off-road biking on their mountain trails. Off-road biking is usually prohibited in wilderness areas and national parks.

In many localities, off-road bikers have organized into clubs. Currently there is an international organization, the International Mountain Bike Association (IMBA), as well as a national organization, the National Off-Road Bicycle Association (NORBA). Through a joint effort of the IMBA, NORBA, the National Ski Patrol, and the Bureau of Land Management, the National Mountain Bike Patrol (NMBP) was recently formed to train volunteers in outdoor emergency care, NMBP procedures, trail etiquette, and environmental issues.

Like road bikers, those who ride mountain bikes are at risk for crashes and serious injuries, but mainly from a loss of control at high speeds or on steep or uneven terrain rather than collisions with motor vehicles. Studies have shown that 80% of recreational mountain bikers will be injured during their careers; the figure is higher for racers. Abrasions are the most common injuries, followed by contusions, lacerations, fractures, and concussions. One of the most commonly fractured bones is the clavicle.

Most off-road bikers are men in their late teens to late 30s. Mountain biking injuries tend to be multiple, with more than half to the lower extremity, most commonly the knee, while about 30% involve the upper extremity. About a third of serious mountain biking injuries involve the trunk, and 12% involve the head and neck. Extensive face injuries and serious chest and abdominal

Documentation Tips

Incident response is a critical phase of incident management. It is the phase in which emergency medical care is initiated, but it also signals the opportunity to preserve evidence and gather the information necessary to compile the appropriate forms, logs, records, and information as soon after an incident as possible. A well-trained investigation team is able to develop information that will provide the resort the greatest understanding of the circumstances surrounding an incident. A delay in compiling this information may result in losing a critical piece of information.

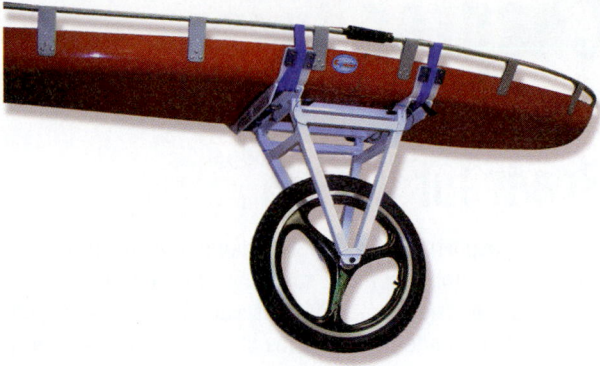

Figure 14-15 On trails, single-wheeled litters with handles at each end are useful and effective.

injuries such as ruptured spleens and pelvic fractures, especially those involving the hip joint, occasionally occur. However, only about a fourth of all injuries are severe enough to require medical care.

Most injuries (almost 90%) occur off-road rather than on paved terrain, and three fourths of them occur when riding downhill, especially during turns. A few involve collisions, half with moving objects such as another bicycle or motor vehicle and half with stationary objects such as rocks and trees. Approximately 80% of collisions involve excessive speed, and riding in unfamiliar terrain contributes to a third of these collisions. In many cases, a deceleration accident throws the rider forward over the handlebars, which tends to result in more serious injuries than crashes in which the rider falls to the side. Alcohol or drugs are involved in less than 3% of mountain biking accidents. Equipment failure (usually of brakes or tires) causes less than 10% of accidents.

Although off-road bicyclists are injured more often than road bicyclists, the number of injuries that require medical care is about the same. The incidence of serious head injury is low, which may be partly due to a high rate of helmet use—90%—compared with 57% in road bicyclists.

Injuries can be reduced by using a helmet; wearing sturdy, leather mountain biking gloves to prevent hand abrasions; avoiding excessive speeds—especially while riding in unfamiliar terrain; and paying strict attention to equipment maintenance. Racers should consider wearing helmets with face protectors; chest and shoulder pads; and elbow, forearm, knee, and shin guards.

Off-road bikers with minor injuries tend to self-evacuate. Techniques and equipment used to transport the more seriously injured cyclists over unpaved roads include the use of four-wheel drive ambulances and six-wheeled all-terrain vehicles equipped with cargo areas that will accommodate a litter. On trails, standard backcountry rescue techniques that use litter-bearers may be needed; single-wheeled litters with handles at each end are useful and effective ▲ **Figure 14-15**. Helicopters are a valuable resource where landing pads are available; at ski areas, properly constructed landing pads can be used during both summer and winter.

Chapter *Sweep*

Ready for Review

While snowsports and mountain biking provide tremendous opportunities for fun, these sports are not accident free. The nature and distribution of injuries vary between snowsports depending on gender, mechanisms of injury, and which parts of the body are involved.

Knee sprains continue to be a common serious ski injury for alpine skiers, while distal radial fractures of the wrist account for the common snowboard injury. Abrasions lead the list for mountain bikers.

Injury prevention begins with staying in good physical condition; using good equipment; and giving the equipment proper, regular maintenance. Eating appropriate food; having the proper clothing for the sport, the environment, and a variety of conditions; and being familiar and aware of your surroundings increase the safety factor. Each individual in the outdoor environment has a responsibility for appropriate behavior for themselves and others.

Vital Vocabulary

acromioclavicular separations The joint between the clavicle and the acromion of the scapula at the point of the shoulder.

acromion The lateral extension of the spine of the scapula that forms the highest point of the shoulder.

anterior cruciate ligament (ACL) Ligament in the knee that runs from the posterior femur to the anterior tibia, preventing forward dislocation of the tibia.

camber The arch that is formed when a ski or snowboard is placed on a flat surface, with the middle of the board higher than the tip and tail.

compression Impact between a body part and a blunt object.

dorsiflexion Upward flexion of the foot.

inversion Reversal of a normal relationship. The turning or rotation of the foot about its long axis so that the sole points inward.

medial collateral ligament Condensation or thickening of the medial joint capsule of the knee, that provides medial stability to the knee joint; most frequently injured knee ligament in snowsports.

nonrotational fall Occurs when a skier falls forward over the ski tips, which tends to bend the leg over the front edge of the boot.

phantom foot syndrome A mechanism responsible for anterior cruciate ligament injury when the tail of the ski acts as a lever pointing in a direction opposite to that of the foot. Occurs when the thigh rotates internally when the knee is hyperflexed, as when novices try to stop by sitting down.

Raynaud's syndrome A disease of the hands and feet, characterized by intermittent spasm of the small arteries of the fingers and toes caused by exposure to cold.

rotational fall A fall that causes the foot to turn outward, forcing the leg outward at the knee.

scaphoid A proximal boat-shaped bone of the carpus (bones of the wrist joint) on the radial side.

shoulder separation Usually caused by a direct blow or hard fall onto the shoulder that forces the acromion part of the scapula forward and tears the ligaments that attach it to the clavicle.

skier's thumb A sprain or fracture of the structures at the base of the thumb that occurs when the thumb is bent backward during a fall.

skier's toe Characterized by pain in the big toe caused by repeated dorsiflexion.

snowboarder's ankle Fracture of the talus (the support structure for both the tibia and fibula).

talus A bone of the foot that forms the distal portion of the ankle joint and supports the tibia and fibula.

tension pneumothorax An expanding collection of air outside the lung that places pressure on the heart and blood vessels.

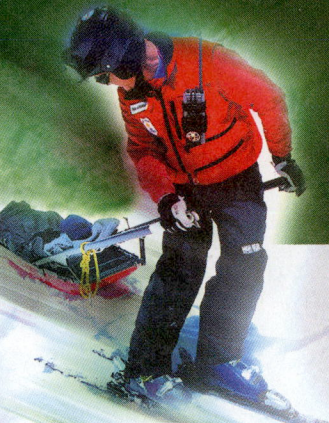

Assessment in Action

A 24-year-old male mountain biker was attempting to bunny-hop a log. The back wheel of the bike failed to clear the log, causing the cyclist to be thrown over the handlebars and hit the ground on his right shoulder. When you arrive, he is alert and sitting on the ground cradling his right arm against his chest. Upon inspection, you find he has tenderness and there is a deformity on the anterior portion of his shoulder.

1. Appropriate assessment for this patient includes performing:
   A. the initial assessment only.
   B. the scene size-up.
   C. a series of decisions about treatment and transport.
   D. a detailed physical exam on the scene.

2. What injuries do you suspect?
   A. Shoulder dislocation
   B. Fractured ulna
   C. Respiratory problems
   D. Sprained ankle

3. What injuries would you rule out before making a transportation decision?
   A. Bleeding and abrasions
   B. Fractured clavicle
   C. Head and neck injuries
   D. Dislocation

4. Assuming his only injury is to the shoulder area, what emergency care would you give?
   A. Transport while the patient holds his arm.
   B. Backboard
   C. Air splint on arm
   D. Sling and swathe

5. Given this circumstance, what function should be checked during assessment, after splinting, and following transport?
   A. Check respirations.
   B. Check nervous, circulatory, and motor function distally.
   C. Check scene for mechanism of injury.
   D. Check number of rescuers to assist.

Points to Ponder

You find a 34-year-old beginner skier who decided to go to the top of the mountain after lunch. She said she caught the inside edge of her downhill ski when she tumbled forward. She said her foot rotated in and her knee popped. She cannot put weight on the knee. What injury do you suspect and why? How would you stabilize her injury if the leg is straight or if the leg is bent? How would you transport her in the toboggan?

Issues Patient Comfort; Scene Management; Best Care for Patient; Incident Investigation; Transport Decisions

Online Outlook

There are many studies on types of injuries for various outdoor sports. Many of these statistics can help focus your training on the injuries that are most prevalent in your sport. These can guide your decisions on types of equipment necessary to best handle these emergencies in the outdoor environment. To improve your knowledge of outdoor sports emergencies, complete Exercise 14 at www.OECzone.com

www.OECzone.com

Environmental Emergencies

Objectives

Cognitive

🌲 **1.** List the signs and symptoms of exposure to cold (p 414).

🌲 **2.** Explain the steps in providing emergency medical care to a patient exposed to cold (p 419).

🌲 **3.** List the signs and symptoms of high altitude illnesses (p 426).

🌲 **4.** Explain the steps in providing emergency care to a patient suffering from a high altitude illness (p 428).

🌲 **5.** Explain the steps in providing emergency care for an avalanche victim (p 441).

6. Describe the various ways that the body loses heat (p 431).

🌲 **7.** List the signs and symptoms of exposure to heat (p 432).

🌲 **8.** Explain the steps in providing emergency care to a patient suffering from heat exposure (p 432).

🌲 **9.** Explain the steps in providing emergency care for a patient who has been struck by lightning or received an electrical injury (p 436).

🌲 **10.** Recognize the signs and symptoms of water-related emergencies (p 437).

11. Describe the complications of near drowning (p 437).

Affective

None.

Psychomotor

🌲 **12.** Demonstrate the assessment and emergency care of a patient with exposure to cold (p 418).

🌲 **13.** Demonstrate the assessment and emergency care of a patient with high altitude illnesses (p 428).

🌲 **14.** Demonstrate the assessment and emergency care of an avalanche victim (p 441).

🌲 **15.** Demonstrate the assessment and emergency care of a patient suffering from heat exposure (p 432).

🌲 **16.** Demonstrate the assessment and emergency care of a patient affected by lightning or electrical exposure (p 436).

17. Demonstrate the assessment and emergency care of a near-drowning patient (p 437).

18. Demonstrate completing a prehospital care report for patients with environmental emergencies (p 77–78).

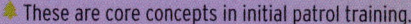 These are core concepts in initial patrol training.

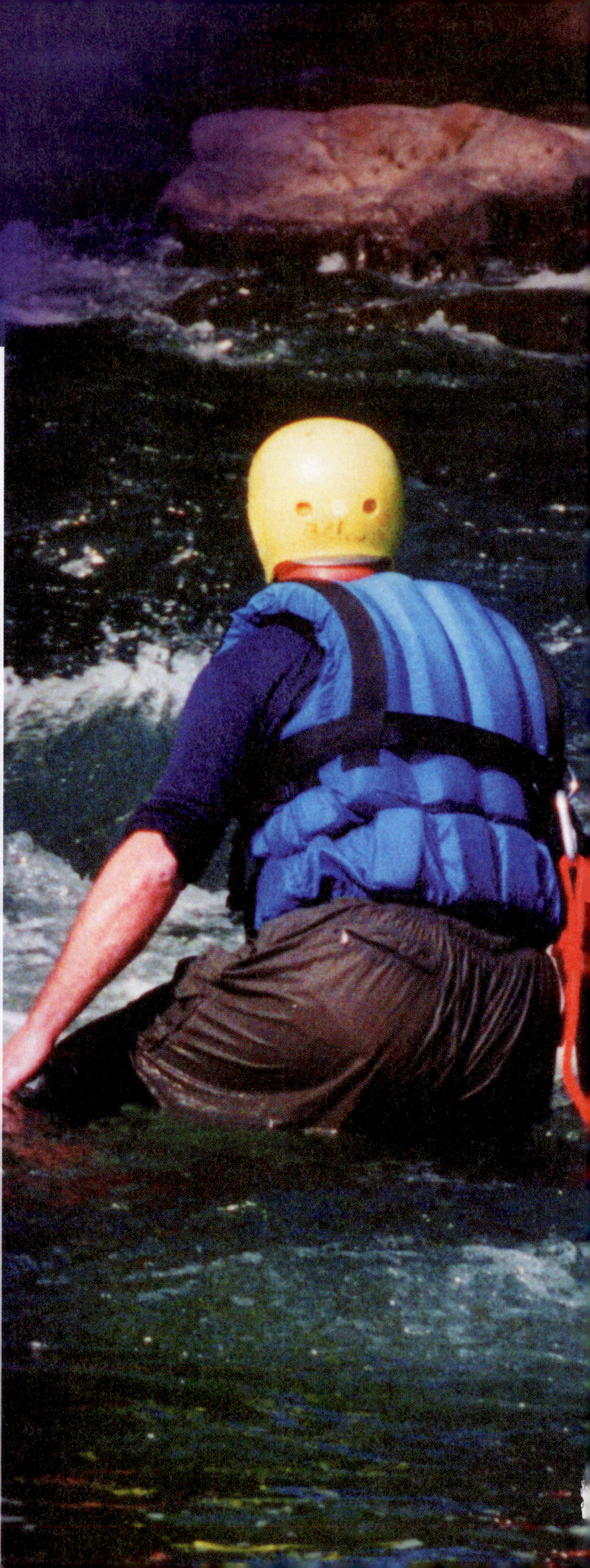

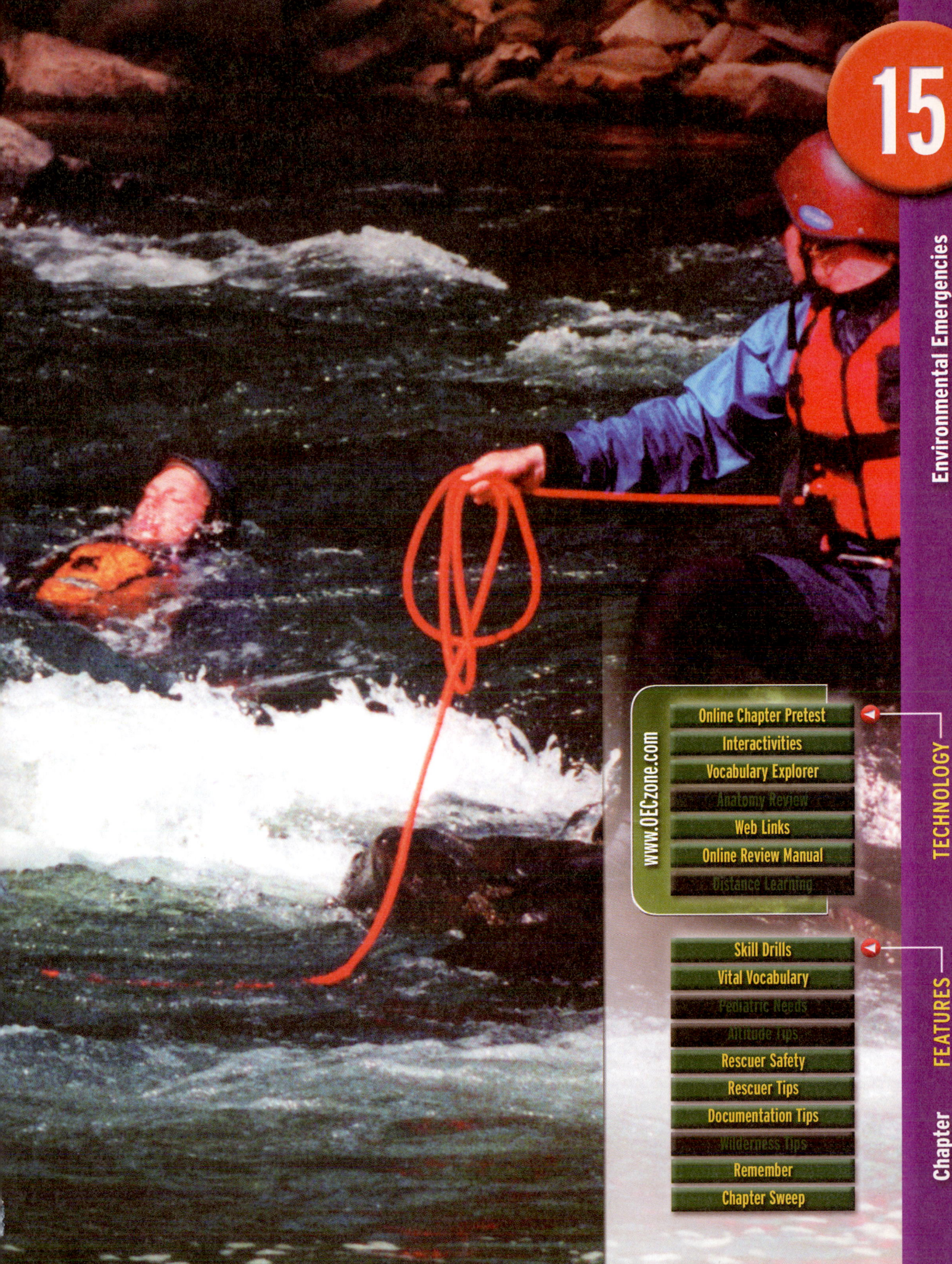

Chapter

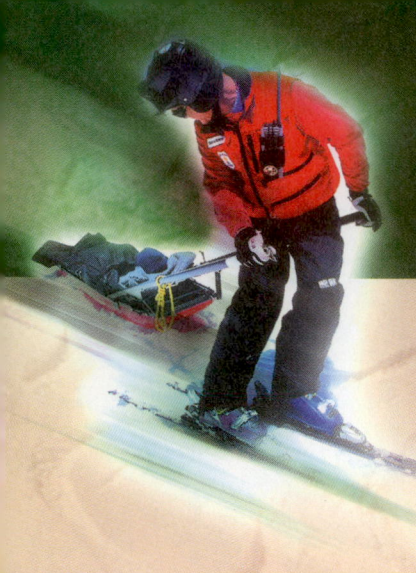

It is 3:25 pm and you are assigned to ski Thruway, an intermediate trail. The day began as a combination of bright sunshine obscured for short periods with heavy snow showers. The temperature has not risen above 28° F and the afternoon winds are blowing in a cold front. Partway down Thruway, you stop to investigate a skier sitting on the side of the trail. As you size up the scene, you observe an approximately 30-year-old man dressed in jeans and a windbreaker. The jeans are damp and the lower legs of the jeans are frozen solid and caked with packed snow. As you get closer to the skier you notice two quarter-size white patches, one on each cheek. The skier does not give any signs to acknowledge your presence. He is only minimally responsive, sitting motionless and staring out into the trail. You introduce yourself and ask to assist him. He responds in slow, slurred speech. It is at this time that you notice the odor of alcohol on the skier's breath.

Regardless of where you work as a rescuer, environmental emergencies will be a part of your regular duties. This chapter will provide information necessary to care for patients with an environmental emergency and help you answer the following questions:

1. How does heat exhaustion differ from heatstroke?

2. Are there differences between the signs and symptoms of a patient with acute hypothermia when compared to a patient with chronic hypothermia?

Environmental Emergencies

Heat and cold both can overwhelm the body's mechanisms for regulating temperature, including sweating and radiation of body heat into the atmosphere. A variety of medical emergencies can result from exposure to heat or cold, particularly when an individual is involved in snowsports and other recreational activities in wilderness and high altitude environments. There is also a range of medical emergencies that arise from water recreation, and these can sometimes be complicated by the cold. These emergencies include localized injuries and systemic illnesses. As a rescuer, you can save lives by recognizing and responding properly to these emergencies, most of which require prompt treatment in the hospital.

This chapter describes how the body regulates core temperature and the ways in which body heat is lost to the environment. It then discusses the various forms of heat-, cold-, high-altitude-, and water-related emergencies, including how to assess and treat hypothermia, hyperthermia, and snow and water injuries.

Cold Exposure

Normal body temperature must be maintained within a very narrow range for the body's chemistry to work efficiently. If the body, or any part of it, is exposed to cold environments, these mechanisms may be overwhelmed. Cold exposure may cause injury to individual parts of the body, such as the feet, hands, ears, or nose, or to

the body as a whole. When the entire body temperature falls, the condition is called **hypothermia**. The process of how the body loses heat is covered in Chapter 2: The Well-Being of the Rescuer.

Hypothermia

Hypothermia, or "exhaustion-exposure," refers to cooling of the central part of the body to a **core temperature** below 95°F (35°C) as determined by a low-reading core thermometer (usually a rectal thermometer). Hypothermia can occur at temperatures well above freezing, and at temperatures below freezing, the patient may suffer frostbite as well. The combination of cold, wind, and water is especially dangerous, as in being stranded in a blizzard at temperatures near or below 32°F (0°C) or falling into a mountain stream. Hypothermia has complicated many natural disasters, such as earthquakes occurring during cold months of the year. In addition, it is a factor in about a third of the 8,000 drowning deaths that occur yearly in the United States.

When the human body temperature falls progressively, all body functions tend to diminish or slow. The initial drop of one to two degrees triggers shivering, followed by clumsiness, stumbling, falling, slow reactions, mental confusion, and difficulty in speaking (▶ Table 15-1). The patient frequently is unaware of what is happening. Impaired use of the hands is very serious because it hampers attempts to put on more clothing, set up shelter, or light a fire. At body temperatures below 90°F (32.2°C), shivering gradually ceases and the muscles become progressively more rigid. The breathing rate and pulse rate slow, and the patient becomes irrational and gradually becomes unresponsive. Death may occur at body temperatures below 80°F (26.6°C).

It is important to consider the possibility of hypothermia when dangerous environmental conditions exist, since hypothermia is an insidious condition that is difficult to recognize in its early stages and death can occur within 2 hours of the onset of symptoms. Other members of a party may not realize that a companion is hypothermic because they are becoming hypothermic themselves. When the body is too cold to be capable of shivering, it cannot warm itself in a cold environment without outside help. Methods for preventing hypothermia are discussed in Chapter 2.

Hypothermia is potentially lethal. The mortality rate is greater than 50% in severe cases and may approach 100% in those complicated by injuries or previous illnesses. The most common cause of death is ventricular fibrillation, which can occur spontaneously at body temperatures of 77°F (25°C) or below, or can be precipitated by a sudden jolt at higher body temperatures. However, with proper emergency care, the mortality rate from hypothermia should be low in otherwise healthy

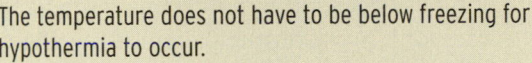

Remember

The temperature does not have to be below freezing for hypothermia to occur.

patients with core (rectal) temperatures at or above 90°F (32.2°C).

A patient with severe hypothermia may appear to be dead, with fixed and dilated pupils, undetectable pulse and breathing, and body rigidity resembling rigor mortis. However, the patient may still be saved with proper emergency care. The dictum "No one is dead until warm and dead" (coined by US Army hypothermia expert Murray Hamlet) emphasizes that rewarming should be considered in any patient with hypothermia.

Patrollers should watch for the development of hypothermia in skiers or snowboarders stranded on stalled chairlifts and persons lying or standing in the snow for long periods, such as accident victims and gatekeepers at ski races. An injury impairs the body's heat conservation mechanisms, making an injured

TABLE 15-1 Signs and Symptoms of Hypothermia

	°F	°C	Signs and Symptoms
Mild Hypothermia	98–95	36.6–35	Patient feels chilly and has some difficulty using his or her hands. Shivering begins.
	95–90	35–32.2	Shivering increases and becomes violent. Patient stumbles and exhibits loss of coordination, weakness, difficulty speaking, slow thinking, and mild confusion.
Severe Hypothermia	90–86	32.2–30	Shivering ceases and muscles become stiff. The patient is incoherent and is unable to stand or walk. Exposed skin is blue or puffy. Movements are jerky. Senses are dulled, but the patient is still able to maintain posture and the appearance of contact with surroundings.
	86–80	30–26.6	Patient exhibits impaired responsiveness and has dilated pupils. Breathing and pulse slow down.
	Below 80	Below 26.6	Patient is unresponsive and rigid. Pulse is unobtainable and breathing is very slow. Ventricular fibrillation, asystole, and death occur.

patient more susceptible to cold injury as well. Cold temperatures and high altitude increase the risk of shock, which predisposes the injured patient to further chilling, making frostbite and hypothermia more likely. One key to care for a hypothermic patient is putting insulating material beneath and over patients and providing protection (shelter) from the wind.

Types of Hypothermia

Hypothermia can be divided according to duration of exposure into three categories: acute (less than an hour), subacute (1 to 24 hours), and chronic (a day or more). These distinctions are somewhat arbitrary but significant, because although at first there is a large difference between the core and shell temperatures, as time passes the core temperature becomes closer to the shell temperature. Also, in acute hypothermia, blood glucose levels are normal or slightly elevated, and the blood electrolyte levels and acid-base balance (pH) are still normal or only slightly disturbed. In subacute and chronic hypothermia, the blood glucose level falls and the patient tends to become acidotic due to shivering and starvation.

Mild Hypothermia

A hypothermic person whose rectal temperature is 90°F (32°C) or above can be rewarmed by any of the previously listed means that are available or can be improvised. Self-warming by shivering in a sleeping bag placed out of the wind is probably the method of choice for the well-nourished patient in good physical condition who can shiver vigorously. However, shivering is a mixed blessing since it uses considerable energy and is exhausting. If body-to-body warming is used, the "heat donor" must be given food and fluids while "working" and should be replaced if he or she becomes cold.

Small devices that concentrate heat, such as canteens of hot water, chemical heating pads, and hot rocks, should be wrapped to prevent burns and placed against areas of high heat loss, such as the sides of the chest, sides of the neck, and the groin ▶ Figure 15-1 .

Rescue groups usually carry some of the more sophisticated rewarming devices. Under more civilized conditions, more active rewarming devices such as a hot tub (at 105°F to 110°F [41°C to 43°C]), an electric blanket, or several electric heating pads can be used. When the patient is able to swallow, give him or her hot, sweet liquids, which not only boost morale but combat dehydration. Avoid giving the patient alcohol and caffeine; being diuretics, they can promote dehydration.

After rewarming, it is best to make camp and allow the patient (and the others in the party) to rest overnight before proceeding.

Severe Hypothermia

The mortality rate outside a hospital is high for patients who have a rectal temperature below 90°F (32°C), mainly because of the frequency of ventricular fibrillation and the development of serious metabolic and electrolyte problems that cannot be detected or treated in the field. Patients who can be cared for in a hospital have a greater chance of survival because personnel can discover, monitor, and treat these problems rapidly and rewarm the patient under controlled conditions in an intensive care unit.

Because serious complications may develop during rewarming, the best field results are obtained by *stabilizing the core temperature by preventing further heat loss and transporting the patient rapidly to medical care* rather than attempting aggressive field rewarming.

Patients with body temperatures below 90°F (32°C) will be relatively stable for a time if treated gently and not allowed to cool further. Prevent additional heat loss by applying heat through one of the slow rewarming methods listed. Do not use fast rewarming methods such as a hot tub or electric blanket set on medium or high.

Individuals with subacute and chronic hypothermia are dehydrated, partly because cooling increases urine

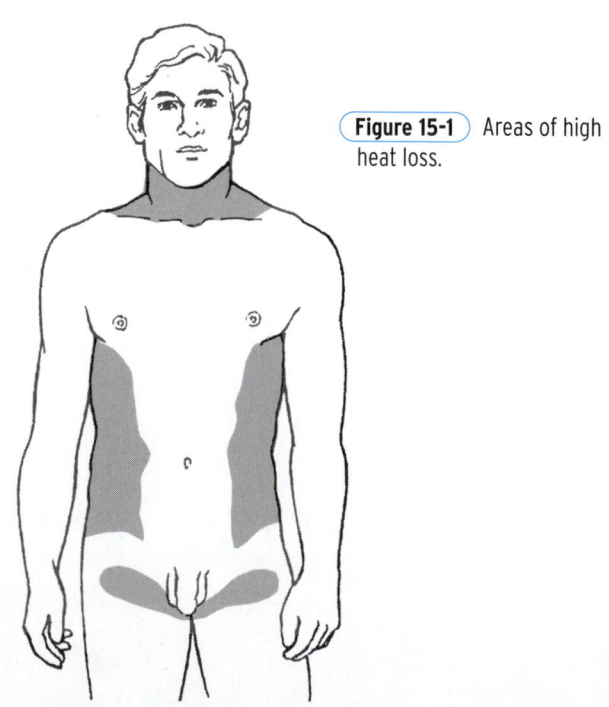

Figure 15-1 Areas of high heat loss.

production. If appropriate equipment and properly trained rescuers are available, give the patient warmed IV fluids, such as 5% glucose in normal saline.

The colder patients will have slow respirations and low blood pressure. Because these signs are "normal" under the circumstances, rescue breathing and aggressive treatment of shock are rarely indicated. Any rescue breathing should be performed via mouth-to-mask rather than via bag-valve-mask because the patient will benefit from the warmth of the rescuer's lungs.

Patients with severe hypothermia may appear to be in cardiac arrest or dead because their pulse and respirations are so difficult to detect. Spend several minutes attempting to find these vital signs before concluding that they are absent.

CPR may actually *precipitate* ventricular fibrillation in a patient with a pulse that is weak or slow enough to be undetectable. Therefore, do not give CPR unless *careful examination* reveals no signs of life, or you strongly suspect ventricular fibrillation because of a sudden event, such as collapse of the patient or loss of a previously detected heartbeat. In very cold patients, CPR may be impossible because the chest is incompressible. In any case, transport to medical care is more important than CPR. An exception to this is the patient with submersion hypothermia, in which case CPR should be started as soon as possible according to standard protocols.

Once begun, CPR should be continued at the normal rate until the patient is hospitalized. Patients who have suffered cardiac arrest due to hypothermia have survived after receiving CPR for several hours. This suggests that they may have a more favorable outlook than patients with cardiac arrest due to other causes.

Before transport, make sure the patient is stable, splint fractures, and treat other injuries using standard methods. Move the patient slowly and carefully, avoiding sudden jolts. Prevent further cooling during transportation by using portable, self-contained, slow rewarming devices that do not require constant monitoring, such as the Heatpac, a battery or propane-operated airway rewarming device, or chemical heating pads.

Obviously, a rapid transport method, such as helicopter evacuation, is preferable to a long, bumpy toboggan or over-snow vehicle ride. If possible, take the patient to a hospital known to have facilities for rewarming patients with severe hypothermia (such as cardiopulmonary bypass capability).

If the party is too small to evacuate a patient with severe hypothermia, send for help and provide slow rewarming in a tent or snow shelter. The best method is probably body-to-body contact in a sleeping bag.

Documentation Tips

Recording specific results of your early assessment is particularly valuable in hypothermic patients. If there is a question about beginning CPR, note where you checked the pulse and for how long. Also note the initial body temperature and where it was taken. These points will be important to hospital staff, and will help protect you if medicolegal issues are ever raised.

Every situation is different, however, and the course of action depends on the weather, the size and physical condition of the party, its equipment, the terrain, and the distance to definitive medical help. Remember that care of a patient with hypothermia requires the combined efforts of several people: one to give body-to-body contact, one to set up shelter, one to build a fire, and at least two to get help. Be sure that other party members do not compound the problem by becoming hypothermic themselves.

Severity of Hypothermia

Hypothermia severity can be classified according to the patient's core temperature as mild (90°F [32.2°C] and above) and severe (below 90°F [32.2°C]). This division is useful because emergency care differs according to severity, as described shortly.

Different types of hypothermia are characterized by the well-recognized settings in which they occur. Following are the various types and their causes.

1. Immersion hypothermia is caused by immersion in cold water. It usually is acute or subacute when seen. This type of hypothermia develops rapidly (over one to several hours) because of the ability of cold water to conduct heat away from the body about 25 times more rapidly than cold air. A similar setting is the combination of cold rain and high wind.

2. Field hypothermia occurs outdoors in previously healthy individuals such as off-area skiers and snowboarders, climbers, and lost hikers and hunters. It is usually subacute or chronic because of the time required for search operations, and may accompany injuries occurring outdoors in cold weather.

3. Urban hypothermia may occur indoors or outdoors in cities and towns. It usually develops in individuals with a physical predisposition, dis-

ability, or illness. Urban hypothermia is usually subacute or chronic when discovered and has a high mortality rate. Predisposing conditions include those that:

- increase heat loss (large surface-area-to-mass ratios in premature and term newborns, infants, and small children; patients with burns or widespread skin disorders).
- interfere with heat production or distribution (malnutrition, anemia, old age, shock, heart disease, diabetes, arteriosclerosis, and endocrine abnormalities such as hypothyroidism).
- interfere with temperature regulation (central nervous system disease and injury, certain drugs).
- interfere with normal judgment (senility, psychosis, drug and alcohol abuse). Homeless people are especially at risk for urban hypothermia during cold spells. Many drugs, including sedatives, tranquilizers, lithium, and beta blockers, can accelerate the development of hypothermia.

4. Submersion hypothermia, a combination of acute hypothermia and hypoxia, is caused by near drowning in cold water. Cooling due to submersion in water of 70°F (21.1°C) or below appears to protect the central nervous system from the effects of hypoxia for a limited period of time; the colder the water, the greater the protection. The more rapid cooling rates of smaller individuals may explain why survival is higher in children and infants than adults. In some rare cases, individuals have survived without neurologic damage after being submerged as long as 66 minutes, usually in very cold (41°F [5°C]) water.

Lastly, don't overlook dehydration, especially in a nordic or backcountry environment, as it is a main contributor to hypothermia.

Assessment of a Patient with Suspected Hypothermia

In the field, it is better to anticipate and watch for hypothermia in patients exposed to dangerous weather conditions so its progression can be halted while the patient is still in its milder stages.

Although hypothermia can be suspected from its signs and symptoms, accurate diagnosis depends on documenting a body core temperature below 95°F (35°C), using a low-reading rectal thermometer

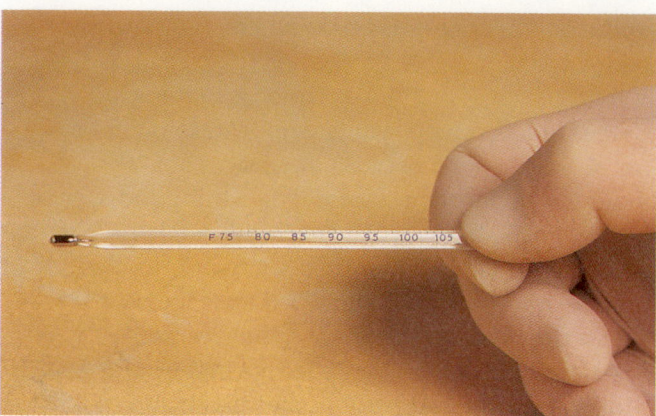

Figure 15-2 A special rectal hypothermia thermometer registers temperatures well below that of a regular thermometer.

▲ **Figure 15-2**). However, for obvious reasons, rescuers are reluctant to take rectal temperatures in the field. An oral temperature may be substituted if the patient is responsive; the thermometer should be left under the tongue for a minimum of 3 minutes. Remember that the temperatures given in this section are rectal temperatures; oral temperatures read 1° lower.

If you do not have a thermometer, the patient's temperature can be estimated by noting his or her mental status and the presence of shivering. If the patient is shivering and capable of appropriate actions such as zipping an open parka and picking up a dropped mitten, the core temperature is probably 90°F (32.2°C) or above. If the patient is no longer shivering and, especially, if responsiveness is altered, the core temperature is likely below 90°F. However, remember that shivering is stressful and will cease after several hours because of a low blood glucose level and exhaustion.

Suspect developing hypothermia when a companion shivers, appears clumsy, stumbles, drops things, has slurred speech, and lags behind. Any person who is found ill, injured, or unresponsive outdoors in cold weather or is removed from cold water should be considered hypothermic until proven otherwise.

An assessment of hypothermia starts with the scene size-up. Upon approaching the patient, consider the following questions. Do conditions predispose to hypothermia? Has the patient obviously been injured? What has probably happened? Does the patient have an altered mental status? Before going further, institute BSI precautions.

Next, perform the initial assessment, assessing the patient's level of responsiveness and ABCs. Remember that in profound hypothermia, the pulse may be weak and very slow and the patient may be breathing only

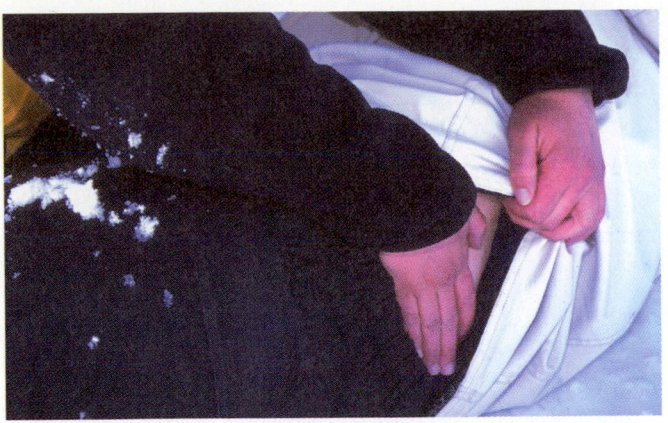

Figure 15-3 If a thermometer is not available, feel the patient's skin inside the clothing.

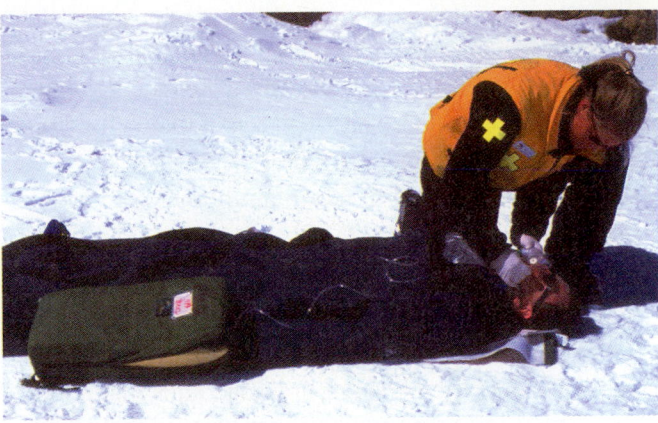

Figure 15-4 Place dry blankets over and under the hypothermia patient; give warm, humidified oxygen; assess the pulse before considering CPR.

a few times a minute. Take more time than you normally would to assess breathing and pulse. Do not start CPR prematurely (as addressed earlier in this chapter). Take the patient's temperature or, if a thermometer is not available, feel the skin of the patient's back inside the clothing (▲ **Figure 15-3**). Cold skin indicates hypothermia.

Before performing the rapid body survey, take measures to stabilize the patient's body temperature and prevent further cooling.

Emergency Care of a Patient with Hypothermia

The principles of emergency care for a patient with hypothermia are as follows:

1. Stabilize the body temperature by preventing further heat loss.

2. Rewarm the patient as safely as possible.

3. Rewarm the body core in advance of the shell, if possible.

4. Treat the patient gently to avoid precipitating ventricular fibrillation.

5. If the patient can swallow, give warm fluids to correct dehydration.

The application of these principles depends on the patient's core temperature, the equipment available, and the presence of complicating factors such as other illnesses or injuries.

The first priority is to stabilize the body temperature and prevent further heat loss by getting the patient out of the wind or water and into a tent or other shelter. If the patient's clothing is wet, gently exchange it for dry clothing if available. Place the patient in a sleeping bag or place a blanket or spare clothing under and over the

patient. Because a great deal of heat can be lost through the head, be sure to cover the patient's head and neck ▲ **Figure 15-4** .

If clothing is wet and no dry clothing is available, wrap something windproof, such as a poncho, around the patient to reduce evaporative cooling. Because of the risk of ventricular fibrillation precipitated by a sudden jolt to a cold, acidotic heart, avoid unnecessary handling and do not allow the patient to sit, stand, or walk until he or she has been rewarmed. It may be better to cut off wet clothing than to undress a severely hypothermic patient, but do not destroy clothing that may be needed later.

Meanwhile, build a fire or light a stove. Further emergency care depends on the patient's measured or estimated body core temperature. (▶ **Table 15-2**) summarizes emergency care of the hypothermic patient.

Rewarming Methods

Because the numbing effects of cold on the nerves in the skin make hypothermic patients less aware of temperature, they are more subject to burns than are uninjured individuals. During rewarming, always monitor the effects of rewarming devices by periodically testing them on yourself.

Rewarming methods, which can be quite limited in the field, are divided into fast and slow methods. Fast methods provide large amounts of heat rapidly and are frequently water-based systems because water has the highest specific heat of any common substance except hydrogen (1 calorie per gram per degree Celsius). This is about five times greater than the specific heat of dry air. Thus, as warm water cools, a large amount of heat is transferred to the body if in contact with the skin. Fast rewarming devices suitable for field use include the following:

1. The "hydraulic sarong," a homemade device in which a backpacking stove is used to heat a pot of water. A bilge pump then circulates the hot water through plastic tubes sewn into a blanket wrapped around the patient's trunk (▶ **Figure 15-5**).

2. Bathtubs (found in mountain homes or cabins) filled with hot water.

3. Electric blankets (using electricity available in campgrounds, mountain cabins, etc).

Fast rewarming is accomplished in hospitals by use of hot tubs, electric blankets, and machines that circulate warmed fluid through a rubber blanket that is wrapped around the patient. Other hospital means of rewarming include devices that blow hot air over the patient, peritoneal dialysis (pumping warmed fluid in and out of the peritoneal cavity), and direct warming of the blood using a heart-lung machine.

Slow methods are more likely to be non–water-based. They provide less heat and therefore rewarm the patient more slowly. In many cases, their main value may be to prevent further cooling.

Means of accomplishing slow rewarming in the field include the following:

1. Allowing a mildly hypothermic patient to rewarm by shivering inside a prewarmed sleeping bag. For more serious cases, wrap the patient in non-binding clothing including head covering; provide plenty of insulation underneath, or wrap the sleeping bag in a tarp or space blanket.

2. Body-to-body contact, in which one or two rescuers get into a sleeping bag with the patient, all stripped to the waist. This method, however, is less effective than vigorous shivering.

3. Canteens filled with hot water placed against the patient's body in areas where heat is lost, and wrapped well to prevent burning.

4. Hot rocks placed against the patient's body in areas where heat is lost, and wrapped well to prevent burning.

5. Chemical heating pads (▶ **Figure 15-6**). Despite their popularity, chemical heating pads deliver little heat (less than 15 kcal per medium-sized pad), but they can help if placed in strategic positions, eg, the side of the neck, over carotid arteries.

6. Devices for delivering heated, humidified air or oxygen to the lungs (▶ **Figure 15-7**).

7. A small, lightweight stove that can deliver 250 watts of heat for several hours using a charcoal cartridge for fuel (▶ **Figure 15-8**).

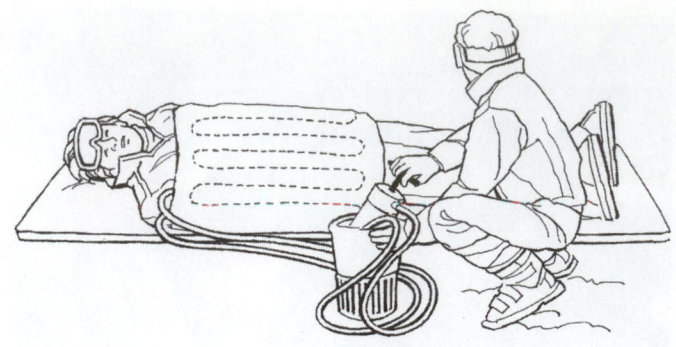

Figure 15-5 The "hydraulic sarong," in which a backpacking stove is used to heat water that is then circulated by a pump through plastic tubes sewn in the blanket.

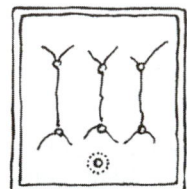

Figure 15-6 Chemical heating pad.

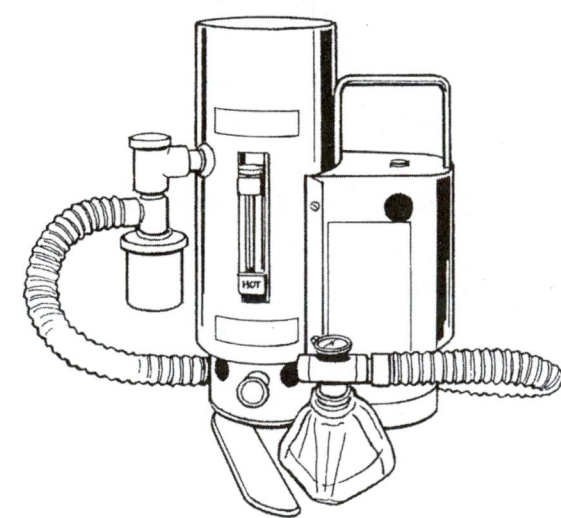

Figure 15-7 Portable device for delivering heated, humidified air or oxygen to the lungs.

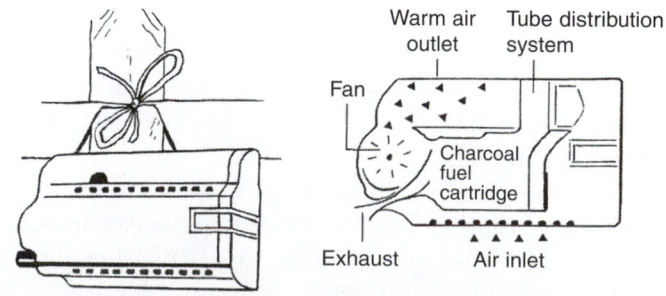

Figure 15-8 A small, lightweight stove that can deliver 250 watts of heat for several hours using a charcoal cartridge for fuel.

Table 15-2 Summary of Emergency Care of a Hypothermic Patient

General measures

1. Stop further heat loss:
   a. Get the patient out of the wind and into a tent or other shelter.
   b. Build a fire or start a stove.
   c. Add insulation beneath and around the patient. Cover the patient's head and neck.
   d. Replace wet clothing with dry clothing.
   e. Watch for hypothermia in other party members.

2. Treat the patient gently. Do not allow the patient to move about until rewarmed.

3. Hydrate with warm, sweet liquids after the patient is alert, awake, and able to swallow.

4. Treat any injuries.

Specific measures for mild hypothermia
(core temperature 90°F [32.2°C] or above, shivering, mental status normal)

1. Raise core temperature by whatever means available:
   a. Self-rewarming by shivering inside a sleeping bag if able to shiver vigorously.
   b. Hot rocks or canteens placed against high heat loss areas, wrapped to prevent burns.
   c. Body-to-body contact in a sleeping bag.
   d. Rescue-team equipment (eg, hydraulic sarong, heating pads, a lightweight stove, airway rewarming devices).
   e. Civilization (eg, hot tub or electric blanket).

Specific measures for severe hypothermia
(core temperature below 90°F [32.2°C], absence of shivering, altered mental status)

1. Prevent further cooling by using one of the slow-rewarming methods. Avoid fast rewarming in the field. Use portable devices such as a lightweight stove, airway rewarming devices, and heating pads during evacuation.

2. Treat dehydration with warm fluids if the patient is able to swallow or warmed IV fluids if equipment and expertise are available.

3. Avoid jostling and jolting the patient during transportation, as ventricular fibrillation can occur.

4. Avoid performing CPR unless ventricular fibrillation occurs. The exception is near-drowning (submersion hypothermia), in which case you should follow standard CPR protocols.

5. If the patient cannot be evacuated, use slow rewarming methods, such as body-to-body heat in a shelter, and send for help.

Although the delivery of heated air or oxygen to the lungs would seem to be an ideal way to rewarm the core of the patient's body, studies have shown that the amount of heat actually delivered is small and the main value of the method is probably to prevent loss of heat from the airway. Nevertheless, its use is supported by considerable field experience, and patients usually report feeling warmer when breathing hot, humidified air or oxygen. If electricity is available, an electric blanket set on low also can rewarm the patient slowly.

Slow methods suitable for hospital use include covering the patient with blankets in a warm room and delivering heated, humidified oxygen to the lungs with a machine designed to administer anesthesia. In a hospital, slow and fast methods usually are combined; for instance, a patient may be given warmed oxygen while a special machine blows warm air over the patient's entire body or the patient is further warmed by fluid circulating through a rubber blanket.

Recreational parties must generally rely on slow, improvised methods of rewarming, such as shivering, canteens filled with hot water, hot rocks, and body-to-body contact in a sleeping bag. Rescue groups can carry a hydraulic sarong, a lightweight stove, chemical heating pads, and devices for airway rewarming.

Regardless of the nature or severity of the cold injury, remember that even an unresponsive patient may be able to hear you. Some patients have told of hearing themselves pronounced dead by someone who had forgotten the old saying: "No one is dead unless he is warm and dead." If you carry an AED, you should consider defibrillation, although a heart that is chilled into ventricular fibrillation cannot be shocked back into its natural rhythm until it is rewarmed to a temperature at which it can function.

Local Cold Injuries

Most injuries from cold are confined to exposed or distal parts of the body. The extremities, particularly the feet, and the exposed ears, nose, and face, are especially vulnerable to cold injury (▼ **Figure 15-9**). When exposed parts of the body become very cold but not frozen, the condition is called frostnip, chilblains, or immersion foot (trench foot). When the parts become frozen, the injury is called **frostbite**.

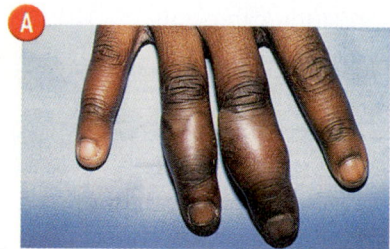
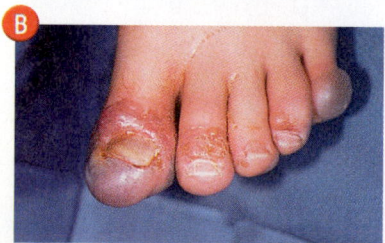
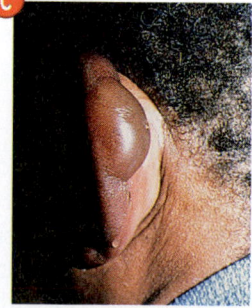

Figure 15-9 The extremities and the ears, nose, and face are particularly susceptible to frostbite.

You should try to find out the duration of the exposure, the temperature to which the body part was exposed, and the wind velocity during exposure. These are important factors in determining the severity of a local cold injury. You should also investigate a number of underlying factors:

- Exposure to wet conditions
- Inadequate insulation from cold or wind
- Restricted circulation from tight clothing or boots or circulatory disease
- Fatigue
- Poor nutrition
- Alcohol or drug abuse
- Hypothermia
- Diabetes
- Cardiovascular disease
- Older age

In hypothermia, blood is shunted away from the extremities in an attempt to maintain the core temperature. This shunting of blood increases the risk of local cold injury to the extremities, ears, nose, and face. Thus, the patient with hypothermia should also be assessed for frostbite or other local cold injury. The reverse is also true. You must remember that both local and systemic cold exposure problems can occur in the same patient.

Frostbite

Frostbite, the actual freezing of a body part, occurs when the heat produced by the part, the heat carried to it by the blood, and the amount of insulation covering it are insufficient to prevent its temperature from falling below the freezing point of body tissue (about 24.8°F, or ¯4°C). The amount of total damage depends on the extent and duration of freezing at the tissue level. The earlier frostbite can be discovered, the better the results of emergency care.

The risk of frostbite is increased by the body's tendency, when exposed to cold, to guard the temperature of vital, internal organs (the core) by restricting the flow of warm blood to the skin, muscles, and extremities (the shell).

Certain body tissues have a higher risk of frostbite than others. The hands, feet, ears, cheeks, nose, and male genitals are all located far from the heart at the periphery of the body and rapidly lose heat because of their large surface area-to-mass ratio (volume) and poorly protected positions.

Other factors that contribute to the development of frostbite include inadequate insulation, high wind, wet clothing, fatigue, poor nutrition, apathy, alcohol and drug use, smoking, and contact with metal or hydrocarbon liquids such as gasoline. Decreased peripheral circulation due to atherosclerosis (seen in patients with diabetes and the elderly), swelling from injury, shock, blood vessel spasm, and tight footwear may also be a contributing factor in some cases.

Frostbite frequently occurs in unprepared persons who are unfamiliar with the hazards of cold, wind, and wetness, and who misinterpret the subtle differences between a painfully cold or numb body part and a frozen one. A positive attitude is apparently a useful force in combating cold-weather injury—partly because the person is more likely not to neglect obvious preventive measures.

As the skin cools, the following progressive changes occur:

1. Blood vessels constrict.

2. Walls of capillaries and other small blood vessels are damaged. This allows plasma to leak into the surrounding tissues, causing swelling and red cell sludging.

3. Blood circulation in the damaged area slows.

4. Extracellular ice crystals form, causing osmotic changes that damage cells through dehydration, shrinkage, and toxic changes in electrolyte concentrations. Proteins and other important substances become denatured (ie, their molecular structure is modified, thus altering their original properties).

5. Nerve injury causes pain followed by numbness.

6. Clots form in small blood vessels, causing further decrease in tissue circulation. A lack of blood supply causes cell damage and, ultimately, tissue death.

Toxic substances produced by injured cells increase tissue damage ▲ **Figure 15-10** . These substances can be found in high concentration in the blister fluid of persons with frostbite.

As frostbite thaws, the appearance of the injured part depends largely on the degree of blood vessel injury. When vessel injury is limited to minor damage to vessel walls, plasma but not red cells leaks out into the surrounding tissues, causing edema in mild cases and large blebs and blisters containing pale or yellow fluid in more extensive cases. More severe vessel

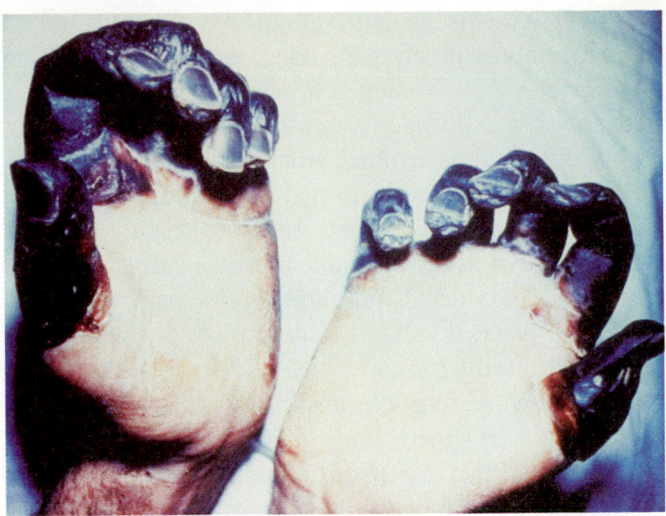

Figure 15-10   Gangrene, or permanent cell death, can occur when tissue is frozen and certain chemical changes occur in the cells.

injury allows red cells to leak out as well, producing smaller blisters containing dark reddish or purple fluid. When there has been extensive spasm and clotting, very little blood can reenter the injured area, blisters are small or absent, and the tissues quickly become gangrenous.

It is difficult to predict the severity of injury when frostbite is first seen. A definitive assessment may require observation over a period of time and special equipment found only in a hospital. Similar to the situation with burns, several levels of damage can exist side by side in an affected body part, ranging from the most superficial to full-thickness freezing of an entire body part.

Types of Frostbite

Frostbite may be hard to classify before a frostbitten area has thawed. The most common, mildest local cold injury is called **frostnip**. This is a cold-induced area of superficial blood vessel constriction. Although there may be a few ice crystals on the skin surface, the skin is still soft and there is no actual freezing of tissue. A patient with frostnip feels a mild tingling or pain followed by numbness. Inspection reveals a gray or yellowish patch of skin, usually on the nose, ear, cheek, finger, or toe. The tissues beneath the area remain soft and pliable. This type of injury is common in poorly dressed schoolchildren, cold-weather joggers, and skiers or snowboarders riding chairlifts on very cold, windy days. After warming, the affected part is tender, pink, warm, and may be shiny or slightly swollen. Since the injury involves only the superficial skin layers, blisters do not form.

True frostbite is actual freezing of a body part and most commonly involves the hands or feet. In superficial frostbite only the skin is frozen; in **deep frostbite** both the skin and underlying tissues are frozen, including muscles, tendons, and bones.

Frostbite should be suspected if a painfully cold part suddenly stops hurting when it obviously is not getting warmer. The skin is not pliable and the affected part is cold, solid, "wooden," and numb, with a pale, waxy color ▶**Figure 15-11**). It resembles a piece of chicken just removed from the freezer.

After thawing, large blisters filled with clear or yellow fluid develop in superficial frostbite and smaller blisters filled with reddish or purple fluid in the less severe cases of deep frostbite. In the worst cases, the skin is puffy and turns dark purple, blisters are absent, and **gangrene** develops within a few days. In milder cases the part is painful; in more severe cases with extensive nerve damage there is complete loss of sensation.

The severe environmental conditions that cause frostbite are also the conditions that make it difficult to discover frostbite early. Because the patient is concerned mainly with survival, mittens, boots, and socks are difficult to remove for assessment and optimal emergency care is a challenge.

Assessment and Emergency Care of Frostbite

Identification of frostnip is based on the findings on inspection and palpation of the involved area and the patient's typical symptoms in a setting where cold injury might be expected. The appropriate emergency care is to apply direct body heat, eg, place a warm hand on an affected cheek or hold an affected finger in an armpit, either the patient's or your own. The heat applied need be no warmer than body temperature. Then, consider why frostnip occurred. The patient may need to add clothing or seek shelter.

Frostbite is a much more serious injury because of the danger of tissue death and permanent damage to surviving tissue. Because the results of emergency care are frequently poor in severe cases, prevention is especially important (see Chapter 2).

Like frostnip, frostbite is also identified by inspection and palpation of the affected body part and the patient's symptoms in a setting where frostbite might be expected. You should also consider the possibility of hypothermia. If the patient is shivering or has an altered mental status, assess as you would for suspected hypothermia (described earlier in this chapter).

Frozen parts rewarmed rapidly recover better than those rewarmed slowly. Therefore, the preferred emer-

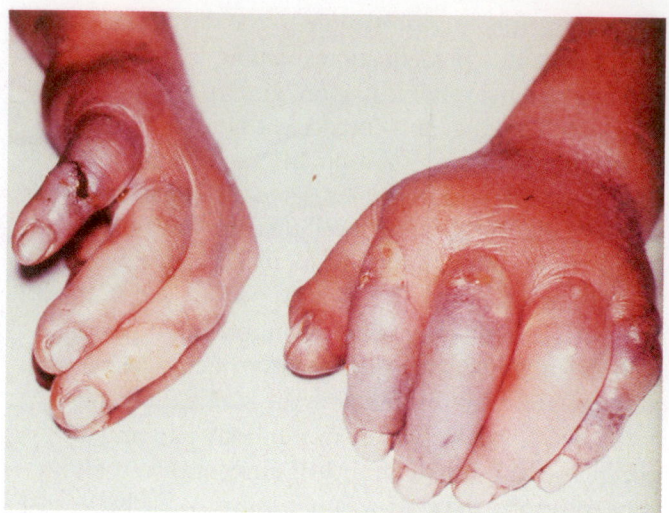

Figure 15-11   Frostbitten parts are hard and usually waxy to touch.

gency care is rapid rewarming in a water bath with the water temperature carefully controlled between 102°F and 108°F (38.8°C and 42.2°C). Cooler water rewarms too slowly; warmer water may burn the tissues.

Rewarming should be done only in a sheltered area where the patient's entire body can be kept warm. You will need a suitable thermometer to test water temperature (a standard clinical thermometer may not read high enough) and a vessel large enough so that the extremity can be immersed without touching the sides of the vessel. A 20-qt pot is a suitable size for rewarming a foot or hand. Remove constricting objects such as rings and bracelets beforehand, as they may compromise circulation when the affected parts begin to swell.

Stir the water occasionally, being careful not to bump the extremity. Monitor the temperature of the bath and, as the water cools, remove the extremity, add hot water, stir, and retest the water temperature before reimmersing the extremity. Continue rewarming for 20 to 30 minutes or until the frozen areas turn deep red or bluish and the color change has progressed distally as far as it will go.

While the frozen part is being rewarmed, give the patient hot drinks and warm the rest of the body to open up circulation to the frostbitten area. Rewarming usually causes severe pain, so you may wish to remind the patient about this and prepare to offer comfort. Patients with frostbite or in danger of frostbite developing should refrain from smoking or chewing tobacco since nicotine interferes with circulation and retards healing.

One of the worst things that can happen to a frostbitten part is for it to refreeze after thawing. *This always leads to gangrene.* Therefore, protect the part from refreezing if at all possible. After thawing, dry the extremity and apply thick layers of sterile dressings held in place by a loosely applied, self-adhering roller bandage. Wrap the part in a parka or blanket, leaving footwear off if the affected part is a foot. Leave blisters unopened, separate digits with nonadhering gauze pads, and elevate the part to reduce swelling. Offer ibuprofen 400 mg (two of the nonprescription tablets) twice daily if it is available.

Unfortunately, frostbite frequently occurs under circumstances in which the party is small and subject to severe environmental stress and where there are no facilities and equipment for proper emergency care. In particular, there may be no suitable thermometer or container large enough for rewarming and, besides, the party's main concern may be to escape alive. In this case, either the patient will have to self-evacuate on foot or the party will have to make camp and send for help, realizing that a frozen foot or hand will likely rewarm spontaneously. It is acceptable to walk out on a freshly thawed foot, if necessary, but all possible efforts must be made to prevent refreezing.

At times, a patient may be unaware that a body part has been frozen until it starts to hurt after thawing. By this time it is too late for rapid rewarming. Assessment of a frostbitten foot requires you to remove the patient's boot, even though it may be difficult to get the boot back on a blistered and swollen thawed foot if the patient must self-evacuate.

The best field care for a patient with frostbite is evacuation to medical care—as fast and as safely as possible. Exercise judgment in deciding whether to rapidly rewarm a frozen extremity in the field. Do not attempt rewarming if the extremity has already rewarmed spontaneously, if you do not have the proper equipment or proper shelter, or if you can obtain medical care within an hour or two. Conversely, rapid field rewarming may be advisable if equipment and shelter are available, if the patient can be carried out or evacuated by vehicle or toboggan, and if there is a good chance the part can be protected from refreezing during evacuation.

In the past, it has been recommended that a patient with a frozen foot try to keep it frozen while walking or skiing out to where it can be rapidly rewarmed under proper conditions. Most experienced authorities disagree with this, based on the difficulty of keeping a foot frozen without putting the entire body in serious danger from hypothermia.

The prevention of frostbite is essentially the process of applying the principles of cold weather survival as outlined in Chapter 2. It is important to be well insu-

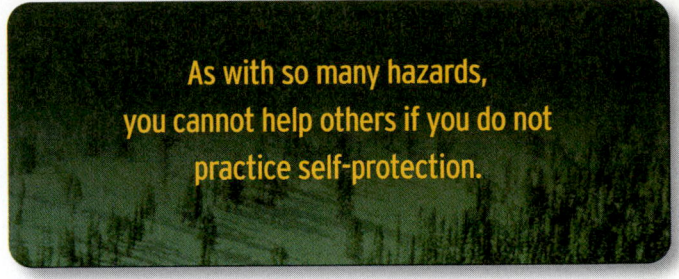

As with so many hazards, you cannot help others if you do not practice self-protection.

lated against the cold and to be rested, well fed, and well hydrated. Do not go out in the cold if you are ill or injured. If conditions become too severe, stop and dig in. Studies suggest that taking 400 mg of ibuprofen twice daily with food may help prevent damage from substances produced by injured tissue, if taken when the frostbite risk is high.

Cold Exposure and You

As a rescuer, you are also at risk for hypothermia if you work in a cold environment. If cold weather search-and-rescue operations are a possibility, you should be thoroughly familiar with local conditions. Be aware of existing and potential weather conditions, and stay on top of changes that are forecast for the area. Make sure proper clothing is available, and wear it whenever appropriate. Your vehicle, too, must be properly equipped and maintained for a cold environment. As with so many hazards, you cannot help others if you do not practice self-protection. Never allow yourself to become a casualty!

High Altitude Illness

With ascent from sea level, solar radiation increases and ambient temperature, partial pressure of oxygen (PO_2), atmospheric pressure, and humidity fall. For every 1,000' (305 m) of altitude, the temperature drops about 3.5°F (1.6°C), the barometric pressure drops about 20 mm Hg, and the amount of ultraviolet radiation increases by about 5%. The percentage of oxygen in the air remains constant at 21%, but the PO_2 drops so that at 10,000' (3,048 m), only two thirds of the sea-level value remains, and at 18,000' (5,486 m), only half remains.

Before reading further in this section, you may wish to review the section on oxygen in Chapter 2.

Ascent to altitude, especially if too rapid to allow acclimatization, has a number of well-recognized effects on the human body. The effects are both acute and chronic. Acute effects produce the signs and symptoms of high altitude illnesses resulting from lack of oxygen.

This lack impairs cell function both directly, through interference with oxygen-requiring chemical reactions, and indirectly, through changes in the circulatory, respiratory, and nervous systems. Administration of oxygen, bringing the patient to lower elevation, or simulating higher atmospheric pressure with a Gamow Bag can modify these changes.

Speed of ascent, altitude reached, and duration of stay are important factors. It makes a difference whether you reach altitude by walking, driving, or flying, how fast you ascend, the altitude reached and length of stay there, how much you exert yourself while there, and how easy it is to go back down. For example, a study of trekkers in the Mt. Everest region of Nepal showed that symptoms developed in twice as many individuals who arrived at the site by air compared to individuals who walked there and had more time to acclimatize. Even at altitudes of 6,500′, **acute mountain sickness (AMS)** can develop if one ascends from sea level. The altitude at which a person sleeps seems to be a more important factor in acclimatizing than the highest altitude reached during the day.

To understand the adverse effects of high altitude, it is useful to view acute high altitude illnesses as a spectrum of illnesses that blend into each other rather than as specific disorders. At one end of the spectrum are the direct effects of lack of oxygen, or hypoxia, which are evident immediately during exposure to air containing low oxygen pressure. In the middle of the spectrum are effects resulting from changes in the brain produced by hypoxia. These changes can take anywhere from 6 hours to 4 days to develop and cause the signs and symptoms of acute mountain sickness. At the other end of the spectrum are two severe, potentially fatal illnesses: **high altitude cerebral edema (HACE)**, which is a complication of AMS, and **high altitude pulmonary edema (HAPE)**. Thus, the headache, breathlessness, and lightheadedness you note immediately when you drive to the top of Colorado's Pike's Peak are due to hypoxia. These symptoms disappear quickly as you drive back down. However, if you stay at the top, brain changes that cause the signs and symptoms of AMS may start to develop. The headache, shortness of breath, and fatigue get worse, and you may lose your appetite, become nauseated, vomit, and have trouble sleeping.

Individuals vary considerably in their tolerance to altitude changes. Some individuals can reach very high altitude with little distress, while others become ill at the moderate altitudes of ski areas, such as in the Colorado Rocky Mountains.

Acute Mountain Sickness

AMS, which is by far the most common altitude illness, seems to be caused by the following body changes:

1. Failure to adequately increase breathing in response to hypoxia.

2. Fluid retention that does not stimulate the normal amount of increase in urinary output.

3. Increased cerebral blood flow, plasma leaking from brain capillaries, and brain swelling. The brain swelling can be seen on computed tomography (CT) and magnetic resonance imaging (MRI) scans taken of affected patients.

Although these changes tend to diminish over one or several days as the person becomes acclimated to the altitude, they occasionally will continue or get worse. If the brain swelling progresses, it can result in HACE accompanied by increased intracranial pressure.

Although AMS can occur without any preceding symptoms of hypoxia, the symptoms of hypoxia may blend into those of AMS.

Signs and Symptoms of Acute Mountain Sickness

Neurologic signs and symptoms are as follows:

- Headache, which is typically generalized, throbbing, worse at night, and aggravated by stooping over

- Apathy

- Insomnia

- Lightheadedness

- Loss of appetite, nausea, vomiting

Other signs and symptoms include the following:

- Pale or ill appearance

- Weakness, fatigue

- Shortness of breath on exertion

- Edema of ankles

- Poor urine output

Retinal hemorrhages develop in many patients with AMS, which suitably trained individuals can see with an ophthalmoscope. The patient usually is not aware of the hemorrhages unless they affect the macula, the part of the retina responsible for sharpest vision.

AMS has been reported at altitudes as low as 6,500′ (1,981 m). Studies have shown that at least a mild degree of AMS develops in up to 20% of skiers or snowboarders who fly from low altitudes to ski resorts at

8,000' to 9,000' in the Rocky Mountains. Mild forms of AMS are also seen in Yellowstone National Park at altitudes of 6,500' to 7,500'.

Predisposing factors of AMS include too rapid of an ascent, overexertion, and exposure to cold. Younger adults seem to be more susceptible than older individuals, but good physical conditioning does not seem to confer immunity to high altitude illness. Individuals who automatically increase their breathing at higher altitudes appear to be less susceptible to AMS. Some high altitude symptoms, such as throbbing headache, can be improved by voluntary hyperventilation.

The prevention of AMS is addressed in Chapter 2.

Signs and Symptoms of High Altitude Cerebral Edema

Signs and symptoms of HACE include the following:

1. Signs and symptoms of AMS, but worse.

2. Ataxia (loss of muscle coordination resulting in difficulty maintaining balance).

3. Altered mental status, which may progress to complete unresponsiveness.

High Altitude Pulmonary Edema

HAPE occurs about 10 times more frequently than HACE. Although HAPE has been recognized in the Andes for years, it was largely ignored in North America until 1960, when Charles Houston, MD, reported a case in a cross-country skier and suggested that some patients diagnosed with pneumonia might have had pulmonary edema instead. Subsequently, extensive studies have been carried out in altitude chambers, by Indian Army physicians in the Himalayas, by Dr. Houston and others on Mount Logan in Canada, and by Peter Hackett, MD, Robert Schoene, MD, Robert Roach, MD, and others on Mount McKinley (Denali).

HAPE appears to be caused by the following hypoxia-induced changes in the lungs:

1. Increased pulmonary artery pressure resulting from narrowing of the small pulmonary blood vessels.

2. Damage to the capillary walls in the lungs.

3. The opening of high-pressure shunts in some parts of the lungs.

These changes result in increased fluid in the alveoli that, if left untreated, will cause pulmonary edema.

Early signs and symptoms of HAPE include the following:

- a dry cough, frequently occurring at night.
- increasing respiratory distress, made worse by exertion.
- mild chest pain, usually perceived as an ache beneath the sternum.
- a decrease in the ability to exercise.

Late signs and symptoms of HAPE include the following:

- cyanosis.
- a cough that produces large amounts of frothy, pink sputum.
- rapid pulse and respirations at rest.
- audible, gurgling sounds during breathing. When a stethoscope or the ear is placed on the naked chest, wet crackling sounds can be heard when the patient breathes.
- severe respiratory distress and frank pulmonary edema.

▼ Table 15-3 summarizes the signs and symptoms of HACE and HAPE.

HAPE and HACE often occur together, and the hypoxia that is caused by the pulmonary edema tends to make the cerebral edema worse. The most important impediment to early recognition of HAPE and HACE is their insidious onset (often 24 to 48 hours to develop). Early signs and symptoms frequently go unrecognized

Table 15-3 Summary of the Signs and Symptoms of HACE and HAPE	
HACE	• Symptoms of AMS, but worse • Ataxia • Altered mental status
HAPE	Early: • Cough, increasing respiratory distress, mild chest pain • Weakness Later: • Cyanosis, severe cough with abundant frothy, pink sputum • Rapid pulse, severe respiratory distress • Audible gurgling sounds in the chest

or are ignored by patients and their companions, who may be suffering from some degree of AMS themselves. By the time a serious problem is suspected, nightfall or bad weather may make evacuation to a lower altitude difficult.

Assessment of a Patient with High Altitude Illness

Again, the starting point of assessment is to do a scene size-up. Consider AMS in anyone who is not feeling well at altitudes of 6,500′ (1,981 m) or higher.

Next, perform the initial assessment. Assess the patient's vital signs, especially the pulse and respiratory rate, and compare them with those of other party members or healthy individuals at the same altitude.

Early recognition of a high altitude illness depends on careful questioning of the patient. Ask about fatigue, headache, loss of appetite, nausea, vomiting, shortness of breath, dizziness, and trouble with balance. Assess the level of responsiveness, and if it is decreased, assess the patient's ability to move and perception of pain and touch.

Listen to the patient's chest with your ear against the patient's bare skin, or use a stethoscope if one is available. Listen for abnormal sounds such as rattles, wheezes, and bubbly sounds. Also, assess for ataxia by seeing if the patient can pass the "drunk driver" test by walking a straight line with one foot in front of the other, toe touching heel; by getting up on the knees from a recumbent position without swaying; or seeing whether the patient can touch the tip of his or her nose with the index finger while his or her eyes are closed.

During the SAMPLE history, ask whether the patient has had previous similar problems at high altitude. Next, perform the rapid body survey.

Be certain to also perform an ongoing assessment. This very important step allows you to detect a progression of symptoms.

Emergency Care of High Altitude Illness

The appropriate emergency care of high altitude illness depends on such variables as the setting and general nature of the outdoor outing. (▶ **Table 15-4**) summarizes emergency care of a patient with high-altitude illness.

Skiing, Trekking, and Climbing Parties at High Altitude

The cornerstone of emergency care for high altitude illness is rapid descent to a lower altitude, and oxygen administration (if available). However, because many patients with mild to moderate symptoms will improve as they become acclimatized, not all patients require descent. Therefore, the crucial practical consideration

Remember

Because supplemental oxygen supplies are always limited, oxygen use should not delay preparations for descent.

is to accurately determine if the patient has AMS, which may improve with rest alone, or early HACE or HAPE, which will require immediate evacuation to a lower altitude.

Mild symptoms appearing early on the first day of reaching altitude are more likely to be due to acute hypoxia. A day or two of rest at the same altitude may be effective treatment for patients with mild AMS, if the following requirements are met: their symptoms are not progressive, help is available to carry them down, and they can be carefully monitored during this time, including during the night.

Signs and symptoms that mandate immediate descent include the following:

- Development of ataxia
- Increasing respiratory distress
- Cyanosis
- Inability to eat or drink because of nausea and vomiting that lasts for more than a few hours
- Altered mental status

The party should descend at least 2,000′ (610 m) and preferably below the altitude at which the initial symptoms of AMS began. You should begin your descent early, when you first start thinking about it, while it is still daylight, and while the patient can still walk. Have someone else carry the patient's pack. If the patient can no longer walk, carry him or her in a sitting position.

These guidelines are not absolute; if there is any question about whether to descend, always descend.

Oxygen causes temporary improvement but is rarely available outside of aid facilities or large expeditions. It is effective even at low flow rates (1 to 2 L/min). However, because supplemental oxygen supplies are always limited, oxygen use should not delay preparations for descent.

Allow the patient to stay in the most comfortable position, usually sitting up or lying with the chest and head elevated. In addition, keep the patient warm and at rest. Avoid any unnecessary exertion.

Treat headache with a nonprescription medication. Aspirin or ibuprofen is preferable to acetaminophen.

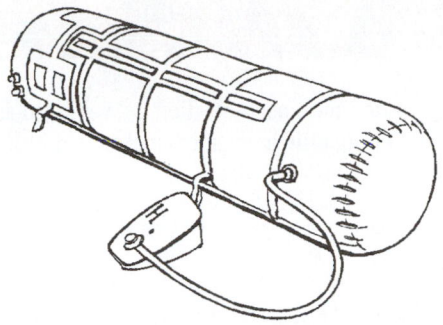

Figure 15-12 Small, portable hyperbaric chambers have been used successfully on high altitude expeditions and at high altitude ski resorts.

You will also want to encourage the patient to eat and, more importantly, to drink fluids.

If the patient becomes unresponsive, provide care for unresponsiveness as described in Chapter 12.

Small, portable, hyperbaric chambers (▲ Figure 15-12) have been used successfully on high altitude expeditions and at high altitude ski resorts. They have been found to be as effective as oxygen administration, producing enough improvement that the patient can frequently descend under his or her own power. These chambers, or Gamow Bags, weigh 15 lb (6.8 kg) or less and are large enough to hold one large or two small patients. The chamber is typically cylindrical and made of airtight nylon, opens with a zipper, and inflates with a foot or hand pump. The patient can be pressurized 2 lb per square inch (PSI) above atmospheric pressure within a few minutes, which is equivalent to a drop in altitude of about 6,000' (1,829 m).

A number of drugs are available that have some value in preventing and treating AMS, but they do not replace the effects of descent. They are discussed in Appendix D.

The risk of severe altitude illness is quite low after the fifth day at a given altitude, but symptoms can still be precipitated by stresses, such as swimming in a cold stream, a hard fall, hypothermia, or a respiratory infection.

High Altitude Ski Areas and Other Resorts

The previously described guidelines also can be applied to patrons of high altitude resorts who have signs and symptoms of AMS and may be seen by emergency care providers. Patients who fall under the immediate-descent guidelines previously listed should be given high-flow oxygen and rapidly transported to medical care. This can be a local physician or hospital emergency department, if available, or to the nearest town with a hospital, one at a lower altitude. Regardless of the destination, high-flow oxygen administration should be continued en route.

Table 15-4 Summary of Emergency Care of a Patient with High Altitude Illness
1. Recognize the problem and stop further ascent.
2. Descend rapidly.
3. Give oxygen, if available, but do not delay descent.
4. Keep the patient in the most comfortable position.
5. Treat headache with mild analgesics.
6. Feed and hydrate.
7. Give care for unresponsiveness, if necessary.

Patients with mild symptoms of AMS can stay for 1 or 2 days at the high altitude if they agree to keep in touch with emergency care providers and can be monitored by reliable companions. Advise these patients to stay warm, rest, get plenty of sleep, eat a light diet, use nonprescription analgesics for headache, avoid sleeping pills and tranquilizers, and return if they feel worse. Alcohol interferes with the normal increased breathing response to high altitude and also should be avoided. Acetazolamide (Diamox®), which requires a physician's prescription, is useful in speeding acclimatization and treating mild AMS. It can also be taken prophylactically prior to ascent.

Patients with more severe symptoms of AMS should be given oxygen and monitored carefully by responsible persons. Many resort hotels have facilities for giving oxygen when necessary. Patients who do not improve in a few days should return to a lower altitude. It is surprising in how many people mild altitude illness develops at mountain resorts higher than 8,000' when they ascend from sea level.

Sunburn, Windburn, and Snow Blindness

Humans are more vulnerable to the harmful effects of solar radiation when at high altitudes, on snow, or on bodies of water. This is because the thin, clear atmosphere at higher altitudes filters out fewer of the harmful, ultraviolet rays, and exposure is increased by reflection of sunlight from snow or water.

Injury to the skin and eyes is more likely to occur on cloudy days when individuals often forget to protect themselves and during the longer days of spring and summer.

Sunburn is a first- or second-degree skin burn caused by ultraviolet (UV) light in the medium-wave range. This consists of UVB rays at a wavelength of 290 to 320 nanometers (nm) and, to a lesser extent, UVA rays at a wavelength of 320 to 400 nm. Repeated sun exposure over many years may lead to chronic degenerative skin changes, such as wrinkling, darkening, and thickening. Localized benign growths, called actinic keratoses, are common and are premalignant. These changes, which resemble accelerated changes of aging, can be delayed by avoiding excessive sun exposure and using proper skin protection.

Cancer researchers have noted increasing rates of epitheliomas (basal cell and squamous cell carcinomas) and malignant melanoma in the past decade. These cancers are associated with high degrees of ultraviolet exposure from the sun and from tanning booths mistakenly recommended in the past as a health measure. Gradual destruction of the ozone layer by chlorofluorohydrocarbons and other processes is expected to increase the amount of ultraviolet exposure that the earth receives.

The skin can be protected by clothing or topical sunscreens. Sunscreen preparations come in two basic types: physical and chemical. Physical sunscreens block sunlight mechanically. They consist of opaque greases containing substances such as zinc oxide, titanium dioxide, or red veterinary petrolatum and are particularly suitable for small areas such as the nose and lips. Chemical sunscreens rely on chemical agents to selectively filter out harmful rays. The most effective products now available against UVB rays contain para-amino-benzoic acid (PABA) and its derivatives (such as Padimate), cinnamates, and salicylates. Products effective against UVA rays contain benzophenones such as oxybenzone, anthranilates, and dibenzoylmethanes (such as Parsol). Some preparations contain both physical and chemical sunscreens. Varieties of chemical sunscreens are available that resist removal by water or perspiration.

Individuals can be classified into the following six groups according to their degree of sun sensitivity:

- Type I (redheaded, fair skin, freckles): always burns, never tans.

- Type II (blond, fair skin): always burns, tans minimally.

- Type III (brunette, darker complexion): burns moderately, tans gradually.

- Type IV (Mediterranean): burns minimally, tans easily.

- Type V (Middle-Eastern, Asian, American Indian): rarely burns, tans easily.

- Type VI (black): never burns, tans deeply.

Most manufacturers of sunscreen creams, lotions, and lip salves now specify the **sun protection factor (SPF)** on the label. This number, usually from 2 to 50, refers to how much longer skin protected with the product can be exposed to the sun before becoming red.

It is important to remember that clothing does not necessarily block out the harmful rays of the sun. An untreated, white cotton T-shirt has an SPF of about 8. Special sun-protective clothing is available (see Chapter 2).

Because there is no such thing as a safe tan, products with an SPF of 15 or greater should be used regularly during sun exposure. For practical purposes, maximal protection is given by topical sunscreens with SPF 30; little or no additional benefit is provided by those with higher numbers. To prevent sunburn, apply sunscreen 1 to 2 hours before sun exposure and reapply it several times during the day, particularly if you are sweating heavily. Sunscreens should not be used on children younger than 6 months because immature skin absorbs more of the chemical agents and is less capable of detoxifying and excreting them.

Because sunscreens with a cream or oil base are better at preventing frostbite and windburn than alcohol-based preparations, they are preferable for use by skiers, snowboarders, high altitude climbers, and others exposed to cold and wind as well as sunlight.

Care for sunburn by removing the patient from exposure and applying cool compresses. Later, moisturizing skin lotions with aloe are useful to control discomfort. Consult a physician if the sunburn is extensive or the skin is blistered.

Windburn is an irritation of the skin that resembles superficial sunburn. It is partly due to the drying effect of the low humidity at high altitudes. It can be prevented to some extent by wearing a facemask or by applying a greasy sunscreen. Treat windburn by applying soothing, greasy ointments or lotions (greasy sunscreens are useful for both prevention and treatment of sunburn).

Snowblindness is sunburn of the conjunctiva of the eye caused by UV radiation and can be prevented by wearing dark glasses or goggles. Because radiation can reach the eye by reflection from the snow, glasses or goggles should have extensions on each side and below, as do ski goggles, "glacier" glasses, or goggles. Dark gray lenses are best; they generally transmit only 10% to 15% of light and should block all UV light up to a wavelength of 380 nm (all UVB and most UVA radiation). They should be made of polycarbonate rather than glass or plastic. Polycarbonate blocks all UV radiation and resists shattering. Goggles should be adequately ventilated and have easily replaceable lenses. A separate set of yellow or red lenses is desirable to increase contrast in flat light.

Symptoms of snow blindness develop 6 to 12 hours after exposure. The eyes are sensitive and feel irritated and are often described as feeling as if there is "sand in the eye." Eye motion produces pain, the conjunctivae are reddened, and the patient experiences excessive tearing, squinting, and swelling around the eye. Emergency care includes covering the eyes or putting the patient in a dark room, applying cool compresses, and using nonprescription pain relievers. In severe cases, the patient should see a physician because medication can be prescribed to relieve the pain and speed healing.

Heat Exposure

Normal body temperature is 98.6°F (37°C). Complicated regulatory mechanisms keep this internal temperature constant, regardless of the ambient temperature, the temperature of the surrounding environment. In a hot environment or during vigorous physical activity, when the body itself produces excess heat, the body will try to rid itself of the excess heat. There are several ways of doing this. The two most efficient are sweating (and evaporation of the sweat) and dilation of skin blood vessels, which brings blood to the skin surface to increase the rate of heat radiation. In addition, of course, the person who becomes overheated can remove clothing and try to find a cooler environment.

Ordinarily, the heat-regulating mechanisms of the body work very well, and individuals are able to tolerate significant temperature changes. When the body is exposed to more heat energy than it loses or generates more heat than it can lose, hyperthermia results. Hyperthermia is a high core temperature, usually 101°F (38.3°C) or more.

Rescuer Safety

Keeping yourself hydrated while on duty is very important, especially during periods of heavy exertion or work in the heat. Drink at least 3 L of water per day, and more when exertion or heat is involved. Urinary color and frequency correlate directly with the body's fluid level.

When the body's mechanisms to decrease body heat are overwhelmed and the body is unable to tolerate the excessive heat, illness develops. High air temperature can reduce the body's ability to lose heat by radiation; high humidity reduces the ability to lose heat through evaporation. Another contributing factor is vigorous exercise, during which the body can lose more than 1 L of sweat an hour, causing loss of fluid and electrolytes. Illness from heat exposure can take the following three forms:

- Heat cramps
- Heat exhaustion
- Heatstroke

All three forms of heat illness may be present in the same patient, since untreated heat exhaustion may progress to heatstroke. Heatstroke is a life-threatening emergency.

Persons at greatest risk for heat illnesses are children; the elderly; patients with heart disease, COPD, emphysema, diabetes, dehydration, and obesity; and those with limited mobility. The elderly, newborns, and infants exhibit poor thermoregulation. Newborns and infants often wear too much clothing. Alcohol and certain drugs, including medications that dehydrate the body or decrease the ability of the body to sweat, also make a person more susceptible to heat illnesses. When you are treating someone for a heat illness, always obtain a medication history.

Heat Cramps

Heat cramps are painful muscle spasms that occur after vigorous exercise. They do not occur only when it is hot outdoors. They may be seen in factory workers and even well-conditioned athletes. The exact cause of heat cramps is not well understood. We know that sweat produced during strenuous exercise, particularly in a warm environment, causes a change in the body's electrolyte, or salt, balance. The result may be a loss of essential electrolytes from the cells. Dehydration may also play a role in the development of muscle cramps. Large amounts of water can be lost from the body as a

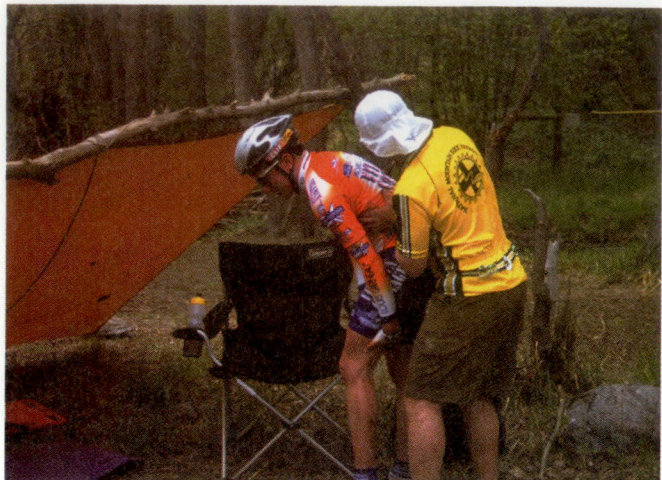

Figure 15-13 A patient with heat cramps should be moved to a cool environment as you begin your assessment and treatment.

result of excessive sweating. This loss of water may affect muscles that are being stressed and cause them to go into spasm.

Heat cramps usually occur in the leg or abdominal muscles. When the abdominal muscles are involved, the pain and muscle spasm may be so severe that the patient appears to have an acute abdominal problem. If a patient with a sudden onset of abdominal cramps has been exercising vigorously in a hot environment, you should suspect heat cramps.

Take the following steps to treat heat cramps in the field (▲ **Figure 15-13**):

1. **Remove the patient** from the hot environment, including sunlight, a source of radiant heat gain. Loosen any tight clothing.

2. **Rest the cramping muscles.** Have the patient sit or lie down until the cramps subside.

3. **Replace fluids by mouth.** Rehydration with water alone may be inadequate. Use an electrolyte solution or a teaspoon of table salt added to a quart of water. With adequate rest and fluid replacement, the body will adjust the distribution of electrolytes, and the cramps will disappear.

If the cramps do not go away after these measures, transport the patient to the hospital.

Once the cramps are gone, the patient may resume activity. For example, an athlete can return to play once the heat cramps have disappeared. However, heavy sweating may cause the cramps to recur. Hydration by drinking a lot of water is the best preventive and treatment strategy.

Heat Exhaustion

Heat exhaustion, also called *heat prostration* or *heat collapse*, is the most common serious illness caused by heat. It is the result of the body's losing so much water and so many electrolytes through very heavy sweating that hypovolemia (fluid depletion) occurs. For sweating to be an effective cooling mechanism, the sweat must be able to evaporate from the body. Otherwise, the body will continue to produce sweat, with further loss of body water. People standing in the hot sun and particularly those wearing several layers of clothing, such as football fans or parade watchers, may sweat profusely but experience little body cooling. High humidity will also decrease the amount of evaporation that can occur. Individuals working or exerting themselves in poorly ventilated areas are unable to release heat through convection. Thus, people who work or exercise vigorously and those who wear heavy clothing in a warm, humid, or poorly ventilated environment are particularly prone to heat exhaustion.

The signs and symptoms of heat exhaustion and those of associated hypovolemia are as follows:

- Onset while working hard or exercising in a hot, humid, or poorly ventilated environment and sweating heavily

- Onset, even at rest, in the elderly and infant age groups in hot, humid, and poorly ventilated environments or extended time in hot, humid environments

- Cold, clammy skin with ashen pallor

- Dry tongue and thirst

- Dizziness, weakness, or faintness, with accompanying nausea or headache

- Normal vital signs, although the pulse is often rapid and the diastolic blood pressure may be low

- Normal or slightly elevated body temperature; on rare occasions, as high as 104°F (40°C)

To treat the patient, follow the steps in
▶ **Skill Drill 15-1**):

1. **Remove any excessive layers of clothing,** particularly around the head and neck **(Step 1)**.

2. **Move the patient promptly** from the hot environment, preferably into an air-conditioned area. If outdoors, move out of the sun.

3. **Give the patient oxygen** if this was not already done as part of the initial assessment.

SkillDrill 15-1   Treating for Heat Exhaustion

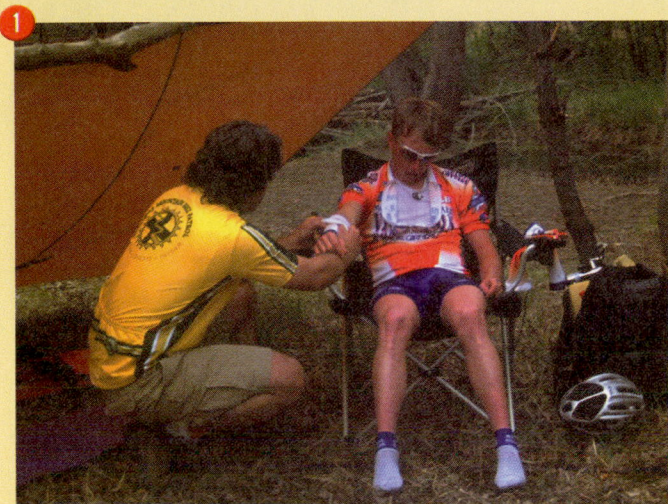

Remove extra clothing.

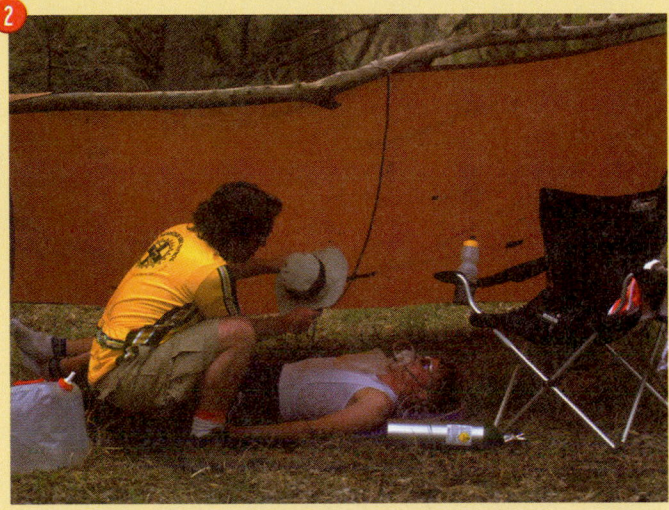

Move the patient to a cooler environment.
Give oxygen.
Place the patient in a supine position, elevate the legs, and fan the patient.

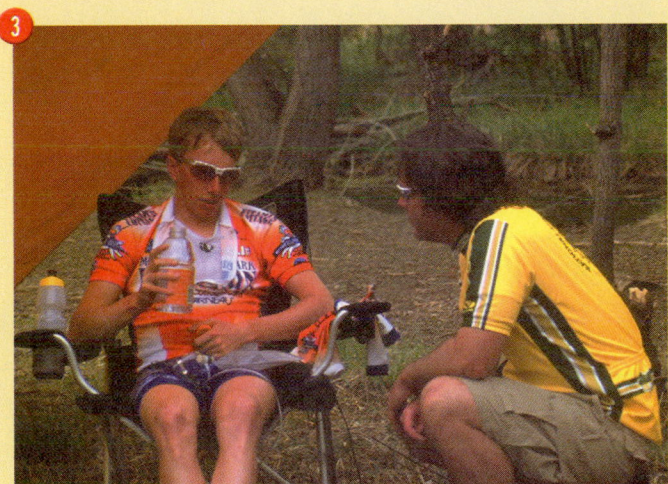

If the patient is fully alert, give an electrolyte solution by mouth.

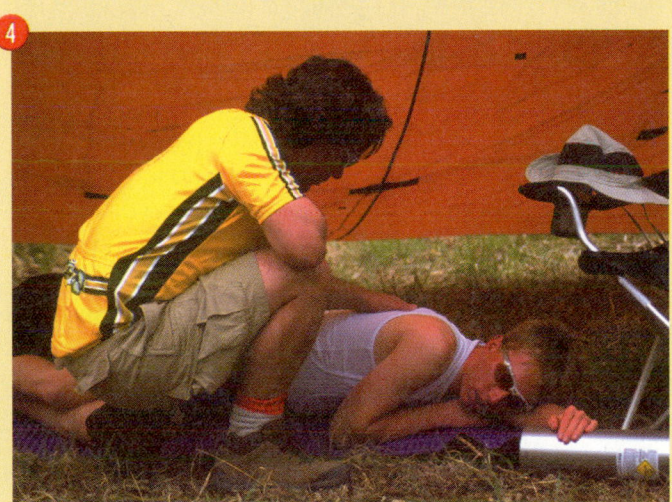

If nausea develops, position the patient on the side.

4. **Encourage the patient to lie down** and elevate the legs (supine position). Loosen any tight clothing and fan the patient for cooling **(Step 2)**.

5. **If the patient is fully alert,** encourage him or her to sit up and slowly drink up to a liter of an electrolyte solution or a solution of table salt and water (1 teaspoon table salt to 1 quart water), as long as nausea does not develop. Never force

fluids by mouth on a patient who is not fully alert, or allow drinking while supine, because the patient could aspirate the fluid into the lungs **(Step 3)**.

If the patient does become nauseated, transport on the side, also to prevent aspiration.

In most cases, these measures will reverse the symptoms, causing the patient to feel better within 30 minutes. But you should prepare to transport the patient to the hospital for more aggressive treatment, such as IV fluid therapy and close monitoring, especially in the following circumstances:

- The symptoms do not clear up promptly.
- The level of consciousness decreases.
- The temperature remains elevated.
- The person is very young, elderly, or has an underlying medical condition, such as diabetes or cardiovascular disease.

6. **Transport the patient on his or her side** if you think the patient may be nauseated and ready to vomit, but make certain that the patient is secured **(Step 4)**.

Heatstroke

Heatstroke, the least common but most serious illness caused by heat exposure, occurs when the body is subjected to more heat than it can handle, and normal mechanisms for getting rid of the excess heat are overwhelmed. The body temperature then rises rapidly to the level at which tissues are destroyed. Untreated heatstroke always results in death.

Heatstroke can develop in patients during vigorous physical activity or when they are outdoors or in a closed, poorly ventilated, humid space. It also occurs during heat waves among individuals (particularly the elderly) who live in buildings with no air conditioning or with poor ventilation. It may also develop in children who are left unattended in a locked car on a hot day.

Many patients with heatstroke have hot, dry, flushed skin because their sweating mechanism has been overwhelmed. However, early in the course of heatstroke, the skin may be moist or wet. Keep in mind that a patient can have heatstroke even if he or she is still sweating. The body temperature rises rapidly in patients with heatstroke. It may rise to 106°F (41°C) or more. As the body core temperature rises, the patient's level of consciousness falls.

Often, the first sign of heatstroke is a change in behavior (eg, irrational, sometimes uncooperative). However, the patient then becomes unresponsive very quickly. The pulse is usually rapid and strong at first, but as the patient becomes increasingly unresponsive, the pulse becomes weaker and the blood pressure falls.

Recovery from heatstroke depends on the speed with which treatment is administered, so you must be able to identify this patient quickly. Emergency treatment has one objective: Get the body temperature down by any means available. Take the following steps when treating a patient with heatstroke:

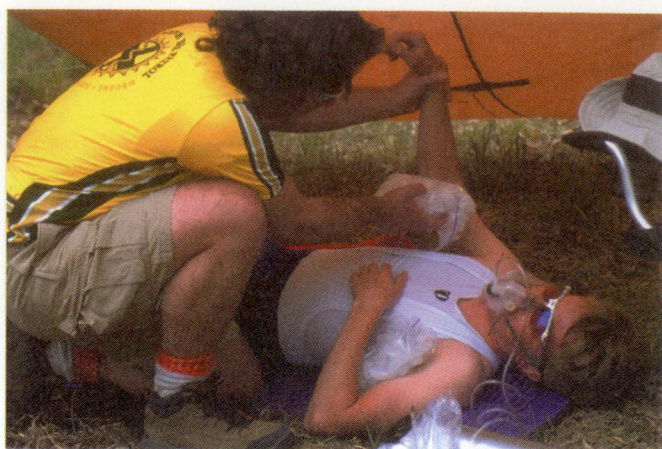

Figure 15-14 As part of treatment of heatstroke, give oxygen and place cool packs about the patient's neck, groin, and armpits.

1. **Call for an ambulance.**
2. **Move the patient** out of the hot environment and into a cool place.
3. **Set the air conditioning (if any)** to maximum cooling.
4. **Remove the patient's clothing.**
5. **Give the patient oxygen** if this was not done as part of the initial assessment.
6. **Apply ice packs** to the patient's neck, groin, and armpits **▲ Figure 15-14**.
7. **Cover the patient** with wet towels or sheets, or spray the patient with cool water and fan him or her to quickly evaporate the dampness on the skin.
8. **Aggressively and repeatedly fan** the patient with or without dampening the skin.
9. **Notify the hospital** as soon as possible so that the staff can prepare to treat the patient immediately on arrival.

An interesting condition has now been described where athletes such as marathoners take in too much fluid during a race, trying to prevent heat illness. This dilutes the electrolytes in the blood and body, potentially causing severe illness from metabolic and electrolyte disturbances.

Lightning and Electrical Injury

High-voltage electrical current represents a significant hazard in modern society because of the large number of electrical appliances and their ubiquitous power sources. Annually, approximately 1,000 deaths occur from electrocution (including 100 to 200 deaths from lightning) in the United States, and many more cases of severe electrical burns occur.

While outdoors, individuals are susceptible to injury from lightning during electrical storms and from high-voltage power lines, which can be found even in remote areas. Ski areas use large amounts of electric power, and chairlifts attract lightning strikes, particularly in late spring.

You need to know how to protect yourself from the dangers of electricity, especially lightning, and how to care for patients injured by electricity.

Ways in Which Electricity Causes Injury

Electricity can cause injury in the following ways:

1. Injury to the respiratory control center in the brain may stop breathing.

2. Cardiac arrest (ventricular fibrillation or cessation of heart activity [asystole]) can occur from a direct effect on the heart. Alternating current tends to cause ventricular fibrillation, while lightning, high-voltage batteries, and other types of direct current cause asystole.

3. Direct effects on the nervous and musculoskeletal systems can cause pain, paralysis, blindness, numbness, weakness, loss of hearing or speech, and unresponsiveness.

4. Direct effects on the skin, muscles, and internal organs can cause severe, deep burns. Because an electric current tends to travel easily along blood vessels, significant internal damage may be overlooked at first if surface burns are unimpressive.

5. The current can cause strong muscular contractions that throw the patient off balance and cause injury resulting from falls.

6. Secondary kidney injury may occur because the kidneys are overloaded with breakdown products of blood and injured muscle.

Lightning is caused by violent vertical air currents associated with the development of cumulonimbus clouds ("thunderheads"). These are huge, billowing vertical clouds with anvil-shaped tops that may tower to 60,000′ or more ▶ **Figure 15-15** . The air currents produce differences of electrical potential between clouds or between a cloud and the earth. Cumulonimbus clouds usually produce large raindrops, huge snowflakes, or hail. They tend to develop during the afternoon or evening in hot, sultry weather but also can be part of an advancing cold front. Lightning can occur when it is snowing.

Lightning causes injury in the same way as any other direct electric current, except that the duration of the

bolt is so short (.0001 to .001 second) that burns are less severe. The fatality rate in lightning strikes is about 30%. An individual who is struck by lightning may sustain a characteristic superficial skin burn with a pattern resembling a fern leaf ▼ **Figure 15-16** .

In addition to direct lightning strikes, individuals may be injured by ground currents and side flashes from nearby strikes. Strikes often cause a person's clothing to explode off the body by instantly converting sweat or other moisture to steam.

An individual who has been injured by electricity and was not thrown clear by the jolt must be removed from the source of the current before emergency care can be given. The only safe way to do this is to shut off the power source. The danger to the rescuer is so great that only those individuals with special training and equipment should attempt to remove a hot wire directly from a patient.

Individuals trapped in a vehicle near a fallen power line are relatively safe as long as they remain inside the vehicle. If the occupants must be evacuated before the power can be shut off, instruct them to jump out, taking care to avoid touching the vehicle and the ground at the same time.

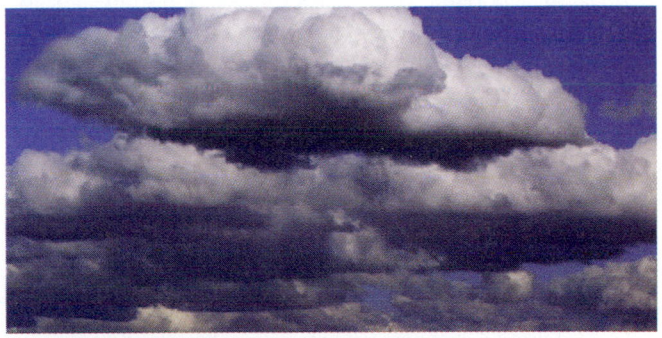

Figure 15-15 Cumulonimbus clouds, "thunderheads," are huge billowing vertical clouds with anvil-shaped tops that may tower to 60,000′ or more.

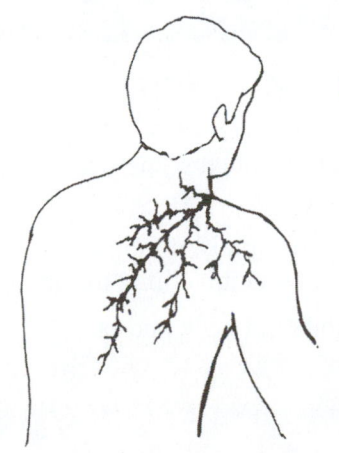

Figure 15-16 An individual who is struck by lightning may sustain a characteristic superficial skin burn with a pattern resembling a fern leaf.

Assessment and Emergency Care of Electrical Injury Patients

Because of possible danger to the rescuer, the scene size-up is important. Initiate BSI. Do not touch the patient until you are sure that *all* live wires are clear.

Considering the high incidence of pulmonary or cardiopulmonary arrest in patients who have sustained electrical burns, the scene size-up, initial assessment, and basic life support measures are critical (see Chapter 7). Assessment should be rapid and rescue breathing or CPR, if necessary, should be started as soon as possible. Spontaneous heart action may return before spontaneous breathing, so prolonged rescue breathing may be necessary.

Open the airway with care because the patient could have a neck injury from a fall. Because damage to the circulatory and respiratory systems usually is temporary and patients may be capable of full recovery, continue CPR or rescue breathing as long as possible. Give high-flow oxygen if available.

CPR and rescue breathing are more successful in patients who have sustained an electric shock, particularly from a lightning strike, than in patients with other types of cardiac and respiratory arrest. Therefore, in contrast to the usual triage process (see Chapter 28), in a multiple-victim electrical accident, patients who are apparently dead should be cared for first.

When caring for a patient who has sustained an electrical injury, the appropriate initial assessment is the same as that for the unresponsive patient, as outlined in Chapters 5, 7, and 12. Special attention should be paid to checking the vital signs, sensation, ability to move, and assessing for burns, wounds, fractures, and other evidence of trauma.

A responsive lightning strike patient may be deaf (burst eardrums) or blind (usually temporary).

Remember

In contrast to the usual triage process, in a multiple-victim electrical accident, patients who are apparently dead should be cared for first.

Give care for altered responsiveness as outlined in Chapter 12.

The next step is to dress burns and other wounds and splint fractures. Perform the detailed physical exam as appropriate, and rapidly transport the patient to definitive care, performing the ongoing assessment en route.

▼ Table 15-5 summarizes emergency care of a patient with electrical injury.

Prevention of Electrical Injury

Most substances can be classified as being either conductors or **insulators**. Conductors transmit electric currents; insulators resist their flow. Most metals and objects that are wet or contain water (including the human body) are good conductors. Because electric currents tend to follow paths of least resistance, a person can be injured when a body part is accidentally positioned in such a way that it aligns with the path, thus completing a circuit. Most urban electrical injuries result from faulty electrical equipment, careless use of appliances, or accidental contact with a power line. Handling an electrical appliance while sitting in a bathtub or standing in a shower is a particularly dangerous practice.

Lightning is the main electrical hazard in remote areas. If caught in an electrical storm, you should avoid standing in or near bodies of water and take shelter away from high points, exposed ridges, solitary trees,

Table 15-5 Summary of Emergency Care of Electrical Injury Patients

1. Be aware of possible dangers, especially live wires.
2. Perform a rapid and thorough scene size-up and initial assessment.
3. Start basic life support rapidly, if indicated. Do not stop CPR or rescue breathing too soon.
4. Consider the possibility of neck and other injuries from falling.
5. Give high-flow oxygen.
6. Give care for altered responsiveness as needed.
7. Perform the focused history and physical exam and take care of additional injuries, if present.
8. Use cervical collar and backboard, if necessary, and transport the patient rapidly to a hospital.
9. Perform the ongoing assessment en route.

and trees taller than surrounding trees, because these all attract lightning strikes. If swimming or in a small boat (especially a sailboat), return to shore at the first threat of a storm. Avoid using telephones and other electrical appliances during storms. Stay out of small caves where body parts are close to the walls or ceiling, because ground currents may flow through the body instead of taking a longer course along the cave wall. Large buildings and enclosed vehicles are usually safe.

To estimate the storm's distance, count the seconds between the lightning and the thunder and divide by 5. The number obtained is the miles between you and the storm. If caught in the open, keep party members well separated, retreat as far down on the side of a ridge or other exposed area as possible, and move away from ice axes, ski poles, and other metal objects. If golfing, remove cleated shoes and keep your distance from your clubs. Squat on your heels until the danger is over. This position shortens the body and minimizes ground contact, decreasing the tendency for the body to act as a lightning rod and making it less likely that ground currents will pass through it.

During electrical storms at alpine ski areas, ski lifts and exposed summit structures should be cleared of occupants. Avoid metal structures such as lift towers.

Drowning and Near Drowning

Drowning is death from suffocation after submersion in water; **near drowning** is defined as survival, at least temporarily (24 hours), after suffocation in water. Drowning is often the last in a cycle of events caused by panic in the water (▶ Figure 15-17). It can happen to anyone who is submerged in water for even a short period of time. Struggling toward the surface or the shore, the person becomes fatigued or exhausted, which leads him or her to sink even deeper. However, drowning also occurs in mop buckets, puddles, bathtubs, and other places where the individual is not completely submerged. Small children can drown in only a few inches of water if unattended.

Inhaling very small amounts of either fresh or salt water can severely irritate the larynx, sending the muscles of the larynx and the vocal cords into spasm, called **laryngospasm**. The average person experiences this to a mild degree when a bit of a drink is inhaled and the patient coughs and seems to be choking for a few seconds. This is the body's attempt at self-preservation, since laryngospasm prevents more water from entering the lungs. But this can be too much of a good thing in severe cases such as water submersion, since the patient's lungs cannot be ventilated when significant

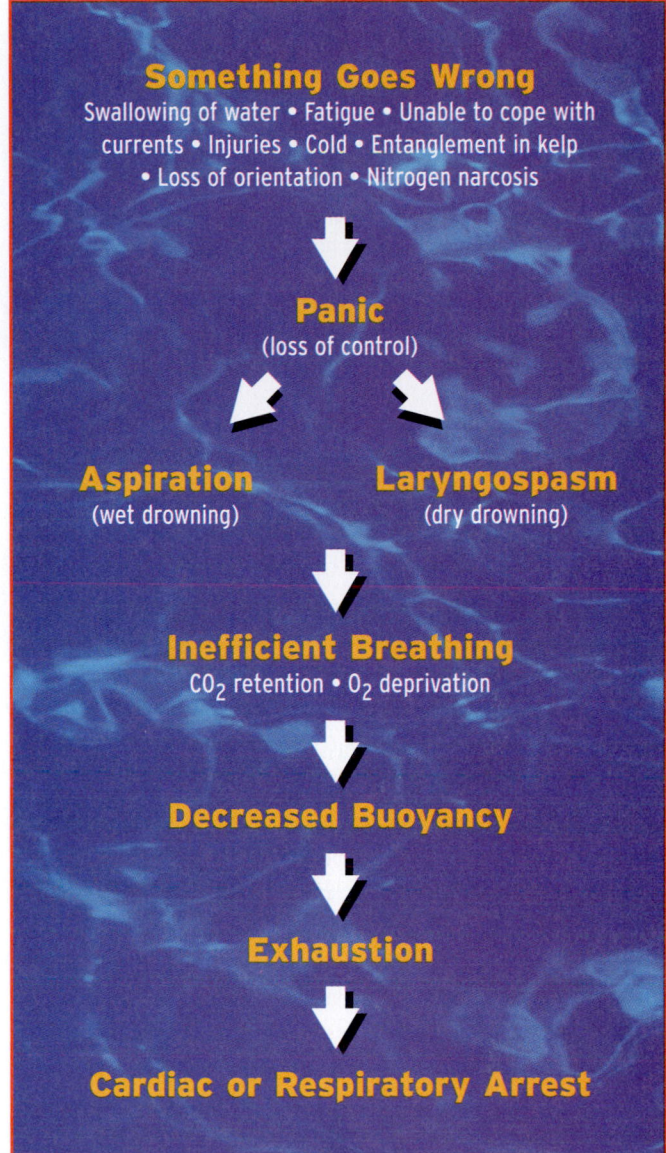

Figure 15-17 Panic in the water often precedes drowning.

laryngospasm is present. Instead, progressive hypoxia occurs until the patient becomes unconscious. At this point, the spasm relaxes, making rescue breathing possible. Of course, if the patient has not already been removed from the water, the patient may now inhale deeply, and more water may enter the lungs. In 85% to 90% of cases, significant amounts of water enter the lungs of the drowning victim.

Emergency Medical Care

Treatment begins with rescue and removal from the water. When necessary, artificial ventilation should begin as soon as possible, even before the victim is removed from the water. At the same time, you must

Rescuer Tips

The cold-water near-drowning patient may require more care than two rescuers can provide by themselves. Airway management and ventilation needs can make it difficult to remove wet clothing, treat hypothermia, or perform further assessment unless additional trained help is available. On this type of response, consider requesting additional help before you encounter the patient.

take care to stabilize and protect the patient's spine when a long fall or dive has occurred (or if this is a possibility when no information is provided). Associated cervical spine injuries are possible, especially in diving mishaps. If the patient does not have a possible spinal injury, you can turn the patient quickly to the left side to allow draining from the upper airway. Note that water will not drain from the lungs. If there is evidence of upper airway obstruction by foreign matter, remove the obstruction manually or, if available, by suction. If necessary, use abdominal thrusts, followed by assisted ventilations. Administer oxygen if this was not done as part of the initial assessment, either by mask for patients who are breathing spontaneously or via BVM device for those requiring assisted ventilation.

Check for a carotid pulse immediately after the patient emerges from the water. It may be difficult to find a peripheral pulse because of constriction of the peripheral blood vessels and low cardiac output. Nevertheless, if the pulse is unmeasurable, start CPR if the patient is unresponsive.

Even if resuscitation in the field appears completely successful, you must always transport near-drowning patients to the hospital. Inhalation of any amount of fluid can lead to delayed complications lasting for days or weeks.

Make sure that the patient is kept warm, especially after cold water immersion. Make sure blankets and protection from the environment are provided as needed. If ventilation equipment is not available but oxygen is, you can breathe the oxygen in yourself and give mouth-to-mask ventilation until rescue equipment arrives. In this method, your expired air will have a higher percentage of oxygen.

Spinal Injuries in Submersion Incidents

Submersion incidents may be complicated by spinal fractures and spinal cord injuries. You must assume that spinal injury exists with the following conditions:

- The submersion has resulted from a diving or surfing mishap, long fall, or collision.
- The patient is unconscious, and no information is available to rule out the possibility of a mechanism causing neck injury.
- The patient is conscious but complains of weakness, paralysis, or numbness in the arms or legs.
- You suspect the possibility of spinal injury despite what witnesses say.

Most spinal injuries in diving incidents affect the cervical spine. When spinal injury is suspected, the neck must be protected from further injury. This means that you will have to stabilize the suspected injury while the patient is still in the water. These are done more easily in calm, shallow water where the rescuer can stand. Follow the steps in (▶ **Skill Drill 15-2**):

1. **Turn the patient supine.** Two rescuers are usually required to turn the patient safely, although in some cases one rescuer will suffice. Always rotate the entire upper half of the patient's body as a single unit. Twisting only the head, for example, may aggravate any injury to the cervical spine **(Step 1)**.

2. **Restore the airway and begin ventilation.** Immediate ventilation is the primary treatment of all drowning and near-drowning patients. As soon as the patient is face up in the water, use a pocket mask if it is available. Have the other rescuer support the head and trunk as a unit while you open the airway and begin artificial ventilation **(Step 2)**.

3. **Float a buoyant backboard under the patient** as you continue ventilation **(Step 3)**.

4. **Secure the head and trunk to the backboard** to eliminate motion of the cervical spine. Do not remove the patient from the water until this is done **(Step 4)**.

5. **Remove the patient from the water, on the backboard (Step 5)**.

6. **Cover the patient with a blanket.** Give oxygen if the patient is breathing spontaneously. Begin CPR if there is no pulse. Effective cardiac compression or CPR is extremely difficult to perform when the patient is still in the water **(Step 6)**.

SkillDrill 15-2   Stabilizing a Patient with a Suspected Spinal Injury in the Water

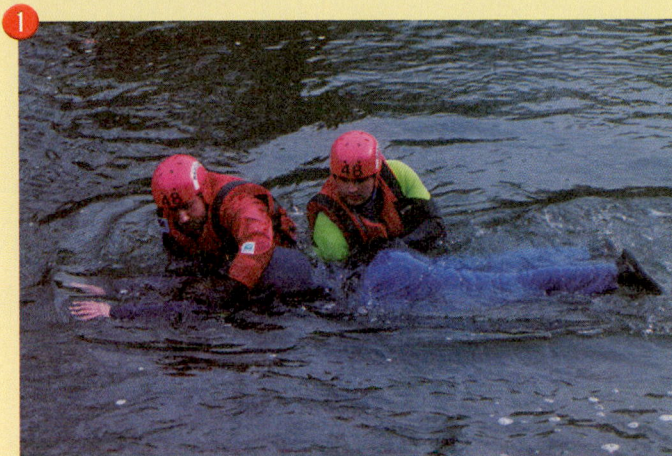

1. Turn the patient to a supine position by rotating the entire upper half of the body as a single unit.

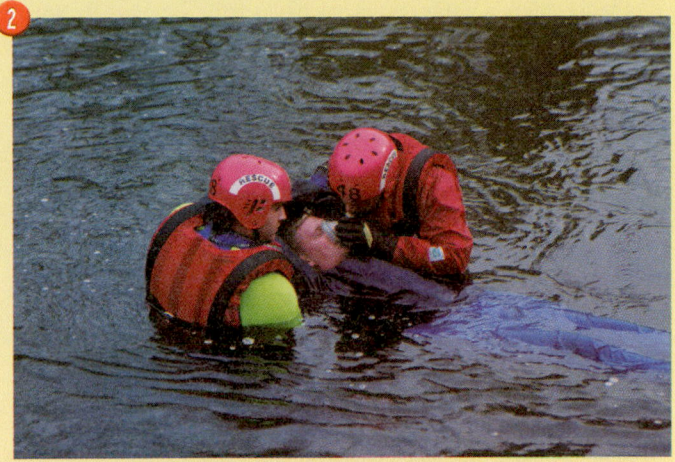

2. As soon as the patient is turned, begin artificial ventilation using the mouth-to-mouth method or a pocket mask.

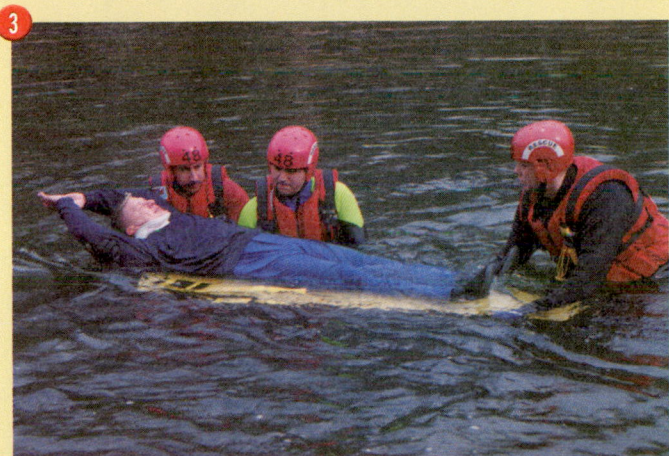

3. Float a buoyant backboard under the patient.

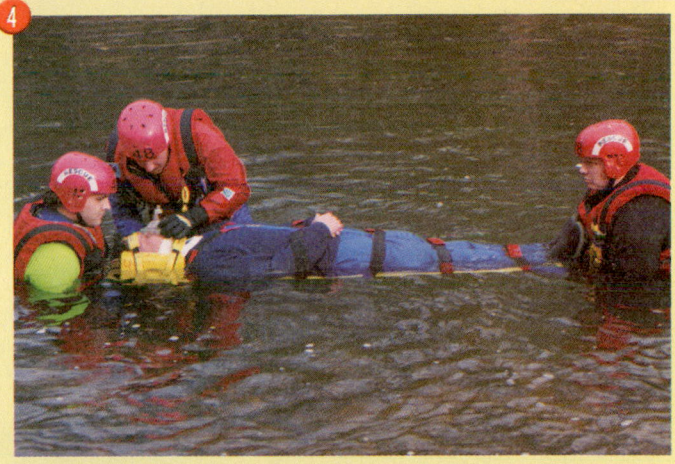

4. Secure the patient to the backboard.

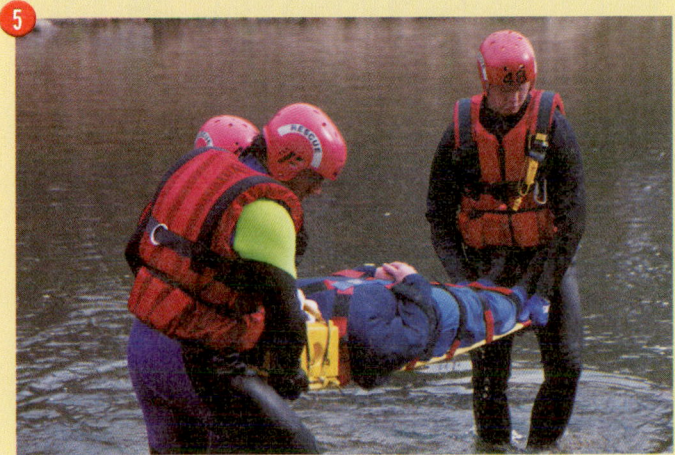

5. Remove the patient from the water.

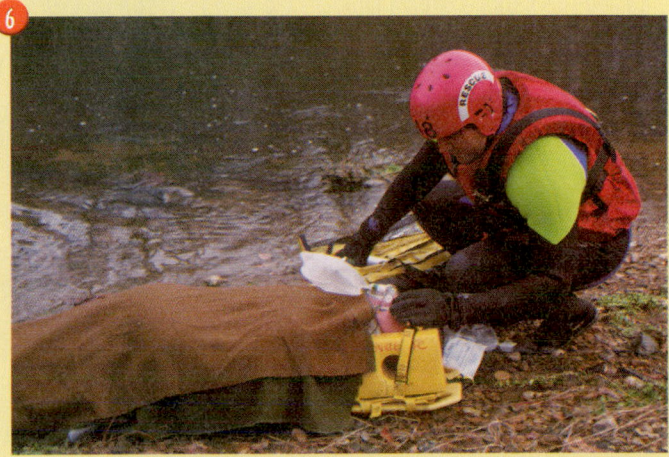

6. Cover the patient with a blanket and apply oxygen if breathing. Begin CPR if breathing and pulse are absent.

Rescuer Safety

You must ensure the safety of rescue personnel before a water rescue can begin. If the patient is conscious and still in the water, you should perform a water rescue. An old saying sums up the basic rule of water rescue: "Reach, throw and row, and *only then go.*" First, try to reach for the patient ▶ **Figure 15-18A**. If that does not work, then throw the patient a rope, a life preserver, or any floatable object that is available ▶ **Figure 15-18B**. For example, an inflated spare tire, rim and all, will float well enough to support two people in the water. Next, use a boat if one is available ▶ **Figure 15-18C**. Do not attempt a swimming rescue unless you are trained and experienced in the proper techniques ▶ **Figure 15-18D**. Even then, you should always wear a helmet and a personal flotation device ▶ **Figure 15-19**. Too many well-meaning individuals have themselves become victims while attempting a swimming rescue. In cold climates or cold water locations, rapid hypothermia is a concern for rescuers as well. Be prepared for this potential event.

If you work in a recreation area near lakes, rivers, or the ocean, you must have a prearranged plan for water rescue. This plan should include access to and cooperation with local personnel who are trained and skilled in water rescue; these personnel should help to develop the protocol for water rescue. Because the success of any water rescue depends on how rapidly the patient is removed from the water and ventilated, make sure you always have immediate access to personal flotation devices and other rescue equipment.

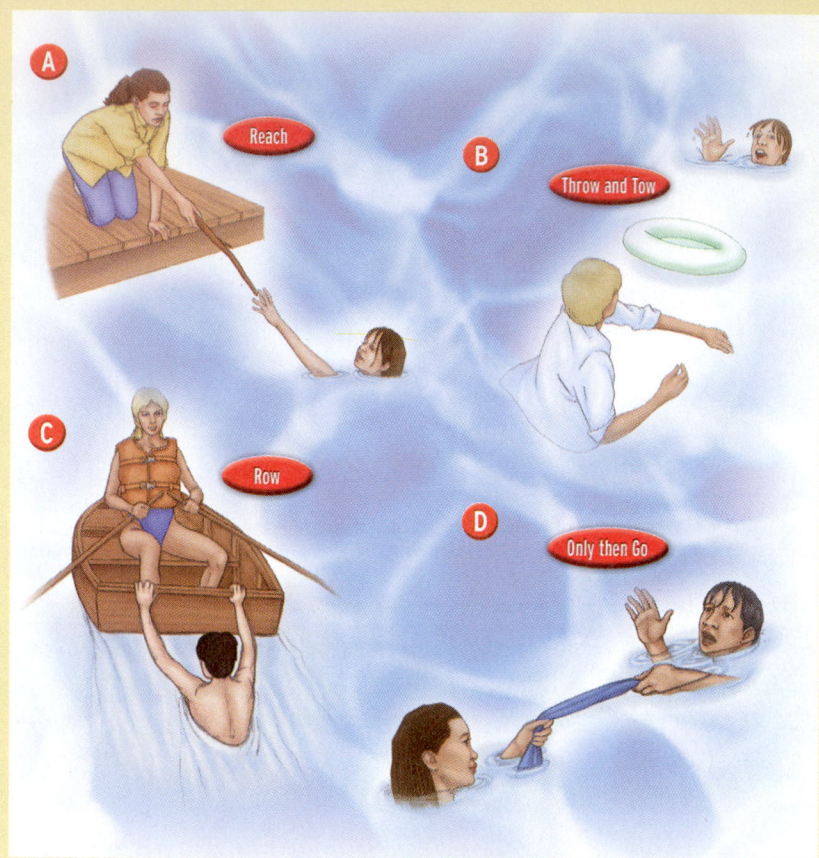

Figure 15-18 Basic rules of water rescue. **A.** Reach the person from shore. If you cannot reach the person from shore, wade closer. **B.** If an object that floats is available, throw it to the person. **C.** Use a boat if one is available. **D.** If you must swim to the person, use a towel or board for him or her to hold onto. Do not let the person grab you.

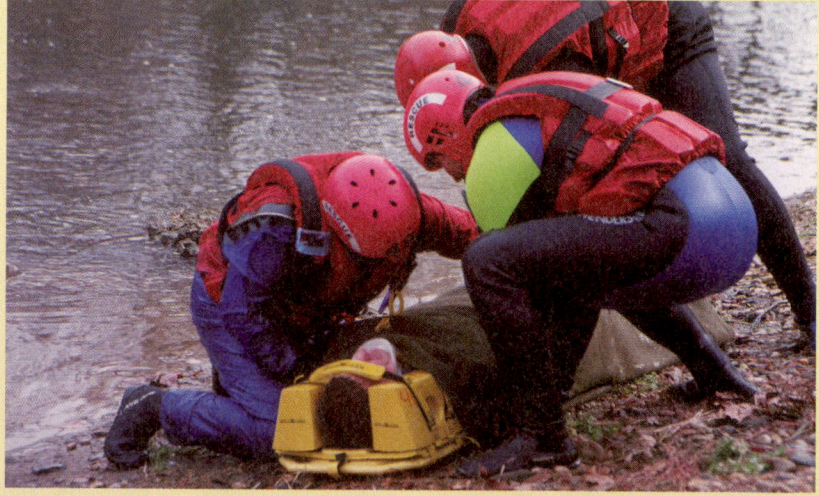

Figure 15-19 When performing a water rescue, you must wear proper personal protective equipment, including a personal flotation device.

Recovery Techniques

On occasion, you may be called to the scene of a drowning and find that the patient is not floating or visible in the water. An organized rescue effort in these circumstances calls for personnel who are experienced with recovery techniques and equipment, including snorkel, mask, and scuba gear. <u>Scuba</u> (self-contained underwater breathing apparatus) gear is a system that delivers air to the mouth and lungs at atmospheric pressures that increase with the depth of the dive.

As a last resort, when standard procedures for recovery are unsuccessful, you may have to use a grappling iron or large hook to drag the bottom for the victim. Although the hook could seriously wound the patient, it may be the only effective way to bring him or her to the surface for resuscitation efforts.

Resuscitation Efforts

You should *never* give up on resuscitating a cold-water drowning victim. When a person is submerged in water that is colder than body temperature, heat will be conducted from the body to the water. The resulting hypothermia can protect vital organs from the lack of oxygen. In addition, exposure to cold water will occasionally activate certain primitive reflexes, which may preserve basic body functions for prolonged periods. In one case, a 2½-year-old girl recovered after being submerged in cold water for at least 66 minutes. Continue full resuscitation efforts until the patient recovers or is pronounced dead by a physician.

Also, whenever a person dives or jumps into very cold water, the **diving reflex**, slowing of the heart rate caused by submersion in cold water, may cause immediate **bradycardia**, a slow heart rhythm. Loss of consciousness and drowning may follow. However, the person may be able to survive for an extended period of time under water, thanks to a lowering of the metabolic rate associated with hypothermia. For this reason, you should continue full resuscitation efforts no matter how long the patient has been submerged.

Avalanche Injuries

Eighty percent of avalanche deaths are caused by asphyxia, 10% to 15% by injuries, and only 5% by hypothermia. If the patient is found alive, he or she will be hypoxic, usually hypothermic, and frequently have injuries and shock.

In a Swiss study of 422 skiers buried in avalanches occurring between 1981 and 1991, Hermann Brugger and Markus Falk found an overall death rate of 57%. The chance of survival was 92% if the victim was uncovered within 15 minutes of burial, but by the 35-minute mark the survival rate dropped to only 30%. Presence of an air pocket increased the chances of survival during the first 90 minutes of burial. According to the study, the more deeply the victim was buried, the less likely the survival—probably because of the longer rescue times involved. Therefore, to have a reasonable chance of surviving, an avalanche victim must be rescued by companions rather than by a ski patrol or other organized rescue team.

With modern avalanche control techniques, there is minimal risk of being caught in an avalanche in the controlled parts of an alpine ski area. Most avalanche victims are backcountry skiers and snowboarders, snowmobilers, or climbers. Each member of a group that ventures into avalanche-prone areas should be trained in avalanche avoidance, proper conduct if caught in an avalanche (including the need to create an air pocket), and rescue techniques. Each should carry a shovel, **avalanche probe** (or ski poles that convert into a probe), and an avalanche transceiver at all times. When in avalanche terrain, skiers should remove pole straps from their wrists and release safety straps. A new device, a backpack-mounted "avalanche airbag," may prove useful in preventing avalanche fatalities among those who wear it.

Ski patrollers and other rescue personnel who may be called upon to help in an avalanche rescue should frequently refresh their training and ability to use an **avalanche transceiver**.

When a rescuer is participating in an avalanche rescue, the priority upon locating the victim is uncovering his or her head and chest (▼ **Figure 15-20**). Note whether the patient has an air pocket around the face and, if so, preserve it. Avoid unnecessary jostling, which may precipitate ventricular fibrillation.

As soon as the patient's head is exposed, open the airway, and start rescue breathing unless the patient is breathing spontaneously. Water, snow, blood, or vomitus

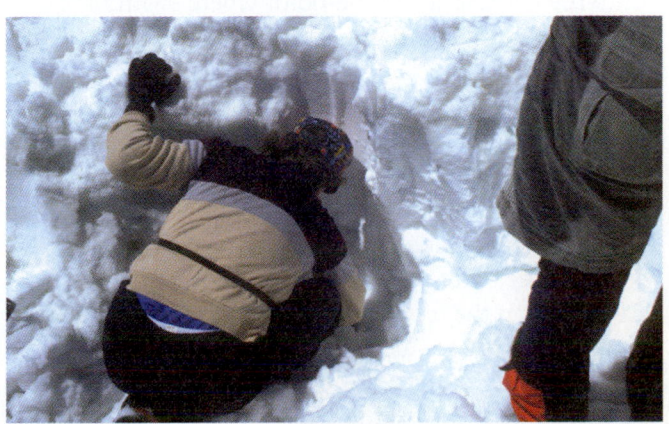

Figure 15-20 Carefully excavate the avalanche victim's head and chest.

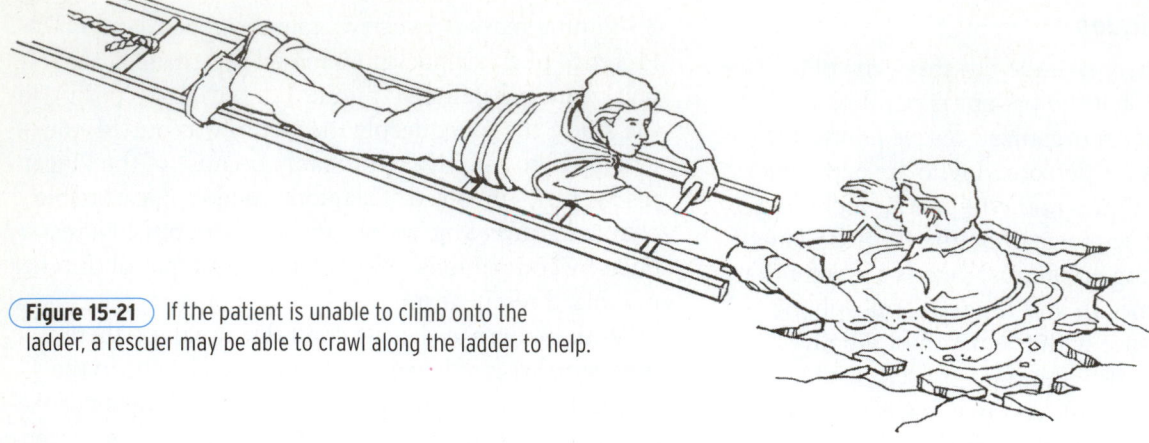

Figure 15-21 If the patient is unable to climb onto the ladder, a rescuer may be able to crawl along the ladder to help.

frequently block the airway. A portable suction unit is useful and should be included in avalanche rescue caches. A patient in cardiac arrest must be fully uncovered or removed from the burial site before CPR can be given.

Upon extrication, add insulating materials under, over, and around the patient to prevent further heat loss. Although the patient is almost always hypothermic, rewarming is usually not possible during CPR. Give high-flow oxygen, if available.

After breathing and circulation have been restored, perform the rapid body survey, manage hypothermia as described previously in this chapter, and treat any fractures or other injuries using the proper techniques.

Ice Rescue

The popularity of ice fishing, ice skating, ice boating, and snowmobiling on frozen lakes increases the likelihood that rescuers may have to aid a person who has broken through the ice. Ice rescue is very hazardous to the rescuer. You should have a healthy respect for thin ice and cold water, and you should remember that it is no help to anyone if you fall through the ice while attempting a rescue. Within minutes, cold water can numb the extremities to the point where swimming and self-extrication are impossible.

To allow a patient to reach the shore or a rescuer to reach the patient, an ice rescue must be performed so that the weight of the patient and any rescue equipment is widely distributed across the ice. All rescuers should wear personal flotation devices.

An excellent rescue device is a lightweight ladder with a lifeline tied to the shore end. The ladder is shoved out on the ice to the patient, who crawls onto the ladder and edges along it to safety. If the patient is unable to climb onto the ladder, a rescuer may be able to crawl along the ladder to help ▲ **Figure 15-21** . If the ice breaks under the ladder, the far end will dip and the

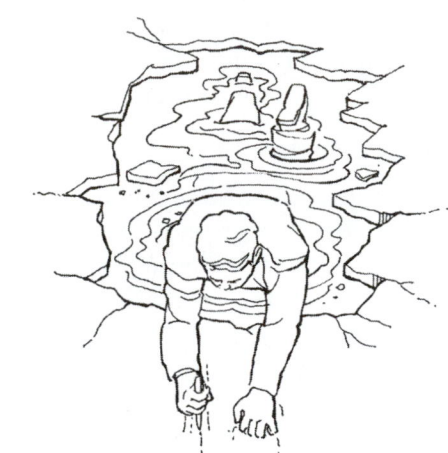

Figure 15-22 A pocketknife, ski pole tip, or any sharp object that will penetrate the surface of the ice can be used to increase traction.

near end will rise, making it easier to pull the ladder back to safety by the lifeline.

If a ladder is unavailable, one or more wide boards or a stout tree branch can be used. Alternative techniques, especially if the ice is too fragile to support these devices, include shoving canoes, rowboats, or rubber rafts out onto the ice or throwing a spare tire or ring buoy to the patient. In addition, a fire hose with the ends capped can be inflated with air to make a semirigid, buoyant device that can be shoved out to the patient much like a long pole. Helicopters have been used successfully, especially in multiple-victim disasters.

An individual who falls through the ice should attempt self-rescue by extending his or her arms forward over the ice and kicking the legs up so that the body is held in a level position. He or she should then work forward onto the ice by kicking and carefully pulling with the forearms, elbows, and hands. A pocketknife, ski pole tip, or any sharp object that will penetrate the surface of the ice can be used to increase traction ▲ **Figure 15-22** . This maneuver can be successful even if the ice continues to break ahead of the patient; it should be continued until he or she reaches firm ice. Once the patient has pulled his or her entire body onto firmer ice, he or she should carefully roll or edge toward shore, distributing body weight as widely as possible.

Falling through the ice while on skis would be unusual, but if it occurs, the individual should release the ski bindings as soon as possible to prevent the skis from acting as a "sea anchor."

All individuals who break through ice are assumed to be hypothermic and should be provided emergency care as described above. Extricate rapidly.

Diving Emergencies

Most serious water-related injuries are associated with dives, with or without scuba gear. Some of these problems are related to the nature of the dive; others result from panic. Panic is not restricted to the person who is frightened by water. It can happen even to the experienced diver or swimmer.

There are more than 3,000,000 scuba sport divers in the United States, and approximately 200,000 new divers being trained annually. Medical problems relating to scuba diving techniques and equipment are becoming increasingly common. These problems are separated into three phases of the dive: descent, bottom, and ascent.

Descent Emergencies

Descent problems are usually due to the sudden increase in pressure on the body as the person dives deeper into the water. Some body cavities cannot adjust to the increased external pressure of the water; the result is severe pain. The usual areas affected are the lungs, the sinus cavities, the middle ear, the teeth, and the area of the face surrounded by the diving mask. Usually, the pain caused by these "squeeze problems" forces the diver to return to the surface to equalize the pressures, and the problem clears up by itself. A diver who continues to complain of pain, particularly in the ear, after returning to the surface should be transported to the hospital.

A person with a perforated tympanic membrane (ruptured eardrum) may have a special problem while diving. If cold water enters the middle ear through a ruptured eardrum, the diver may lose his or her balance and orientation. The diver may then shoot to the surface and run into ascent problems.

Emergencies at the Bottom

Problems related to the bottom of the dive are rarely seen. They include inadequate mixing of oxygen and

> Panic is not restricted to the person who is frightened by water. It can happen even to the experienced diver or swimmer.

carbon dioxide in the air the diver breathes and accidental feeding of poisonous carbon monoxide into the breathing apparatus. Both are the result of faulty connections in the diving gear. These situations can cause drowning or rapid ascent; they require emergency resuscitation and transport of the patient.

Ascent Emergencies

Most of the serious injuries associated with diving are related to ascending from the bottom and are referred to as *ascent problems*. These emergencies usually require aggressive resuscitation. Two particularly dangerous medical emergencies are *air embolism* and *decompression sickness* (also called "the bends").

Air Embolism

The most dangerous, and most common, emergency in scuba diving is **air embolism**, a condition involving bubbles of air in the blood vessels. Air embolism may occur on a dive as shallow as 6'. The problem starts when the diver holds his or her breath during a rapid ascent. The air pressure in the lungs remains at a high level while the external pressure on the chest decreases. As a result, the air inside the lungs expands rapidly, causing the alveoli in the lungs to rupture. The air released from this rupture can cause the following injuries:

- Air may enter the pleural space and compress the lungs (a pneumothorax).
- Air may enter the mediastinum (the space within the thorax that contains the heart and great vessels), causing a condition called *pneumomediastinum*.
- Air may enter the bloodstream and create bubbles of air in the vessels called *air emboli*.

Pneumothorax and pneumomediastinum both result in pain and severe dyspnea. An air embolus will act as a plug and prevent the normal flow of blood and oxygen to a specific part of the body. The brain and spinal cord are the organs most severely affected by air embolism because they require a constant supply of oxygen.

The following are potential signs and symptoms of air embolism:

- Blotching (mottling of the skin)
- Froth (often pink or bloody) at the nose and mouth
- Severe pain in muscles, joints, or abdomen
- Dyspnea and/or chest pain
- Dizziness, nausea, and vomiting
- Dysphasia (difficulty speaking)
- Difficulty with vision
- Paralysis and/or coma
- Irregular pulse and even cardiac arrest

Decompression Sickness

Decompression sickness, commonly called the bends, occurs when bubbles of gas, especially nitrogen, obstruct the blood vessels. This condition results from too rapid an ascent from a dive. During the dive, nitrogen that is being breathed dissolves in the blood and tissues because it is under pressure. When the diver ascends, the external pressure is decreased, and the dissolved nitrogen forms small bubbles within those tissues. These bubbles can lead to problems similar to those that occur in air embolism (blockage of tiny blood vessels, depriving parts of the body of their normal blood supply), but severe pain in certain tissues or spaces in the body is the most common problem.

The most striking symptom is abdominal and/or joint pain so severe that the patient literally doubles up or "bends." Dive tables and computers are available to show the proper rate of ascent from a dive, including the number and length of pauses that a diver should make on the way up. However, even divers who stay within these limits can suffer the bends.

Even after a "safe dive," decompression sickness can occur from driving a car up a mountain or flying in an unpressurized airplane that climbs too rapidly to a great height. However, the risk of this diminishes after 24 to 48 hours. The problem is exactly the same as ascent from a deep dive: a sudden decrease of external pressure on the body and release of dissolved nitrogen from the blood that forms bubbles of nitrogen gas within the blood vessels.

You may find it difficult to distinguish between air embolism and decompression sickness. As a general rule, air embolism occurs immediately on return to

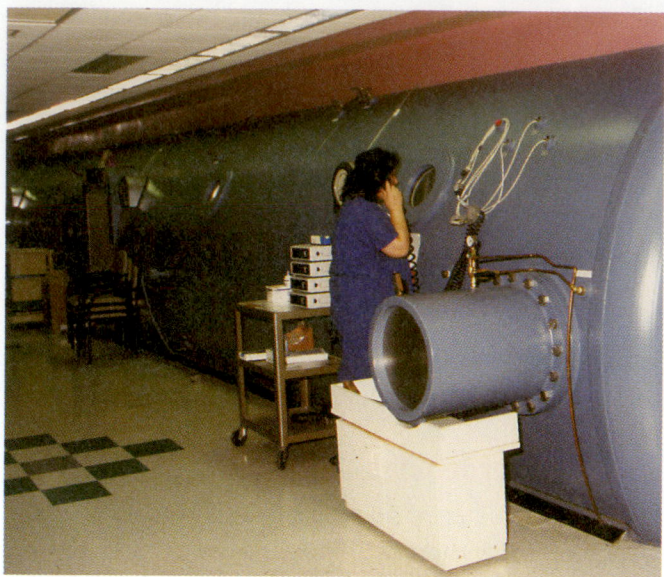

Figure 15-23 A hyperbaric chamber, usually a small room, is pressurized to more than atmospheric pressure and used to treat decompression sickness and air embolism.

the surface, whereas the symptoms of decompression sickness may not occur for several hours. The emergency treatment is the same for both. It consists of BLS followed by recompression in a **hyperbaric chamber**, a chamber or a small room that is pressurized to more than atmospheric pressure **▲ Figure 15-23** . Recompression treatment allows the bubbles of gas to dissolve into the blood and equalizes the pressures inside and outside the lungs. Once these pressures are equalized, gradual decompression can be accomplished under controlled conditions to prevent the bubbles from re-forming.

In treating patients who are suspected of having air embolism or decompression sickness, you should follow these accepted treatment steps:

1. Remove the patient from the water. Try to keep the patient calm.
2. Begin BLS and administer oxygen.
3. Place the patient in a left lateral recumbent position with the head down.
4. Provide prompt transport to the nearest recompression facility for treatment.

Injury from decompression sickness is usually reversible with proper treatment. However, if the bubbles block critical blood vessels that supply the brain or spinal cord, permanent central nervous system injury may result. Therefore, the key in emergency management of these serious ascent problems is to recognize that an emergency exists and treat as soon as possible. Administer oxygen and provide rapid transport.

Other Water Hazards

You must pay close attention to the body temperature of a person who is rescued from cold water. Treat hypothermia caused by immersion in cold water the same way you treat hypothermia caused by cold exposure. Prevent further heat loss from contact with the ground, stretcher, or air, and transport the patient promptly.

A person swimming in shallow water may suffer from **breath-holding syncope**, a loss of consciousness caused by a decreased stimulus for breathing. This happens to swimmers who breathe in and out rapidly and deeply before entering the water in an effort to expand their capacity to stay underwater. While increasing the oxygen level, this hyperventilation lowers the carbon dioxide level. Because an elevated level of carbon dioxide in the blood is the strongest stimulus for breathing, the swimmer may not feel the need to breathe even after using up all the oxygen in his or her lungs. The emergency treatment of breath-holding syncope is the same as that for a drowning or near drowning.

Injuries caused by boat propellers, sharp rocks, water skis, or dangerous marine life may be complicated by immersion in cold water. In these cases, remove the patient from the water, taking care to protect the spine, and administer oxygen. Apply dressings and splints if indicated, and monitor the patient closely for any signs of immersion or cold injury.

You should be aware that a child who is involved in a drowning or near drowning may be the victim of child abuse. Although it may be difficult to prove, such incidents should be handled according to the rules set up for suspected child abuse.

Swimmer's Ear

Swimmer's ear is an infection of the outer ear canal and is seen in swimmers and divers whose ears are continually wet. Symptoms include pain and tenderness associated with the ear, a white or yellow discharge, and partial deafness.

The individual should see a physician for specific treatment. Swimmer's ear can be prevented by putting several drops of a solution of vinegar diluted to half strength with rubbing alcohol or tap water in both ears after swimming. Commercial preparations containing 2% acetic acid in propylene glycol are available.

Associated Injuries

Kayaking, rafting, canoeing, sailing, windsurfing, motor boating, water skiing, and surfing all can cause injuries. Whitewater sports are particularly hazardous because the patient may be far from medical help. The additional complication of submersion is always a danger.

The patient should be moved to calm, shallow water or must be removed from the water before assessment and emergency care can be performed and provided effectively. Conduct the initial assessment and care for urgent problems and soft-tissue, bone, and joint injuries as outlined in previous chapters. Rigid collars, extremity splints, cylindrical leg splints, and pillow splints can be improvised from life jackets, paddles, kayak float bags, and camping equipment such as pack straps and air mattresses.

The emergency care of injuries caused by hazardous marine life is discussed in Chapter 13.

Chapter *Sweep*

Ready for Review

Cold illness can be either a local or a systemic problem. Local cold injuries include frostbite, frostnip, and immersion foot. Frostbite is the most serious because tissues actually freeze with this injury. All patients with a local cold injury should be removed from the cold and protected from further exposure. You can rewarm frostnipped parts, including immersion foot, with your warm hands or breath. On the other hand, you can cause further damage to a frostbitten part by attempting to rewarm it in the field. If this is necessary because you cannot transport the patient to the hospital, immerse the part in water at a temperature between 100° and 112°F (38° and 44.5°C).

Patients who are exposed to the cold can also become hypothermic. The key to treating such patients is to stabilize vital functions and prevent further heat loss. Do not attempt to rewarm patients who have moderate to severe hypothermia, because they are prone to developing arrhythmias unless handled very carefully. Even if you cannot find a pulse, do not consider a patient dead until he or she is "warm and dead." Local protocol will dictate whether or not such patients receive CPR or defibrillation in the field.

The body's regulatory mechanisms normally maintain body temperature within a very narrow range around 98.6°F (37°C). The body can increase its core temperature by increasing its metabolism, for example, by shivering. In general, however, body temperature is regulated by losing heat to the atmosphere. The very young and the very old, as well as patients with certain diseases and medication regimens, are at increased risk of heat or cold injuries because their regulatory mechanisms are not as efficient as those of other patients.

Emergency care of a patient with high-altitude illness includes recognizing the problem and stopping further ascent. Give oxygen if available; however, if not available, do not delay the descent. Treat headache with mild analgesics. Feed and hydrate the patient. Likewise, humans are more vulnerable to the harmful effects of solar radiation when at high altitudes, on snow, or on bodies of water. Precautions need to be taken against these environmental elements to avoid injuries to the skin and eyes. Patients with sunburn, windburn, or snowblindness need to be removed from the sun's exposure. Care for sunburn and snowblindness include applying cool compresses and using nonprescription pain relievers. Windburn should be treated with greasy ointments or lotions.

Heat illness can take three forms: heat cramps, heat exhaustion, and heatstroke. Heat cramps are painful muscle spasms that occur with vigorous exercise. They usually go away if you remove the patient from the hot environment, rest the affected muscles, and replace lost fluids (by drinking a lot of water).

Heat exhaustion, a more systemic illness, is essentially a form of hypovolemic shock. It occurs when the body loses so much water and so many electrolytes that it becomes dehydrated. Patients with heat exhaustion may be cold and clammy, weak or faint, confused, and have a headache. As with other patients in shock, the pulse is often rapid. Body temperature can be high, and the patient may or may not still be sweating. Treatment includes removing the patient, if feasible, from the heat and treating for mild hypovolemic shock, usually with oral fluids. More often, intravenous fluids will be necessary.

Heat exhaustion can progress to heatstroke. This is a life-threatening emergency, usually fatal if untreated. Patients with heatstroke may or may not still be sweating, but they will usually be dry and will have high body temperatures. Changes in mental status can include coma. Rapid lowering of the body temperature in the field can save the life of a patient with heatstroke. Fanning dampened skin and placement of cold packs around the neck, armpits, and groin are key.

In the outdoors, people are susceptible to injury from lightning during electrical storms, metal structures in resort areas, and high-voltage power lines in remote areas. Understanding how to protect yourself and others in these circumstances is paramount to emergency care. Scene size-up and initial assessment are important and need to be rapid. Institute BSI precautions and rapidly provide rescue breathing or CPR, if necessary. Patients who are apparently dead should be cared for first.

Drowning and near-drowning incidents can occur even in areas that are not associated with water recreation. The first rule in caring for victims of such incidents is to be sure not to become a victim yourself. Take care to protect the spine when removing patients from the water, since spinal cord injuries, especially cervical spine injuries, are often involved in drownings. Be aware of the possibility of hypothermia, especially in cold water immersions.

Although avalanches kill people in many ways, most fatalities are due to suffocation, cardiac problems, hypothermia, and internal injuries. Treatment for suffocation includes clearing the air passages and making room for chest expansion; extending the head; and, for all suffocation and cardiac problems, providing resuscitation by use of mouth-to-mask, plastic airway, BVM device, or CPR. Treating hypothermia includes preventing further loss by providing dry clothes, providing internal heating by using warmed and humidified oxygen, supplying external heat or covering the core of the body with a prewarmed sleeping bag, giving warm drinks, treating the patient for shock, and transporting the person to a hospital. Treating internal injuries requires detailed patient assessment, providing indicated emergency care and rapid transport to definitive care.

While some injuries associated with scuba diving are immediately apparent, others may show up hours later. Most significant injuries occur during ascent. Patients with air embolism or decompression sickness may have pain, paralysis, or altered mental status. Be prepared to transport such patients to a recompression facility with a hyperbaric chamber.

www.OECzone.com

Vital Vocabulary

acute mountain sickness (AMS) A condition that can occur at altitudes above 6,500′, caused by lack of oxygen. Among the signs and symptoms of AMS are a throbbing headache, apathy, lightheadedness, nausea, vomiting, weakness, fatigue, shortness of breath, and a generally ill appearance.

air embolism Air bubbles in the blood vessels.

ambient temperature The temperature of the surrounding environment.

avalanche probe A long pole used to search for a body buried in the snow.

avalanche transceiver An electronic device that can emit a signal and also receive a signal from another transceiver. Worn by people in avalanche-prone terrain to assist rescue in the event of avalanche burial.

bradycardia Slow heart rate.

breath-holding syncope Loss of consciousness caused by a decreased breathing stimulus.

core temperature The temperature of the central part of the body (eg, the heart, lungs, and vital organs).

decompression sickness A painful condition seen in divers who ascend too quickly, in which gas, especially nitrogen, forms bubbles in blood vessels and other tissues; also called "the bends."

deep frostbite A full- or partial-thickness freezing of a body part, most commonly the hands and feet.

diving reflex Slowing of the heart rate caused by submersion in cold water.

drowning Death from suffocation after submersion in water.

electrolytes Certain salts and other chemicals that are dissolved in body fluids and cells.

frostbite Damage to tissues as the result of exposure to cold; frozen body parts.

frostnip A mild cold injury caused by cold-induced superficial blood vessel constriction.

gangrene Tissue death followed by bacterial invasion and putrification; usually caused by loss of blood supply.

heat cramps Painful muscle spasms usually associated with vigorous activity in a hot environment.

heat exhaustion A form of heat injury in which the body loses significant amounts of fluid and electrolytes because of heavy sweating; also called heat prostration or heat collapse.

heatstroke A life-threatening condition of severe hyperthermia caused by exposure to excessive natural or artificial heat, marked by warm, dry skin; severely altered mental status; and often irreversible coma.

high altitude cerebral edema (HACE) A serious complication of acute mountain sickness, characterized by swelling of the brain, ataxia, and altered mental status.

high altitude pulmonary edema (HAPE) A type of high-altitude illness characterized by the lungs filling with edema fluid.

hyperbaric chamber A chamber, usually a small room, pressurized to more than atmospheric pressure.

hyperthermia A condition in which core temperature rises to 101°F (38.3°C) or more.

hypothermia A fall in body core temperature to below 95°F (35°C).

insulators Materials that resist transmission of electricity, heat, or sound.

laryngospasm A severe constriction of the larynx and vocal cords.

near drowning Survival, at least temporarily, after suffocation in water.

rewarm To raise the body temperature of a patient with hypothermia, or to raise the temperature of a part affected with frostbite.

scuba A system that delivers air to the mouth and lungs at various atmospheric pressures, increasing with the depth of the dive; stands for *self-contained underwater breathing apparatus*.

snowblindness Sunburn of the conjunctiva of the eye.

sun protection factor (SPF) A number that refers to how much longer skin protected by a sunscreen can be exposed to the sun before becoming red (compared to unprotected skin).

sunburn A superficial or partial-thickness burn caused by ultraviolet light in the medium-wave range (UVB) with a wavelength of 290 to 320 nanometers.

windburn Irritation of the skin caused by exposure to wind; resembles superficial sunburn.

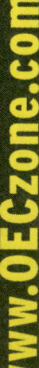

Assessment in Action
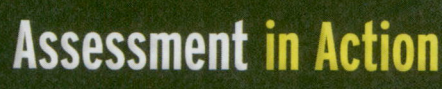

It is early July in the Green Mountains of Vermont. You and your husband have decided to hike a section of the Appalachian Trail that winds its way over the highest peak of the ski area at which you patrol during the ski season. It is a very warm and humid Saturday and the forecast is calling for late afternoon showers. You begin your hike at Route 11 and head north toward the peak. It should take about 2 hours to reach the summit. As you ascend the trail you begin to realize that there is an overabundance of hikers on the trail today. You reach the peak in a little over the expected time and set up for a leisurely lunch and well-deserved rest. The sky is becoming very ominous in a spectacular sort of way, heralding the rapid approach of a cold front. You opt to cut your lunch short and begin to pack. The sky is darkening, the wind is beginning to howl, and you can feel the temperature plummet. Suddenly, you are startled by an ear-shattering crack and a blinding flash. You realize that lightning has struck the peak just above you. There are a number of people shouting for help. You and your husband rush to see if you can offer assistance.

As you size up the scene, you observe six adults on the ground. Three of the adults are trying to stand, two of the adults are moving, and one is motionless. You move toward the adult who is motionless and find a man in his 30s. He is unresponsive, his skin and clothing are smoldering, and he is in respiratory and cardiac arrest.

1. Which of the following actions should you take first?
   A. Initiate CPR on the unresponsive patient.
   B. Immediately head for the lift.
   C. Tend to the patients who are moving and need assistance.
   D. Take triage tags out of your pack.

2. To estimate the storm's distance, count the seconds between the lightning and the thunder and divide by:
   A. 2.
   B. 3.
   C. 4.
   D. 5.

3. What possible action should the other adults take to prevent further lightning-induced injuries?
   A. Congregate near a large rock.
   B. Disperse and move off the summit.
   C. Move under a tall tree.
   D. Walk quickly and closely spaced down the ridge.

Challenging Questions

4. Which is an acronym for the system used at a multiple-casualty incident (MCI) scene to deal effectively with multiple patients?
   A. DCAP
   B. AVPU
   C. START
   D. SAMPLE

5. In a triage situation caused by a lightning strike, you should:
   A. consider the unresponsive patient as BLACK—deceased or soon to become deceased.
   B. tend to only the patients who are responsive.
   C. activate EMS if possible, and initiate CPR on the unresponsive patient who is still very salvageable and may need CPR for an extended period of time.
   D. wait for additional responders before taking action.

Points to Ponder

While hiking at altitude as a part of multi-day educational trip, one of the members of your group begins to complain of mild headaches and a feeling of lightheadedness. You stop and question the student, who seems tired and a bit slow to respond. His tent mate tells you that "Frank" didn't sleep well the night before and tossed and turned a lot. This is your third day above 10,000' and you had planned to take the students on a summit hike today and another tomorrow as a part of your mountain travel course. What illness do you think is affecting Frank? If you continue with your climbing plan, what other symptoms might be noted, and could this condition worsen? What treatment plan should be considered? With self-evacuation the only option, how would you deal with a sick patient?

Issues Altitude Illnesses, Care in the Back Country, Alternate Planning, Transport Decisions.

Online Outlook

Hypothermia can develop either quickly, as when someone is immersed in cold water, or more gradually, as when a lost hunter is exposed to the cold environment for several hours or more. To learn more about preventing and treating hypothermia, complete Exercise 15 at www.OECzone.com.

Behavioral Emergencies

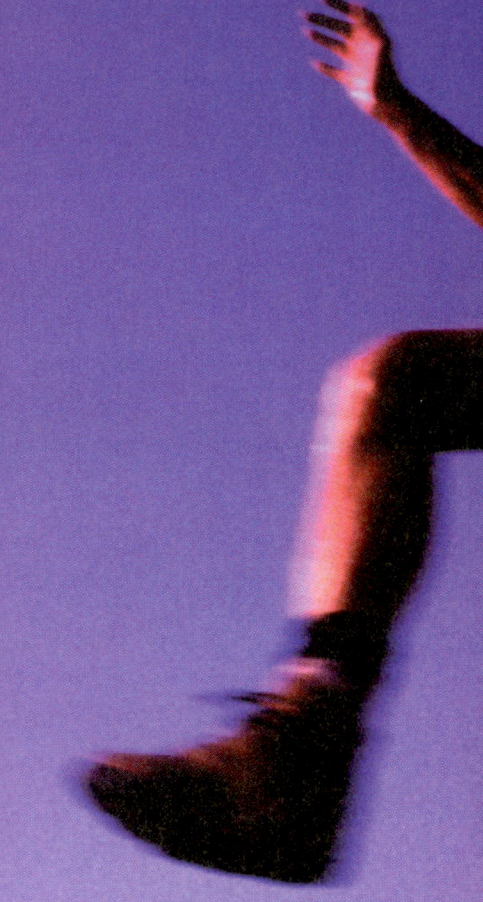

Objectives

Cognitive

🌲 1. Define behavioral emergencies (p 452).

🌲 2. Discuss the general factors that may cause an alteration in a patient's behavior (p 453).

3. State the various reasons for psychological crises (p 453).

4. Discuss special medicolegal considerations for managing behavioral emergencies (p 456).

🌲 5. Discuss the special considerations for assessing a patient with behavioral problems (p 455).

6. Discuss the general principles of an individual's behavior which suggest that the patient is at risk for violence (p 457).

7. Discuss methods to calm behavioral emergency patients (p 454).

Affective

🌲 8. Explain the rationale for learning how to modify your behavior toward the patient with a behavioral emergency (p 452).

Psychomotor

🌲 9. Demonstrate the assessment and emergency medical care of the patient experiencing a behavioral emergency (p 455).

🌲 These are core concepts in initial patrol training.

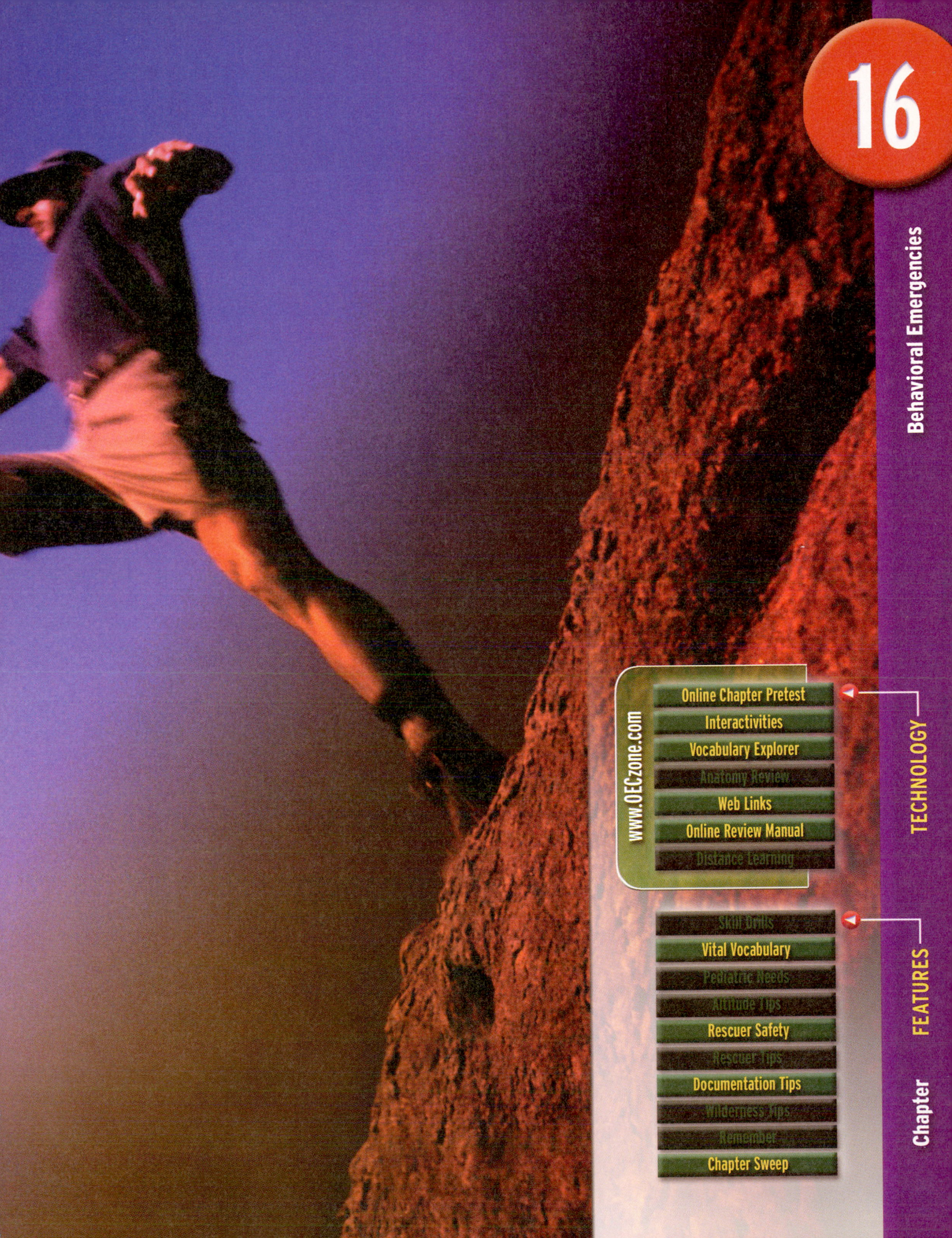

www.OECzone.com

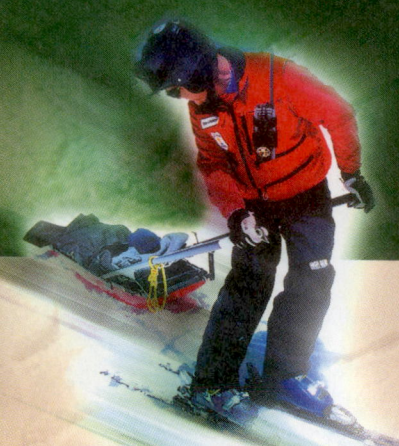

You are skiing down an intermediate run when you come across a young woman sitting in the snow. She seems disoriented and does not know what day it is or where she is.

Behavioral emergencies can be very challenging calls for a variety of reasons. This chapter will give you insights into how you can safely and effectively manage these calls in addition to helping you answer the following questions:

1. How can you differentiate between the two types of altered mental status—organic and functional?

2. Is this an important distinction? Why?

Behavioral Emergencies

As a rescuer, you can expect to deal often with patients undergoing a psychological or behavioral crisis. The crisis may be due to the emergency situation, mental illness, mind-altering substances, stress, or many other medical causes. This chapter discusses various kinds of behavioral emergencies, including those involving overdoses, violent behavior, and mental illness. You will learn how to assess a person who exhibits signs and symptoms of a behavioral emergency and what kind of emergency care may be required in these situations. The chapter also covers legal concerns in dealing with disturbed patients. Finally, it describes how to identify and manage the potentially violent patient, including the use of restraints.

Myth and Reality

Everyone has emotional problems at some point in life, some more severe than others. Perfectly healthy people may have some of the symptoms and signs of mental illness from time to time. Therefore, you should not jump to the conclusion that you are mentally disturbed when you behave in certain ways that are discussed in this chapter. For that matter, you also should not jump to this conclusion about a patient in any given situation.

The most common misconception about mental illness is that if you are feeling "bad" or "depressed," you must be "sick." That is simply untrue. There are many perfectly justifiable reasons for feeling depressed, including divorce, loss of a job, and the death of a relative or friend. For the teenager who just broke up with his girlfriend of 12 months, it is altogether normal to withdraw from ordinary activities and to feel "blue." This is a normal reaction to a crisis situation. However, when a person finds that Monday morning blues last until Friday, week after week, he or she may indeed have a psychiatric disorder, coupled with difficulty functioning.

Many people believe that all individuals with mental health disorders are dangerous, violent, or otherwise unmanageable. This is untrue. Only a small percentage of those with mental health problems fall into these categories. As an OEC technician, you may occasionally see a violent patient. After all, you are seeing people who are, by definition, considered to be having an emergency; otherwise, you probably would not be seeing them. You are there because family members or friends felt unable to manage the patient by themselves. This may be a result of the use or abuse of drugs or alcohol. It may be that the patient has a long history of mental illness and is reacting to a particularly stressful event.

While you cannot determine what has caused a person's behavioral problem, you may be able to predict that the person will become violent. The ability to predict violence is an important assessment tool for the rescuer.

Defining Behavioral Emergencies

Behavior is what you can see of a person's response to the environment: his or her actions. Sometimes, it is obvious what a person is responding to: a person is punched, and he or she runs away or bursts into tears or hits back. Sometimes, it is less clear, as when someone is depressed for very complex reasons.

Most of the time, individuals respond to the environment in reasonable ways. Over the years, they have learned to adapt to a variety of situations in daily life, including stresses and strains. This is called adjustment. There are times, however, when the stress is so great that the normal ways of adjusting do not work. When this happens, a person's behavior is likely to change, even if only temporarily. The new behavior may not be appropriate, or normal.

The definition of a **behavioral crisis** or emergency is any reaction to events that interferes with the **activities** of daily living (ADL) or has become unacceptable to the patient, family, or community. For example, when someone experiences an interruption of the daily routine, such as washing, dressing, and eating, chances are his or her behavior has become a problem. For that person, at that time, a behavioral emergency may exist. If the interruption of daily routine tends to recur on a regular basis, the behavior is also considered a mental health problem. It is then a pattern, rather than an isolated incident.

For example, a person who experiences a panic attack after having a heart attack is not necessarily mentally ill. Likewise, you would expect a person who is fired from a job to have some sort of reaction, often sadness and depression. These behavioral problems are short-term and isolated events. However, the person who reacts with a fit of rage, attacking people and property or going on a "bender" for a week, has gone beyond what society considers appropriate or normal behavior. That person is clearly undergoing a behavioral emergency. Usually, if an abnormal or disturbing pattern of behavior lasts for at least a month, it is regarded as a matter of concern from a mental health standpoint. For example, chronic depression, a persistent feeling of sadness and despair, may be a symptom of a mental or physical disorder. This type of long-term problem would be labeled a mental health disorder.

A person who is no longer able to respond appropriately to the environment may be having what is called a psychological or psychiatric emergency. When a psychiatric emergency arises, the patient may show agitation or violence or become a threat to himself, herself, or others. This is more serious than a more typical behavioral emergency that causes inappropriate behavior such as interference with ADL or intolerable actions. An immediate threat to the person involved or to others in the immediate area, including family, friends, bystanders, and rescuers should be considered a psychiatric emergency. For example, a person might respond to the death of a spouse by attempting suicide. Disruption can take many forms; not all involve violence nor are they all psychiatric emergencies.

The Magnitude of Mental Health Problems

According to the National Institutes of Mental Health, at one time or another, one in five Americans has some type of mental disorder, an illness with psychological or behavioral symptoms that may result in an impairment in functioning. It can be caused by a social, psychological, genetic, physical, chemical, or biologic disturbance.

Documentation Tips

The medicolegal issues associated with behavioral emergencies put added emphasis on thorough and specific documentation. Record detailed, objective findings that support the conclusion of abnormal behavior (withdrawn, won't talk, crying uncontrollably) and quote the patient's own words when appropriate. ("Life isn't worth it any more," or "The voices are telling me to kill people.") Avoid judgmental statements; these create the impression that you based your care on personal bias rather than the patient's needs.

Pathology: Causes of Behavioral Emergencies

Although sudden grief, emotional conflicts, and other psychological problems can cause behavioral emergencies, sudden illness, recent trauma, drug or alcohol intoxication, and diseases of the brain, such as Alzheimer's disease, can produce abnormal behavior as well. Likewise, altered mental status can arise from low levels of blood glucose, lack of oxygen, inadequate blood flow to the brain, and excessive heat or cold. As a rescuer, you are not responsible for diagnosing the underlying cause of a behavioral or psychiatric emergency. However, you should know the two basic categories of diagnosis a physician will use: organic (physical) and functional (psychological).

Organic brain syndrome is a temporary or permanent dysfunction of the brain caused by a disturbance in the physical or physiologic functioning of brain tissue, such as the disturbances listed above. That is, something has gone wrong in the way the organ itself is working. For example, low levels of blood glucose could cause organic brain syndrome.

A functional disorder is one in which the abnormal operation of an organ cannot be traced to an obvious change in the actual structure, or physiology, of the organ. Something has gone wrong, but the root cause cannot be identified as the working of the organ itself. Schizophrenia and bipolar disorder are the two most common psychotic conditions. A psychotic individual is unable to differentiate between reality and his or her subjective state. Because of this, these individuals do not reason as a normal person would. Many psychotic people can be treated with medications and function in the "real" world. However, if they forget or quit taking their medication, they can become acutely psychotic. If you determine the patient to be psychotic, you must recognize that the patient may not understand what has happened, what you are saying, or what you want to do to help him or her. The rescuer must show extreme *patience*

You should know the two basic types of underlying causes of behavioral emergencies: organic (physical) and functional (psychological).

and understanding. It can be very difficult to communicate with an acutely psychotic individual.

These two types of disorders can look very much alike. An **altered mental status**, or a change in the way a person thinks or behaves, is one indicator of central nervous system disease. A patient displaying bizarre behavior may turn out to have an acute medical illness that is the cause, or a partial cause, of the behavior. Recognizing this possibility may allow you to save a life.

Safe Approach to a Behavioral Emergency

All the regular prehospital care skills—assessment, providing care, patient approach, history taking, and patient communication—are used in behavioral emergencies. However, other management techniques also come into play. There is not room in this chapter for a full discussion of these techniques, but you should follow general guidelines to ensure your safety at the scene of a behavioral emergency (▼ Table 16-1).

TABLE 16-1 Safety Guidelines for Behavioral Emergencies

- **Be prepared to spend extra time.** It may take longer to assess, listen to, and prepare the patient for transport.

- **Have a definite plan of action.** Decide who will do what. If restraint is needed, how will it be accomplished?

- **Identify yourself calmly.** Try to gain the patient's confidence. If you begin shouting, the patient is likely to shout louder or become more excited. A low, calm voice is often a quieting influence.

- **Be direct.** State your intentions and what you expect of the patient.

- **Assess the scene.** If the patient is armed or has potentially harmful objects in his or her possession, have these removed by law enforcement personnel before you provide care.

- **Stay with the patient.** *Do not let the patient leave the area, and do not leave yourself unless law enforcement personnel can stay with the patient.* Otherwise, the patient may go to another room and obtain weapons, lock himself or herself in the bathroom, or take pills.

- **Encourage purposeful movement.** Help the patient to get dressed and gather appropriate belongings to take to the hospital.

- **Express interest in the patient's story.** Let the patient tell you what happened or what is going on now in his or her own words. However, do not play along with auditory or visual disturbances.

- **Do not get too close to the patient;** everyone needs personal space. Furthermore, you want to be sure you can move quickly if the patient becomes violent or tries to run away. Do not physically talk down to or directly confront the patient. A squatting, 45° angle approach is usually not confrontational but may hinder your movements. Do not allow the patient to get between you and the exit.

- **Avoid fighting with the patient.** You do not want to get into a power struggle. Remember, the patient is not responding to you in a normal manner; he or she may be wrestling with internal forces over which neither of you has control. You and others may be stimulating these inner forces without knowing it. If you can respond with understanding to the feeling that the patient is expressing, whether this is anger, fear, or desperation, you may be able to gain his or her cooperation. If it is necessary to use force, be sure you have adequate help and move toward the patient quietly and with assured firmness.

- **Be honest and reassuring.** If the patient asks whether he or she has to go to the hospital, the answer should be, "Yes, that is where you can receive medical help."

- **Do not judge.** You may see behavior that you dislike. Set those feelings aside and concentrate on providing emergency medical care.

Assessing a Behavioral Emergency

In evaluating a situation that is considered a behavioral emergency, the first things to consider are your safety and how the patient is responding to the environment (▼ Table 16-2). Is the situation unduly dangerous to you and your fellow rescuers? Do you need immediate law enforcement backup? Does the patient's behavior seem typical or normal in the circumstances? For example, a patient who has just been assaulted has good reason to be fearful of other people, including you. On the other hand, if you ask a person, "Do you know where you are?" and he or she replies, "The planet Venus" (and does not seem to be joking), you may conclude that the person is disoriented, regardless of the cause.

A behavioral crisis puts tremendous stress on a person's coping mechanisms, including natural abilities and training. The person is actually incapable of responding reasonably to the demands of the environment. This state may be temporary, as in an acute illness, or longer-lived, as in a complex, chronic mental illness. In either case, the patient's perception of reality may be compromised or distorted.

Sometimes a patient in a behavioral or psychiatric emergency will not respond at all to your questions. In those cases, you may be able to tell quite a lot about the patient's emotional state from facial expressions, pulse, and respirations. Tears, sweating, and blushing may be significant indicators of state of mind. Also, make sure

---

TABLE 16-2   Questions to Ask in Evaluating a Behavioral Crisis

- How does the patient relate to you?

- Does the patient answer your questions appropriately?

- Is the patient withdrawn or detached?

- Is the patient hostile or friendly? Too friendly?

- Does the patient understand why you are there?

- How is the patient dressed? Is the dress appropriate for the time of year and occasion? Are the clothes clean or dirty?

- Are the patient's movements coordinated or jerky and awkward? Does he or she appear to be agitated?

- Are the patient's movements purposeful? Are the movements helping to accomplish a task, such as sitting down and putting on a pair of shoes, or do they appear to be aimless, such as rocking back and forth in the chair?

- Has the patient harmed himself or herself? Is there damage to the surroundings?

- What are the patient's facial expressions? Are they bland and flat or expressive? Does the patient show joy, fear, or anger as appropriate? To what degree?

- Does the patient appear relaxed, or stiff and guarded?

- Are the patient's vocabulary and expressions what you would expect under the circumstances? Are they in line with the patient's social and educational background?

- Is the patient easily distracted?

- Are the patient's responses to what is going on around him or her appropriate?

- Is the patient's memory intact? Check orientation to time, place, person: Do you know what day/month/year it is? Do you know where you are? Do you know who I am?

- Is the patient alert and able to talk logically and coherently?

- What is the patient's mood? Does he or she seem agitated, elated, abnormally depressed?

- Does the patient appear fearful or worried?

- Does the patient express disordered thoughts, delusions, or hallucinations? That is, does he or she appear to be seeing, hearing, or responding to people or situations that are not present?

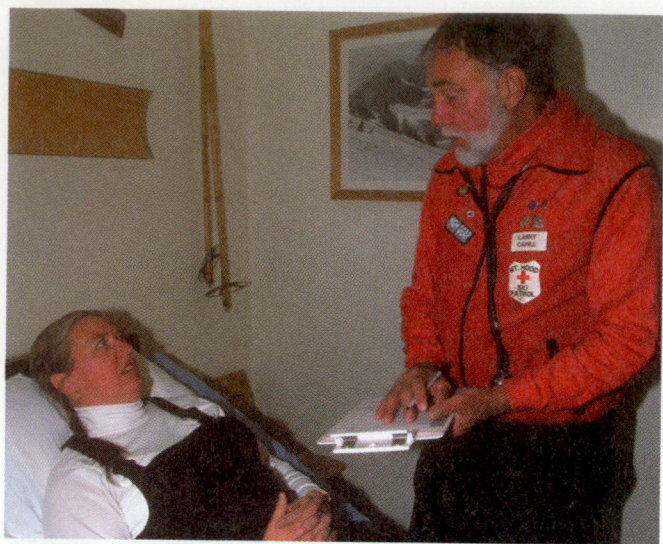

Figure 16-1 Making eye contact with a patient can provide useful clues about a patient's emotional state.

that you look at the patient's eyes; a patient who has a blank gaze or rapidly moving eyes may be experiencing CNS depression or some type of extra stress **▲ Figure 16-1** .

In trying to determine the reason for the patient's state, you should consider three major areas as possible contributors:

- Is the patient's central nervous system functioning properly? For example, the patient may be experiencing diabetic problems, particularly hypoglycemia. He or she may have been poisoned or may be responding to a physical trauma of some sort. Any of these situations could cause the patient to behave in an unusual or irrational fashion.

- Are hallucinogens or other drugs or alcohol a factor? Does the patient see strange things? Is everything distorted? Do you smell alcohol on the patient's breath?

- Are **psychogenic** circumstances, symptoms, or illness (caused by mental rather than physical factors) involved? These might include the death of a loved one, severe depression, a history of mental illness, threats of suicide, or some other major interruption of ADL.

Family, friends, and observers may be of great help in answering these questions. Together with your observations and interaction with the patient, they should provide enough data for you to assess the situation. This assessment has two primary goals: recognizing major

threats to life and reducing the stress of the situation as much as possible.

Medicolegal Considerations

The medical and legal aspects of emergency medical care become more complicated when the patient is undergoing a behavioral or psychiatric emergency. Nevertheless, legal problems are greatly reduced with the emotionally disturbed patient who consents to care. Gaining that patient's confidence is therefore a critical task for the rescuer.

Mental incapacity can take many forms: unconsciousness (as a result of hypoxia, alcohol, or drugs), temporary but severe stress, or depression. Once you have determined that a patient has impaired mental capacity, you must decide whether he or she requires immediate emergency medical care. A patient who is mentally unstable may resist your attempts to render care. Nevertheless, you must not leave this patient alone. Doing so may expose you to civil action for abandonment or negligence. In such situations, you should request that law enforcement personnel handle the patient. Another reason for seeking law enforcement support is for the patient who resists treatment; such a patient will often threaten rescuers and others.

Consent

When a patient is not mentally competent to grant consent for emergency medical care, the law assumes that there is implied consent. For example, the consent of an unconscious patient is implied if life or health is at risk. The law refers to this as the emergency doctrine: consent is implied because of the necessity for immediate emergency treatment. In a situation that is not immediately life threatening, emergency medical care or transportation may be delayed until the proper consent is obtained.

In cases involving psychiatric emergencies, however, the matter is not always clear-cut. Does a life-threatening emergency exist or not? If you are not sure, you should request the assistance of law enforcement personnel.

Limited Legal Authority

As a rescuer, you have limited legal authority to require or force a patient to undergo emergency medical care when no life-threatening emergency exists. Patients have the right to refuse care. However, most states have legal statutes regarding the emergency care of mentally ill and drug-impaired individuals. These statutory provisions permit law enforcement personnel

When a patient is not mentally competent to grant consent for emergency medical care, the law assumes that there is implied consent.

to place such a person in protective custody so that emergency care can be rendered. You should be familiar with your local and state laws regarding these situations.

The typical provision states that "any police officer who has reasonable cause to believe that a person is mentally ill and dangerous to himself, herself, or others or gravely disabled...may take such person into custody and take or cause such person to be taken to a general hospital for emergency examination..." Again, since these provisions vary, you should become familiar with those in your state.

The general rule of law is that a competent adult has the right to refuse treatment, even if lifesaving care is involved. In psychiatric cases, however, a court of law would probably consider your actions in providing lifesaving care to be appropriate, particularly if you have a reasonable belief that the patient would harm himself, herself, or others without your intervention.

The Potentially Violent Patient

Violent patients make up only a small percentage of those undergoing a behavioral or psychiatric crisis. However, the potential for violence by such a patient is always an important consideration for the rescuer.

Use the following list of risk factors to assess the level of danger:

- **Past history.** Has the patient previously exhibited hostile, overly aggressive, or violent behavior? Ask individuals at the scene, or request this information from law enforcement personnel or family.

- **Posture.** How is the patient sitting or standing? Is the patient tense, rigid, or sitting on the edge of his or her seat? Such physical tension is often a warning signal of impending hostility.

- **The scene.** Is the patient holding or near potentially lethal objects such as a knife, gun, glass, poker, or bat (or near a window or glass door)?

- **Vocal activity.** What kind of speech is the patient using? Loud, obscene, erratic, and bizarre speech patterns usually indicate emotional distress. Someone using quiet, ordered speech is not as likely to strike out as someone who is yelling and screaming.

- **Physical activity.** The motor activity of a person undergoing a psychiatric crisis may be the most telling factor of all. The patient who has tense muscles, clenched fists, or glaring eyes; is pacing; cannot sit still; or is fiercely protecting personal space requires careful watching. Agitation may predict a quick escalation to violence.

Other factors to consider in assessing a patient's potential for violence include the following:

- Poor impulse control
- A history of truancy, fighting, and uncontrollable temper
- Low socioeconomic status, unstable family structure, or inability to keep a steady job
- Tattoos, especially those with gang identification or statements such as "Born to Kill" or "Born to Lose"
- Substance abuse
- Depression, which accounts for 20% of violent attacks
- Functional disorder (If the patient says that voices are telling him or her to kill, believe it.)

Chapter Sweep

Ready for Review

Behavioral emergencies can present the rescuer with great difficulties in patient management. Your major responsibility in these situations is to defuse potentially life-threatening incidents and reduce the impact of the stressful condition without exposing yourself to unnecessary risks. While only a small percentage of individuals with mental health disorders are dangerous to themselves or others, you may be exposed to a higher proportion of violent individuals in your daily activities. There are a number of warning signs of violence, including a past history of hostile behavior, rigidity, loud and erratic speech patterns, agitation, and depression.

A behavioral emergency is any reaction to events that interferes with activities of daily living. A person who is no longer able to respond appropriately to the environment may be having a more serious psychiatric emergency. Not all behavioral emergencies involve a mental health problem, however. Some emergencies are a temporary response to a traumatic event.

Assessing a person who may be having a behavioral crisis involves observing the person, talking with the person, and talking with friends, family members, and witnesses to the person's behavior. It also involves proper patient assessment for other possible physical causes or medical conditions. You are looking for indications that the person's thoughts, feelings, and reactions are inappropriate for the circumstances.

Consider contributing factors in three areas: central nervous system functioning, drug or alcohol use, and psychogenic circumstances such as the death of a loved one or other major interruption of normal life.

As a rescuer, you have limited legal authority to require a patient to undergo emergency medical care in the absence of a life-threatening emergency. However, most states have provisions allowing law enforcement personnel to place mentally impaired persons in custody so that such care can be provided. You should always involve law enforcement personnel any time you are called to assist a patient in a severe behavioral or psychiatric crisis.

In providing emergency medical care for a patient having a behavioral emergency, be direct, honest, and calm; have a definite plan of action; stay with the patient at all times, but don't get too close; express interest in the patient's story, but do not judge his or her behavior. Always treat such patients with respect.

Vital Vocabulary

activities of daily living (ADL) The basic activities a person usually accomplishes during a normal day, such as eating, dressing, and washing.

altered mental status A change in the way a person thinks and behaves that may signal disease in the central nervous system.

behavior How a person functions or acts in response to his or her environment.

behavioral crisis The point at which a person's reactions to events interfere with activities of daily living.

depression A persistent mood of sadness, despair, and discouragement; depression may be a symptom of many different mental and physical disorders, or it may be a disorder on its own.

functional disorder A disorder in which there is no known identifiable physiologic reason for the abnormal functioning of an organ or organ system.

mental disorder An illness with psychological or behavioral symptoms and/or impairment in functioning, caused by a social, psychological, genetic, physical, chemical, or biologic disturbance.

organic brain syndrome Temporary or permanent dysfunction of the brain, caused by a disturbance in the physical or physiologic functioning of brain tissue.

psychogenic A symptom or illness that is caused by mental or emotional factors as opposed to physical ones.

www.OECzone.com

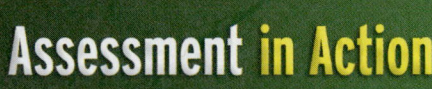

Assessment in Action

It is late afternoon in the resort lounge. You notice a man who is obviously upset talking to a woman. Suddenly he screams, "I can't take it, you're all against me!" He stands and gets louder. He is sputtering and his speech is slightly slurred. He picks up a wine bottle.

1. Which of the following characterize this patient's behavior?
   A. Psychosis
   B. Hallucination
   C. Drug dependence
   D. Depression

2. In assessing the patient's potential for violence, which of the following factors would concern you the most?
   A. The patient is talking to you while lying on a couch.
   B. The patient yells at you when you ask him about the comment he made.
   C. A family member at the scene reports that the patient has no history of violence.
   D. The patient has a medium physical build and does not appear to have a weapon.

3. An appropriate way to communicate with this patient includes:
   A. using a low, calm voice.
   B. responding to the yelling with a loud voice.
   C. using a commanding tone.
   D. responding with a disinterested, detached voice.

4. Assessment of this patient includes:
   A. taking his shirt off to observe chest rise.
   B. evaluating movement of all four extremities.
   C. gathering more information.
   D. obtaining a complete set of vital signs.

5. You invite him to the patrol room to rest. On the way he starts screaming at you. While you try to verbally calm him, he turns and physically attacks you. You have the right to:
   A. physically strike him in return.
   B. demand his ID.
   C. use reasonable force to protect yourself.
   D. do whatever it takes to restrain him.

6. Which would be most helpful in the assessment of this patient?
   A. A complete set of vital signs
   B. History from the patient
   C. Information from the woman with him
   D. AVPU

Challenging Questions

7. Head injuries, diabetic reactions, and hypoxia can all result in behaviors that appear to be psychotic in nature. What do they all have in common that cause this?

8. When documenting a patient care run for an emotionally disturbed patient, it is helpful to also list the names of those who were in attendance, including police officers, security guards, nurses, etc. Why is this necessary?

Points to Ponder

You have responded to a lodge call for an incident that has resulted in a bleeding problem. You find that a man and his girlfriend have been drinking and are now shouting at each other. The man is holding his bleeding right hand. As you walk up to him, you see the woman brandishing a broken beer bottle. She turns toward you and makes a threatening gesture with the broken glass. What is your first concern? What other resources should you consider? How should you approach the woman?

Issues Safety Concerns, Willingness to Protect Yourself and Your Partner, Legal and Safety Issues of Domestic Disputes, Use of Law Enforcement, Personal Feelings about Spouse Abuse.

Online Outlook

Any time you encounter a patient with behavioral issues in a setting that would require initial transport of this patient from a remote area to a location for access to EMS services, you must be concerned with legal and safety issues for rescuers, the patient, and other bystanders. To learn more about dealing with a behavioral emergency, complete Exercise 16 at www.OECzone.com.

www.OECzone.com

Obstetrics and Gynecological Emergencies

Objectives

Cognitive

♠ 1. Identify the following structures: uterus, vagina, fetus, placenta, umbilical cord, amniotic sac, perineum (p 462).

♠ 2. Identify and explain the use of the contents of an obstetrics kit (p 466).

♠ 3. Identify predelivery emergencies (p 463).

♠ 4. State indications of an imminent delivery (p 465).

♠ 5. Differentiate the emergency medical care provided to a patient with predelivery emergencies from a normal delivery (p 463).

6. State the steps in the predelivery preparation of the mother (p 465).

♠ 7. Establish the relationship between body substance isolation and childbirth (p 466).

♠ 8. State the steps to assist in the delivery (p 467).

9. Describe care of the baby as the head appears (p 467).

♠ 10. Describe how and when to cut the umbilical cord (p 470).

11. Discuss the steps in the delivery of the placenta (p 471).

12. List the steps in the emergency medical care of the mother postdelivery (p 470).

13. Summarize neonatal resuscitation procedures (p 472).

14. Describe the procedures for the following abnormal deliveries: breech birth, prolapsed cord, limb presentation (p 474).

15. Differentiate the special considerations for multiple births (p 476).

16. Describe special considerations of meconium (p 469).

17. Describe special considerations of a premature baby (p 477).

♠ 18. Discuss the emergency medical care of a patient with a gynecological emergency (p 478).

Affective

19. Explain the rationale for understanding the implications of treating two patients (mother and baby) (p 470).

Psychomotor

20. Demonstrate the steps to assist in the normal cephalic delivery (p 467).

21. Demonstrate necessary care procedures of the fetus as the head appears (p 467).

22. Demonstrate infant neonatal procedures (p 467).

23. Demonstrate postdelivery care of infant (p 470).

24. Demonstrate how and when to cut the umbilical cord (p 469).

25. Attend to the steps in the delivery of the placenta (p 471).

26. Demonstrate the postdelivery care of the mother (p 471).

27. Demonstrate the procedures for the following abnormal deliveries: vaginal bleeding, breech birth, prolapsed cord, limb presentation (p 474).

28. Demonstrate the steps in the emergency medical care of the mother with excessive bleeding (p 476).

♠ These are core concepts in initial patrol training.

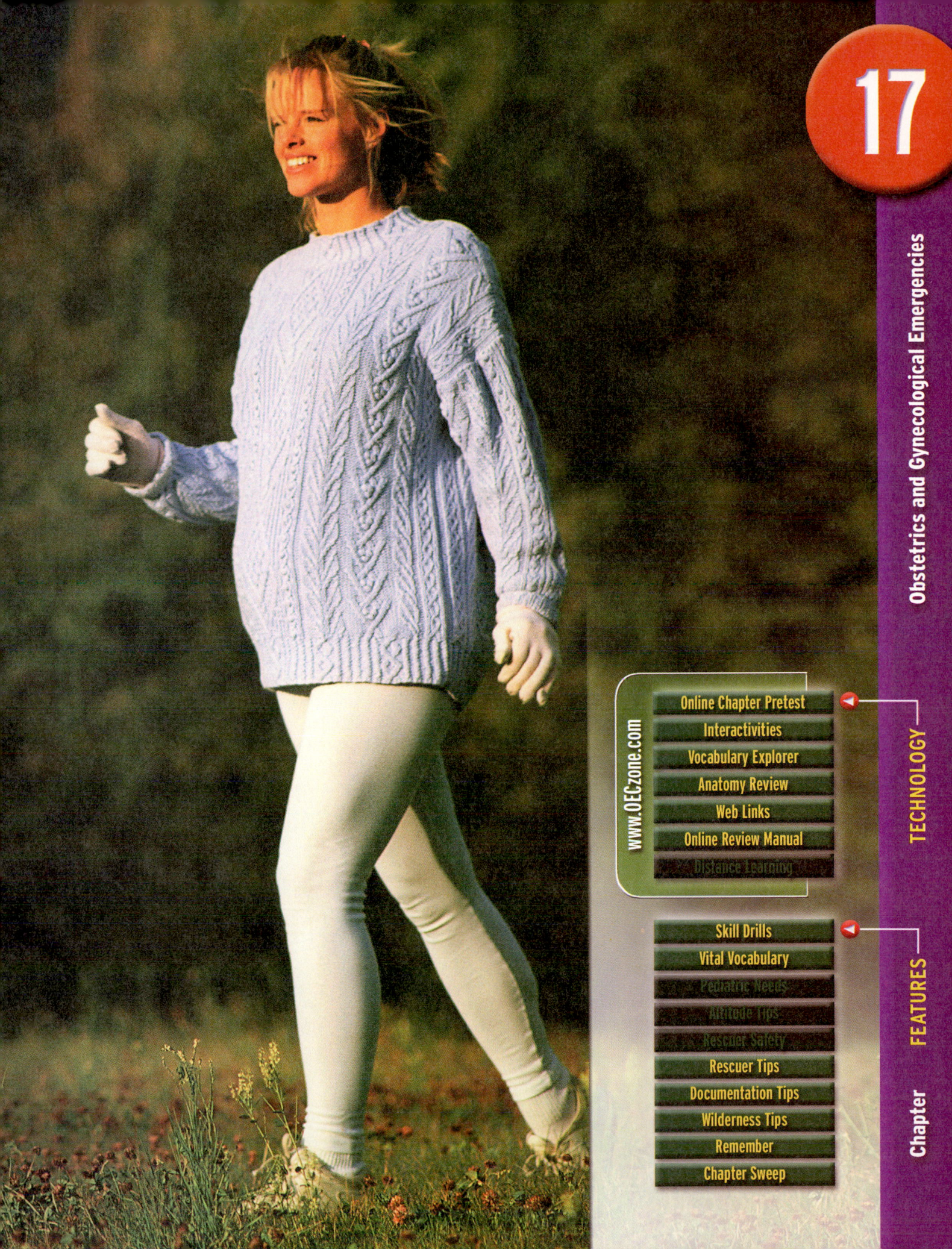

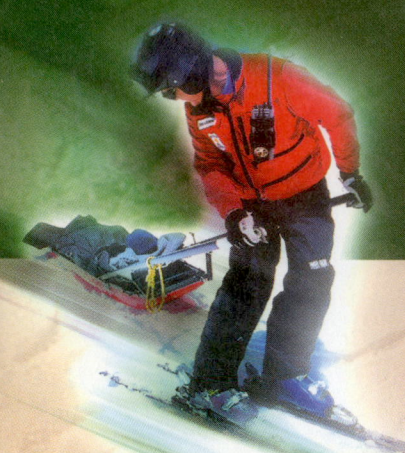

You are the rescuer

A woman walks into your patrol facility carrying her 2-year-old child. She appears pregnant, close to full term, and tells you she has gone into labor. The family is visiting for the day. Her husband and son are somewhere on the slopes and are supposed to meet her in the resort cafeteria for lunch.

While most births are uneventful and require little or no medical intervention, others may be life threatening to both the mother and baby. This chapter will help prepare you for emergency deliveries and will also help you answer the following questions:

1. What are the most common indicators that birth is imminent?

2. How does the care provided during a normal delivery differ from that provided to an expectant mother experiencing a predelivery emergency?

Obstetrics and Gynecological Emergencies

Most infants in the United States are delivered in a hospital, with doctors and nurses in attendance to care for not only the mother, but also the newborn infant. Today, more and more women are exercising regularly throughout their pregnancy and participating in recreational sports in the outdoor environment. Most deliveries in the outdoor environment will be unexpected and more likely to be early or complicated, and you will find yourself with a decision to make: Should you stay on the scene and deliver the infant or arrange to transport the patient to the hospital? This chapter will tell you how to make this decision and how to proceed if on-scene delivery is necessary. It describes the normal process of childbirth and discusses common complications so that you will be prepared to handle both normal and abnormal deliveries. Next, it describes the evaluation and care of the newborn. Finally, the chapter discusses gynecological emergencies unrelated to childbirth.

Anatomy of the Female Reproductive System

The **fetus** is the developing, unborn infant that grows inside the mother's uterus for approximately 9 months. The **uterus**, or womb, is the muscular organ where the fetus grows (▶ **Figure 17-1**). It is responsible for contractions during labor and ultimately helps to push the infant through the birth canal. The **birth canal** is made up of the vagina and the lower one third or neck of the uterus, called the **cervix**. The cervix contains a mucous plug that seals the uterine opening, preventing contamination from the outside world. When the cervix begins to dilate, this plug is discharged as pink-tinged mucus,

or a **bloody show**. This "show" may signal the first stage of labor.

The **vagina** is the outermost cavity of a woman's reproductive system and forms the lower part of the birth canal. It is about 8 to 12 cm in length, begins at the cervix, and ends as an external opening of the body. Essentially, the vagina completes the passageway from the uterus to the outside world for the delivering infant. The **perineum** is the area of skin between the vagina and the anus. During birth, as the infant moves through the birth canal, the perineum will begin to bulge significantly.

As the fetus grows, it requires more and more nourishment. The **placenta**, a disk-shaped structure, is body tissue that attaches to the inner lining of the wall of the uterus and is connected to the fetus by the umbilical cord. After delivery, the placenta, or afterbirth, separates

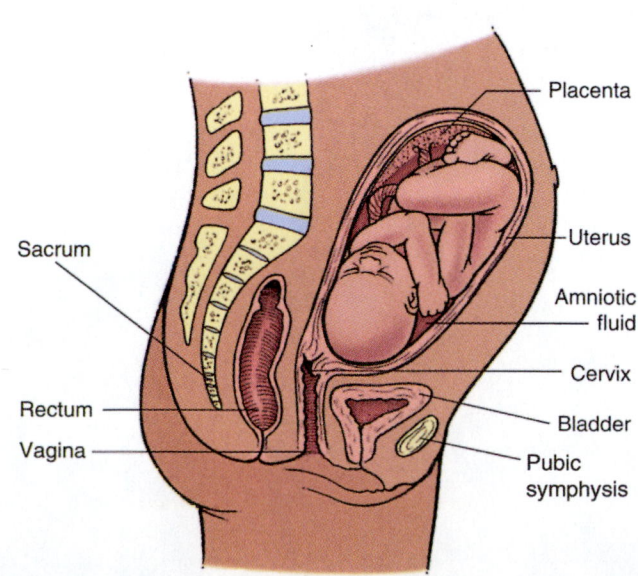

Figure 17-1 Anatomic structures of the pregnant woman.

from the uterus and is delivered. The **umbilical cord** is the infant's lifeline, connecting mother and infant through the placenta. The umbilical cord contains two arteries and one vein. These vessels supply blood to the fetus: the vein carries blood toward the heart (baby) and the arteries carry blood away from the heart (baby). Oxygen and other nutrients cross from the mother's circulation through the placenta and then along the umbilical cord to support the fetus as it grows. Carbon dioxide and waste products travel the same route in the opposite direction. The remarkable thing about this exchange is that the mother's blood and that of the fetus do not mix during the process.

The fetus develops inside a fluid-filled, baglike membrane called the **amniotic sac**, or bag of waters. The sac contains about 500 to 1,000 mL of amniotic fluid, which helps to insulate and protect the floating fetus as it develops. Released in a gush when the sac ruptures, usually at the onset of labor, this fluid helps to lubricate the birth canal and remove bacteria.

A full-term pregnancy is from 36 to 40 weeks, counting from the first day of the last menstrual cycle. The pregnancy is divided into 3 trimesters of about 3 months each. Deliveries before 36 weeks are considered premature. Toward the end of the third trimester, the head of the fetus normally descends through the broad upper inlet of the mother's pelvis, positioning itself for the delivery.

Stages of Labor

There are three stages of labor: dilation of the cervix, expulsion of the baby, and delivery of the placenta. The first stage begins with the onset of contractions and ends when the cervix is fully dilated. Because the cervix has to be stretched thin by uterine contractions until the opening is large enough for the infant to pass through into the vagina, the first stage is usually the longest, lasting an average of 16 hours for a first delivery. You will usually have time to transport the mother during the first stage of labor.

The onset of labor starts with contractions of the uterus. Other signs of the beginning of labor are the bloody show and the rupture of the amniotic sac, called breaking of the water. These events may occur before the first labor pain or later in the first stage of labor. The uterine contractions may not come at regular intervals at first. The mother may think that she simply has a nagging backache. The frequency and intensity of true labor increase with time. The uterine contractions become more regular and last about 30 to 60 seconds each. The length of labor varies greatly. As a general rule, it is longer in a **primigravida**, a woman

who is experiencing her first pregnancy, and becomes shorter in a **multigravida**, a woman who has experienced previous pregnancies. (Two similar terms refer to the outcomes of those pregnancies. A **multipara** is a woman who has had more than one baby born alive, and a **primipara** has had one live birth.)

The second stage of labor begins when the cervix is fully dilated and ends when the infant is born. During this stage, you will have to make a decision about helping the mother to deliver on scene or providing transport to the hospital. Because the infant has to move through the birth canal during this stage, the uterine contractions are usually closer together and last longer. Pressure on the rectum may make the mother feel as if she needs to have a bowel movement. Under no circumstances should you let the mother sit on the toilet. She may also have the uncontrollable urge to push down. The perineum will begin to bulge significantly, and the top of the infant's head should begin to appear at the vaginal opening. This is called **crowning** ▼ Figure 17-2 .

The third stage begins with the birth of the infant and ends with the delivery of the placenta. This may take up to 30 minutes. Usually, the mother is not transported during that time. It is important that you always follow BSI precautions, to protect yourself, the baby, and the mother from exposure to body fluids. There is a high potential of exposure due to body fluids released during childbirth.

Emergencies Prior to Delivery

Most pregnant women are healthy, but some may be ill when they conceive or become ill during pregnancy. You may safely use oxygen to treat any heart or lung disease in the mother without harm to the fetus.

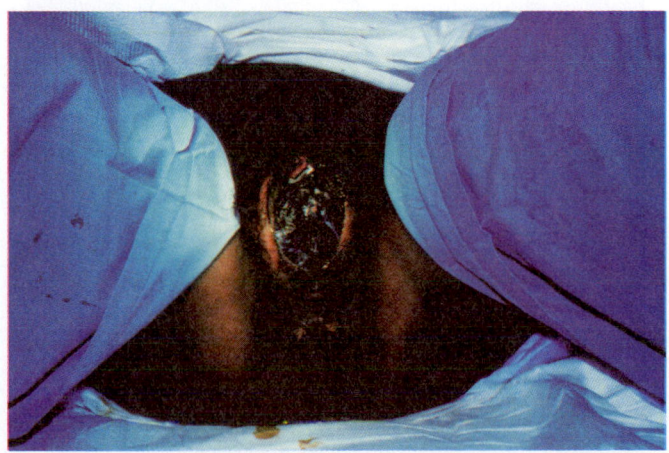

Figure 17-2 Crowning occurs when the infant's head appears at the vaginal opening.

As the time for delivery nears, certain complications can occur. One of these is preeclampsia, or **pregnancy-induced hypertension**, a condition that can develop after the 20th week of gestation, most commonly in primigravidas. This condition is characterized by the following signs and symptoms:

- Headache
- Seeing spots
- Swelling in the hands and feet
- Anxiety
- High blood pressure

Another condition is **eclampsia**, convulsions that result from severe hypertension. To treat eclampsia, lay the mother on her side, maintain an airway, and provide supplemental oxygen; if vomiting occurs, suction the airway. Transport a pregnant patient with convulsions promptly. As usual, size up the situation and perform your initial assessment, history, and physical exam, and assess the baseline vital signs. Provide treatment based on signs and symptoms.

If the patient is hypotensive, position her on the left side. Positioning the mother in this way can prevent **supine hypotensive syndrome**, a problem in which low blood pressure develops when the mother lies supine resulting from compression by the weight of the fetus onto the inferior vena cava.

Hemorrhage from the vagina that occurs before labor begins may be very serious; call for ALS. In early pregnancy, it may be a sign of a spontaneous abortion, or miscarriage. Bleeding may be a sign of an **ectopic pregnancy**, a pregnancy that develops outside the uterus, most often in a fallopian tube. Ectopic pregnancy occurs about once in every 200 pregnancies. The leading cause of maternal death in the first trimester is internal hemorrhage into the abdomen following rupture of an ectopic pregnancy. For this reason, you should consider the possibility of an ectopic pregnancy in women who have missed a menstrual cycle and complain of sudden stabbing and usually unilateral pain in the lower abdomen. A history of pelvic inflammatory disease, tubal ligations, or previous ectopic pregnancies should heighten your suspicions for a possible ectopic pregnancy.

In the later stages of pregnancy, hemorrhage may indicate problems with the placenta. In **placenta abruptio**, the placenta separates prematurely from the wall of the uterus (▼ Figure 17-3). In **placenta previa**, the placenta develops over and covers the cervix (▼ Figure 17-4).

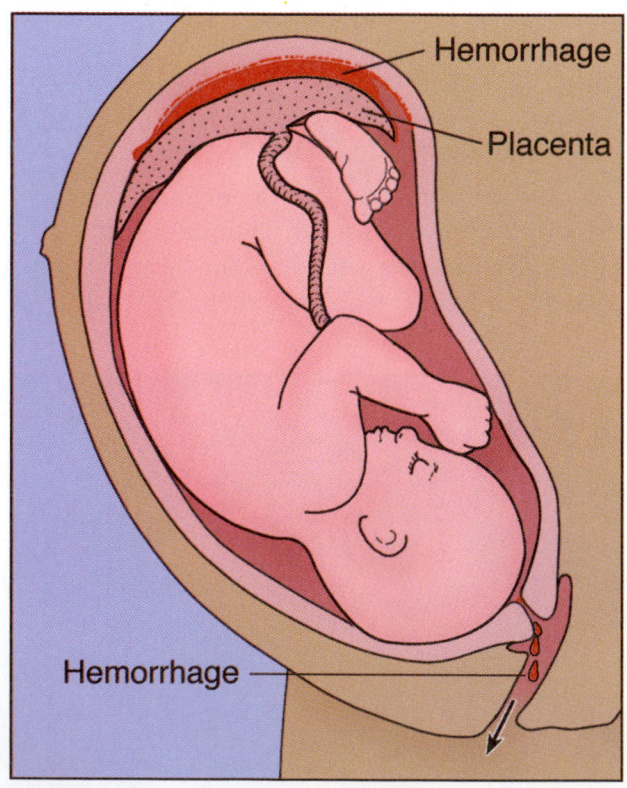

Figure 17-3 In placenta abruptio, the placenta separates prematurely from the wall of the uterus.

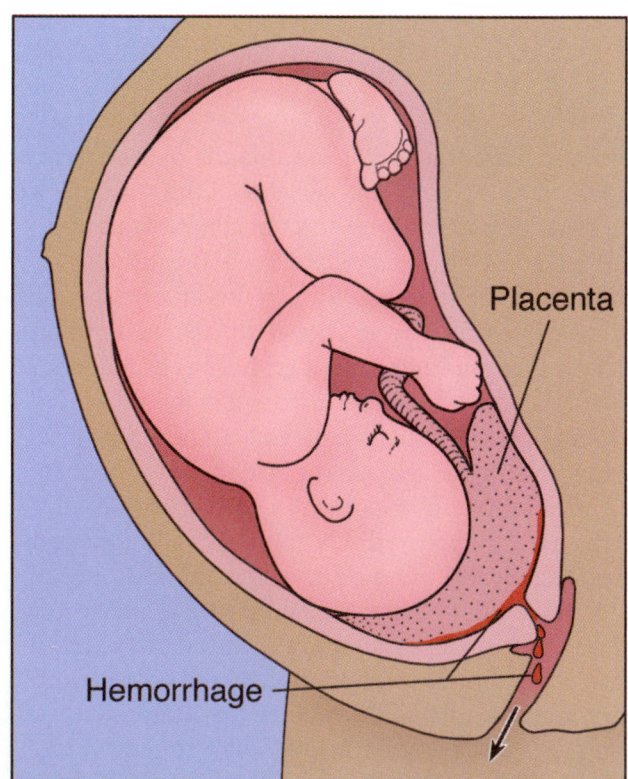

Figure 17-4 In placenta previa, the placenta develops over and covers the cervix.

Any bleeding from the vagina in a pregnant woman is a serious sign and should be treated in the hospital promptly. If the mother shows signs of shock, have her lie on her left side, and give her high-flow oxygen. Place a sterile pad or sanitary napkin over the vagina, and replace it as often as necessary. Save the pads so that hospital personnel can estimate how much blood she has lost. Also save any tissue that may be passed from the vagina. Do not put anything into the vagina.

When a pregnant woman sustains blunt abdominal trauma, severe hemorrhage may occur from injuries to the pregnant uterus. The resulting oxygen deprivation can cause grave injury to the fetus. Promptly evaluate a pregnant trauma victim; support the airway, and if there is any sign of bleeding, administer high-flow oxygen. Arrange for immediate evacuation and ALS transportation. Have the mother lie on her left side rather than on her back; this will relieve the pressure of the uterus on intra-abdominal organs, especially the inferior vena cava and abdominal aorta. Pregnant women have an increased amount of blood volume. Therefore, a pregnant trauma patient may have a significant amount of blood loss before showing signs of shock. However, the infant may be in trouble well before this. Often, if the mother has sustained serious trauma, the blood supply to the fetus is reduced so that the body can supply an adequate amount of blood to the mother. In most cases, the only chance to save the infant is to adequately resuscitate the mother.

Preparing for Delivery

Consider delivering the patient at the scene in the following circumstances:

- When delivery can be expected within a few minutes
- When a natural disaster, bad weather, or some other type of catastrophe makes it impossible to reach the hospital
- When no transportation is available

How do you determine whether delivery is going to occur within a few minutes? First, look for crowning. Second, ask the mother these questions:

- How long have you been pregnant?
- When are you due?
- Is this your first baby?
- Are you having contractions? How far apart are the contractions? How long do the contractions last?

> In the first trimester, the leading cause of maternal death is internal hemorrhage into the abdomen, resulting from a ruptured ectopic pregnancy.

- Do you feel as though you have to strain or move your bowels?
- Have you had any spotting or bleeding?
- Have you had any gushing of fluid from the vagina?
- Were any of your previous children delivered by cesarean section?

Also consider asking the following questions:

- Have you had a complicated pregnancy in the past?
- Do you use drugs, drink alcohol, or take any medications?
- Is there any possibility that this is a multiple birth?
- Does your doctor expect any complications?

If this is not the patient's first child, she may be able to tell you whether she is about to deliver. If she says that she is, make immediate preparations for delivery. Otherwise, does she have a rock-hard abdomen? Does she say that she has to move her bowels or feels the need to push? If so, the infant's head is probably pressing on the rectum, and delivery is about to occur. At this point, you should inspect the vagina to determine whether crowning has occurred; if so, delivery is imminent. Do not touch the vaginal area until you are sure that delivery is, in fact, imminent. In general, do not touch vaginal areas except during delivery (under certain circumstances) and when an additional rescuer is present. Spread the mother's legs apart gently, explaining that you are doing so to decide whether the baby should be delivered immediately or if she should be transported to the hospital for the delivery.

Once labor has begun, there is no way it can be slowed down or stopped. Never attempt to hold the mother's legs together. To do so would only complicate the delivery. Do not let her go to the bathroom. Instead, reassure her that the sensation of needing to move her bowels is normal and that it means she is about to deliver.

Wilderness Tips

If delivery is imminent and the mother is outdoors, seek shelter and arrange for a clean, flat surface for delivery of the infant.

If you decide to deliver at the scene, remember that you are only *assisting* the mother with the delivery. Your part is to help, guide, and support the infant as it is born. Remember to use BSI precautions at all times. Try to limit distractions for yourself and for the mother. You want to appear calm and reassuring while protecting the mother's modesty. Most important, recognize when the situation is beyond your level of training. The decision and means to transport a woman in labor from the outdoor environment to a location where there is access to the local EMS system is difficult. In general, consider evacuation to a location with access to EMS if:

- it can be reached within 20 minutes
- the head is not visible during contraction, or in the case of a primigravida, is visible but smaller than a 50 cent piece
- the umbilical cord or any part of the infant other than the head is visible through the vaginal opening
- the woman has been told that she has a breech presentation or that a cesarean section will be necessary

Disposable sterile emergency OB kits are available for purchase (▶ **Figure 17-5**), but the outdoor or back-country environment may require improvisation. Items that need to be assembled for an emergency delivery—

potentially without sterile supplies—are listed in (▼ **Table 17-1**).

Remember to size up the situation, perform your initial assessment, focused history, and physical exam, assess baseline vital signs, and provide treatment based on signs and symptoms.

PATIENT POSITION. The mother's clothing should be pushed up to her waist or, if she is wearing trousers and undergarments, removed. Remember to limit the mother's exposure and preserve her modesty as much as you can while helping her to move into a semi-Fowler's position. Place the mother on a firm surface that is padded with blankets, folded sheets, or towels. Put a pillow or blankets beneath her hips to elevate them about 2" to 4". It is sometimes better to put a pillow under one hip to allow the mother to turn to one side. This may also make it easier to suction the infant once it is born. Support the mother's head, neck, and upper back with pillows and blankets.

If the emergency delivery is occurring, you should move the mother to a sturdy flat surface. You will find it easier to work on a firm surface than on a bed. Elevate

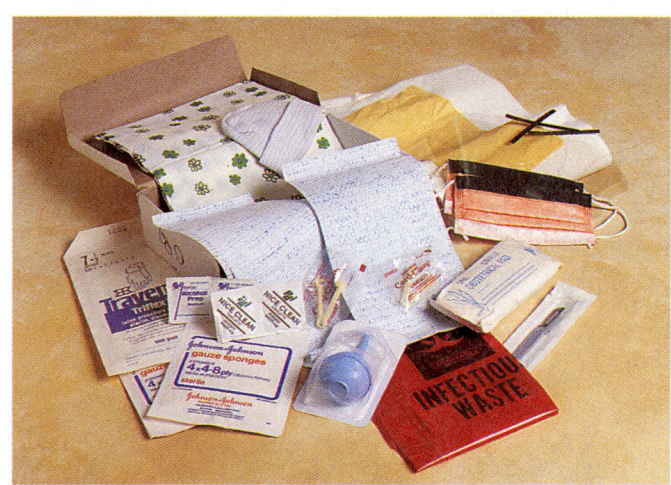

Figure 17-5 Disposable sterile OB kit.

Table 17-1 Suggested Supplies for an Emergency Delivery		
• Clean sheets and towels	• Sanitary napkins	• Two sterile 12" pieces of white cloth tape; or
• Sterile disposable gloves	• 4" × 4" gauze sponges	
• Face shield with eye protection	• Plastic (biohazard) bag	• Two clean white cotton shoelaces, sterilized by boiling
• Scissors or razor blade	• Infant blanket	
	• Soft rubber bulb syringe	

the mother's hips, and support her head with one or two pillows. Have her keep her legs and hips flexed, with her feet flat on the surface beneath her and her knees spread apart. Track the progression of the delivery closely at all times; you do not want an abrupt delivery, when the crowning head pops out uncontrollably, to occur.

PREPARING THE DELIVERY FIELD. Take the following steps to prepare the area where the infant will be born:

1. As time allows, place towels or sheets on the floor around the delivery area to help soak up the amniotic fluid that will be released when the amniotic sac ruptures (▶ **Figure 17-6A**). Note that the amniotic sac may have ruptured before you arrived. Elevate the mother's hips, and support her head with one or two pillows.

2. Open the OB kit carefully so that its contents remain sterile. Assemble equipment necessary if an OB kit is not available.

3. Put on the sterile gloves.

4. Use clean, preferably sterile sheets and towels to make a sterile delivery field. Place one sheet or towel under the mother's buttocks, and unfold it toward her feet. The other sheet should be draped over her abdomen and upper legs. Alternatively, you can use three sheets: (1) folded under the buttocks, (2) placed between the legs, just below the vagina, and (3) placed across the abdomen (▶ **Figure 17-6B**).

Delivering the Baby

A second rescuer should be at the mother's head to comfort, soothe, and reassure her during the delivery. The mother may want to grip someone's hand. She may yell, cry, or say nothing at all. It is not uncommon for mothers to become nauseated, and some may vomit. If this occurs, have your assistant turn the mother's head to the side so that her mouth and airway can be cleared manually or with suction, as needed.

You must continually assess the mother for crowning. Do not allow an abrupt delivery to occur. Position yourself so that you can see the vagina at all times. Time the mother's contractions from the beginning of one to the beginning of the next to determine the frequency of the contractions. In addition, time the duration of each contraction. You do this by feeling the mother's abdomen from the moment the contraction begins (uterus/abdomen tightening) to the moment it ends (uterus/abdomen relaxing). Remind the patient to

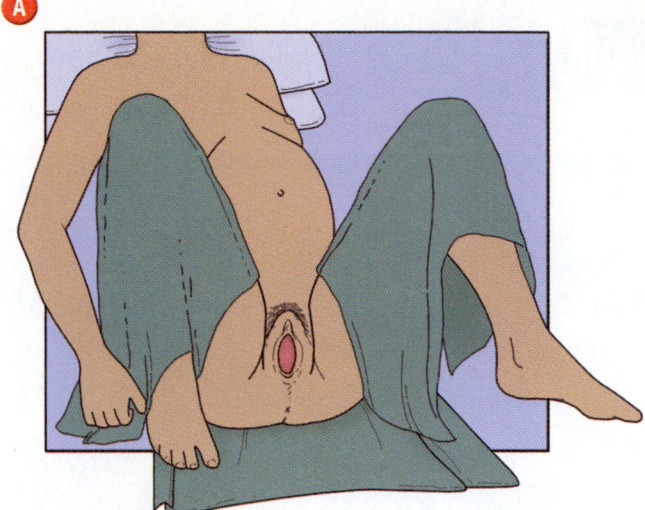
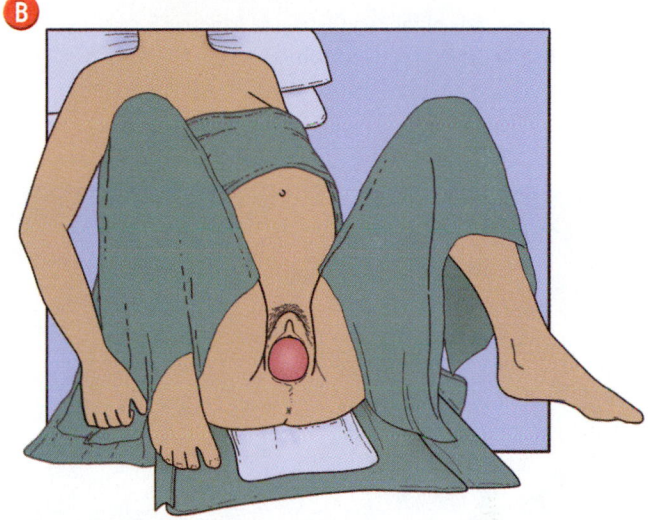

Figure 17-6 Preparing the delivery field. **A.** Place sheets or towels under the mother, elevate the mother's hips, and support her head with one or two pillows. **B.** Use sterile sheets and towels from the OB kit to make a clean delivery field. Place one sheet under the buttocks, drape the other over the abdomen, and place drapes over the thighs.

take quick, short breaths during each contraction but not to strain. In between contractions, encourage the mother to rest and breathe deeply through her mouth.

Follow the steps in (▶ **Skill Drill 17-1**) to deliver the baby. These steps are described in more detail.

1. Allow the mother to push the head out. Support it as it emerges, **placing your gloved hand over its bony parts. Suction fluid from the mouth first, then the nostrils (Step 1).**

2. **Feel at the neck to see if the cord is wrapped** around it. If it is, gently lift it over the baby's head without pulling hard on the cord.

SkillDrill 17-1 Delivering the Baby

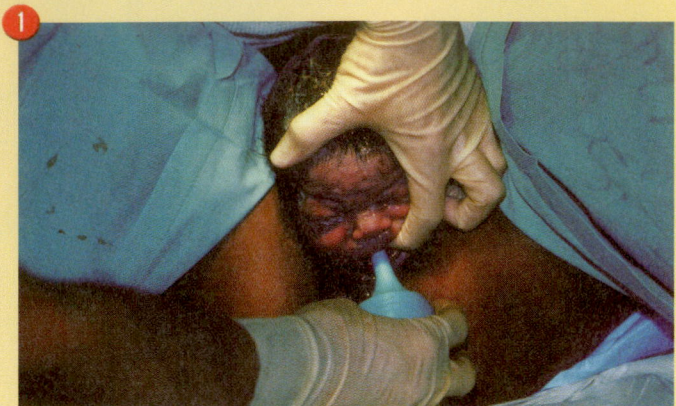

1 Support the bony parts of the head with your hands as it emerges. Suction fluid from the mouth, then nostrils.

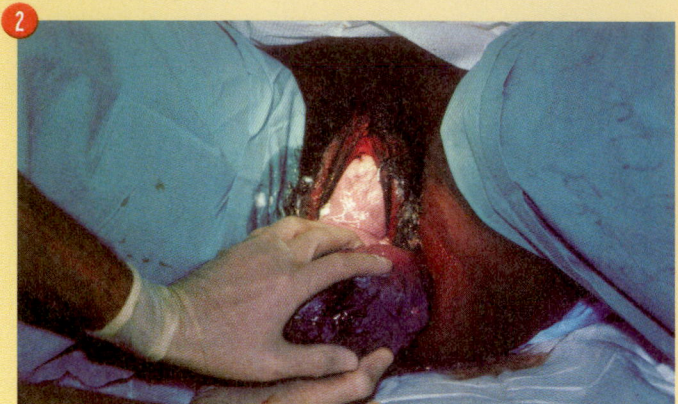

2 As the upper shoulder appears, guide the head down slightly, if needed to deliver the shoulder.

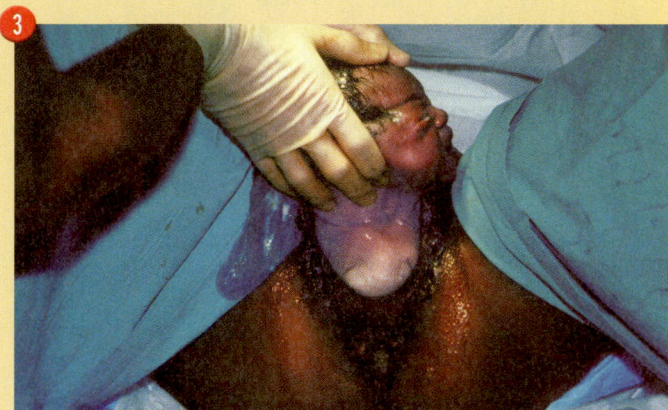

3 Support the head and upper body as the lower shoulder delivers, guiding the head up if needed.

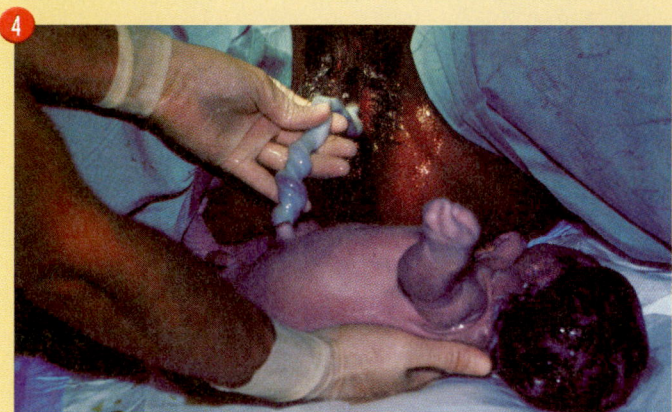

4 Handle the slippery delivered infant firmly but gently, keeping the neck in neutral position to maintain the airway.

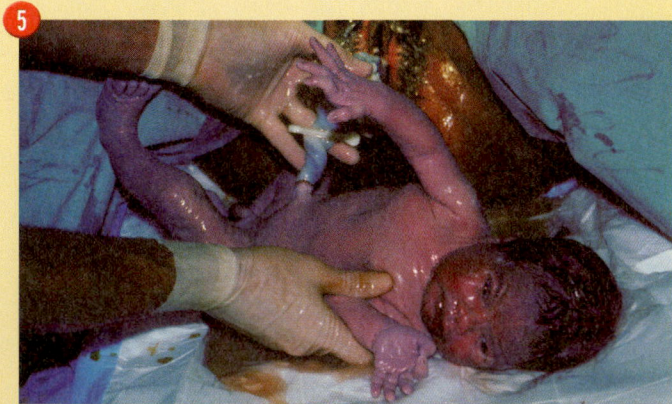

5 Place clamps 2" to 4" apart and cut between them.

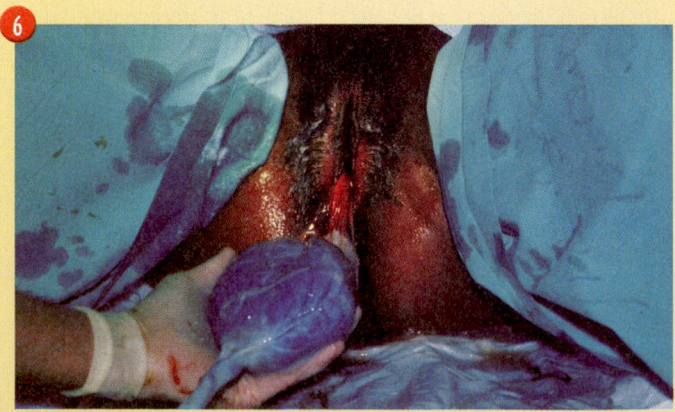

6 Allow the placenta to deliver itself. Do not pull on the cord to speed delivery.

3. Once the head is delivered, the upper shoulder will be visible. **Guide the head down slightly, if needed to help that shoulder deliver (Step 2)**.

4. **Support the head and upper body as the shoulders deliver.** You may need to guide the head up slightly to deliver the lower shoulder **(Step 3)**.

5. Once the body is delivered, handle the infant firmly but gently. It will be slippery. **Make sure the baby's neck is in a neutral position to keep the airway open (Step 4)**.

6. If transport to a medical facility or EMS access location will be delayed more than 20 minutes, the umbilical cord will need to be cut. **Place the clamps or tie the strips of cloth tape about 2″ to 4″ apart**, about four fingerwidths from the infant's body. Once they are firmly in place, cut between the clamps **(Step 5)**.

7. **The placenta delivers itself,** usually within 30 minutes of birth. Never pull on the end of the umbilical cord in an attempt to speed delivery of the placenta **(Step 6)**.

Delivering the Head

Watch the head as it begins to exit the vagina, as it must be supported as it emerges. It may take two, three, or more contractions for the delivery of the head to occur from the time it begins to crown. Once it is obvious that the head is coming out farther with each contraction, you should place your gloved hand over the emerging bony parts of the head and exert very gentle pressure on it, decreasing the pressure slightly between contractions. This will allow the head to come out smoothly and prevent it and the rest of the infant from suddenly popping out during a strong contraction, possibly causing injury. You may want to move the patient's feet so that you are between the patient's legs during the delivery. Be careful that you do not poke your fingers into the infant's eyes or

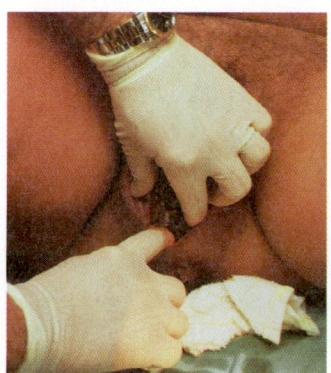

into the two soft spots, called *fontanels*, on the head. One fontanel is located at the front of the head, near the brow, and one is near the back of the head. The brain is covered only by skin and membranes at these spots.

Gentle pressure, exerted horizontally across the perineum, may reduce the risk of tearing as the infant is emerging **◄ Figure 17-7** . Also be prepared for the possi-

Figure 17-7 Applying gentle pressure on the perineum may reduce the risk of tearing as the infant emerges.

bility that feces may come out because of the pressure on the rectum.

UNRUPTURED AMNIOTIC SAC. Usually, the amniotic sac will break or rupture at the beginning of labor. The sac may also rupture during contractions. If the amniotic sac has not ruptured by this point, it will appear as a fluid-filled sac (like a water balloon) emerging from the vagina. This situation is serious, as the sac will suffocate the baby if it is not removed. If it has not spontaneously ruptured, tear it with your fingers or carefully remove it with a scissor blade directed away from the baby's face, only as the head is crowning, not before. As the sac is punctured, amniotic fluid will gush out. Push the ruptured sac away from the infant's face as the head is delivered. Clear the baby's mouth and nose immediately, using the bulb syringe and gauze sponge. If the amniotic fluid is greenish instead of clear or has a foul odor (meconium staining), make note of this in the information you will relay to medical control. Meconium is a sign of two possible problems: a newborn with airway obstruction or an abnormally slow pulse, respirations, poor tone, or color. Thick meconium can clog the airway of the newborn. Aggressive suctioning of the baby's mouth and oropharynx before delivery of the body may prevent meconium aspiration and respiratory distress. Once the head has been delivered, it usually rotates to one side or the other rather than straight up and down.

UMBILICAL CORD AROUND THE NECK. As soon as the head is delivered, use the index finger of your other hand to feel whether the umbilical cord is wrapped around the neck. This commonly is called a **nuchal cord**. A nuchal cord that is wound tightly around the neck could cause the infant to strangle. It must therefore be released from the neck immediately **▼ Figure 17-8** . Usually, you can

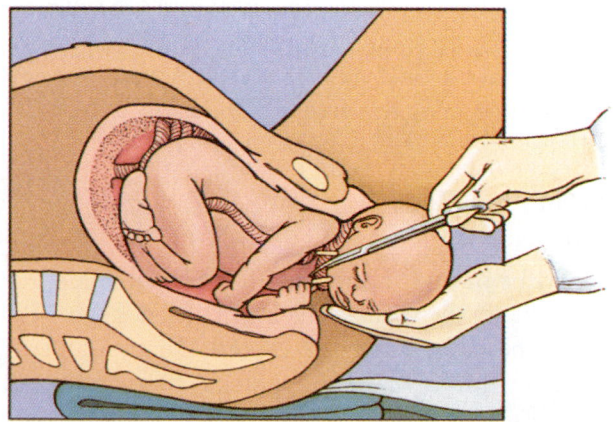

Figure 17-8 If the umbilical cord is wound tightly around the baby's neck, it must be released immediately by either slipping it gently over the infant's delivered head or, if necessary, by placing two clamps or ties about 2″ apart on the cord and cutting between the clamps.

If the infant is held higher than the vagina, blood will be siphoned from the infant through the umbilical cord back into the placenta.

As a baby delivers, you must divide your attention between two patients. This can keep two rescuers busy, even when things go well. To ensure that special care needs do not result in neglecting one patient, designate one rescuer to pay primary attention to each patient. Call for help early if you suspect that both will need special care, or that one will require resuscitation.

slip the cord gently over the infant's delivered head (or over the shoulder, if necessary). If not, you must cut it by placing two clamps or ties about 2″ apart on the cord and cutting the cord between the clamps. If the cord is wrapped more than once around the neck, a rare event, you have to clamp and cut only once; then you can unwrap the cord from around the neck. Handle the cord very carefully; it is fragile and easily torn. Fortunately, the cord is usually not wrapped around the infant's neck and does not have to be cut until after the entire infant has been delivered. However, you must always check for a nuchal cord.

Now that you have delivered the infant's head and verified that no nuchal cord is present, you will need to suction the amniotic fluids from the infant's airway before the delivery proceeds. You must ask the mother not to push while you are doing this, although her desire to do so will be very strong. While supporting the infant's head with one hand, quickly and efficiently suction the fluid from the mouth first and then the nostrils. If you suction the nostrils first, you may stimulate the infant to aspirate the fluid in the mouth or pharynx; since infants are nose breathers, any stimulation of the nose will cause a gasping response. In suctioning the airway, fully compress the bulb syringe before it is inserted 1″ to 1½″ into the infant's mouth, then release the bulb to suction fluids and mucus into the syringe. Make sure the syringe does not touch the back of the mouth. Discard the fluid into a towel, and repeat the procedure, suctioning the mouth and nostrils two or three times each, or until they are clear.

Delivering the Body

By the time you are finished suctioning, the mother will most likely be pushing again, and the upper shoulder will be visible in the vagina. The infant's head is the largest part of the body. Once it is born, the rest of the infant usually delivers easily. Support the head and upper body as the shoulders deliver. Do not pull the infant from the birth canal. The abdomen and hips will appear; once these deliver, support them with your other hand. Grasp the infant's feet as they are born.

Now the infant is being well supported with both hands. Handle the infant firmly but carefully. It will be slippery with a white, cheesy substance, called vernix caseosa.

Postdelivery Care

As soon as the entire infant is born, dry the baby off and wrap it immediately in a blanket or towel, and place it on one side, with the head slightly lower than the rest of its body. Wrap the baby so that only the face is exposed, making sure that the top of the head is covered. Also make sure that the baby's neck is in a neutral position so the airway remains open. Newborn babies are very sensitive to cold, so if it is at all possible, you should keep the blanket or towel warm before you use it. Use a sterile gauze pad to wipe the infant's mouth, and once again suction the mouth and nose. Suctioning the nose is particularly important, since babies breathe through their noses. If you prefer, you can pick up and cradle the infant in your arm at the level of the mother's vagina while doing this, but always keep the head slightly downward to help prevent aspiration. After suctioning, keep the infant at the same level as the mother's vagina until the umbilical cord is cut. If the infant is higher than the vagina, blood will be siphoned from the infant through the umbilical cord back into the placenta.

A newborn's body temperature can drop very quickly, so dry and wrap the infant as soon as possible. Only then will you clamp and cut the umbilical cord.

Once the infant is born, the umbilical cord is of no further use to either mother or infant. Postdelivery care of the umbilical cord is important, as infection is easily transmitted through the cord to the baby. Using two cloth ties or clamps, tie or clamp the cord somewhere between the mother and the infant, preferably four fingers' width from the infant. Place the ties or clamps about 2″ to 4″ apart. Ties should be clean, preferably sterile cotton tape or shoelaces that have been sterilized in boiling water. Tighten the tape slowly so that it does

Documentation Tips

Recording time of birth will ensure that the information is available for the birth certificate. It also provides you with a starting point from which to time the intervals for Apgar scores. This is even more important with multiple births. You will be busy; consider asking a family member to act as "timekeeper."

not cut the cord, and then secure it with a square knot. Do not use ordinary string or twine, which will cut through the soft, fragile tissues of the cord. Once the ties or clamps are firmly in place, carefully cut the cord between them with the scissors or a razor blade that has been sterilized by boiling. Remember, the cord is fragile; if handled too roughly, it could be torn from the infant's abdomen, resulting in a fatal hemorrhage. Once the ties or clamps are in place, there is no need to rush.

If you use clamps, after you have cut the cord, be sure to tie off the cord between the clamp and the baby, about 1" nearer to the infant than to the clamp. Cut the ends of the tape, but do not remove either clamp. The part of the cord that is coming out of the mother's vagina is attached to the placenta and will be delivered when the placenta delivers.

By now, the infant should be pink and breathing on its own. Give the infant, wrapped in a warm blanket, to your assistant; he or she can monitor the infant and complete its initial care. Alternatively, you can give the infant to the mother if she is alert and in stable condition. The mother may want to begin breastfeeding at this time. You need to return your attention to the mother and the delivery of the placenta.

Delivery of the Placenta

The placenta is attached to the end of the umbilical cord that is coming out of the mother's vagina. Again, you need only assist. Like the infant, the placenta delivers itself, usually within a few minutes of the birth, though it may take as long as 30 minutes. Never pull on the end of the umbilical cord in an attempt to speed delivery of the placenta. You may tear the cord, the placenta, or both and cause serious, perhaps life-threatening, hemorrhage.

The normal placenta is round, about 7" in diameter and about 1" thick. One surface is smooth and covered with a shiny membrane; the other surface is rough and divided into lobes (▶ **Figure 17-9**). Wrap the entire placenta and cord in a towel, place them into a plastic bag, and be sure it accompanies the mother and infant to the

hospital. Hospital personnel will examine the placenta and the cord to make certain that the entire placenta has been delivered. If a piece of the placenta has been retained inside the mother, it could cause persistent bleeding or infection.

After delivery of the placenta and before transport, place a sterile pad or sanitary napkin over the vagina and straighten the mother's legs. You can help to slow bleeding by gently massaging the mother's abdomen with a firm, circular motion. The abdominal skin will be wrinkled and very soft. You should be able to feel a firm, grapefruit-sized mass in the lower abdomen. This is called the fundus. As you massage the fundus, the uterus will contract and become firmer. You can also place the infant at the mother's breast to nurse, which stimulates the uterus to contract. Both massaging the uterus and having the baby stimulate the mother's nipples will cause a production of oxytocin, which is a hormone that will help to contract the uterus and slow bleeding. Before taking her, the infant, and the placenta to the hospital, take a minute to congratulate the mother and thank anyone who assisted. Be sure to record the time of birth for the birth certificate.

Some bleeding, usually less than 500 mL, occurs before the placenta delivers. The following are emergency situations:

- More than 30 minutes elapse, and the placenta has not delivered.

- There is more than 500 mL of bleeding before delivery of the placenta.

- There is significant bleeding after the delivery of the placenta.

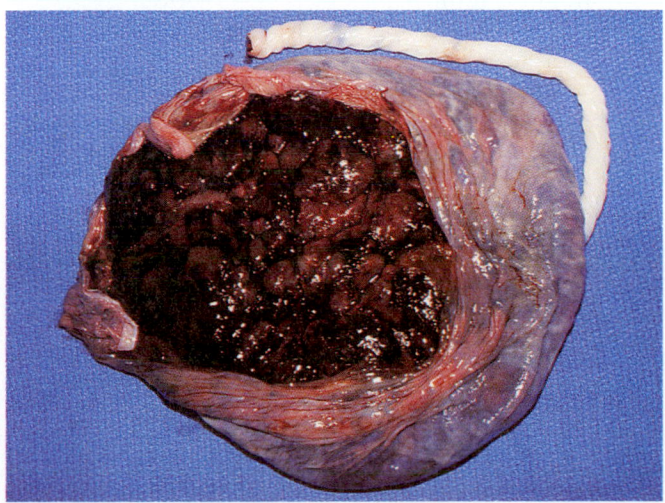

Figure 17-9 The normal placenta is round, about 7" in diameter and 1" thick. One surface is smooth; the other is rough and divided into lobes.

If one or more of these events occur, the mother and infant will require prompt evacuation to an ALS access location or medical facility. Place a sterile pad or sanitary napkin over the mother's vagina, place her in Trendelenburg's (shock) position, administer oxygen, and monitor her vital signs closely. Never put anything into the vagina.

Neonatal Evaluation and Resuscitation

Remember that before you handle a newborn infant, put on gloves and follow BSI precautions. As soon as the infant is born, you must complete an initial assessment. A newborn infant will usually begin breathing spontaneously within 15 to 20 seconds after birth. If not, gently tap or flick the soles of the feet or rub the baby's back to stimulate breathing. If the baby does not breathe after 10 to 15 seconds, begin resuscitation efforts. You should use the same scoring system that physicians in hospitals use to assess the status of the infant: the **Apgar score**. This system assigns a number value (0, 1, or 2) to each of five areas of activity of the newborn infant:

- **Appearance.** Shortly after birth, the skin of a light-skinned infant and the mucous membranes of a dark-skinned infant should turn pink. Infants often have cyanosis of the extremities for a few minutes after birth, but hands and feet should "pink up" quickly. Blue skin all over or blue mucous membranes signal a central cyanosis.

- **Pulse.** If a stethoscope is unavailable, you can measure pulsations in the umbilical cord with your fingers. Obviously, the infant with no pulse requires immediate CPR.

- **Grimace or irritability.** Grimacing, crying, or withdrawing in response to stimuli is normal in a newborn and indicates that the infant is doing

well. The way to test this is to snap a finger against the sole of the infant's foot.

- **Activity or muscle tone.** The degree of muscle tone indicates the oxygenation of the infant's tissues. Normally, the hips and knees are flexed at birth, and, to some degree, the infant will resist attempts to straighten them out. A newborn should not be floppy or limp.

- **Respirations.** Normally, the newborn's respirations are regular and rapid, with a good strong cry. If the respirations are slow, shallow, or labored or if the cry is weak, the infant may have respiratory insufficiency and need assistance with ventilations. Complete absence of respirations or crying is obviously a very serious sign; in addition to assisted ventilations, CPR may be necessary.

The total of the five numbers is the Apgar score. A perfect score is 10. The Apgar score should be calculated at 1 minute and 5 minutes after birth. Most infants will have a score of 7 or 8 at 1 minute and a score of 8 to 10 at 5 minutes. ▶ **Table 17-2** shows how to calculate an Apgar score.

Consider the following delivery situation. You have assisted a delivery or arrived to find that a delivery has already taken place. You now have two patients who need assessment and care: the mother and the infant. Follow these steps in assessing the infant:

1. **Quickly calculate the Apgar score** to establish a baseline for the infant's vital functions.

2. **Suctioning and stimulation** should result in an immediate increase in respirations. If they do not, you must begin artificial ventilation. Unlike adults, who may have a sudden cardiac arrest, infants who get into trouble usually have a respiratory arrest first. Therefore, it is essential to keep the infant ventilating and oxygenating well.

3. **If the infant is breathing well,** you should next check the pulse rate by feeling the brachial pulse or the pulsations in the umbilical cord. The pulse rate should be at least 100 beats/min. If it is not, begin artificial ventilation. This alone may increase the infant's heart rate. Reassess respirations and heart rate at least every 30 seconds to make sure that the pulse rate is increasing and that respirations are becoming spontaneous.

Remember

APGAR scoring system

- Appearance
- Pulse
- Grimace or irritability
- Activity or muscle tone
- Respirations

TABLE 17-2 Apgar Scoring System

Area of Activity	Score		
	2	1	0
Appearance	Entire infant is pink.	Body is pink, but hands and feet remain blue.	Entire infant is blue or pale.
Pulse	More than 100 beats/min	Fewer than 100 beats/min	Absent pulse
Grimace or Irritability	Infant cries and tries to move foot away from finger snapped against its sole.	Infant gives a weak cry in response to stimulus.	Infant does not cry or react to stimulus.
Activity or Muscle Tone	Infant resists attempts to straighten out hips and knees.	Infant makes weak attempts to resist straightening.	Infant is completely limp, with no muscle tone.
Respiration	Rapid respirations	Slow respirations	Absent respirations

4. **Assess the infant's skin color.** You are looking for central cyanosis. Central cyanosis is a bluish discoloration of the face and trunk that indicates a lack of oxygen in the infant's bloodstream. If you find it, administer high-flow oxygen (10 to 15 L/min) through oxygen tubing held close to the infant's face.

5. **Remember, you now have two patients.** As soon as you determine that the infant is having problems, you will need to arrange for rapid evacuation for ALS access.

In situations in which assisted ventilations are needed, you should use an infant BVM device
▶ **Figure 17-10**). Cover the infant's mouth and nose with the mask and begin ventilations with high-flow oxygen at a rate of 40 to 60 breaths/min. Make sure you have a good mask-to-face seal. Using gentle pressure, make the chest rise with each breath. Initially, it may be necessary to bypass the pop-off valve to accomplish this.

Assisted ventilation has been successful if you see both sides of the chest rise and hear breath sounds. After 15 to 30 seconds of adequate ventilations, assess the heart rate. If the heart rate is at least 100 beats/min and the infant is breathing spontaneously, you can stop the assisted ventilations. Do not stop suddenly. Instead, gradually decrease the rate and pressure of the assisted ventilations to determine whether the infant will continue to breathe adequately on its own. If not,

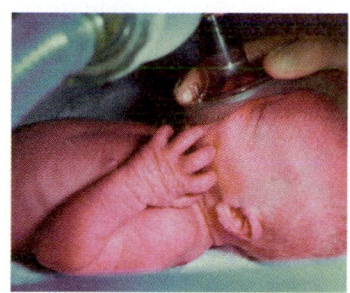

Figure 17-10 Use an infant bag and mask, ensuring that you cover both the infant's nose and mouth. Ventilate with high-flow oxygen at a rate of 40 to 60 breaths/min.

continue assisted ventilations until it does. You may find that gently stimulating the infant by rubbing it will help it to maintain its respirations.

If the heart rate is less than 80 beats/min or between 80 and 100 beats/min and not coming up with ventilations, continue assisted ventilations and start cardiac compressions. Even though this infant has a pulse, the rate and blood output from the heart are not adequate for the needs of a newborn.

Skill Drill 17-2   Giving Chest Compressions to an Infant

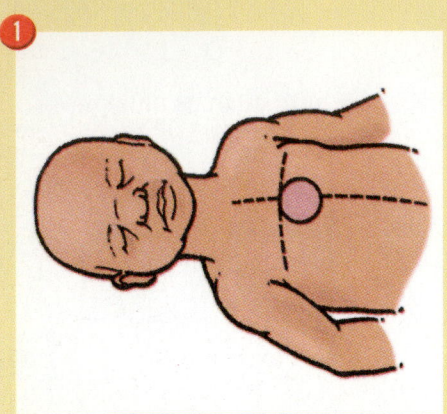

Find the proper position: just below nipple line, on the middle third of the sternum.

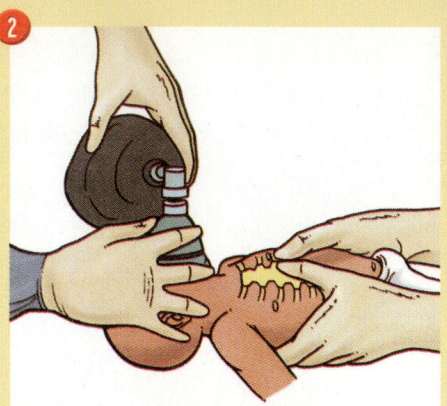

Wrap your hands around the body, with your thumbs resting at that position.

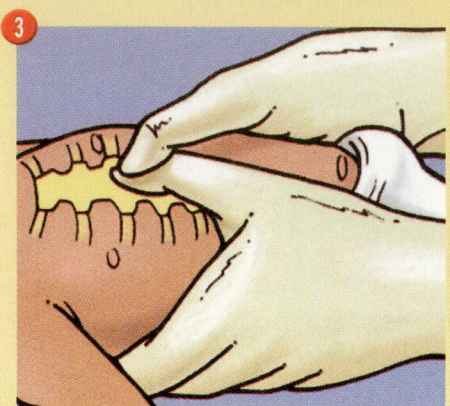

Press your thumbs gently against the sternum, compressing $1/2$" to $3/4$" deep.

There are two ways to give chest compressions to an infant. For the preferred method, follow the steps in ▲ Skill Drill 17-2 :

1. **Find the proper position:** one finger width below an imaginary line drawn between the nipples on the middle third of the sternum **(Step 1)**.

2. On a normal, full-term-sized infant, **place both hands around the infant so that your thumbs are side by side,** resting on the middle third of the sternum, and the rest of your fingers encircle the thorax. In premature or very small infants, you may have to place one thumb over the other to perform chest compressions **(Step 2)**.

3. **Press the two thumbs gently against the sternum.** The newborn's chest is easy to compress. Use only enough force to compress the sternum $1/2$" to $3/4$" **(Step 3)**.

If your hands are too small to encircle the chest, you should use the middle and ring fingers of one hand to provide the compressions while your other hand supports the infant's back.

BVM ventilation is performed during the pause after every third compression. You should deliver a combined total of 120 ventilations and compressions per minute, 90 compressions to 30 ventilations. Keep in mind that ventilation is absolutely crucial to the successful resuscitation of the neonate.

If the infant does not begin breathing on its own or does not have an adequate heart rate, continue CPR. Once CPR has been started, do not stop until the infant responds with adequate respirations and heart rates or is pronounced dead by a physician. Do not give up! Many infants have survived without brain damage after prolonged periods of effective CPR. If the infant presents in distress, you should not wait to measure the Apgar score, but begin appropriate care measures immediately.

Abnormal or Complicated Delivery Emergencies

Breech Delivery

The **presentation** is the position in which an infant is born, the part of the body that comes out first. Most infants are born head first, in what is called a vertex presentation. Occasionally, the buttocks come out first. This is called a **breech presentation** ▶ Figure 17-11 . With a breech presentation, the infant is at great risk for delivery trauma. In addition, prolapsed cords are more common. Breech deliveries are usually slow, so there may be time to get the mother to the hospital. However, if the buttocks have already passed through the vagina, delivery is underway, and you should follow emergency procedures and call for ALS backup. In general, if the mother does not deliver within 10 minutes of the buttocks presentation, apply high-flow oxygen and immediately evacuate her to an ALS access location or medical facility. If ALS cannot be easily accessed, use a cell phone or radio, if possible, to contact medical control via 9-1-1 to guide you through this difficult situation.

The preparations for a breech delivery are the same as those for a vertex delivery. Position the mother, assemble an emergency delivery kit, and place yourself and your assistant as you would for a normal delivery. Allow the buttocks and legs to deliver spontaneously, supporting them with your hand to prevent rapid expulsion. The buttocks will usually come out easily. Let the legs dangle on either side of your arm while you support the trunk and chest as they are delivered. The head is almost always face down and should be allowed to deliver spontaneously. As the head is delivering, you should keep the infant's airway open: Make a "V" with your gloved fingers, and then place them into the vagina to keep the walls of the vagina from compressing the airway. *This is one of only two circumstances in which you should put your fingers into the vagina.*

Rare Presentations

On very rare occasions, the presenting part of the infant is neither the head nor buttocks, but a single arm, leg, or foot. This is called a **limb presentation** (▼ **Figure 17-12**). You cannot successfully deliver such a

presentation in the field. These infants usually must be delivered surgically. If you are faced with a limb presentation, you must immediately arrange for transportation of the mother to the hospital. If a limb is protruding, cover it with a sterile towel. Never try to push it back in, and never pull on it. Place the mother on her back, with head down and pelvis elevated. Since both mother and infant are likely to be physically stressed in this situation, remember to place the mother on high-flow oxygen.

Prolapse of the umbilical cord, a situation in which the umbilical cord comes out of the vagina before the infant (▶ **Figure 17-13**), is another rare presentation that must be handled in the hospital. This situation is very dangerous, because the infant's head will compress the cord during birth and cut off circulation to the infant, depriving it of oxygenated blood. Do not attempt to push the cord back into the vagina. Prolapse of the umbilical cord usually occurs early in labor when the amniotic sac ruptures. As a result, there is time to get the mother to the hospital. Your job is to try to keep the infant's head from compressing the cord.

Place the mother on a backboard in Trendelenburg's position, with her hips elevated on a pillow or folded sheet. Alternatively, the mother may be placed in a knee-chest position: kneeling and bent forward, face

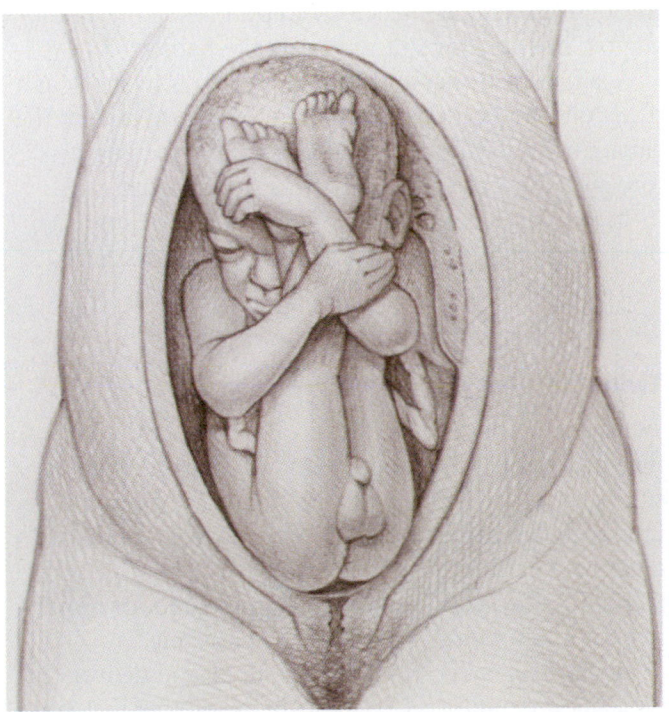

Figure 17-11 An infant in a breech presentation presents with the buttocks first. Breech deliveries are usually slow, so you will often have time to arrange for transportation of the mother to the hospital.

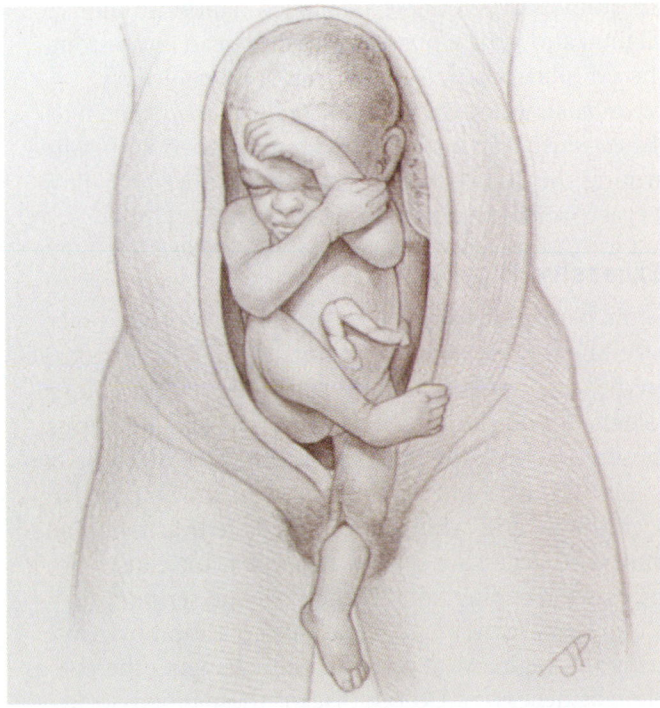

Figure 17-12 In very rare instances, an infant's limb, usually a single arm or leg, presents first. This is a very serious situation, and you must arrange for prompt transport for hospital delivery.

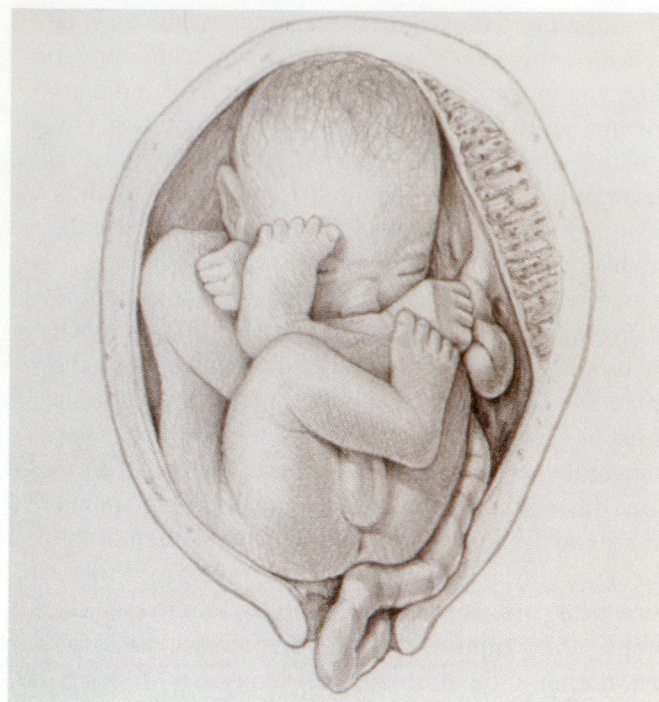

Figure 17-13 A prolapsed umbilical cord, another rare situation, is very dangerous and must be cared for at the hospital.

Place the mother in Trendelenburg's position, administer oxygen, monitor vital signs frequently, and continue to massage the uterus while awaiting transportation to the hospital. Never hold the mother's legs together in an effort to stop the bleeding, and never pack the vagina with gauze pads in an attempt to control bleeding.

Abortion (Miscarriage)

Delivery of the fetus and placenta before 20 weeks is called **abortion**, or miscarriage. Abortions may be spontaneous, without any obvious known cause, or deliberate. Deliberate abortions may be self-induced, by the mother herself or by someone else, or planned and performed in a hospital or clinic. Regardless of the reasons for the abortion, it may cause complications that you may be called upon to treat.

The most serious complications of abortion are bleeding and infection. Bleeding can result from portions of the fetus or placenta being left in the uterus (incomplete abortion) or from injury to the wall of the uterus (perforation of the uterus and possibly the adjacent bowel or bladder). Infection can result from such perforation, as well as from the use of nonsterile instruments. If the mother is in shock, treat and arrange for prompt transportation to the hospital. Collect and send to the hospital any tissue that passes through the vagina. Never try to pull tissue out of the vagina; instead, cover it with a sterile pad.

Again, as you encounter a patient who is in shock as a result of complications of abortion, be sure to size up the situation, perform your initial assessment, focused history and physical exam, and assess baseline vital signs.

In rare instances of abortion, massive bleeding may occur and cause severe hypovolemic or hemorrhagic shock. In these instances, treat and arrange for immediate transport to the emergency department.

Twins

Twins occur about once in every 80 births. Sometimes, there is a family history of twins. The mother may suspect that she is having twins because she has an unusually large abdomen. Usually, however, twins are diagnosed early in pregnancy with modern ultrasound techniques. With twins, always be prepared for more than one resuscitation, and call for assistance.

Twins are smaller than single infants, and delivery is typically not difficult. Consider the possibility that you are dealing with twins any time the first infant is small or the mother's abdomen remains fairly large after the birth. If twins are present, the second one will usually

down. Either of these positions is meant to help keep the weight of the infant off the prolapsed cord. Carefully insert your sterile gloved hand into the vagina, and gently push the infant's head away from the umbilical cord. *Note that this is the only other occasion on which you should actually place a hand into the vagina.* Wrap a sterile towel, moistened with saline, around the exposed cord. Give the mother high-flow oxygen, and evacuate her rapidly.

Excessive Bleeding

Some bleeding always occurs with delivery. However, bleeding that exceeds approximately 500 mL is considered excessive. Although up to 500 mL of blood loss is tolerated, you should continue to massage the uterus. Be sure to check the massage technique if bleeding continues. If the mother appears to be in shock, treat her accordingly and arrange for immediate evacuation and transport. There are several other possible causes of excessive bleeding, all of which may be serious and require emergency care. Treat this condition by covering the vagina with a sterile pad, changing the pad as often as necessary. Do not discard these blood-soaked pads; hospital personnel will use them to estimate the amount of blood that the mother has lost. Also save any tissue that may have passed from the vagina.

> Premature infants need special
> care to survive. Often, they require
> resuscitation, which should be done unless
> it is physically impossible.

be born within 45 minutes of the first. About 10 minutes after the first birth, contractions will begin again, and the birth process will repeat itself.

The procedure for delivering twins is the same as that for single infants. Clamp and cut the cord of the first infant as soon as it has been born and before the second infant is delivered. The second infant may deliver before or after the first placenta. There may be only one placenta, or there may be two. When the placenta has been delivered, check whether there is one umbilical cord or two. If two cords are coming out of one placenta, the twins are called identical. If only one cord is coming out of the placenta, then the twins are called fraternal, and there will be two placentas. Occasionally, the two placentas of fraternal twins are fused, so you might think that you are dealing with identical twins. Remember, if you see only one umbilical cord coming out of the first placenta, there is still another placenta to be delivered. However, if both cords are attached to one placenta, the delivery is over. Identical twins are of the same gender; fraternal twins may be of different genders, or they may be the same.

Record the time of birth of each twin separately. Twins may be so small in weight that they look premature; handle them very carefully and keep them warm.

Premature Infant

The usual *gestational period,* the period of prenatal development, is 9 calendar months, or 40 weeks. A normal, single infant will weigh approximately 7 lb at birth. Any infant that delivers before 8 months (36 weeks of gestation) or weighs less than 5 lb at birth is considered *premature.* This determination is not always easy to make. Often, the exact gestation time cannot be determined. Since you probably have no scale to weigh the infant, you will have to use physical guidelines. A premature infant is smaller and thinner than a full-term infant, and its head is proportionately larger in comparison with the rest of its body (▶ **Figure 17-14**). The *vernix caseosa,* a cheesy white coating on the skin that is found

on the full-term infant, will be missing on the premature infant or will be very minimal. There will also be less body hair.

Premature infants need special care to survive. Often, they require resuscitation, which should be done unless it is physically impossible. With such care, infants as small as 1 lb have survived and developed normally. Follow these procedures when you are handling a premature infant:

1. **Keep the infant warm.** Dry the infant as soon as it is born, and then remove the wet towels. Wrap it in a warm blanket, exposing the face but covering the head.

2. **Keep the mouth and nose clear of mucus.** The small nasal passages can easily be obstructed. Use the bulb syringe to suction the mouth and nostrils frequently. Handle the infant very gently.

3. **If the cord has to be cut, carefully observe** the cut end of the cord attached to the infant, and be sure that it is not bleeding. The loss of even a few drops of blood can be very serious.

4. **Give oxygen.** Open the valve on your oxygen cylinder slowly to give a steady stream of oxygen (about 70 to 100 bubbles per minute through the water bottle that is attached to the oxygen tank). Direct the stream of oxygen not into the infant's mouth, but into a small tent over the infant's head; you can use a blanket or a piece of aluminum foil to make the tent. Although there is some danger to a premature infant from receiving

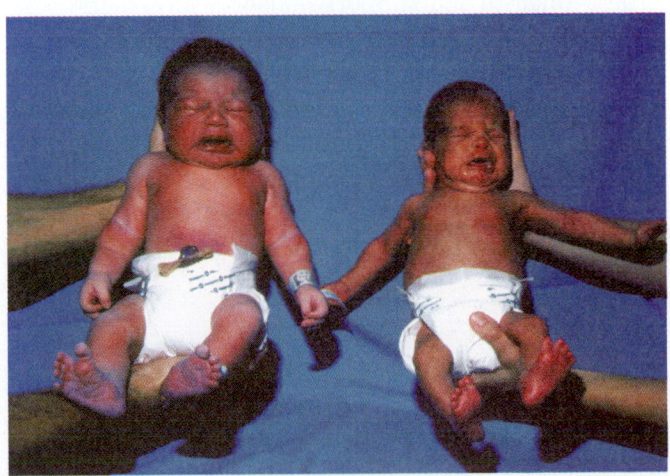

Figure 17-14 A premature infant (right) is smaller and thinner than a full-term infant (left).

very high concentrations of oxygen, there is no danger if it is given over a short period of time in this manner.

5. **Do not infect the infant.** Premature infants are very susceptible to infection. Protect them from contamination. Do not breathe directly into the infant's face. A mask will help to create a barrier. Keep everyone else as far away from the infant as possible.

6. **Notify the hospital.** A neonatal (newborn) transport team with specialized personnel and equipment for the care of premature and sick newborn infants may be available to meet and care for the infant at the ALS access location. If so, be sure to contact the hospital before leaving the scene so that medical control can decide whether to call in the team. If not, you should still notify the hospital as soon as possible so that staff can be ready to receive the premature infant and mother. Avoid unnecessary on-scene delays.

You must keep the premature infant warm with additional blankets, thermal packets, and a warmed patient environment. Any delays will lower the infant's body temperature.

Fetal Demise

Unfortunately, you may find yourself delivering an infant that has died in the mother's uterus before labor. This will be a true test of your medical, emotional, and social abilities. Grieving parents will be emotionally distraught and perhaps even hostile, requiring all your professionalism and support skills.

The onset of labor may be premature, but labor will otherwise progress normally in most cases. If an intrauterine infection has caused the demise, you may note an extremely foul odor. The delivered infant may have skin blisters, skin sloughing, and a dark discoloration, depending on the stage of decomposition. The head will be soft and perhaps grossly deformed.

Do not attempt to resuscitate an obviously dead infant. However, do not confuse such an infant with those who have had a cardiopulmonary arrest as a complication of the birthing process. You must attempt to resuscitate normal-appearing infants.

Delivery Without Sterile Supplies

On rare occasions, you may have to deliver an infant without a sterile OB kit. Even if you do not have a sterile kit, you should always have goggles and sterile gloves with you. These are for your own protection as well as that of the mother and infant. Carry out the delivery as if sterile supplies were on hand. If you can, use clean sheets and towels that have not been used since they were laundered. As soon as the infant is born, wipe the inside of its mouth with your finger to clear away blood and mucus. Without an OB kit, you should not cut or tie the umbilical cord. Instead, as soon as the placenta delivers, wrap it in a clean towel or put it in a plastic bag and transport it with the infant and mother to the hospital. Always keep the placenta and the infant at the same level so that blood does not drain from the infant into the placenta. Be sure to keep the infant warm. As in the case of other deliveries, note the presence of green-tinged fluid or secretions (meconium staining).

Gynecological Emergencies

Occasionally, women who are not pregnant will have major gynecological problems requiring urgent medical care. These include excessive bleeding and soft-tissue injuries to the external genitalia. These genital parts have a rich nerve supply, making injuries very painful.

Treat lacerations, abrasions, and tears with moist, sterile compresses, using local pressure to control bleeding and a diaper-type bandage to hold the dressings in place. Leave any foreign bodies in place after stabilizing them with bandages. Under no circumstances should you ever pack or place dressings in the vagina. Continue to assess these patients while arranging for transportation to the emergency department. Contusions and other blunt trauma will require careful in-hospital evaluation.

Although you might not know the exact cause of a gynecological emergency, you should treat these individuals as you would any other victim of blood loss: observe BSI precautions, ensure maintenance of the airway, give oxygen, take and document vital signs, and treat for shock while arranging for prompt transport. Always have a second rescuer present, preferably a woman, when treating gynecological emergencies.

Environmental Stresses and Pregnancy

Although pregnancy is considered a relative contraindication to wilderness or backcountry travel, more and more women are recognizing the benefit of regular exercise and are engaging in outdoor sporting activities well into their third trimester. Some athletes find that the physiologic changes that accompany pregnancy—such as improved flexibility and a higher, more anterior center of gravity—actually enhance the sporting experience. On the down side, women participating in strenuous sports may be at risk for blunt abdominal trauma and subsequent hemorrhage from uterine injury, fetal demise, or premature labor. In addition, environmental conditions place unique stresses on the mother and fetus.

For example, pregnant women are more susceptible to altitude sickness and are more likely to develop severe symptoms. A longer period of adjustment to high altitude is required before engaging in any exertional activities. At higher altitude, lower circulating fetal oxygen levels and maternal dehydration may endanger the fetus. Therefore, a pregnant woman must stay well-hydrated, progress gradually to higher altitudes, and limit activity in order to minimize symptoms of altitude sickness and to allow the fetus to compensate. Once acclimatized, most pregnant women find that their endurance and ability to participate in strenuous activities at altitude remain limited due to fetal oxygen requirements.

A potentially hazardous sport for pregnant women is scuba diving. The fetus is placed at risk from nitrogen bubbles released in the fetal-placental tissue during ascent. Increasing abdominal girth, buoyancy, and difficulty breathing also create problems for the mother and may lead to panic, even in the experienced diver. Pregnancy is thus considered by many to be a contraindication to this sport.

It is significantly harder for pregnant women to acclimatize to high ambient temperatures and humidity. This may be dangerous to the fetus, since the fetus depends on the mother to eliminate excess heat. Pregnant women participating in summertime outdoor sporting events or exercise need to stay well hydrated and consider exercising during cooler times of the day. Hyperthermia—particularly when combined with dehydration and electrolyte disturbances—increases the risk of premature labor.

Chapter *Sweep*

Ready for Review

Inside the uterus, the developing fetus floats in the amniotic sac. The umbilical cord connects mother and infant through the placenta. Eventually, the uterus will propel the infant through the birth canal. The first stage of labor, dilation, begins with the onset of contractions and ends when the cervix is fully dilated. The second stage, expulsion of the baby, begins when the cervix is fully dilated and ends when the infant is born. The third stage, delivery of the placenta, begins with the birth of the infant and ends with the delivery of the placenta.

Once labor has begun, it cannot be slowed or stopped; however, there is usually time to transport the patient to the hospital during the first stage. During the second stage, you must decide whether to deliver the baby at the scene or transport the mother. During the third stage, once the infant has been born, you will probably not transport until the placenta has delivered.

Use an infant BVM device to assist ventilations, starting with high-flow oxygen at a rate of 40 to 60 breaths/min. If the infant starts to breathe on its own, attach an oxygen tubing mask and watch for signs of adequate oxygenation. If the heart rate is less than 80 beats/min, start cardiac compressions, using only enough force to compress the sternum $1/2$" to $3/4$". Perform a combined total of 120 ventilations and compressions per minute, 90 compressions to 30 ventilations.

Abnormal or complicated deliveries include breech deliveries (buttocks first), limb presentations (arm, leg, or foot first), and prolapse of the umbilical cord (umbilical cord first). Quickly transport the patient with a limb presentation or prolapsed umbilical cord to the hospital. The only times you should place a finger or hand into the vagina are to keep the walls of the vagina from compressing the infant's airway during a face-down breech presentation or to push the infant's head away from the cord in a prolapse situation.

Excessive bleeding is a serious emergency. Cover the vagina with a sterile pad; change the pad as often as necessary, and send all used pads to the hospital for examination.

Use local pressure and a diaper-type bandage to hold dressings in place when treating nonobstetric injuries to the external genitalia. Never place dressings in the vagina. Treat patients with these injuries as you would any other victim of blood loss.

Vital Vocabulary

abortion Delivery of the fetus and placenta before 20 weeks; miscarriage.

amniotic sac The fluid-filled, baglike membrane in which the fetus develops.

Apgar score A scoring system for assessing the status of a newborn that assigns a number value to each of five areas of assessment.

birth canal The vagina and cervix.

bloody show A plug of pink-tinged mucus that is discharged when the cervix begins to dilate.

breech presentation Delivery in which the buttocks come out first.

cervix The lower one-third, or neck, of the uterus.

crowning The appearance of the infant's head at the vaginal opening during labor.

eclampsia Convulsions (seizures) resulting from severe hypertension in the pregnant woman.

ectopic pregnancy A pregnancy that develops outside the uterus, typically in a fallopian tube.

fetus The developing, unborn infant inside the uterus.

limb presentation A delivery in which the presenting part is a single arm, leg, or foot.

multigravida A woman who has had previous pregnancies.

multipara A woman who has had more than one live birth.

nuchal cord An umbilical cord that is wrapped around the infant's neck.

perineum The area of skin between the vagina and the anus.

placenta Tissue attached to the uterine wall that nourishes the fetus through the umbilical cord.

placenta abruptio Premature separation of the placenta from the wall of the uterus.

placenta previa A condition in which the placenta develops over and covers the cervix.

pregnancy-induced hypertension A condition of late pregnancy that also involves headache, visual changes, and swelling of the hands and feet; also called preeclampsia.

presentation The position in which an infant is born; the part of the infant that appears first.

primigravida A woman who is experiencing her first pregnancy.

primipara A woman who has had one live birth.

prolapse of the umbilical cord A situation in which the umbilical cord comes out of the vagina before the infant.

supine hypotensive syndrome Low blood pressure resulting from compression of the inferior vena cava by the weight of the fetus when the mother is supine.

umbilical cord The conduit connecting mother to infant via the placenta; contains two arteries and one vein.

uterus The muscular organ where the fetus grows, also called the womb; responsible for contractions during labor.

vagina The outermost cavity of a woman's reproductive system; the lower part of the birth canal.

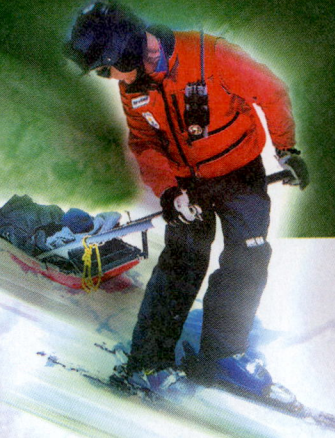

Assessment in Action

You are a member of a small nordic patrol located in a state park. A group of cross-country skiers approach you, calling for help. A member of their group is 7 months pregnant and has gone into premature labor. She is located in an overnight camping shelter 2 miles away, accompanied by her sister. After contacting the park ranger by radio, you and a fellow patroller proceed on skis to the hut. Inside, you find a 22-year-old woman lying on the floor with a small puddle of blood under her buttocks.

The patient tells you she has been having contractions for several hours but thought they were false labor pains. When her water broke, she realized the situation was serious and she sent her husband and companions for help. She has had an uneventful pregnancy to date and as an athlete, she has remained physically active. You check and find the baby's head at the vaginal opening. While you are getting the history and checking the patient, your fellow patroller obtains baseline vital signs, including a pulse of 138 beats/min, respirations of 32 breaths/min, and a blood pressure of 118/68 mm Hg. The closest hospital is 50 minutes away.

1. The most important assessment finding for this patient at this time is:
   A. vital signs.
   B. visualizing the presenting part.
   C. absence of prenatal care.
   D. presence of contractions.

2. This patient states her "bag of waters" has broken. What is the medical term for the "bag of waters"?
   A. Uterus
   B. Amniotic sac
   C. Cervix
   D. Placenta

3. This patient was found lying in a puddle of blood under her buttocks. Some of that was from the amniotic fluid and some was blood from capillaries breaking. A normal amount of blood that can be expected prior to delivery of the placenta is about:
   A. 250 mL.
   B. 500 mL.
   C. 750 mL.
   D. 1,000 mL.

4. From the assessment findings of this patient, what is her stage of labor?
   A. First stage
   B. Transition from first to second stage
   C. Second stage
   D. Third stage

5. As you prepare for the birth of this infant, it is very important to ask which one of the following?
   A. Do you feel as though you have to have a bowel movement?
   B. Do you feel pressure in the small of your back?
   C. When is your due date or how long have you been pregnant?
   D. Have you had any gushing of fluid or spotting?

6. She tells you that she didn't think the baby was due for another month and a half. How does this change what you will be doing?
   A. The mother will need more oxygen.
   B. There is more likelihood of bleeding.
   C. The baby will be easier to care for.
   D. The baby may need more resuscitation.

7. The baby should be suctioned as soon as the:
   A. baby is completely out of the vagina.
   B. baby begins to cry.
   C. head emerges from the vagina.
   D. umbilical cord is clamped.

8. As the baby is being delivered, you discover the cord is wrapped around the baby's neck. What should you do?
   A. Nothing, delivery of the baby will straighten it out.
   B. Try to ease the cord over the baby's head or shoulders.
   C. Stop the delivery and immediately transport.
   D. Attempt to reinsert the baby to loosen the cord.

Challenging Questions

9. Why is it important to find out how many times this mother has been pregnant?

10. Resuscitating a newborn includes drying, warming, suctioning, and stimulating. Why are these so important?

Points to Ponder

You respond to a woman who has fallen while skiing. She is 5 months' pregnant and landed on her abdomen when she fell. She is complaining of severe abdominal pain and believes she is leaking fluid from her vagina. The man with her states that they are Jehovah's witnesses and that they had planned a home delivery. He would like his wife transported off the slope so he can get her into their car and return home. He insists that they do not want or require further medical care. The woman appears scared and confused. This is their first child. How would you deal with this situation? What questions should you ask the mother to help assess her health and to prepare for a possible delivery emergency?

Issues Dealing with Bystanders, Patient Confidentiality, Personal Feelings about Miscarriage, Optional Answers to Difficult Questions.

Online Outlook

Watch how the fetus grows from conception through delivery from actual ultrasound images and review postdelivery care by completing Exercise 17 at **www.OECzone.com**.

Trauma

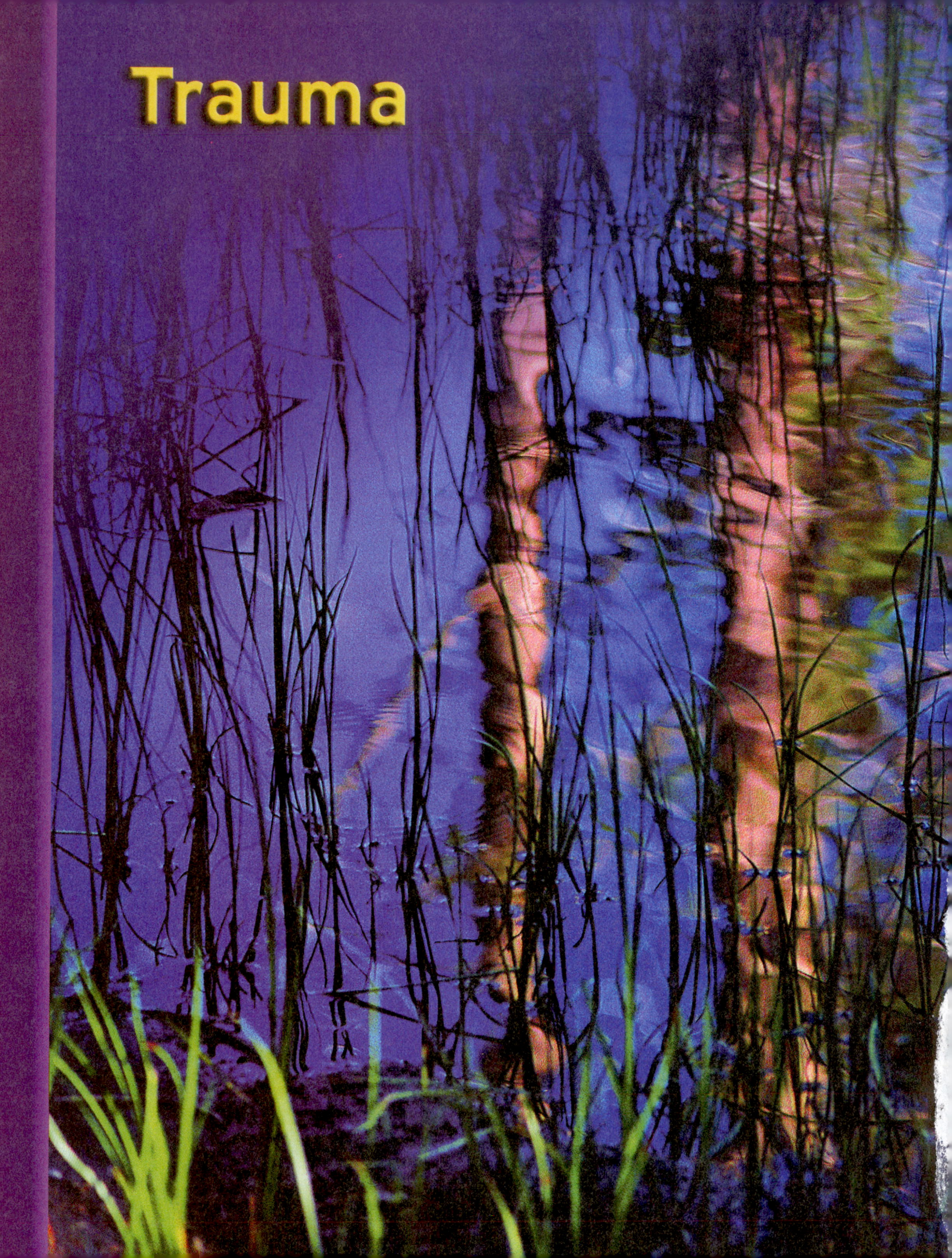

5

Section

Mechanisms and Patterns of Injury

Cognitive

♠ **1.** Describe what is meant by "mechanism of injury" (p 486).

♠ **2.** Discuss the importance of kinetic energy in producing injuries (p 487).

♠ **3.** Describe the types of trauma and give examples of injuries produced by each type (p 488).

♠ **4.** List some significant mechanisms of injury (p 488).

Affective

♠ **5.** Relate how the characteristics of the human body tissues and organs and the laws of physics apply to trauma injuries (p 488).

6. List some ways in which injuries related to kinetic injury can be prevented (p 487).

♠ **7.** Describe the process of using the mechanism of injury to predict injuries (p 491).

Psychomotor

None

♠ These are core concepts in initial patrol training.

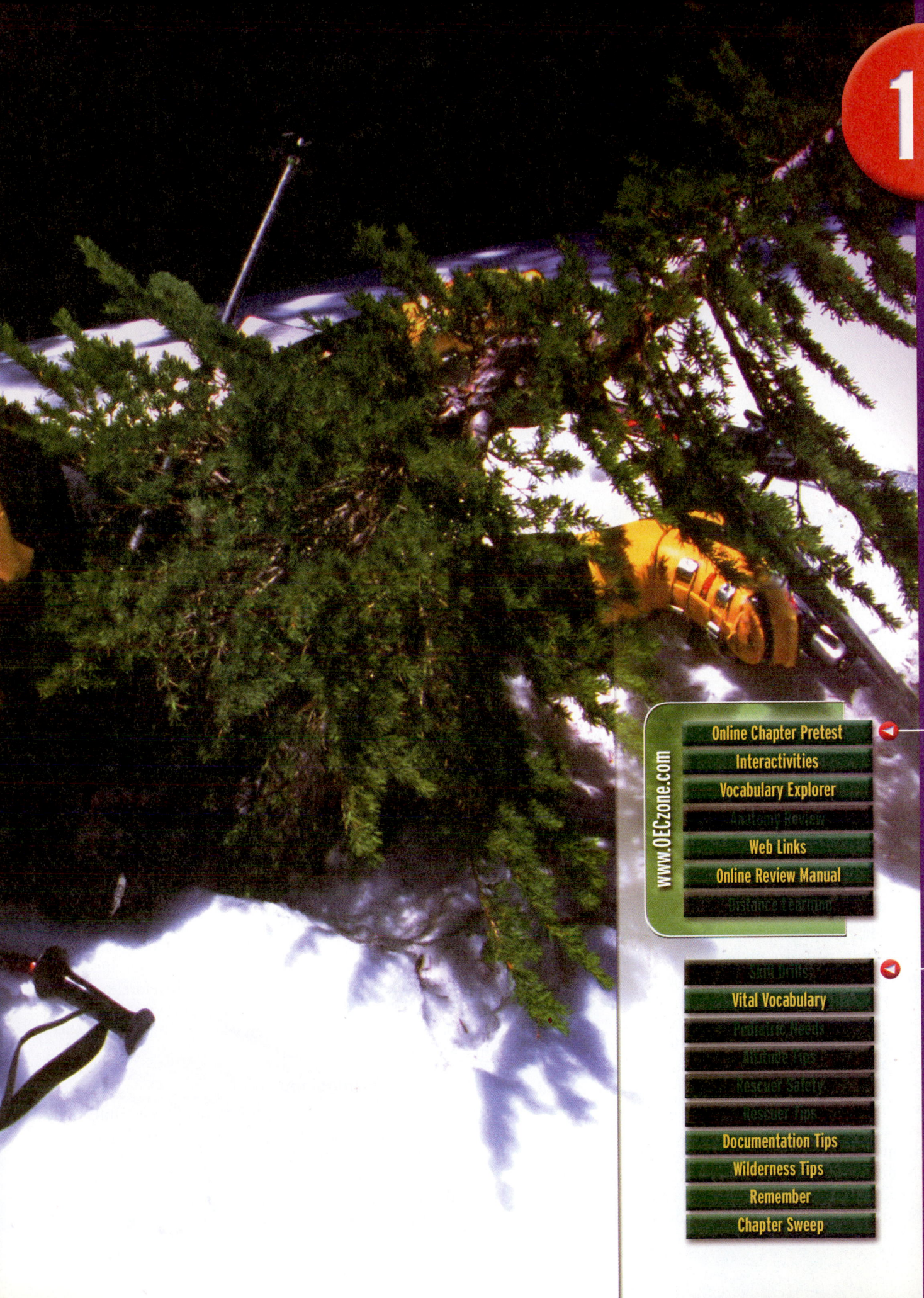

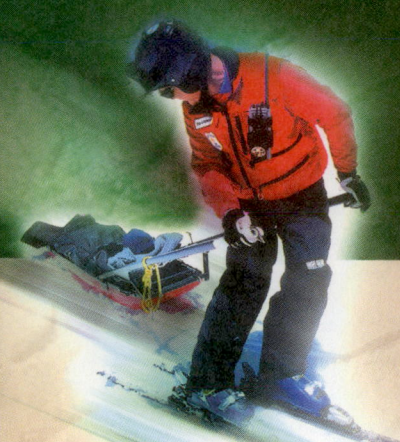

You are called to tower 12 of Windsong Lift to care for a skier who has fallen out of a chair into deep powder snow. When you arrive, the skier is sitting up in a large hole in the snow. He fell about 20'. He is alert, oriented, and complaining of a painful right knee.

Your careful assessment discloses a tender knee but no pain, tenderness, swelling, or deformity of his neck or back. The patient says he wants to continue skiing.

1. Is the mechanism of injury important in determining what your emergency care will be in this case? Why or why not?

2. In addition to caring for his knee, should you suspect a spinal injury and call for a backboard, immobilize him, and transport him to the aid room? Why or why not?

Mechanisms and Patterns of Injury

Injuries in the outdoors are not random events. Their nature is governed by specific anatomic and physiologic characteristics of the human body and by basic laws of physics. All of these factors, taken together and used to analyze a given injury or injuries, are referred to as the **mechanism of injury (MOI)**. This process allows us to:

- *Understand* how injuries occur and why some injuries are more common than others.
- *Predict* the types, numbers, locations, and severity of injuries likely to have resulted from an emergency, based on observation of the scene and assessment of the patient.
- *Anticipate* the development of life-threatening complications.

Tissue Characteristics

Tissue characteristics determine the ease with which human body parts are injured, the mechanics of their construction, their location, and the manner and frequency of their use. A soft, elastic tissue such as the skin will deform when a force is applied to it. At first, this occurs without injury (for example, when you pinch a fold of skin). As the force increases, however, the *threshold of injury* will eventually be exceeded, and the skin will be contused, torn, or avulsed. A harder, less elastic tissue such as bone is more resistant to cuts and punctures but less resistant to breakage from deforming forces than skin. Solid organs such as the spleen and liver are more likely to rupture than hollow, more pliable organs such as the stomach or bladder.

This is not the case, however, when a hollow organ is distended with fluid, such as the bladder, which may be as easily injured as a solid organ. Flexible organs that are rigidly anchored, such as the spleen or kidney, are more susceptible to injury from displacing forces than loosely attached, flexible organs that can move within body cavities, such as the intestines.

Organs that are protected by parts of the skeletal system, such as the spinal cord and the organs of the chest and pelvic cavities, are less prone to injury from equivalent forces than less-protected organs, such as those of the abdominal cavity.

The activities of daily life injure the extremities more often than the trunk. The extremities are prone to injury because they are frequently in motion, are located more distally, have less protection, and are often used to protect the trunk from injury, as when you extend your arms to break a fall. The shoulder joint, which has a shallow cup and a wide range of motion, is more often dislocated than the hip joint, which has a deep cup and a more narrow range of motion.

Most injuries are associated with *motion*, either motion of the human body itself, or motion of an object that has an impact on the body, or both. Therefore, rescuers should be familiar with the physical laws of motion and with the kinetic energy equation discussed in (▶ **Figure 18-1**).

Mechanism Terminology

Understanding mechanisms of injury requires learning a few new definitions used in physics. The term **force**, for example, is used for any action that changes the state of rest or motion of a body to which it is applied. A **body** is *any* mass of matter that is distinct from other masses of matter (when the *human* body is specified, it will be identified accordingly in this chapter). **Energy** is the capacity for doing work. It can be either **potential energy**, which is derived from the position of a body in a gravity field with respect to its own parts or to another body, or **kinetic energy**, which is energy associated with **motion**, the action or process of a change of position.

The terms **trauma** and **injury** are often used interchangeably. Both refer to damage to the human body by an external force. In this chapter, however, trauma refers to the end effect of a force applied to the human body, and injury refers to the actual type and extent of human body damage produced by this end effect.

Newton's Laws of Motion

Newton's First Law of Motion states that a body at rest will tend to remain at rest and a body in motion will tend to remain in motion unless acted upon by an outside force. For example, a moving skier will continue to move in a straight line unless he or she applies energy through the leg muscles to produce a turning motion (▶ **Figure 18-2**).

The **Law of Conservation of Energy** states that energy can neither be created nor destroyed but may be changed from one form to another. For example, the energy of a moving object that strikes the human body does not just disappear; it *disperses* as it deforms and injures the tissues. The amount of injury is roughly proportional to the amount of kinetic energy that must be dispersed.

The most important aspect of kinetic energy is its relationship to **velocity**, or speed. The speed of a moving object is more important than its mass, or weight, since while the amount of kinetic energy produced goes up in *direct* portion as the mass increases, it goes up in proportion to the *square* of the speed as the speed increases. For example, if the speed of the object *doubles*, the amount of kinetic energy produced increases *four times*. Therefore, hitting a tree at 30 mph can theoretically cause four times as much damage as hitting a tree at 15 mph. (However, remember that you can be just as dead after a 15-mph collision as after a 30-mph collision).

Figure 18-1 Kinetic energy of a body in motion.

The amount of kinetic energy of a body in motion is equal to one-half the product of the mass of the body times the velocity squared. Thus, when E_k = kinetic energy, M = mass, and V = velocity, then E_k = M/2 X V^2. For example, a 100-lb (45-kg) skier traveling at 15 miles per hour (24 kilometers per hour) has a kinetic energy of approximately 1,000 joules (1 joule = 1 kg/m²/second²). A skier who weighs 50% more (150 lb, or 67 kg) and is traveling at the same speed has a kinetic energy that is 50% greater (1,500 joules). However, a 100-lb skier traveling *twice* as fast (30 miles per hour/48 kilometers per hour) has *four times* (not twice) the kinetic energy (4,000 joules). If such a skier hits a tree, a large part of the kinetic energy is dispersed by crushing or tearing the skier's body.

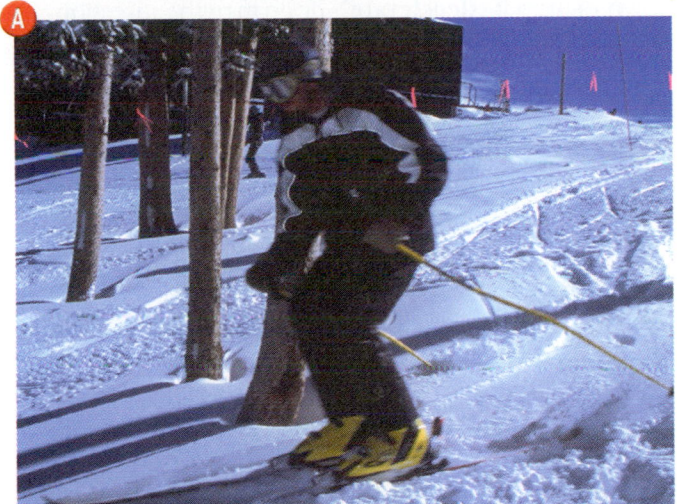

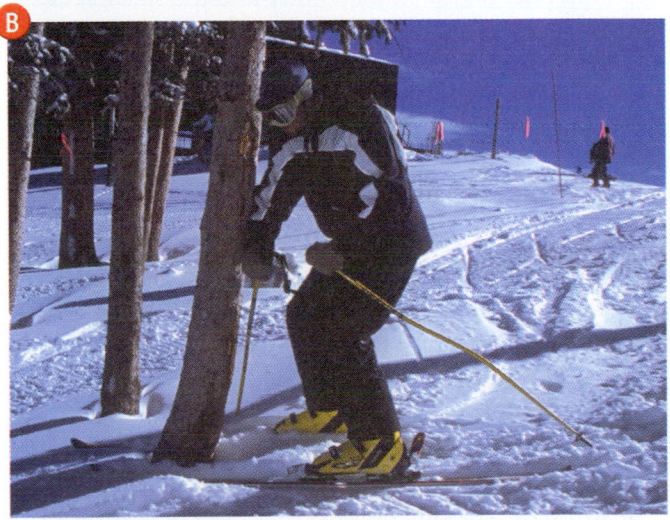

Figure 18-2 A moving skier will travel in a straight line unless he or she applies energy to turn (**A**) or collides with an object (**B**).

Another important type of kinetic energy is the energy of a falling body. Because of the force of gravity, a falling body (specified as at sea level at 45° latitude), regardless of its mass (weight), increases its speed by 32′ per second every second (976 cm per second every second). This means that a free-falling climber will build up kinetic energy very rapidly. However, the speed of a falling body does not increase infinitely. A final falling speed of about 200′ (61 m) per second, called the **terminal velocity**, is reached when the air resistance equals the pull of gravity. This varies to some extent depending on the shape of the body, the position in which it is falling, and the density of the air.

Kinetic energy causes injury because it is applied to the human body in the form of a force, which has both **magnitude** (strength) and **direction** (a route, course, or path). Forces act on the human body to move it from a resting position, speed it up (**accelerate**), slow it down or stop it (**decelerate**), or change the direction of its motion.

Types of Trauma and Resulting Injuries

Forces can lead to the following types of trauma: penetration, compression (blunt), bending, rotational, and distraction (stretching). Bending trauma is further divided into hyperflexion and hyperextension. Examples of injuries caused entirely by one force and one type of trauma are unusual because most serious injuries involve more than one force and more than one type of trauma.

The specific injury depends on the magnitude and direction of the force or forces, the type of trauma, and the human body part involved. The type of surface also has an impact on the human body and the rate of deceleration or acceleration. For example, a skier who lands in deep powder snow after a fall experiences less trauma than one who lands on ice or concrete. Likewise, the occupants of a car that runs into a soft snowbank or a stand of small trees experience less trauma than those in a car that hits a brick wall or a large tree at the same speed.

The effects of trauma can be modified by such things as controlling velocity (ie, avoiding higher speeds), using protective devices such as helmets, seat belts, and air bags, and slowing the rate of deceleration (such as by trying to tuck and roll when falling forward rather than landing head-on and skidding).

Penetration and compression traumas are caused by similar forces. The difference is that in **penetration trauma**, the size, shape, and sharpness of the wounding

> ### Remember
>
> **Types of Trauma**
>
> | | | |
> |---|---|---|
> | Penetration | Compression | Deceleration |
> | Acceleration | Bending | Distraction |
> | Rotational | | |

object and its speed and direction (or the speed and direction of the moving human body that has an impact on it) are great enough to drive the object through the skin. This may cause a laceration or puncture wound in addition to damage to deeper tissues. Penetration trauma can be caused by sharp objects moving at moderate to high speeds, such as bullets, knives, ice axes, ski pole tips, and arrows. It can also be caused when a moving human body strikes an object such as a sharp rock or broken tree limb.

In **compression (blunt) trauma**, the object involved tends to be larger in diameter and less sharp, or the force is weaker or the direction different, so that the skin may not be broken (▼ **Figure 18-3**). Compression trauma frequently damages tissues beneath the skin, however, causing a closed wound such as a contusion or hematoma as well as damage to internal organs. If compression trauma is great, a bone under the skin may break.

The types of trauma and the various actions of forces are further illustrated by several common injury pat-

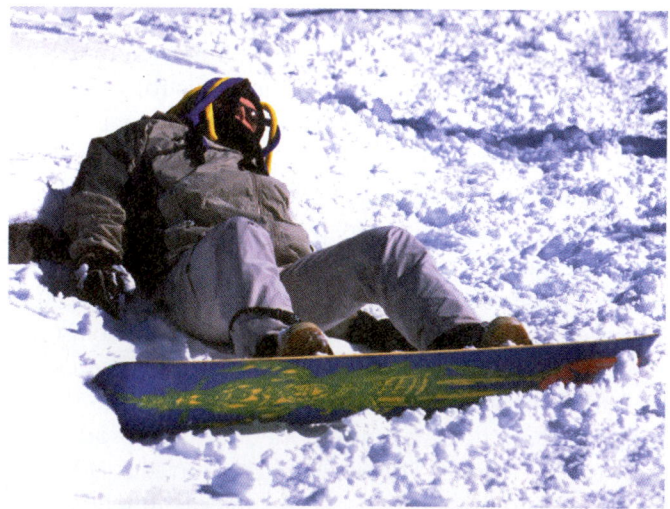

Figure 18-3 A mechanism of compression trauma is collision with a blunt object such as a rock.

terns. An example of the action of a decelerating force is a full-impact collision between a snowrider and a tree. When the rider's body comes to an abrupt halt against the tree, kinetic energy is dispersed through the production of various types of trauma to the rider (▼ **Figure 18-4**) and damage to the tree. The specific types of trauma depend on the rider's speed, the rider's body position as it strikes the tree, the angle of impact, the rate of deceleration, the rider's physical condition, the number and strength of layers of clothing worn, and whether the rider is wearing a helmet.

The parts of the rider's body that have a direct impact on the tree trunk are subject to compression trauma, which squeezes the soft tissues, rupturing blood vessels and producing contusions and hematomas. Compression trauma can also break underlying bones, such as the skull and ribs, bruise or rupture internal organs, or cause rigidly fixed organs and structures to rupture. A glancing impact with the tree can produce a shearing type of penetration trauma (produced by one object moving parallel to another object) such as a laceration or abrasion. Full impact with a sharp part of the

tree, such as a broken branch, can produce a puncture type of penetration trauma, such as an open chest wound, abdominal wound, or impalement.

In a **hyperextension** type of **bending trauma**, a skier or rider may fall on a steep, icy slope, start to slide backwards, and hit a tree with the middle of his back. The impact tends to reverse the normal forward curve of the spine momentarily, and—in addition to contusions and lacerations—can cause fractures or fracture-dislocations of the back and even rupture the aorta.

In a **hyperflexion** type of bending trauma, a skier or rider may strike the tree at an angle that has an impact on the anterior midtorso and bends the upper and lower parts of the body like a horseshoe around the tree (▼ **Figure 18-4A**). This type of trauma can cause wedge-shaped vertebral compression fractures with the narrow side anterior (▼ **Figure 18-4B**) or fracture-dislocations of the spine as well as the types of compression and penetration trauma described earlier.

The hyperflexion type of bending trauma can also result in a wedge-shaped compression fracture of one or more thoracic or lumbar vertebrae when the human

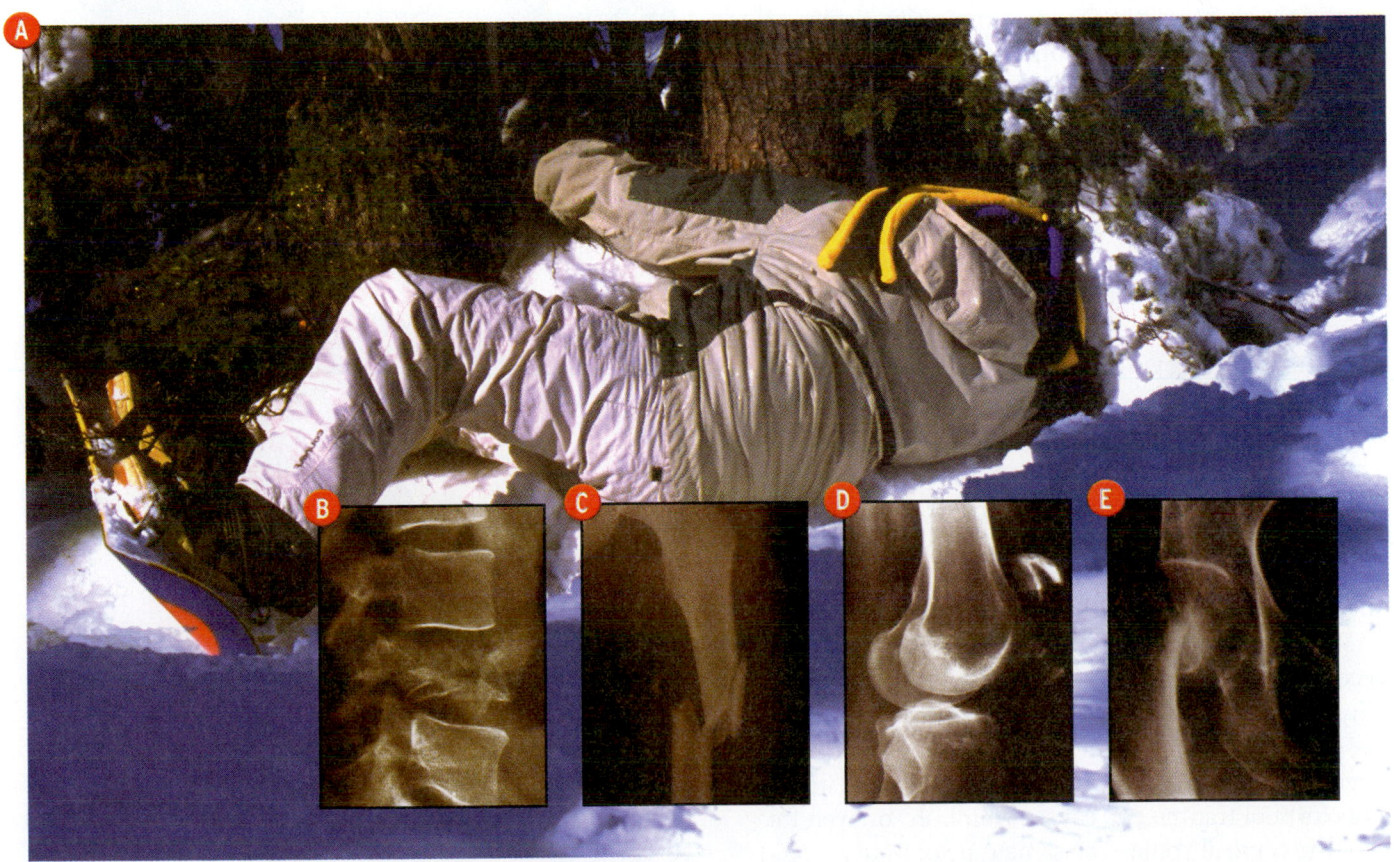

(**Figure 18-4**) Types of injuries produced by a collision. **A.** Hyperflexion type of bending trauma can result in **B.** compression fractures or fracture-dislocation of the spine, **C.** femoral shaft fractures, **D.** patellar fracture, or **E.** fracture-dislocation of the hip.

body is forced into forward flexion by a decelerating force. This can occur when a climber falls, lands hard on the feet, and pitches forward. Stronger forces of this type can cause a fracture-dislocation of the spine.

If a skier or rider strikes a tree with the midthigh, hyperflexion trauma can produce a fracture of the middle part of the femoral shaft ◄ **Figure 18-4C** . If a bent knee strikes the tree, the skier's thigh and leg may come to a sudden halt (deceleration type of compression trauma) while the pelvis and the rest of the body continue to move forward. This situation, also common in automobile crashes when an occupant's knee strikes the dashboard, can cause a patellar fracture ◄ **Figure 18-4D** , femur fracture, or fracture-dislocation of the hip joint ◄ **Figure 18-4E** as the force is transmitted up the femur and exits through the rear of the acetabulum, or socket.

If the skier's other foot is wedged under a log for half an hour or longer before it is freed, the resulting tissue damage is a slowly developing type of compression trauma called a **crushing injury**. A crushing injury involves both direct tissue injury and secondary injury when pressure on the blood vessels interferes with circulation. Crushing injuries are common in victims of building collapses, mine tunnel collapses, river rafting, motor vehicle crashes with ejection, motor vehicle crashes where a patient is pinned against a structure, when a force (car, person) lands on the patient, and natural disasters such as avalanches, earthquakes, and hurricanes.

Because many organs are somewhat free to move inside the cavities of the human body, they can be injured by secondary collisions. When the human body suddenly stops moving (decelerates), internal organs continue to move forward until they collide with the body wall or until their movements are stopped by the tightening of their attachments. At times the attachments will tear, causing severe bleeding. Secondary collisions can injure the brain within the cranial cavity, the heart and aorta within the chest cavity, and the liver, spleen, and intestines within the abdominal cavity.

When an automobile is struck from the rear by an accelerating force, its speed suddenly increases, causing a hyperextension type of bending trauma to the neck of the occupant. This type of injury may be prevented to a large extent if a properly positioned headrest is in place. This form of trauma can cause "whiplash" or even fracture the cervical spine. The same type of injury would occur to a snow slider struck from behind by a fast-moving person.

A skier who catches a pole basket in a tree while wearing the pole strap around the wrist may dislocate a shoulder due to a decelerating force. Because of hyperextension and **distraction trauma**, the shoulder joint is rotated externally, hyperabducted, and pulled apart by the resulting forces ▼ **Figure 18-5** . Distraction trauma caused by an accelerating force occurs when a person with long hair is scalped after the hair is caught in moving machinery such as a surface tow lift.

Rotational trauma is well known to ski patrollers, who are familiar with the twisting type of deceleration

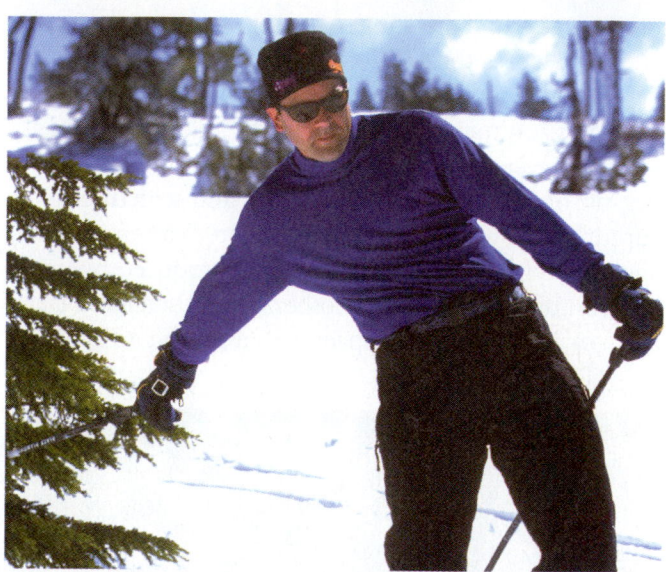

Figure 18-5   A ski pole basket that catches on a tree can cause hyperextension to the shoulder and stretching traumas.

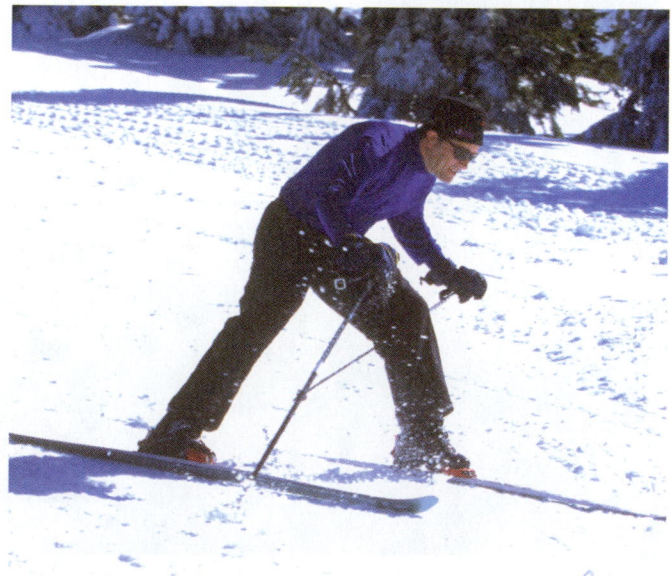

Figure 18-6   A twisting fall can produce rotational trauma.

fall that can cause a knee sprain or a spiral fracture of the tibia (◄ **Figure 18-6**).

Accidents frequently cause multiple injuries, partly because of the continued action of forces over time. The rider who experiences a hard fall may fracture both heel bones on landing (▼ **Figure 18-7**) and also the pelvis and

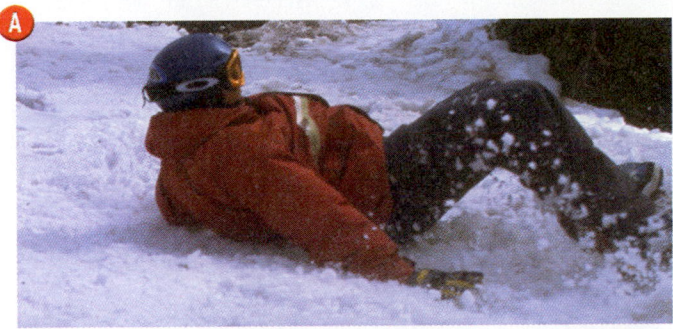

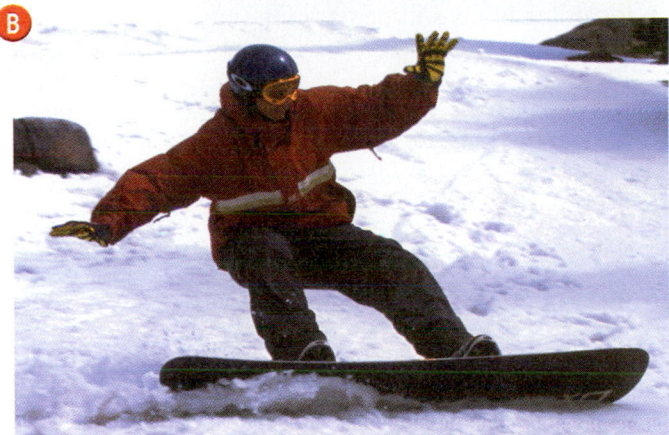

Figure 18-7 Injuries can result from **A.** pitching backward after **B.** landing on the feet after a hard fall.

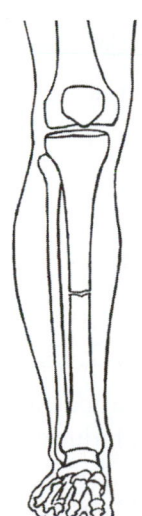 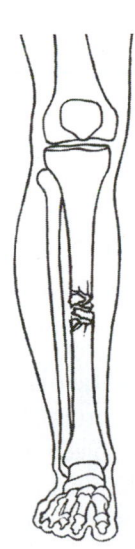

Figure 18-8 Simple tibia fracture.

Figure 18-9 Comminuted tibia fracture.

spine as the decelerating force is transmitted toward the head. Then, as energy continues to disperse, the rider may pitch backward, landing on outstretched hands and fracturing the wrists, forearms, or clavicles, and possibly even dislocating one or both shoulders.

The amount of damage is proportional to the amount of energy involved. For example, if ski bindings do not release, an easy fall may produce a simple fracture of the tibia (▼ **Figure 18-8**), while a fall at high speed may cause a comminuted fracture of the tibia (▼ **Figure 18-9**). Similarly, a high-velocity rifle bullet causes much more internal damage and a larger exit wound than a low-velocity pistol bullet of the same caliber.

Direct and Indirect Injuries

Injuries can be either direct or indirect. In a direct injury, the trauma occurs at the place where the force meets the human body, for example, the contusion produced by compression trauma when a skier falls and hits a rock. In an indirect injury, the force meets the human body in such a way that energy is transmitted to another part of the human body where the trauma is concentrated and the injury occurs, for example, the dislocated shoulder or fractured clavicle caused by falling forward on an outstretched hand.

An important complication of indirect injuries is the development of a **fulcrum point**—the hinge-like point about which a lever turns—which allows an extremity or equipment item such as a ski to function as a lever. This fulcrum can focus forces and multiply them many times.

Patterns of Injury

One of the most valuable benefits of being able to analyze and understand the mechanism(s) of injury (MOI) and incorporate this information into your initial and ongoing assessments is that these skills help you predict potential injuries, particularly *internal* injuries (► **Table 18-1**). These skills are important when caring for the patient with compression trauma, where visible signs of injury on the body surface may be minimal, and the signs and symptoms of serious internal injury may not have had time to develop. A blow to the head, for example, may produce only a minor scalp wound but may cause serious intracranial bleeding due to torn blood vessels. In the chest, in addition to causing a compression injury of the chest wall with contusions and multiple broken ribs, a decelerating force may shear off the movable aortic arch from the more fixed thoracic aorta. This type of chest injury can also injure the heart by squeezing it

Table 18-1   Recognizing Developing Problems in Trauma Patients

Airway Obstruction	Significant bleeding into the mouth, back of the throat, or nose
	Swelling or bleeding following blunt or penetrating trauma to the face
	Swelling about the neck (may compress the airway) following blunt or penetrating trauma to the neck
	Inability to swallow, resulting in possible choking on secretions
Breathing Problems	Significant chest pain following blunt trauma
	Any penetrating trauma to the chest, unless it is a superficial cut (remember to check the back, too.)
	Object hit by torso is bent or crushed, indicating blunt trauma to the chest
Hidden Blood Loss	Bruising or obvious trauma to the upper abdomen
	Significant mechanism of injury, including blunt and penetrating trauma
	Obvious bruising in the area of the pelvis
	Tenderness on gentle palpation of the pelvis
Damage to Major Vessels	Blunt or penetrating trauma to the neck, chest, or groin area (which could tear the major vessels in these areas)
	Object hit by torso is bent or crushed, indicating blunt trauma to the chest
Damage to the Heart	Object hit by torso is bent or crushed, indicating blunt trauma to the chest
Brain Injury	History of losing consciousness, inability to recall what happened, dazed appearance, confusion, disorientation, combativeness after the traumatic incident
	Slurred speech
	Difficulty moving the extremities
	Severe headache, especially if accompanied by nausea and vomiting
	Obvious blunt or penetrating trauma to the head, other than superficial cuts
	Appearance of intoxication, as signs and symptoms (especially head trauma) may be masked by the effects of alcohol
Possible Spinal Injury	Severe neck or back pain
	History of difficulty moving or feeling the extremities

between the sternum and the spine. Such a cardiac contusion can cause the pumping function of the heart to fail or can tear the heart muscle and cause bleeding into the sac around the heart (pericardial tamponade, see Chapter 11).

In the abdomen and pelvis, compression trauma can fracture the pelvic bones, and the sharp ends of the bones can lacerate the bladder and pelvic blood vessels (▶ Figure 18-10). Decelerating and shearing forces can also rupture abdominal organs—particularly the pancreas, spleen, liver, and kidneys—producing serious intra-abdominal bleeding.

Injuries tend to occur in predictable types and combinations. Those caused by automobile crashes tend to group according to the vehicle's velocity, the seat the injured person was occupying, whether the seat belt was fastened, whether the air bag(s) (if any) deployed, whether the impact was direct or rotational, and whether it came from the front, rear, or side. In motor vehicle (especially automobile) collisions, the location and amount of damage to the vehicle give an indication of the amount of kinetic energy involved and provide clues about where the occupant(s) struck the vehicle's interior and the extent of the impact(s). A broken windshield, especially with a "star" pattern, suggests that one or more occupants struck the windshield with the head, raising the possibilities of head and neck injuries. A broken steering wheel or bent steering column indicates the possibility of a fractured sternum, crushed chest, flail chest, or injuries to the heart and lungs. A bent dashboard may indicate a deceleration injury to a lower extremity, as well as head and neck injuries. A vehicle hit from the side indicates the possibility of head, upper extremity, lateral chest, abdominal, pelvic, hip, femur, and other injuries.

Most nonvehicular outdoor injuries are related to the type of terrain and the mode of transportation. Because skiing, snowboarding, and snowmobiling involve increasing velocity, they are more dangerous than walking and snowshoeing. The person has less time to make decisions, and high-speed collisions and falls can result. Skiing- and snowboard-related accidents are discussed in detail in Chapter 14.

Hikers who slip or fall are subject to decelerating forces that can cause compression and penetration trauma, producing lacerations, abrasions, contusions, sprains, and fractures. Less frequently, falling trees and limbs cause injuries. Mountain hiking and technical mountaineering introduce the possibility of rock-fall and falls from heights with serious multiple injuries. As a rule of thumb, a fall from three times or more a person's height will cause critical injury, depending to some extent on the softness of the landing surface and whether the person strikes intervening objects (such as ledges) on the way down. Avalanches present a danger for a multitude of traumatic injuries as well as asphyxiation.

Water sports introduce a different type of terrain and mode of transportation. The kinetic energy of rapidly moving water *must be experienced to be appreciated*; it can pin a person in a canoe or kayak against rocks, fallen

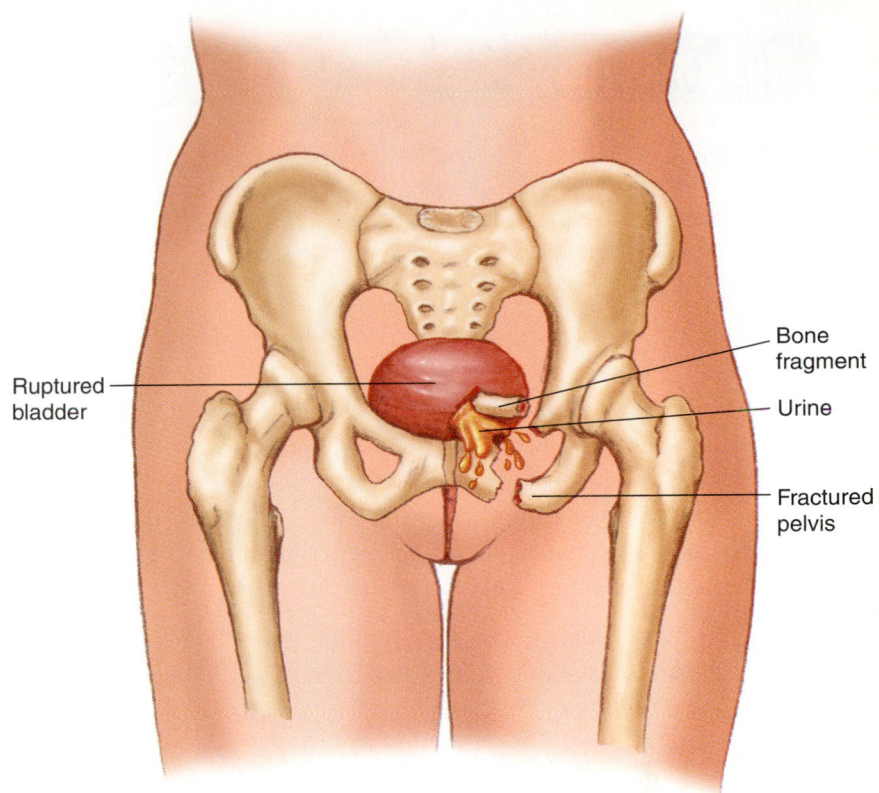

Figure 18-10   Fractured pelvic bones can lacerate the bladder and pelvic blood vessels.

Ruptured bladder

Bone fragment

Urine

Fractured pelvis

trees, and other obstacles. Compression and penetration trauma can be caused by collisions with sharp prows of watercraft or with rocks and other stationary objects. Underwater obstacles that entrap extremities can cause fractures due to bending trauma (as well as pin the victim underwater and cause drowning). Compression and bending trauma focused on the head and neck can result from diving into water that is too shallow.

In determining the MOI, it is important to ask yourself the following questions:

1. How much kinetic energy was involved? Consider the estimated speed of travel, the distance of the fall, or the speed of the striking object. Were the forces produced strong enough to cause fractures and serious internal injuries, or were they weak enough so that you anticipate finding less serious injuries?

2. What are the characteristics of the ground or any other surface involved? Is the surface smooth or rough, hard or soft, compressible or rigid?

3. What forces and body parts were involved? Were the forces accelerating or decelerating? What was the patient's body position upon impact?

Wilderness Tips

In the wilderness, or in any setting where prolonged transport to care is an issue, you need to be concerned with not only what you can see to be an obvious problem, but with what could reasonably develop, given the signs, symptoms, and environment.

4. On the basis of the previously mentioned factors, your assessment of the patient, and your knowledge of the patterns of injury, what types of trauma were or could have been involved (penetration, compression, bending [hyperflexion or hyperextension], rotational, or distraction)?

5. On the basis of the type(s) of trauma, what *visible* injuries would you expect to see? Do you see them?

6. On the basis of the type(s) of trauma and your knowledge of surface anatomy and the location of underlying organs, what types of *internal* injuries might have occurred? Is there any pain, tenderness, swelling, ecchymosis, or other signs or symptoms that suggest the presence of these injuries?

7. Are there any signs of internal bleeding, such as shock developing in the absence of obvious external bleeding in a patient with compression trauma to the torso? If not, could it be too soon for signs and symptoms to have developed?

8. On the basis of your analysis of the MOI, is there any likelihood of a spine injury?

Remember that determining and considering the MOI is part of the scene size-up that you register as you arrive at the scene. It is also part of the patient assessment—your first impression and the detailed physical exam—as you search for less obvious, additional injuries. A patient, when first seen, may be free of symptoms and have a normal or unremarkable assessment despite having experienced a serious injury that is potentially fatal or permanently disabling. Therefore, by acquiring experience and a feel for the types of injuries likely to have been produced based on the mechanism of injury, you will increase your chances of discovering *all* of the patient's injuries, even those that are not immediately obvious.

Early recognition of internal bleeding may depend on your alertness and careful patient monitoring based on an understanding of the MOI and its significance. When the MOI suggests a possible spinal cord injury, you should immobilize the patient on a backboard, even if pain is minimal and paralysis or loss of sensation is absent. Neck fractures and internal injuries of the head, chest, abdomen, or pelvis are notorious for initially appearing to be minor.

You can identify significant MOIs based on a combination of the estimated kinetic energy produced, the amount of protection present, and the human body area involved (▶ **Table 18-2**). Any significant mechanism of injury should raise the rescuer's index of suspicion regarding the possible resulting injuries. In general, you should care for all patients with significant MOIs as though they have spinal cord injuries and internal injuries involving the head, chest, abdomen, or pelvis. Make arrangements for rapid transport to medical care as soon as possible.

Table 18-2 Significant Mechanisms of Injury

Anticipate **multiple** or **serious injuries** if the patient:

1. fell from a height of two and a half to three times his or her own height (or less if horizontal motion was involved, eg, with a moving chairlift).

2. was involved in a moderate- to high-speed vehicle collision.
   a. automobile, motorcycle, bicycle, snowmobile, or all-terrain vehicle.
   b. vehicle collision in which another occupant of the vehicle was killed.
   c. automobile crash while unrestrained (no seat belt or air bag); in the case of a young child, no child seat).
   d. ejected from a vehicle or in a vehicle that rolled over during a crash.
   e. passenger in a car whose front end or front axle was displaced rearward 20" or more by a crash.
   f. motorcycle, bicycle, snowmobile, or all-terrain vehicle crash, especially when no helmet was worn.

3. as a pedestrian or bicyclist, was hit by an automobile going 25 mph (40 km/h) or faster.

4. while skiing or snowboarding, collided at high speed with another skier or snowboarder or an immobile object such as a tree or lift tower.

5. has a gunshot wound or other penetrating injury of the head, neck, chest, abdomen, or pelvis.

6. is in shock or respiratory distress and there is no external explanation for it (such as external bleeding). This is especially true of compression trauma to the chest, abdomen, or pelvis.

7. is unresponsive due to a head injury.

8. was buried in an avalanche or involved in a cave-in or explosion.

9. was struck by a rock, tree, or other falling object.

10. received significant electrical shock (see Chapter 15).

Chapter *Sweep*

Ready for Review

Obtaining information about the mechanism of injury (MOI)—that is, how the injuries occurred and what forces were likely involved—can be just as important as obtaining vital signs in assessing the patient. This information can help the OEC technician as well as the EMS and hospital staff to focus their attention on damage that may not be immediately obvious.

The specific injury depends on the magnitude and direction of the force or forces, the type of trauma, and the human body part involved. On the basis of these parameters, you can identify serious mechanisms of injury (MOI). Take the necessary steps to treat these as serious trauma injuries.

Vital Vocabulary

acceleration The process of increasing speed; the rate of change of velocity with respect to time.

bending trauma An impact that tends to momentarily reverse the normal forward curve of the spine.

body In physics, any mass of matter that is distinct from other masses of matter.

compression (blunt) trauma Trauma caused by an impact between a body part and a blunt object; impact may cause injury without penetrating soft tissues or internal organs and cavities.

crushing injury An injury caused by compression that involves both direct tissue injury and injury caused by circulation disturbance resulting from pressure on blood vessels.

deceleration The process of decreasing speed; eg, when a skier's body abruptly loses speed upon colliding with a tree.

direction Route, course, path.

distraction trauma Trauma caused by stretching.

energy The capacity for doing work.

force Any action that changes the state of rest or motion of a body to which that force is applied.

fulcrum point The hinge-like point about which a lever turns.

hyperextension Extreme or abnormal extension.

hyperflexion Extreme or abnormal flexion.

injury A specific damage or wound.

kinetic energy Energy associated with motion.

Law of Conservation of Energy In physics, the law that holds that energy can be neither created nor destroyed but may be changed from any form to any other form.

magnitude Great size, strength, or extent.

mechanism of injury (MOI) The mechanical forces coupled with the environmental conditions or obstacles involved in producing an injury.

motion The action or process of change of position.

Newton's First Law of Motion A body at rest will tend to remain at rest and a body in motion will tend to remain in motion unless acted upon by an outside force.

penetration trauma Trauma caused by a sharp object moving at a moderate to high speed that penetrates the skin, or by a moving body striking a narrow, pointed object.

potential energy The position of a body in a gravity field with respect to its own parts or another body.

rotational trauma Trauma caused by a twisting force.

terminal velocity A final speed of fall reached when the air resistance equals the pull of gravity.

trauma The effect of a force applied to the body; often used interchangeably with injury; a physical or psychological wound or injury.

velocity Speed. The magnitude of velocity is the body's speed, and the direction of velocity is the body's direction of motion.

www.OECzone.com

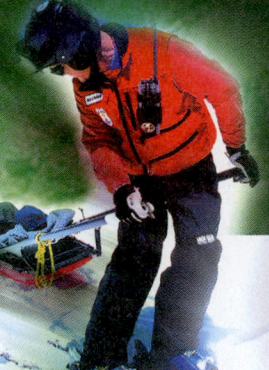

Assessment in Action

A skier was going down the slope at a good rate of speed when he fell and slammed into a tree. He rebounded off of the tree and slid a little way down the hill. He is lying on his back, complaining of pain in the hip area. His skis are off, and he is conscious and alert.

The patient deteriorates over time despite careful handling, due to internal bleeding. Pulse when found is 92 beats/min and respirations are 18 breaths/min. Both rapidly progress to a pulse of 140 beats/min and respirations of 26 breaths/min. Pain in the area of the pelvic injury is significant, and you know that mishandling would accelerate the deterioration of the general condition of the patient.

1. Given the fact that this was a collision, which of the following would be of greatest importance in determining the severity of injury?
   A. The speed of the skier
   B. The skier hitting a fixed object
   C. The distance of the slide
   D. Whether or not the surface was smooth

2. Given the mechanism of injury, the skier is at greatest risk for which of the following injuries?
   A. Sternal bruising
   B. Hollow organ rupture
   C. Head and spine injury
   D. Fractured pelvis

3. Which is the key decision to be made on the slope?
   A. When to take the blood pressure
   B. Recognizing the load-and-go situation
   C. Correctly identifying the patient's condition
   D. Requesting needed equipment

4. What skills need to be completed before transport?
   A. Spinal stabilization
   B. Oxygen administration
   C. Universal precautions
   D. All of the above

Challenging Question

5. Your adult patient jumped approximately 20' from a tree, landing feet first then falling forward on his hands. Which bones/joints may be injured?

6. A car heading up the narrow road to a ski resort goes off the road and rolls over. You arrive to find both occupants still in the upside-down car, seat-belted in. How does a basic understanding of physics as it relates to "kinetic energy" contribute to improving the care you provide to trauma patients?

7. Your 24-year-old patient received a puncture wound in the right side of his back as he careened down a rock face. He is complaining of difficulty breathing. At the hospital, the physician tells you this patient sustained a collapsed lung. How did that happen?

Points to Ponder

While watching a GS race, you observe a racer miss the gate at a tremendous rate of speed. He spins and swirls in a cloud of snow, striking his head on the left side two times. You ski over to him and find that he has collided with a horizontal, rigid metal pipe and is doubled over on it. One ski released and the other is still on. This injury will be severe. Both legs are broken. What kind of trauma should you suspect? Seeing the patient doubled over a pipe tells you he may have suffered what kind of injury? The pipe that the skier struck has caused what kind of trauma to the pelvic area?

Issues: Dealing with the Press, Others Watching and Critiquing Your Care, BSI Precautions, Responsibility to Patient and Area, Patient's Privacy

Online Outlook

Injuries in the outdoors are not random examples of the work of capricious Fate, nor are they the deliberate actions of malevolent gods. The nature of injuries is governed by specific anatomic and physiologic characteristics of the human body and by basic laws of physics. To learn more about the mechanisms and patterns of injury, complete Exercise 18 at www.OECzone.com.

www.OECzone.com

Soft-Tissue Injuries

Objectives

Cognitive

1. State the major functions of the skin (p 501).
2. List the layers of the skin (p 500).
♣ 3. Establish the relationship between body substance isolation (BSI) and soft-tissue injuries (p 506).
♣ 4. List the types of closed soft-tissue injuries (p 502).
♣ 5. Describe the emergency medical care of the patient with a closed soft-tissue injury (p 503).
♣ 6. State the types of open soft-tissue injuries (p 503).
♣ 7. Describe the emergency medical care of the patient with an open soft-tissue injury (p 506).
♣ 8. Discuss the emergency medical care considerations for a patient with a penetrating chest injury (p 507).
♣ 9. State the emergency medical care considerations for a patient with an open wound to the abdomen (p 508).
10. Differentiate the care of an open wound to the chest from an open wound to the abdomen (p 507).
♣ 11. List the classification of burns (p 511).
♣ 12. Define superficial burn (p 512).
♣ 13. List the characteristics of a superficial burn (p 512).
♣ 14. Define partial-thickness burn (p 512).
♣ 15. List the characteristics of a partial-thickness burn (p 512).
♣ 16. Define full-thickness burn (p 512).
♣ 17. List the characteristics of a full-thickness burn (p 512).
♣ 18. Describe the emergency medical care of the patient with a superficial burn (p 513).
♣ 19. Describe the emergency medical care of the patient with a partial-thickness burn (p 513).
♣ 20. Describe the emergency medical care of the patient with a full-thickness burn (p 513).
♣ 21. List the functions of dressing and bandaging (p 518).
22. Describe the purpose of a bandage (p 519).
♣ 23. Describe the steps in applying a pressure bandage (p 506).
♣ 24. Establish the relationship between airway management and the patient with chest injury, burns, and blunt and penetrating injuries (p 506).
25. Describe the effects of improperly applied dressings, splints, and tourniquets (p 519).
♣ 26. Describe the emergency medical care of a patient with an impaled object (p 509).
27. Describe the emergency medical care of a patient with an amputation (p 510).
♣ 28. Describe the emergency care for a chemical burn (p 516).
♣ 29. Describe the emergency care for an electrical burn (p 518).

♣ These are core concepts in initial patrol training.

Affective

None

Psychomotor

♣ 30. Demonstrate the steps in the emergency medical care of closed soft-tissue injuries (p 503).
♣ 31. Demonstrate the steps in the emergency medical care of open soft-tissue injuries (p 506).
♣ 32. Demonstrate the steps in the emergency medical care of a patient with an open chest wound (p 507).
♣ 33. Demonstrate the steps in the emergency medical care of a patient with open abdominal wounds (p 508).
♣ 34. Demonstrate the steps in the emergency medical care of a patient with an impaled object (p 509).
35. Demonstrate the steps in the emergency medical care of a patient with an amputation (p 510).
36. Demonstrate the steps in the emergency medical care of an amputated part (p 510).
♣ 37. Demonstrate the steps in the emergency medical care of a patient with superficial burns (p 513).
♣ 38. Demonstrate the steps in the emergency medical care of a patient with partial-thickness burns (p 513).
♣ 39. Demonstrate the steps in the emergency medical care of a patient with full-thickness burns (p 513).
40. Demonstrate the steps in the emergency medical care of a patient with a chemical burn (p 516).
41. Demonstrate completing an incident report for patients with soft-tissue injuries (p 77-78).

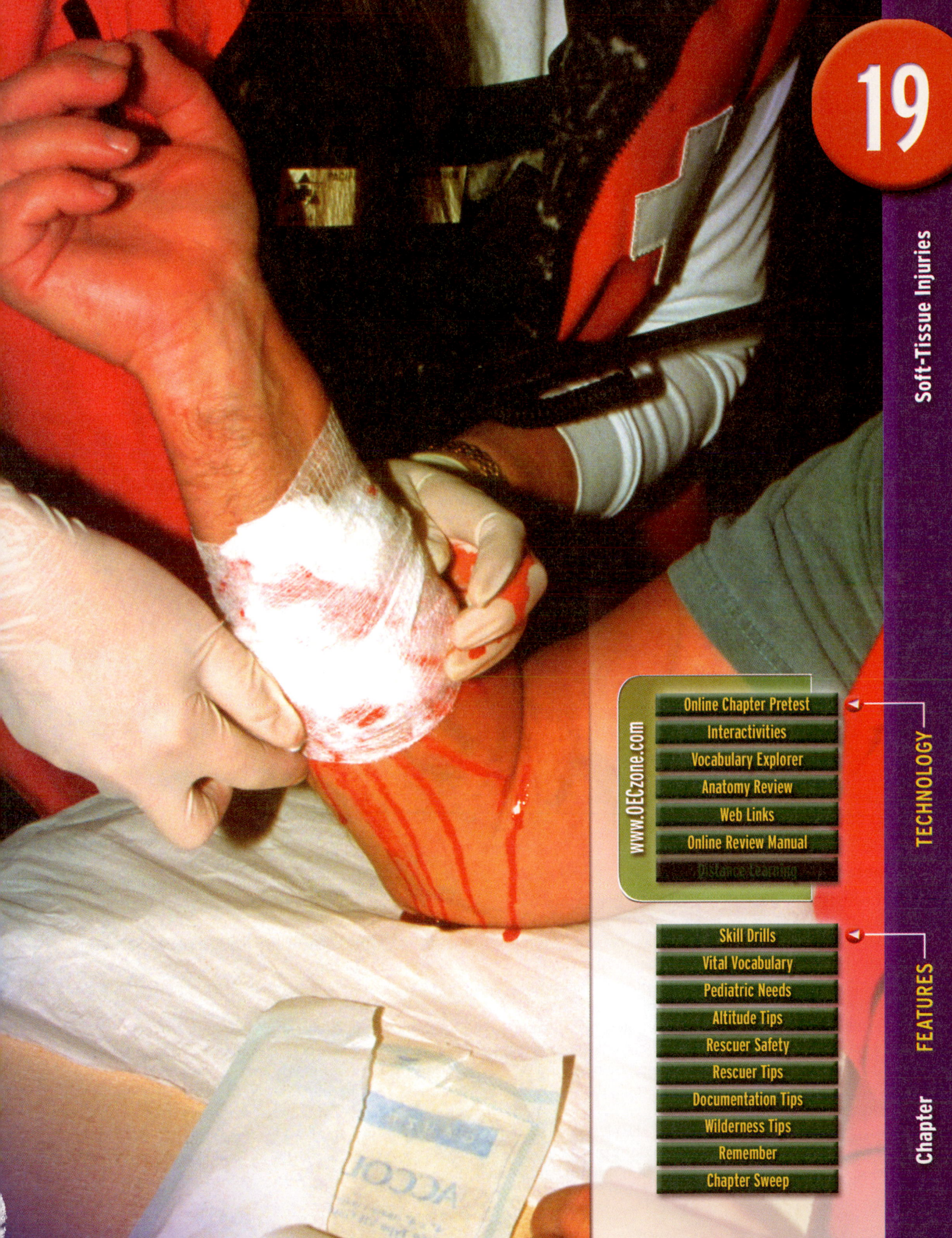

19

Soft-Tissue Injuries

TECHNOLOGY

Online Chapter Pretest
Interactivities
Vocabulary Explorer
Anatomy Review
Web Links
Online Review Manual
Distance Learning

FEATURES

Skill Drills
Vital Vocabulary
Pediatric Needs
Altitude Tips
Rescuer Safety
Rescuer Tips
Documentation Tips
Wilderness Tips
Remember
Chapter Sweep

Chapter

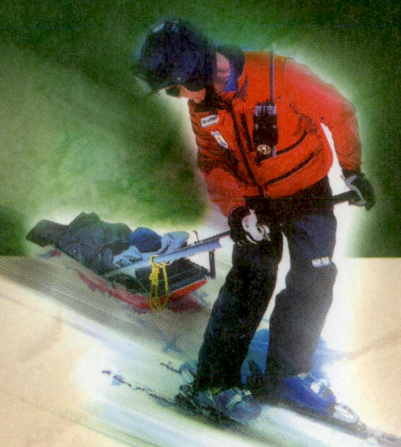

On a warm and sunny April day, a skier in shorts, a halter top, and a visor falls on a steep, icy slope coming to rest against an exposed rock. Her extremities are red and bloody, and she has an enlarged left thigh.

Such falls produce significant soft-tissue injuries. This chapter will help prepare you to properly care for these injuries as well as help you answer the following questions:

1. What is the difference between a dressing and a bandage?

2. Is there a difference in the care for chemical burns and electrical burns? Please describe it.

Soft-Tissue Injuries

Injuries to skin, subcutaneous tissue, and muscle are termed soft-tissue injuries. They range from simple bruises and abrasions to serious lacerations and amputations. Exposure and injury to blood vessels, nerves, and bone may be associated, as well as entry into body cavities with major organ injury. In all instances, you must control bleeding, prevent further contamination, and protect wounds and tissue from further damage. Therefore, you must be able to apply appropriate dressings and bandages to all parts of the body.

The Anatomy and Function of the Skin

The skin is the largest organ in the body, and is the first line of defense against external forces. The skin varies in thickness depending on age and location; it is thinner in children and older people than in young adults, thicker on the scalp, back and soles of the feet, and thinner on the eyelids, lips, and ears. Thin skin is more easily damaged than thick skin.

Anatomy of the Skin

The skin has two principal layers: the **epidermis** and the **dermis** (▶ Figure 19-1). The epidermis is the tough, external layer that forms a watertight covering for the body. The epidermis is itself composed of several layers. The cells on the surface layer of the epidermis are constantly worn away. They are replaced by cells that are pushed to the surface when new cells form in the germinal layer at the base of the epidermis. Deeper cells in the germinal layer contain pigment granules. Along with blood vessels in the dermis, these granules produce skin color.

The dermis is the inner layer of the skin. It lies below the germinal cells of the epidermis. The dermis contains the structures that affect skin function and

> ### Remember
>
> The skin plays several crucial protective and regulatory roles. Remember the importance of this organ in protecting against infection and maintaining internal temperature and fluid balance. These functions are critical in the outdoor setting.

appearance: hair follicles, sweat glands, and sebaceous glands. The sweat glands act to cool the body. They discharge sweat onto the surface of the skin through small pores, or ducts, that pass through the epidermis. Sebaceous glands produce sebum, the oily material that waterproofs the skin and keeps it supple. Sebum travels to the skin's surface along the shaft of adjacent hair follicles. Hair follicles are small organs that produce hair. There is one follicle for each hair, each connected with a sebaceous gland and a tiny muscle. This muscle pulls the hair erect whenever you are cold or frightened.

Blood vessels in the dermis provide the skin with nutrients and oxygen. Small branches reach up to the germinal cells, but no blood vessels penetrate farther into the epidermis. There are also specialized nerve endings within the dermis.

The skin covers all external surfaces of the body. The various openings in our body, including the mouth, nose, anus, and vagina, are not covered by skin. Instead, these openings are lined with **mucous membranes**. These membranes are similar to skin in that they, too, provide a protective barrier against bacterial invasion. But mucous membranes differ from skin in that they secrete a watery substance that lubricates the openings. Therefore, mucous membranes are moist, while skin is dry.

Functions of the Skin

The skin serves many functions. It protects the body by keeping bacteria out and water in. The nerves in the skin report to the brain on the environment and on many sensations such as temperature, touch, and pain.

The skin is also the body's major organ for regulating temperature. In a cold environment, the blood vessels in the skin constrict, diverting blood away from the skin and decreasing the amount of heat that is radiated from the body's surface. In hot environments, the vessels in the skin dilate. The skin becomes flushed or red, and heat radiates from the body's surface. Also, sweat glands secrete sweat. As the sweat evaporates from the skin's surface, your body temperature drops, and you begin to cool down.

Any break in the skin allows bacteria to enter and raises the possibilities of infection, fluid loss, and loss of temperature control. Any one of these problems can cause serious illness and even death.

Types of Soft-Tissue Injuries

Soft tissues are often injured because they are exposed to the environment. There are three types of soft-tissue injuries:

Wilderness Tips

Being sun safe every day can help keep your skin healthy. Practice positive health habits to reduce exposure to ultraviolet radiation and protect the skin and eyes from sunburn and permanent damage. Apply sunscreen before heading out and reapply often. You should use a sunscreen with a minimum rating of SPF 15.

- **Closed injuries**, in which soft-tissue damage occurs beneath the skin or mucous membrane but the surface remains intact.

- **Open injuries**, in which there is a break in the surface of the skin or the mucous membrane, exposing deeper tissue to potential contamination.

- **Burns**, in which the soft tissue receives more energy than it can absorb without injury. The source of this energy can be thermal heat, frictional heat, toxic chemicals, electricity, or nuclear radiation.

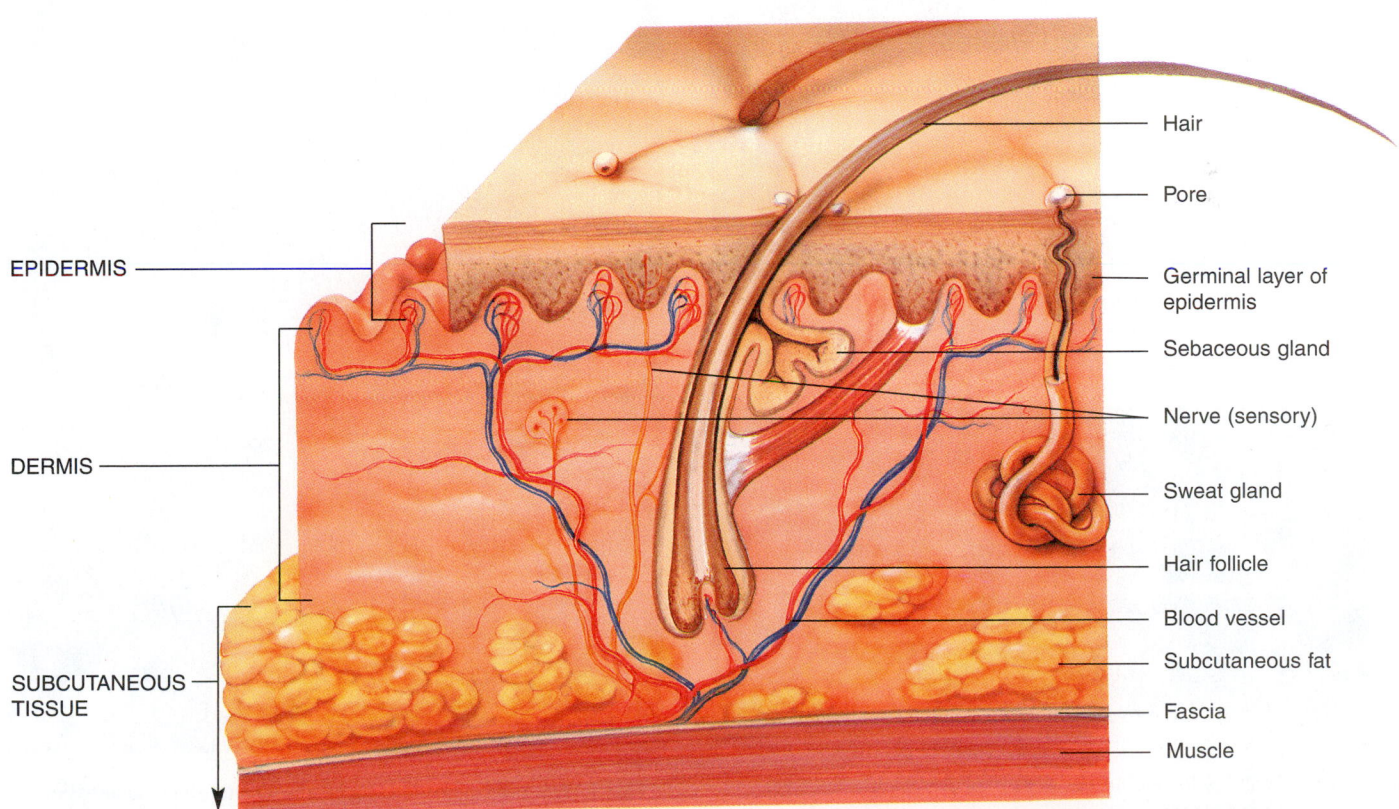

EPIDERMIS

DERMIS

SUBCUTANEOUS TISSUE

Hair

Pore

Germinal layer of epidermis

Sebaceous gland

Nerve (sensory)

Sweat gland

Hair follicle

Blood vessel

Subcutaneous fat

Fascia

Muscle

Figure 19-1 The skin is composed of a tough external layer called the epidermis and a vascular inner layer called the dermis.

Closed Injuries

Closed soft-tissue injuries are characterized by a history of blunt trauma, pain at the site of injury, swelling beneath the skin, and discoloration. Such injuries can vary from mild to quite severe.

A contusion, or bruise, results from blunt force striking the body. The epidermis remains intact, but cells within the dermis are damaged, and small blood vessels are usually torn. The depth of the injury varies, depending on the amount of energy absorbed. As fluid and blood leak into the damaged area, the patient may have swelling and pain. The buildup of blood produces a characteristic blue or black discoloration called ecchymosis (▼ Figure 19-2).

A hematoma is a pool of blood that has collected within damaged tissue or in a body cavity (▼ Figure 19-3). It occurs whenever a large blood vessel is damaged and bleeds rapidly. It is usually associated with extensive tissue damage. A hematoma can result from a soft-tissue injury, a fracture, or any injury to a large blood vessel. In severe cases, the hematoma may contain more than a liter of blood.

A crushing injury occurs when a great amount of force is applied to the body for a long period of time (▼ Figure 19-4). The extent of the damage depends on just how long that period is. In addition to causing some direct soft-tissue damage, continued compression of the soft tissues will cut off their circulation, producing further tissue destruction. For example, if a patient's legs are trapped under a collapsed pile of rocks, damage to the leg tissues will continue until the rocks are removed.

Another form of compression can result from the swelling that occurs whenever tissues are injured. The cells that are injured leak watery fluid into the spaces between the cells. If swelling is excessive or occurs in a confined space such as the skull, the tissue pressure will increase to dangerous levels. The pressure of the fluid may become great enough to compress the tissue and cause further damage. This is especially true if the blood vessels become compressed, cutting off blood flow to the tissue. This condition is called compartment syndrome. Excessive swelling often follows injury of the brain, the spinal cord, and the extremities.

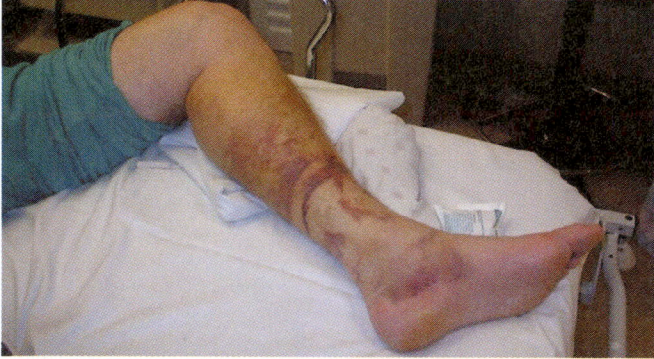

Figure 19-2 Contusions, more commonly known as bruises, occur as a result of a blunt force striking the body. The buildup of blood produces a characteristic blue or black discoloration (ecchymosis).

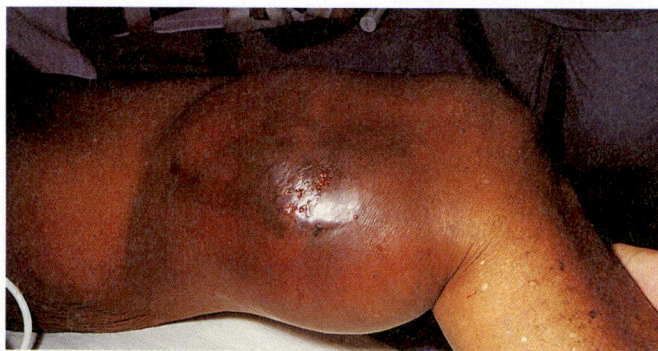

Figure 19-3 A hematoma develops whenever a large blood vessel is damaged and bleeds rapidly.

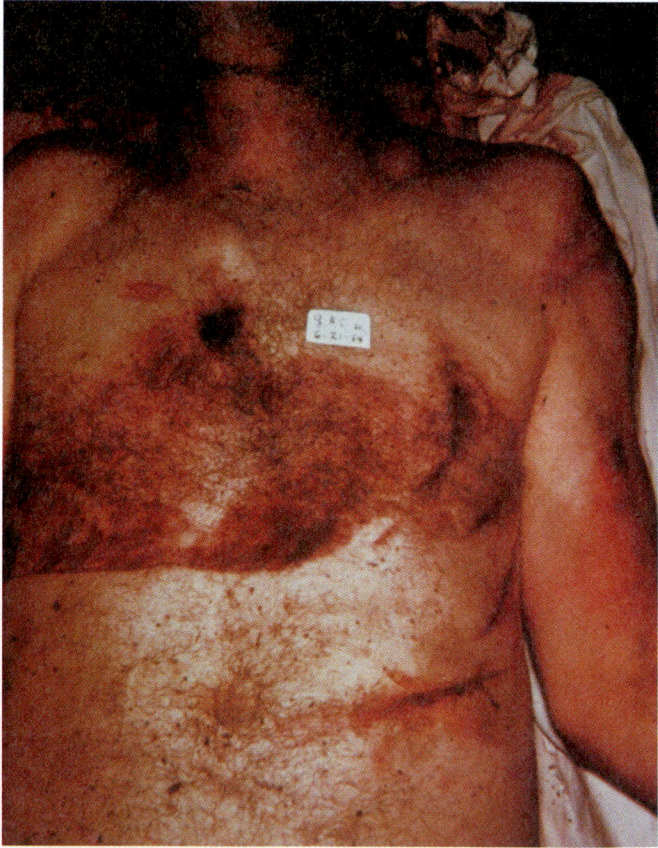

Figure 19-4 The damage associated with a crush or compression injury varies depending on the direct damage to the soft tissues and on how long the tissue was cut off from circulation.

Severe closed injuries can also damage internal organs. The greater the amount of energy absorbed from the blunt force, the greater is the risk of injury to deeper structures. Therefore, you must assess all patients with closed injuries for more serious hidden injuries. Remain alert for signs of shock or internal bleeding, and begin treatment of these conditions if necessary.

Emergency Medical Care

Small contusions require no special emergency medical care. More extensive closed injuries may involve significant swelling and bleeding beneath the skin, which could lead to hypovolemic shock. Before treating a closed injury, make sure to follow BSI precautions. Wear gloves as you work with the patient.

Soft-tissue injuries may look rather dramatic. However, you must still focus on airway and breathing first. Always provide oxygen and maintain the airway in patients who need it. If the patient has difficulty breathing, you may have to assist ventilations.

Treat a closed soft-tissue injury by applying the acronym RICES:

- **Rest** the patient and the injured part.
- **Ice** (or a cold pack) slows bleeding by causing blood vessels to constrict and also reduces pain.
- **Compression** over the injury site slows bleeding by compressing the blood vessels.
- **Elevation** of the injured part just above the level of the patient's heart decreases swelling.
- **Splinting** decreases bleeding and also reduces pain by immobilizing a soft-tissue injury or an injured extremity.

In addition to using these measures to control bleeding and swelling, you should also be alert for signs of developing shock, including increased heart rate, increased respiratory rate, cool or clammy skin, and decreased blood pressure. Any or all of these signs may indicate internal bleeding, resulting from injuries to internal organs. If the patient appears to be in shock, you should elevate his or her legs, give supplemental oxygen, and provide prompt transport to the hospital.

Open Injuries

Open injuries differ from closed injuries in that the protective layer of skin is damaged. This can produce more extensive bleeding. More important, however, a break in the protective skin layer or mucous membrane means that the wound is contaminated and may become infected. **Contamination** means that infective organisms or foreign bodies, such as dirt, gravel, or metal, are present. You must address these two problems in your treatment of open soft-tissue wounds. There are four types of open soft-tissue wounds that you must be prepared to manage: abrasions, lacerations, avulsions, and penetrating wounds.

An **abrasion** is a wound of the superficial layer of the skin, caused by friction when a body part rubs or scrapes across a rough or hard surface. An abrasion usually does not penetrate completely through the dermis, but blood may ooze from the injured capillaries in the dermis. Known by a variety of names, including road rash, road burn, strawberry, and mat burn, abrasions can be extremely painful ▼ Figure 19-5 .

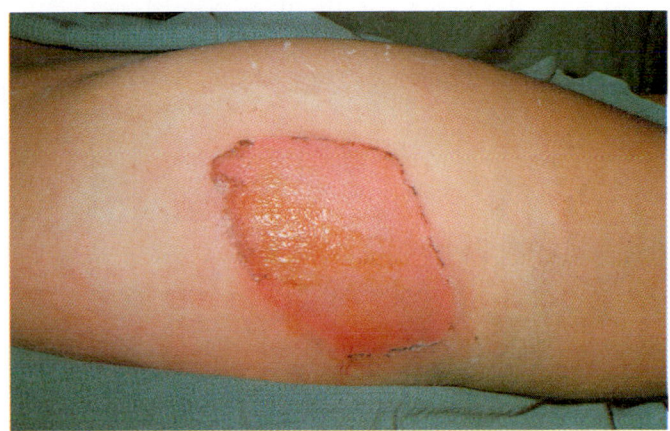

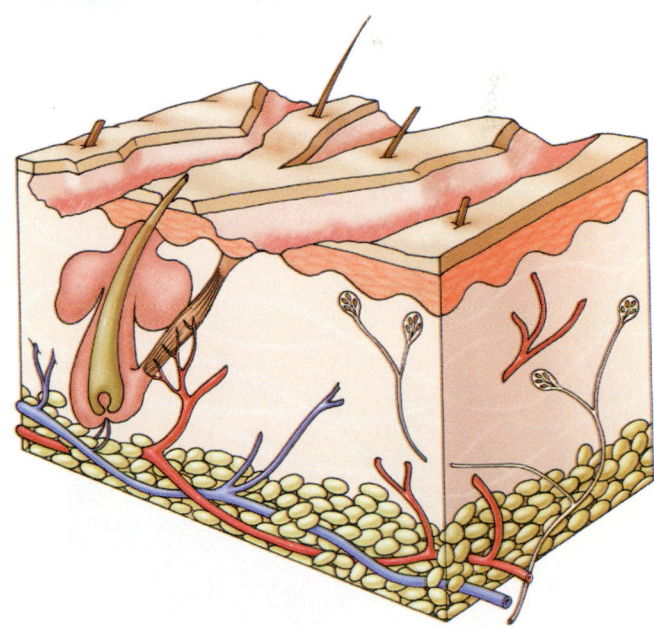

Figure 19-5 Abrasions usually do not penetrate completely through the dermis, but blood may ooze from the capillaries. These wounds are typically superficial and result from rubbing or scraping across a hard surface.

A <u>laceration</u> is a smooth or jagged cut caused by a sharp object or a blunt force that tears the tissue. The depth of the injury can vary, extending through the skin and subcutaneous tissue even into the underlying muscles and adjacent nerves and blood vessels ▼ Figure 19-6 . A laceration may appear linear (regular) or stellate (irregular) and may occur along with other types of soft-tissue injury. Lacerations that involve cut arteries may result in severe bleeding.

An <u>avulsion</u> is an injury that separates various layers of soft tissue (usually between the subcutaneous layer and fascia) so that they are either completely unattached (amputation) or hanging as a flap ▼ Figure 19-7 . Usually, there is significant bleeding. If the avulsed tissue is hanging from a small piece of skin, the circulation through the flap may be at risk. If you can, clean the

area by pouring clean water or saline over the avulsed flap to remove debris and replace the flap in its original position. If this causes increased bleeding, apply a sterile bandage. If an avulsion is complete, you should wrap the separated tissue in sterile gauze and bring it with you to the emergency department.

We usually think of amputations as involving the upper and lower extremities. But other body parts, such as the scalp, ear, nose, penis, or lips, may also be totally avulsed, or amputated. You can easily control the bleeding from some amputations, such as the fingers, with pressure dressings. But if an avulsion involves a large area of muscle mass, such as a thigh, there may be massive bleeding. In this situation, you need to treat the patient for hypovolemic shock. The use of pressure points may also be necessary to control bleeding not

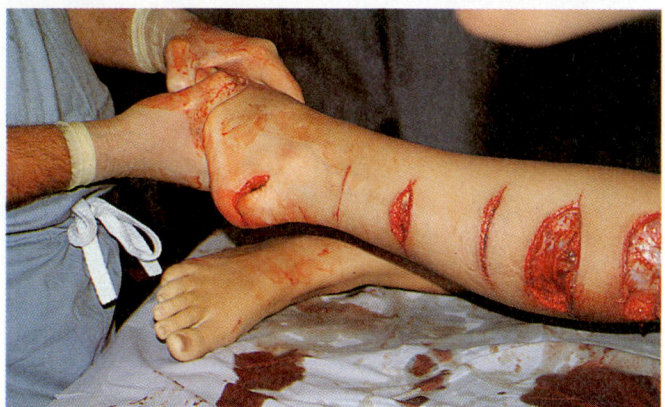

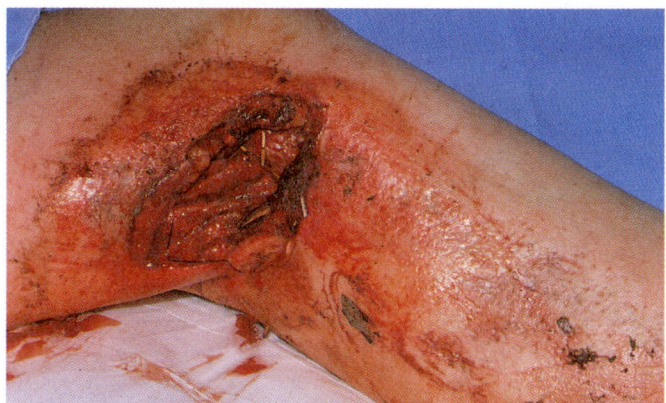

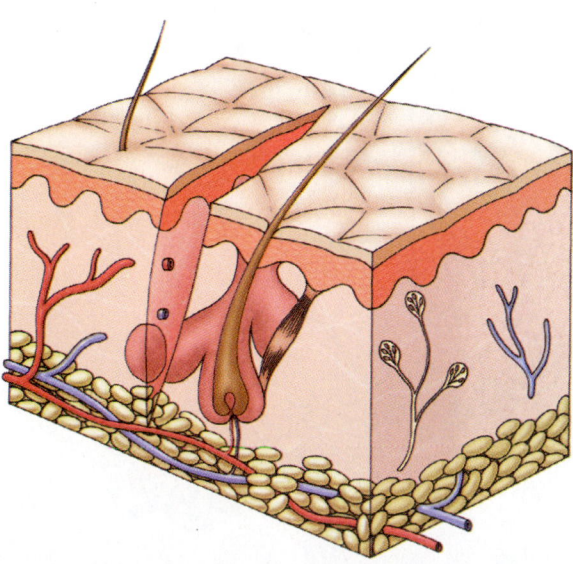

Figure 19-6 Lacerations vary in depth and can extend through the skin and subcutaneous tissue to the underlying muscles, nerves, and blood vessels. These wounds can be smooth or jagged as a result of a cut by a sharp object or a blunt force that tears the tissue.

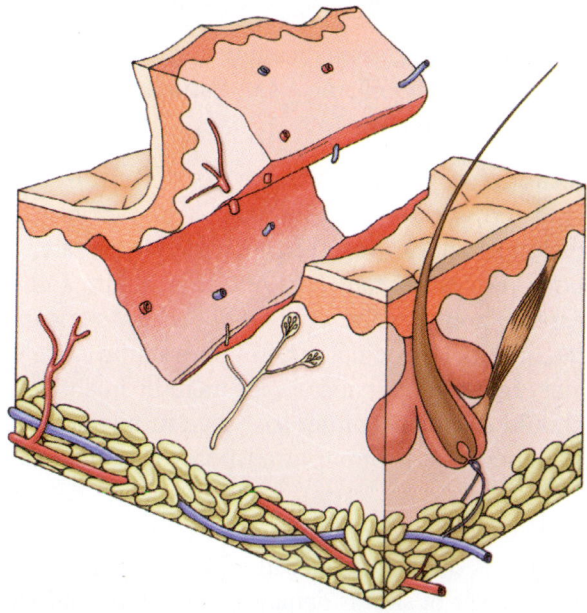

Figure 19-7 Avulsions are injuries characterized by either complete separation of tissue or tissue hanging as a flap. Significant bleeding is common.

controlled with a pressure dressing (see Skill Drill 8-1 in Chapter 8).

A <u>penetrating wound</u> is an injury resulting from a sharp, pointed object, such as a knife, ice pick, splinter, or bullet. Such objects leave relatively small entrance wounds, so there may be little external bleeding (▼ **Figure 19-8**). However, these objects can damage structures deep within the body. If the wound is in the chest or abdomen, the injury can cause rapid, fatal bleeding. Assessing the amount of damage a puncture wound has created is very difficult. Generally, rapid transport to the hospital is necessary.

Stabbings and shootings often result in multiple penetrating injuries. You must assess these patients carefully to identify all wounds. Since a penetrating object can pass completely through the body, always look for both entrance and exit wounds, especially with gunshot wounds. An entrance wound is usually smaller than an exit wound. A gun shot at close range will leave an entrance wound with powder burns around the edges (▼ **Figure 19-9**). Because of its larger size, an exit wound may bleed excessively.

Gunshot wounds have some unique characteristics that require special care. The amount of damage from a gunshot wound is directly related to the speed of the bullet. Thus, it is important to find out the type of gun that was used in the shooting. Sometimes, the patient or bystanders can tell you how many rounds were fired. This information can help hospital personnel to better care for the patient. Shotgun wounds create multiple paths of missiles (shot) and create a larger surface area and volume of tissue damage.

Most shootings end up in court at some point, and you may be called to testify. For this reason, you must carefully document the circumstances surrounding any gunshot injury, the patient's condition, and the treatment you give.

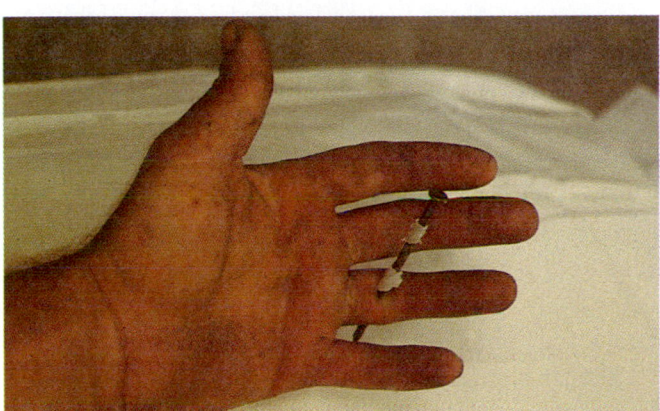

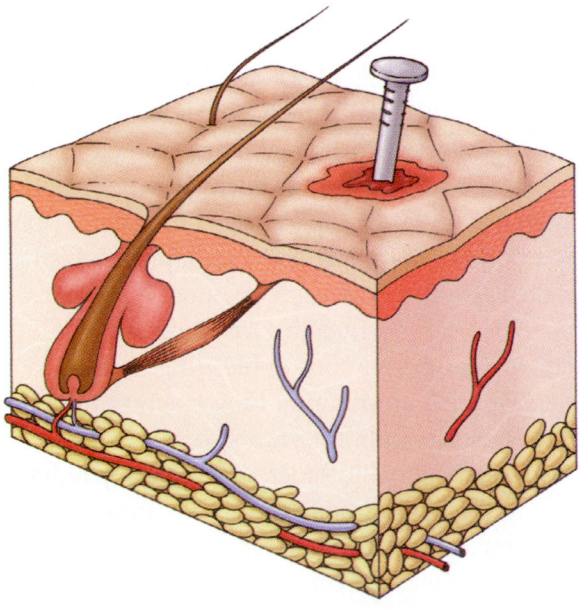

Figure 19-8 Penetrating wounds often cause very little external bleeding but can damage structures deep within the body.

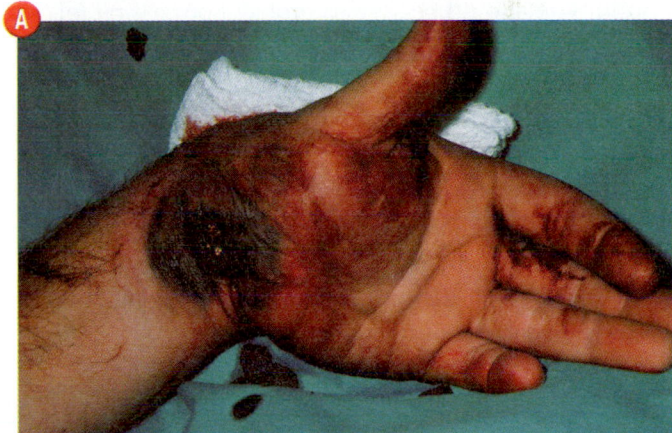

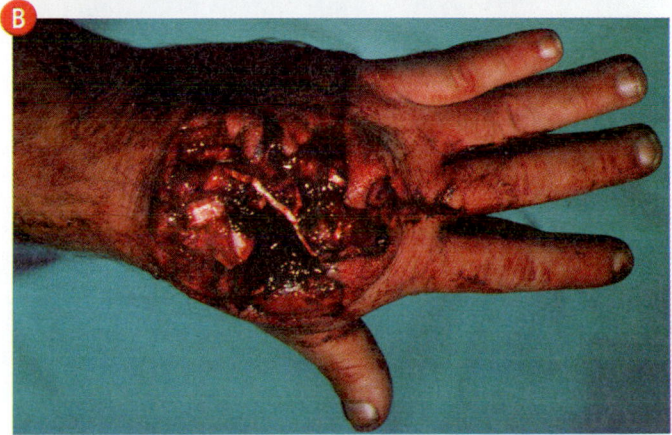

Figure 19-9 **A.** An entrance wound from a gunshot may have burns around the edges. **B.** An exit wound is larger and results in greater damage to soft tissues.

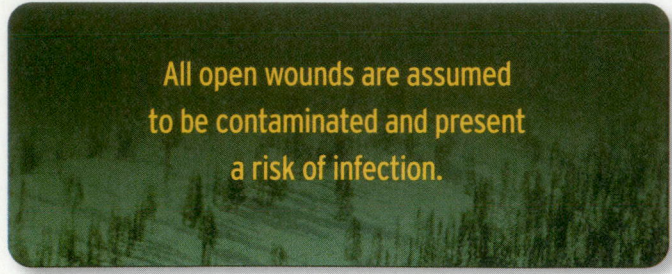

All open wounds are assumed to be contaminated and present a risk of infection.

As with closed wounds caused by crushing, open wounds caused by crushing may involve damaged internal organs or broken bones, as well as extensive soft-tissue damage (**▼ Figure 19-10**). While external bleeding may be minimal, internal bleeding may be severe, even life-threatening. The crushing force damages soft tissues, as well as vessels and nerves. This frequently results in a painful, swollen, deformed area.

Emergency Medical Care

Before you begin caring for a patient with an open wound, you should be sure to protect yourself by following BSI precautions. Wear gloves, eye protection, and, if necessary, a gown. Remember that you must be sure the patient has an open airway and administer oxygen if necessary before caring for the wound. Then assess the severity of the wound, removing any clothing that may be covering it.

Your treatment priority is ABC, including controlling the bleeding, which can be extensive and severe. Follow the steps in (**▶ Skill Drill 19-1**):

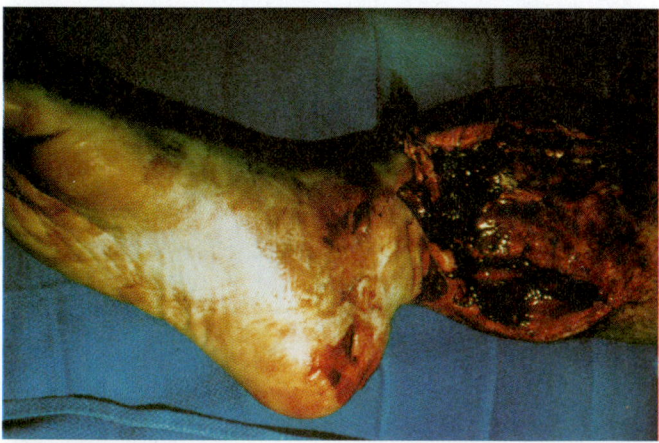

Figure 19-10 A crushing open wound is characterized by extensive tissue damage and deformity that is often accompanied by swelling and extreme pain.

1. **Apply a dry, sterile dressing** over the entire wound. Apply pressure to the dressing with your gloved hand **(Step 1)**.

2. **Maintain the pressure** and secure the dressing with a roller bandage **(Step 2)**.

3. **If bleeding continues or recurs, leave the original dressing in place.** Apply a second dressing on top of the first, and secure it with another roller bandage and apply pressure to the corresponding arterial pressure point **(Step 3)**.

4. **Splint the extremity** to stabilize the injury, even if there is no suspected fracture, to help minimize movement, further control the bleeding, and keep the dressing in place **(Step 4)**.

Assessment of the patient for further signs of injury follows the DCAP-BTLS method: inspect and palpate for Deformities, Contusions, Abrasions, Punctures/ Penetrations, Burns, Tenderness, Lacerations, Swelling, and Crepitation. It is important not to focus all of your attention on the obvious open wound and neglect a systematic evaluation of the entire patient in this manner. If you follow this systematic approach, you are unlikely to miss other significant injuries that the patient may have sustained.

All open wounds are assumed to be contaminated and present a risk of infection. If hospital treatment is available in 1 hour or less, do not clean an open wound. Rubbing, brushing, or washing an open wound will only cause additional bleeding. However, should there be a delay of 2 hours or more before hospital treatment can be provided, carefully remove loose foreign material and clean the wound with soap and water, antiseptic solution, or pressure washing, and apply a sterile dressing. To prevent the wound from drying, you may apply sterile dressings moistened with sterile saline solution, if possible, then cover the wound with a dry, sterile dressing.

Often, you can better control bleeding from open soft-tissue wounds by splinting the extremity, even if there is no fracture. Splinting can also help you to keep the patient calm and quiet, as it typically reduces pain. In addition, splinting keeps sterile dressings in place, minimizes damage to an already injured extremity, and makes moving the patient easier.

Keep in mind that a patient who is bleeding significantly from an open wound is at risk for hypovolemic shock. You must be alert for this possibility and provide treatment, as needed.

SkillDrill 19-1   Controlling Bleeding from a Soft-Tissue Injury

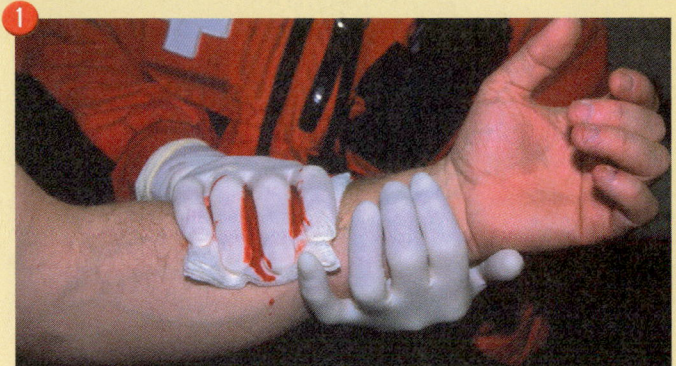

Apply direct pressure with a sterile bandage.

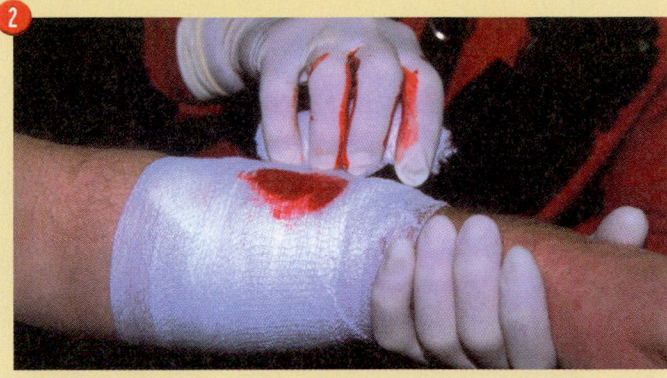

Maintain pressure with a roller bandage.

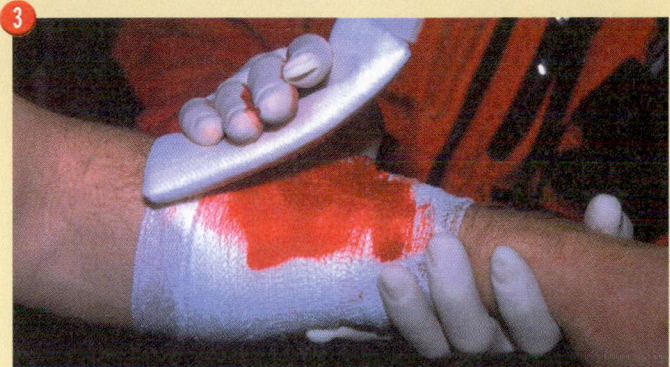

If bleeding continues, apply a second dressing and roller bandage over the first, and apply pressure to the corresponding arterial pressure point.

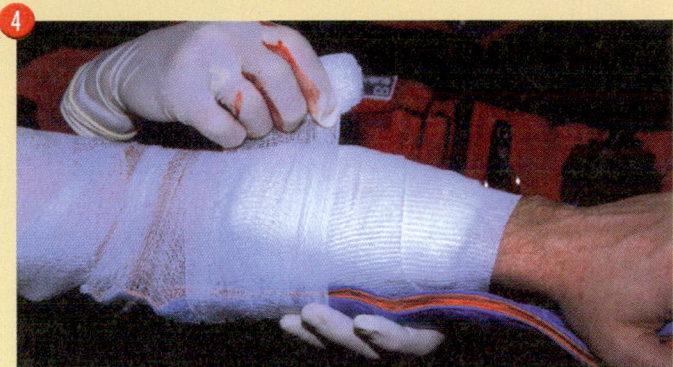

Splint the extremity.

Chest Wounds

A penetrating wound to the chest may cause air to enter the pleural space (**pneumothorax**) or blood to collect in the chest (**hemothorax**) (▶ **Figure 19-11**). Ordinarily, the pressure inside the chest cavity is slightly lower than the pressure of the atmosphere. Inhalation further reduces this pressure, so air will move through a wound just as easily as it moves through the nose and mouth during normal breathing. The air that enters through the wound remains in the pleural space, and the lung does not expand; when the patient exhales, air passes back through the wound. Such "sucking chest wounds" reduce the ability of the lungs to provide fresh oxygen to the blood.

Initial emergency care should include giving supplemental oxygen, sealing the wound, and transporting the patient promptly to the nearest hospital. Follow the steps in (▶ **Skill Drill 19-2**) for care of a sucking chest wound.

1. **Keep the patient supine and administer oxygen.** The buildup of blood in the chest can result in difficulty breathing and shock. The patient may be placed in a position of comfort if no spinal injury is suspected **(Step 1)**.

2. **Seal the wound** with an **occlusive dressing** large enough that it is not pulled or sucked into the chest cavity. An occlusive dressing prevents air from being sucked into the chest through the wound. Several sterile materials, including aluminum foil, Vaseline gauze, or a folded universal dressing, may be used for this purpose **(Step 2)**.

3. **Depending on your local protocol, you may seal the dressing on all four sides,** or you may seal only three sides to create a flutter valve, which is a one-way valve that allows air to leave the chest cavity but not return **(Step 3)**.

SkillDrill 19-2 Sealing a Sucking Chest Wound

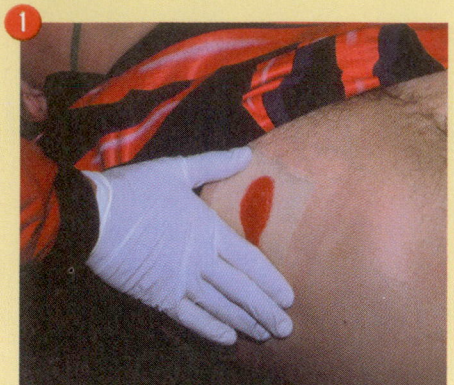

1 Keep the patient supine and give oxygen.

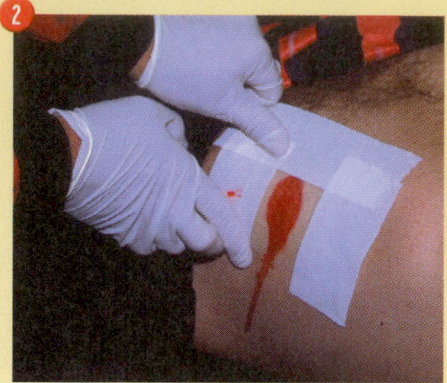

2 Seal the wound with an occlusive dressing.

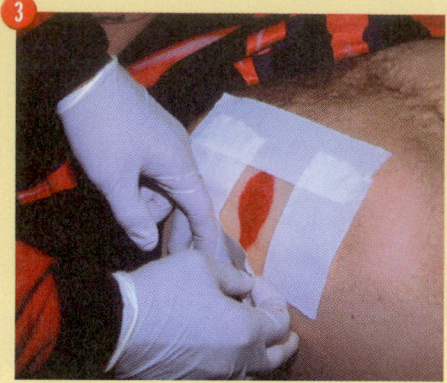

3 Follow local protocol regarding sealing or leaving open the dressing's fourth side.

Abdominal Wounds

An open wound in the abdominal cavity may expose internal organs. In some cases, the organs may even protrude through the wound, an injury called an **evisceration** (▼ Figure 19-12). Do not touch or move the exposed organs. Rather, cover the wound with sterile gauze compresses moistened with sterile saline solution and secured with a sterile dressing (▶ Figure 19-13). Because the open abdomen radiates body heat very effectively, and because exposed organs lose fluid rapidly, you must keep the organs moist and warm. If you do not have gauze compresses, you may use moist sterile dressings, covered and secured in place with a bandage and tape. Do not use any material that is adherent or loses its substance when wet, such as toilet paper, facial tissue, paper towels, or absorbent cotton. If the patient's legs and knees are uninjured, flex them to relieve pressure on the abdomen. Most patients with abdominal wounds require immediate transport to a trauma center, depending on the local protocol.

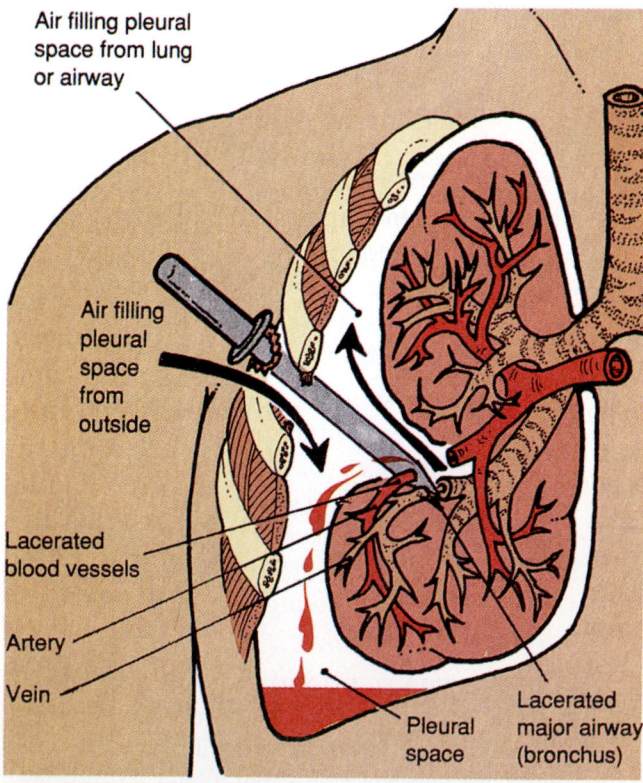

Air filling pleural space from lung or airway

Air filling pleural space from outside

Lacerated blood vessels

Artery

Vein

Pleural space

Lacerated major airway (bronchus)

Figure 19-11 Penetrating wounds can cause air to enter the chest or blood to collect in the chest.

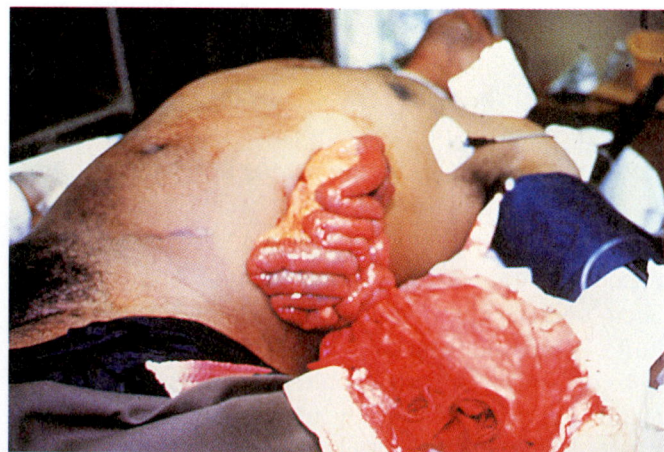

Figure 19-12 An abdominal evisceration is an open wound to the abdomen in which organs protrude through the wound.

SkillDrill 19-3   Stabilizing an Impaled Object

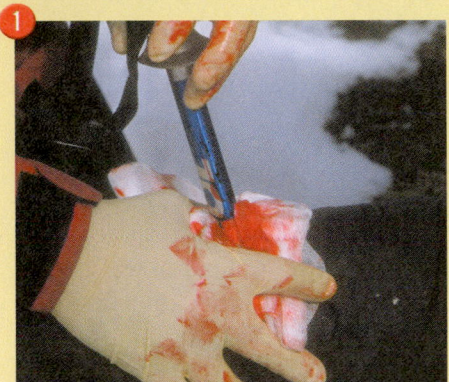

Do not attempt to move or remove the object.

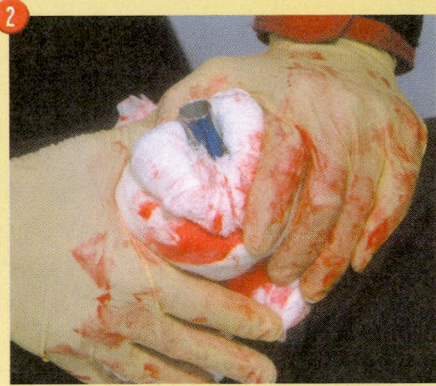

Control bleeding and stabilize the object in place using soft dressings, gauze, and/or tape.

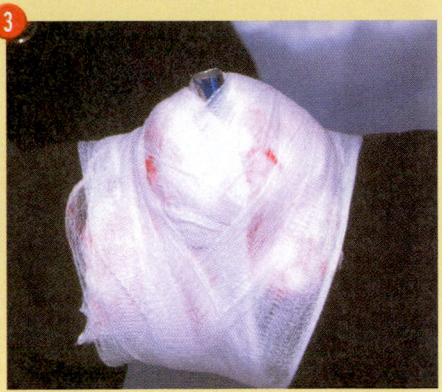

Add bulky dressings to stabilize and protect the impaled object during transport.

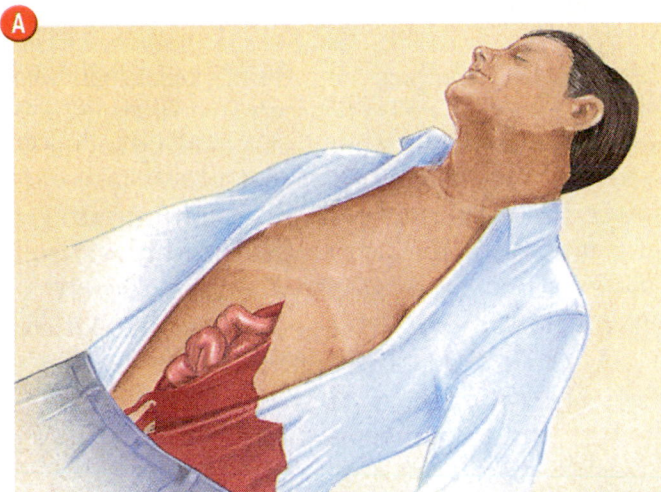

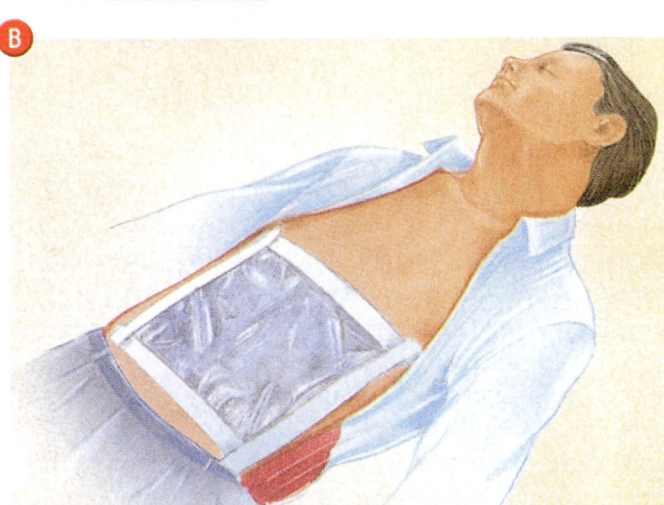

Figure 19-13   **A.** Cover exposed organs with sterile gauze compresses moistened with sterile saline solution. **B.** Place a dressing over the compresses, and secure it in place by taping all four sides.

In the rare case where evisceration has occurred in an extreme cold environment with transport and evacuation requiring longer than 1 hour, it is appropriate (using BSI) to place the exposed organs back into the abdominal cavity as best as possible. If available, applying warm moist saline gauze bandages over the wound is appropriate. Rapidly transport the patient.

Impaled Objects

Occasionally, a patient will have an object, such as a ski pole, knife, fishhook, wood splinter, or piece of glass, impaled in his or her body. To treat this, follow the steps in (▲ Skill Drill 19-3):

1. **Do not attempt to move or remove the object** unless it is impaled through the cheek and interferes with breathing. In most cases, a surgeon will have to remove the object; moving it in the field may damage nerves, blood vessels, or muscles within the wound **(Step 1)**.

2. **Remove any clothing covering the injury. Control bleeding, and apply a bulky dressing** to stabilize the object. Some combination of soft dressings, gauze, and tape may be effective, depending on the location and size of the object. To prevent further injury, manually secure the object by incorporating it into the dressing **(Step 2)**.

3. **Protect the impaled object** from being bumped or moved during transport by adding multiple dressings. If available, a rigid item such as a plastic cup or a section of a plastic water bottle can be taped over the stabilized object and its bandaging **(Step 3)**.

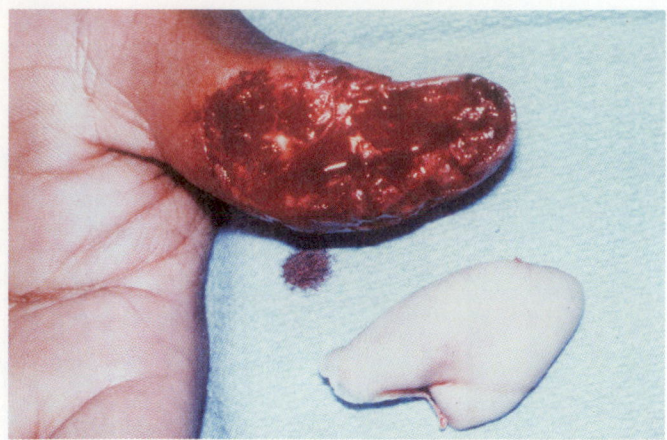

Figure 19-14 Amputated parts can often be reimplanted, so you should make every attempt to find the part and transport it to the emergency department along with the patient.

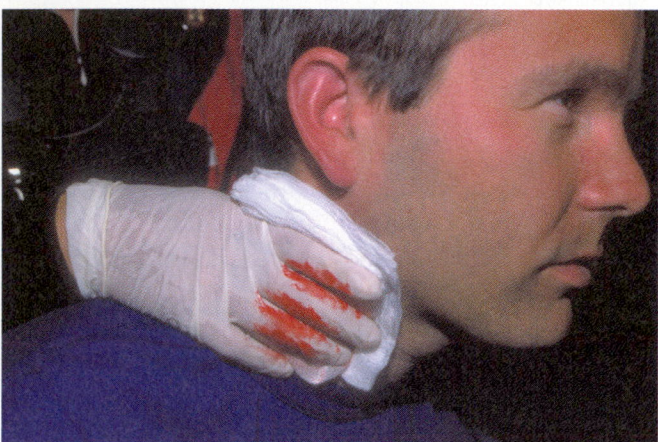

Figure 19-15 Open injuries to the neck can be very dangerous. If veins are open to the environment, they can suck in air, resulting in a potentially fatal condition called air embolism.

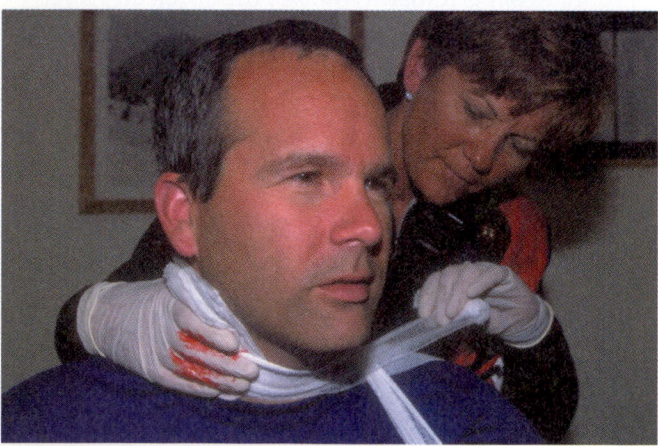

Figure 19-16 Cover neck wounds with an airtight dressing, and apply manual pressure. Be sure that you do not compress both carotid arteries at the same time, as this may impair circulation to the brain.

The only exception to the rule of not removing an impaled object is an object in the cheek that obstructs breathing. In this situation, restoring the airway takes priority. If the object is very long, cut off (shorten) the exposed portion, first securing it to minimize motion and thus internal damage and pain. Once the object is secured and the bleeding is under control, provide prompt transport.

Sometimes an impaled object prevents transport or moving a patient who is severely injured and in shock. For example, a heavy steel rod welded onto a large piece of equipment is impaled, with no immediate way to cut off the rod. Wasting valuable time waiting for a cutting torch is inappropriate. Remove the patient from the impaled object and transport.

Amputations

Surgeons today can often reimplant an amputated part (◀ **Figure 19-14**). However, correct prehospital care of the amputated part is vital to successful reattachment. With partial amputations, make sure to immobilize the part with bulky compression dressings and a splint to prevent further injury. Do not sever any partial amputations; this may make it impossible to reimplant the part.

With a complete amputation, make sure to wrap the part in a sterile dressing and place it in a plastic bag. Follow your local protocols regarding how to preserve amputated parts. In some areas, dry, sterile dressings are recommended for wrapping amputated parts; in other areas, dressings moistened with sterile saline are recommended. Put the bag in a cool container filled with $\frac{1}{4}$ ice and $\frac{3}{4}$ water. The goal is to keep the part cool without allowing it to freeze or develop frostbite. The amputated part should be transported with the patient.

Neck Injuries

An open neck injury can be life-threatening. If the veins of the neck are open to the environment, they may suck in air (◀ **Figure 19-15**). If enough air is sucked into a blood vessel, it can actually block the flow of blood in the lungs, sending the patient into cardiac arrest. This condition is called air embolism. To control bleeding and prevent the possibility of air embolism, cover the wound with an occlusive dressing. Apply manual pressure, but do not compress both carotid vessels at the same time; if you do, this may impair circulation to the brain (◀ **Figure 19-16**). Secure a pressure dressing over the wound by wrapping roller gauze loosely around the neck and then firmly through the opposite axilla.

Burns

As a rescuer, you will often provide care to patients who have been burned. Burns account for over 6,000 deaths a year. Burns are also among the most serious and painful of all injuries. A burn occurs when the body, or a body part, receives more energy than it can absorb without injury. Potential sources of this energy include heat, toxic chemicals, electricity, and UV radiation from the sun. The proper emergency care of a burn may increase a patient's chances of survival and decrease the risk or duration of a long-term disability. Although a burn may be the patient's most obvious injury, you should always perform a complete assessment to determine whether there are other serious injuries.

Burn Severity

The seriousness of a burn may influence medical control's choice of a treatment facility. Five factors will help you to determine the severity of a burn:

1. What is the depth of the burn?

2. What is the extent of the burn?

These first two factors are the most important. After gauging these, ask yourself the remaining questions:

3. Are any critical areas (face, upper airway, hands, feet, genitalia) involved?

4. Are there any preexisting medical conditions or other injuries?

5. Is the patient younger than age 5 years or older than age 55 years?

If the answer to any of these last three questions is yes, you should upgrade the burn's classification ► **Table 19-1**) .

Table 19-1 Classification of Burns in Adults

Critical Burns

- Full-thickness burns involving the hands, feet, face, upper airway, or genitalia

- Full-thickness burns covering more than 10% of the body's total surface area

- Partial-thickness burns covering more than 30% of the body's total surface area

- Burns associated with respiratory injury (smoke inhalation)

- Burns complicated by fractures

- Burns on patients younger than age 5 years or older than age 55 years that would be classified as "moderate" on young adults

Moderate Burns

- Full-thickness burns involving 2% to 10% of the body's total surface area (excluding hands, feet, face, genitalia, or upper airway)

- Partial-thickness burns covering 15% to 30% of the body's total surface area

- Superficial burns covering more than 50% of the body's total surface area

Minor Burns

- Full-thickness burns covering less than 2% of the body's total surface area

- Partial-thickness burns covering less than 15% of the body's total surface area

- Superficial burns covering less than 50% of the body's total surface area

DEPTH. Burns are first classified according to their depth (▼ Figure 19-17). You must be able to identify the following three types of burns:

- **Superficial (first-degree) burns** involve only the top layer of skin, the epidermis. The skin turns red but does not blister or actually burn through. The burn site is painful. A sunburn is a good example of a superficial burn.

- **Partial-thickness (second-degree)** burns involve the epidermis and some portion of the dermis. These burns do not destroy the entire thickness of the skin, nor is the subcutaneous tissue injured. Typically, the skin is moist, mottled, and white to red. Blisters are common. Partial-thickness burns cause intense pain.

- **Full-thickness (third-degree) burns** extend through all skin layers and may involve subcutaneous layers, muscle, bone, or internal organs. The burned area is dry and leathery and may appear white, dark brown, or even charred. Some full-thickness burns feel hard to the touch. Clotted blood vessels or subcutaneous tissue may be visible under the burned skin. If the nerve endings have been destroyed, a severely burned area may have no feeling. However, the surrounding, less severely burned areas may be extremely painful.

A pure full-thickness burn is unusual. Severe burns are typically a combination of superficial, partial-thickness, and full-thickness burns. Superficial burns heal well without scarring.

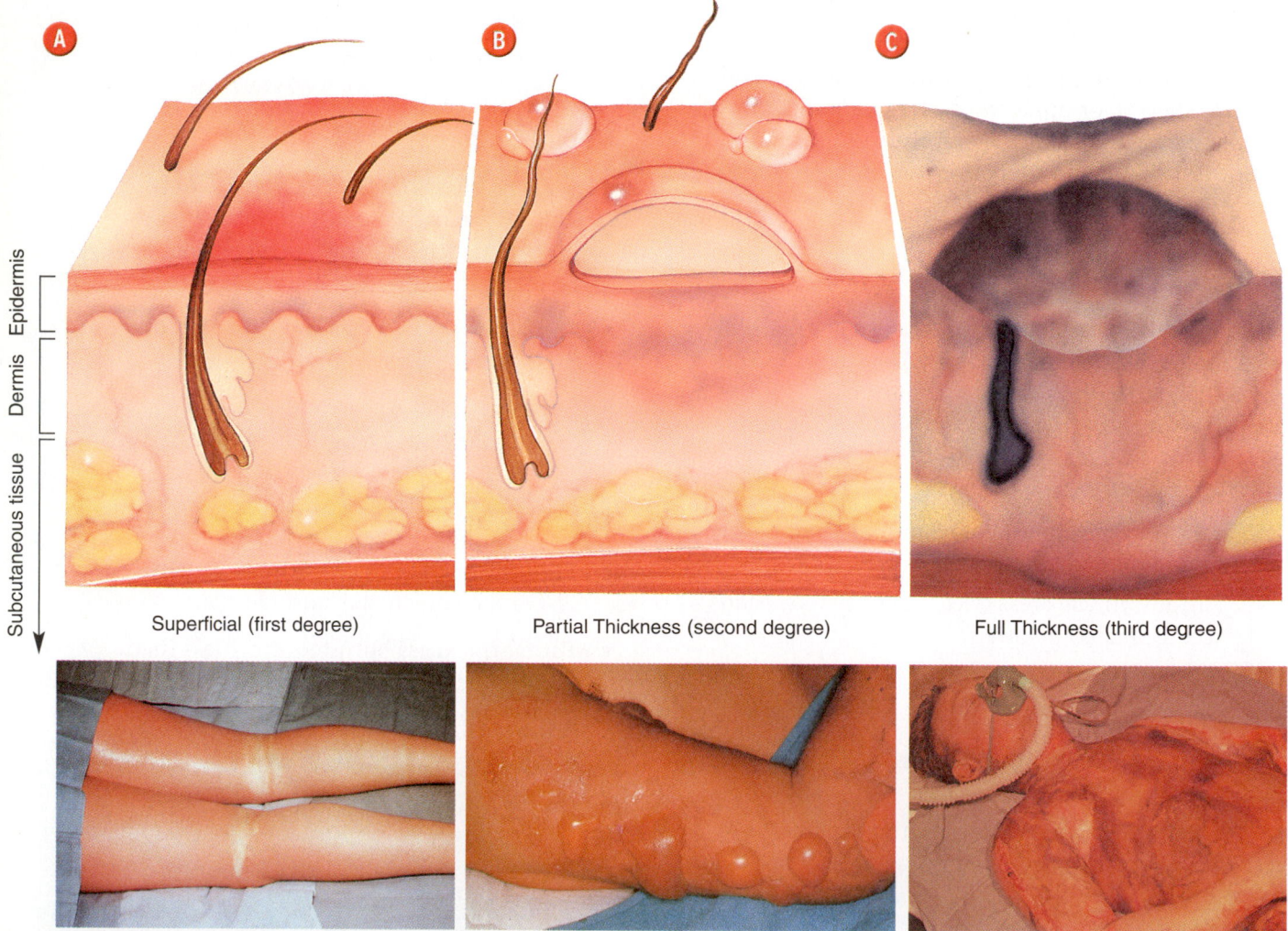

Superficial (first degree)   Partial Thickness (second degree)   Full Thickness (third degree)

Figure 19-17   Classification of burns. **A.** Superficial or first-degree burns involve only the epidermis. The skin turns red but does not blister or actually burn through. **B.** Partial-thickness or second-degree burns involve some of the dermis, but they do not destroy the entire thickness of the skin. The skin is mottled, white to red, and is often blistered. **C.** Full-thickness or third-degree burns extend through all layers of the skin and may involve subcutaneous tissue and muscle. The skin is dry, leathery, and often either white or charred.

Documentation Tips

It can be difficult documenting the location and severity of a patient's burn. If in doubt, sketch an outline of the human body and shadow in the affected areas on the drawing. Don't forget to add a sketch of the patient's back as well.

Pediatric Needs

Burns to children are generally considered more serious than burns to adults (▼ **Table 19-2**). This is because infants and children have more surface area relative to total body mass, which means greater fluid and heat loss. In addition, children do not tolerate burns as well as adults do. Children are also more likely to go into shock, develop hypothermia, and experience airway problems.

Many burns in infants and children result from child abuse. The classic burn resulting from deliberate immersion involves the hands and wrists, as well as the feet, lower legs, and buttocks. Similarly, burns around the genitals and multiple cigarette burns should be viewed as possible abuse. You should report all suspected cases of abuse to the proper authorities (Chapter 30).

TABLE 19-2 Classification of Burns in Infants and Children

Critical Burns
- Full-thickness or partial-thickness burns covering more than 20% of the body's total surface area
- Burns involving the hands, feet, face, airway, or genitalia

Moderate Burns
- Partial-thickness burns covering 10% to 20% of the body's total surface area

Minor Burns
- Partial-thickness burns covering less than 10% of the body's total surface area

Small partial-thickness burns also heal without scarring. However, deep partial-thickness burns and all full-thickness burns are best managed surgically.

Significant airway burns may be associated with singeing of the hair within the nostrils, soot around the nose and mouth, hoarseness, or hypoxia.

It may be impossible to accurately estimate the depth of a particular burn. Even experienced burn surgeons sometimes underestimate or, more commonly, overestimate the extent of a particular burn.

EXTENT. One quick way to estimate the surface area that has been burned is to compare it to the size of the patient's palm, which is roughly equal to 1% of the patient's total body surface area. Another useful measurement system is the **Rule of Nines**, which divides the body into sections, each of which is approximately 9% of the total surface area (▶ **Figure 19-18**). Remember that the head of an infant or child is relatively larger than the head of an adult, and the legs are relatively smaller.

Emergency Medical Care

Your first responsibility in caring for a patient with a burn is to stop the burning process and prevent additional injury. (▶ **Skill Drill 19-4**) presents the steps in caring for a burn patient:

1. **Follow BSI precautions.** Because a burn destroys the patient's protective skin layer, always wear gloves and eye protection when treating a burn patient.

2. **Move the patient away from the burning area.** If any clothing is on fire, wrap the patient in a blanket or follow specific guidelines outlined by your local fire department protocol to put out the flames, then remove any smoldering clothing and/or jewelry.

3. **Immerse the area in cool, sterile water or saline solution,** or cover with a clean, wet, cool dressing, if the skin or clothing is hot. This not only stops the burning, it also relieves pain. However, immersion increases the risk of infection and hypothermia. For this reason, you should not keep the affected part under water for more than 10 minutes. If the burning has stopped before you arrive, *do not immerse it at all.* As an alternative to immersion, irrigation of the burned area until the burning stops may also be used, followed by the application of a sterile dressing **(Step 1)**.

4. **Give oxygen if the patient has a critical burn.** Also remember that more fire victims die from

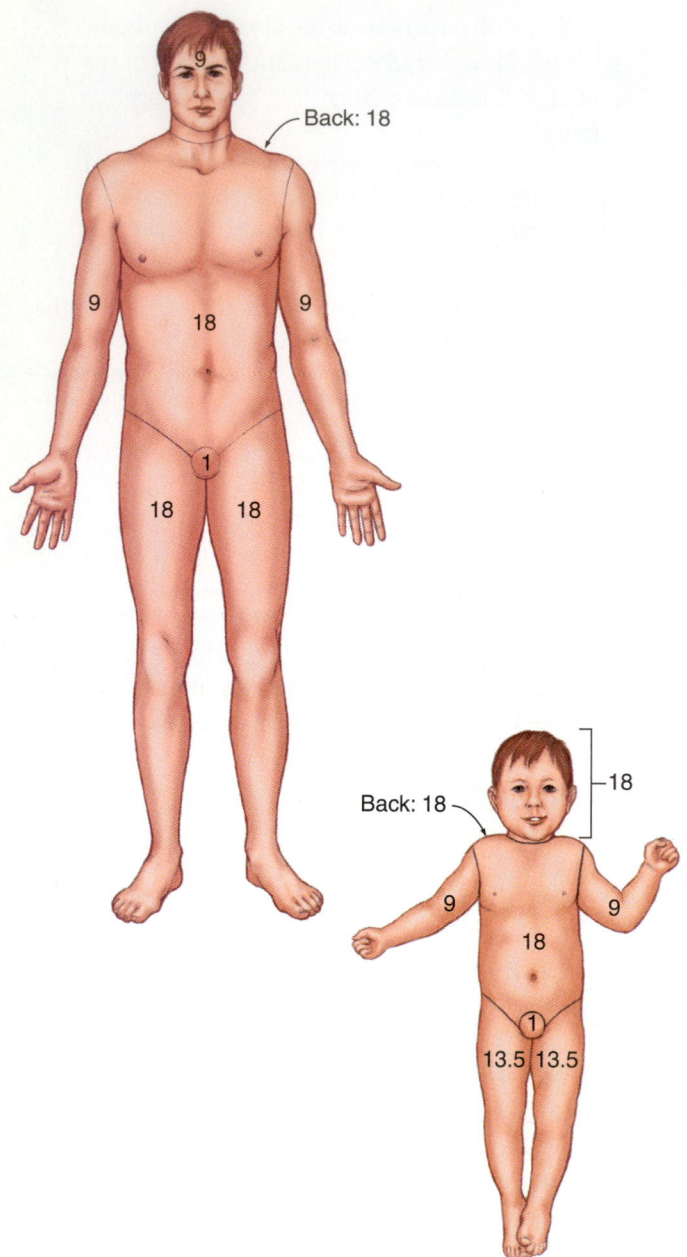

Figure 19-18 The Rule of Nines is a quick way to estimate the amount of surface area that has been burned. It divides the body into sections, each approximately 9% of the total body surface area.

Therefore, you must continually assess the airway for possible problems.

5. **Rapidly estimate the burn's severity.** Then cover the burned area with a dry, sterile dressing to prevent further contamination. Sterile gauze is best if the area is not too large. You may cover larger areas with a clean, white sheet. Most important, do not put anything else on the burned area. Use only a dry, sterile dressing, sterile burn sheet, or clean, white sheet. Never use ointments, lotions, or antiseptics of any kind. In addition, do not intentionally break any blisters.

6. **Check for traumatic injuries** or other medical conditions that may be more immediately life-threatening. Most patients who have been burned have normal vital signs and can communicate at first, which will make your assessment easier **(Step 2)**.

7. **Treat the patient for shock** if necessary, and prepare for transport **(Step 3)**.

8. **An extensive burn can produce hypothermia** (loss of body heat). Prevent further heat loss by covering the patient with warm blankets.

9. **Provide prompt transport** by local protocol. Do not delay transport to do a prolonged assessment or to apply coverings to burns in a critical patient **(Step 4)**.

Chemical Burns

A chemical burn can occur whenever a toxic substance contacts the body. Most chemical burns are caused by strong acids or strong alkalis. The eyes are

smoke inhalation than from skin burns. A patient who has burns about the face or has inhaled smoke or fumes may develop respiratory distress. Therefore, you should give oxygen to these patients as well. Keep in mind that a patient who appears to be breathing well at first may suddenly develop severe respiratory distress.

SkillDrill 19-4 Caring for Burns

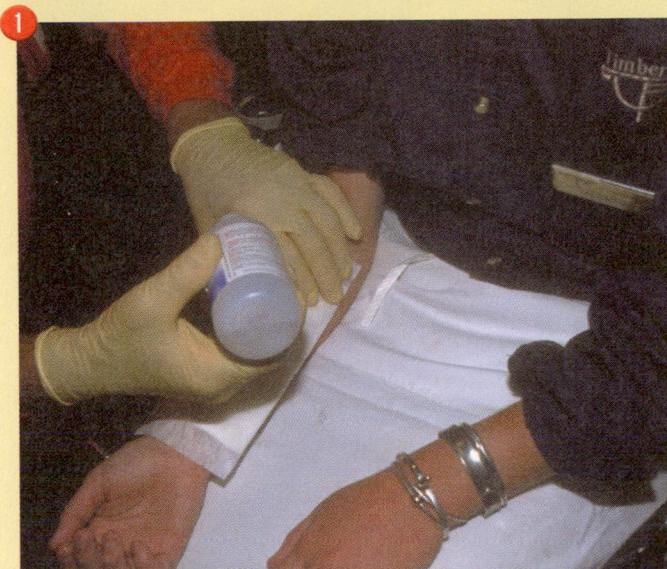

1. Follow BSI precautions to help prevent infection.

Remove the patient from the burning area; extinguish or remove hot clothing and jewelry as needed.

If the wound(s) is still burning or hot, immerse the hot area in cool, sterile water, or cover with a wet, cool dressing.

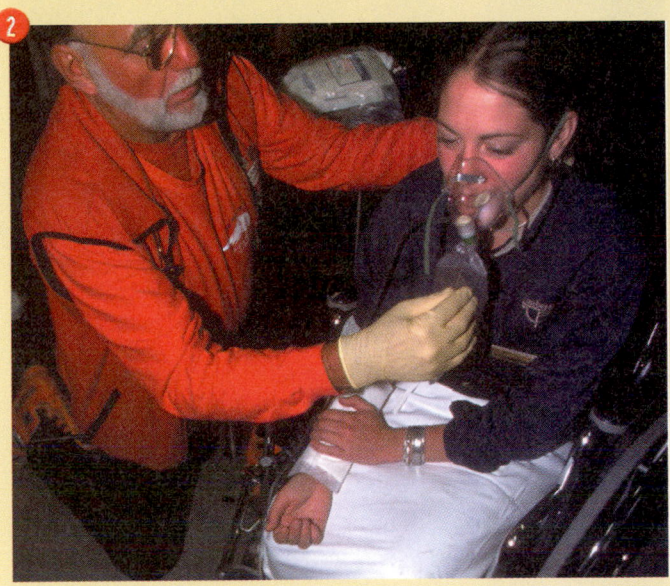

2. Give supplemental oxygen and continue to assess the airway.

Estimate the severity of the burn, then cover the area with a dry, sterile dressing or clean sheet.

Assess and treat the patient for any other injuries.

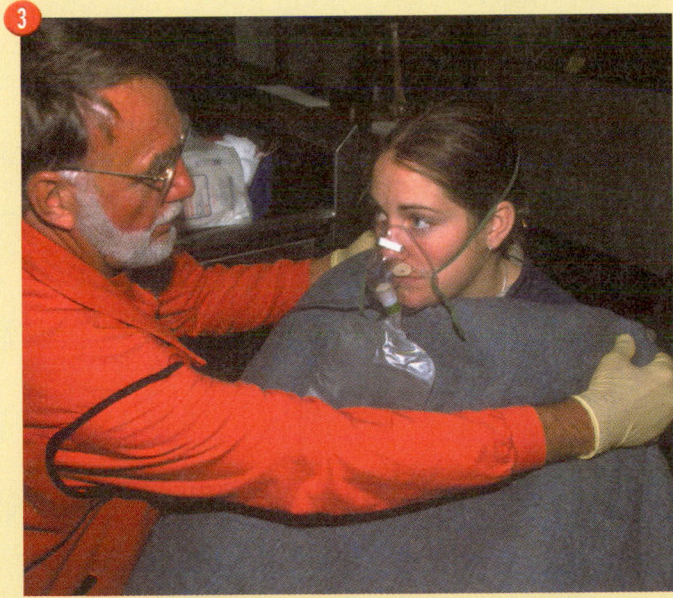

3. Prepare for transport.

Treat for shock if needed.

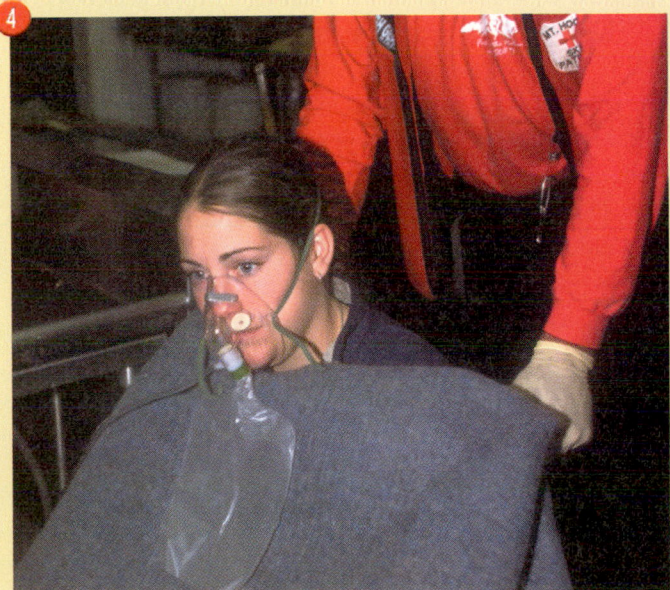

4. Cover the patient with blankets to prevent loss of body heat.

Transport promptly.

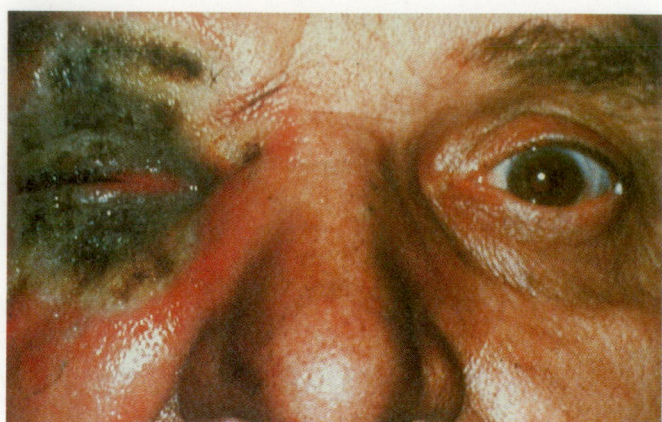

Figure 19-19   The eyes are particularly vulnerable to chemical burns.

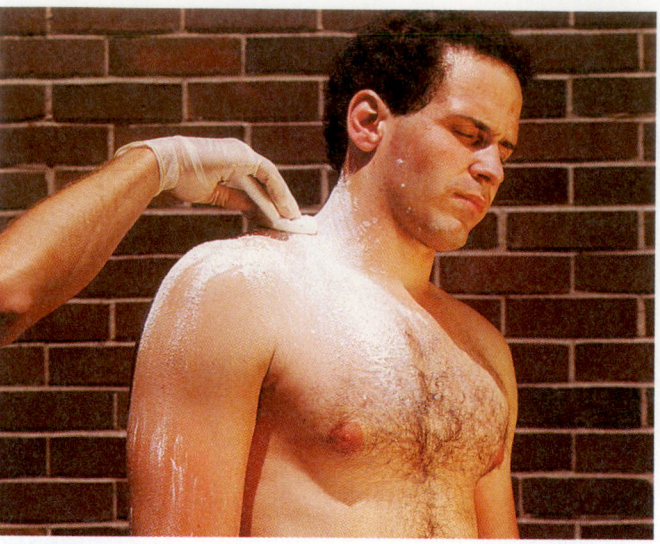

Figure 19-20   Brush dry chemicals off the patient before you flush the burned area with water.

particularly vulnerable to chemical burns ▲ **Figure 19-19** . Sometimes, simply the fumes of strong chemicals can cause burns, especially to the respiratory tract.

To prevent exposure to hazardous materials, you must wear the appropriate gloves and eye protection whenever you are caring for a patient with a chemical burn. Be particularly careful not to get any chemical, dry or liquid, on yourself or on your uniform; consider wearing a protective gown when this is a possibility. Remember that exposure risk is also present when you are cleaning up after the call. In cases of severe chemical burns or exposure, consider mobilization of the HazMat team, if appropriate.

The emergency care of a chemical burn is basically the same as that for a thermal burn. To stop the burning process, remove any chemical from the patient. A dry chemical that is activated by contact with water may damage the skin more when it is wet than when it is dry. Therefore, always brush dry chemicals off the skin and clothing before flushing the patient with water ▲ **Figure 19-20** . Remove the patient's clothing, including shoes, stockings, and gloves, because there may be small amounts of chemicals in the creases.

Immediately begin to flush the burned area with large amounts of water ▶ **Figure 19-21** , taking care not to contaminate uninjured areas or make the patient hypothermic. Never direct a forceful stream of water from a hose at the patient; the extreme water pressure may mechanically injure the burned skin. Continue flooding the area with gallons of water for 15 to 20 minutes after the patient says the burning pain has stopped. If an eye has been burned, hold the eyelid open while flooding the eye with a gentle stream of water ▶ **Figure 19-22** . Continue flushing the contaminated area on the way to the hospital. Make sure the Material Safety Data Sheets (MSDS) go with the patient to definitive care.

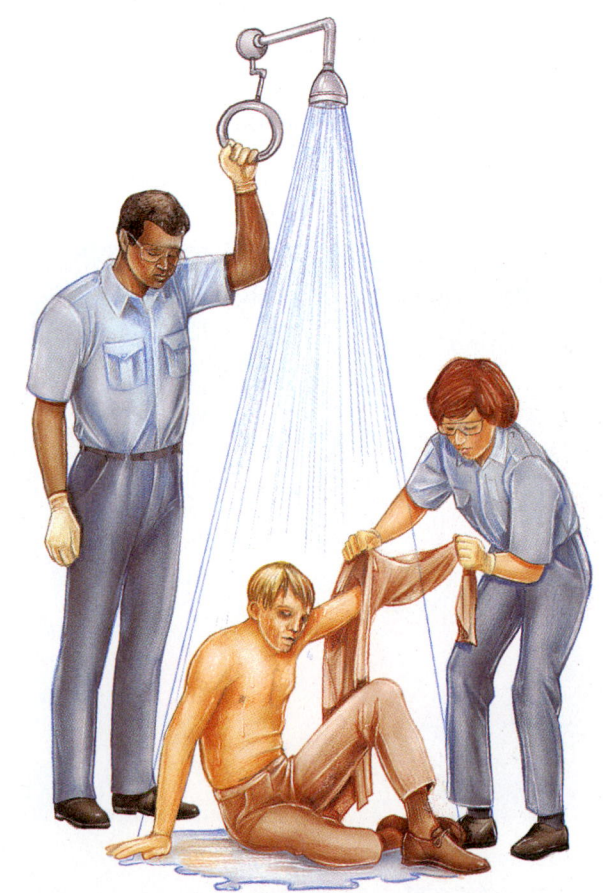

Figure 19-21   Flush the burned area with large amounts of water for 15 to 20 minutes after the patient says that the burning pain has stopped. Be careful to avoid contaminating uninjured areas.

Electrical Burns

Electrical burns may be the result of contact with high- or low-voltage electricity. High-voltage burns may occur when utility workers make direct contact with power lines. However, ordinary household current is powerful enough to cause severe burns.

For electricity to flow, there must be a complete circuit between the electrical source and the ground. Any substance that prevents this circuit from being completed, such as rubber, is called an insulator. Any substance that allows a current to flow through it is called a conductor. The human body, which is primarily water, is a good conductor. Thus, electrical burns occur when the body, or a part of it, completes a circuit connecting a power source to the ground (▼ **Figure 19-23**).

Your safety is of particular importance when you are called to the scene of an emergency involving electricity. Obviously, you can be fatally injured by coming into contact with power lines. But you can also be fatally injured by touching a patient who is still in contact with a live power line or any other electrical source. For this reason, you must never attempt to remove someone from an electrical source unless you are specially trained to do so. Likewise, you should never move a downed power line unless you have the special training and equipment necessary for the job or unless you are absolutely certain that the line is not live. Before even approaching someone who may still be in contact with a power line or an electrical appliance, make certain that

the power is turned off. Always assume that any downed power line is live.

There is always a burn injury where the electricity entered the body (an entrance wound) and another where it exited (an exit wound). The entrance wound may be quite small (▶ **Figure 19-24A**), but the exit wound can be extensive and deep (▶ **Figure 19-24B**). Always look for both entrance and exit wounds. There are two dangers specifically associated with electrical burns. First, there may be a large amount of deep tissue injury. Electrical burns are always more severe than the external signs indicate. The patient may have only a

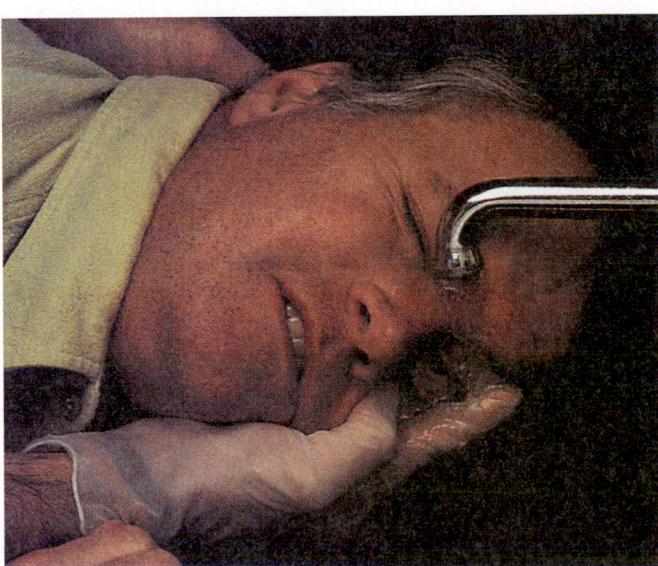

Figure 19-22 Flood the affected eye with a gentle stream of water. Hold the eyelids open, a challenging task because the patient's reflex is to keep the eye shut. Take care to prevent any of the chemical from getting into the other eye during flushing.

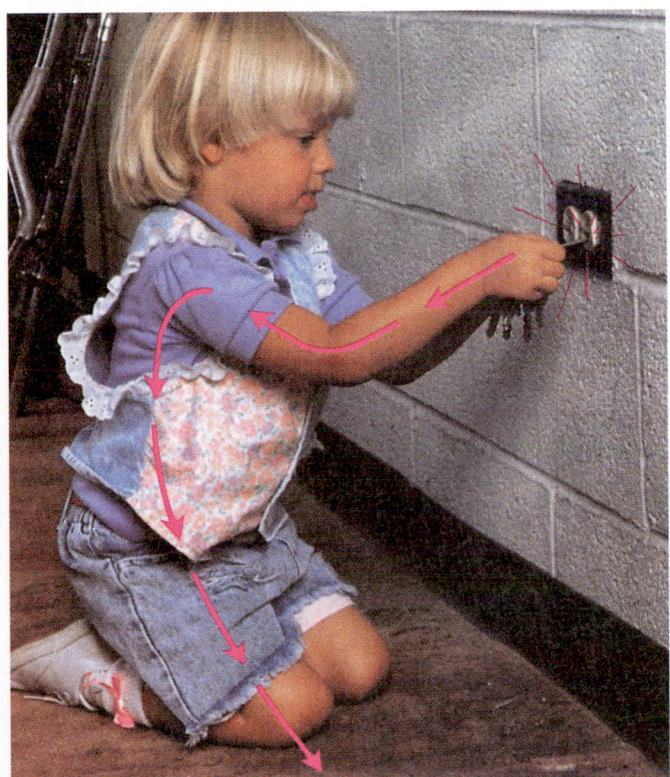

Figure 19-23 The human body is a good conductor of electricity. An electrical burn usually occurs when the body, acting as a conductor, completes a circuit.

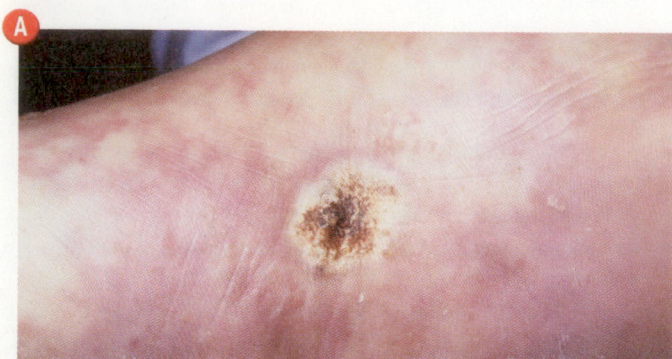

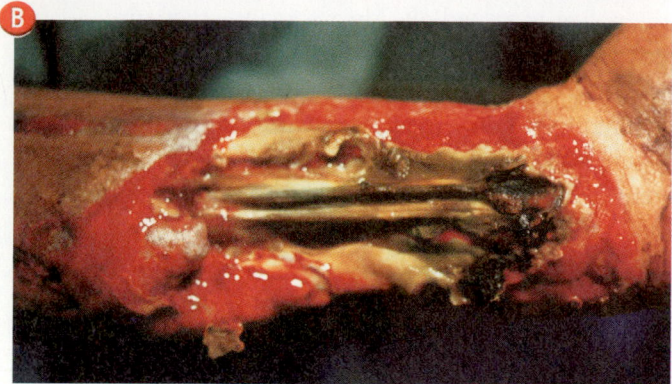

Figure 19-24 Electrical burns, like gunshot wounds, have entrance and exit wounds. **A.** An entrance wound is often quite small. **B.** The exit wound can be extensive and deep.

small burn to the skin but have massive damage to the deeper tissues ▼ **Figure 19-25**. Second, the patient may go into cardiac arrest from the electric shock.

If indicated, begin CPR and apply the AED. Although CPR may need to be quite prolonged in electrical burn cases, it has a high success rate if started promptly. You should be prepared to defibrillate if necessary. If neither CPR nor defibrillation is indicated, give supplemental oxygen, and monitor the patient closely for respiratory and cardiac arrest. Treat the soft-tissue injuries by placing dry, sterile dressings on all burn wounds and splinting suspected fractures. Provide prompt transport; all electrical burns are potentially severe injuries that require further treatment in the hospital.

Dressing and Bandaging

All wounds require bandaging. In most instances, splints help to control bleeding and provide firm support for the dressing. There are many different types of dressings and bandages ▶ **Figure 19-26**. You should be familiar with the function and proper application of each.

In general, dressings and bandages have three primary functions:

- To control bleeding
- To protect the wound from further damage
- To prevent further contamination and infection

Figure 19-25 External signs of an electrical burn may be deceiving. The entrance wound may be a small burn, while the damage to deeper tissue may be massive.

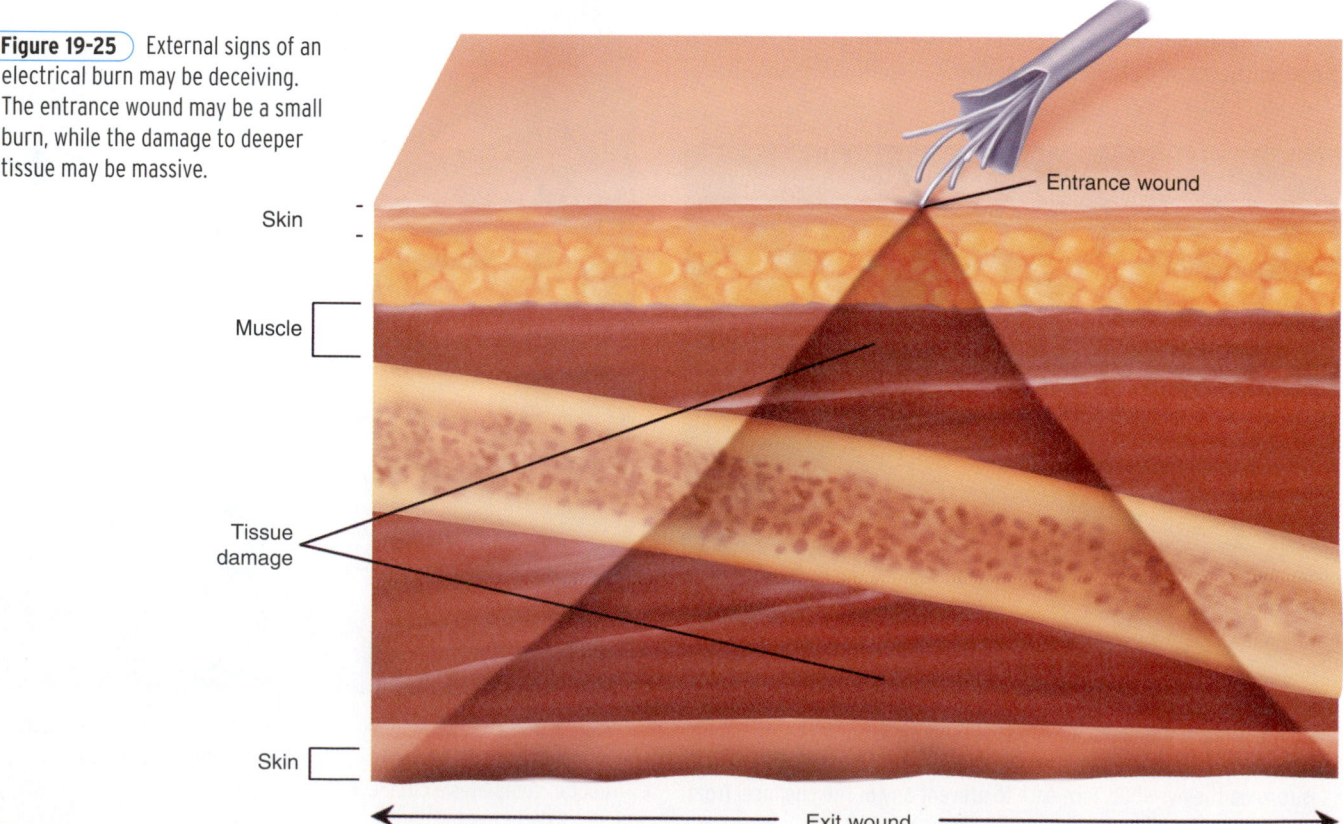

Skin

Muscle

Tissue damage

Skin

Entrance wound

Exit wound

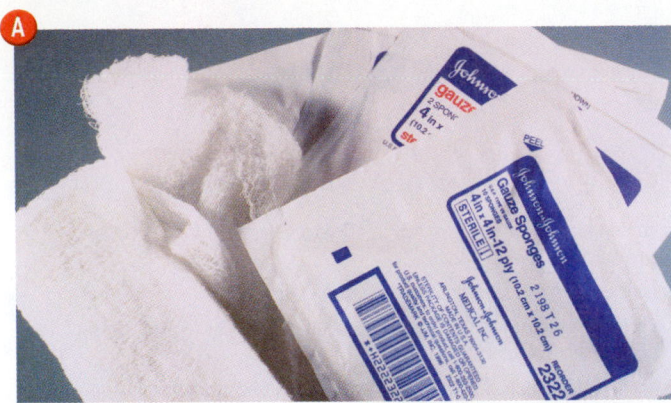

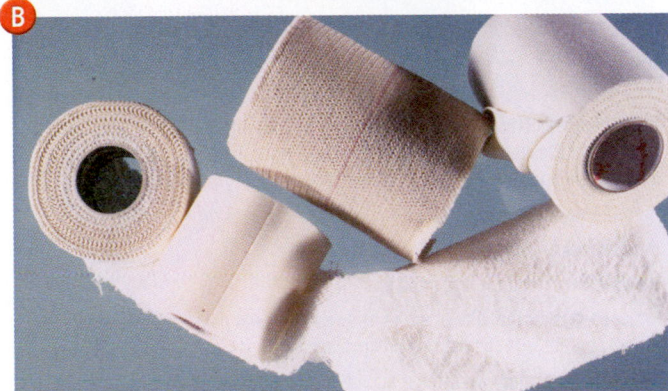

Wilderness Tips

Consult Appendix D for specific bandaging techniques useful in the outdoor setting.

Figure 19-26 **A.** Many types of sterile dressings are used for covering open wounds, including universal dressings, gauze pads, adhesive dressings, and occlusive dressings. **B.** Bandages keep dressings in place and include soft roller bandages, triangular bandages, and adhesive tape. Splints may also be used to hold dressings in place.

Sterile Dressings

Universal dressings, conventional 4" × 4" and 4" × 8" gauze pads, and assorted small adhesive-type dressings and soft self-adherent roller dressings will cover most wounds.

Measuring 9" × 36" and made of thick, absorbent material, the universal dressing is ideal for covering large open wounds. It also makes an efficient pad for rigid splints. These dressings are available in compact, commercially sterilized packages. The universal dressing material is also available in 20-yd rolls, which some rescuers cut into 3′ lengths, package, and sterilize themselves.

Gauze pads are appropriate for smaller wounds, and adhesive-type dressings are useful for minor wounds. Occlusive dressings, made of Vaseline gauze, aluminum foil, or plastic, prevent air and liquids from entering (or exiting) the wound. They are used to cover sucking chest wounds, abdominal eviscerations, and neck injuries.

Bandages

To keep dressings in place during transport, you can use soft roller bandages, rolls of gauze, triangular bandages, or adhesive tape. The self-adherent, soft roller bandages are probably easiest to use. They are slightly elastic, which makes them easy to apply, and you can tuck the end of the roll into a deeper layer to secure it in place. The layers adhere somewhat but should not be applied too tightly to one another.

Adhesive tape holds small dressings in place and helps to secure larger dressings. Some people, however, are allergic to adhesive tape. If you know that a patient has this problem, use paper or plastic tape instead.

Do not use elastic bandages to secure dressings. If the injury swells, the bandage may become a tourniquet and cause further damage. Any improperly applied bandage that impairs circulation can result in additional tissue damage or even the loss of a limb. For this reason, you should always check a limb distal to a bandage for signs of impaired circulation or loss of sensation. Air splints are useful in stabilizing broken extremities, and they can be used with dressings to help control bleeding from soft-tissue injuries.

Chapter Sweep

Ready for Review

The skin has two principal layers: the tough outer layer, called the epidermis, and the inner layer, called the dermis, which contains the hair follicles, sweat glands, and sebaceous glands. The functions of the skin are to keep bacteria out and water in, to report to the brain on the environment, and to regulate body temperature.

There are three types of soft-tissue injuries: closed injuries, open injuries, and burns. Closed injuries include contusions, hematomas, and crushing injuries. They can be treated by applying RICES (rest, ice, compression, elevation of the injured part, and splinting). Open injuries produce more extensive bleeding and may become infected. There are four types of open injuries: abrasions, lacerations, avulsions, and penetrating wounds. In treating these injuries, you must first control bleeding. Use a dry, sterile dressing, covered by a roller bandage, a second pressure dressing (if necessary), and a splint. Do not try to clean out an open wound unless there will be a delay of 2 hours or more before definitive treatment is available.

Burns are one of the most serious and painful of soft-tissue injuries. They can occur from heat (thermal), chemicals, electricity, and radiation. Burns are classified primarily by the depth and extent of the burn, the body area involved, and are either superficial, partial-thickness, or full-thickness.

Treatment for burns includes BSI precautions, stopping the burning process, caring for the burn wounds, and treating the patient for shock (oxygen and prevention of further heat loss).

Dressings and bandages are designed to control bleeding, protect the wound from further damage, and prevent further contamination and infection. Use universal dressings for large open wounds, gauze pads for smaller wounds, adhesive-type dressings for minor wounds, and occlusive dressings for sucking chest wounds and abdominal eviscerations. Use soft roller bandages, rolls of gauze, triangular bandages, or adhesive tape to keep dressings in place. Do not use elastic bandages. Always check a limb distal to a bandage for signs of impaired circulation.

Vital Vocabulary

abrasion Loss or damage of the superficial layer of skin as a result of a body part rubbing or scraping across a rough or hard surface.

avulsion An injury in which soft tissue either is torn completely loose (amputation) or is hanging as a flap.

burns An injury in which the soft tissue receives more energy than it can absorb without injury, from thermal heat, frictional heat, toxic chemicals, electricity, or nuclear radiation.

closed injury Injury in which damage occurs beneath the skin or mucous membrane but the surface remains intact.

compartment syndrome Swelling in a confined space that produces dangerous pressure; may cut off blood flow or damage sensitive tissue.

contamination The presence of infective organisms or foreign bodies such as dirt, gravel, or metal.

contusion A bruise without a break in the skin.

dermis The inner layer of the skin, containing hair follicles, sweat glands, nerve endings, and blood vessels.

ecchymosis Discoloration associated with a closed wound; signifies bleeding.

epidermis The outer layer of skin that acts as a watertight protective covering.

evisceration The displacement of organs outside the body.

full-thickness (third-degree) burn A burn that affects all skin layers and may affect the subcutaneous layers, muscle, bone, and internal organs, leaving the area dry, leathery, and white, dark brown, or charred.

hematoma Blood collected within the body's tissues or in a body cavity.

hemothorax Collection of blood in the chest.

laceration A smooth or jagged open wound.

mucous membrane The lining of body cavities and passages that are in direct contact with the outside environment.

occlusive dressing Dressing made of Vaseline gauze, aluminum foil, or plastic, that prevents air and liquids from entering or exiting a wound.

open injury An injury in which there is a break in the surface of the skin or the mucous membrane, exposing deeper tissue to potential contamination.

partial-thickness (second-degree) burn A burn affecting the epidermis and some portion of the dermis but not the subcutaneous tissue, characterized by blisters and skin that is white to red, moist, and mottled.

penetrating wound An injury resulting from a sharp, pointed object.

pneumothorax Entry of air into the pleural space.

Rule of Nines A system that assigns percentages to sections of the body, allowing calculation of the amount of skin surface involved in the burn area.

superficial (first-degree) burn A burn affecting only the epidermis, characterized by skin that is red but not blistered or actually burned through.

Points to Ponder

You are working at a junior race at your local ski area and notice a racer twist his knee during a practice run. His coach has evaluated the knee and when the racer stands, his knee collapses. His parents wave for you to come over. You hear that the racer and the coach believe he can still compete, but the parents want your opinion. You have recently completed the OEC course and your protocol would be to splint and transport. The coach is pushing for an answer as to whether the skier can participate in the race. Would you assess the racer? Would you make a decision to allow him to continue? What would you tell the parents? Once the parents call you over, can you not treat the patient?

Issues Legal Liability, Training Standards and Protocols, Refusing Treatment, Use of Non-EMT Skills and Outside Knowledge.

www.OECzone.com

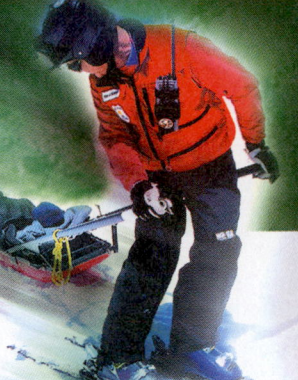

Assessment in Action

It's a beautiful summer Saturday on your mountain, and your patrol is providing coverage for a downhill mountain bike race. A cyclist, out of control, has left the course and crashed over a small cliff, falling about 10′. He slides into a rock and rolls off into the remains of a downed tree.

The broken end of a branch leaves a 1″ hole under his right scapula. The wound is still bubbling with each breath when you arrive. The patient is alert and articulate and appears pale. He tells you that the reason he stayed motionless by the creek edge was because it "hurt too bad" to move. He has numerous contusions and abrasions, primarily to his right side. He also has a large avulsion to his right calf that is bleeding freely. Vital signs include a pulse of 126 beats/min, shallow respirations of 40 breaths/min, and a blood pressure of 134/70 mm Hg.

1. Your first step in caring for this patient is to:
   A. check his pulse, sensation, and function in all four extremities.
   B. apply oxygen and cover the open chest wound and stop the bleeding.
   C. ask him to identify what he thinks is the biggest problem.
   D. ask him if he has any allergies or is on any medication.

2. The most appropriate method to manage bleeding from his avulsion injury is to:
   A. separate the layers of tissue with sterile gauze and bandage.
   B. apply a wide-band tourniquet and loosen regularly.
   C. apply sterile gauze over the injury with an elastic bandage.
   D. replace the tissue and apply direct pressure over the bleeding site.

3. The patient's right shoulder and upper arm are both quite swollen with an extensive contusion. This is an indicator of which of the following?
   A. Nerve damage
   B. Systemic infection
   C. Internal bleeding
   D. Allergic reaction

4. If this patient were to survive his first couple of days, because of the nature of his injuries, he would still be at high risk for:
   A. infection.
   B. infarction.
   C. malnutrition.
   D. hypertension.

5. During your care you note that this patient is becoming confused. Which of the following must you immediately assess?
   A. Ability to obey commands
   B. Movement, pulse, and sensation of the distal extremity
   C. Respirations, pulse, and BP
   D. Pupil reaction

6. It is important to continue to assess vital signs and assess for hypoperfusion because of this patient's penetrating injury. Which of the following explanations for this is most correct?
   A. The spleen is located in that area.
   B. The liver is located in that area.
   C. The heart is located in that area.
   D. The pancreas is located in that area.

Later, you are called to a camping area where a camper has tried to light a campfire with lighter fluid. He has burns to the anterior surface of his arms, face, and upper chest to the nipple line. He is screaming in pain. The burned areas are red with some blistering of his hands and lower arms. His eyebrows have been singed and blisters are forming on his chin. The following questions apply to this patient.

7. What do you know about this patient's airway?
   A. Nothing until you check his respiratory rate.
   B. His airway is intact because he is screaming.
   C. His respirations are inadequate because he is screaming.
   D. Nothing until you check his mucous membranes and tongue.

8. This patient has signs of possible respiratory involvement. Without looking at his mucous membranes and tongue, how can you tell?
   A. His mental status
   B. His pulse
   C. The blisters on his face
   D. His respiratory rate

9. This patient has burns over the anterior surface of both his arms, upper chest to the nipple line, and face. What approximate percentage of body surface area burn should you report to the receiving hospital?
   A. 18%
   B. 23%
   C. 27%
   D. 32%

Challenging Question

10. If both arms of your patient are burned, how can you obtain a blood pressure?

Online Outlook

Because the soft tissues are exposed to the environment, they are often injured. Test your ability to identify different soft-tissue injuries by completing Exercise 19 at www.OECzone.com.

Eye Injuries

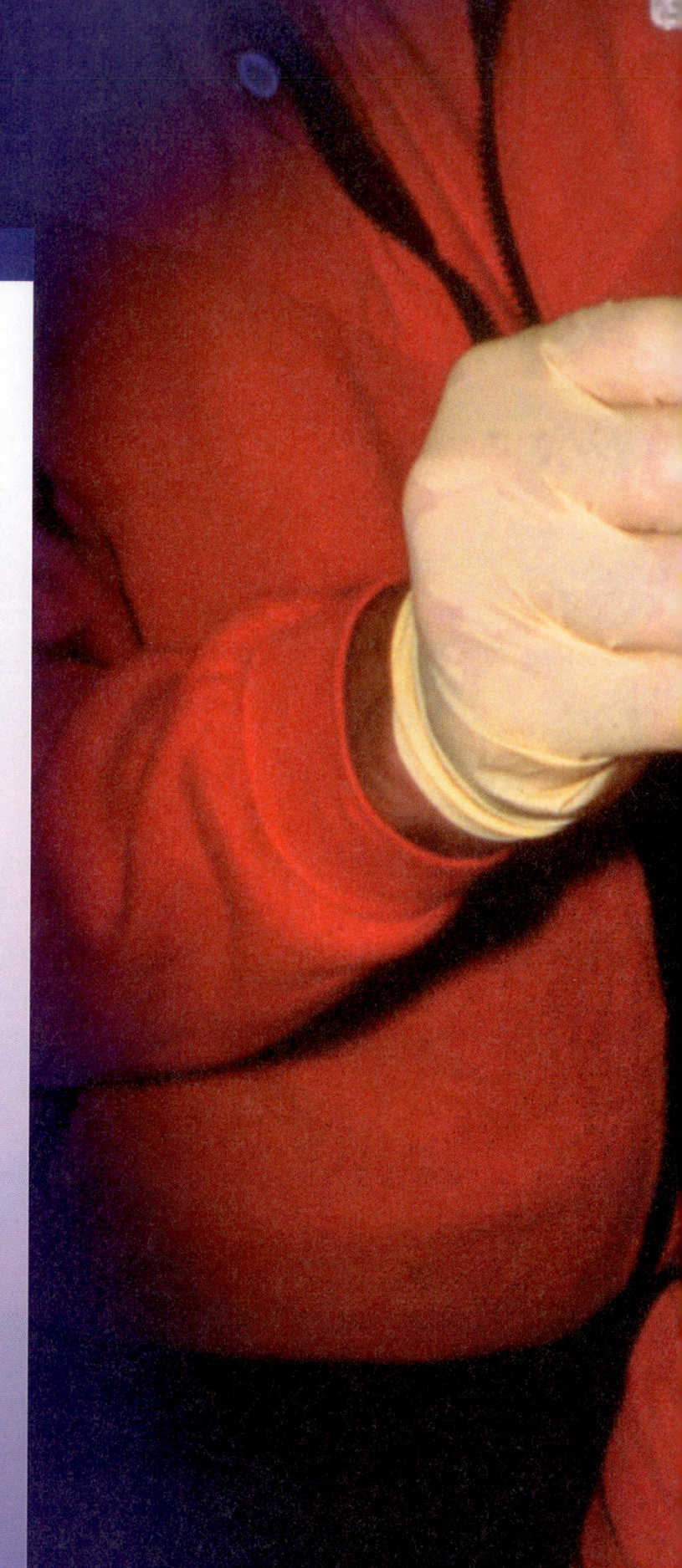

Objectives

Cognitive

1. List the main anatomical features of the eye (p 524).
2. Describe the principal functions of the eye (p 524).
3. Describe the signs and symptoms of eye injuries (p 525).
4. List the steps necessary to assess eye injuries (p 525).
5. Describe the steps for managing foreign objects in the eye (p 526).
6. Describe the steps for managing puncture wounds to the eye (p 526).
7. Describe how to manage burns to the eye (p 528).
8. Describe how to remove contact lenses from the eye (p 532).
9. Recognize abnormalities of the eyes that may indicate underlying head injury (p 532).
10. Recognize and manage a patient with an artificial eye (p 533).

Affective

None

Psychomotor

11. Demonstrate the use of irrigation to flush out foreign bodies lying on the surface of the eye (p 526).
12. Demonstrate the care of the patient with chemical burns to the eye (p 528).
13. Demonstrate the steps in the emergency care of the patient with lacerations of the eyelids, ruptured globe, and impaled foreign body (p 530).
14. Demonstrate the stabilization of a foreign object impaled in the eye (p 527).

These are core concepts in initial patrol training.

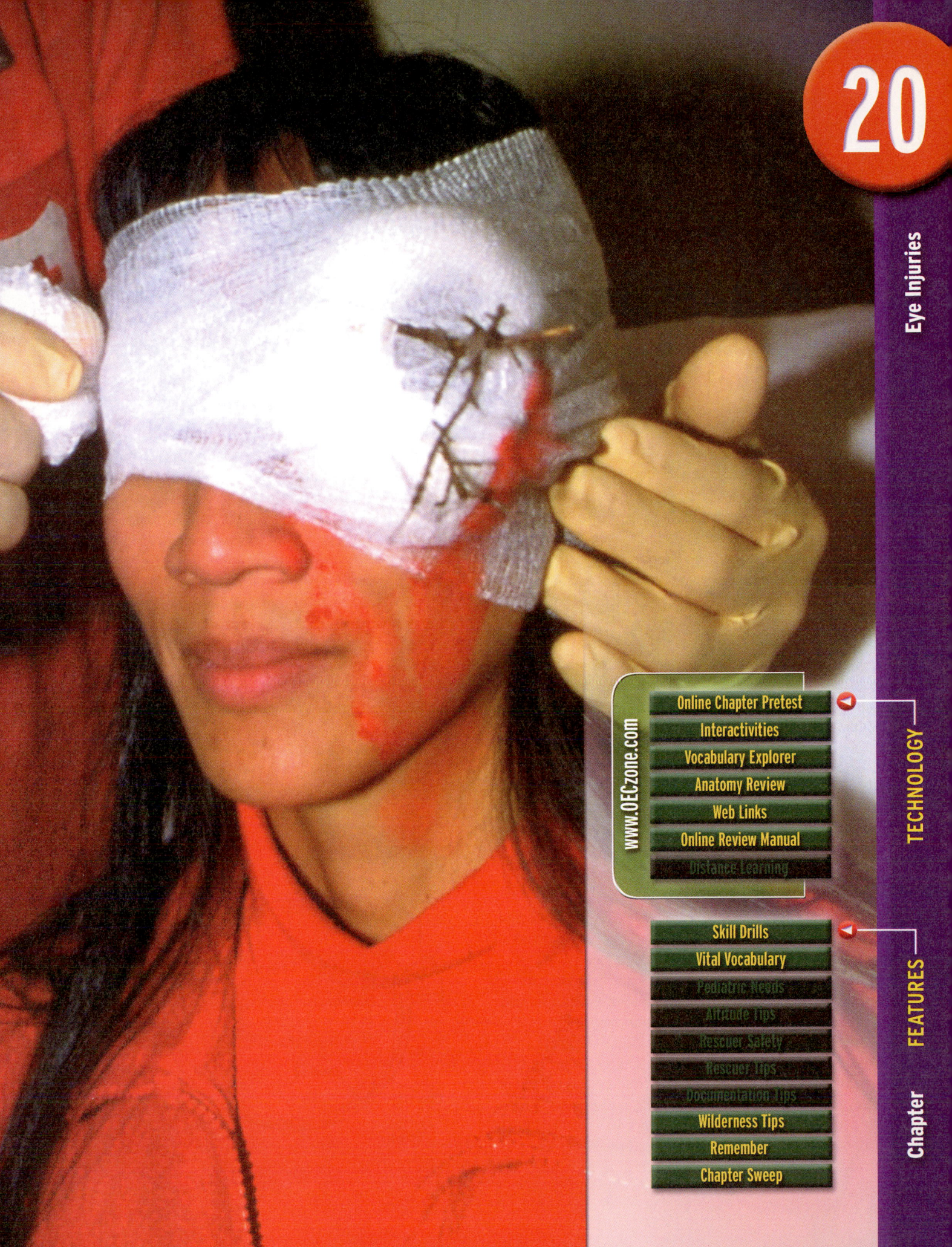

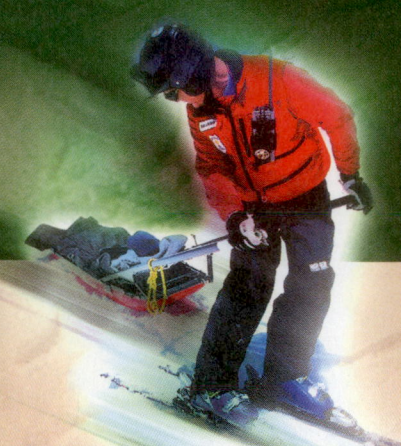

A hiker has slipped off the trail and rolled over an embankment. During the fall, he hit a tree branch with his face. As a result, a branch about the size of a pencil is impaled in his eye. He is in a great deal of pain, and he is hysterical.

The possible loss of sight is a frightening event, making calls involving eye injuries very stressful for both patients and care providers. This chapter will present practical information about caring for these fragile organs and will also help you answer the following questions:

1. Why is it important to bandage both eyes in cases where only one eye is injured?

2. When is it appropriate to remove contact lenses from your patient's eyes?

Eye Injuries

Injuries to the eye are common, and you will encounter many in your work as a rescuer. Proper emergency medical care for these injuries can minimize damage, which can often be severe. Fortunately, most eye injuries are relatively minor, such as foreign objects in the eye, corneal abrasions, and contusions. Some injuries are more serious, such as rupture of the globe, which requires immediate expert management. This chapter first reviews the structure and function of the eye and then looks at the different types of eye injuries, describing the emergency management of each. The handling of contact lenses and artificial eyes is also discussed.

Anatomy and Physiology of the Eye

The eye is globe-shaped, approximately 1" in diameter, and located within a bony socket in the skull called the **orbit** (▶ Figure 20-1). The orbit is composed of the adjacent bones of the face and skull; the roof of the orbit forms the base of the floor of the cranial cavity, and directly above it are the frontal lobes of the brain. In the adult, more than 80% of the eyeball is protected within this bony orbit. Between and below the orbits are the nasal bones and the sinuses, respectively. Therefore, any severe injury to the face or head can potentially damage the eyeball or the muscles attached to the eyeball that cause the eye to move.

The eyeball, or **globe**, keeps its global shape as a result of the pressure of the fluid contained within its two chambers. The clear, jellylike fluid near the back of the eye is called the vitreous humor. If the globe is ruptured and this gel leaks out, it cannot be replaced. In front of the lens is a clear fluid called the aqueous humor, named for its watery appearance; in Latin,

aqua means "water." In penetrating injuries of the eye, aqueous humor can also leak out, but with time and good medical treatment, the body can make more.

The inner surface of the eyelids and the exposed surface of the eye itself, which are covered by a delicate membrane, the **conjunctiva**, are kept moist by fluid produced by the **lacrimal glands**, often called tear glands (▶ Figure 20-2). Humans blink unconsciously many times per minute. This action sweeps fluid from the lacrimal glands over the surface of the eye, cleaning it. The tears drain on the inner side of the eye through two lacrimal (tear) ducts into the nasal cavity. This is why, when people cry, they sometimes need to blow their nose.

The white of the eye, called the **sclera**, extends over the surface of the globe. This is extremely tough, fibrous tissue that helps to maintain the eye's globular shape

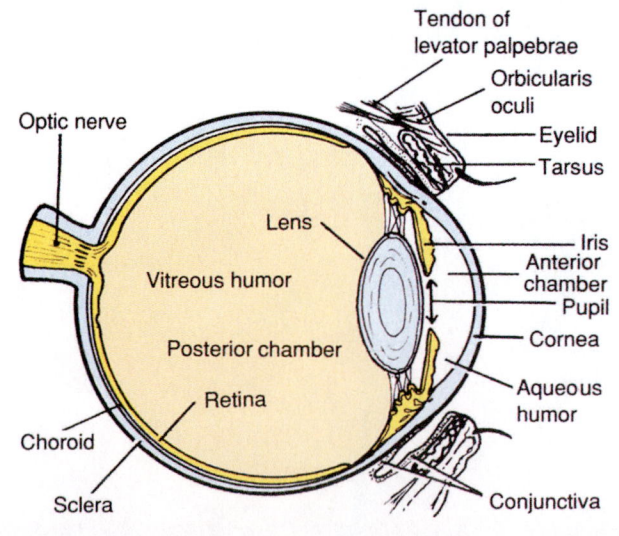

Figure 20-1   The major components of the eye.

and protect the more delicate inner structures. On the front of the eye, the sclera is continuous with a clear, transparent tissue called the <u>cornea</u>, which allows light to enter the eye. A circular muscle lies behind the cornea with an opening in its center. Like the shutter in a camera, this muscle adjusts the size of the opening to regulate the amount of light that enters the eye. This circular muscle and surrounding tissue are called the <u>iris</u>. The iris is pigmented, giving the eye its characteristic brown, green, or blue color.

The opening in the center of the iris, which allows light to move to the back of the eye, is called the <u>pupil</u>. Normally, the pupil appears black. Like the aperture in a camera, the pupil becomes smaller in bright light and larger in dim light. The pupil also becomes smaller and larger when the person is looking at objects near at hand and farther away; these adjustments occur almost instantaneously. Normally, the pupils in both eyes are equal in size. A difference between them may indicate injury to the eye or to the brain.

Behind the iris is the <u>lens</u>. Like the lens of a camera, this lens focuses an image on the light-sensitive area at the back of the globe, called the <u>retina</u>. You can think of the retina as the film in the camera. Within the retina are numerous nerve endings, which respond to light by transmitting nerve impulses through the <u>optic nerve</u> to the brain. In the brain, the impulses are interpreted as vision.

The retina is nourished by a layer of blood vessels between it and the sclera at the back of the globe. This layer is called the choroid. If, as sometimes happens, the retina detaches from the underlying choroid and sclera, the nerve endings are not nourished, and the patient then experiences blindness. This may be partial blindness, depending on how much of the retina is separated. This condition is called <u>retinal detachment</u>.

Common Eye Injuries

Eye injuries are common, particularly in sports. An eye injury can produce severe complications, including blindness. Proper emergency treatment will minimize pain and may very well help to prevent permanent loss of vision.

Treatment starts with a thorough examination to determine the extent and nature of any damage. Always perform your examination using BSI precautions, taking great care to avoid aggravating the problem. You are looking for specific abnormalities or conditions that may suggest the nature of the problem (▼ Figure 20-3). For example, blunt or penetrating injuries can produce swollen or lacerated eyelids. Bleeding soon after irritation or injury can result in a bright red conjunctiva. A damaged cornea quickly loses its smooth, wet appearance.

In a normal, uninjured eye, the entire circle of the iris is visible. The pupils are round, equal in size, and react equally when exposed to light (▶ Figure 20-4). Both eyes move together in the same direction when following your moving finger. After an injury, pupil reaction or shape and eye movement are often disturbed. Any of these conditions should cause you to suspect an injury of the globe or its associated tissues. Remember, though, that abnormal pupil reactions sometimes are a sign of brain injury rather than eye injury.

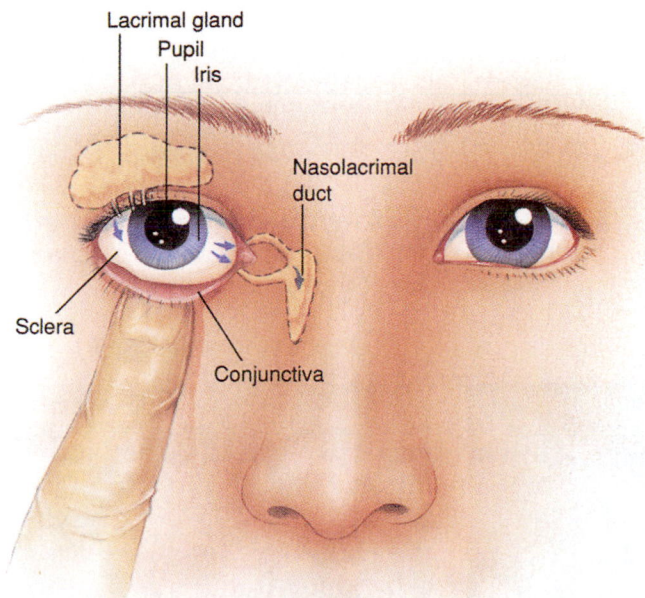

Lacrimal gland
Pupil
Iris
Nasolacrimal duct
Sclera
Conjunctiva

Figure 20-2   The lacrimal system consists of tear glands and ducts. Tears act as lubricants and keep the front of the eye from drying out.

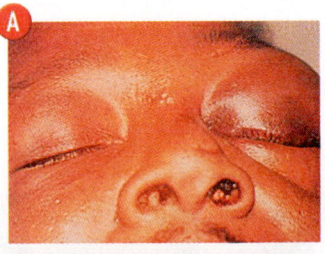
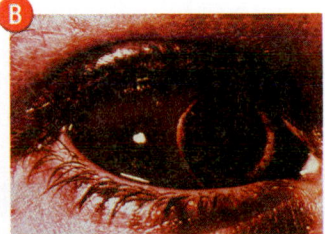
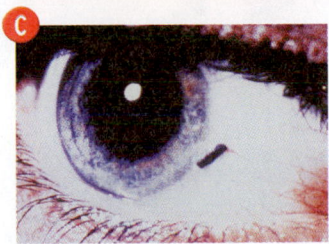

Figure 20-3   Injuries to the eyes are easily detected by **A.** swelling, **B.** bleeding, and **C.** the presence of foreign objects in the eye.

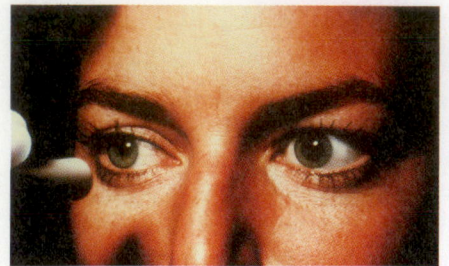

Figure 20-4 Normally, the pupils are round, equal in size, and equally reactive when exposed to light.

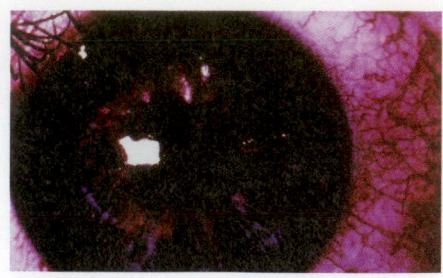

Figure 20-5 Conjunctivitis is often associated with the presence of a foreign object in the eye.

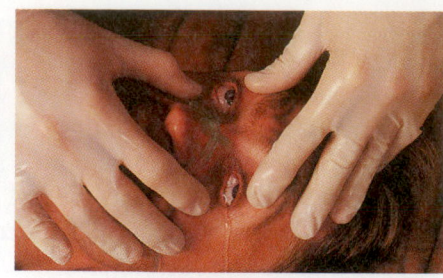

Figure 20-6 One method of irrigation is to direct saline into the injured eye using a round nasal airway or cannula. Always flush from the nose side of the eye toward the outside to avoid flushing material into the other eye.

Certain elements of the patient's history are particularly important. Therefore, as you perform your assessment, always note and record the patient's signs and symptoms, including their severity and duration, the details of how the injury occurred, were glasses or contact lenses in place, any reported changes in vision, the use of any eye medications, and any history of eye surgery, including refractive surgery.

Foreign Objects

Large objects are prevented from penetrating the eye by the protective orbit that surrounds it. However, moderate-sized and smaller foreign objects of many different types can enter the eye and cause significant damage. Even a very small foreign object, such as a grain of sand lying on the surface of the conjunctiva, may produce severe irritation (▲ **Figure 20-5**). The conjunctiva becomes inflamed and red—a condition known as <u>conjunctivitis</u>—almost immediately, and the eye begins to produce tears in an attempt to flush out the object. Irritation of the cornea or conjunctiva causes intense pain. The patient may have difficulty keeping the eyelids open, because the irritation is further aggravated by bright light.

If a small foreign object is lying on the surface of the patient's eye, you should use a normal saline solution to gently irrigate the eye. Irrigation with 500 to 1,000 mL of sterile saline solution will frequently flush away loose, small particles. If a small bulb syringe is at hand, you

can use this, or a nasal airway or cannula, to direct the saline into the affected eye (▲ **Figure 20-6**). Always flush from the nose side of the eye toward the outside to avoid flushing material into the other eye. After it is flushed away, a foreign body will often leave a small abrasion on the surface of the conjunctiva. For this reason, the patient will complain of irritation even when the particle itself is gone.

Gentle irrigation usually will not wash out foreign bodies that are stuck to the cornea or lying under the upper eyelid. To examine the undersurface of the upper eyelid, pull the lid upward and forward. If you spot a foreign object, you may be able to remove it with a moist, sterile, cotton-tipped applicator. (Never attempt to remove a foreign body that is stuck to the cornea.)

► **Skill Drill 20-1**

1. **Tell the patient to look down** while you grasp the lashes of the upper eyelid with your thumb and index finger. Gently pull the eyelid away from the eyeball **(Step 1)**.

2. **Gently place a cotton-tipped applicator** horizontally along the center of the outer surface of the upper eyelid **(Step 2)**.

3. **Pull the eyelid forward and up,** which causes it to roll or fold back over the applicator, exposing the undersurface of the eyelid **(Step 3)**.

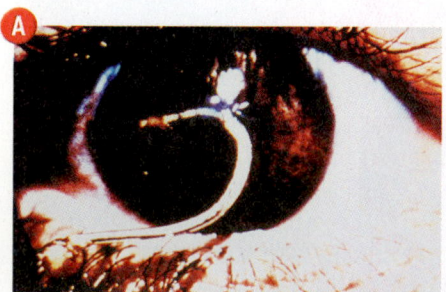

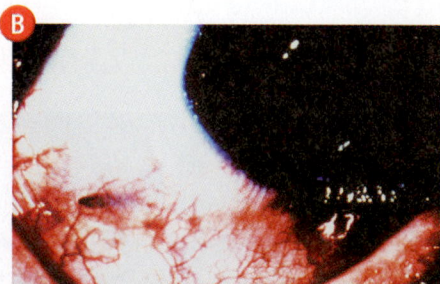

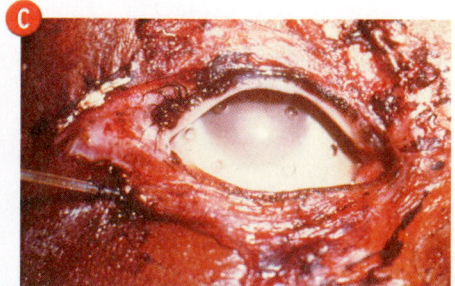

Figure 20-7 Any number of objects can become impaled in the eye. **A.** Fishhook. **B.** Sharp, metal sliver. **C.** Knife blade.

Skill Drill 20-1 Removing a Foreign Object from Under the Upper Eyelid

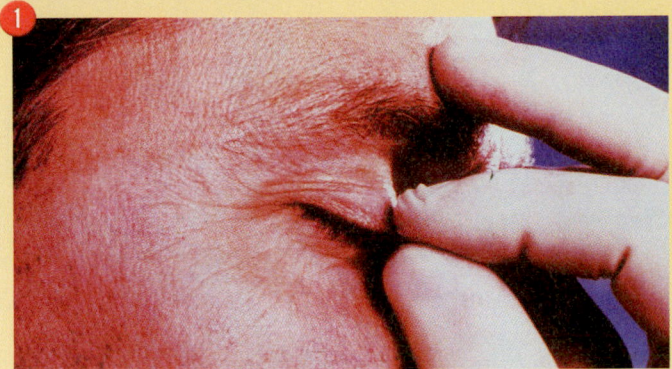

Have the patient look down, grasp the upper lashes, and gently pull the lid away from the eye.

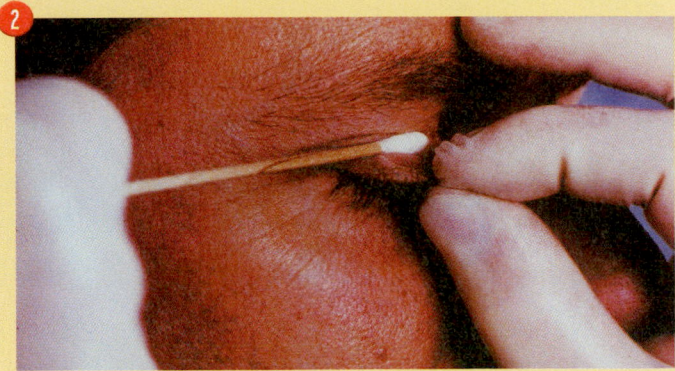

Place a cotton-tipped applicator on the upper lid, ½" from the lashes.

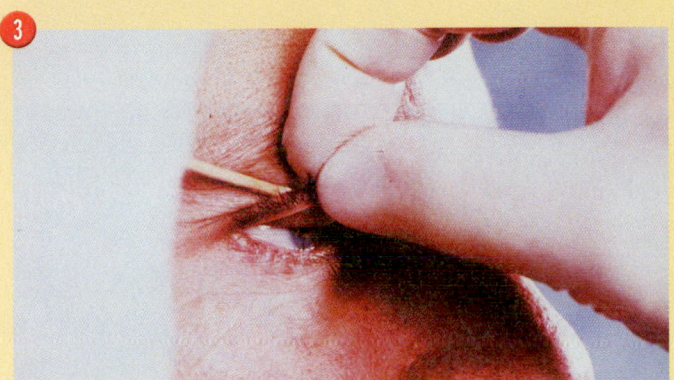

Pull the lid forward and up, folding it back over the applicator.

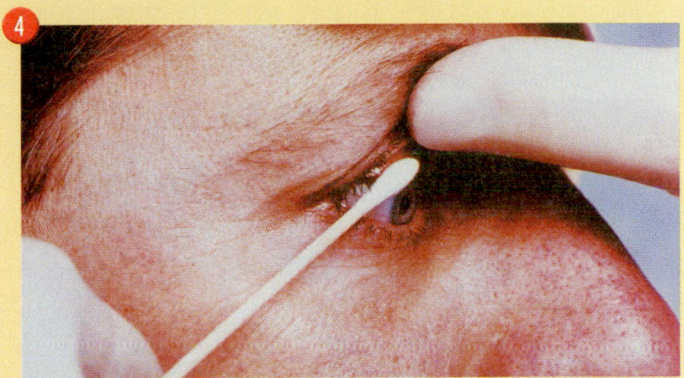

Gently remove the foreign object with a moistened, sterile applicator.

4. **If you see a foreign object, gently remove it** with a moistened, sterile, cotton-tipped applicator **(Step 4)**.

Foreign bodies ranging in size from a pencil to a sliver of metal may be impaled in the eye (◀ **Figure 20-7**). These objects must be removed by a physician. Your care involves stabilizing the object and preparing the patient for transport to definitive care. The greater the length of foreign object you can see sticking out of the eye, the more important stabilization becomes in avoiding further damage. Bandage the object in place to support it. Cover the eye itself with a moist, sterile dressing, and then surround the object with a doughnut-shaped collar made from roller gauze or a small gauze pack. Follow the steps in ▶ **Skill Drill 20-2**):

1. **Begin to prepare the doughnut ring** by wrapping a 2" gauze roll around your fingers and thumb enough times to make a thick dressing layer. You can adjust the inner diameter of what will become the ring by spreading your fingers or squeezing them together **(Step 1)**.

2. **Remove the gauze** from your hands and start wrapping the remainder of the gauze roll around this ring that you have created **(Step 2)**.

3. **Work your way around the ring** until you have wrapped all the way around it and finished the "doughnut" **(Step 3)**.

4. **Carefully place the ring over the eye** and impaled object, without bumping the object. You can then stabilize the object and the gauze collar with a roller bandage surrounding the head. Bandage both the injured and uninjured eyes to minimize eye movement and prevent further damage to the globe, since both eyes move in concert **(Step 4)**.

Skill Drill 20-2   Stabilizing a Foreign Object Impaled in the Eye

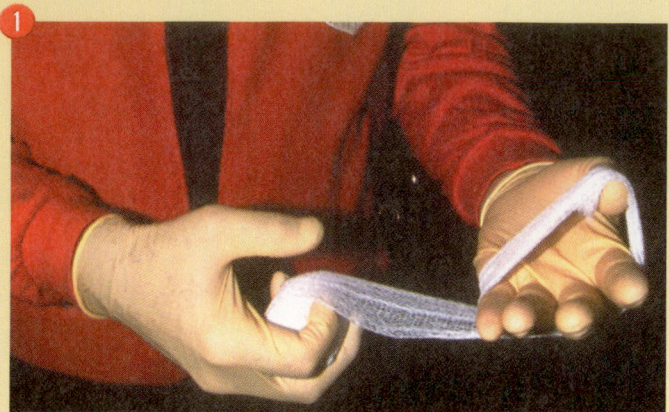

To prepare a doughnut ring, wrap a 2" gauze roll around your fingers and thumb seven or eight times. Adjust the diameter by spreading your fingers.

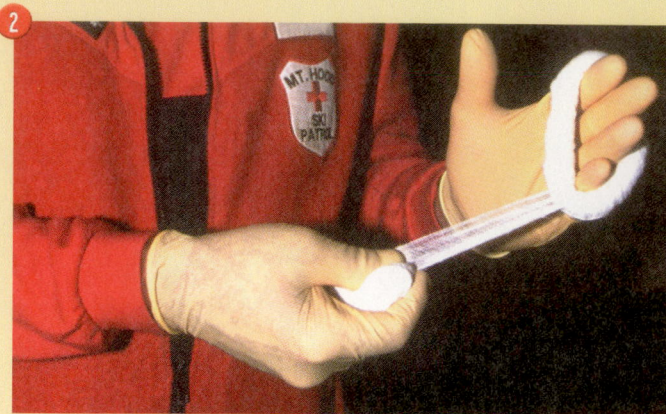

Wrap the remainder of the roll, . . .

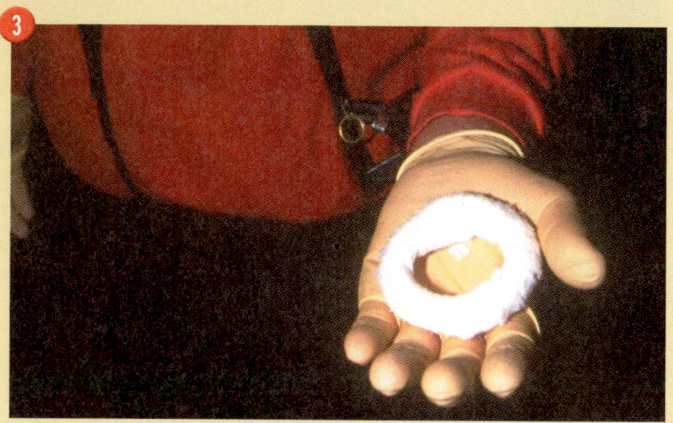

. . . working around the ring.

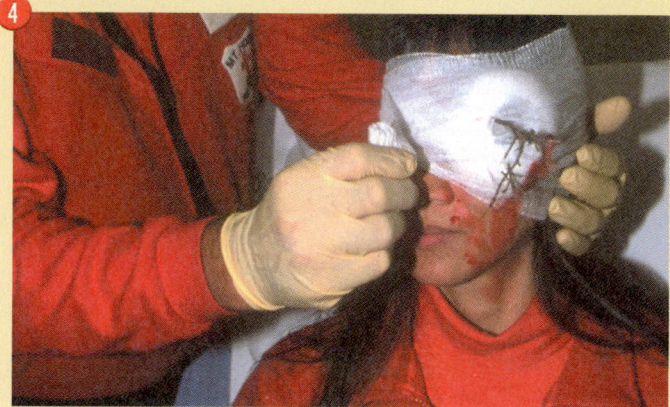

Place the dressing over the eye to hold the impaled object in place, then secure it with a gauze dressing.

Sometimes, foreign bodies, particularly small metal fragments, become completely embedded within the eye itself. The patient may not even be aware of the cause of the problem. Suspect such an injury when the history includes metal work (eg, hammering, exposure to splinters, vigorous filing) and when there are other signs of ocular injury. This type of injury must be handled by an ophthalmologist on an urgent basis. It may require X-rays and special equipment to find the foreign body.

Burns of the Eye

Chemicals, heat, and light rays all can burn the delicate tissues of the eye, often causing permanent damage. Your role is to stop the burn and prevent further damage.

CHEMICAL BURNS. Chemical burns, usually caused by acid or alkaline solutions, require immediate emergency care ▶ Figure 20-8 . This consists of flushing the eye with water or a sterile saline irrigation solution. If sterile saline is not available, you can use any clean water.

The idea is to direct the greatest amount of solution or water into the eye as gently as possible ▶ Figure 20-9 . Because opening the eye spontaneously may cause the patient pain, you may have to force the lids open to irrigate the eye adequately. Ideally, you will use a bulb or irrigation syringe, a nasal cannula, or some other device that will allow you to control the flow. IV fluid and tubing can be used. In some circumstances, you may have to resort to pouring water into the eye by holding the patient's head under a gently running faucet. You

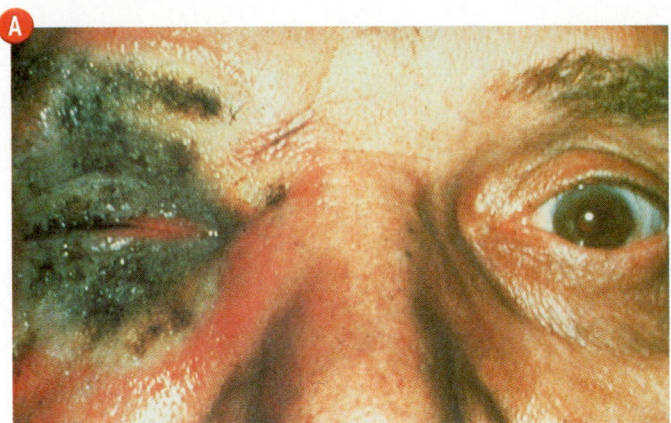

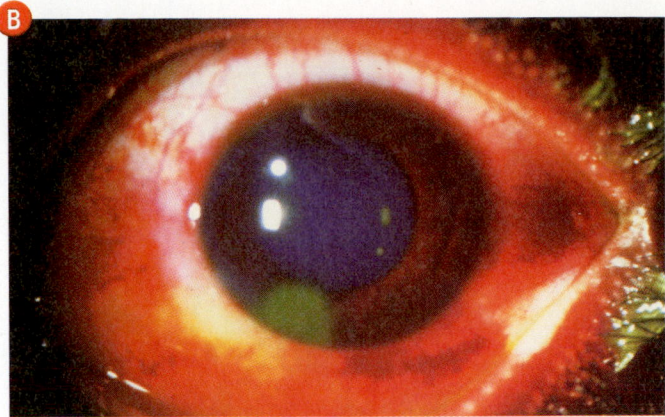

Figure 20-8   **A.** Chemical burns typically occur when an acid or alkali is splashed into the eye.   **B.** This figure shows a chemical burn from lye, an alkaline solution. Because lye can continue to damage the eye even when diluted, fast action is needed.

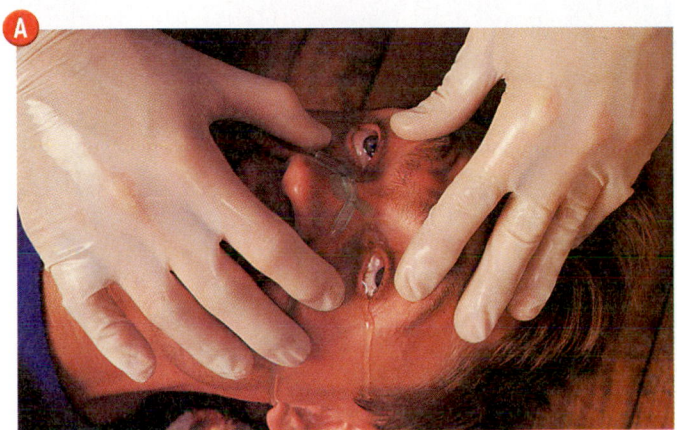

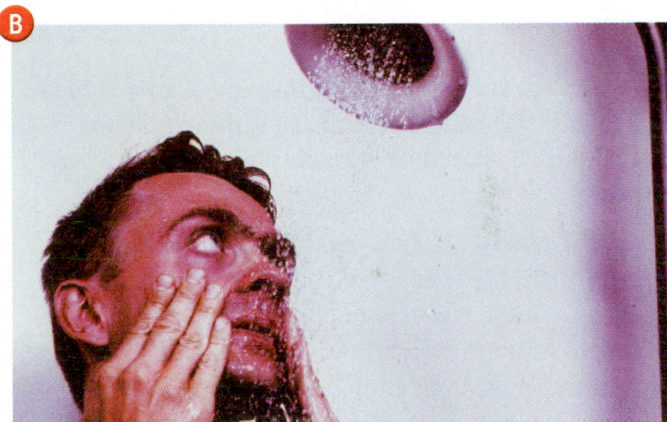

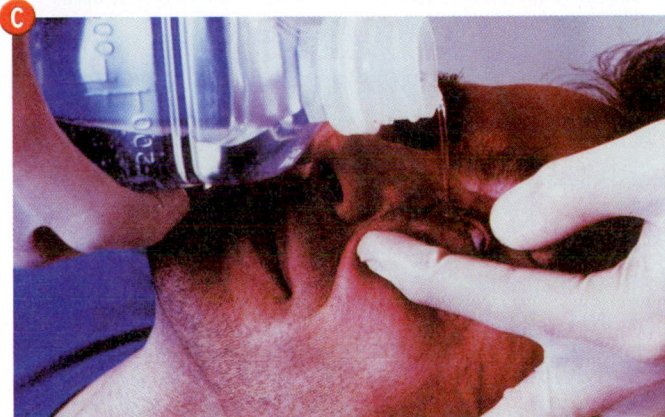

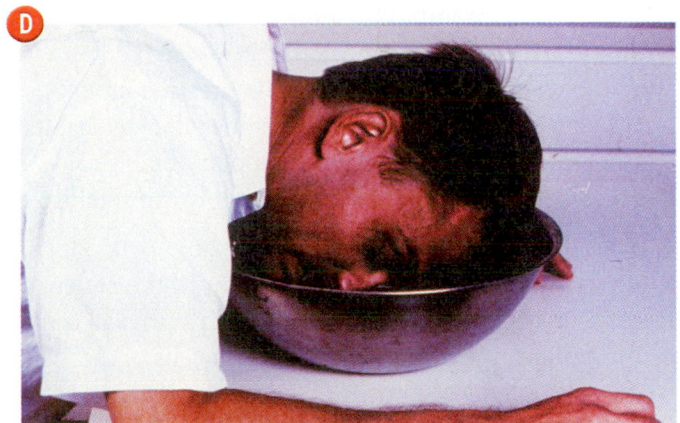

Figure 20-9   The following are four ways to effectively irrigate the eye.   **A.** Nasal cannula connected to IV fluid bag.   **B.** Shower.   **C.** Bottle.   **D.** Basin. Remember, you must protect the uninjured eye from the irrigating solution.

can even have the patient immerse his or her face in a large pan or basin of water and rapidly blink the affected eyelid. If only one eye is affected, care must be taken to avoid contaminated water getting into the unaffected eye.

Irrigate the eye for at least 5 minutes. If the burn was caused by an alkali or a strong acid, you should irrigate the eye for 20 minutes. Strong acids and all alkaline solutions can penetrate deeply, requiring a prolonged flush. Again, always take care to protect the uninjured eye and prevent irrigation fluid from running into it.

After you have completed irrigation, apply a clean, dry dressing to cover the eye, and transport the patient

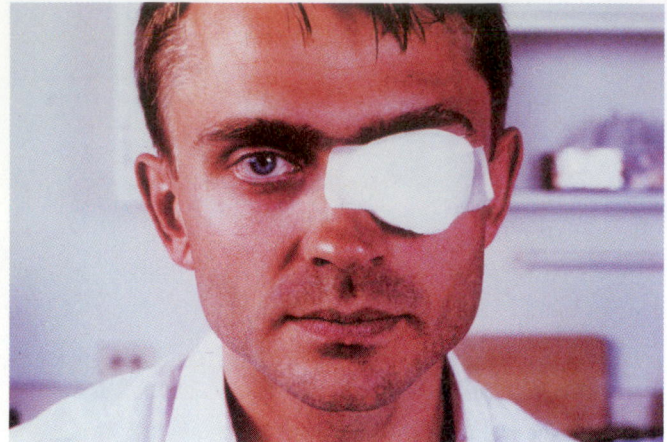

Figure 20-10 Apply a clean, dry dressing over the closed eye after you have finished irrigation.

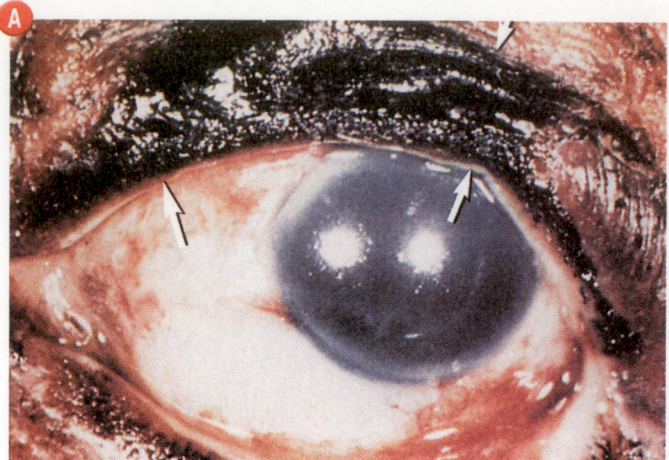

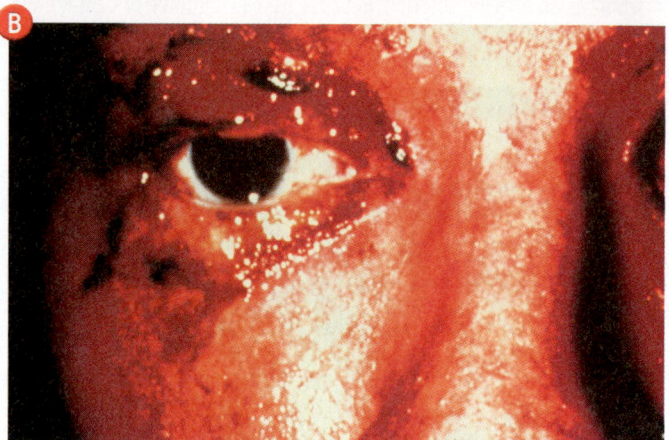

Figure 20-11 Thermal burns occasionally cause significant damage to the eyelids. **A.** Arrows show some full-thickness burns. **B.** Burns of the eyelids require immediate hospital care.

promptly to the hospital for further care ▲ **Figure 20-10**. If the irrigation can be carried out satisfactorily in the ambulance, it should be done during transport to save time.

THERMAL BURNS. When a patient is burned in the face during a fire, the eyes usually close rapidly because of the heat. This reaction is a natural reflex to protect the eye from further injury. However, the eyelids remain exposed and are frequently burned ▶ **Figure 20-11**. Burns of the eyelids require very specialized care. It is best to provide prompt transport for these patients without further examination. First, however, you should cover both eyes with a sterile dressing moistened with sterile saline. If sterile saline is not available, use clear tap water to which ½ teaspoon of table salt has been added per quart. You may apply eye shields over the dressing.

LIGHT BURNS. Infrared rays, eclipse light (if the patient has looked directly at the sun), and laser burns all can cause significant damage to the sensory cells of the eye when rays of light become focused on the retina. Retinal injuries that are caused by exposure to extremes of light are generally not painful but may result in permanent damage to vision.

Superficial burns of the eye can result from ultraviolet rays from an arc welding unit, light from prolonged exposure to a sunlamp, or reflected light from a bright snow-covered area (snow blindness). This kind of burn often is not painful at first but may become so 3 to 5 hours later, as the damaged cornea responds to the injury. A severe conjunctivitis with redness, swelling, and excessive tear production usually develops. You can ease the pain from these corneal burns by covering each eye with a sterile pad moistened with sterile saline and an eye shield. Have the patient lie down during transport to the hospital, and protect him or her from further exposure to bright light. This patient should be examined by a physician as soon as possible.

Lacerations

Lacerations of the eyelids require very careful repair to restore both appearance and function ▶ **Figure 20-12**. Bleeding may be heavy, but it usually can be controlled by gentle, manual pressure. If there is a laceration of the globe itself, apply no pressure to the eye; compression can interfere with the blood supply to the back of the eye and result in loss of vision from damage to the retina. Furthermore, pressure may squeeze the vitreous humor, iris, lens, or even the retina out of the eye and cause irreparable damage or blindness.

Follow these three important guidelines in treating penetrating injuries of the eye:

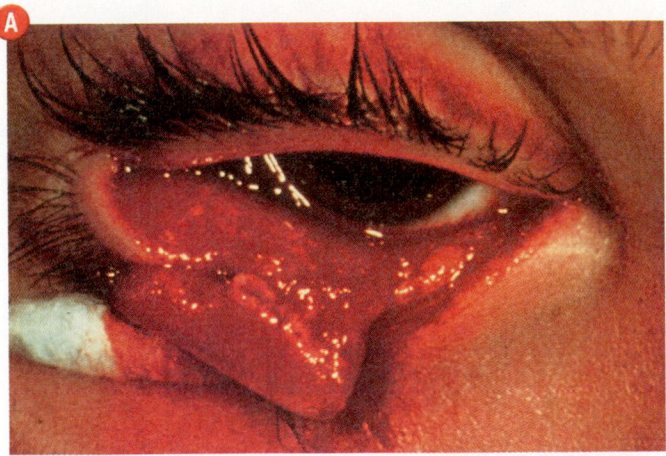

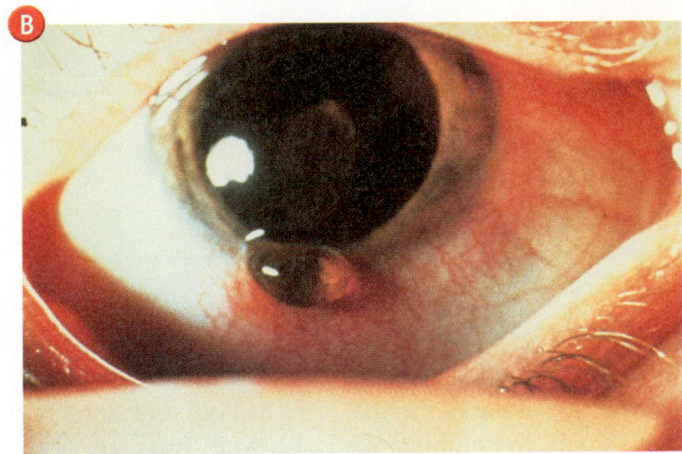

Figure 20-12 Lacerations are serious injuries that require prompt transport. **A.** While bleeding can be heavy, never exert pressure on the eye. **B.** Pressure may squeeze the vitreous humor, iris, lens, or even the retina out of the eye.

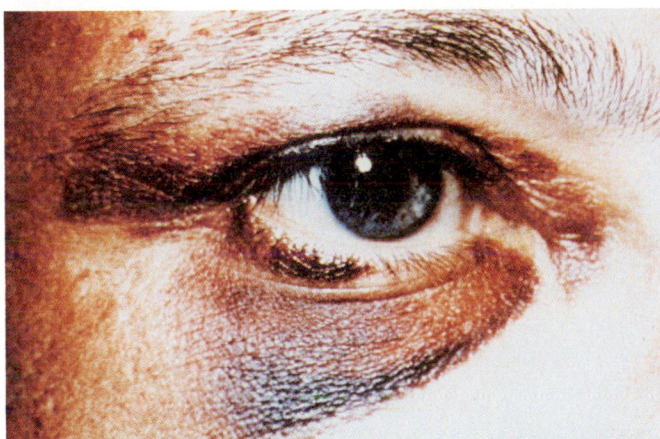

Figure 20-13 The typical "black eye" is caused by bleeding into the tissue around the orbit.

1. **Never exert pressure** on or manipulate the injured eye (globe) in any way.

2. **If part of the eyeball is exposed,** gently apply a sterile dressing moistened with sterile saline to prevent drying.

3. **Cover the injured eye** with a protective metal eye shield or sterile dressing.

On rare occasions following a serious injury, the eyeball may be displaced out of its socket. Do not attempt to reposition it. Simply cover the eye, and stabilize it with a moist, sterile dressing. Have the patient lie in a supine position while en route to the hospital.

Blunt Trauma

Blunt trauma can cause a number of serious injuries of the eye. These range from the ordinary "black eye," a result of bleeding into the tissue around the orbit

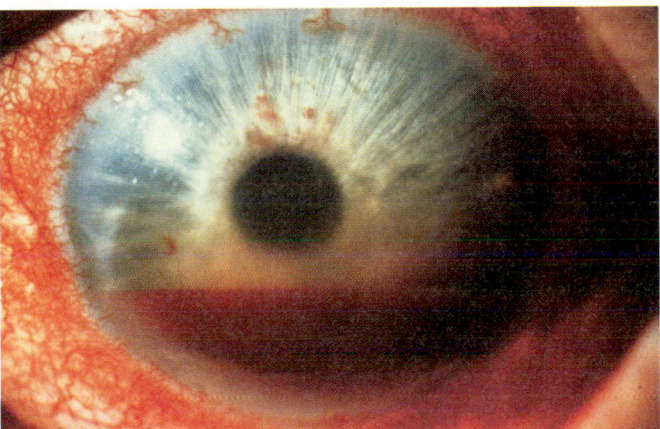

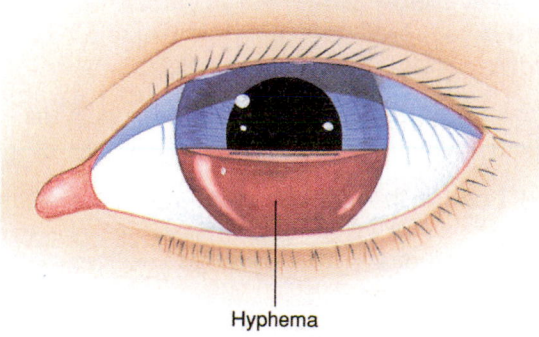

Hyphema

Figure 20-14 A hyphema, characterized by bleeding into the anterior chamber of the eye, is common following blunt trauma to the eye. This condition may seriously impair vision.

(▲ **Figure 20-13**), to a severely damaged globe. You may see an injury called <u>hyphema</u>, or bleeding into the anterior chamber of the eye, that obscures part or all of the iris (▲ **Figure 20-14**). This injury is common in blunt trauma and may seriously impair vision. It may also be a sign of a more serious injury to the globe.

Blunt trauma can also cause a fracture of the orbit, particularly of the bones that form its floor and support the globe. This injury is called a **blowout fracture**. The fragments of fractured bone can entrap some of the muscles that control eye movement, causing double vision ▶ **Figure 20-15** . Any patient who reports pain, double vision, or decreased vision following a blunt injury about the eye should be placed on a stretcher and transported promptly to the emergency department. Protect the eye from further injury with a metal shield; cover the other eye to minimize movement on the injured side.

Another possible result of blunt eye injury is retinal detachment. This injury is often seen in sports, especially boxing. It is painless but produces flashing lights, specks, or "floaters" in the field of vision and a cloud or shade over the patient's vision. Because the retina is separated from the nourishing choroid, this injury requires prompt medical attention to preserve vision in that eye.

Eye Injuries Following Head Injury

Abnormalities in the appearance or function of the eyes often occur following a closed head injury. Any of the following eye findings should alert you to the possibility of a head injury:

- One pupil larger than the other ▶ **Figure 20-16**

- The eyes not moving together or pointing in different directions

- Failure of the eyes to follow the movement of your finger as instructed

- Bleeding under the conjunctiva, which obscures the sclera (white portion) of the eye

- Protrusion or bulging of one eye

Record any of these observations, along with the time that you make them. For an unconscious patient, remember to keep the eyelids closed; drying of the ocular tissue can cause permanent injury and may result

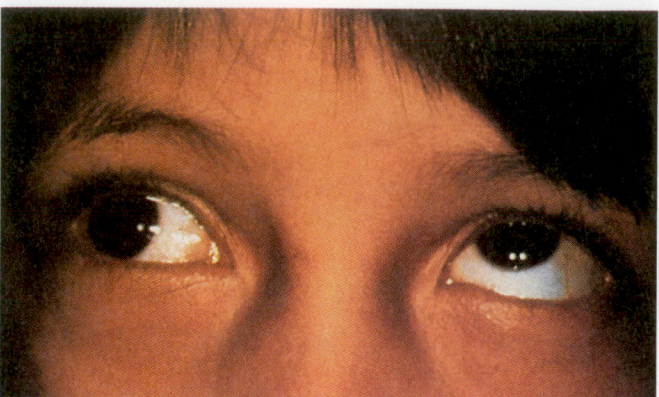

Figure 20-15 A patient with a blowout fracture will not move his or her eyes together because of muscle entrapment. The patient therefore sees double images of any object.

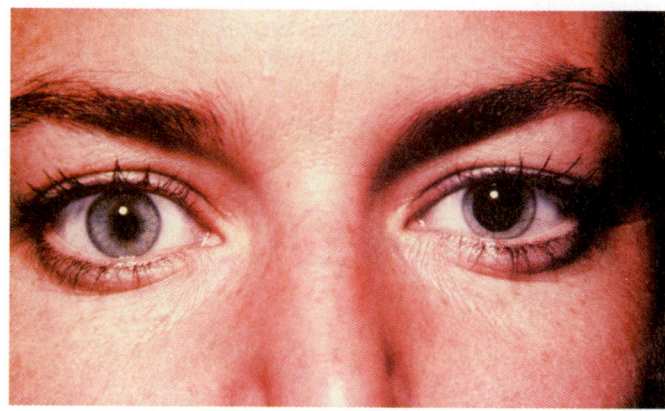

Figure 20-16 Variation of pupil size may indicate a head injury.

in blindness. Cover the lids with moist gauze, or hold them closed with clear tape. Normal tears will then keep the tissues moist.

Contact Lenses and Artificial Eyes

Small, hard contact lenses usually are tinted, making them relatively easy to see. Large, soft ones are clear and can be very difficult to see. In general, you should not attempt to remove either kind of lens from a patient. However, with an unresponsive patient, hard contact lenses should be removed if it will take more than 3 hours to transport the patient to the hospital. In any case, the eyes of such a patient should be taped shut if necessary to keep the eyes closed. You should never attempt to remove a lens from an eye that has been— or may have been—injured, since manipulating the lens can aggravate the problem. The only time that contact lenses should be removed immediately in the field is in the case of a chemical burn of the eye. In

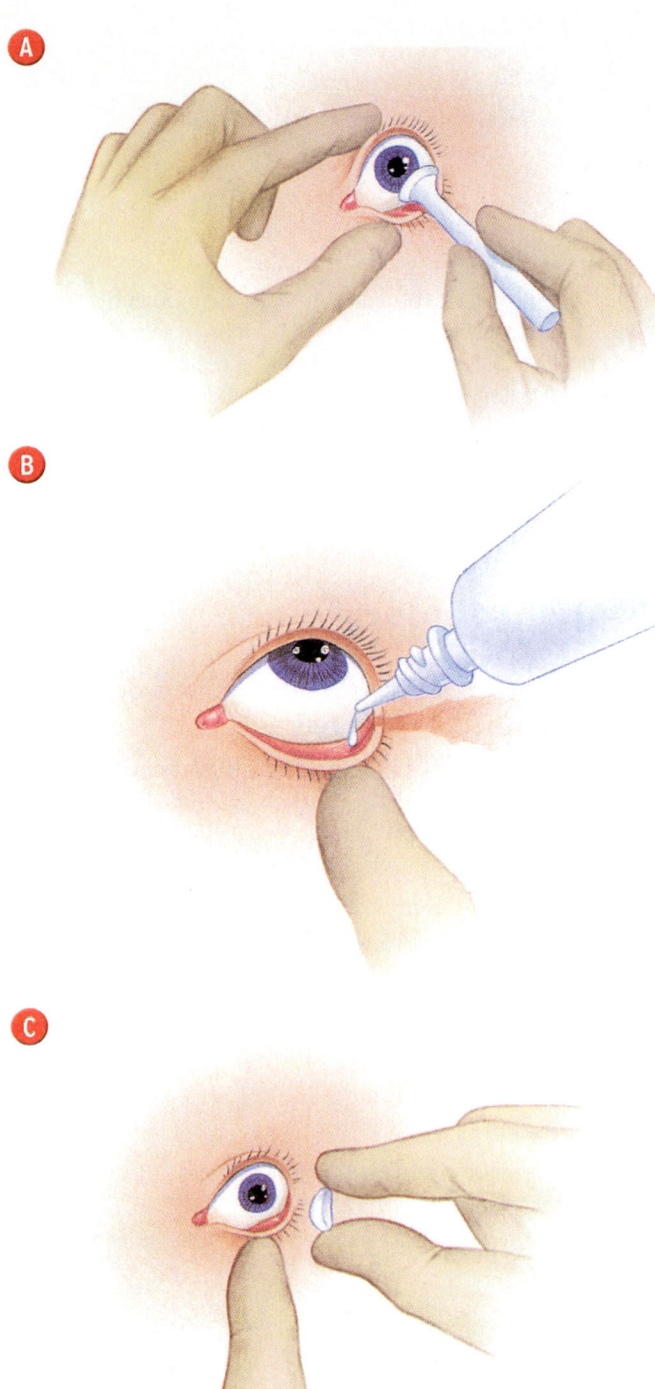

Wilderness Tips

With an unresponsive patient, hard contact lenses should be removed if it will take over three hours to transport the patient to the hospital. In any case, the eyes of such a patient should be taped shut if necessary to keep the eyes closed.

this situation, the lens can trap the chemical and make irrigation difficult.

If it is necessary to remove a hard contact lens, use a small suction cup, moistening the end with saline ◀ **Figure 20-17A** . To remove soft lenses, place one to two drops of saline onto the lens ◀ **Figure 20-17B** , gently pinch it between your thumb and index finger, and lift it off the surface of the eye ◀ **Figure 20-17C** .

Always advise the area clinic, EMS, and/or emergency department staff if a patient is wearing contact lenses so that the patient can be properly cared for at the hospital.

Occasionally, you may find yourself caring for a patient who is wearing an eye prosthesis, an artificial eye. Many people are surprised to find that it can be difficult to distinguish a prosthesis from a natural eye. You should suspect an eye of being artificial when it does not respond to light, move in concert with the opposite eye, or appear quite the same as its mate. If you think that a patient may have an artificial eye but you are not sure, go ahead and ask about it. Although no harm will be done if you care for an artificial eye as you would a normal one, you need to be totally clear about the patient's eye function.

Figure 20-17 Removing contact lenses should be limited to patients with burn injuries. **A.** To remove hard contact lenses, use a specialized suction cup moistened with sterile saline solution. **B.** To remove soft contact lenses, instill one or two drops of saline or irrigating solution. **C.** Next, pinch off the lens with your thumb and index finger.

Chapter Sweep

Ready for Review

The eye is globe-shaped, about 1" in diameter, and located within a bony socket called the orbit, which is actually part of the skull. Any severe injury to the face or head can potentially damage the eyeball or eye muscles. The fluid in the back of the eye is called the vitreous humor and cannot be replaced; the fluid in the front of the eye is called the aqueous humor and can be replaced with proper medical treatment. The eye works like a camera, with the iris and pupil making adjustments to light and the retina acting like film. Nerve endings in the retina send impulses through the optic nerve to the brain, which interprets them as vision.

In assessing a patient with a possible eye injury, look for swollen or lacerated eyelids, a bright red conjunctiva, irregular pupil reactions or eye movements, and a cornea that no longer appears wet and smooth. Foreign bodies on the surface of the eye should be irrigated gently with a normal saline solution; always flush from the nose side of the eye toward the outside. If a foreign body is on the undersurface of the lid, remove it with a moist, cotton-tipped applicator. Do not remove foreign bodies that are stuck to the cornea. If a foreign body is impaled in the eye, bandage the object in place, using roller gauze to create a collar around it, until it can be removed by a physician. Small metal fragments that are entirely embedded within the eye must be treated by an ophthalmologist.

Chemicals, heat, and light rays can all burn the eyes, causing permanent damage. Irrigate chemical burns with saline solution or clean water for at least 5 minutes, then apply a clean, dry dressing to the eye and transport the patient promptly. Transport the patient with heat burns of the eyelid immediately, covering both eyes with a sterile, moist dressing. Superficial burns of the eye resulting from exposure to ultraviolet rays or a sunlamp can become very painful after several hours. You can ease the pain from these corneal burns by covering the eyes with a sterile, moist pad and eye shield; the patient should lie down during transport.

Use gentle manual pressure to control bleeding from a lacerated eyelid, but do not apply pressure to a laceration of the globe itself. Instead, apply a moist, sterile dressing to prevent drying, cover the injured eye with a protective metal shield, cover the opposite eye, and transport the patient. Never attempt to reposition a displaced eyeball. Blunt trauma can cause a range of injuries, including hyphema, retinal detachment, and blowout fractures. Any patient who complains of pain, double vision, or decreased vision following a blunt injury about the eye should be placed on a stretcher and transported promptly to the emergency department.

Suspect a head injury if the patient has one pupil larger than the other, eyes not moving together, bleeding under the conjunctiva, or protrusion or bulging of one eye. Keep the eyelids closed if the patient is unconscious so that the eyes do not dry out.

Never remove contact lenses from an injured eye unless the injury is a chemical burn.

Vital Vocabulary

blowout fracture Fracture of the orbit or of the bones that support the floor of the orbit.

conjunctiva The delicate membrane that lines the eyelids and covers the exposed surface of the eye.

conjunctivitis Inflammation of the conjunctiva.

cornea The transparent tissue layer in front of the pupil and iris of the eye.

globe The eyeball.

hyphema Bleeding into the anterior chamber of the eye, obscuring part or all of the iris.

iris The muscle and surrounding tissue behind the cornea that dilate and constrict the pupil, regulating the amount of light that enters the eye; pigment in this tissue gives the eye its color.

lacrimal glands The glands that produce fluids to keep the eye moist; also called tear glands.

lens The transparent part of the eye through which images are focused on the retina.

optic nerve A cranial nerve that transmits visual information to the brain.

orbit The bony eye socket.

pupil The circular opening in the middle of the iris that admits light to the back of the eye.

retina The light-sensitive area of the eye where images are projected; a layer of cells at the back of the eye that changes the light image into electrical impulses, which are carried by the optic nerve to the brain.

retinal detachment Separation of the retina from its attachments at the back of the eye.

sclera The tough, fibrous white portion of the eye that protects the more delicate inner structures.

snow blindness Sunburn to the cornea of the eye.

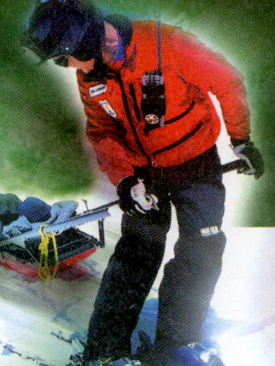

Assessment in Action

There has been a flash fire explosion, cause unknown, in which a camper has sustained burns to the face, neck, and hands. After stumbling into a fellow camper, the injured camper falls onto his face but remains conscious.

Assessment reveals superficial and partial-thickness burns on the left side of his face involving his ear, left cheek, nose, and lips. His left eye appears swollen, with bruising appearing on both his upper and lower eyelids. His left eye appears to be tearing; the tears appear clear. A section of his hair is singed as is his left eyebrow and eyelashes. He also has smoke residue on the left side of his face. As you progress through your assessment, you cannot convince the patient to open his eye because "it hurts too much." He does not know if he could see out of that eye immediately after the incident. Vital signs include a pulse of 134 beats/min, respirations of 26 breaths/min, and a blood pressure of 124/82 mm Hg.

1. Excessive tearing from his left eye may indicate which of the following?
   A. The eye is irritated.   **B.** He has lacerated the globe.
   C. A hyphema is present.   **D.** The lens has ruptured.

2. The purpose of tearing is to:
   A. express emotions such as sadness or happiness.
   B. flush the eye of any foreign material.
   C. prevent any mucus from clouding the eye.
   D. provide nourishment to the conjunctiva.

3. Which of the following should be done for this patient's eyes immediately?
   A. Patching both eyes to prevent any unnecessary movement of the eye itself
   B. Attempting to visualize his eye to determine appropriate treatment
   C. Irrigating his eyes immediately; visualization is not necessary
   D. Applying direct pressure with dry, sterile dressings for 3 to 5 minutes

4. You attempt to look at the patient's eye and discover that the conjunctiva of his eye is extremely red and irritated. You notice black powder located on the right half of his globe. You also note a hyphema is present. Appropriate treatment includes which of the following?
   A. Immediate patching of both eyes
   B. Applying a moist, sterile dressing over the injured eye
   C. Covering the injured eye with a protective metal eye shield
   D. Irrigating the eye to remove the powder

5. Which of the following is the appropriate method to use to irrigate this patient's eye?
   A. Running water from the right eye to the left eye
   B. Running water from the left eye to the right eye
   C. Squirting water under high pressure into the left eye
   D. Flushing from the nasal side of the eye to the lateral side

6. Your patient is complaining of seeing a very bright light prior to the explosion and now has pain and excessive tearing. After irrigating his eye, the best method of treatment en route to the hospital includes:
   A. shutting off all interior lights and maintaining a calm atmosphere.
   B. patching both eyes with sterile, moist pads and transport supine.
   C. transporting in a sitting position and keep him warm en route.
   D. not patching the eyes but protecting them from bright lights.

7. Because this was an explosion from an unknown source that occurred in close proximity to the patient, what other injuries should you suspect?
   A. Ruptured eardrums   **B.** Lung damage
   C. Ruptured abdominal   **D.** Ruptured abdominal solid
      hollow organs   organs

Challenging Questions

8. On arrival at the hospital, your patient starts to have a nosebleed. The physician tells you the bleeding is coming from the patient's eye. How could this be?

9. Why should patients with traumatic eye injuries be transported in a supine position?

10. What is the advantage of having both eyes patched?

Points to Ponder

It was one of the most glorious days you have ever had climbing. The weather was clear, the snow firm, and your partner strong. After spending a couple hours on the summit shooting pictures and celebrating your uneventful descent to high camp, you turn in and fall asleep with a broad grin. The next morning your first attempt to open your eyes is met with agony. Any light is painful, and just moving your eyes from side to side produces tears. What injury are you experiencing and how might you begin to treat yourself?

Issues Dealing with Disabling Injuries, Safety, Partner Relationships, Admitting Mistakes, Transportation

Online Outlook

Injuries to the eye are very common, and you will encounter many in your work as a rescuer. Proper emergency medical care for these injuries can minimize damage, which can often be severe. Review your knowledge of different types of eye injuries by completing Exercise 20 at www.OECzone.com.

Face and Throat Injuries

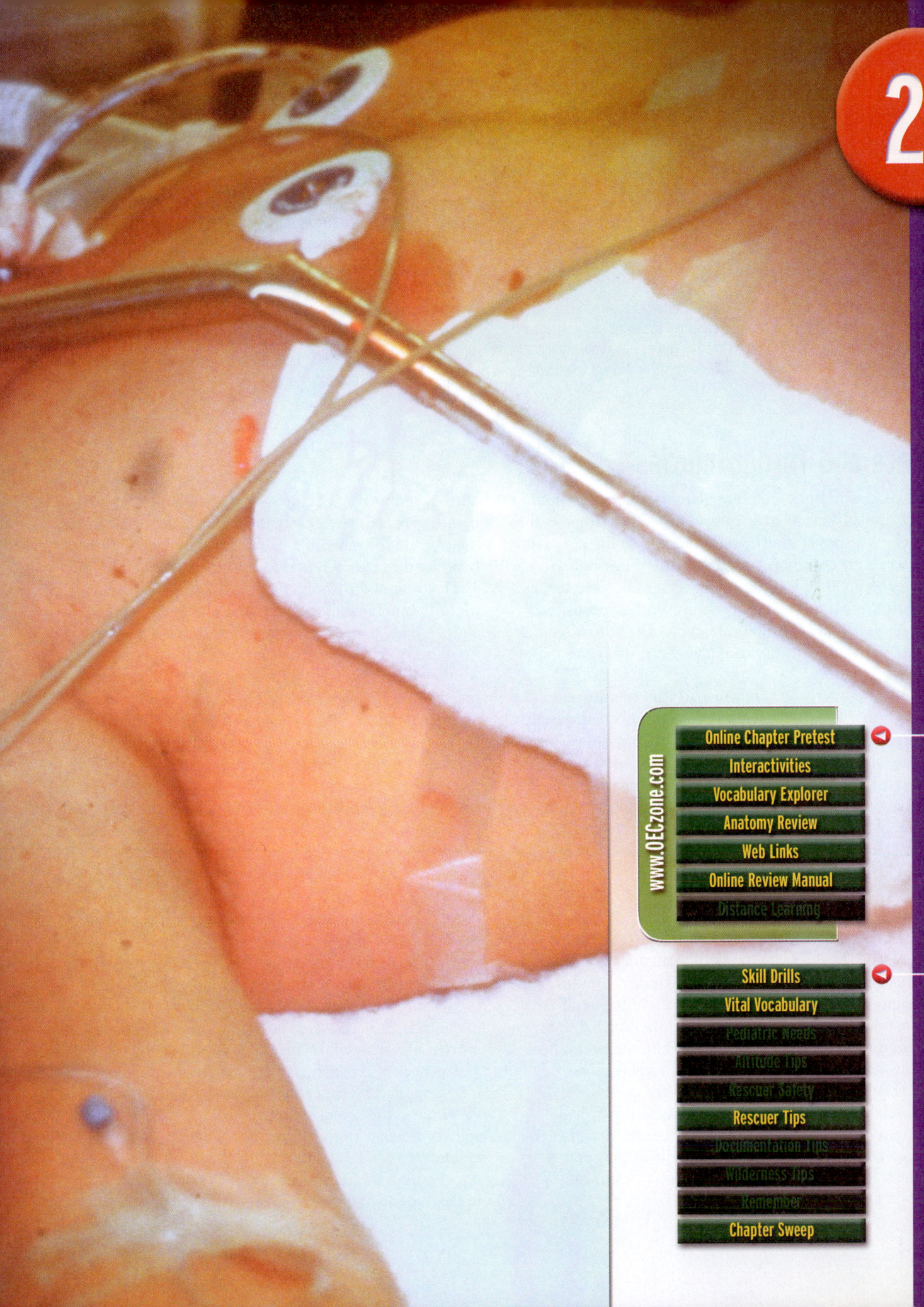

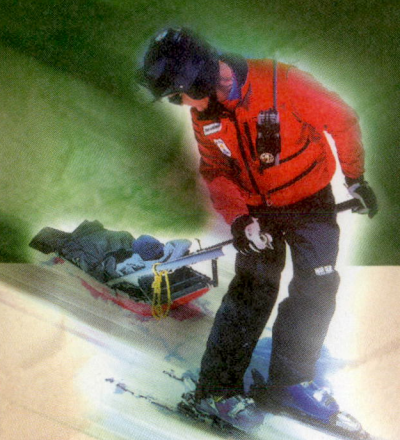

You are the rescuer

You respond to a call where a 19-year-old female skier has collided with a snowboarder. She was hit in the throat by the snowboard and is having difficulty breathing.

Because of the associated airway management implications, injuries to the face and/or throat must be carefully assessed and managed. This chapter offers information that you will need to know to manage these injuries appropriately. It will also help you answer the following questions:

1. What are some of the physical findings you'd expect when caring for a patient with a suspected facial fracture?

2. Can you list at least two possible causes of airway obstruction for a patient with facial injuries?

Face and Throat Injuries

The face and neck are particularly vulnerable to injury because of their relatively unprotected positions on the body. Soft-tissue injuries and fractures to the bones of the face are common and vary greatly in severity. Some are potentially life-threatening, and many leave disfiguring scars if not treated properly. With appropriate prehospital and hospital care, what may at first seem to be a devastating injury can have a surprisingly good outcome.

As a rescuer, your objective is to prevent further injury, particularly to the cervical spine, to manage any acute airway problems, and to control bleeding. This chapter first reviews the anatomy of the head and neck, then examines the factors that can produce upper airway obstruction. A discussion of outdoor emergency care of soft-tissue wounds of the face, nose, and ear; facial fractures; penetrating injuries of the neck; and dental injuries follows.

Anatomy of the Head and Neck

The head is divided into two parts: the cranium and the face. The **cranium**, or skull, contains the brain, which connects to the spinal cord through the **foramen magnum**, a large opening at the base of the skull. The most posterior portion of the cranium is called the **occiput**. On each side of the cranium, the lateral portions are called the temples or temporal regions. Between the temporal regions and the occiput lie the parietal regions. The forehead is called the frontal region. Just anterior to the ear, in the temporal region, you can feel the pulse of the superficial temporal artery. The thick skin covering the cranium, which usually bears hair, is called the scalp.

The face is composed of the eyes, ears, nose, mouth, cheeks, and jowls. Six bones—the nasal bone, the two **maxillae** (upper jawbones), the two zygomas (cheekbones), and the mandible (jawbone)—are the major bones of the face (▶ Figure 21-1).

The orbit of the eye is composed of the lower edge of the frontal bone of the skull, the zygoma, the maxilla, and the nasal bone. The bony orbit protects the eye from injury. By viewing the face from the side, you can see the eyeball recessed in the orbit. Only the proximal one third of the nose—the bridge—is formed by bone. The remaining two thirds is formed by cartilage. Unlike the nose, the exposed portion of the ear is composed entirely of cartilage that is covered by skin. The external, visible part of the ear is called the **pinna** (▶ Figure 21-2). The earlobes are the fleshy portions at the bottom of each ear. The **tragus** is a small, rounded, fleshy bulge immediately anterior to the ear canal. The superficial temporal artery can be palpated just anterior to the tragus. About 1″ posterior to the external opening of the ear is a prominent bony mass at the base of the skull called the **mastoid process**.

The **mandible** forms the jaw and chin. Motion of the mandible occurs at the **temporomandibular joint (TMJ)**, which lies just in front of the ear on either side of the face. Below the ear and anterior to the mastoid process, the angle of the mandible is easily palpated.

The neck also contains many important structures. It is supported by the cervical spine, or the first seven vertebrae in the spinal column (C1 through C7). The spinal cord exits from the foramen magnum and lies within the spinal canal formed by the vertebrae. The upper part of the esophagus and the trachea lie deep in the midline of the neck. The carotid arteries may be

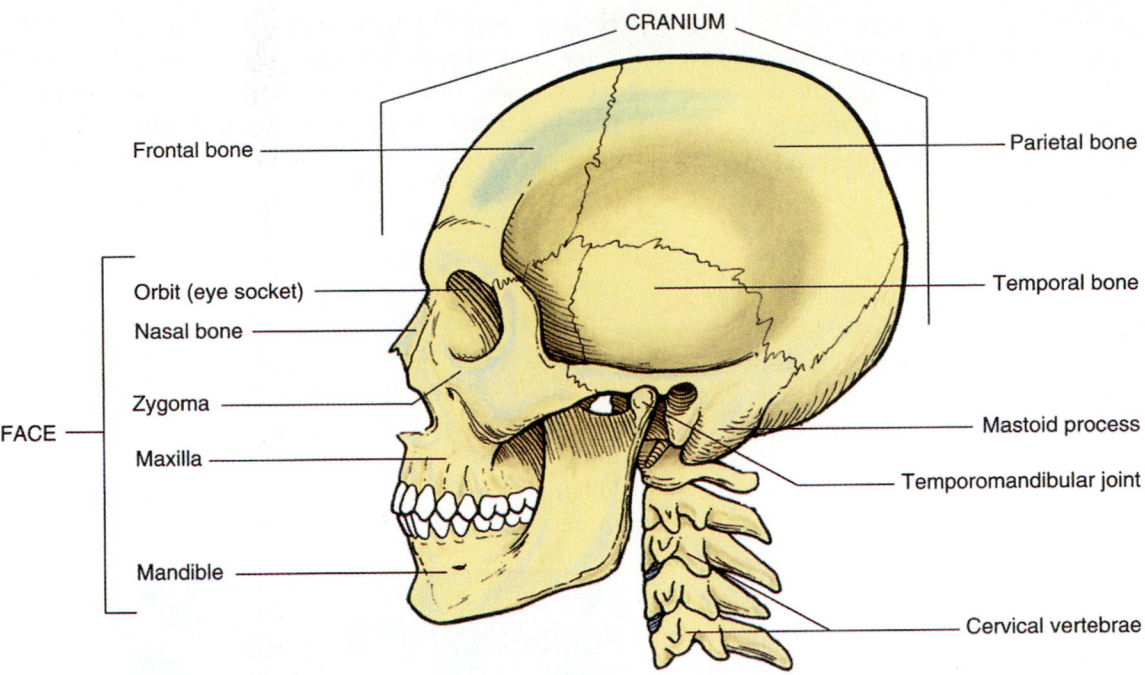

CRANIUM

Frontal bone

Parietal bone

Orbit (eye socket)

Nasal bone

Temporal bone

FACE

Zygoma

Maxilla

Mastoid process

Temporomandibular joint

Mandible

Cervical vertebrae

Figure 21-1 The face is composed of six bones: the nasal bone, two maxillae, two zygomas, and the mandible.

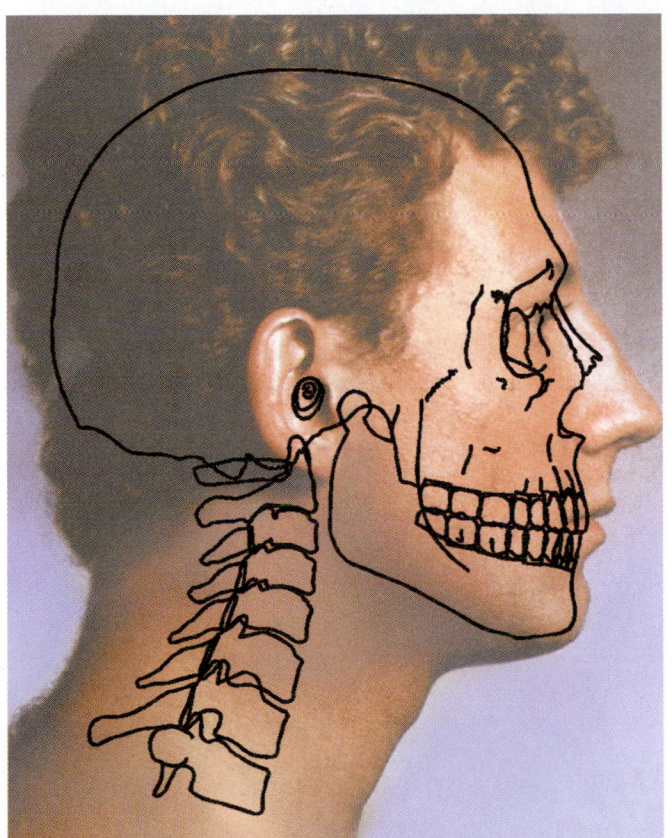

Figure 21-2 Principal features of the head and neck include the pinna, the tragus, the mastoid process, the occiput, the seventh cervical vertebra, and the temporomandibular joint.

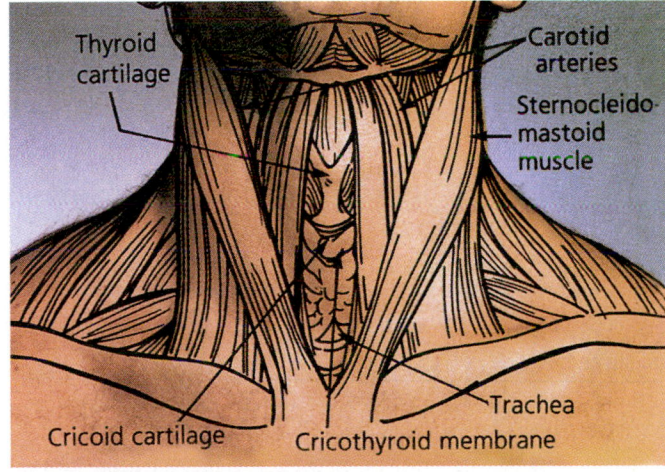

Thyroid cartilage

Carotid arteries

Sternocleido-mastoid muscle

Trachea

Cricoid cartilage

Cricothyroid membrane

Figure 21-3 Important landmarks in the neck include the cricoid cartilage, the thyroid cartilage, the carotid arteries, the cricothyroid membrane, and the sternocleidomastoid muscles.

found on either side of the trachea, along with the jugular veins and several nerves.

Several useful landmarks can be palpated and seen in the neck ◄ **Figure 21-3** . The most obvious is the firm prominence in the center of the anterior surface commonly known as the **Adam's apple**. Specifically, this prominence is the upper part of the larynx, formed by the thyroid cartilage. It is more prominent in men than in women. The other portion of the larynx is the cricoid cartilage, a firm ridge of cartilage inferior to the thyroid cartilage, which is somewhat more difficult to palpate. Between the thyroid cartilage and the cricoid cartilage in the midline of the neck is a soft depression, the cricothyroid membrane. This is a thin sheet of connective tissue (fascia) that joins the two cartilages. The cricothyroid membrane is covered at this point only by skin.

Inferior to the larynx, several additional firm ridges are palpable in the anterior midline. These ridges are the cartilage rings of the trachea. The trachea connects the larynx with the main air passages of the lungs (the bronchi). On either side of the lower larynx and the upper trachea lies the thyroid gland. Unless it is enlarged, this gland is usually not palpable.

Pulsations of the carotid arteries are easily palpable in a groove 1 to 2 cm lateral to the larynx. Lying immediately adjacent to these arteries, but not palpable, are the internal jugular veins and several important nerves. Lateral to these vessels and nerves lie the **sternocleido-mastoid muscles**. These muscles originate from the mastoid process of the cranium and insert into the medial border of each collarbone and the sternum at the base of the neck. They allow movement of the head.

A series of bony prominences lie posteriorly, in the midline of the neck. They are the spines of the cervical vertebrae. The lower cervical spines are more prominent than the upper ones. They are more easily palpable when the neck is in flexion. At the base of the neck posteriorly, the most prominent spine is the seventh cervical vertebra.

Injuries of the Face

Injuries about the face often lead to partial or complete obstruction of the upper airway. Several factors may contribute to the obstruction. Bleeding from facial injuries can be very heavy, producing large blood clots in the upper airway. These clots can lead to complete obstruction, particularly in a patient who is not fully conscious. In particular, direct injuries to the nose and mouth, the larynx, or the trachea are often the source of significant bleeding. In addition, as a result of an injury, loosened teeth or dentures may become dislodged into the throat, where they may be swallowed or aspirated. The swelling that often accompanies injury to the soft tissues in these areas can also contribute to the obstruction.

The airway may also be affected when the patient's head is turned to the side, as so often is the case with a patient who has an altered level of consciousness or is unconscious. Other factors that interfere with normal respirations include possible injuries to the brain and/or

cervical spine that may be associated with facial injuries. If the great vessels in the neck are injured, significant bleeding and pressure on the upper airway are common; these result in airway obstruction as well.

Soft-Tissue Injuries

Soft-tissue injuries of the face and scalp are very common. The skin and underlying tissues in these areas have a rich blood supply, so bleeding from penetrating injuries may be heavy. Indeed, even minor soft-tissue wounds of the face and scalp may bleed a great deal. A blunt injury that does not break the skin may cause a break in a blood vessel wall, leading blood to collect under the skin; this is called a **hematoma** (▼ **Figure 21-4**). Often, a flap of skin is peeled back, or **avulsed**, from the underlying muscle and fascia (▼ **Figure 21-5**).

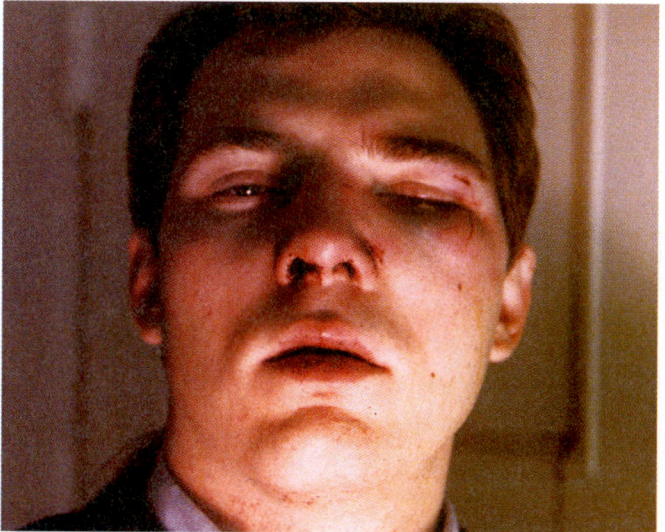

Figure 21-4 Facial hematoma. These injuries are often caused by hitting the ground during a "faceplant" or by interpersonal altercations.

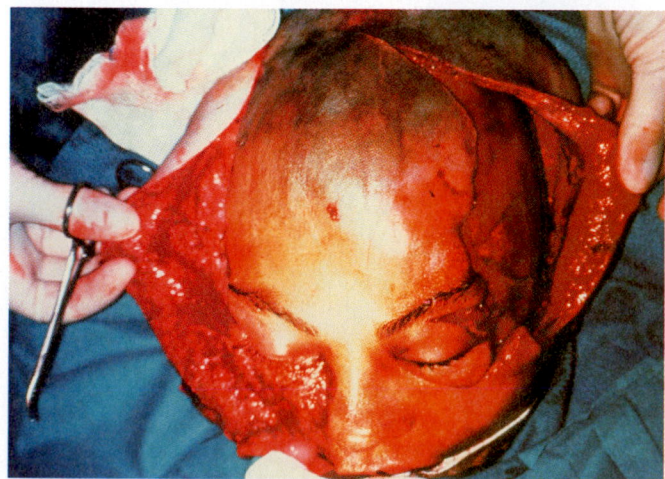

Figure 21-5 A major avulsion injury is characterized by a large flap of skin that is peeled back from the underlying muscle and tissue.

The emergency care of soft-tissue injuries to the face and scalp is the same as treatment of soft-tissue injuries elsewhere on the body. You should assess the ABCs and care for any life threats first. Remember also to follow BSI precautions in all cases.

Your first step is to open and clear the airway. Remember that blood draining into the throat can produce vomiting and airway obstruction. Take appropriate precautions if you suspect that the patient has sustained a cervical spine injury; be sure to avoid moving the neck. Use the jaw-thrust to open the patient's airway, and then suction the mouth. Once the patient is immobilized in a cervical collar and on a backboard, you can turn the backboard to one side to allow any blood or vomitus to drain out of the mouth rather than pool in the pharynx and obstruct the airway.

Control bleeding by applying direct manual pressure with a dry, sterile dressing. Use roller gauze, wrapped around the circumference of the head, to hold a pressure dressing in place ▼ **Figure 21-6** . Do not apply excessive pressure if there is a possibility of underlying skull fracture. When an injury exposes the brain, eye, or other structures, cover the exposed parts with a moist, sterile dressing to protect them from further damage ▶ **Figure 21-7** . For injuries in which the skin is not broken, apply ice locally to help control the swelling of bruised tissues.

For soft-tissue injuries around the mouth, you should always check for bleeding inside the mouth. Broken teeth and lacerations to the tongue may cause profuse bleeding and obstruction of the upper airway ▼ **Figure 21-8** . Often, the patient will swallow the blood from lacerations inside the mouth, so the hemorrhage may not be apparent. You should also inspect the

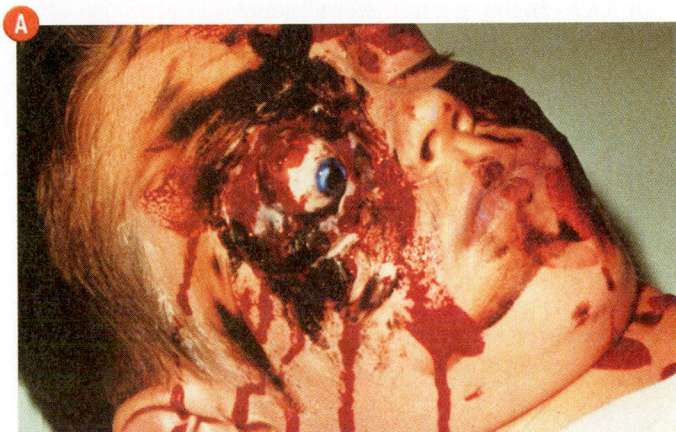

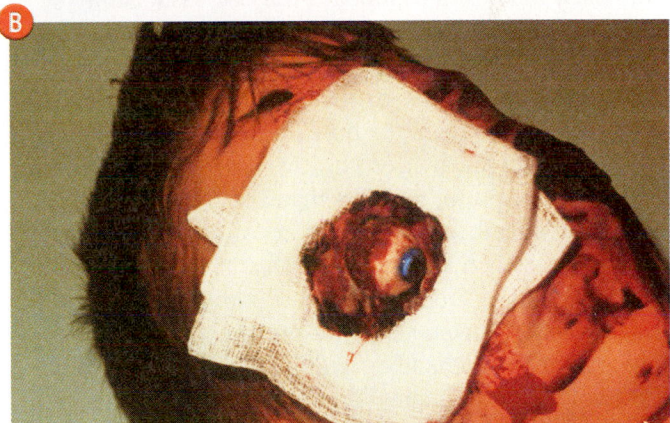

Figure 21-7   An injury that exposes the brain, eye, or other structures (A) should be covered with a moist, sterile dressing to prevent further damage (B).

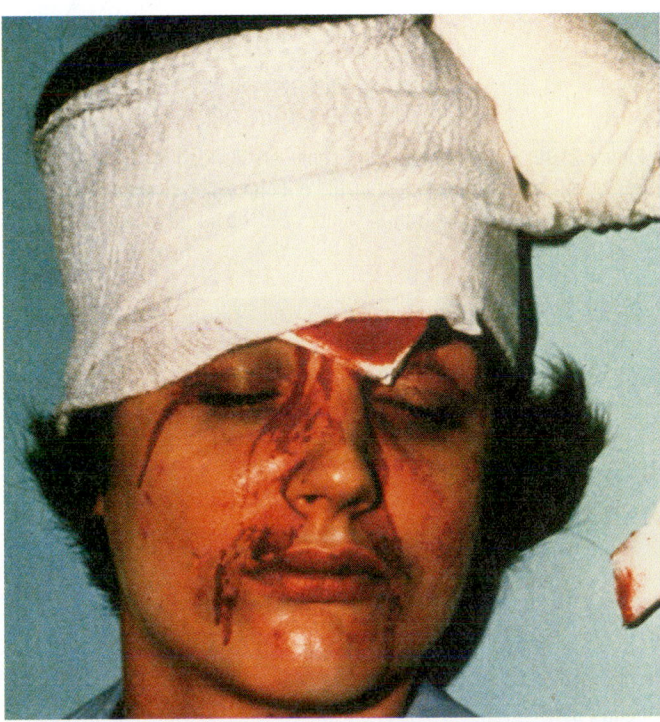

Figure 21-6   Use roller gauze, wrapped around the circumference of the head, to hold a pressure dressing in place.

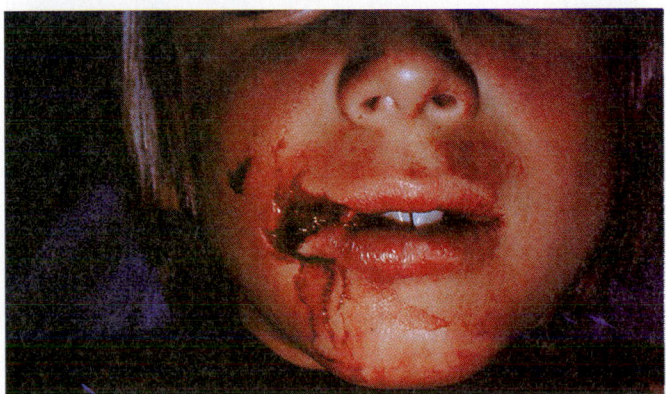

Figure 21-8   Soft-tissue injuries around the mouth can be associated with profuse bleeding inside the mouth and obstruction of the airway.

inside of the mouth for bleeding and hidden injuries in patients who have sustained facial trauma. Remember that patients who swallow blood are prone to vomiting.

Often, physicians will be able to graft a piece of avulsed skin back into the appropriate position. For this reason, if you find portions of avulsed skin that have become separated, you should wrap them in a sterile dressing, place them in a plastic bag, and keep them cool. Deliver the bag to the emergency department along with the patient. In many avulsion injuries, the skin will still be attached in a loose flap ▼ **Figure 21-9** . Rinse the flap and the bed where the flap originated with clean water or saline. Place the flap in a position that is as close to normal as possible, and hold it in place with a dry, sterile dressing. These steps will help to increase the patient's chances of being restored to normal appearance.

Injuries of the Nose

The nose often takes the brunt of deliberate physical assaults and car crashes. Blunt injuries to the nose caused by a fist or a dashboard may be associated with fractures and soft-tissue injuries of the face, head injuries, and/or injuries to the cervical spine.

In assessing injuries involving the nose, it helps to picture the inside of the nose itself ▶ **Figure 21-10** . The nasal cavity is divided into two sections or chambers by the nasal septum, which is made of cartilage. Within each nasal chamber, there are layers of bone called the **turbinates**, which are covered with a moist lining. Both chambers have a superior turbinate, a middle turbinate, and an inferior turbinate. As we breathe, the air moves through the nasal chambers and is humidified as it passes over the turbinates. Directly above the nose are the frontal sinuses and, on either side, the orbit of the eye.

All these structures should be assessed for injury. In cases of severe injury, there may also be injury to the

cervical spine. Keep in mind that cerebrospinal fluid (CSF) may escape down through the nose (or ears) following a fracture at the base of the skull. If blood or drainage contains CSF, a characteristic staining of the dressing will occur.

You can control bleeding from abrasions and lacerations to the nose by applying a sterile dressing. If the patient is bleeding heavily from the nose, place the patient in a sitting position, leaning forward, and pinch the nostrils together ▼ **Figure 21-11** . For a detailed

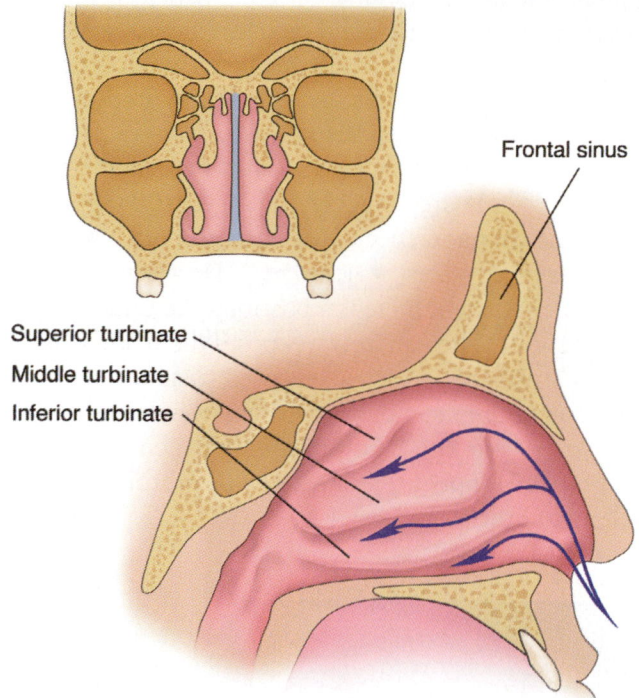

Frontal sinus

Superior turbinate
Middle turbinate
Inferior turbinate

Figure 21-10   The nose has two chambers, divided by the septum. Each chamber is composed of layers of bone called turbinates. Above the nose are the frontal sinuses and, on either side, the orbit of the eye.

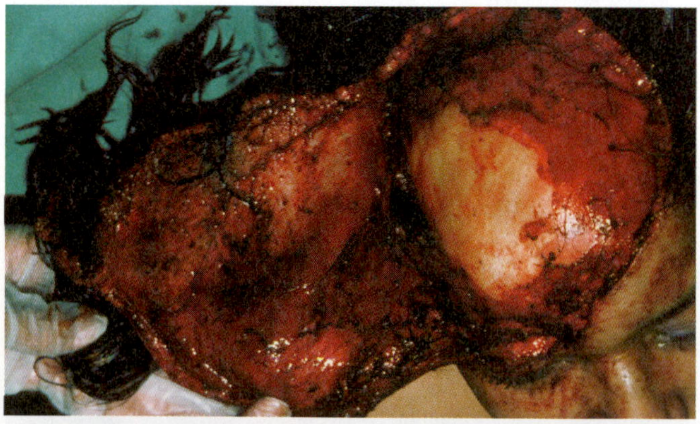

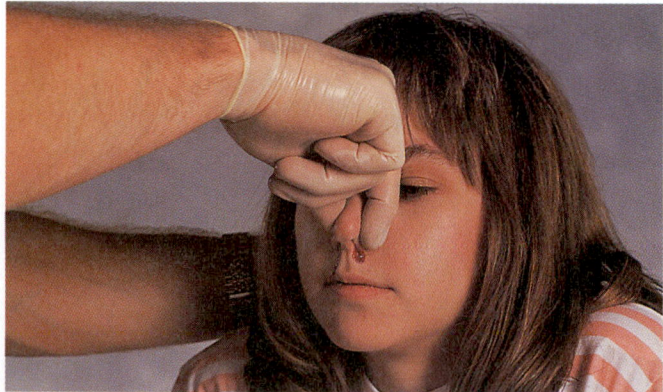

Figure 21-9   If avulsed skin is still attached, place the flap in a position that is as close to normal as possible, and hold it in place with a dry, sterile dressing.

Figure 21-11   Control bleeding from the nose by pinching the nostrils together.

discussion of the care for epistaxis, see Skill Drill 8-3 in Chapter 8, Bleeding.

Injuries of the Ear

The ear is a complex organ that is associated with both hearing and balance. The ear is divided into three parts ▼ Figure 21-12 . The external ear is composed of the pinna, or auricle, which is the part lying outside of the head, and the **external auditory canal**, which leads in toward the **tympanic membrane**, or eardrum. The middle ear contains three small bones (the hammer, anvil, and stirrup) that move in response to sound waves hitting the tympanic membrane. This is the mechanism by which we appreciate sounds. The middle ear is connected to the nasal cavity by the **eustachian tube**, which is the internal auditory canal. This connection permits equalization of pressure in the middle ear when external atmospheric pressure changes. The inner ear is composed of bony chambers filled with fluid. As the head moves, so does the fluid. In response, fine nerve endings within the fluid send impulses to the brain indicating both the position of the head and the rate of change of position.

Ears are often injured, but they usually do not bleed very much. If local pressure does not control the bleeding, you can apply a roller dressing ▶ Figure 21-13 . First, however, you should place a soft, padded dressing

between the ear and the scalp, as bandaging the ear against the tender underlying scalp is extremely painful. In the case of an ear avulsion, you should wrap the avulsed part in a moist sterile dressing and put it in a plastic bag. Often, avulsed tissue from the ear can be reattached.

The external auditory canal is a favorite place for children to place foreign bodies such as peanuts or candy. All such items should be removed by a physician in the emergency department. Never try to manipulate the foreign body, as you may press it further into the auditory canal and cause permanent damage to the tympanic membrane.

Again, you should note any clear fluid coming from the ear of a severely injured patient, since this may indicate a fracture at the base of the skull.

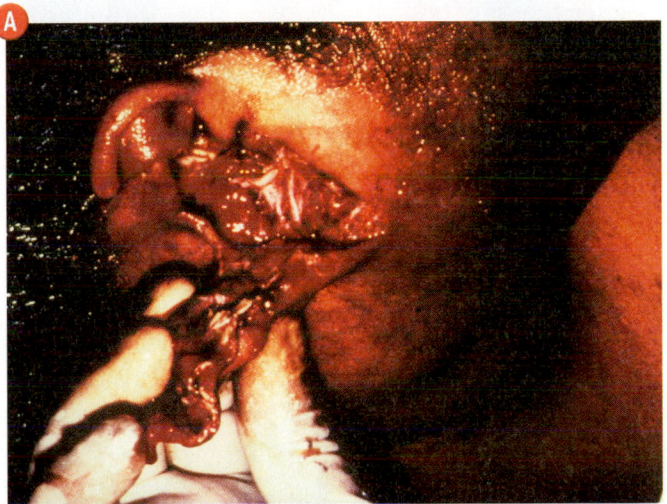
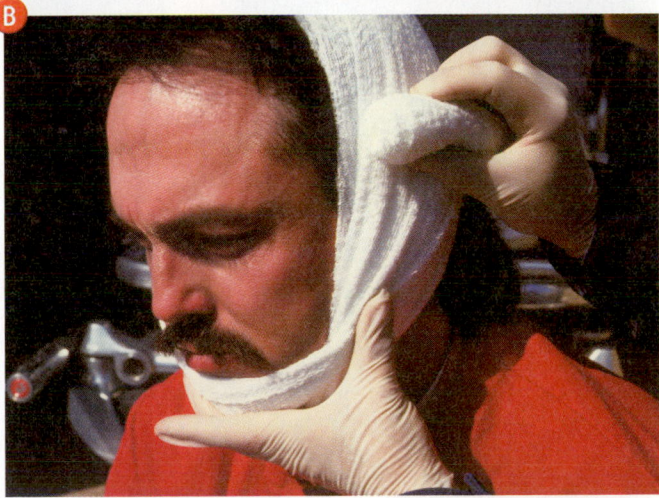

Figure 21-13 **A.** A major laceration of the ear is shown. **B.** Proper treatment includes use of a soft, sterile pad behind the ear, between it and the scalp. Then wrap a roller gauze dressing around the head to include the entire ear.

Figure 21-12 The ear has three principal parts: the external ear, composed of the pinna, external auditory canal, and tympanic membrane; the middle ear, including the hammer, anvil, and stirrup; and the inner ear, composed of bony chambers filled with fluid.

Facial Fractures

Fractures of the facial bones typically result from blunt impact. For example, the patient's head collides with a tree, lift tower, or windshield in a snowmobile or is hit by a snowboard or falling rocks from a climb. You should assume that any patient who has sustained a direct blow to the mouth or nose has a facial fracture. Other clues to the possibility of fracture include bleeding in the mouth, inability to swallow or talk, absent or loose teeth, and/or loose or movable bone fragments. Patients may also report that "it doesn't feel right" when they close their jaw, signaling an irregularity of bite.

Facial fractures alone are not acute emergencies unless there is serious bleeding (▼ Figure 21-14). Such bleeding

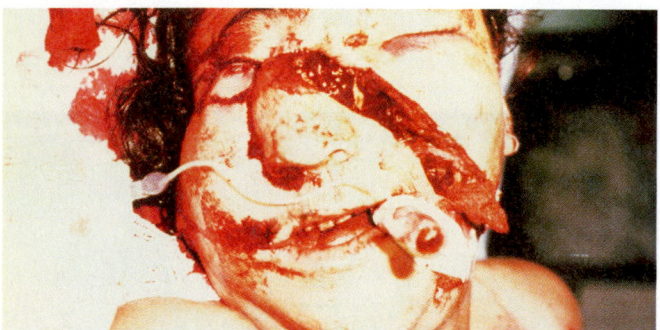

Figure 21-14 Bleeding following a crush injury to the face can be life-threatening because, in addition to the external hemorrhage, blood clots in the airway can cause a complete obstruction.

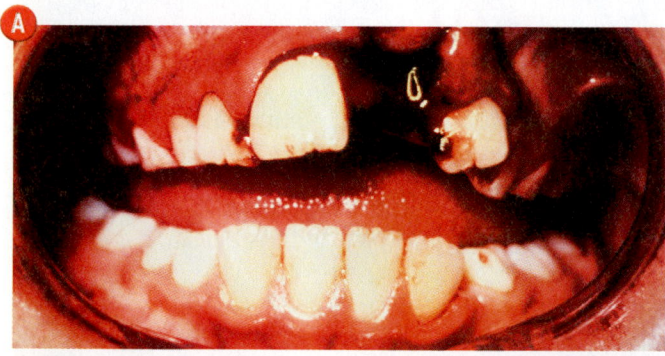

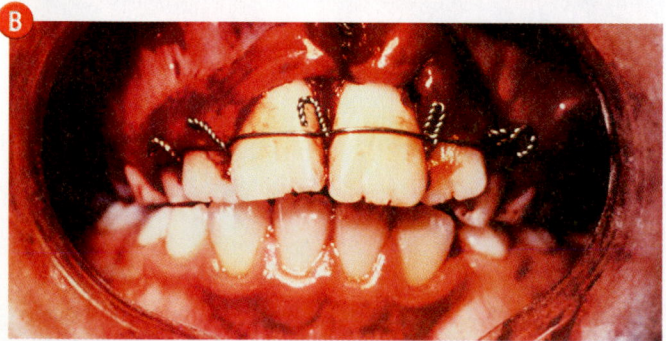

Figure 21-15 **A.** Save any lost teeth or bone fragments following an injury to the mouth. **B.** Even with traumatic loss of a tooth, the possibility of successful reimplantation is very good.

can be life-threatening. In addition to external hemorrhage, there is the danger of blood clots in the upper airway, leading to obstruction of the upper airway. Fractures around the face and mouth can also produce deformity and loose bone fragments. However, plastic surgeons can repair the damage perfectly as long as 7 to 10 days after the injury. Be sure to remove and save loose teeth or bone fragments from the mouth; it is often possible to reimplant them (◄ Figure 21-15). Remove dentures and dental bridges to protect against airway obstruction.

Another source of potential airway obstruction is swelling, which can be extreme within the first 24 hours after injury. If you notice swelling during assessment or at any time while the patient is under your care, you should check for airway obstruction.

Replacing a whole dislodged tooth back into the socket within the first 30 minutes with correct front-to-back orientation is best. First, hold the tooth by the usually exposed part, and rinse off the root (do not scrub it). Then insert it into the socket. If you are unable to do this, or in the unconscious patient who you are worried about aspiration, put the tooth in a container of (in order of effectiveness) milk, saline, water, or saliva.

Injuries of the Neck

The neck contains many structures that are vulnerable to injury either by blunt trauma, such as from a steering wheel in a car crash, or by penetrating injury, such as a stab or gunshot wound. These structures include the upper airway, the esophagus, the carotid arteries and jugular veins, the thyroid cartilage or Adam's apple, the cricoid cartilage, and the upper trachea. Any injury to the neck is serious and should be considered life-threatening until proven otherwise in the emergency department.

Blunt Injuries

Any crushing injury of the upper part of the neck is likely to involve the larynx or trachea. Examples

SkillDrill 21-1 Controlling Bleeding from a Neck Injury

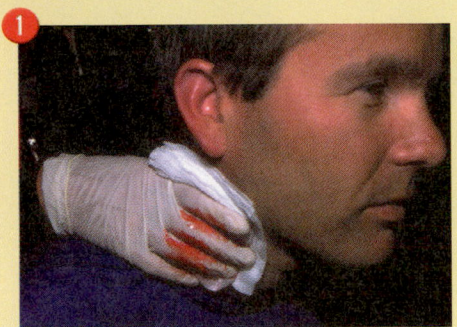
Apply direct pressure to control bleeding.

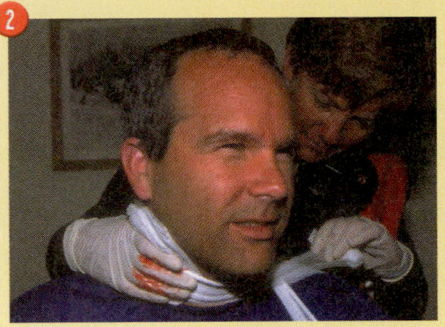
Use a roller gauze to secure a dressing in place.

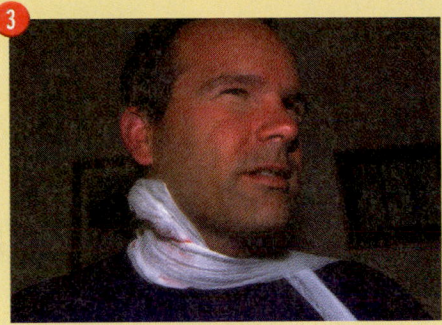
Wrap the bandage around and under the patient's shoulder.

include a collision with a steering wheel, an attempt to ski under a rope at a slope closure, and hitting a tree limb while riding a mountain bike. Once the cartilages of the upper airway and larynx are fractured, they do not spring back to their normal position. Such a fracture can lead to loss of voice, severe and sometimes fatal airway obstruction, and leakage of air into the soft tissues of the neck ▼ Figure 21-16 . The presence of air in the soft tissues is called **subcutaneous emphysema**. Palpation produces a characteristic crackling sensation. If you feel this sensation when you palpate the neck, you should maintain the airway as best you can and provide immediate transport. Be aware that complete airway obstruction can develop very rapidly in these patients as a result of swelling or bleeding into underlying tissues. It may be very difficult to manage the airway in patients; some will require a surgical airway at the hospital. You should also keep in mind that an incident involving an injury to the throat may also have caused a c-spine injury.

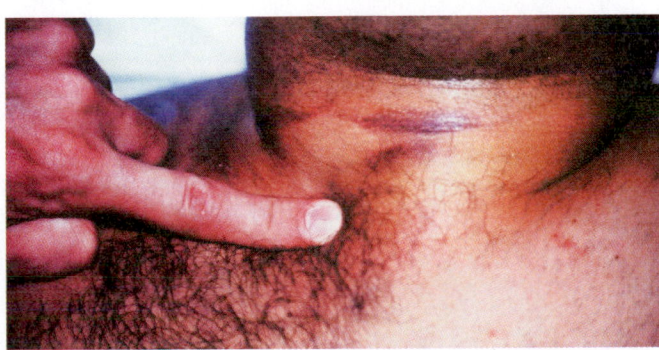
Figure 21-16 Fractures of the larynx or trachea can cause air to leak from the airway into the subcutaneous tissues. The presence of air in the soft tissues, called subcutaneous emphysema, produces a crackling sensation.

Penetrating Injuries

Penetrating injuries to the neck can cause profuse bleeding from laceration of the great vessels in the neck, either the carotid artery or the jugular veins. The airway, the esophagus, and even the spinal cord can also be damaged by a penetrating injury.

Direct pressure over the bleeding site will control most neck bleeding. Follow the steps in
▲ Skill Drill 21-1 :

1. **Apply direct pressure** to the bleeding site using your gloved fingertips and a sterile dressing **(Step 1)**.

2. **Secure the dressing in place** with roller gauze adding more dressing if needed **(Step 2)**.

3. **Wrap the gauze around and under the patient's shoulder.** Do not wrap the gauze around the neck to avoid possible airway and circulation problems **(Step 3)**.

However, the tissues within the neck may still bleed and compress the upper airway, so you should look for signs of airway obstruction. If a vein has been opened, air may be sucked through it to the heart, a clinical situation called **air embolism**. A large amount of air in the right atrium and right ventricle can lead to cardiac arrest.

You might find it necessary to apply pressure both above and below the penetrating wound to control life-threatening bleeding from the carotid artery (above) and the jugular vein (below). You may also need to treat the patient for shock.

Always maintain cervical spine immobilization, and with the patient fully immobilized to a backboard, provide prompt transport. Ensure that the airway remains open en route and apply high-flow oxygen.

Chapter Sweep

Ready for Review

Soft-tissue injuries and fractures to the bones of the face and neck are common and vary in severity. Proper emergency care can improve the patient's chances of making a complete recovery in health and appearance. Your priorities are to prevent further injury, especially to the cervical spine, and to manage any acute airway problems. These problems can result from heavy bleeding, swelling, and injuries to the brain or cervical spine that interfere with normal respiration.

To control the often heavy bleeding from soft-tissue injuries to the face and scalp, use direct manual pressure with a dry, sterile dressing, unless you suspect a skull fracture. Use a moist, sterile dressing for exposed parts of the brain or eye. Always check for bleeding inside the mouth. Open and clear the airway in all patients with facial injuries. Save any pieces of avulsed skin for possible attachment later; hold any avulsed flaps in place with a dry, sterile dressing. If the patient is bleeding heavily from an injury to the nose, apply a sterile dressing.

Injuries to the ear usually do not bleed very much. If local pressure does not control the bleeding, you can apply a roller dressing. Remember to place padding between the ear and the scalp, as bandaging the ear against the tender underlying scalp is extremely painful. Often, avulsed tissue from the ear can be reattached, so save any avulsed tissue. Always leave foreign bodies in the ear for a physician to remove. Watch for clear fluid coming from the ear or nose; this may indicate a basal skull fracture.

Assume that any patient who has sustained a direct blow to the nose or mouth has a facial fracture. Signs of fracture include irregularity of bite, inability to swallow or talk, and bleeding in the mouth. Check for airway obstruction if you notice swelling or if there is serious bleeding.

Both blunt and penetrating injuries to the neck can be life-threatening. With blunt injuries, you should palpate the neck and feel for the characteristic crackling associated with subcutaneous emphysema; patients with this sign may be in danger of complete airway obstruction within minutes. Direct pressure over the bleeding site will control most neck bleeding. However, bleeding may still occur within the tissues of the neck and compress the upper airway. If a vein has been lacerated, be alert for the possibility of air embolism. You may have to apply pressure both above and below the penetrating wound to control life-threatening bleeding from the carotid artery and jugular vein. Patients with a neck injury require spinal immobilization and prompt transport.

Vital Vocabulary

Adam's apple The firm prominence in the upper part of the larynx formed by the thyroid cartilage.

air embolism The presence of air in the veins, which can lead to cardiac arrest if it enters the heart.

avulse To pull or tear away.

cranium The skull.

eustachian tube The internal auditory canal that connects the middle ear to the nasal cavity.

external auditory canal The ear canal; leads to the tympanic membrane.

foramen magnum The large opening at the base of the skull through which the brain connects to the spinal cord.

hematoma The collection of blood in a space, tissue, or organ due to a break in the wall of a blood vessel.

mandible The bone of the lower jaw.

mastoid process The prominent bony mass at the base of the skull about 1" posterior to the external opening of the ear.

maxilla The bone that forms the upper jaw on either side of the face and contains the upper teeth, the orbit of the eye, the nasal cavity, and the palate.

occiput The most posterior portion of the skull.

pinna The external, visible part of the ear.

sternocleidomastoid muscles Muscles on either side of the neck that allow movement of the head.

subcutaneous emphysema The presence of air in soft tissue; palpation produces a characteristic crackling sensation.

temporomandibular joint (TMJ) The joint formed where the mandible and cranium meet, just in front of the ear.

tragus The small, rounded, fleshy bulge that lies immediately anterior to the ear canal.

turbinates Layers of bone within the nasal cavity.

tympanic membrane The eardrum, which lies between the external and middle ear.

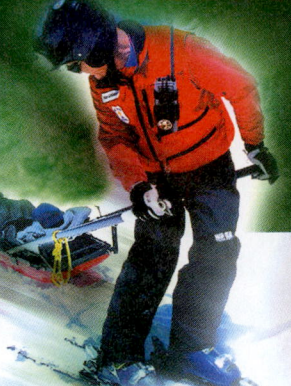

Assessment in Action

You respond to a call from a restaurant at your mountain where a diner, carrying a tray of food, tripped and hit his head on a glass decorative panel. He is reported to have head and neck lacerations with a lot of associated bleeding. The patient is 31 years old, in good health, and not taking any medication.

When his wife saw him bleeding on the floor, she applied pressure over her husband's wound with a large cloth napkin. She states that he did not lose consciousness. Your assessment reveals that the man is alert and oriented. He is talking in complete sentences, but is spitting blood. He has multiple lacerations to the face and neck. He has a 2" long laceration to the right cheek and a 4" long laceration to the right side of his neck, just below the ear, and down the shoulder. The bleeding from the neck appears to be controlled, but there is a large quantity of blood on the napkin that the wife used to apply pressure to the wound. Vital signs include a pulse of 110 beats/min, respirations of 22 breaths/min, and a blood pressure of 132/82 mm Hg.

1. What is the highest priority in caring for this patient?
   A. Administering low concentrations of oxygen.
   B. Treating potential or actual airway obstruction.
   C. Applying sterile dressings and bandaging the wound.
   D. Providing complete stabilization to a long backboard.

2. Which of the following interventions is acceptable for controlling bleeding of his neck injury?
   A. A wide band as a tourniquet
   B. A circumferential pressure dressing
   C. Direct pressure with a sterile dressing
   D. A pressure point

3. In most cases, a patient who sustains trauma to the face or throat should be placed in which of the following positions?
   A. Prone
   B. Supine
   C. Sitting up
   D. Turned to the side

4. Which of the following tools is considered an essential treatment adjunct for this patient, who has sustained face and neck trauma and is spontaneously breathing?
   A. AED
   B. BVM device
   C. Portable suction
   D. Hemostats

5. Which of the following statements about airway obstruction related to blunt trauma to the neck is true in this patient situation?
   A. Immediate transport is necessary because of the danger of possible obstruction.
   B. Airway obstruction is not likely to develop for at least 2 to 3 hours after the injury.
   C. Complete airway obstruction secondary to trauma is easily managed in the field by EMT-Bs.
   D. Airway obstruction rarely occurs as a complication of blunt trauma to the neck.

6. Additional injuries that you should suspect in this patient include:
   A. internal abdominal injuries.
   B. head and spinal injuries.
   C. injury to the respiratory system.
   D. disturbance with hearing and sight.

7. Assessment of this patient's neck should involve which of the following?
   A. Palpation for subcutaneous emphysema
   B. Palpation of the anterior cervical vertebra
   C. Listening over the carotid artery for abnormal sounds
   D. Listening over the wound site for subcutaneous emphysema

Challenging Questions

8. Every effort should be taken to prevent this patient from swallowing blood. Why is this important?

9. This patient is at risk for an air embolism if a major vein has been lacerated. How would you know if an air embolism occurred?

10. How would you appropriately bandage this patient's neck wound?

Points to Ponder

You respond to a call to find a skier who has been hit in the throat with a ski pole. The patient's throat is quite swollen, he is cyanotic, and he appears unable to breathe. You apply a cold pack to his throat and prepare to transport. Before you are able to get him loaded into the ambulance, he loses consciousness. You are not trained to perform a cricothyrostomy (create an artificial opening in his throat), but you have seen it done in the hospital twice. Would you ask medical control for permission to perform a cricothyrostomy? Why or why not? If medical control authorized the procedure, who would be liable for any damages that might occur? What other treatments might you try?

Issues Advanced Airway Management, EMT/Paramedic Relationships, Reporting Procedures, Impact of Reporting Treatment Issues.

Online Outlook

Soft-tissue injuries and fractures to the bones of the face and neck are common and vary in severity. Your priorities are to prevent further injury, especially to the cervical spine, and to manage any acute airway problems. Review your knowledge of these priorities by completing Exercise 21 at www.OECzone.com.

www.OECzone.com

Chest Injuries

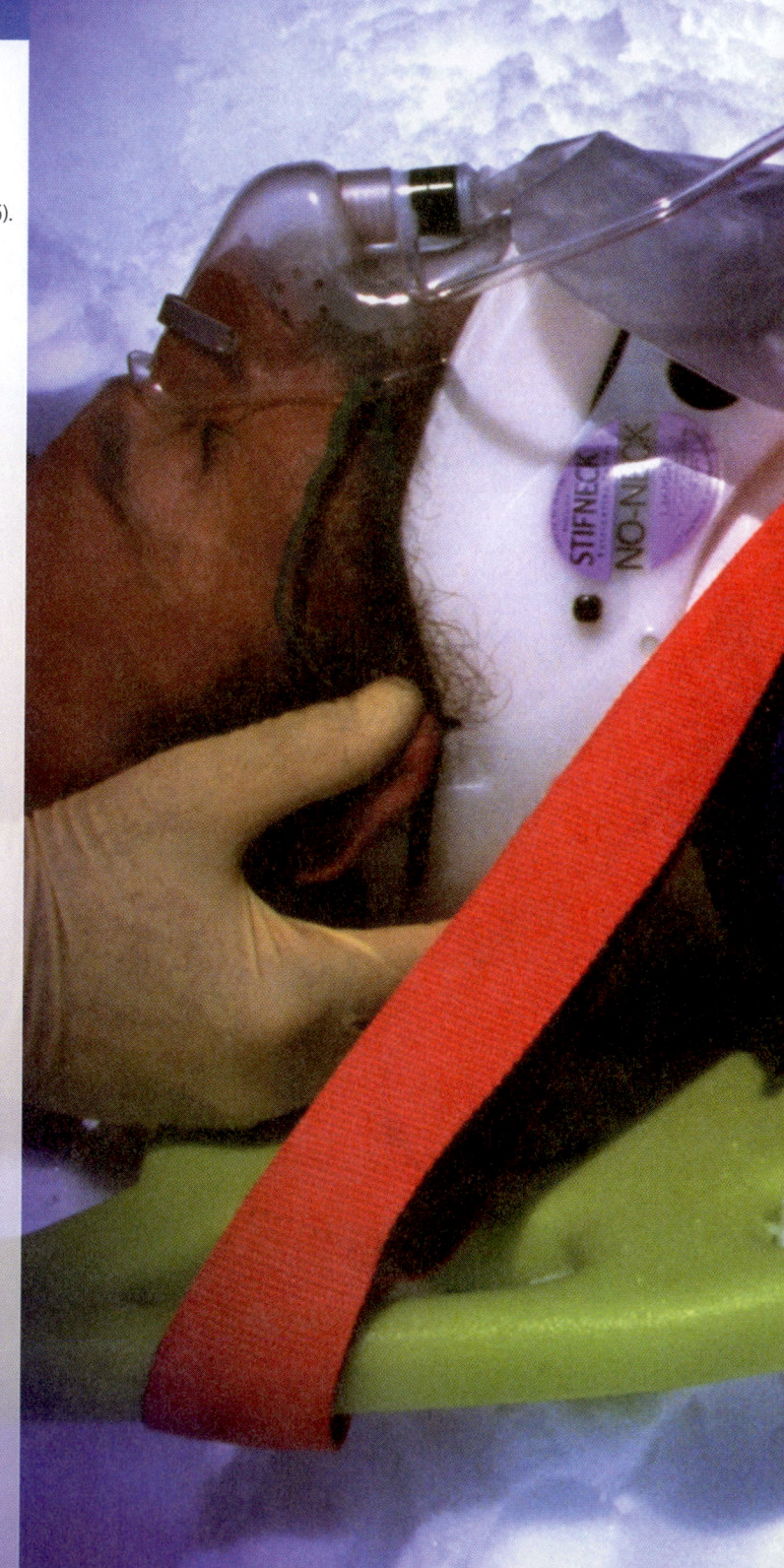

Objectives

Cognitive

♠ **1.** Differentiate between a pneumothorax, a hemothorax, a tension pneumothorax, and a sucking chest wound (p 553).

♠ **2.** Describe the emergency medical care of a patient with a flail chest (p 555).

♠ **3.** Describe the emergency medical care of a patient with a sucking chest wound (p 553).

4. Discuss the complications that can accompany chest injuries (p 553).

Affective

None

Psychomotor

♠ **5.** Demonstrate the steps in the emergency medical care of a sucking chest wound (p 553).

♣ These are core concepts in initial patrol training.

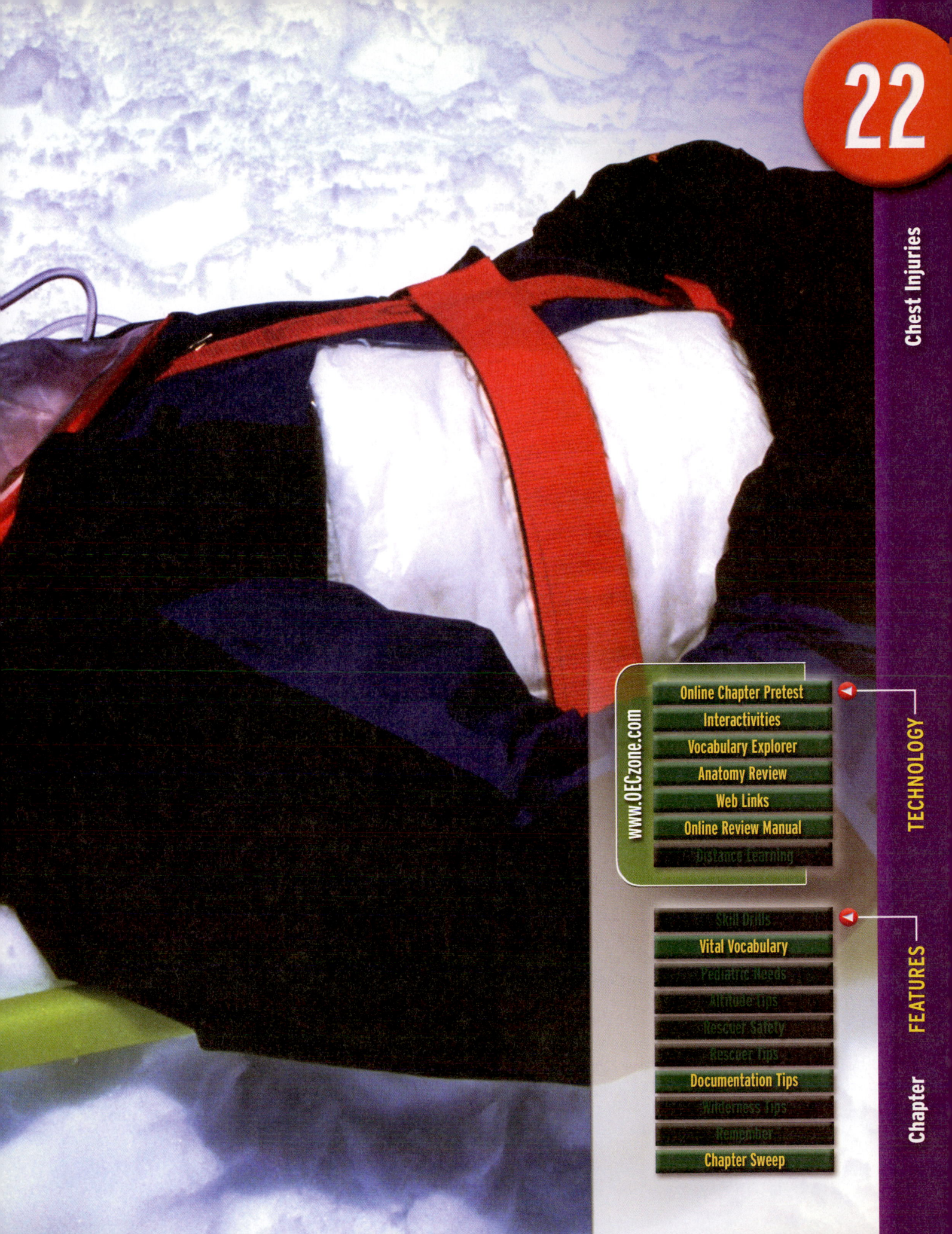

TECHNOLOGY

www.OECzone.com

- Online Chapter Pretest
- Interactivities
- Vocabulary Explorer
- Anatomy Review
- Web Links
- Online Review Manual
- Distance Learning

FEATURES

- Skill Drills
- Vital Vocabulary
- Pediatric Needs
- Altitude Tips
- Rescuer Safety
- Rescuer Tips
- Documentation Tips
- Wilderness Tips
- Remember
- Chapter Sweep

Chapter

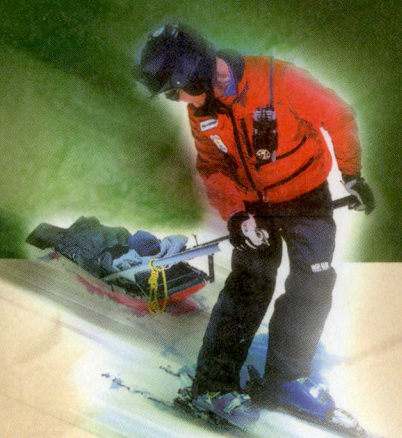

"Patrol 4, respond to a skier at the bottom of the first chute in the high bowl who has hit a tree and has a penetrating injury to his chest from a tree branch."

Many of the organs essential for life itself are found in the chest cavity. Injuries to this area of the body are therefore challenging. This chapter will provide you with the knowledge you'll need to care for these injuries, along with helping you answer the following questions:

1. Why is it important to seal open chest wounds as quickly as possible?

2. What are some of the possible consequences of a blunt injury to the heart? A penetrating injury?

Chest Injuries

Chest injuries are both common and, given the likelihood of damage to the heart, lungs, or great blood vessels, potentially very serious. Any injury that interferes with normal breathing must be treated without delay to prevent permanent damage to tissues that depend on a continuous supply of oxygen. Another major problem with chest injuries may be internal bleeding. Blood from lacerations of the thoracic organs or major blood vessels can collect in the chest cavity, compressing the lungs. Also, air can collect in the chest and prevent the lungs from expanding. Your ability to act quickly to care for patients with these injuries can make the difference between a successful outcome and death.

This chapter begins with a review of the anatomy of the chest and the physiology of respiration. It then describes the common signs and symptoms of chest injuries and the proper emergency medical treatment for specific injuries.

Anatomy and Physiology of the Chest

To understand and evaluate chest injuries in the prehospital setting, you must first understand the anatomy of the chest and the mechanism by which gases are exchanged during breathing. A quick review will help you to appreciate the logic in both the emergency treatment of chest injuries and the potential complications of that treatment.

The chest (thoracic cage) extends from the lower end of the neck to the diaphragm (▶ Figure 22-1). In an individual who is lying down or who has just completed exhalation, the diaphragm may rise as high as the nipple line. Thus, a penetrating injury to the chest, such as a

gunshot or stab wound, may penetrate the lung and diaphragm and injure the liver, stomach, or spleen.

The contents of the chest are partially protected by the ribs, which are connected in the back to the vertebrae and in the front, through the costal cartilages, to the sternum (▶ Figure 22-2). The trachea, which is in the middle of the neck, divides into the left and right mainstem bronchi, which supply air to the lungs. Of course, the thoracic cage also contains the heart and the great vessels: the aorta, the right innominate and left subclavian arteries and their branches, and the superior and inferior venae cavae. The esophagus runs through the back of the chest, connecting the pharynx above with the stomach and the abdomen. At the bottom of the chest, the diaphragm is a muscle that separates the thoracic cavity from the abdominal cavity.

When you inhale, the intercostal muscles between the ribs contract, elevating the rib cage. At the same time, the diaphragm contracts and pushes the contents of the abdomen down. The pressure inside the chest decreases, and air enters the lungs through the nose and mouth. When you exhale, the intercostal muscles and diaphragm relax, and the tissues move back to their normal positions, allowing air to be exhaled. Note that the nerves supplying the diaphragm (the phrenic nerves) exit the spinal cord at C3, C4, and C5. A patient whose spinal cord is injured at the C5 level or below will lose the power to move his or her intercostal muscles, but the diaphragm will still contract. The patient will still be able to breathe because the phrenic nerves remain intact. Patients with spinal cord injuries at C3 or above can lose their ability to breathe entirely (▶ Figure 22-3).

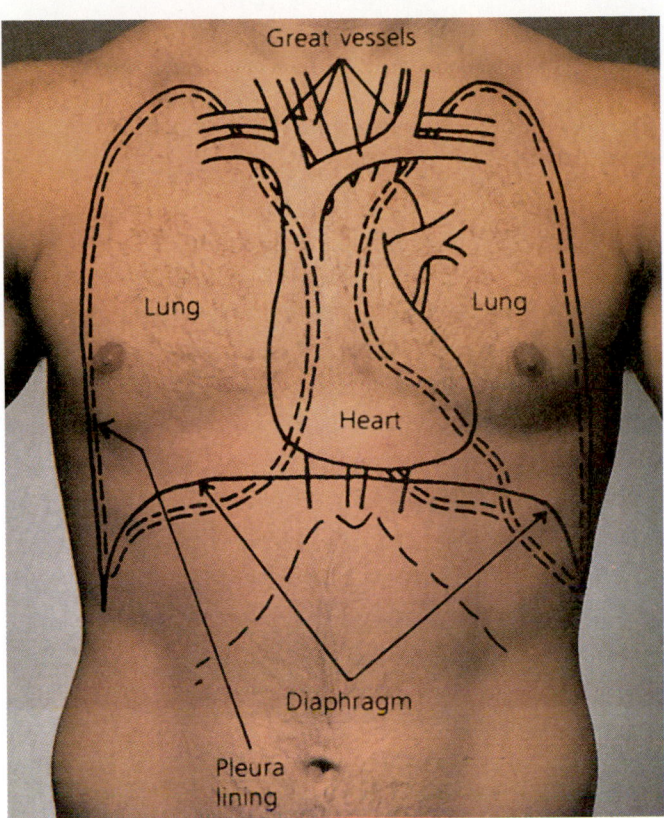

Figure 22-1 A view of the anterior aspect of the chest shows the major organs beneath the surface.

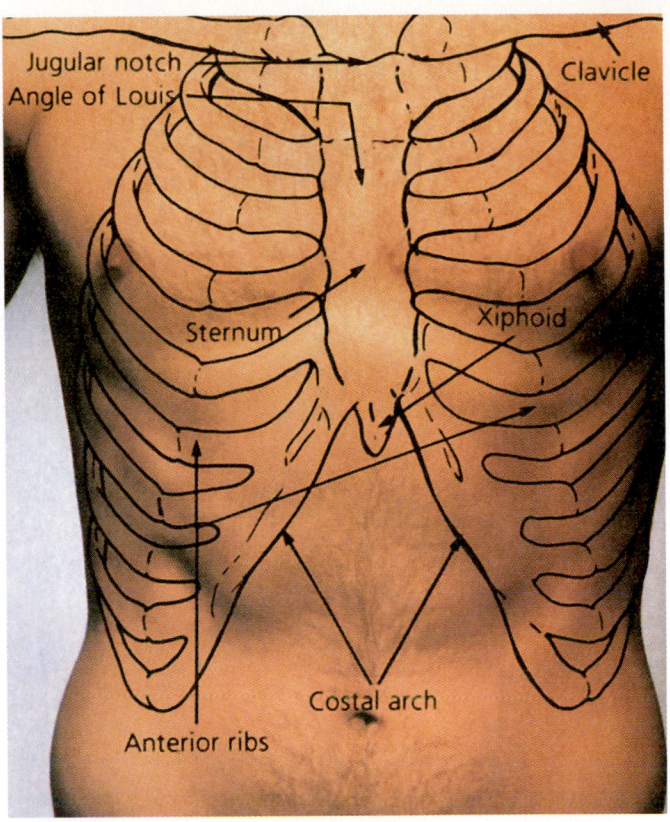

Figure 22-2 The organs within the chest are protected by the ribs, which are connected in back to the vertebrae and in the front, through the costal cartilages, to the sternum.

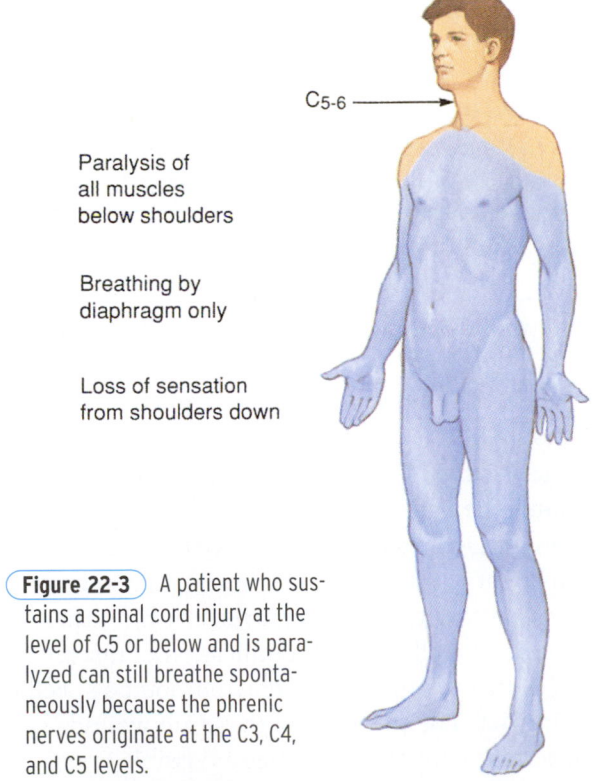

C5-6

Paralysis of all muscles below shoulders

Breathing by diaphragm only

Loss of sensation from shoulders down

Figure 22-3 A patient who sustains a spinal cord injury at the level of C5 or below and is paralyzed can still breathe spontaneously because the phrenic nerves originate at the C3, C4, and C5 levels.

Injuries of the Chest

There are two basic types of chest injuries: open or closed. As the name implies, a **closed chest injury** is one in which the skin is not broken. This type of injury is generally caused by blunt trauma, such as a full-impact collision between a skier and a tree or when a person is struck by a falling object ▶ **Figure 22-4** . In **open chest injuries**, the chest wall itself is penetrated by some object such as a tree branch, ski pole, or the broken end of a fractured rib ▶ **Figure 22-5** .

In blunt trauma, a blow to the chest may fracture the ribs, the sternum, or whole areas of the chest wall, bruise the lungs and the heart, and even damage the aorta. Almost one-third of people who are killed immediately in car crashes die as a result of traumatic rupture of the aorta. Although the skin and chest wall are not penetrated in a closed injury, the contents of the chest may be lacerated by broken ribs. Indeed, vital organs can actually be torn from their attachment in the chest cavity without any break in the skin.

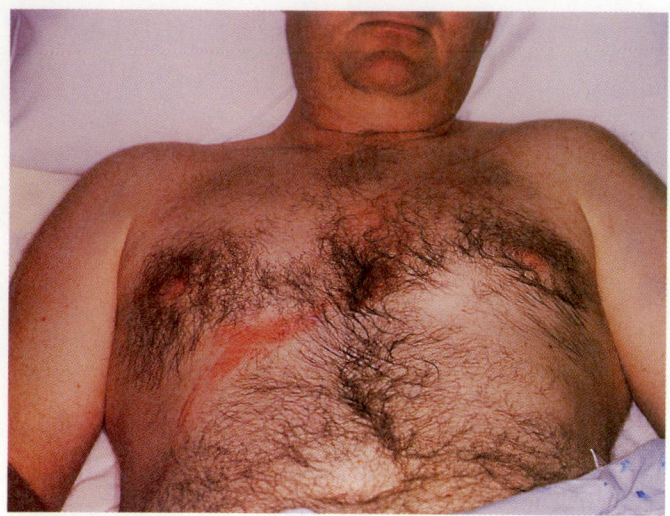

Figure 22-4 Closed injuries usually result from blunt trauma, such as when a patient strikes a fixed object (like a tree) in a crash or is struck by a falling object.

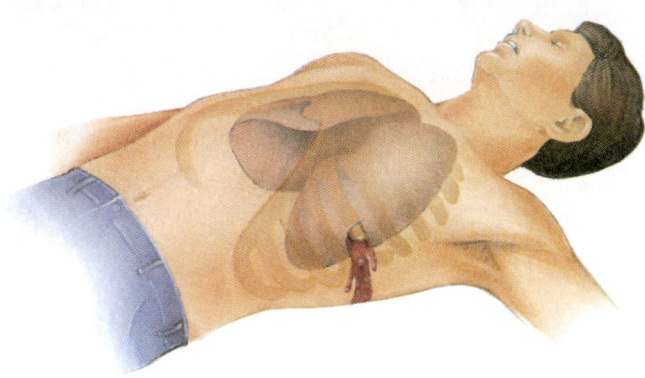

Figure 22-5 Open injuries occur when the chest wall is penetrated by some type of object or the broken end of a fractured rib.

Signs and Symptoms

Important signs and symptoms of chest injury include the following:

- Pain at the site of injury
- Pain localized at the site of injury that is aggravated by or increased with breathing
- Dyspnea (difficulty breathing, shortness of breath)
- Hemoptysis (coughing up blood)
- Failure of one or both sides of the chest to expand normally with inspiration
- Rapid, weak pulse and low blood pressure
- Cyanosis (a bluish discoloration of the skin), most marked in the lips and fingernails

After a chest injury, any change in normal breathing is a particularly important sign. A healthy, uninjured adult usually breathes from 12 to 20 times per minute without difficulty and without pain. Respirations of fewer than 8/min or more than 24/min may indicate abnormal breathing. Patients with chest injuries often have **tachypnea** (rapid respirations) and shallow respirations because it hurts to take a deep breath.

As with any other injury, pain and tenderness are common at the point of impact as a result of a bruise or fracture. Pain is usually aggravated by the normal process of breathing. Irritation of or damage to the pleural surfaces causes a characteristic sharp or sticking pain with each breath when these normally smooth surfaces slide on one another. This sharp pain is called *pleuritic pain* or *pleurisy*.

In an injured patient, **dyspnea** (difficulty with breathing) has many causes, including airway obstruction, damage to the chest wall, improper chest expansion due to the loss of normal control of breathing, or lung compression because of accumulated blood or air. Dyspnea in an injured patient indicates significant compromise of lung function; prompt, vigorous support and rapid transport are required.

Patient Assessment

After your initial assessment, in which you quickly evaluate the patient's ABCs and treat potential life threats, carefully observe the patient's chest wall. If the chest wall does not expand on each side when the patient inhales, the chest muscles may have lost their ability to work appropriately. Loss of muscle function may be the result of a direct injury to the chest wall, or it may be related to an injury of the nerves that control those muscles. Check also for paradoxical motion, an abnormality associated with multiple fractured ribs, in which one segment of the chest wall moves opposite of the remainder of the chest, ie, out with expiration and in with inspiration.

Rapid assessment using DCAP-BTLS is mandatory to determine the nature and extent of thoracic injury. Inspection for Deformities, such as asymmetry of the left versus right chest or shoulder girdle, may reveal the presence of multiple rib fractures, crush injuries, or significant chest wall injury. Identification of discrete areas of Contusion or Abrasion may pinpoint a specific point of impact. The presence of Puncture wounds or other penetrating injuries indicates a possible open chest injury, which should be managed accordingly. Be alert for associated Burns, which may alter respiratory mechanics. Palpate for Tenderness to localize the injury and the presence of fractures. Look for Lacerations and local Swelling. Application of this systematic approach to patient assessment minimizes the chance of missing significant injury.

Hemoptysis, the spitting or coughing up of blood, usually indicates that the lung itself or the air passages have been damaged. With a laceration of the lung, blood can enter the bronchial passages and is coughed up as the patient tries to clear the airway.

A rapid, weak pulse and low blood pressure are the principal signs of hypovolemic shock, which can result from extensive bleeding from lacerated structures within the chest cavity. Shock following a chest injury may also result from insufficient oxygenation of the blood by the poorly functioning lungs.

Cyanosis in a patient with a chest injury is a sign of inadequate respiration. The classic blue appearance around the lips and fingernails indicates that blood is not being oxygenated sufficiently. Patients with cyanosis are unable to provide a sufficient supply of oxygen to the blood through the lungs and require immediate respiratory support and supplemental oxygen.

Many of these signs and symptoms occur simultaneously. When any one of them develops as a result of a chest injury, the patient requires prompt hospital care. Remember that the principal reason for concern about a patient who has a chest injury is that his or her body has no means of storing oxygen; it is supplied and used continuously, even during sleep. Any interruption in this supply can be rapidly lethal and must be treated aggressively.

Complications of Chest Injuries

Pneumothorax

In any chest injury, damage to the heart, lungs, great vessels, and other organs in the chest can be complicated by the accumulation of air in the pleural space. This is a dangerous condition called a **pneumothorax**. In this condition, air enters through a hole in the chest wall or the surface of the lung as the patient attempts to breathe, causing the lung on that side to collapse (▲ **Figure 22-6**). As a result, any blood that passes through the lung is not oxygenated, and hypoxia will develop. Depending on the size of the hole and

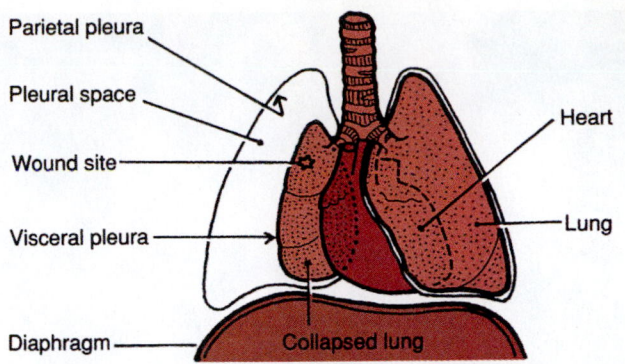

Figure 22-6 Pneumothorax occurs when air leaks into the space between the pleural surfaces from an opening in the chest wall or the surface of the lung. The lung collapses as air fills the pleural space.

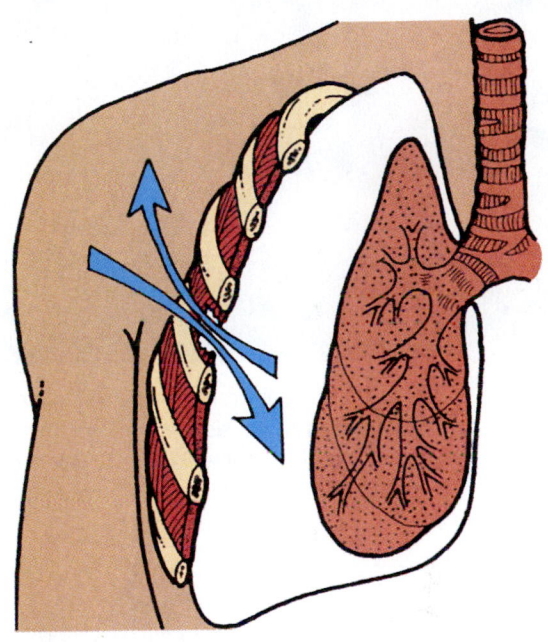

Figure 22-7 With a sucking chest wound, air passes from the outside into the pleural space and back out with each breath, creating the sucking sound.

the rate at which air fills the cavity, the lung may collapse in a few seconds or a few hours. If the hole is in the chest wall, you can actually hear this condition in the form of a sucking sound as the patient inhales and the sound of rushing air as he or she exhales. For this reason, an open or penetrating wound to the chest wall is often called a **sucking chest wound** (▲ **Figure 22-7**).

This type of open pneumothorax is a true emergency requiring immediate emergency medical care and transport. Initial emergency care, after clearing and maintaining the airway and then providing

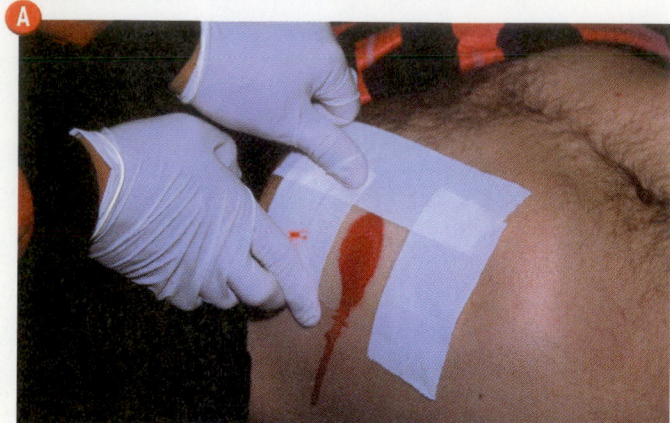

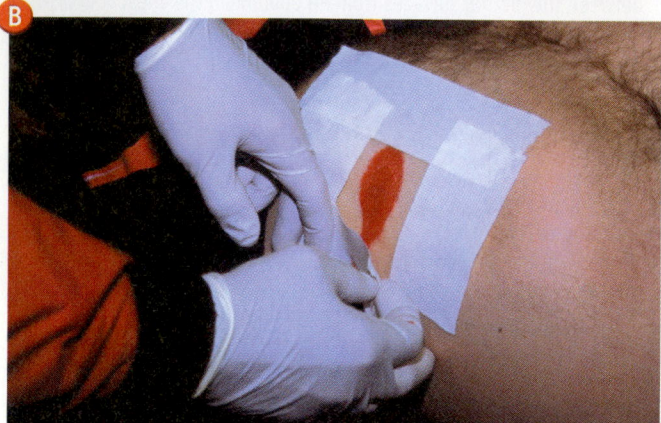

Figure 22-8 A sucking chest wound can be sealed with a large air-tight dressing that either seals all four sides (**A**), or seals three sides with the fourth left open as a flutter valve (**B**). Your local protocol will dictate the way you are to care for this injury.

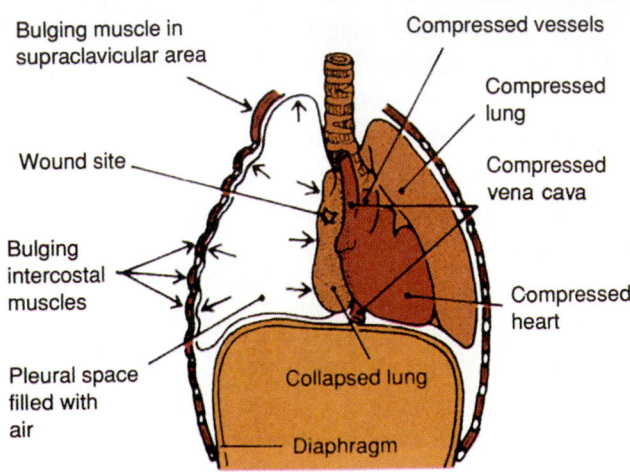

Bulging muscle in supraclavicular area

Compressed vessels

Compressed lung

Wound site

Compressed vena cava

Bulging intercostal muscles

Compressed heart

Pleural space filled with air

Collapsed lung

Diaphragm

Figure 22-9 A tension pneumothorax can develop if a penetrating chest wound is bandaged tightly and air from a damaged lung cannot escape. The air then accumulates in the pleural space.

oxygen, is to rapidly seal the open wound with a sterile <u>occlusive dressing</u> (▲ **Figure 22-8**). The purpose of the dressing is to seal the wound and prevent air from being sucked into the chest through the wound. Several sterile materials, including Vaseline gauze, aluminum foil, plastic wrap, or a folded universal dressing, may be used to seal the wound. Use a large enough dressing so that it is not pulled or sucked into the chest cavity. Depending on your local protocol, you may tape the dressing down on all four sides, or you may create a <u>flutter valve</u>, a one-way valve that allows air to leave the chest cavity but not return, by taping only three sides of the dressing.

SPONTANEOUS PNEUMOTHORAX. Some individuals are born with or develop weak areas on the surface of the lungs. Occasionally, such a weak area will rupture spontaneously, allowing air to leak into the pleural space. Usually, this event, called <u>spontaneous pneu-</u>

<u>mothorax</u>, is not related to any major injury but simply happens with normal breathing. The patient experiences sudden sharp chest pain and increasing difficulty in breathing. The affected lung collapses, losing its ability to expand normally. The amount of pneumothorax that develops varies, as does the amount of respiratory distress the patient experiences.

You should suspect a spontaneous pneumothorax in a patient who experiences sudden chest pain and shortness of breath without a specific known cause. The prehospital treatment that you can provide for this type of pneumothorax is the same as that for a traumatic pneumothorax.

TENSION PNEUMOTHORAX. A <u>tension pneumothorax</u> (▲ **Figure 22-9**) can occur when there is significant ongoing air accumulation in the pleural space. This air gradually increases the pressure in the chest, first causing the complete collapse of the affected lung and then pushing the mediastinum (the central part of the chest containing the heart and great vessels) into the opposite pleural cavity. This prevents blood from returning through the venae cavae to the heart and can cause shock and cardiac arrest.

A tension pneumothorax can also occur as a result of closed, blunt injury of the chest with, or without, a rib fracture. The lung surface, or a bronchus, may be lacerated by a fractured rib, or simply by the forces of blunt trauma without a fractured rib—both may result in an air leak into the pleural space and result in a tension pneumothorax. Very rarely, a tension pneumothorax may arise spontaneously. This might happen in a young adult as a result of a spontaneous pneumothorax.

The common signs and symptoms of tension pneumothorax include increasing respiratory distress, distended neck veins, deviation of the trachea to the side of the chest opposite from the tension pneumothorax, tachycardia, low blood pressure, cyanosis, and decreased breath sounds on the side of the pneumothorax.

Relieving a tension pneumothorax due to a blunt trauma in a patient is often done by inserting a needle through the rib cage into the pleural space; however, this procedure must be performed by ALS personnel or emergency department staff.

If signs and symptoms of a tension pneumothorax develop after sealing an open chest wound, you should partly remove the dressing to relieve the tension. As you do so, you may hear a rush of air out of the chest cavity, although this does not occur in all cases.

Hemothorax

In both blunt and penetrating chest injury, blood can collect in the pleural space from a bleeding rib cage, lung, or great vessel. This condition is called a **hemothorax** (▲ **Figure 22-10**). You should suspect a hemothorax if the patient has signs and symptoms of shock or decreased breath sounds on the affected side, an indication that the lung is being compressed by the blood. The presence of both air and blood in the pleural space is known as a hemopneumothorax.

Rib Fractures

Rib fractures are very common in the elderly, whose bones are brittle, but relatively uncommon in the very young, whose bones are much more supple. Because the upper four ribs are well protected by

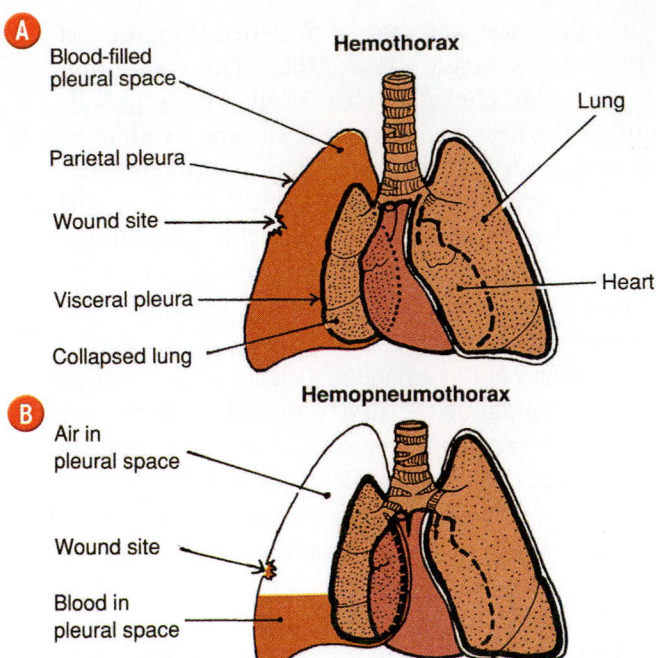

Figure 22-10) **A.** A hemothorax is a collection of blood in the pleural space produced by bleeding within the chest. **B.** When both blood and air are present, the condition is a hemopneumothorax.

the bony girdle of the clavicle and scapula, a fracture of one of these upper ribs is a sign of a very severe mechanism of injury.

Be aware that blunt trauma, with or without rib fractures, may lacerate the surface of the lung, causing a pneumothorax, a tension pneumothorax, a hemothorax or a hemopneumothorax. One sign of this development can be a crackly feeling to the skin in the area (also called *subcutaneous emphysema*), which indicates that air escaping from a lacerated lung is leaking into the chest wall. Be sure to relay this finding to the hospital.

Patients with one or more cracked ribs will report localized tenderness and pain on breathing. The pain is the result of broken ends of the fracture rubbing against each other with each inspiration and expiration. Patients will tend to avoid taking deep breaths, breathing rapidly and shallowly instead. They will often hold the affected portion of the rib cage in an effort to minimize the discomfort. These patients should receive supplemental O_2 during assessment and transport.

Flail Chest

Ribs may be fractured in more than one place. If three or more ribs are fractured in two or more places, or if the sternum is fractured along with several ribs, a segment of chest wall may be detached from the rest of the thoracic cage (▶ **Figure 22-11**). This condition is known as <u>flail chest</u>. In what is called <u>paradoxical motion</u>, the detached portion of the chest wall moves opposite of normal: in instead of out during inhalation, out instead of in during expiration. This occurs because of negative pressure inside the thorax during inspiration. Breathing with a flail chest can be extremely painful and often does not allow for adequate oxygenation.

Your treatment of a patient with a flail chest should include maintaining the airway, providing respiratory support if necessary, giving supplemental oxygen, and performing ongoing assessments for possible pneumothorax or other respiratory complications. Treatment may also include positive pressure ventilation with a bag-valve-mask device.

The patient may find it easier and less painful to breathe if the flail segment is immobilized. You can tape a bulky pad against that segment of the chest for this purpose, although taping too tightly will also prevent adequate ventilation (▶ **Figure 22-12**). Keep in mind that while flail chest is itself a serious condition, it suggests an injury that was forceful enough to cause other serious internal damage as well.

Other Chest Injuries

Pulmonary Contusion

In addition to fracturing ribs, any severe blunt trauma to the chest can also injure the lung. The pulmonary alveoli become filled with blood, and fluid accumulates in the injured area, leaving the patient hypoxic. Severe <u>pulmonary contusion</u>, bruising of the lung, should always be suspected in patients with a flail chest and usually develops over a period of hours. If you believe that a patient may have a pulmonary contusion, you should provide respiratory support and supplemental oxygen to ensure adequate ventilation.

Traumatic Asphyxia

Sometimes, a patient will experience a sudden, severe compression of the chest, which produces a rapid increase in pressure within the chest. This may occur during a sudden crush injury to the chest, such as when a skier hits his or her chest on a tree, rock, or lift tower at high speed. The sudden increase in intrathoracic pressure results in a very characteristic appearance, including distended neck veins, cyanosis in the face and neck, and hemorrhage into the sclera of the eye,

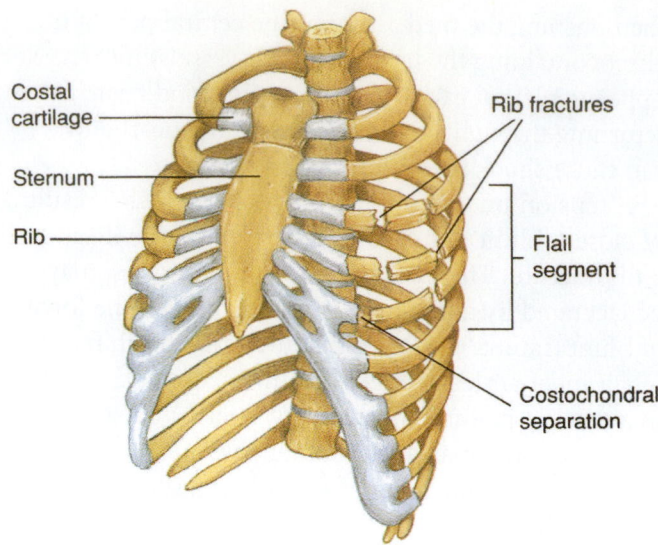

Figure 22-11 When three or more adjacent ribs are fractured in two or more places, a flail chest results. A flail segment will move paradoxically when the patient breathes.

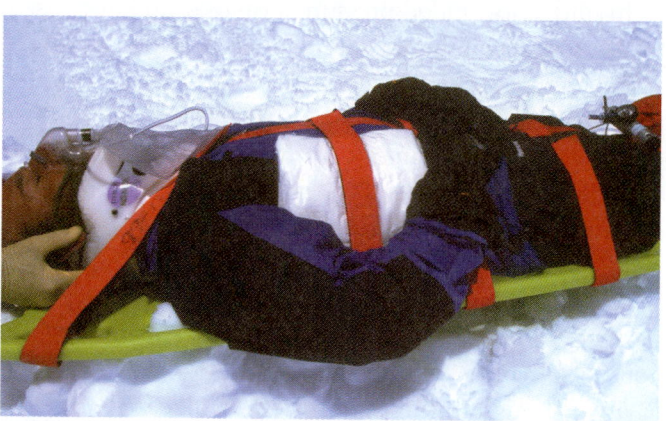

Figure 22-12 A flail anterior chest wall segment can be stabilized by securing (or having the patient hold) a pillow firmly against the chest wall.

signaling the bursting of small blood vessels in the skin. These findings suggest an underlying injury to the heart and pulmonary contusions. You should provide ventilatory support with supplemental oxygen and monitor the patient's vital signs, as you provide immediate transport.

Blunt Myocardial Injury

Blunt trauma to the chest may injure the heart itself, making it unable to maintain adequate blood pressure. There is much debate in the medical literature over how to assess <u>myocardial contusion</u>, or bruising of the heart muscle. Often, the pulse rate is irregular, but dangerous rhythms such as ventricular tachycardia and ventricular fibrillation are uncommon. There is no specific diagnostic test at this time, and there is no prehospital treatment for the condition. Still, you should suspect myocardial contusion in all cases of severe, blunt injury to the chest. Check the patient's pulse carefully, and note any irregularities. Provide supplemental oxygen and transport immediately.

Pericardial Tamponade

In <u>pericardial tamponade</u>, blood or other fluid collects in the <u>pericardium</u>, the fibrous sac surrounding the heart (▼ **Figure 22-13**). This prevents the heart from filling during the diastolic phase, causing a decrease in the amount of blood pumped to the body and decreased blood pressure. Ultimately, as blood accumulates within the pericardial cavity, it compresses the heart until it can no longer function and the patient goes into cardiac arrest. Signs and symptoms of pericardial tamponade include very soft and faint heart tones, often called muffled heart sounds, a weak pulse, low blood pressure, a decrease in the difference between the systolic and the diastolic blood pressure, jugular vein distention (JVD), and shock.

In a trauma situation, even a small amount of fluid in the pericardial sac is enough to cause fatal pericardial tamponade. (Occasionally, fluid in surprisingly large amounts may collect in the pericardial sac as a chronic condition.) Pericardial tamponade is relatively uncommon, seen more often with penetrating injuries to the heart itself than with blunt injuries to the chest.

> Open chest injuries are usually the result of some penetrating trauma, while closed chest injuries occur following blunt or compressive trauma. Both can cause life-threatening injuries that may not be readily apparent during assessment.

If you suspect this life-threatening condition, provide appropriate respiratory support, supplemental oxygen, and prompt transport.

Laceration of the Great Vessels

The chest contains several large blood vessels: the superior vena cava, the inferior vena cava, the pulmonary arteries, four main pulmonary veins, and the aorta, with its major branches distributing blood throughout the body. Injury to any of these vessels may be accompanied by massive, rapidly fatal hemorrhage. Any patient with a chest wound who shows signs of shock may have an injury to one or more of these vessels. Frequently, blood loss is not obvious, because it remains within the chest cavity.

Emergency treatment for these patients includes CPR, if appropriate, ventilatory support, and supplemental oxygen. Here, particularly, immediate transport to the hospital may be critical. For some of these patients, a few minutes can mean the difference between life and death.

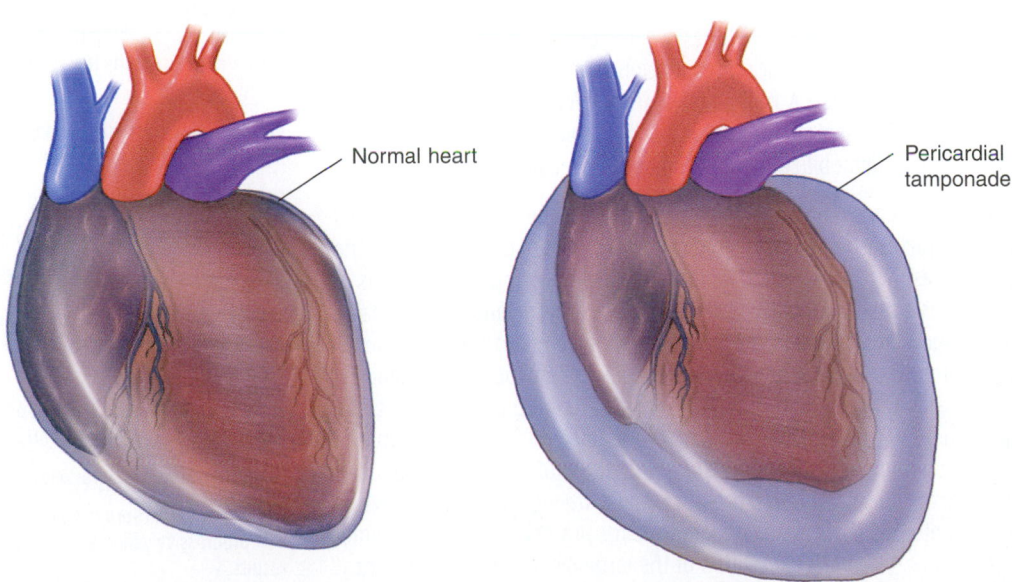

Figure 22-13 Pericardial tamponade is a potentially fatal condition in which fluid builds up within the pericardial sac, causing compression of the heart's chambers and dramatically impairing its ability to pump blood to the body.

Normal heart

Pericardial tamponade

Chapter *Sweep*

Ready for Review

There are two types of chest injuries: penetrating, or open, injuries and blunt, or closed, injuries. In blunt trauma, a blow to the chest may fracture the ribs, the sternum, or whole areas of the chest wall. Other problems include bruising of the lungs and the heart and possible damage to the aorta. Even if the skin and chest wall are not broken, the contents of the chest may be injured.

A sucking chest wound can result in an open pneumothorax, in which air entering through the wound accumulates in the pleural space, causing the lung to collapse. You should seal the wound with a sterile dressing, either taping it down on all four sides or creating a flutter valve by sealing only three sides. Sealing all four sides may create a tension pneumothorax, in which air leaking from a lacerated lung is unable to escape and the lung collapses. Eventually, this air may push the mediastinum into the opposite pleural cavity and prevent blood from returning to the heart. Cardiac arrest results. A tension pneumothorax can also occur in a closed, blunt injury of the chest when a fractured rib or the forces of blunt trauma lacerate the lung surface.

Look for increasing respiratory distress, shock, and decreased breath sounds on one side. You may need to partly remove the dressing to relieve the underlying tension in the chest. The accumulation of blood in the chest is called a hemothorax; the collection of both blood and air is called a hemopneumothorax.

A fractured rib may lacerate the surface of the lung, causing some type of pneumothorax. One sign of this is a crackly feeling to the skin in the area. Multiple rib fractures, with or without a fracture of the sternum, often result in a condition called flail chest, in which a portion of the chest wall is detached from the thoracic cage and moves during respiration in a fashion that is the opposite of normal. A flail chest causes very painful breathing and requires respiratory support and supplemental oxygen. It may help to immobilize the flail segment with a pad.

Other chest injuries include contusions of the lungs and heart and traumatic asphyxia, in which a sudden, severe compression of the chest produces a rapid increase in intrathoracic pressure. Signs of this condition include distended neck veins, cyanosis in the face, and hemorrhage in the sclera. Provide ventilatory support, monitor vital signs, and provide immediate transport. In pericardial tamponade, blood collects in the pericardium, preventing the heart from filling during the diastolic phase and eventually causing cardiac arrest. Signs include muffled heart sounds, a weak pulse, low blood pressure, and distended neck veins. Here as well, you should provide vigorous respiratory support and immediate transport. Laceration of the large blood vessels in the chest can cause a fatal hemorrhage. Suspect such a wound in any patient with a chest wound who shows signs of shock, even if you see little blood; it may be collecting within the chest cavity. This person needs ventilatory support, supplemental oxygen, immediate transport, and possibly CPR.

Vital Vocabulary

closed chest injury Injury to the chest in which the skin is not broken, usually due to blunt trauma.

dyspnea Difficulty with breathing.

flail chest A condition in which three or more ribs are fractured in two or more places, or in association with a fracture of the sternum, so that a segment of chest wall is effectively detached from the rest of the thoracic cage.

flutter valve A one-way valve that allows air to leave the chest cavity but not return. Formed by taping three sides of an occlusive dressing to the chest wall, leaving the fourth open as the valve.

hemoptysis The spitting or coughing up of blood.

hemothorax A collection of blood in the pleural cavity.

myocardial contusion A bruise of the heart muscle.

occlusive dressing Dressing made of Vaseline gauze, aluminum foil, or plastic that prevents air and liquids from entering or exiting a wound.

open chest injury Injury to the chest in which the chest wall itself is penetrated by a fractured rib or some external object.

paradoxical motion The motion of the portion of the chest wall that is detached in a flail chest; the motion—in during inhalation, out during exhalation—is exactly the opposite of normal chest wall motion during breathing.

pericardial tamponade Compression of the heart due to a buildup of blood or other fluid in the pericardial sac.

pericardium The fibrous sac that surrounds the heart.

pneumothorax An accumulation of air or gas in the pleural space.

pulmonary contusion A bruise of the lung.

spontaneous pneumothorax Pneumothorax that occurs when a weak area on the lung ruptures in the absence of major injury, allowing air to leak into the pleural space.

sucking chest wound An open or penetrating chest wall wound through which air passes during inspiration and expiration, creating a sucking sound.

tachypnea Rapid respirations.

tension pneumothorax An accumulation of air or gas in the pleural cavity that progressively increases the pressure in the chest with potentially fatal results.

www.OECzone.com

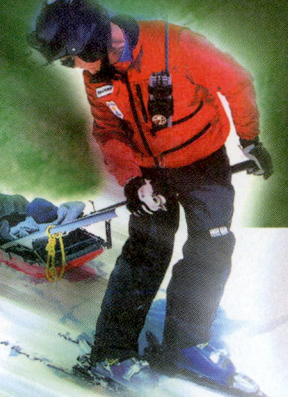

Assessment in Action

You are the first responder to a 22-year-old male snowboarder who was observed losing control and launching off the edge of a ridge, hitting a thick stand of aspen trees at mid-height while airborne. His jacket is torn open with visible blood in the left lateral chest wall and a sucking sound is coming from the area with each inspiration.

During your initial assessment, you are unable to palpate a radial pulse, but you manage to find a fast, weak carotid pulse. Between the patient's moaning and crying, you determine that he has respirations of more than 40 breaths/min.

1. From this information, you know that the patient has:
   A. normal air exchange.
   B. an open and clear airway.
   C. adequate circulation.
   D. adequate perfusion.

2. Your first step in caring for this patient is to:
   A. initiate CPR.
   B. cover the wound, give oxygen, and prepare to transport.
   C. obtain a complete set of vital signs and then check breath sounds.
   D. complete a detailed physical examination and prepare to transport.

3. Appropriate care for his chest wound includes:
   A. leaving it open to drain freely.
   B. packing it with gauze to control bleeding.
   C. covering it with an airtight dressing.
   D. inserting a drain to aid removal of body fluids.

4. Appropriate materials to use for an airtight dressing include Vaseline gauze, aluminum foil, or:
   A. a 4″ x 4″ piece of gauze.
   B. a washcloth.
   C. part of a sheet.
   D. a piece of plastic.

5. The patient has no breath sounds on the left side, appears to be very anxious, and seems to be struggling to breathe. He is becoming cyanotic despite administration of oxygen. His neck veins are distended, and his pulse is so fast and weak that it is almost imperceptible. These signs and symptoms suggest:
   A. a pneumothorax.
   B. an abdominal injury.
   C. a tension pneumothorax.
   D. pericardial tamponade.

6. At this point, the best treatment for this patient is to communicate your findings to the patrol dispatch and:
   A. tape a bulky dressing to the left chest.
   B. keep the patient warm.
   C. loosen the dressing over his wound.
   D. begin positive-pressure ventilation.

Challenging Questions

7. A deviated trachea is listed as one of the signs of a tension pneumothorax. But it is rarely seen in the field. Why?

8. A flail chest is an extremely painful injury for a patient. How can you effectively manage the pain of a flail segment in a conscious patient?

9. The most serious damage from a flail segment is not the broken ribs. What is it?

Points to Ponder

You are assessing a middle-aged woman with chest injury and difficulty breathing. She has cyanosis around her lips, her respirations are 44 breaths/min, and they are shallow and labored. She hit a lift tower with her chest during a high-speed fall. During the trauma assessment, you ask if you can carefully unzip her ski suit and lift up her turtleneck in order to look at her bare chest for discoloration, deformity, or paradoxical breathing because you suspect a flail chest. You assure her that you will do this as efficiently as possible with a blanket over her to keep her warm. The patient refuses to allow you to lift up her turtleneck to expose her chest for visual inspection. You ask whether one of the female ski patrol members could look for you, and the patient refuses to allow that also.

Issues Weather Concerns, Risk Management, Transportation Decisions, Documentation

Online Outlook

Chest injuries are both common and, given the likelihood of damage to the heart, lungs, or great blood vessels, very serious. Test your ability to anticipate and identify different chest injuries by completing Exercise 22 at www.OECzone.com.

www.OECzone.com

Abdomen and Genitalia Injuries

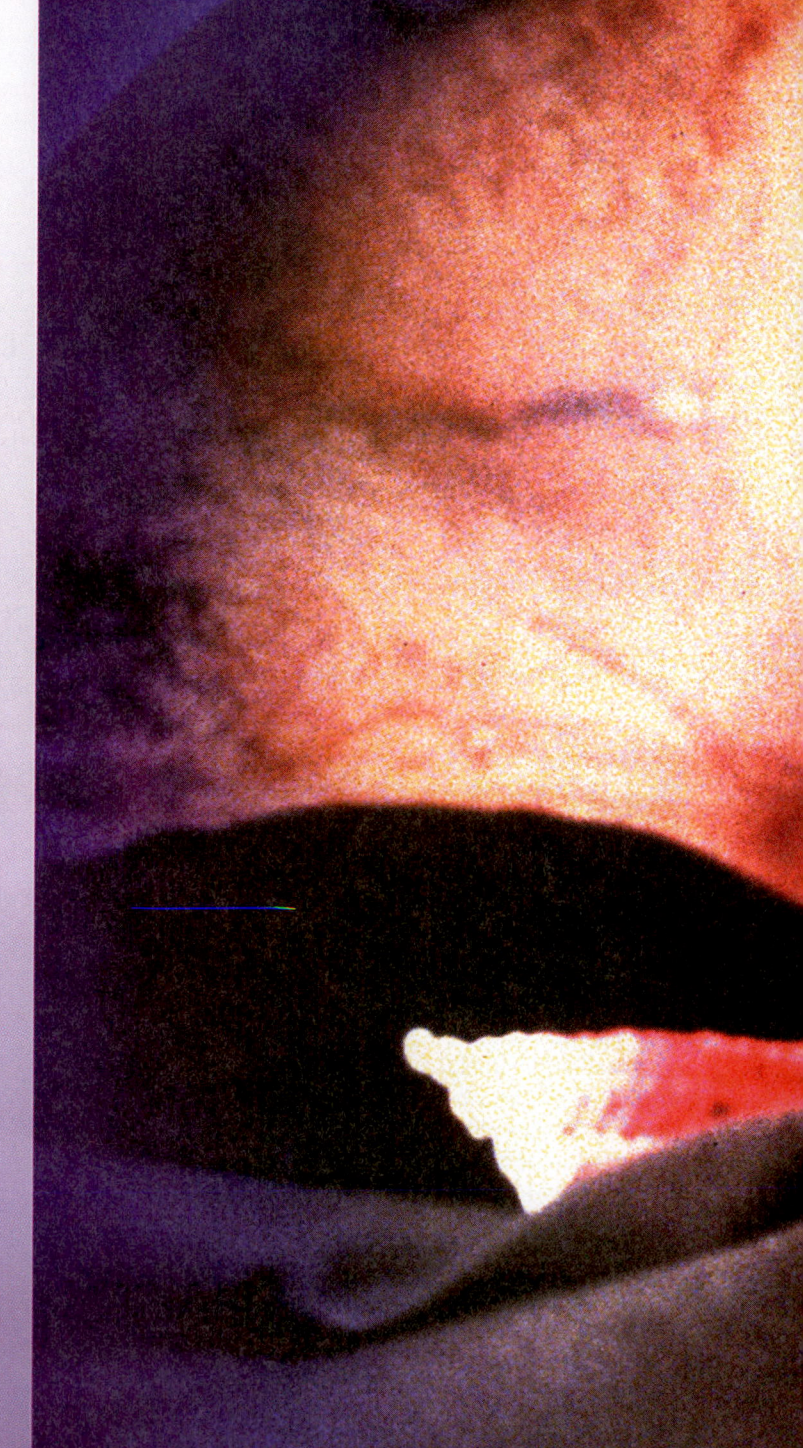

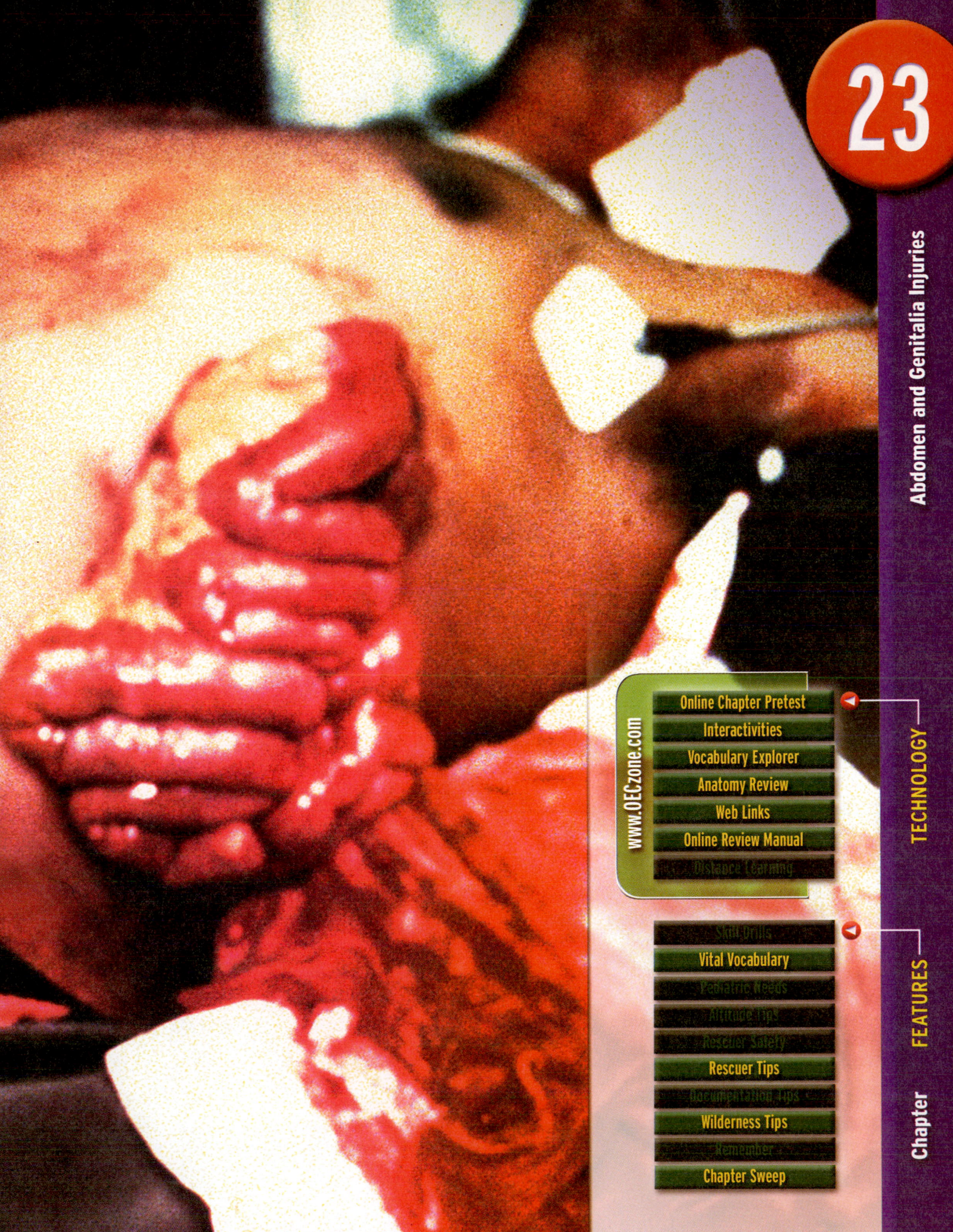

TECHNOLOGY

www.OECzone.com

- Online Chapter Pretest
- Interactivities
- Vocabulary Explorer
- Anatomy Review
- Web Links
- Online Review Manual
- Distance Learning

FEATURES

- Skill Drills
- Vital Vocabulary
- Pediatric Needs
- Altitude Tips
- Rescuer Safety
- Rescuer Tips
- Documentation Tips
- Wilderness Tips
- Remember
- Chapter Sweep

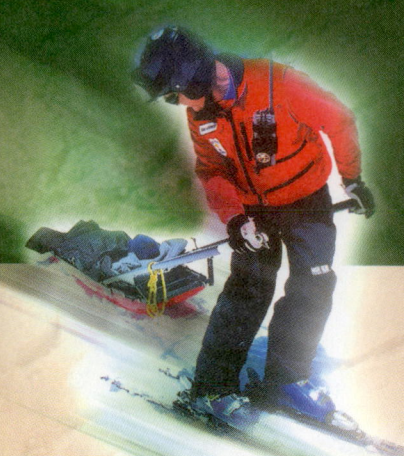

You are the rescuer

A hiker slips and tumbles on some scree down a difficult slope, making a windmill-type fall. In one of the tumbles, the hiker rolls over his backpack and another large object that jabs him hard in the left upper quadrant of his abdomen. He is lying on the snow guarding his abdomen and is in considerable pain.

Injuries to the abdomen, either open (penetrating) or closed (blunt), can be painful and stressful. This chapter will present content relative to both abdominal and genitalia injuries and will also help you answer the following questions:

1. How would you manage a patient who has suffered a laceration to the abdomen that has left approximately 14" of intestine exposed?

2. What would be the appropriate care for a patient with a ski pole impaled in the abdomen?

Abdomen and Genitalia Injuries

The abdomen is the lower of the two major body cavities, extending from the diaphragm to the pelvis. It contains several organs that make up the digestive, urinary, and genitourinary systems. Although any of these organs may be injured, some are better protected than others. You must know where these organs are located within the abdominal or pelvic cavities. You must also understand their functions so that when an illness or injury occurs, you can assess its seriousness.

This chapter begins with a brief review of the anatomy of the abdomen, followed by a discussion of common types of abdominal injuries. Next, patient assessment strategies are discussed, followed by a description of specific abdominal injuries that you are likely to encounter and how to treat each. The genitourinary system is then described, and common injuries and treatment are discussed.

The Anatomy of the Abdomen

The abdomen contains both hollow and solid organs, any of which may be damaged. **Hollow organs**, including the stomach, intestines, ureters, and bladder, are actually structures through which materials pass (▶ **Figure 23-1**). They usually contain food that is in the process of being digested, urine that is being passed to the bladder for release, or bile. When ruptured or lacerated, these organs spill their contents into the **peritoneal cavity** (the abdominal cavity), causing an intense inflammatory reaction called **peritonitis**. The first signs of peritonitis are severe abdominal pain, tenderness, and muscular spasm. Later, normal bowel sounds diminish or disappear

as the bowel stops functioning. A patient may feel nauseous and may vomit; the abdomen may become distended and firm to touch.

The **solid organs**, as their name suggests, are solid masses of tissue. They include the liver, spleen, pancreas, and kidneys (▶ **Figure 23-2**). It is here that much of the chemical work of the body—digestion, excretion, and energy production—takes place. Solid organs have

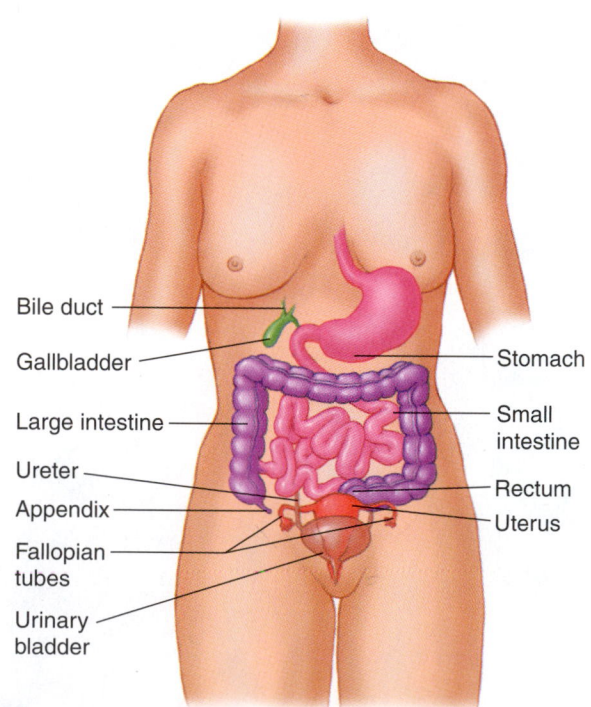

Bile duct
Gallbladder
Large intestine
Ureter
Appendix
Fallopian tubes
Urinary bladder
Stomach
Small intestine
Rectum
Uterus

Figure 23-1 The hollow organs in the abdominal cavity are structures through which materials pass.

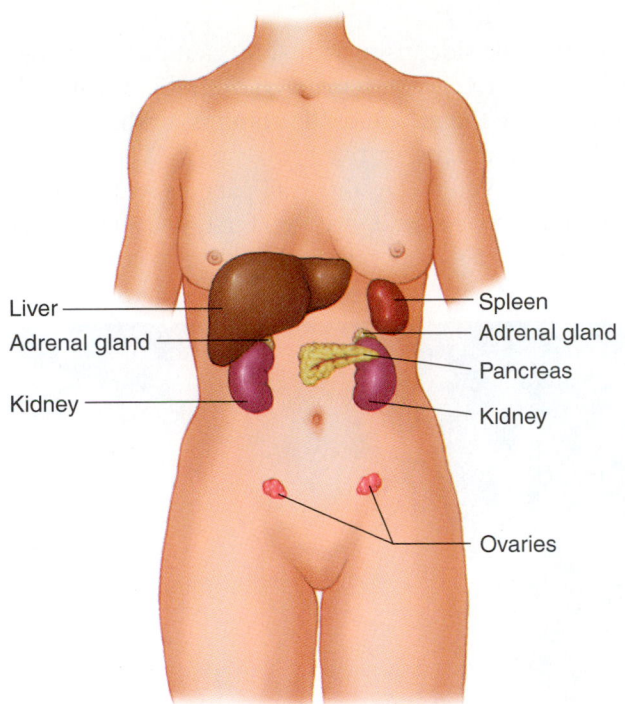

Figure 23-2 The solid organs are solid masses of tissue that do much of the chemical work in the body.

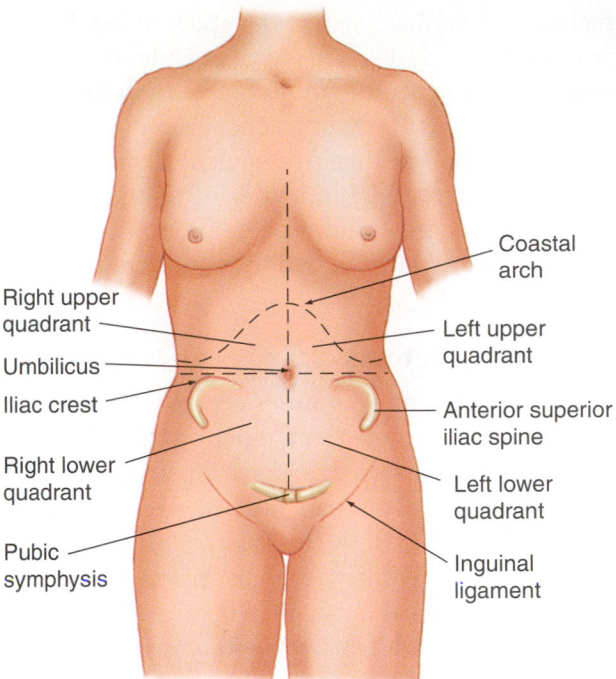

Figure 23-3 The abdominal cavity is divided into four quadrants, which serve as your means of identifying and reporting problems in the abdomen.

a rich blood supply, so injury can cause severe hemorrhage. The same is true of the aorta or inferior vena cava, whether the injury is open or closed. Unlike gastric juices and bacteria, blood within the peritoneal cavity initially produces less of an inflammatory response. Therefore, the absence of pain and tenderness does not necessarily mean the absence of major bleeding in the abdomen.

The bony landmarks in the abdomen include the pubic symphysis, the costal arch, the iliac crests, and the anterior superior iliac spines. The major soft-tissue landmark is the umbilicus, which overlies the fourth lumbar vertebra. The abdomen is divided arbitrarily into quadrants by two perpendicular lines that intersect at the umbilicus (▲ **Figure 23-3**). These quadrants provide a frame of reference for identifying and reporting abdominal signs and symptoms.

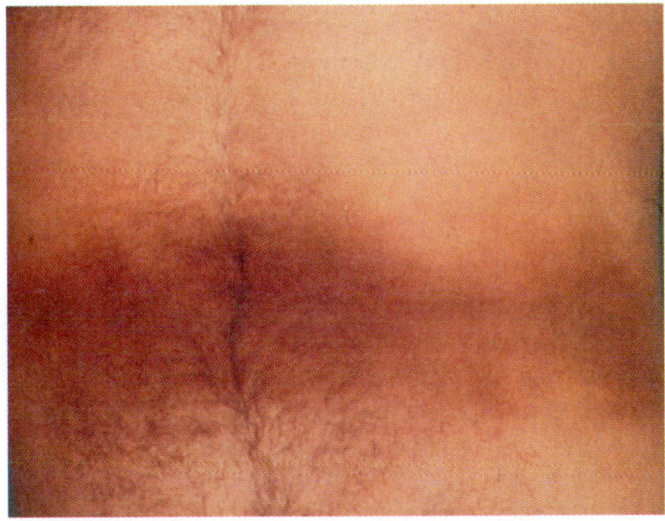

Figure 23-4 Blunt trauma to the abdomen can occur when a patient strikes the steering wheel of an automobile as a result of a crash.

Injuries of the Abdomen

Abdominal injuries may be as obvious as loops of intestines protruding from a stab wound or as subtle as a laceration to the liver or spleen. Remember to follow BSI precautions as you begin your initial assessment; these injuries often bleed profusely, and even if they do not, some blood or other body fluid is likely to be present. Injuries of the abdomen are considered open

or closed and can involve hollow and/or solid organs. Closed abdominal injuries are those in which a severe blow damages the abdomen without breaking the skin; these are also known as blunt injuries. Such a blow might come from the patient's striking the handlebar of a bicycle or the steering wheel of a car (▲ **Figure 23-4**). Open abdominal injuries are those in which a foreign object enters the abdomen and opens the peritoneal cavity to the outside; these are also known as penetrating injuries (▶ Figure 23-5). Open injuries might not go deeper than the wall of the abdomen, but this is difficult to determine. Therefore, you must assume the worst—that organs have been damaged—and provide prompt transport. Stab wounds and gunshot wounds are examples of open injuries.

Signs and Symptoms

Patients with abdominal injuries generally have one principal complaint: pain. But other significant injuries may mask the pain at first, and some patients may not be able to tell you about pain because they are unconscious or unresponsive, such as after a head injury or drug or alcohol overdose. The most common sign of significant abdominal injury is tachycardia. Later signs are those of shock: decreased blood pressure and pale, cool, moist skin. In some cases, the abdomen may become distended from the accumulation of blood and fluid. As a rescuer, you must look for other clues. Blunt injuries include bruises or other visible marks, whose location should guide your attention to underlying structures (▶ Figure 23-6). For example, bruises in the right upper quadrant, left upper quadrant, or flank might suggest an injury to the liver, spleen, or kidney, respectively.

The signs of abdominal injury are usually more definite than the symptoms, including firmness on palpation of the abdomen, obvious entry and exit wounds, bruises, and altered vital signs such as increased pulse rate, increased respiratory rate, decreased blood pressure, and shallow respirations (although this might not appear until later). Common symptoms include abdominal tenderness, particularly localized tenderness, and difficulty with movement because of pain.

Evaluating Abdominal Injuries

Your goal in initial assessment is to evaluate the patient's ABCs and then immediately care for any life threats. You should then begin the focused history and physical exam to determine the type of abdominal injury (open or closed), the extent of the damage, and the presence of shock. Note that patients may or may not be able to tell you about the severity and location of their pain. However, they may report that they feel nauseous, and they may vomit. Remember to keep the airway clear of vomitus so that it is not aspirated into the lungs, especially in a patient who is unresponsive or has an altered level of consciousness. Turn the

patient to one side, using spinal precautions if necessary, and try to clear any material from the throat and mouth. Note the nature of the vomitus: undigested food, blood, mucus, or bile.

Normally, you will evaluate all patients with abdominal injuries in the same manner. First, you should place the patient in a supine position with the knees slightly

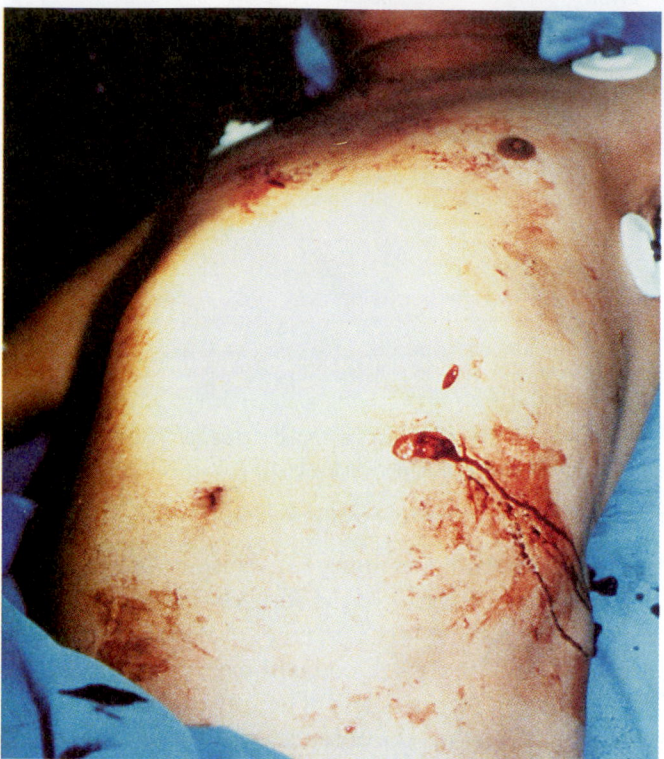

Figure 23-5 Because it is difficult to know how deep a penetrating injury is, assume organ damage and transport promptly.

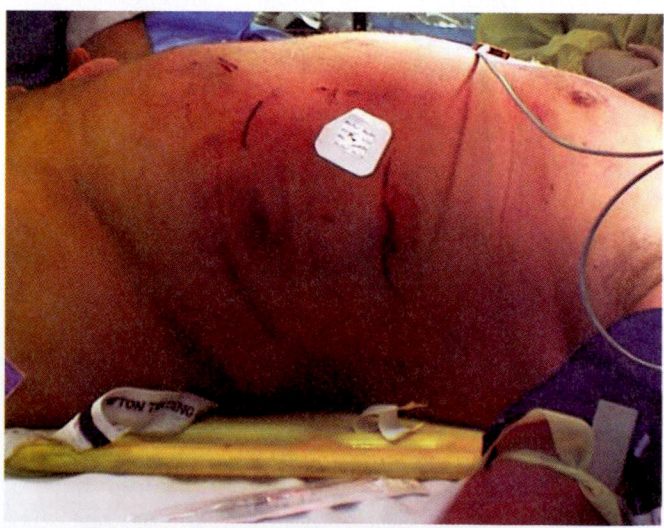

Figure 23-6 Bruising on the abdomen can provide clues to the possible injury of underlying organs.

flexed and supported (▼ **Figure 23-7**). Remove or loosen clothes. Then, before you do anything else, assess and record baseline vital signs. Many abdominal emergencies, aside from those that cause severe bleeding, can cause a rapid pulse and low blood pressure. Your record of vital signs, made as early as possible and periodically thereafter, will be of tremendous help to physicians in evaluating the problem when the patient arrives in the emergency department.

Further assessment follows the DCAP-BTLS sequence: Inspect and palpate the abdomen for the presence of **D**eformity, which may be subtle in abdominal injuries. Look for the presence of **C**ontusions and **A**brasions, which can help localize focal points of impact and may indicate significant internal injury. Puncture wounds and other **P**enetrating injuries must not be overlooked, as the intra-abdominal extent of these injuries may be life-threatening. The presence of **B**urns must be noted and managed appropriately. Palpate for **T**enderness and attempt to localize to a specific quadrant of the abdomen. Identify and treat any **L**acerations with appropriate dressings. **S**welling may involve the abdomen globally and indicate significant intra-abdominal injury.

Quickly assess the patient's condition with a simple inspection, noting the manner in which he or she is lying. Movement of the body or the abdominal organs irritates the inflamed peritoneum, causing additional pain. To minimize this pain, patients will lie still, usually with the knees drawn up, and breathe rapid and shallow. For the same reason, they will contract their abdominal muscles, a sign called **guarding**.

Next, inspect the skin of the abdomen for holes through which bullets, knives, or other missile-type

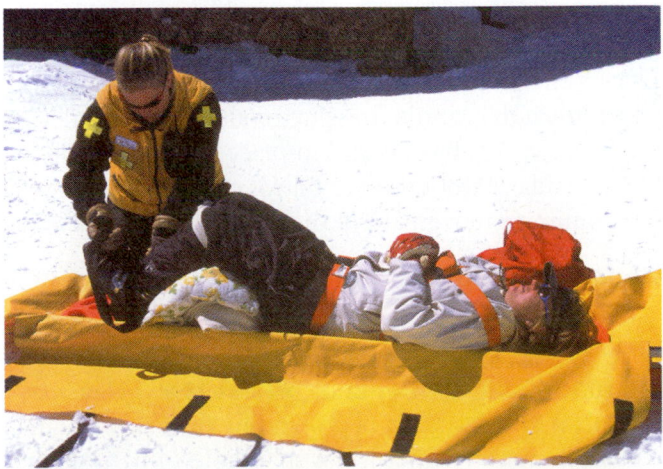

Figure 23-7   Patients with abdominal injuries should be placed in a supine position with the knees slightly flexed and supported.

Wilderness Tips

Abdominal injuries are often associated with fractures or traumatic brain injuries. The rescuer must have a high index of suspicion and perform a very thorough physical exam. Abdominal distention is secondary to bleeding and will never present before shock and cardiovascular collapse. Remember to examine the lower part of the chest and back following palpation of the spine while the patient is supine.

foreign bodies may have passed. Keep in mind that the size of the wound does not necessarily indicate the extent of underlying injuries. If you find an entry wound, you must always check for a corresponding exit hole in the patient's back or sides. If the injury was caused by a very high-velocity missile from a rifle, you may see a small, harmless-looking entrance wound with a large, gaping exit wound. Do not attempt to remove any object that is impaled in the patient. Instead, stabilize the object with supportive bandaging. Bruises or other visible marks are important clues to the cause and severity of any blunt injury. Compression traumas such as hard falls and collisions produce characteristic patterns of bruising on the abdomen or chest.

Always examine the patient's flanks and back for wounds, bruises, abrasions, tenderness, etc.

Types of Abdominal Injuries
Blunt Abdominal Wounds

A patient with a blunt abdominal wound may have one or some combination of the following:

- Severe bruises of the abdominal wall
- Laceration of the liver and spleen
- Rupture of the intestine, stomach, or any hollow organ
- Tears in the mesentery, membranous folds that attach the intestines to the walls of the body, and injury to blood vessels within them
- Rupture of the kidneys, or tearing of the kidneys from their arteries and veins
- Rupture of the bladder, especially in a patient who had been drinking and therefore had a full and distended bladder at the time of the injury
- Severe intra-abdominal hemorrhage
- Peritoneal irritation and inflammation in response to the rupture of hollow organs

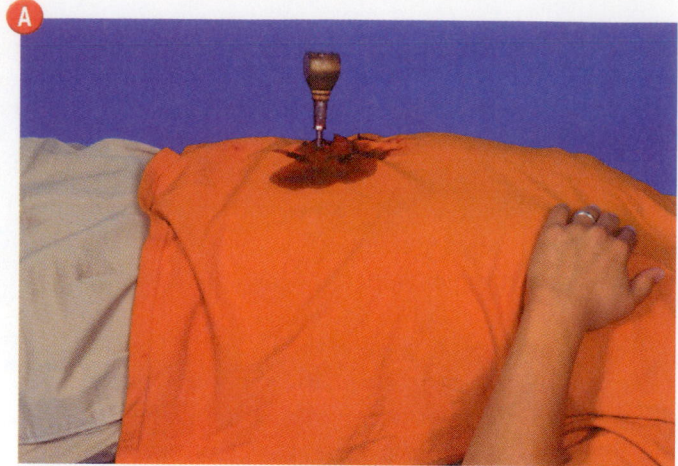

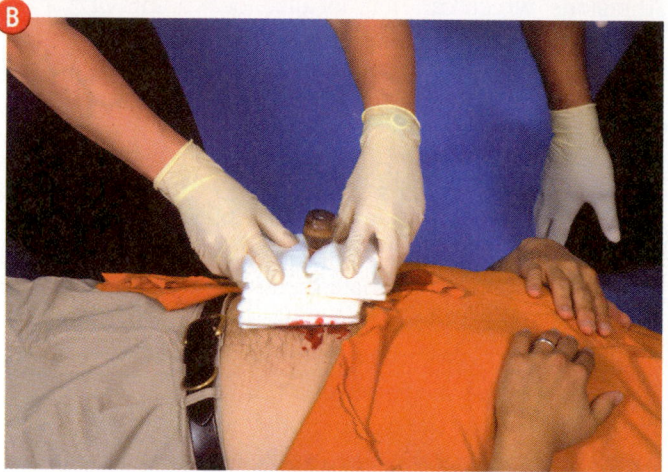

A patient who has sustained a blunt abdominal injury should be log rolled to a supine position on a backboard. Ensure that you protect the spine as you do so. If the patient vomits, turn him or her to one side and clear the mouth and throat of vomitus. Monitor the patient's vital signs for any indication of shock such as pallor; cold sweat; rapid, thready pulse; or low blood pressure. If you see any of these signs, administer supplemental oxygen via nonrebreathing mask, and take all the appropriate measures to treat for shock. Keep the patient warm with blankets, and provide prompt transport to the emergency department.

If there is no spine injury, the patient may be more comfortable with his or her knees slightly bent.

Penetrating Abdominal Injuries

Patients with penetrating injuries generally have obvious wounds and external bleeding ▶ Figure 23-8A . A large wound may have bowel, fat, or a fold of peritoneum protruding from it. In addition to pain, these patients often report nausea and vomiting. Patients with peritonitis generally prefer to lie very still with their legs drawn up because it hurts to move or straighten their legs. They may complain about every bump during transport.

Some penetrating injuries go no deeper than the abdominal wall, but the severity of the injury can be hard to determine. Only a surgeon can accurately assess the damage. Therefore, as you care for a patient with this type of wound, you should assume that the object has penetrated the peritoneum, entered the abdominal cavity, and possibly injured one or more organs even if there are no immediate obvious signs.

If major blood vessels are cut or solid organs are lacerated, bleeding may be rapid and severe. Other signs of intra-abdominal injuries may develop slowly, particularly in penetrating wounds to hollow organs. Once such an organ is punctured and its contents are discharged into the abdominal cavity, peritonitis may develop, but this may take several hours.

Figure 23-8   **A.** Penetrating injuries have obvious wounds and may also have external bleeding. **B.** If the penetrating object is still in place, use a roller bandage to stabilize the object and to control bleeding.

In caring for a patient with a penetrating abdominal wound, follow the general procedures described above for care of a blunt abdominal wound, as well as the following specific steps for the penetrating wound. Inspect the patient's back and sides for exit wounds, and apply a dry, sterile dressing to all open wounds. If the penetrating object is still in place, apply a stabilizing bandage around it to control external bleeding and minimize movement of the object ▲ Figure 23-8B .

Abdominal Evisceration

Severe lacerations of the abdominal wall may result in an **evisceration**, in which internal organs or fat protrude through the wound ▶ Figure 23-9 . Never try to replace an organ that is protruding from an abdominal laceration, whether it is a small fold of peritoneum or nearly all of the intestines. Instead, cover it with sterile gauze compresses moistened with sterile saline

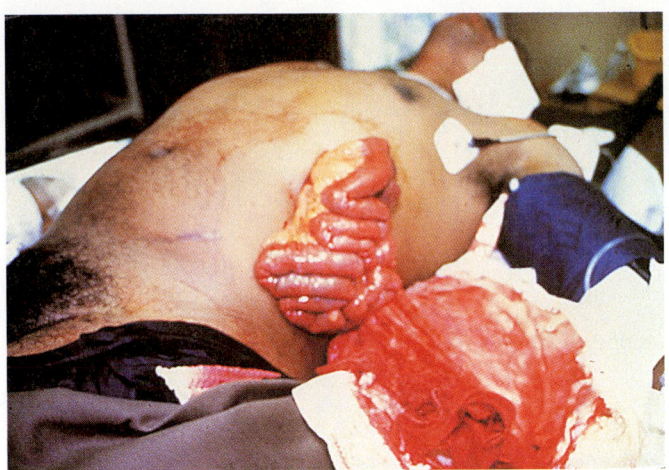

Figure 23-9 An abdominal evisceration is an open abdominal wound from which internal organs or fat protrude.

solution, and secure them with a sterile dressing. The exception to this rule of leaving exposed contents outside the abdominal wall is when a long transport time is required in a cold environment. If there is a possibility that the exposed organs will freeze, a gentle attempt (using BSI precautions) to replace organs into the body should be tried. The typical protocol calls for an occlusive dressing over the organs, secured by trauma dressings.) Because the open abdomen radiates body heat very effectively, and because exposed organs lose fluid rapidly, you must keep the organs moist and warm. If you do not have gauze compresses, you may use moist, sterile dressings, covered and secured in place with a bandage and tape ▼ **Figure 23-10** . Do not use any material that is adherent or loses its substance when wet, such as toilet paper, facial tissue, paper towels, or absorbent cotton.

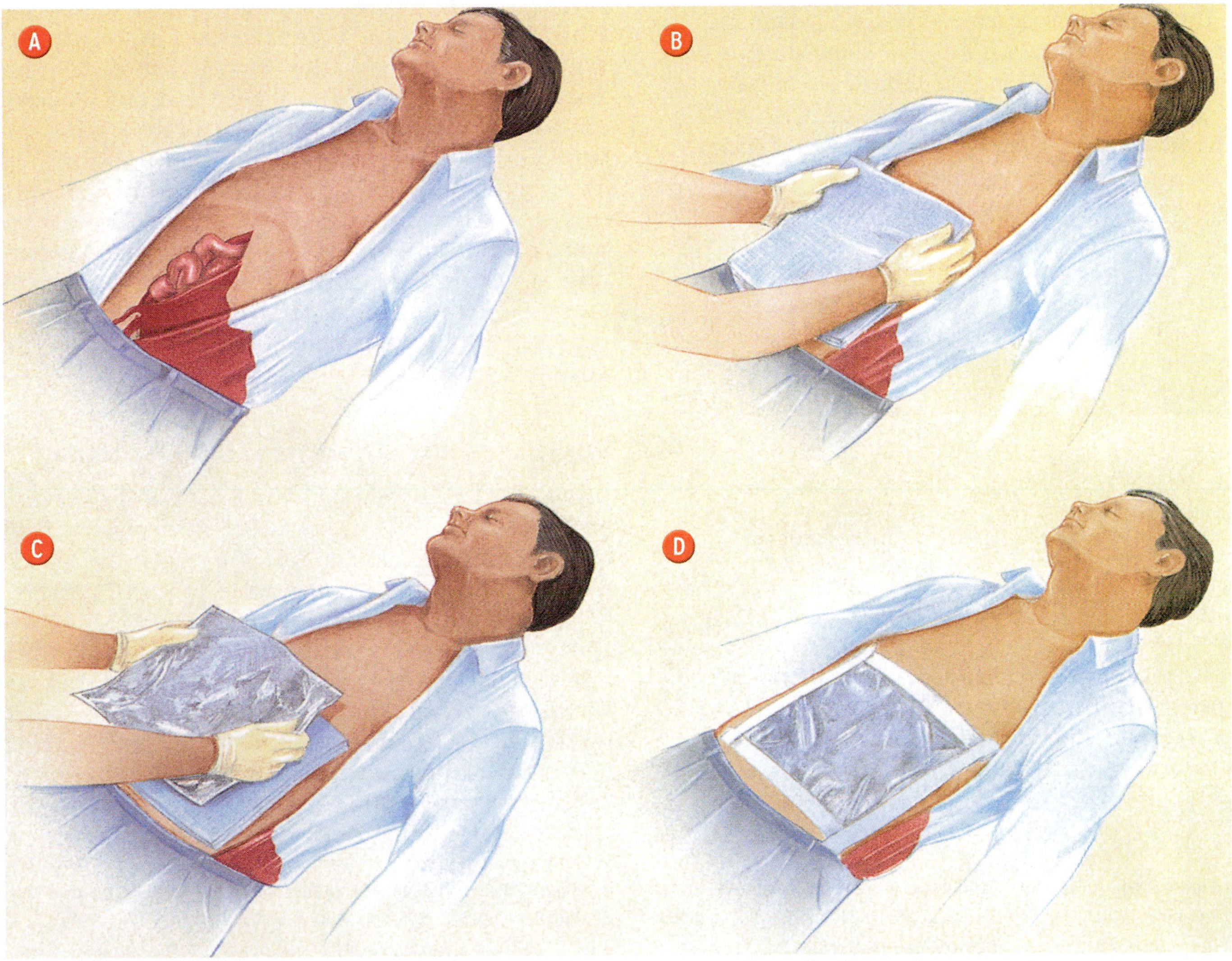

Figure 23-10 **A.** The open abdomen radiates body heat rapidly and must be covered. **B.** Cover the wound with moistened sterile gauze, or with an occlusive dressing, depending on local protocol. **C.** Secure the dressing with a bandage. **D.** Secure the bandage with tape.

Once you have covered the extruding organ, you should provide other emergency care as necessary and arrange for prompt transport to the emergency department.

Anatomy of the Genitourinary System

The genitourinary system controls both the reproductive functions and the waste discharge system, which are generally considered together.

The urinary system controls the discharge of certain waste materials filtered from the blood by the kidneys. In the urinary system, the kidneys are solid organs; the ureters, bladder, and urethra are hollow organs ▶ **Figure 23-11**.

The genital system controls the reproductive processes from which life is created. The male genitalia, except for the prostate gland and the seminal vesicles, and parts of the urethra lie outside the pelvic cavity ▼ **Figure 23-12**. The female genitalia, except for the vulva, clitoris, and labia, are contained entirely within the pelvis ▼ **Figure 23-13**. The male and female reproductive organs have certain similarities and, of course, basic differences. They allow for the production of sperm and egg cells and appropriate hormones, the act of intercourse, and, ultimately, reproduction.

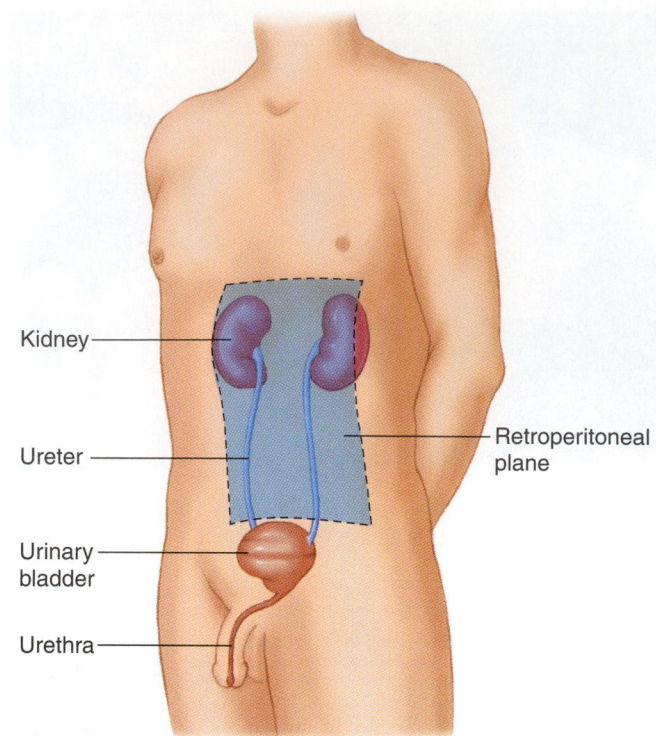

Figure 23-11   The urinary system lies in the retroperitoneal space behind the digestive tract. The kidneys are solid organs; the ureter, bladder, and urethra are hollow organs.

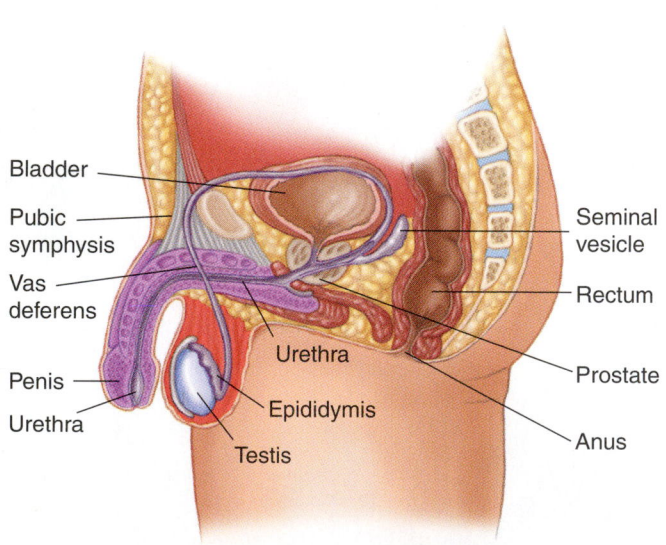

Figure 23-12   The male reproductive system includes the testicles, vasa deferentia, seminal vesicles, prostate gland, urethra, and penis.

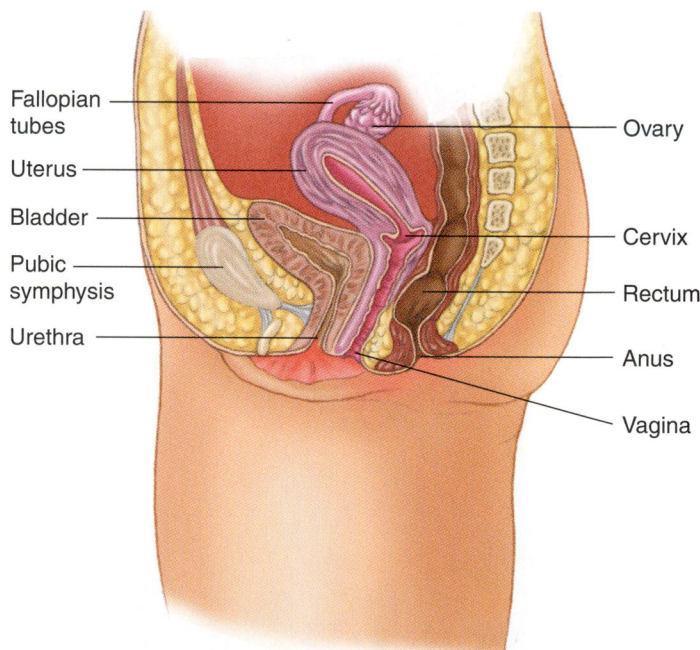

Figure 23-13   The female reproductive system includes the ovaries, fallopian tubes, uterus, cervix, and vagina.

Wilderness Tips

If an unstable pelvic fracture associated with rectal and vaginal injuries is the predominate reason for the evacuation decision in a wilderness setting, this takes priority over doing a rectal or vaginal examination.

Injuries of the Genitourinary System
Injuries of the Kidney

Injuries of the kidney are not unusual and rarely occur in isolation. This is because the kidneys lie in such a well-protected area of the body. A penetrating wound that reaches the kidneys almost always involves other organs. The same is true with blunt injuries. A blow that is forceful enough to cause significant kidney damage almost always damages other intra-abdominal organs, often fracturing a rib as well. Less significant injuries to the kidneys may result from a direct blow or even from a tackle in football. Suspect kidney damage if the patient has a history or physical evidence of any of the following findings:

- An abrasion, laceration, or contusion in the flank

- A penetrating wound in the region of the lower rib cage (the flank) or the upper abdomen

- Fractures on either side of the lower rib cage or of the lower thoracic or upper lumbar vertebrae

- Blood in the urine

Damage to the kidneys may not be obvious on inspection of the patient. You may or may not see bruises or lacerations on the overlying skin. However, you will see signs of shock if the injury is associated with significant blood loss. Because one of the functions of the kidney is the formation of urine, another sign of kidney damage is blood in the urine, called **hematuria**. Treat shock and associated injuries in the appropriate manner. Arrange for prompt transport to the hospital, monitoring the patient's vital signs carefully en route.

Injuries of the Urinary Bladder

Injury of the urinary bladder, either blunt or penetrating, may result in its rupture. When this happens, urine spills into the surrounding tissues, and any urine that passes through the urethra is likely to be bloody. Blunt injuries of the lower abdomen or pelvis often cause rupture of the urinary bladder, particularly when the bladder is full and distended. Sharp, bony fragments from a fracture of the pelvis often perforate the urinary bladder ▼ Figure 23-14 . Penetrating wounds of the lower midabdomen or the perineum (the pelvic floor and associated structures that occupy the pelvic outlet) can directly involve the bladder. In the male, sudden deceleration from a motor vehicle or motorcycle crash can literally shear the bladder from the urethra.

Suspect a possible injury of the urinary bladder if you see blood at the urethral opening or physical signs of trauma on the lower abdomen, pelvis, or perineum. There may be blood at the tip of the penis or a stain on the patient's underwear.

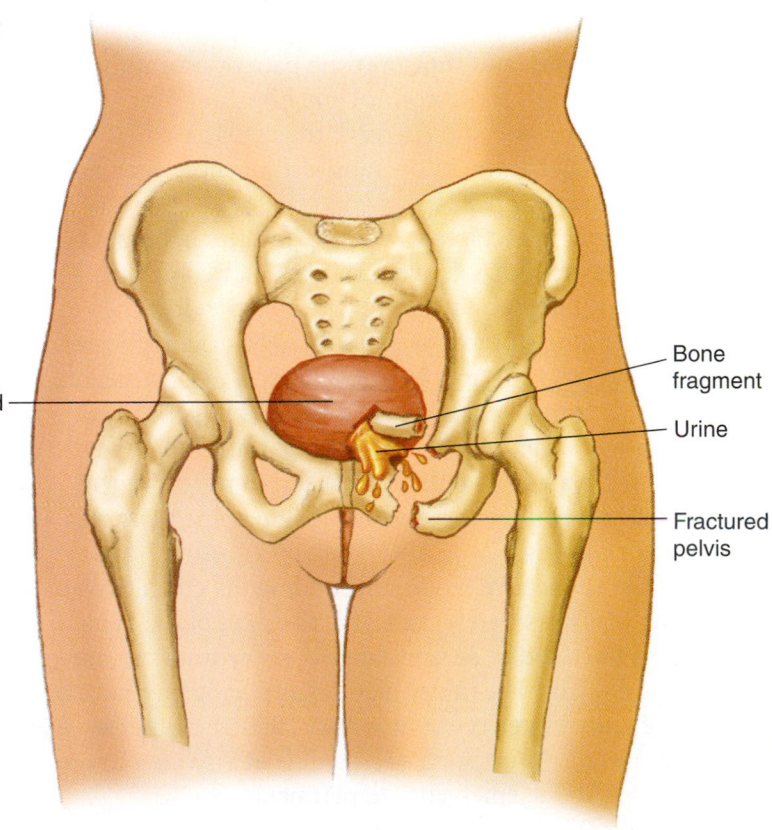

Ruptured bladder

Bone fragment

Urine

Fractured pelvis

Figure 23-14 Fracture of the pelvis can result in a laceration of the bladder by the bony fragments. Urine then leaks into the pelvis.

The presence of associated injuries or of shock will dictate the urgency of transport. In most instances, provide prompt transport, and monitor the patient's vital signs as frequently as possible.

Injuries of the External Male Genitalia

Injuries of the external male genitalia include all types of soft-tissue wounds. Although these injuries are uniformly painful and generally a source of great concern to the patient, they are rarely life-threatening. Avulsion (tearing away) of the skin of the penis can occur, particularly in the uncircumcised male. If you encounter a patient with such an injury, wrap the penis in a soft, sterile dressing moistened with sterile saline solution, and transport the patient promptly. Use direct pressure to control any bleeding. You should try to save and preserve the avulsed skin, but do not delay treatment or transport for more than a few minutes to do so.

Managing blood loss is your top priority in amputation of the penile shaft, whether partial or complete. You should use local pressure with a sterile dressing on the remaining stump. Never apply a constricting device to the penis to control bleeding. Surgical reconstruction of even a completely amputated penis is possible if you can locate the amputated part. Wrap it in a moist, sterile dressing; place it in a plastic bag; and transport it in a cooled container without allowing it to come in direct contact with ice.

If the connective tissue surrounding the erectile tissue in the penis is severely damaged, the shaft of the penis can be fractured or severely angled, sometimes requiring surgical repair. The injury may occur during particularly active sexual intercourse. It is associated with intense pain, bleeding into the tissues, and fear. Provide prompt transport to the emergency department.

Accidental laceration of the skin about the head of the penis usually occurs when the penis is erect and is associated with heavy bleeding. The injury usually appears worse than it actually is; once the penis becomes flaccid, the size of the laceration decreases. Local pressure with a sterile dressing is usually sufficient to stop the hemorrhage.

It is not uncommon for the skin of the shaft of the penis or the foreskin to get caught in the zipper of pants. If a small segment of the zipper is involved (one or two teeth), you can try to unzip the pants. If a longer segment is involved or the patient is agitated, use heavy scissors to cut the zipper away from where it is closed on the penis to make the patient more comfortable during transport. Be sure to explain what the scissors are for before you begin cutting.

Urethral injuries in the male are uncommon. Lacerations of the urethra can result from straddle injuries, pelvic fractures, or penetrating wounds of the perineum. These injuries may bleed quite a lot, although this may not be evident externally. Direct pressure with a dry, sterile dressing usually controls any external hemorrhage. Because the urethra is the channel for urine, it is very important to know whether the patient can urinate and whether hematuria is present. For this reason, you should save any voided urine for later examination at the hospital. Any foreign bodies that may be protruding from the urethra will have to be removed in a surgical setting.

Avulsion of the skin of the scrotum may damage the scrotal contents. If possible, preserve the avulsed skin in a moist, sterile dressing for possible use in reconstruction. Wrap the scrotal contents or the perineal area with a sterile, moist compress, and use a local pressure dressing to control bleeding. Transport this patient promptly to the emergency department.

A straddle injury or direct blow to the scrotum can result in the rupture of a testicle or significant accumulation of blood around the testes. In either case, temporarily stabilize the injury with clothing or an athletic supporter-like swathe made of triangular bandages. You should apply an ice pack to the scrotal area while transporting the patient.

A few general rules apply to the treatment of injuries involving the external male genitalia:

- These injuries are very painful and embarassing. Make the patient as comfortable as possible.

- Use sterile, moist compresses to cover areas that have been stripped of skin.

- Apply direct pressure with dry, sterile gauze dressings to control bleeding.

- Never move or manipulate impaled instruments or foreign bodies in the urethra.

- If possible, always identify and send avulsed parts to the hospital with the patient.

- If urine is obtained, send it to the hospital.

Remember, these are rarely life-threatening injuries and should not be given priority over other, more severe wounds.

Injuries of the Female Genitalia

INTERNAL FEMALE GENITALIA. The uterus, ovaries, and fallopian tubes are subject to the same kinds of injuries as any other internal organ. However, they are rarely damaged because they are small, deep in the pelvis, and well protected by the pelvic bones. Unlike the bladder, which lies adjacent to the bony pelvis, they are usually not injured in a pelvic fracture.

An exception is the pregnant uterus. As pregnancy progresses, the uterus enlarges substantially and rises out of the pelvis, becoming vulnerable to both penetrating and blunt injuries. These injuries can be particularly severe because the uterus has a rich blood supply during pregnancy. You must also keep in mind that

another life—that of the unborn child—is at risk. You can expect to see the signs and symptoms of shock with these patients; be prepared to provide all necessary support and prompt transport. Note that contractions may begin as well. If possible, ask the patient when she is due, and report this information to the hospital.

In the last trimester of pregnancy, the uterus is large and may obstruct the vena cava, decreasing the amount of blood returning to the heart, if the patient is placed in a supine position (**supine hypotensive syndrome**). As a result, blood pressure may decrease. The patient should be carefully placed on her *left* side so that the uterus will not lie on the vena cava. If the patient is secured to a backboard, tilt the board to the *left*.

EXTERNAL FEMALE GENITALIA. The external female genitalia include the vulva, the clitoris, and the major and minor labia (lips) at the entrance of the vagina. Injuries of the external female genitalia can include all types of soft-tissue injuries. Because these genital parts have a rich nerve supply, injuries are very painful. Lacerations, abrasions, and avulsions should be treated with moist, sterile compresses. Use local pressure to control bleeding and a diaper-type bandage to hold dressings in place. Under no circumstances should you pack or place dressings into the vagina. Leave any foreign bodies in place after you stabilize them with bandages.

In general, although these injuries are painful, they are not life-threatening. Bleeding may be heavy, but it can usually be controlled by local compression. Contusions and other blunt injuries all require careful in-hospital evaluation. However, the urgency of the need for transport will be determined by associated injuries, the amount of hemorrhage, and the presence of shock.

Chapter *Sweep*

Ready for Review

Abdominal injuries are classified as either open (penetrating) or closed (blunt) in origin. Either type can damage both hollow organs, such as the stomach and ureters; and solid organs, such as the liver, spleen, and kidneys. Penetrating injuries are most frequently caused by impaled tree limbs or ski poles; blunt injuries are often the result of a collision with a rock or tree. Both types of injury cause pain, although this may be masked at first.

These injuries are evaluated in a similar fashion. Place the patient in a supine position, assess and record vital signs, and perform a visual inspection. Always assume that major damage has occurred to abdominal organs, even if there are no obvious signs. Look for bruises or other marks that may point you toward underlying damage: a firm abdomen, difficulty in moving, abdominal tenderness and guarding, obvious entry and exit wounds, and altered vital signs. If hollow organs have spilled their contents into the peritoneal cavity, peritonitis will develop. In an effort to minimize the pain of this condition, patients will want to lie still with their knees drawn up. Treat for shock as necessary, keep the throat clear of vomitus, keep the patient warm, and provide rapid transport to definitive care.

Do not replace an eviscerated organ unless you expect a long transport time in cold weather where the organs could freeze. Keep the organ warm and moist with sterile gauze compresses. Injuries to the kidneys or bladder will not have obvious external signs, but there are usually more subtle clues such as lower rib pain or a possible pelvic fracture. The external genitalia in both males and females can sustain injuries that can be extremely painful, but these are rarely life-threatening. Never pack dressings into the vagina.

Vital Vocabulary

closed abdominal injury Any injury of the abdomen caused by a nonpenetrating instrument or force, in which the skin remains intact; also called blunt abdominal injury.

evisceration The displacement of organs outside of the body.

guarding Contracting the stomach muscles to minimize the pain of abdominal movement; a sign of peritonitis.

hematuria The presence of blood in the urine.

hollow organs Structures through which materials pass, such as the stomach, small intestine, large intestine, ureters, and bladder.

open abdominal injury An injury of the abdomen caused by a penetrating or piercing instrument or force, in which the skin is lacerated or perforated and the cavity is opened to the atmosphere; also called penetrating injury.

peritoneal cavity The abdominal cavity.

peritonitis Inflammation of the peritoneum.

solid organs Solid masses of tissue where much of the chemical work of the body takes place (eg, the liver, spleen, pancreas, and kidneys).

supine hypotensive syndrome A drop in blood pressure caused when the heavy uterus of a supine, third-trimester pregnant patient obstructs the vena cava, lowering blood return to the heart.

Assessment in Action

It's a hot, humid July evening, and you and your partner are covering the local rodeo. The bull-riding competition begins and the bull twists and turns out of the chute, launching the rider into the air and tossing him onto a fence. The 27-year-old cowboy falls on the other side of the fence, well away from the bull.

Assessment reveals a large bruise developing across his abdomen. He states that, while he is having difficulty breathing, his chief complaint is abdominal pain. Vital signs include a pulse of 140 beats/min, respirations of 32 breaths/min, and a blood pressure of 138/92 mm Hg. His skin is flushed and moist, and his pupils are equal and reactive to light.

1. Given the patient's mechanism of injury, manual immobilization of the cervical spine should be applied:
   A. immediately after the airway is secured.
   B. after the detailed physical examination is completed.
   C. when the patient is being loaded into the ambulance.
   D. after the patient is in the ambulance and ready to transport.

2. Which of the following steps is the most important part of your examination of the patient's abdomen?
   A. Flexion
   B. Inspection
   C. Massage
   D. Auscultation

3. This patient needs to have breath sounds evaluated. In this situation, when should this be done?
   A. Immediately after scene size-up
   B. As soon as the airway is open
   C. After your initial assessment
   D. Once you have immobilized the patient

4. The bruising over his abdomen is becoming more prominent, and the abdomen is beginning to feel tight, suggesting:
   A. a punctured lung.
   B. rapidly spreading infection.
   C. decreasing oxygen levels.
   D. continued internal bleeding.

5. Appropriate care for this patient includes oxygen, immobilization, and:
   A. keeping him warm.
   B. elevating his head.
   C. elevating his feet.
   D. turning him on his side.

6. En route to the hospital, your patient becomes restless. His skin is cool and moist. Repeat vital signs show a pulse of 146 beats/min, respirations of 32 breaths/min, and a blood pressure of 116/76 mm Hg. You suspect that the patient may:
   A. have a head injury with increasing intracranial pressure.
   B. have a pneumothorax with a buildup of pressure on that side.
   C. be developing another problem unrelated to his injury.
   D. be developing progressive shock as a result of his injuries.

7. Why is a ruptured solid organ more easily recognized in the field?
   A. Ruptured solid organs bleed, and shock is more easily recognized.
   B. Ruptured solid organs have more pain than ruptured hollow organs.
   C. Ruptured hollow organs do not cause much of a problem in the field.
   D. Solid organs swell more than hollow organs, so they can be seen more easily.

Challenging Questions

8. Why should an evisceration be covered immediately?

9. Why should one suspect that a trauma patient with unexplained signs of shock and good lung sounds is bleeding in the abdomen?

10. Patients who have an inflamed peritoneum will prefer to lie on their side with their knees drawn up. Why does this reduce pain?

Points to Ponder

A 9-year-old girl skis off the trail and into a tree. She lands in such a way that she is not easily accessible. When the rescuer arrives on the scene, the girl is lying on her side complaining that her "stomach" hurts. She is frightened and repeatedly asks for her parents to be found. For the first few minutes, the patient shows fairly normal vital signs; then they elevate significantly and signs of shock come on rapidly.

Issues Gender Issues of Patient Care, Modesty, Treating Minors, Genital Injuries, Locating a Responsible Adult, Extrication Concerns to "Load and Go."

Online Outlook

The abdomen is the lower of the two major body cavities, extending from the diaphragm to the pelvis. You must know where the organs are located within the abdominal or pelvic cavities. Review your knowledge by completing Exercise 23 at www.OECzone.com.

www.OECzone.com

Principles of Musculoskeletal Injuries

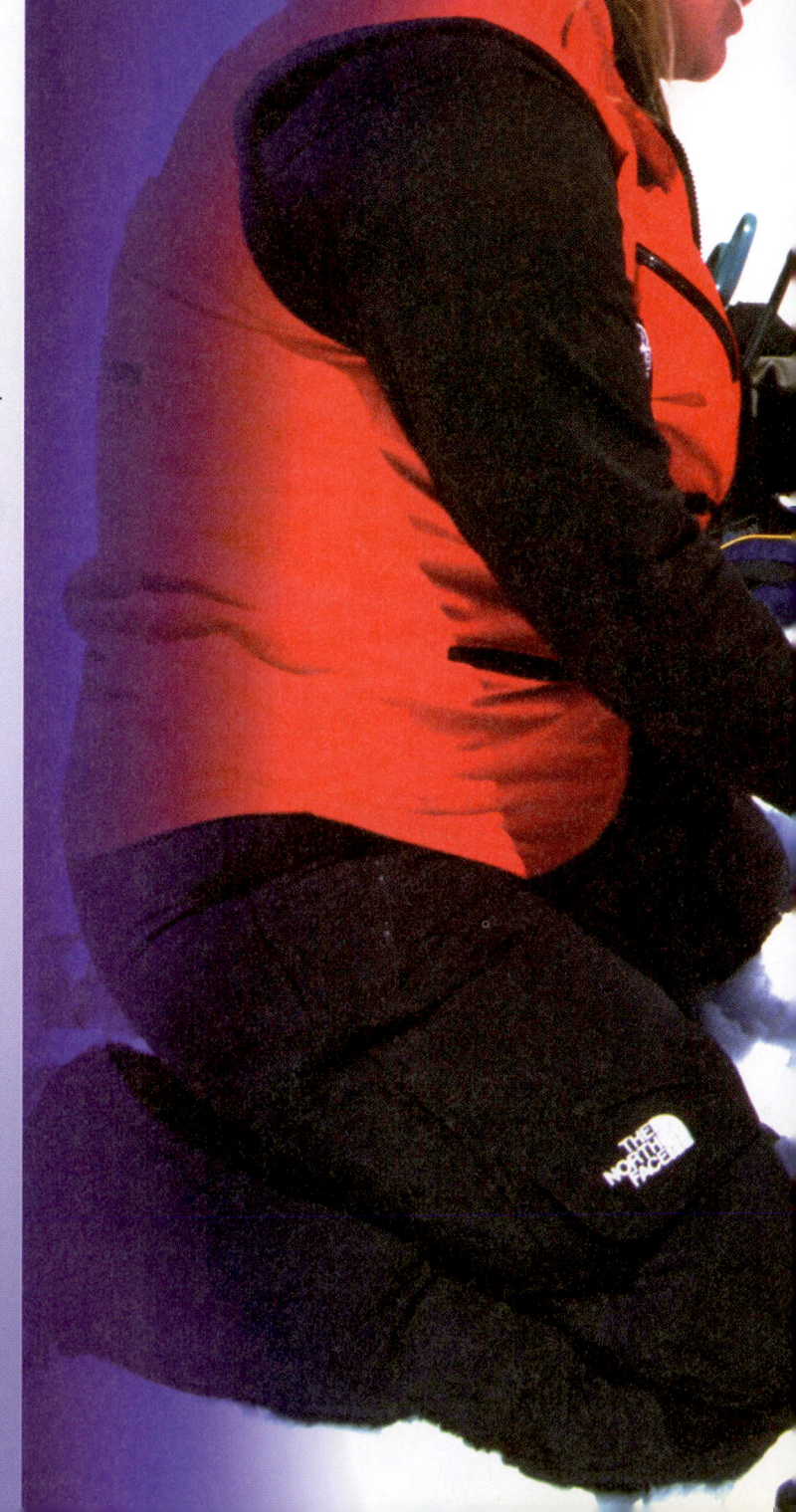

Objectives

Cognitive

♣ **1.** Describe the function of the muscular system (p 576).

♣ **2.** Describe the function of the skeletal system (p 577).

♣ **3.** List the major bones or bone groupings of the spinal column, the thorax, the upper extremities, and the lower extremities (p 577).

♣ **4.** Differentiate between an open and closed painful, swollen, deformed extremity (fracture) (p 580).

♣ **5.** State the reasons for splinting (p 588).

♣ **6.** List the general rules of splinting (p 588).

♣ **7.** List the complications of splinting (p 590).

Affective

♣ **8.** Explain the rationale for splinting at the scene versus load and go (p 588).

Psychomotor

♣ **9.** Demonstrate the emergency medical care principles for injured extremities (p 588).

♣ **10.** Demonstrate the basic principles of applying the three basic splint types: rigid fixation, soft fixation, and traction splints (p 590).

♣ These are core concepts in initial patrol training.

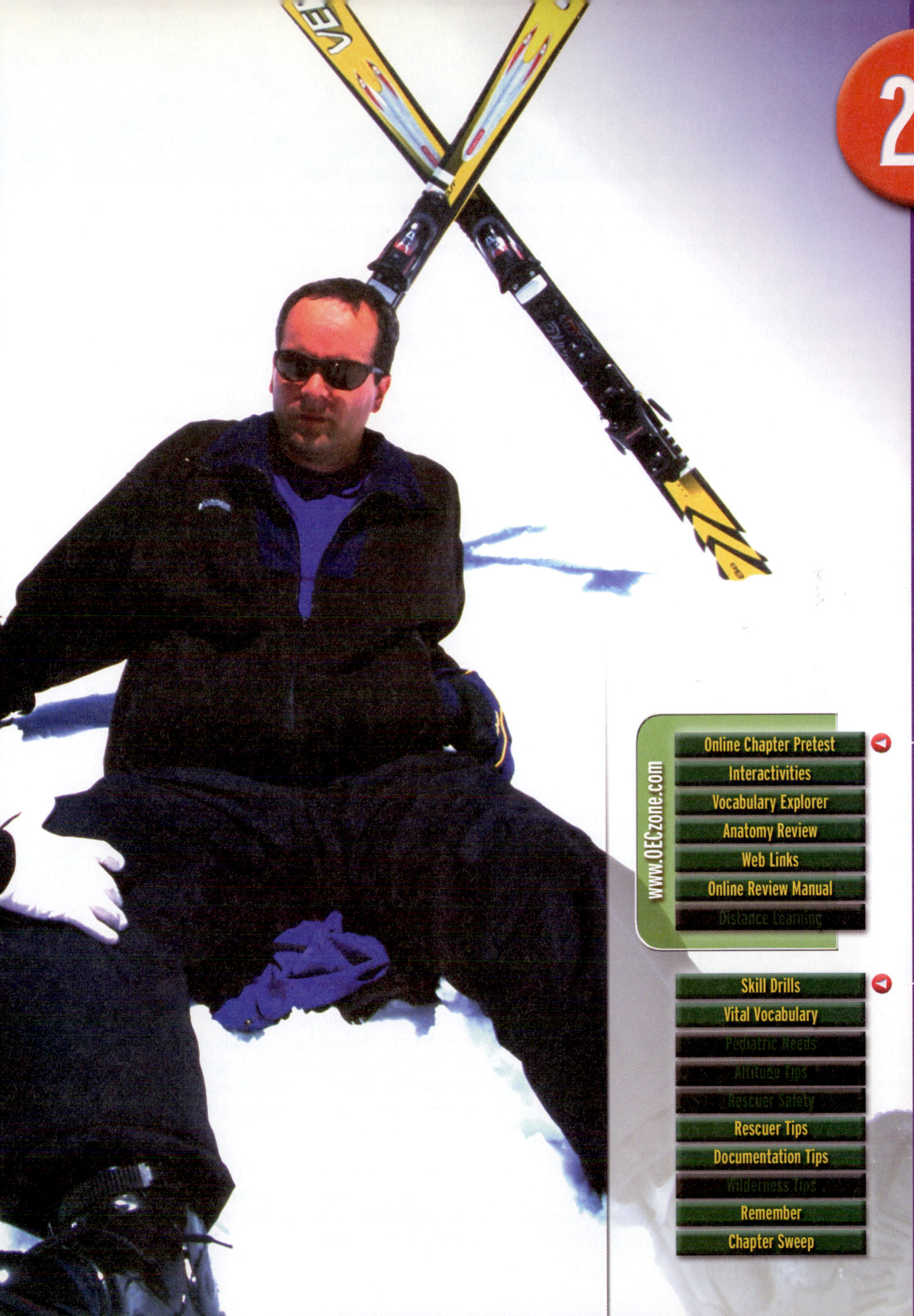

24

Principles of Musculoskeletal Injuries

TECHNOLOGY

www.OECzone.com

Online Chapter Pretest
Interactivities
Vocabulary Explorer
Anatomy Review
Web Links
Online Review Manual
Distance Learning

Skill Drills
Vital Vocabulary
Pediatric Needs
Altitude Tips
Rescuer Safety
Rescuer Tips
Documentation Tips
Wilderness Tips
Remember
Chapter Sweep

Chapter   FEATURES

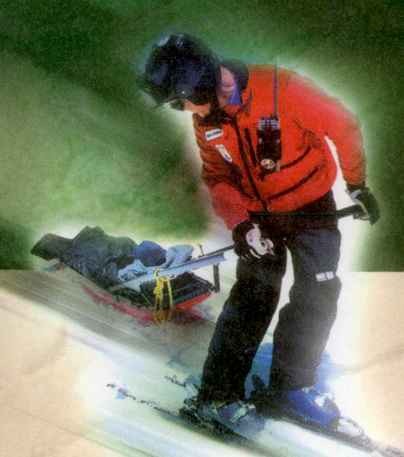

A quick inventory of the equipment in your aid room reminds you of their necessity in the outdoor environment for specific musculoskeletal injuries and the application techniques required for each piece of equipment.

With the increasing popularity of many outdoor recreational activities from the snowsports industry, mountain biking, skateboarding and in-line skating, hiking, climbing, river rafting, kayaking, and many other sports throughout the country, OEC technicians are frequently called to handle the varied musculoskeletal injuries in their given environment before an EMS response team arrives or ALS care can be implemented. This chapter will present the principles of care using a variety of equipment and techniques relative to musculoskeletal injuries in addition to helping you answer the following questions:

1. Why use one technique or piece of equipment over another?
2. Why is the emergency care given in the outdoor/wilderness environment so important for patients with musculoskeletal injuries?

General Principles of Musculoskeletal Injuries

The human body is a well-designed system whose form, upright posture, and movement are provided by the musculoskeletal system, which also protects the vital internal organs of the body. As its combination form suggests, the term "musculoskeletal" refers to the bones and voluntary muscles of the body. However, the bones and muscles themselves are susceptible to external forces that can cause injury. Also at risk are the tendons that attach muscles to bones, the joints that form wherever two bones come into contact, and the ligaments that hold the bone ends of a joint together.

As a rescuer, you must be familiar with the basic anatomy of the body's musculoskeletal system. Although muscles are technically soft tissue, they are discussed in this chapter because of their close relationship to the skeleton. Therefore, the chapter begins with a review of the musculoskeletal anatomy. Various types and causes of musculoskeletal injuries in general are identified, and the assessment and emergency care for each is explained, followed by a detailed discussion of splinting.

Anatomy and Physiology of the Musculoskeletal System
Muscles

The musculoskeletal system is composed of three types of muscles: skeletal, smooth, and cardiac. **Skeletal muscle**, also called striated muscle because of its characteristic stripes, attaches to the bones and usually crosses at least one joint, forming the major muscle mass of the body. This type of muscle is also called voluntary muscle, because it is under direct voluntary control of the brain, responding to commands to move specific body parts. Usually, movement is the result of several muscles contracting and relaxing simultaneously.

All skeletal muscles are supplied with arteries, veins, and nerves. Blood from the arteries brings oxygen and nutrients to the muscles ▶ Figure 24-1 . Waste products, including carbon dioxide and lactic acid, are carried away in the veins. Disease or trauma can result in the loss of a muscle's nervous impulses; this, in turn, can lead to *atrophy*, or a wasting of the muscle. Muscle tissue is directly attached to the bone by tough, ropelike fibrous structures known as **tendons** (muscle to bone), which are extensions of the fascia that covers all skeletal muscle.

Smooth muscle, also called **involuntary muscle**, performs much of the automatic work of the body. This type of muscle is found in the walls of most tubular structures of the body, such as the gastrointestinal tract and the blood vessels. Smooth muscle contracts and relaxes to control the movement of the contents of these structures.

The cardiac muscle neither looks nor acts like skeletal or smooth muscle. It is a specially adapted involuntary muscle with its own regulatory system.

The remainder of this chapter is concerned exclusively with skeletal muscle.

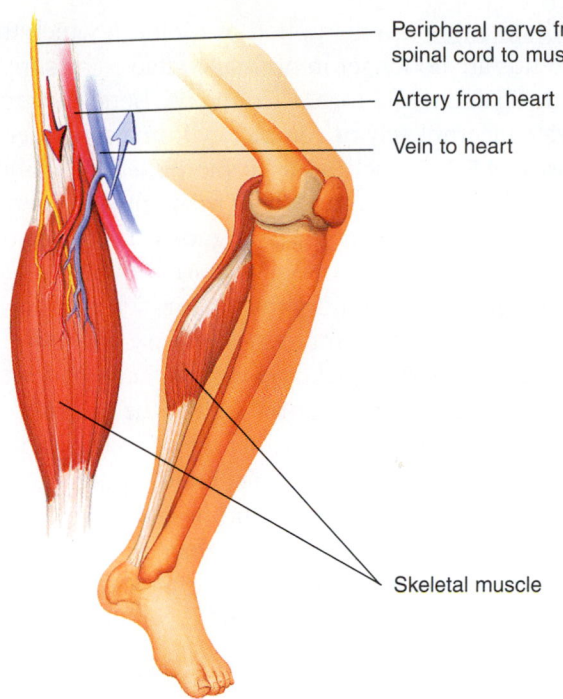

Peripheral nerve from spinal cord to muscle

Artery from heart

Vein to heart

Skeletal muscle

Figure 24-1 Skeletal muscles are supplied with arteries, veins, and nerves that bring oxygen and nutrients, carry away waste products, and supply nervous stimuli.

The Skeleton

The skeleton, which gives us our recognizable human form, protects our vital internal organs, and allows us to move, is made up of approximately 206 bones **▶ Figure 24-2** . The bones in the skeleton also produce blood cells (in the bone marrow) and serve as a reservoir for important minerals and electrolytes.

The skull surrounds and protects the brain. The thoracic cage protects the heart, lungs, and great vessels; the lower ribs protect the liver and spleen. The bony spinal canal encases the spinal cord. The upper extremity extends from the shoulder to the fingertips and is composed of the shoulder, arm, elbow, forearm, wrist, hand, and fingers. The arm extends from the shoulder to the elbow. The forearm extends from the elbow to the fingers. The pelvis supports the body weight and protects the structures within the pelvis: the bladder, rectum, and female reproductive organs. The lower extremity consists of the hip, thigh, leg, and foot. The joint between the pelvis and the thigh is the hip; the joint between the thigh and lower leg is the knee, and the joint between the lower leg and foot is the ankle.

The bones of the skeleton provide a framework to which the muscles and tendons are attached. Bone is a living tissue that contains nerves and receives oxygen and nutrients from the arterial system. Therefore, when

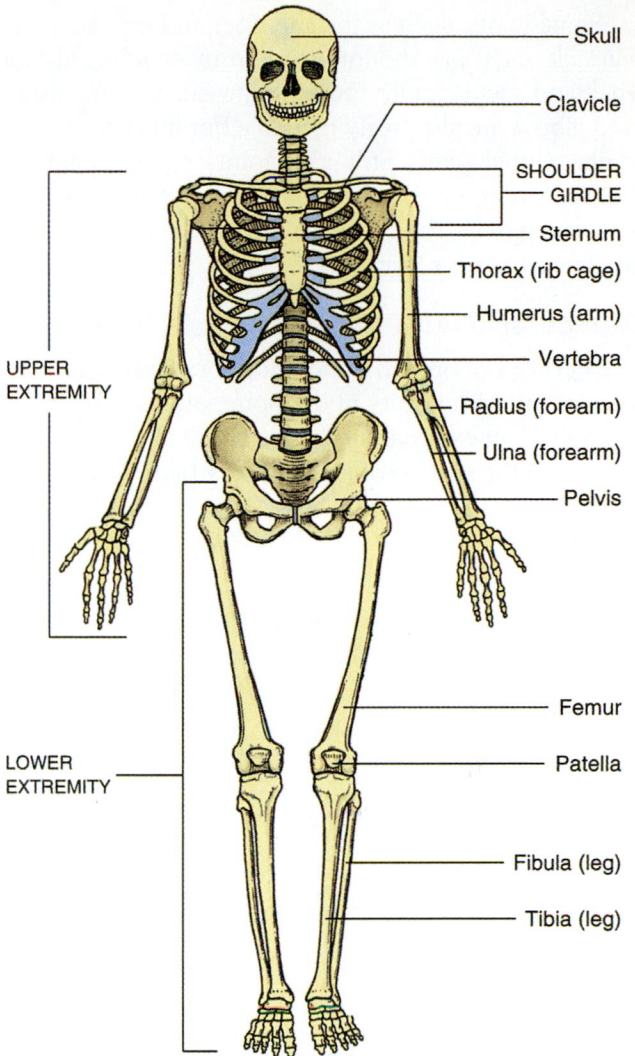

Skull

Clavicle

SHOULDER GIRDLE

Sternum

Thorax (rib cage)

Humerus (arm)

Vertebra

Radius (forearm)

Ulna (forearm)

Pelvis

Femur

Patella

Fibula (leg)

Tibia (leg)

UPPER EXTREMITY

LOWER EXTREMITY

Figure 24-2 The human skeleton, consisting of approximately 206 bones, gives us our form and protects our vital organs.

a bone breaks, a patient typically experiences severe pain and bleeding around the fracture site. Bone marrow, located in the center of each bone, is constantly producing red blood cells to provide oxygen and nourishment to the body and remove waste.

A **joint** is formed wherever two bones come into contact. The sternoclavicular joint, for example, is where the sternum and the clavicle come together. Joints are held together in a tough fibrous structure known as a capsule, which is supported and strengthened in certain key areas by bands of fibrous tissue called **ligaments** (bone to bone). In moving joints, the ends of the bones are covered with a thin layer of cartilage known as **articular cartilage**. This cartilage is a pearly substance that allows the ends of the bones to glide easily. Joints are bathed and lubricated by joint fluid (synovial fluid).

Some joints, such as the shoulder and hip, are *freely movable* and allow motion to occur in a circling fashion (ball and socket joint). Other joints, such as the knee and elbow, are also freely movable but function as hinges (hinge joint). Still other joints, such as joints between vertebra, are *slightly movable*. Certain joints, such as those in the sacroiliac area of the pelvis or skull, are *immovable* ▼ **Figure 24-3** .

Musculoskeletal Injuries

A **fracture** is a broken bone. More precisely, it is a break in the continuity of the bone, often occurring as a result of an external force. The break can occur anywhere on the surface of the bone ▼ **Figure 24-4** .

A **dislocation** is a disruption of a joint in which the bone ends are no longer in normal contact. The supporting ligaments are torn, allowing the bone ends to separate incompletely or completely from each other ▶ **Figure 24-5** . A fracture-dislocation is a combination injury of bone and joint in which the joint is dislocated and there is a fracture of the contiguous end of one or more of the dislocated bones ▶ **Figure 24-6** .

A **sprain** is a joint injury that occurs when there is both some partial or complete temporary dislocation of the bone ends and partial or complete tearing of the supporting ligaments. After the injury, the joint surfaces generally fall back into alignment, so the joint does not remain significantly displaced. Sprains can range from mild to severe, depending on the amount of damage done to the supporting ligaments. The most severe sprains involve temporary complete dislocation of the joint and are very serious; mild sprains typically heal rather quickly.

A **strain**, or muscle pull, is a stretching or tearing of muscle fibers, causing pain, swelling, and bruising of

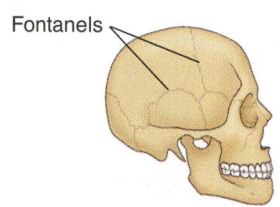

No motion

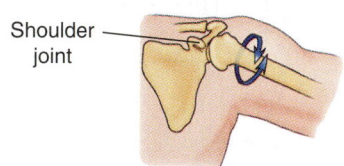

Circular motion

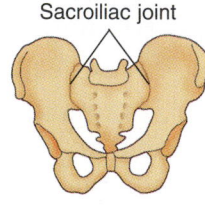
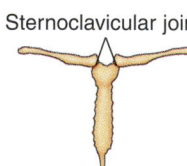

Minimal motion

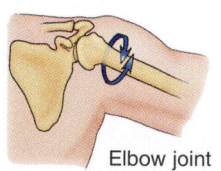
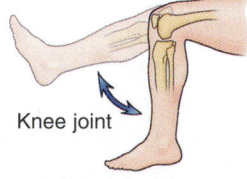

Hinge motion

Figure 24-3 Joints have many functions. Some joints are movable and allow for motion to occur in a circular fashion; others act as hinges. Still others allow only slight motion, while others are immovable and allow no motion at all.

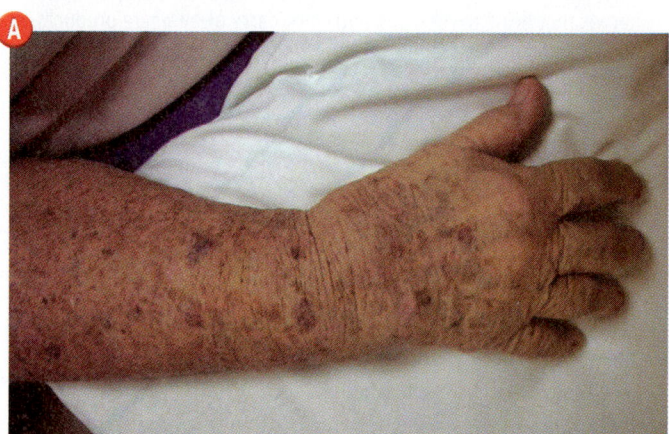

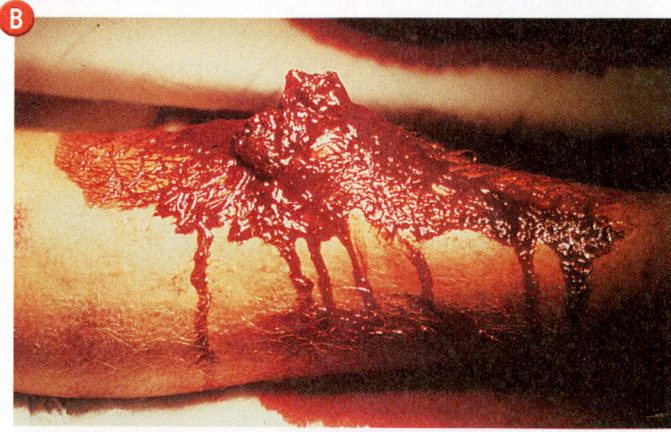

Figure 24-4 A fracture can occur anywhere on the surface of a bone and may be **A.** closed (no break in the skin) or **B.** open (overlying skin is broken).

the soft tissues in the area. Unlike a sprain, no ligament or joint damage occurs.

Injury to bones and joints is often associated with injury to the surrounding soft tissues, especially to the adjacent nerves and blood vessels. The entire area is known as the zone of injury ▶ Figure 24-7 . Depending on the amount of kinetic energy the tissues absorb from

forces acting on the body, the zone may extend to a distant point from the injury site. For this reason, you should not focus on a patient's obvious injury without first completing an initial assessment to check for associated injuries, which may be even more serious. This is especially true when assessing collision injuries or injuries caused by falls from a height.

Mechanism of Injury

Significant force is generally required to cause a fracture or dislocation. This force may be applied to the limb in any of the following ways ▶ Figure 24-8 :

- Direct blows
- Indirect forces
- Twisting forces
- High-energy injury

A direct blow fractures the bone at the point of impact. An example is the **patella** (kneecap) that fractures when it strikes the dashboard in an automobile crash.

Indirect force may cause a fracture or dislocation at a distant point, as when a person falls and lands on an

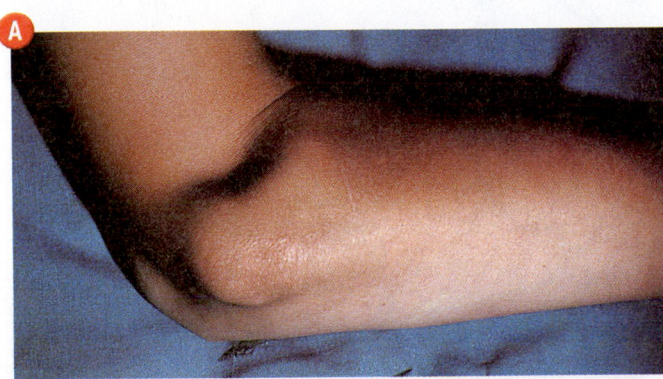

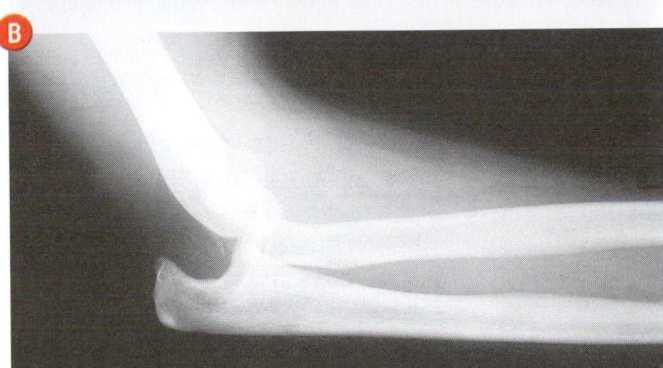

Figure 24-5 A dislocation is a disruption of a joint in which the bone ends are no longer in normal contact. **A.** The clinical appearance of an elbow dislocation. **B.** X-ray appearance of the same elbow.

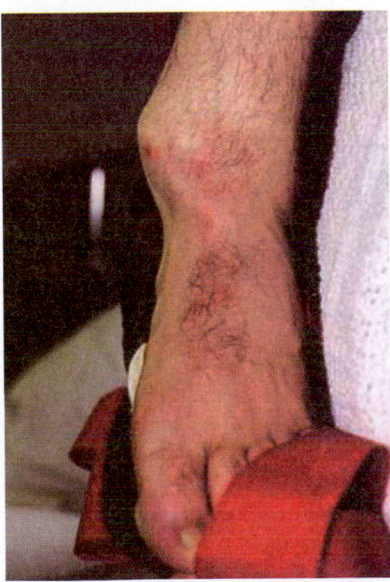

Figure 24-6 Fracture-dislocation of the ankle.

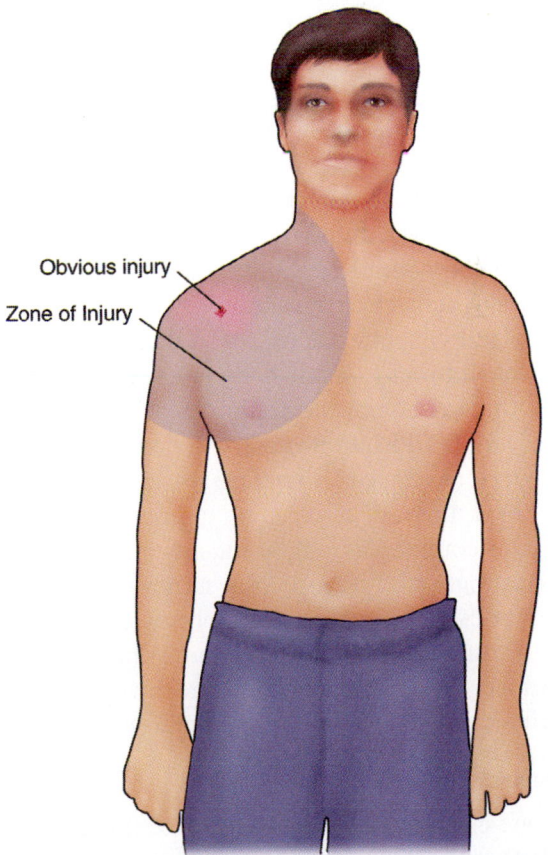

Obvious injury

Zone of Injury

Figure 24-7 The zone of injury is the area of soft tissue, including the adjacent nerves and blood vessels, that surrounds the obvious injury of a bone or joint.

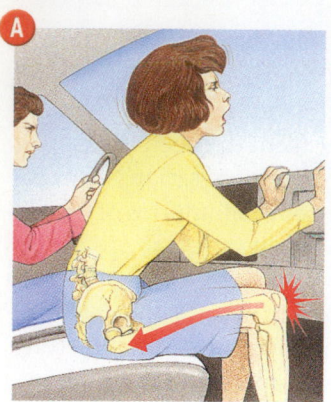 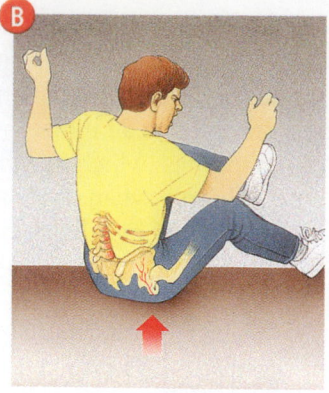 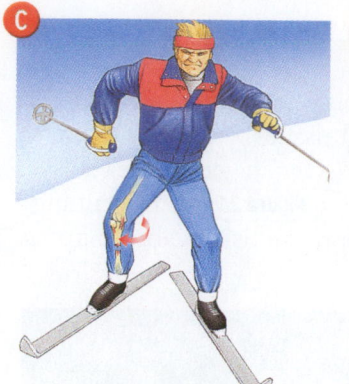 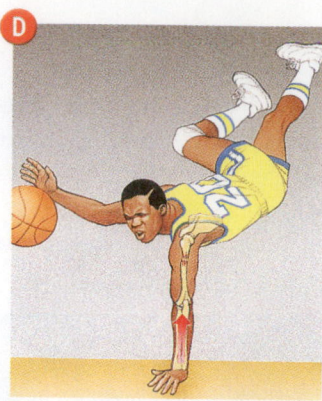

Figure 24-8 Significant force is required to cause fractures or dislocations. Among these are **A.** direct blows, **B.** high-energy injuries, **C.** twisting forces, and **D.** indirect forces.

outstretched hand. The direct impact may cause a wrist fracture, but the indirect force can cause dislocation of the elbow or a fracture of the forearm, humerus, or even clavicle. Therefore, when caring for patients who have fallen, you must identify the point of contact and the mechanism of injury so that you will not overlook associated injuries.

Twisting forces are a common cause of musculoskeletal injury, especially to the anterior cruciate ligament at the knee. Skiing injuries often happen this way. A ski becomes caught, and the skier falls, applying a twisting force to the lower extremity, sustaining a spiral tibial fracture.

High-energy injuries, such as those that occur in skiing into a lift tower, automobile crashes, falls from heights, gunshot wounds, and other extreme forces, produce severe damage to the skeleton, surrounding soft tissues, and vital internal organs. A patient may have multiple injuries to many body parts, including more than one fracture or dislocation in a single limb.

A significant MOI is not necessary to produce a fracture. A slight force can easily fracture a bone that is weakened by a tumor or *osteoporosis*, a generalized bone disease that is common among postmenopausal women. In elderly patients with osteoporosis, minor falls, simple twisting injuries, or even a muscle contraction can cause a fracture, most often of the wrist, spine, or hip. You should suspect the presence of a fracture in any older patient who has sustained even a mild injury.

Fractures

Fractures are classified in several ways. The first designation is whether the fracture is closed or open. In assessing and treating patients with possible fractures or dislocations, a major priority is to determine whether the overlying skin has been violated. If there has been no break in the skin, the patient has a **closed fracture**.

Remember

Suspect a fracture in any older patient with even a mild injury.

However, making this determination is not always as easy as it sounds. With an **open fracture**, there is an external wound, caused either by the same force that fractured the bone or by the broken bone ends lacerating the skin. The wound may vary in size from a very small puncture to a gaping tear that exposes bone and soft tissue **▼ Figure 24-9**. Regardless of the extent and severity of the damage to the skin, you should treat any apparent fracture injury that breaks the skin within the same anatomic segment (ie, arm, forearm, thigh, etc.) as a possible open fracture. External blood loss and a higher likelihood of infection, possibilities that you must try to prevent, tend to occur with open fractures. As a ski or snowboard patroller, you must try to prevent or minimize these possible complications.

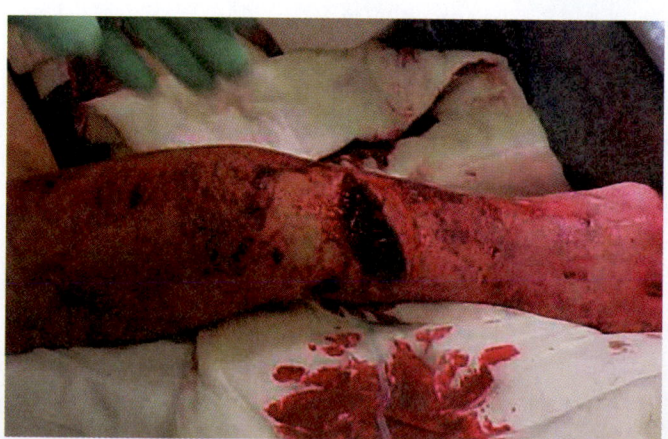

Figure 24-9 Open fracture of the radius and ulna.

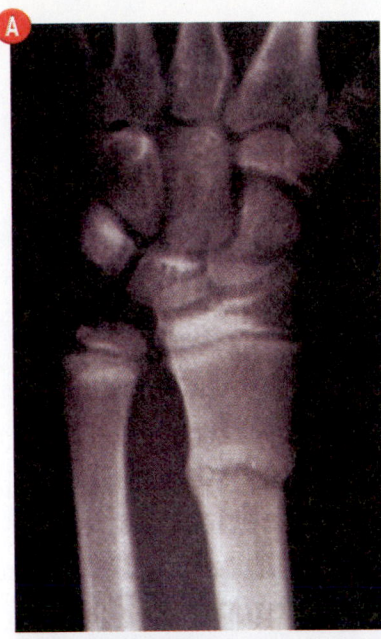

Figure 24-10 **A.** Incomplete torus fracture of the distal radius. **B.** Complete comminuted midshaft fracture of the femur.

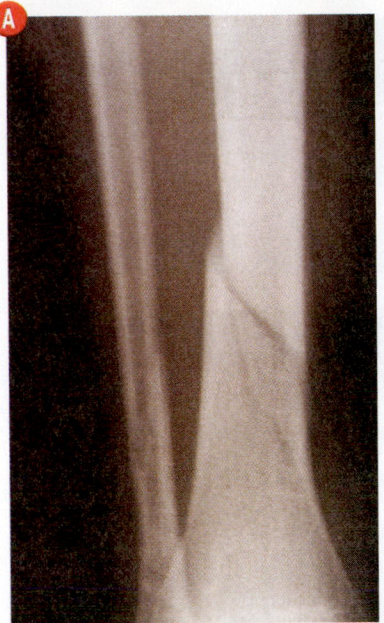

Figure 24-11 **A.** Nondisplaced fracture of the distal tibia and fibula. **B.** Displaced, midshaft fracture of the radius and ulna.

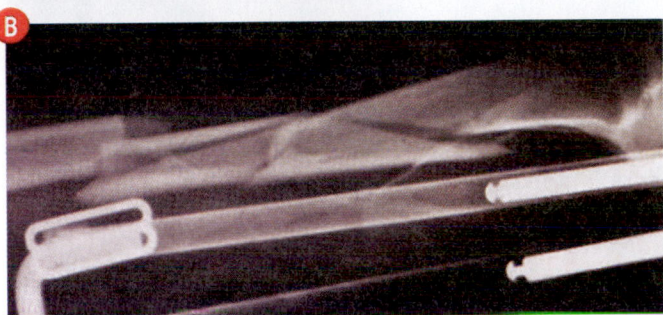

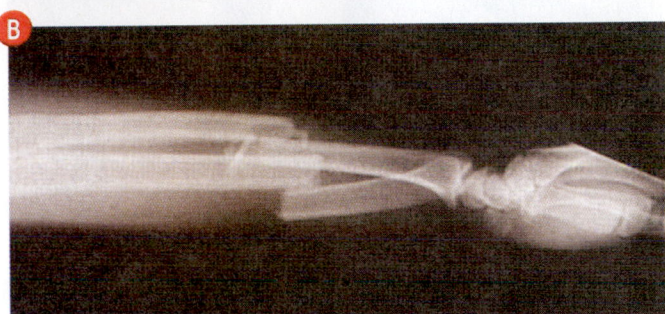

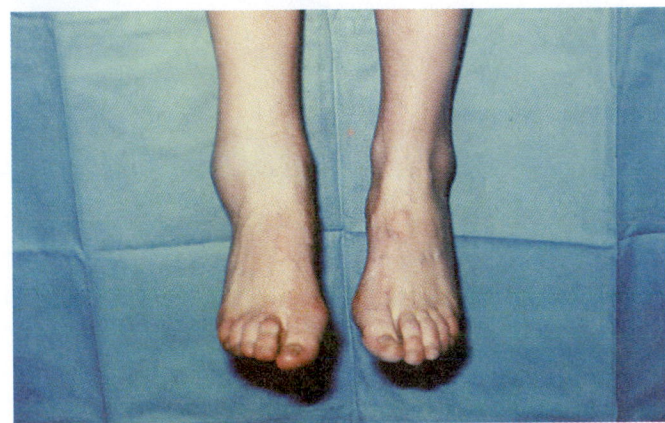

Figure 24-12 Always compare the injured limb with the uninjured limb when checking for deformity.

Another fracture classification depends on whether the injured bone is broken completely through. An *incomplete fracture* (▲ **Figure 24-10A**) describes a break in the bone where the injury does not result in two or more fracture fragments. Conversely, a *complete fracture* (▲ **Figure 24-10B**) is an injury situation where complete disruption of the bone has occurred, and two or more fracture segments have been produced.

A third fracture classification depends on whether the injury force has caused the bone to move from its normal position. A **nondisplaced fracture** (also known as a hairline fracture) is an injury to the bone that may be difficult to distinguish from a sprain or simple contusion (▲ **Figure 24-11A**). In fact, X-rays are usually required for hospital personnel to diagnose a nondisplaced fracture. A **displaced fracture** produces actual deformity, or distortion, of the limb by shortening, rotating, or angulating it (▲ **Figure 24-11B**). Often, the deformity is very obvious and is associated with crepitus; however, in some cases, the deformity is minimal. Be sure to look for differences between the injured limb and the opposite uninjured limb in any patient with a suspected fracture of an extremity (▶ **Figure 24-12**).

Rescue and medical personnel often use several other special terms to describe particular types of fractures (▶ **Figure 24-13**):

- **Greenstick fracture.** An incomplete fracture that passes only partway through the shaft of a bone that occurs in children; may be nondisplaced, or severely angulated.

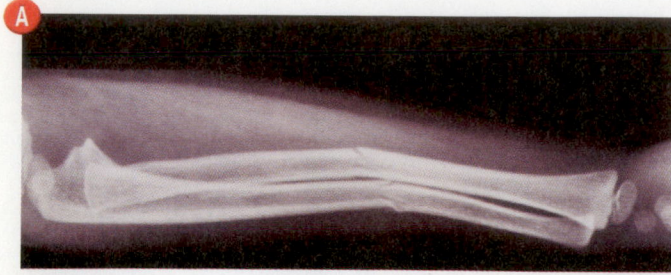

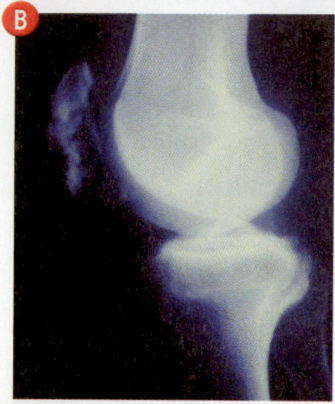

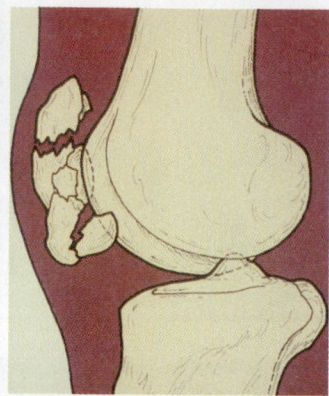

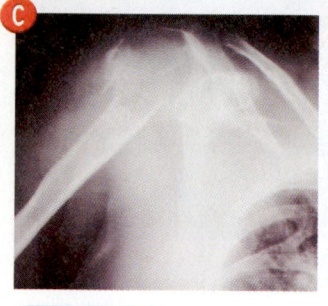

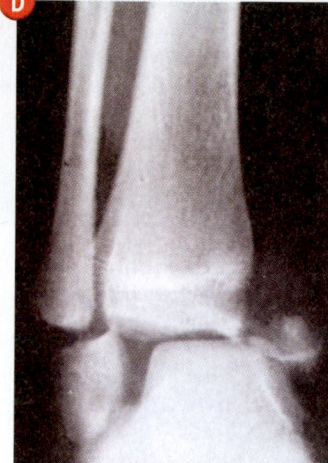

Figure 24-13   Special terms to describe fractures.
A. Greenstick fracture.
B. Comminuted fracture.
C. Pathologic fracture.
D. Epiphyseal fracture.

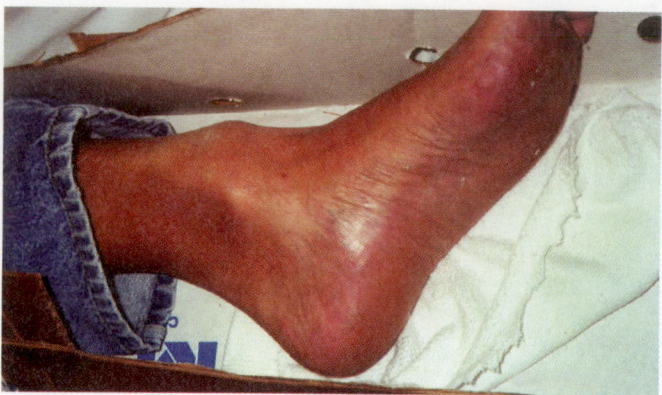

Figure 24-14   Obvious deformity, shortening, rotation, or angulation suggests a fracture. Remember to compare the injured limb with the opposite, uninjured limb.

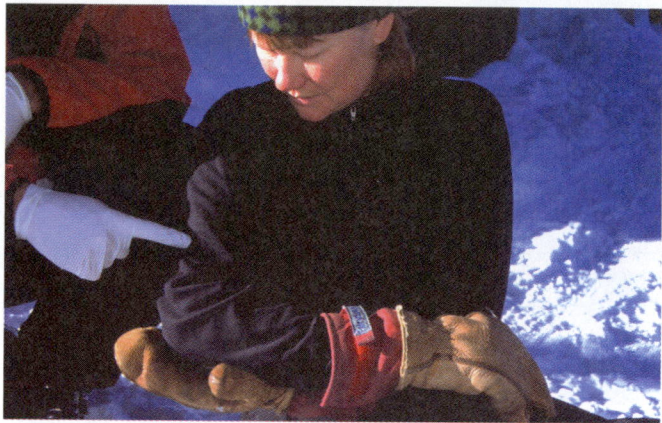

Figure 24-15   Point tenderness is the sensitive spot at the site of injury that can be located by gentle palpation along the bone with the tip of your finger.

- **Comminuted fracture.** A fracture in which the bone is broken into more than two fragments.

- **Pathologic fracture.** A fracture of weakened or diseased bone, seen in patients with osteoporosis or cancer; generally produced by minimal force.

- **Epiphyseal fracture.** A fracture that occurs in the growth zone of a child's bone, which may prematurely stop growth if not properly treated.

The symptoms of pain usually occur with every fracture. You should suspect a fracture if one or more of the following signs is present in any patient who has a history of injury and reports pain.

DEFORMITY. The limb may appear to be shortened, rotated, or angulated at a point where there is no joint
▲ **Figure 24-14** . Always use the uninjured opposite limb as a mirror image for comparison.

TENDERNESS. **Point tenderness** or pain on palpation in the zone of injury is the most reliable indicator of an underlying fracture, although it does not tell you the type of fracture ▲ **Figure 24-15** . If possible, always ask the patient to "point with one finger" to the area that hurts the most. Be sure to wear gloves during any patient contact, especially if there are any open wounds.

GUARDING. An inability to use the extremity is the patient's way of immobilizing it to minimize pain
▶ **Figure 24-16** . The muscles around the fracture contract in an attempt to prevent any movement of the broken bone. Guarding does not occur with all fractures; some patients may continue to use the injured part for a period of time. Occasionally, nondisplaced

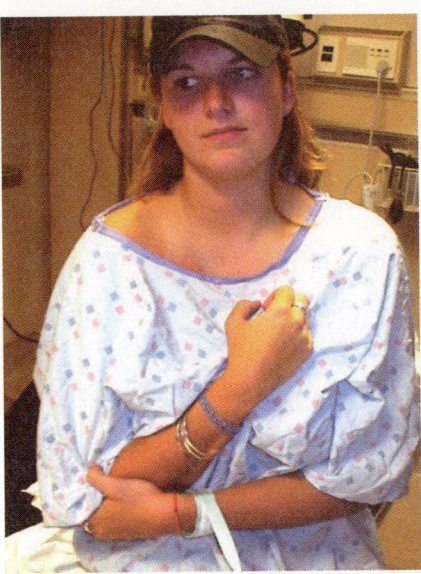

Figure 24-16 Protecting the extremity close to the body is the patient's way of immobilizing it to minimize pain.

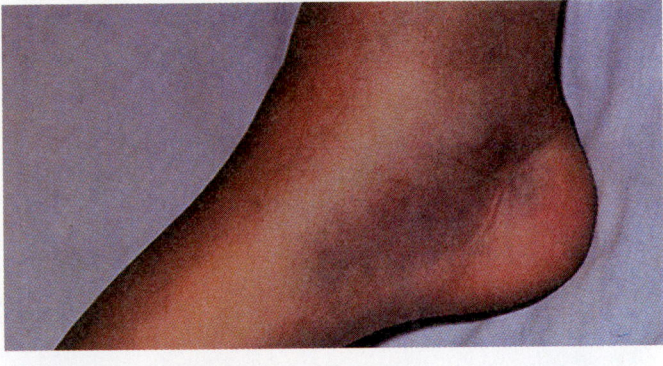

Figure 24-17 Swelling that occurs in association with a fracture can often mask deformity of the limb.

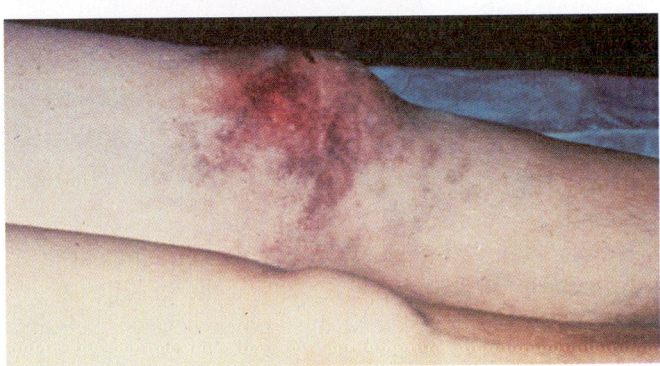

Figure 24-18 Fractures almost always have associated bruising into the surrounding soft tissue.

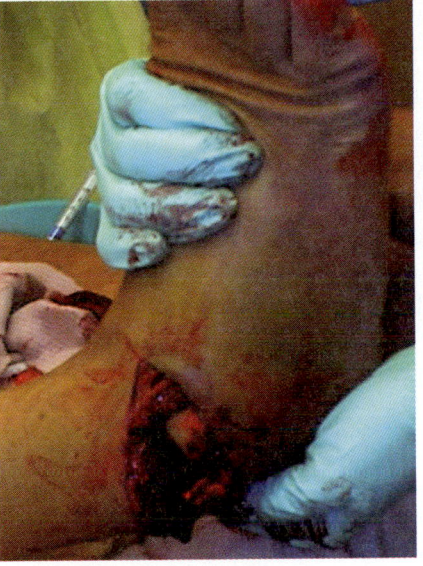

Figure 24-19 Bone ends may protrude through the skin or be visible within the wound of an open fracture.

fractures are not very painful, and there is minimal soft-tissue damage.

SWELLING. Rapid swelling usually indicates bleeding from a fracture site and is typically followed by severe pain. Often, if the swelling is severe enough, it may mask deformity of the limb ▶ **Figure 24-17** . Generalized swelling from fluid buildup may not occur until several hours after an injury.

BRUISING. Fractures are almost always associated with ecchymosis (bruising) of the surrounding soft tissues ▲ **Figure 24-18** . Bruising may be present after almost any injury; it is not specific for bone or joint injuries.

CREPITUS. A grating or grinding sensation known as **crepitus** can be felt and sometimes even heard when fractured bone ends rub together.

FALSE MOTION. Motion at a point in the limb where there is no joint is a positive indication of a fracture.

EXPOSED FRAGMENTS. In open fractures, bone ends may protrude through the skin or be visible within the wound ▲ **Figure 24-19** .

LOCKED JOINT. A joint that is locked into position makes any attempt to move the joint both difficult and painful.

Keep in mind that the signs of crepitus and false motion appear only when a limb is moved or manipulated and are associated with injuries that are extremely painful. Do not manipulate the limb excessively in an effort to elicit these signs.

Dislocations

A dislocated joint sometimes will spontaneously **reduce** itself (return to its normal position) before your assessment. In this situation, you will be able to confirm the dislocation only by taking a patient history. Often, however, injury to the supporting ligaments and

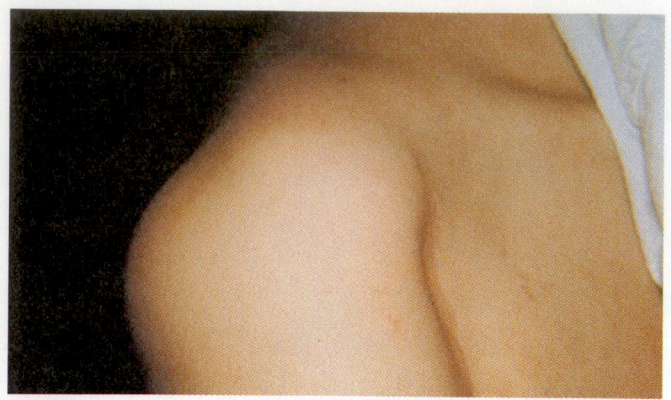

Figure 24-20 Joint dislocations, such as this shoulder, are characterized by deformity, swelling, pain with any movement, tenderness, locking, and sometimes impaired distal circulation.

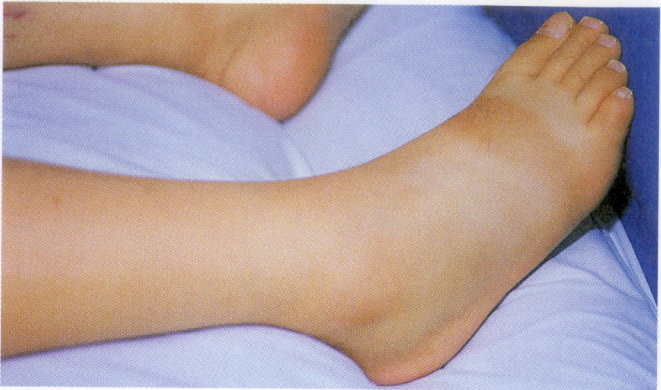

Figure 24-21 Sprains most often occur in the knee, shoulder, or ankle and are characterized by swelling, bruising, point tenderness, pain, and joint instability.

capsule is so severe that the joint surfaces remain partially or completely separated from one another. A dislocation that does not spontaneously reduce is a serious problem. As noted above, the ends of the bone are locked in the displaced position, making any attempt at motion of the joint very difficult and very painful. The most commonly dislocated joints are the fingers, shoulder, elbow, hip, and ankle.

The signs and symptoms of a dislocated joint are similar to those of a fracture ▲ **Figure 24-20** :

- Marked deformity
- Swelling
- Pain that is aggravated by any attempt at movement
- Tenderness on palpation
- Virtually complete loss of normal joint motion (locked joint)
- Occasionally, numbness or impaired circulation in the limb distal to the dislocation

Sprains

A sprain occurs when a joint is twisted or moved beyond its normal range of motion. As a result, the supporting capsule and ligaments are torn. A sprain should be considered a temporary partial dislocation (subluxation). The joint alignment generally returns to a fairly normal position after the injury, although there may be some continued displacement. Note that severe persistent deformity does not typically occur with a sprain. Sprains most often occur in the knee, shoulder, and ankle, but a sprain can occur in any joint. The following signs and symptoms often indicate that the patient may have a sprain ▲ **Figure 24-21** :

- Point tenderness can be elicited over the injured ligaments.
- Swelling and ecchymosis appear at the point of injury to the ligament as a result of torn blood vessels.
- Pain prevents the patient from moving or using the limb normally.
- Instability of the joint is indicated by increased abnormal motion, especially at the knee; however, this may be masked by severe swelling and guarding.

A fracture can look like a sprain, and vice versa. Frequently, you will not be able to distinguish a nondisplaced fracture from a sprain at the accident scene. Therefore, remember to document the apparent mechanism of injury, as certain sprains and fractures occur more consistently with certain mechanisms. This is especially true at the ankle. In general, your approach should always be to try to rule out the possibility of fracture first. *The basic principles of field management for sprains, dislocations, and fractures are essentially the same.*

Assessing Musculoskeletal Injuries

As a rescuer (OEC technician), you will often be "first on" in the team approach to trauma patients. Therefore, your assessment, ability to stabilize patients, and skills splinting extremity injuries are very important. Look at the big picture, evaluating the overall complexity of the situation. Always carefully assess the mechanism of injury to try to determine the amount of kinetic energy that an injured limb has absorbed.

Assessment of patients with uncomplicated musculoskeletal injuries should include an initial assessment

Always assess the mechanism of injury to determine the amount of kinetic energy absorbed.

of the patient; followed by a focused physical exam of the painful, swollen, deformed extremity; including evaluation of neurovascular function. Be sure to follow BSI precautions. If oxygen is indicated and you have not already called for it, be sure to do so.

For musculoskeletal trauma, use the DCAP-BTLS approach. Identify any extremity **D**eformities that likely represent significant musculoskeletal injury and stabilize appropriately. **C**ontusions and **A**brasions may overlie more subtle injuries and should prompt you to carefully evaluate the stability and neurovascular status of the limb. The presence of **P**uncture wounds or other signs of penetrating injury should alert you to the possibility of an open fracture. Associated **B**urns must be identified and treated appropriately. Palpate for **T**enderness, which, like contusions or abrasions, may be the only significant sign of an underlying musculoskeletal injury. When **L**acerations are present on an extremity, open fracture must be considered, bleeding controlled, and dressings applied. Careful inspection for **S**welling with attention to comparison with the opposite limb may also reveal occult musculoskeletal injury.

When patients often have multiple injuries, you must initially assess their overall condition, stabilize the ABCs, and control any serious bleeding before further treating the injured extremity. In a critically injured patient with persistent unstable vital functions (other than CPR), you should secure the patient to a long spine board to rapidly immobilize the spine, pelvis, and extremities and provide prompt transport to the aid room (load and go). In this situation, extensive evaluation and splinting of limb injuries on the hill are a waste of valuable time.

If the patient has no life-threatening injuries while awaiting transport, you may take extra time at the scene to stabilize the patient's overall condition and more completely evaluate the injured extremity. During the detailed physical exam, you can also inspect and gently palpate the other extremities and the spine to identify areas of possible point tenderness

that may indicate additional underlying fractures, dislocations, or sprains. Remember to compare the injured limb with the opposite, uninjured limb. If possible, gently and carefully remove the patient's clothing to look for open fractures or dislocations, severe deformity, swelling, and/or ecchymosis.

Again, it is not necessarily critical that you distinguish among fractures, dislocations, and sprains since their emergency care on the hill is very similar. In most instances, your assessment will be reported as an "injury to the limb." However, you should be able to distinguish mild injuries from severe injuries, since some severe injuries may compromise neurovascular function in the limb.

If your assessment turns up no external signs of injury, ask the patient to move each limb through a range of motion carefully, stopping immediately if a movement causes pain. Skip this step in your evaluation if the patient reports neck or back pain; even the slightest motion could cause permanent damage to the spinal cord.

Assessing Pulse, Motor, and Sensory Function

Many important blood vessels and nerves lie close to the bone, especially around the major joints. Therefore, any injury or deformity of a bone or joint may have associated vessel or nerve injury. For this reason, you should assess neurovascular function initially and during the detailed physical exam, repeating it every 5 to 10 minutes, depending on the patient's condition, until the patient is at the aid room. Always recheck the neurovascular function before and after you splint or otherwise manipulate the limb. Movement at the fracture site can cause a bone fragment to press against or impale an adjacent nerve or blood vessel. Failure to restore circulation in this type of situation can lead to death of the limb. Always give priority to patients with impaired circulation or neurologic deficit resulting from fracture fragment impingement.

SkillDrill 24-1 Assessing Pulse, Motor, and Sensory Function

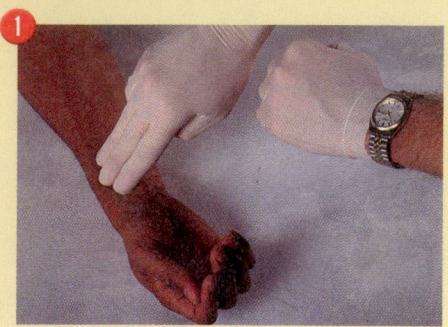

1 Palpate the radial pulse in the upper extremity.

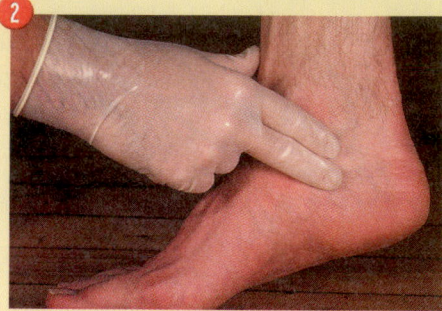

2 Palpate the posterior tibial pulse in the lower extremity. Remember to palpate the dorsalis pedis pulse as well.

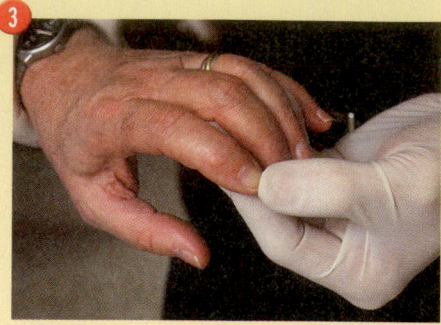

3 Assess capillary refill by blanching a fingernail or toenail.

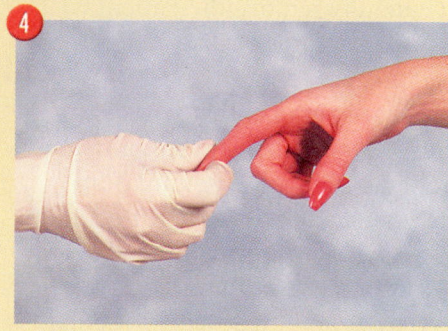

4 Assess sensation on the flesh near the tip of the index finger and thumb, and the little finger as well.

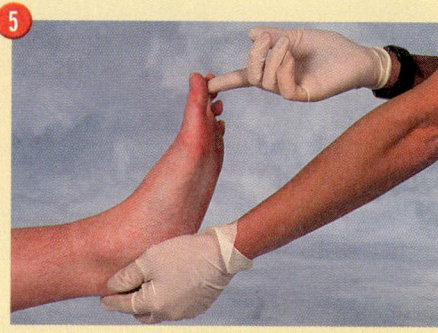

5 On the foot, first check sensation on the flesh near the tip of the great toe.

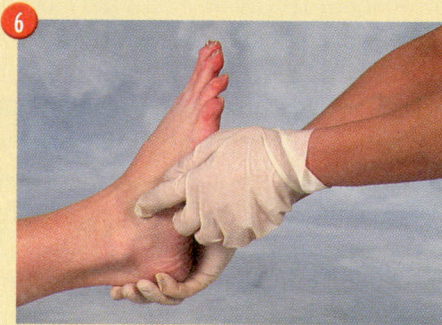

6 Also check foot sensation on the lateral side.

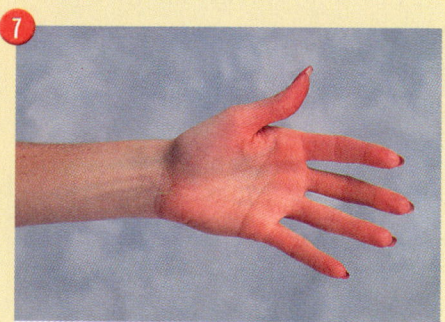

7 Evaluate motor function by asking the patient to open the hand. (Perform motor tests only if the hand or foot is not injured. Stop a test if it causes pain.)

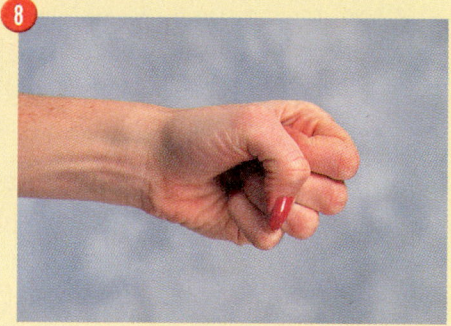

8 Also ask the patient to make a fist.

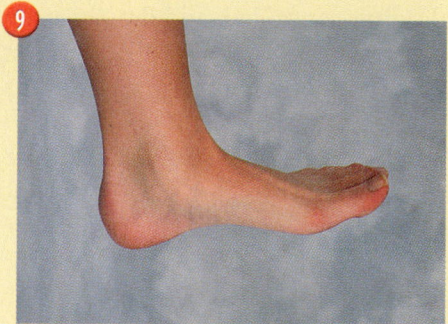

9 To evaluate motor function in the foot, ask the patient to extend (dorsiflex) the foot.

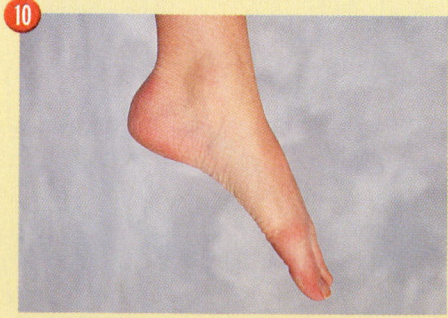

10 Also have the patient flex (plantar flex) the foot and wiggle the toes.

Examination of the injured limb should include assessment of four major signs that are good indicators of circulatory and nerve function distal to the injury: pulse, capillary refill, motor function, and sensory function. Follow the steps in ◄ Skill Drill 24-1 :

1. **Pulse.** Palpate the pulse distal to point of injury.
   - Palpate the radial pulse in the upper extremity **(Step 1)**.
   - In the lower extremity, palpate the posterior tibial and dorsalis pedis pulses **(Step 2)**.

2. **Capillary refill.** Note and record the skin color and temperature, identifying any pallor, cyanosis, or coolness. Then apply firm pressure to the tip of the fingernail or toenail, which will cause the skin to blanch (turn white). If normal color does not return within 2 seconds after you release the nail, you can assume that circulation is impaired. This test is typically recommended for use in children only and is very unreliable in the cold environment **(Step 3)**.

3. **Sensation.** On the hand, check the feeling on the flesh near the tip of the index finger and thumb, as well as the little finger **(Step 4)**. On the foot, check the feeling on the flesh of the big toe **(Step 5)** and on the lateral side of the foot **(Step 6)**. The patient's ability to sense light touch in the fingers or toes distal to the site of a fracture is a good indication that the nerve supply is intact.

4. **Motor function.** Evaluate muscular activity when the injury is proximal to the patient's hand or foot.

Ask the patient to open and close a fist for an upper extremity injury and to wiggle the toes and move the foot up and down at the ankle for a lower extremity injury **(Steps 7-10)**. Sometimes, an attempt at motion will produce pain at the injury site. If this happens, do not continue this part of the examination. To avoid causing pain, do not perform this test at all if the injury involves the hand or foot itself.

Because many of the steps described above require patient cooperation, you will not be able to assess sensory and motor function in an unconscious patient, but you can still evaluate the limb for deformity, swelling, ecchymosis, false motion, and crepitus. If a patient is unconscious, first perform an initial assessment and then examine the extremities. Assume that an unconscious patient has a spinal fracture, and immobilize the spine.

Assessing the Severity of Injury

You must become skilled at quickly and accurately assessing the severity of an injury. The Golden Hour is critical not just for life, but for limb as well. In an extremity with anything less than complete circulation, prolonged hypotension can cause significant damage. For this reason, any suspected open fracture or vascular injury is considered a medical emergency, especially in a patient with multiple trauma.

Remember that most extremity injuries are not critical; you can identify critical injuries by using the musculoskeletal injury grading system shown in ▼ Table 24-1 .

TABLE 24-1 Musculoskeletal Injury Grading System

Minor Injuries
- Minor sprains
- Fractures or dislocations of digits

Moderate Injuries
- Open fractures of digits
- Nondisplaced long bone fractures
- Nondisplaced pelvic fractures
- Major sprains of a major joint

Serious Injuries
- Displaced long bone fractures
- Multiple hand and foot fractures
- Single open long bone fractures
- Displaced pelvic fractures
- Dislocations of major joints
- Multiple digit amputations
- Laceration of a major nerve

Severe, Life-Threatening Injuries (survival is probable)
- Multiple closed fractures
- Limb amputations
- Laceration of a major blood vessel

Critical Injuries (survival is uncertain)
- Multiple open fractures of the limbs
- Pelvic fractures with hemodynamic instability

General Principles of Emergency Medical Care for Injured Extremities

Your first steps in providing care for any patient are the initial assessment and stabilizing the patient's ABCs. After you have done so, you can focus on specific injuries. Remember to always follow BSI precautions.

Follow the steps in ▶ **Skill Drill 24-2** when caring for patients with musculoskeletal injuries:

1. **Completely cover open wounds** with a dry, sterile dressing, and apply local pressure to control bleeding. Once you have applied a sterile dressing, treat an open fracture in the same way as a closed fracture. Assess circulation, motor, and sensory functions (CMS) before the application of splints **(Step 1)**.

2. **Apply the appropriate splint,** and elevate the extremity. Patients with lower extremity injuries should be placed supine with the limb elevated about 6″ to minimize swelling. For any patient, be sure to position the injured limb slightly above the level of the heart. Never allow the injured limb to flop about or dangle from the edge of the backboard or over the edge of a toboggan **(Steps 2 and 3)**.

3. **If swelling is present,** apply cold packs or snow to the area; however, avoid placing cold packs directly on the skin or other exposed tissues. Placing a cold pack on top of a quick splint will not help to reduce swelling.

4. **Prepare the patient for transport.** Reassess the distal circulation, motor, and sensory functions after the application of splints. A patient with an isolated extremity injury will most likely be more comfortable in a semiseated position rather than lying flat; however, either position is acceptable. Ensure that the extremity is elevated above the level of the heart and secured so that it does not dangle from the edge of the toboggan **(Step 4)**.

5. **Always inform rescue squad personnel** about all wounds that have been dressed and splinted.

Splinting

A <u>splint</u> is a flexible or rigid device that is used to protect and maintain the position of an injured extremity ▶ **Figure 24-22** . Unless your life and/or the patient's life is in immediate danger, you should splint all fractures, dislocations, and sprains before moving the patient. By preventing movement of fracture fragments, bone ends, a dislocated joint, or damaged soft tissues, splinting reduces pain and makes it easier to transfer and trans-

port the patient. In addition, splinting will help to prevent the following:

- Further damage to muscles, the spinal cord, peripheral nerves, and blood vessels from fractured bone ends

- Laceration of the skin by broken bone ends. One of the primary indications for splinting is to prevent a closed fracture from becoming an open fracture (conversion)

- Restriction of distal blood flow resulting from pressure of the bone ends on blood vessels

- Excessive bleeding of the tissues at the injury site caused by broken bone ends

- Increased pain from movement of bone ends

- Paralysis of extremities resulting from a damaged spinal column

A splint is simply a device to prevent motion of the injured part. It can be made from almost any material on occasions when you need to improvise. However, a patrol should always have an adequate supply of standard commercial splints.

GENERAL PRINCIPLES OF SPLINTING. The following principles of splinting apply to most injury situations:

1. **Remove or cut clothing from the area** of any suspected fracture or dislocation so that you can inspect extremity for DCAP-BTLS.

2. **Note and record the patient's neurovascular status** distal to the site of the injury, including pulse, circulation, motor function, and sensation. Continue to monitor the neurovascular status until the patient is transferred to your rescue squad.

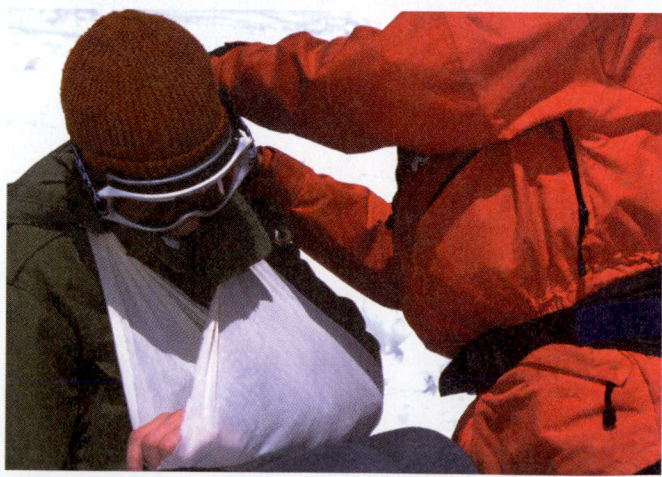

Figure 24-22 Splinting reduces pain and prevents additional damage to the injured extremity.

Skill Drill 24-2   Caring for Musculoskeletal Injuries

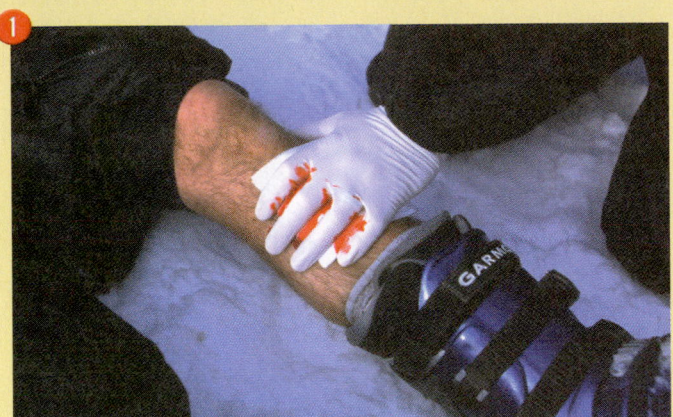
Cover open wounds with a dry, sterile dressing, and apply pressure to control bleeding. Assess distal CMS functions.

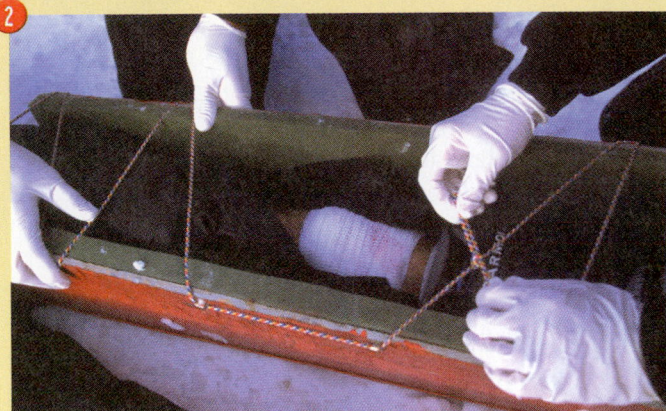
Apply a quick splint.

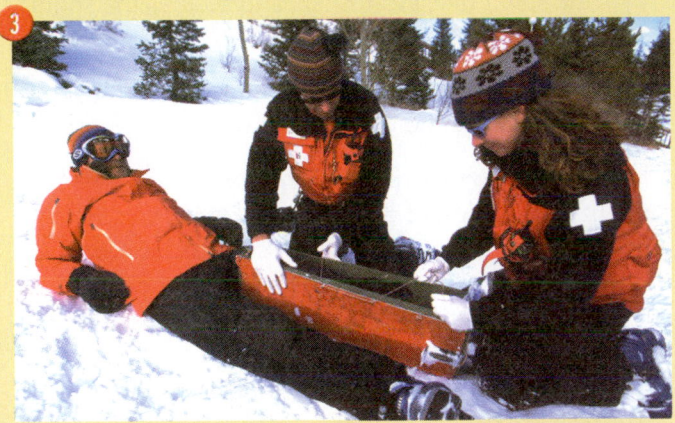
Elevate the extremity and position the patient for transport.

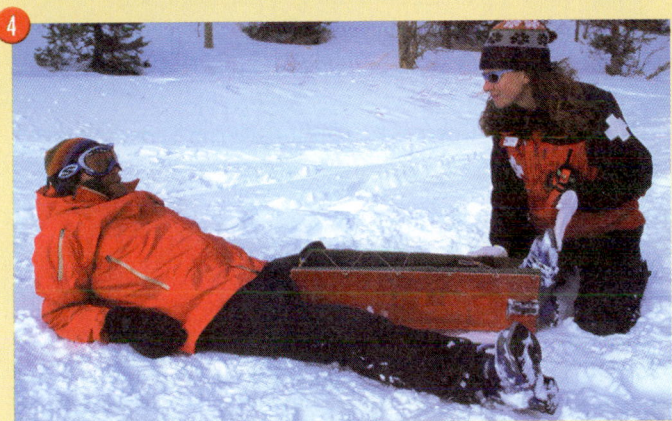
Assess distal CMS functions and position the patient for transport.

3. **Cover all wounds with a dry, sterile dressing** before splinting. Be sure to follow BSI precautions. Do not intentionally push protruding bones back inside the wound. Notify the accepting rescue squad of all open wounds.

4. **Do not move the patient before splinting** an extremity unless there is an immediate hazard to the patient or yourself or the patient's general condition requires immediate transport.

5. In a suspected fracture of the shaft of any bone, be sure to **immobilize the joints** above and below the fracture site.

6. With injuries in and around the joint, be sure to **immobilize the bones** above and below the injured joint.

7. **Pad all rigid splints** to prevent local pressure and discomfort to the patient.

8. While another patroller is applying the splint, **maintain manual immobilization** to minimize movement of the limb and to support and stabilize the injury site.

9. If fracture of a long bone shaft has resulted in severe deformity, **use constant, gentle longitudinal traction** to align the limb so that it can be splinted. This is especially important if the distal part of the injured extremity is cyanotic or pulseless.

10. **Expect to encounter increased pain and some patient resistance** when attempting to realign a fractured limb. If you encounter major resistance, splint the limb in its deformed position.

Remember

The three basic types of splints are rigid fixation, soft fixation, and traction splints.

Documentation Tips

Straightening or splinting an injured limb can compromise distal functions, just as the initial injury can. Record the status of distal circulation, motor, and nervous function (neurovascular status) both before *and* after splinting. At a minimum, your written record should describe these functions before splinting, and confirm that they were the same immediately after splinting and upon rescue squad transfer. For any but the shortest on-the-hill transports, also indicate the results of reassessments as part of your ongoing assessment.

11. **Immobilize all suspected spinal injuries** in a neutral in-line position on a backboard.

12. **If the patient has signs of shock** (hypoperfusion), attempt to align the limb to its normal anatomic position on a spine board and provide rapid transport (total body immobilization).

13. **When in doubt, splint.**

As mentioned above, many different materials can be used as splints if necessary. When no splinting materials are available, or if the patient's general situation demands load and go, *an injured arm can always be splinted to the chest wall, and an injured leg secured to the uninjured leg.*

The three basic types of splints are rigid fixation, soft fixation, and traction splints.

Rigid Fixation Splints

Rigid splints are made from firm materials and are applied to the sides, front, and/or back of an injured extremity to prevent motion at the injury site. Common examples of rigid fixation splints are plywood quick splints and cardboard splints for injuries to the lower extremities, and wire, ladder, board, and malleable metal splints for injuries to the upper extremities.

Quick splints are made of plywood padded with foam and are designed for quick application on a ski hill so the chilled patient can be transported rapidly. It usually takes two patrollers, or a patroller and a bystander, to apply a quick splint to a leg or a knee injury.

To put on the splint, follow the steps in
▶ **Skill Drill 24-3** .

1. **Open the splint flat** next to the patient's injured extremity **(Step 1)**.

2. **Grasp the booted foot** with one hand using slight longitudinal traction, and place the other hand just below the knee or under the lower thigh to support the extremity **(Step 2)**.

3. The **"pant-leg pinch-lift"** is another useful method for lifting and supporting the injured extremity **(Step 3)**.

4. **Have the second rescuer slide the splint** underneath the leg while you gently lower the injured extremity into the splint **(Step 4)**.

5. **The second rescuer then folds up the sides** of the splint like a clamshell, and secures the splint firmly **(Step 5)**.

6. A **neurovascular check** is performed before and after application of the splint **(Step 6)**.

There are two situations in which you must splint the limb in the position of deformity: (1) when the deformity is severe, as is the case with many dislocations; or (2) when you encounter major resistance or extreme pain while attempting to realign the fracture of a long bone. In either situation, you should splint the injured limb in the position found, with whatever splint material is applicable.

CARDBOARD SPLINTS. Cardboard splints are a favorite of ski patrols because they are effective, easy to apply, inexpensive, and disposable. These splints are especially useful when large numbers of patients with lower extremity injuries are treated daily. A quick splint applied on the ski hill will frequently be replaced with a cardboard splint before the patient leaves the aid room. This allows the boot to be removed and CMS to be assessed directly in a warm environment. However, use judgment in deciding whether to subject the patient to a splint change. You may not want to change the splint if the patient has a very painful fracture, a bandaged open fracture, multiple injuries, or a fracture accompanied by shock.

You can either purchase cardboard splints or make them from sturdy single-corrugation packing box cardboard. A convenient size is 15″ × 42″. For rigidity, cut the splint so that the corrugations run lengthwise.

SkillDrill 24-3 Applying a Quick Splint

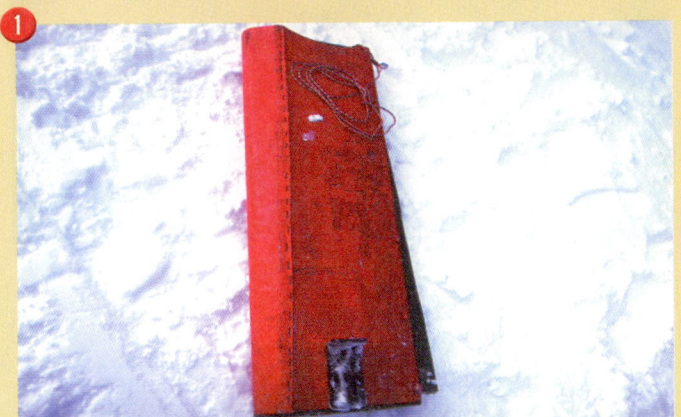

1 Open the quick splint flat next to the patient's injured extremity.

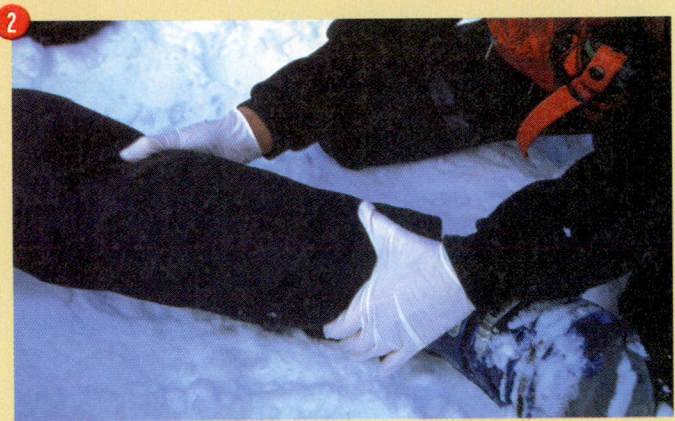

2 Grasp the booted foot with one hand, using slight longitudinal traction, and place the other hand just below the knee or under the lower thigh to support the extremity.

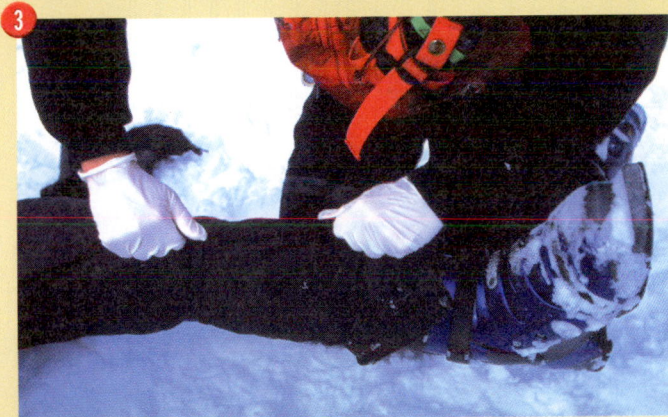

3 The "pant-leg pinch lift" is another useful method for lifting and supporting the injured extremity.

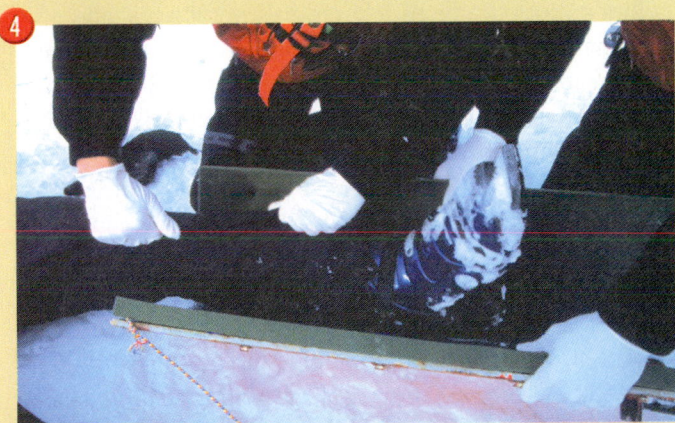

4 Have a second rescuer slide the splint underneath the leg while you gently lower the injured extremity into the splint.

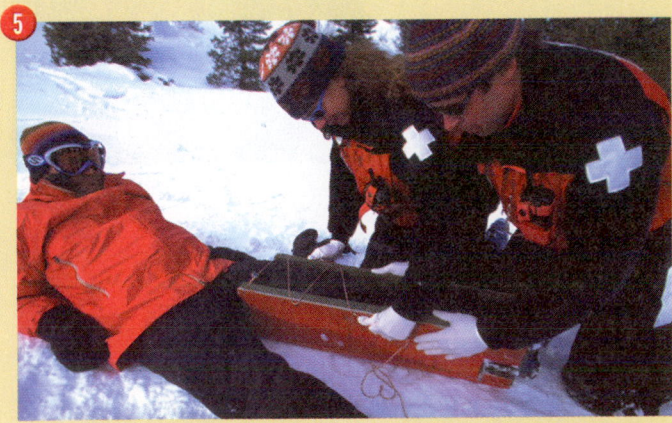

5 The second rescuer then folds up the sides of the splint like a clamshell, and secures the splint straps firmly.

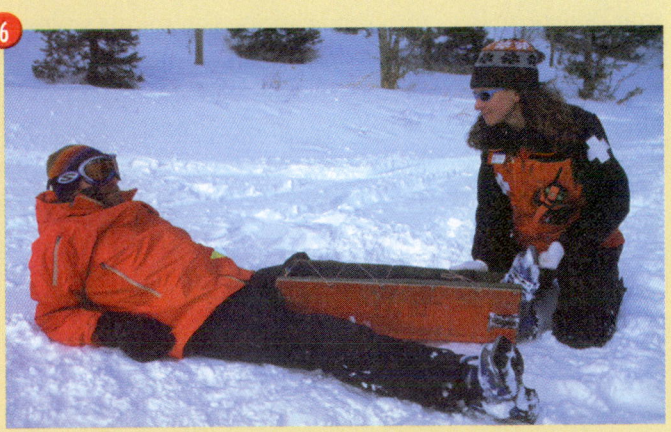

6 Reassess neurovascular function.

Cardboard splints are individually fitted to each patient, using the uninjured extremity as a guide. The splint should extend three quarters of the way or more from the knee to the groin and be deep enough to contain the leg. If the splint is too long, you can cut off part at one end. Mark the bottom of the patient's heel on the splint and cut the edges of the splint so you can bend the end almost to a right angle under the sole of the foot.

After removing the patient's boot in the aid room, lift the injured extremity and slide the splint into position under it in the same manner as for the quick splint. Bend the end of the splint into position and anchor it with staples or tape. Padding makes the splint fit better, protects exposed bony areas, and therefore makes the patient more comfortable, so protect the sides of the knee and ankle with padding and place padding under the knee to keep it slightly flexed. Fold up the sides of the splint and secure them in position with adhesive tape ▶ **Figure 24-23** .

WIRE SPLINTS AND LADDER SPLINTS. Wire splints and ladder splints can be purchased in several sizes, and the smaller sizes are compact enough to fit into an emergency care belt. Commercial ladder splints (3″ × 31″) are available with widely spaced rungs that allow X-rays to be taken with the splint in place ▶ **Figure 24-24** .

You can also construct wire splints from ⅛″ or ¼″ wire mesh. Practical sizes for homemade wire splints are 7″ × 36″ and 18″ × 36″. The smaller splint can be rolled into a 2″ × 7″ cylinder. Fold 1″ adhesive tape over all raw edges to avoid injury from the sharp ends of the wire.

Pad all wire and ladder splints, and cut or bend them to fit the extremity. Lay the splints along the long axis of the extremity, bend them so that all joints are in the position of function, and secure them with self-adhering roller bandages or cravats. Depending on the size and strength of the splints, one or two may be required to immobilize an extremity. You can use the splints singly or doubled on one side of an extremity, place them singly or doubled on either side of the extremity, or apply them like a "sugar tong." For example, two small wire splints can be doubled over to increase their strength and used one on each side to splint upper arm or forearm fractures. You can also use two large wire splints to immobilize a leg or an ankle, one on each side or two together posteriorly.

MALLEABLE METAL SPLINTS. Malleable metal splints have largely replaced wire and ladder splints, especially for the upper extremity. These splints are made of soft sheet metal prepadded with thin sheets of foam that have been glued to one or both sides ▶ **Figure 24-25** .

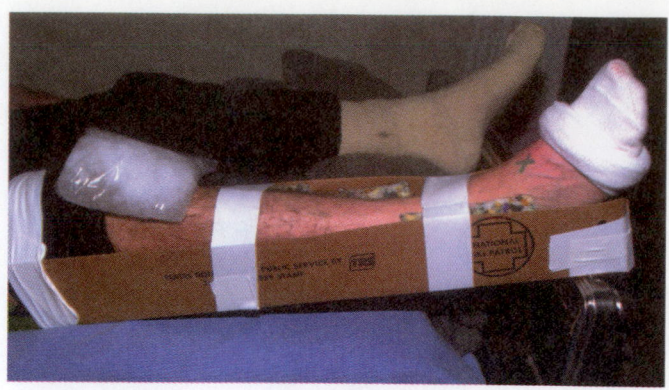

Figure 24-23 Cardboard splint applied to an injured leg.

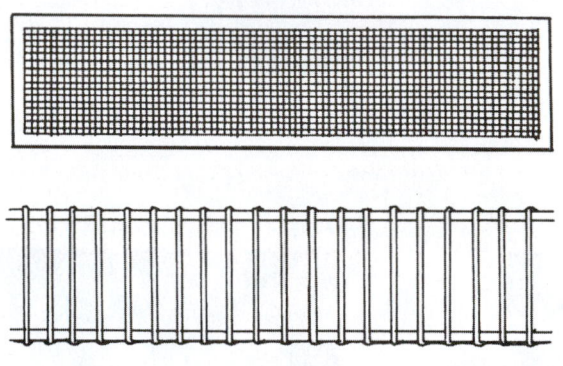

Figure 24-24 Ladder and wire fixation splints.

Figure 24-25 SAM splint.

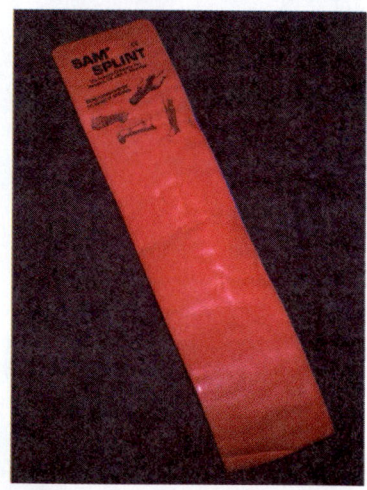

The SAM splint is a popular and versatile model that comes with detailed instructions. It measures 4¼″ × 35½″ and rolls into a 3″ × 4¼″ cylinder. It can be used singly or doubled, rounded sideways into a trough-like shape to fit an extremity, or bent into a sugar-tong shape. If nothing better is available, it can also be used to improvise a rigid cervical collar. The material is soft enough to be cut with shears if necessary.

A small wooden board, a rigid aluminum splint, or a fiberglass splint can be substituted for the malleable metal splint in the aid room, in the same way that a cardboard splint replaces a quick splint.

Soft fixation splints. The most common soft splint used by rescue squads is the precontoured, inflatable, clear plastic air splint. These are available in a variety of sizes and shapes, with or without a zipper that runs the length of the splint. Always inflate the splint after applying it. The air splint is comfortable, provides uniform contact, and has the added advantage of applying firm pressure to a bleeding wound. Air splints are used to immobilize injuries below the elbow or below the knee.

While these splints are probably the best fixation splint for most wilderness rescue groups and nordic ski patrols because of their light weight and collapsibility, their relatively high cost and poor durability make them less practical for alpine ski patrols with high injury volume. In cold weather, the plastic becomes stiff and nonmalleable. Significant changes in the weather affect the pressure of the air in the splint, decreasing as the environment grows colder (outside) and increasing as the environment grows warmer (in the aid room). The same thing happens when there are changes in altitude, which can be a problem with helicopter transport of patients. Therefore, air splints should not be used for alpine ski patrol emergency care.

Other soft fixation splints include vacuum splints, pillow splints, a sling and swathe, and the blanket roll splint for an anterior dislocation of the shoulder.

Vacuum splints. Vacuum splints are also closed, shaped, airtight bags, but unlike the air splint, a vacuum splint is filled with many tiny plastic pellets. After the splint is put in place, the air inside it is evacuated with a suction pump, which draws the plastic pellets close together to form a rigid encasement around the injured part.

Vacuum splints are light, comfortable, work well, and, although expensive, they are a good choice for backcountry and mountain rescue. They also provide good insulation in cold weather. Several types and shapes of large- and small-extremity splints and whole-body splints (for spine injuries) are available. One type of extremity splint (the LOTS splint) includes a femur-traction attachment. However, remember that if a vacuum splint gets a hole in it, it will not work properly.

Sling and swathe. A sling and swathe immobilizes upper extremity injuries by using the chest wall as a splint and is readily available in a rescuer's aid pack. To apply a sling and swathe, follow the directions in ▶ **Skill Drill 24-4** :

1. **Bend the patient's elbow to just under a 90° angle and lay a triangular bandage on the chest wall under the injured arm.** The bandage's long edge should be at the opposite mid-clavicular line just medial to the fingertips of the injured arm, and the upper corner should pass over the opposite shoulder. The apex of the triangle should be just beyond the elbow of the injured arm **(Step 1)**.

2. **Bring the lower corner of the bandage anteriorly around the forearm and up and over the shoulder on the injured side.** Tie the two ends together at the side of the neck. Bring the apex forward and pin it to the front of the sling, or tie a knot in the apex **(Step 2)**.

3. The tips of the fingers should be visible, and the forearm should be cradled in the sling with the weight of the forearm evenly distributed. To make the swathe, fold a second triangular bandage to make a cravat 3″ to 6″ wide. **Wrap the cravat around the patient's chest, include the upper arm on the injured side, and tie it snugly (Step 3)**.

4. **Alternatively, to avoid pressure on an injured shoulder or fractured clavicle, tie the sling as follows:** bring the upper corner across the patient's chest and over the uninjured shoulder—as before. Now bring the lower corner up around the forearm then under the near axilla, where you tie it to the opposite upper corner behind the patient's back. Tie the swathe around the patient's chest and forearm rather than arm **(Step 4)**.

The sling and swathe is used for clavicle fractures, acromioclavicular joint sprains, fractures of the proximal humerus, and—together with a rigid splint—for injuries of the arm, elbow, forearm, wrist, and hand.

The blanket roll splint. The blanket roll splint for an anterior dislocation of the shoulder is easy to make and efficient. The traditional airplane splint, while useful in some situations, often is cumbersome in cold weather, especially when snow becomes packed in the tightening mechanism. Splinting a dislocated shoulder in itself is often difficult because of the mechanics and position of the injury.

To create and apply a blanket roll splint, follow the directions in ▶ **Skill Drill 24-5** :

1. **Open a blanket on the snow,** then fold it longitudinally in thirds or fourths, depending on the angle of the abduction deformity of the injured shoulder **(Step 1)**.

Skill Drill 24-4   Applying a Sling and Swathe

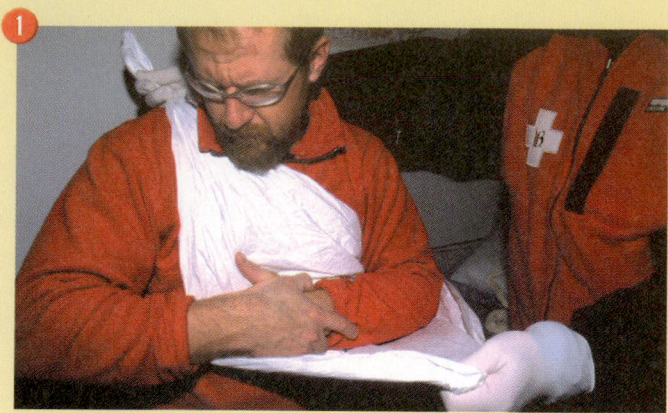

Bend the patient's elbow to just under a 90° angle and lay a triangular bandage on the chest wall under the injured arm. The injured forearm lays across the chest.

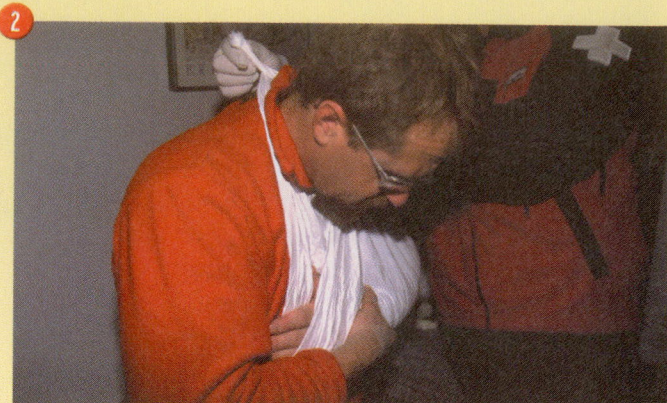

Tie the two ends together at the side of the neck. Bring the apex forward and pin it to the front of the sling, or tie a knot in the apex.

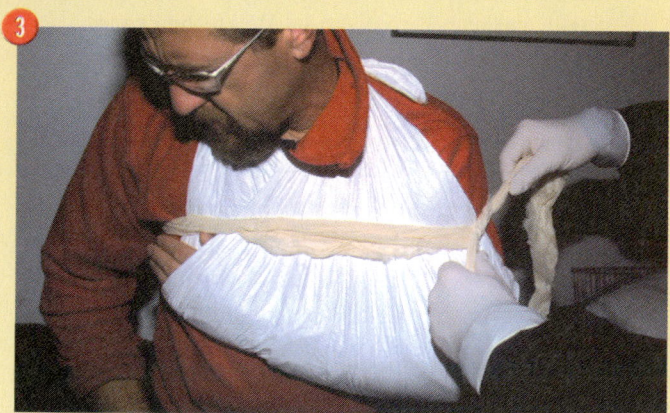

Wrap a swathe around the patient's chest, include the upper arm on the injured side, and tie it snugly under the opposite armpit.

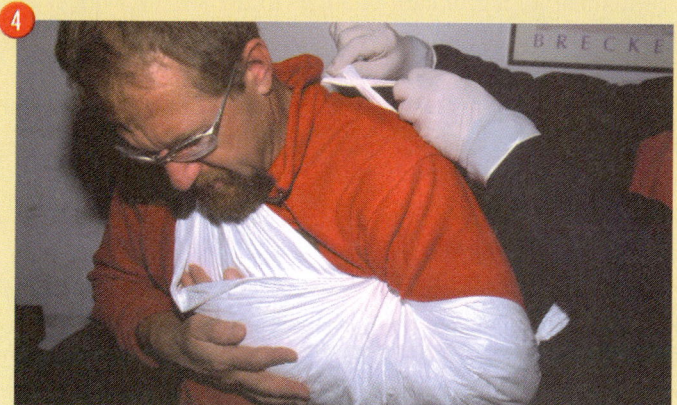

To avoid pressure on an injured shoulder or fractured clavicle, bring the lower corner of the sling under the near axilla. Tie it to the opposite corner behind the patient's back.

2. **Tie single cravats, or two cravats, end to end, and lay them across the blanket.** Tie knots in the two ends of one cravat(s) for identification purposes later **(Step 2)**.

3. **The blanket is rolled firmly,** then snugly positioned and held in the abduction angle of the dislocated shoulder **(Step 3)**.

4. **A second patroller ties one of the cravats over the opposite shoulder,** and the other around the injured person's waist **(Step 4)**.

5. **The hand of the injured arm is then stabilized as comfortably as possible—in a sling and swathe (Step 5)**. A CMS check on the injured extremity hand is carried out before transport, the latter usually being accomplished in a sled with the patient in the semisitting position.

Improvised Fixation Splints

Improvised fixation splints can be made out of boards and other rigid or semirigid materials of the proper size and shape. You can make a suitable splint for an injured forearm by laying branches side-by-side and

Skill Drill 24-5   Forming and Applying a Blanket Roll Splint

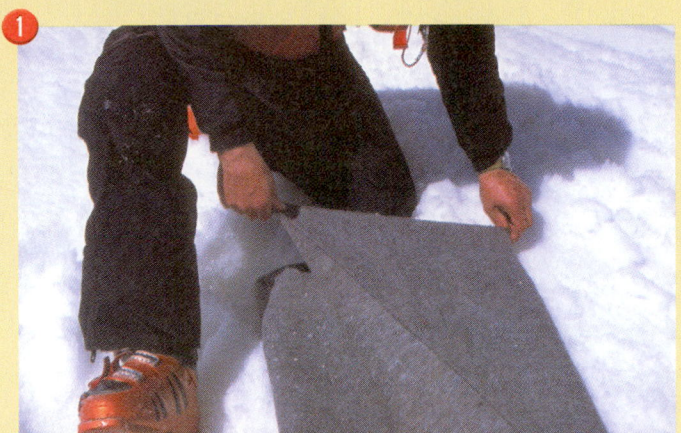

Fold a blanket longitudinally in thirds.

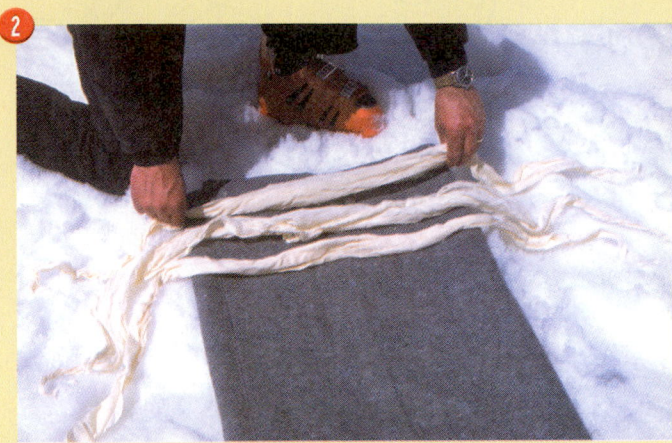

Lay cravats across the blanket. Tie knots in the two ends of one cravat(s) for identification purposes later.

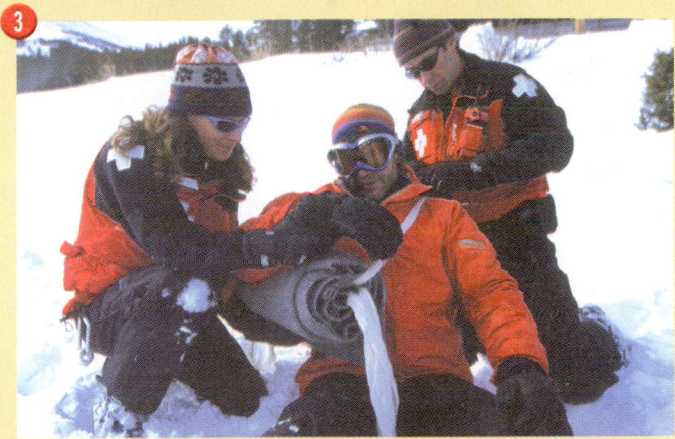

Position the rolled blanket snugly and in the abduction angle of the dislocated shoulder.

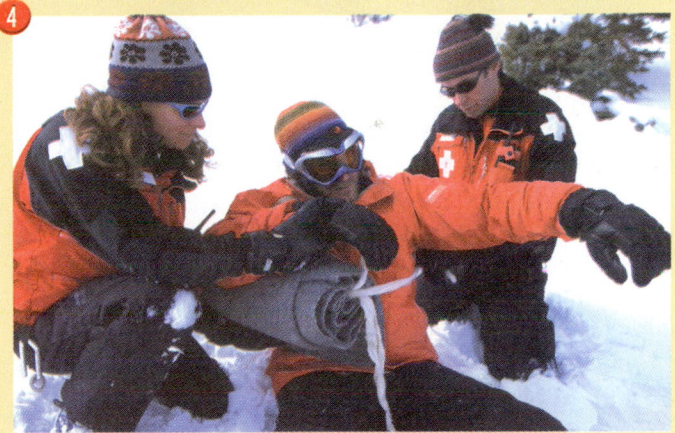

Securely tie the cravats around the neck and waist.

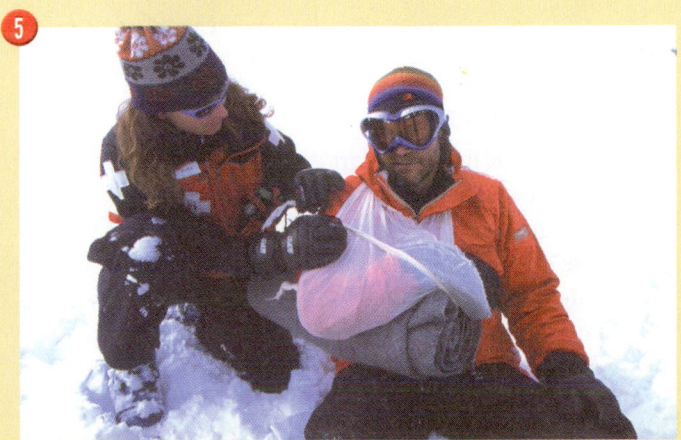

Secure the injured arm with a sling and swathe.

Figure 24-26 Improvised fixation splints.

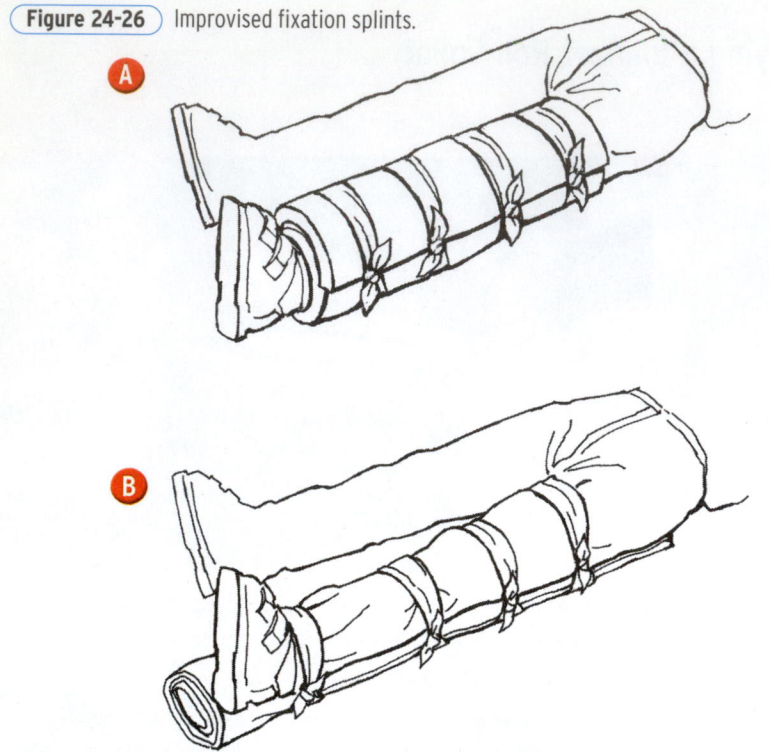

A

B

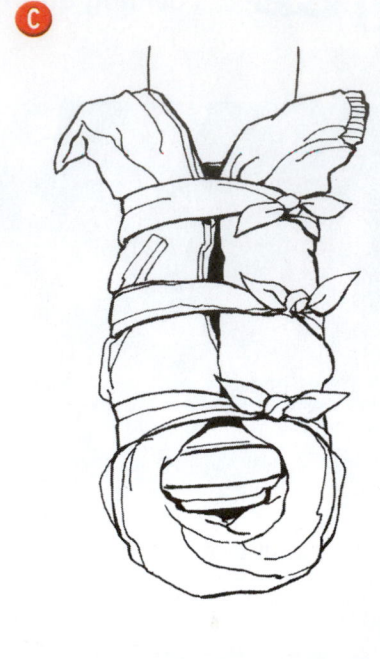

C

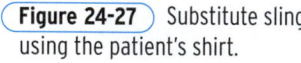

Figure 24-27 Substitute sling using the patient's shirt.

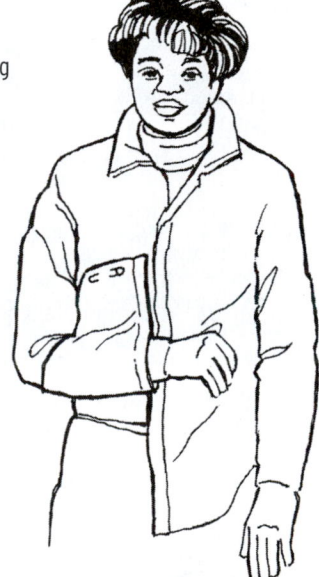

wrapping them with tape. Padded pack straps, rolled newspapers and magazines also make good upper extremity splints.

You can fashion a lower extremity splint out of an inflatable mattress (such as the Therm-A-Rest), a piece of Ensolite, or the removable foam pad from a pack. Roll the material around the extremity and secure it in place ▲ Figure 24-26A . A tightly rolled blanket is a useful splint to place on the posterior aspect of a lower extremity ▲ Figure 24-26B , and a folded pillow or tightly rolled jacket serves as an excellent splint for an injured ankle ▲ Figure 24-26C . If necessary, you can reinforce semirigid and soft improvised splints with branches; ax, shovel, or hammer handles; or ice tools.

Uninjured, nearby parts of the body can also be used as splints. For example, an injured finger or toe can be taped to its neighbor, and, as mentioned earlier, an injured hip or lower extremity can be splinted by tying the lower extremity to the opposite extremity (be sure to pad between the knees and ankles), and the chest wall can be used to splint upper extremity fractures.

A substitute for a sling can be made from a long-sleeved shirt or jacket by fastening the sleeve to the side of the garment with safety pins, or by pulling up the front part of the tail of the shirt around the forearm and pinning it to the shirt breast ▶ Figure 24-27 .

Improvised splints are used primarily in the wilderness setting when more commonly used splints are unavailable.

Traction Splints

In-line, longitudinal <u>traction</u> is the act of exerting a pulling force on a body structure in the direction of its normal alignment. It is the most effective way to realign a fracture of the shaft of a long bone so that the limb can be splinted more effectively. Excessive traction can be very harmful to an injured limb. When applied correctly, however, traction stabilizes the bone fragments and improves the overall alignment of the limb. You should not attempt to "reduce" a fracture or force all the bone fragments back into their normal anatomic alignment. This is the treating physician's responsibility. In the field, the goals of longitudinal traction are as follows:

1. To stabilize the fracture fragments to prevent excessive movement

2. To align the limb sufficiently to allow it to be placed in a splint

3. To avoid potential neurovascular compromise

In emergency care, the classic indication for a traction splint is a fracture of the midshaft (middle half to three fourths) of the femur. A traction splint is not used for fractures of the upper end of the femur, fractures of the lower end of the femur and tibia, or for any upper extremity injury. Several different types of lower extremity traction splints are commercially available, such as the Thomas half-ring splint, the Sager splint, the Kendrick traction device, and the Hare splint. Application of the Thomas, Sager, and Hare traction splints are described later in this chapter. Some rescue groups use a modified quick splint (Steven's Pass splint) to apply traction.

The original traction splint is the Thomas splint, developed during World War I by Sir Hugh Owen Thomas, a famous British surgeon. It was a revolutionary device that dramatically reduced mortality from fractured femurs during that war, probably because it reduced bleeding and minimized shock. The original device had a full ring but was later modified to make the familiar half-ring splint. For simplicity, in the following pages of this textbook, the term "Thomas splint" is used generically to refer to Thomas types of half-ring splints, both commercial and improvised (▶ **Figure 24-28**).

The following principles apply to the application of any traction splint discussed in this text (▶ **Skill Drill 24-6**):

1. At least two rescuers are needed to apply a traction splint. In addition, a third rescuer or bystander may be needed to stabilize the patient on the snow or ground to keep him or her from sliding in the direction of the traction exerted on the injured leg. If a bystander or friend is used, he or she must be properly directed by one of the rescuers. Usually this can be accomplished by grasping the patient under both armpits while kneeling alongside or behind the patient.
   - **An angulated fracture must be realigned before the splint can be applied. One rescuer manually stabilizes the fracture site (Step 1)**.
   - **Expose the injury site,** removing overlying clothes by cutting or ripping along a seam. Many ski pants have zippers that run the length of each leg and can make this task easier. **Care for any wounds discovered** as described previously.

Figure 24-28 Keller-Blake modification of the Thomas splint.

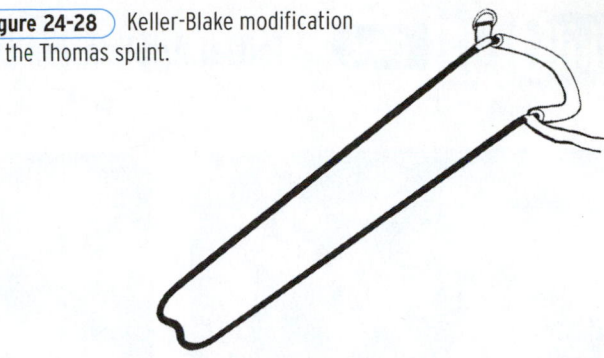

2. When all is ready (adequate personnel on scene and the splint is prepared), **a second rescuer stabilizes the boot on the injured leg and removes the ski or snowboard.** The second rescuer should then begin the assessment of CMS functions at this time **(Step 2)**. Some local protocols allow the boot to remain on the patient at this point.

3. **The first rescuer then firmly grasps the injured leg below the knee with both hands and straightens (realigns) the fracture angulation using manual, longitudinal traction.** *At this point manual traction must be maintained until mechanical traction (exerted by the splint) takes over.* As the first rescuer applies axial traction, the injured leg should remain supported on the snow until it is necessary to lift the leg when applying the splint **(Step 3)**. Some local protocols call for the removal of the boot before placing the injured leg in a traction splint. While in-line manual traction is maintained, the second rescuer can remove the ski or snowboard boot. The sock should be left on after assessing the extremities' CMS status.

4. **The second rescuer readies the splint and ankle hitch. The ankle hitch should be applied at this time** and can be used to manually exert traction **(Step 4)**.

5. **The leg is placed in or on the splint and it is secured** around the upper thigh and seated snugly against the ischial tuberosity. At this time the rescuers can gradually replace manual traction with the mechanical traction of the splint **(Step 5)**.

6. After all straps have been applied, **the CMS status of the injured leg should be reassessed (Step 6)**.

7. The patient should be log rolled onto the **uninjured side and placed on a long backboard (Step 7).** Secure the patient and splint to the backboard in a manner that prevents movement of the splint during evacuation and transport.

Skill Drill 24-6   Initial Application of All Traction Splints

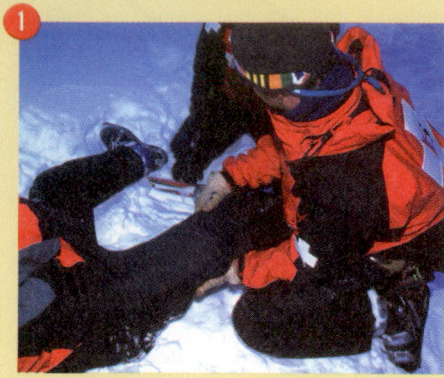

1. One rescuer manually stabilizes the fracture site.

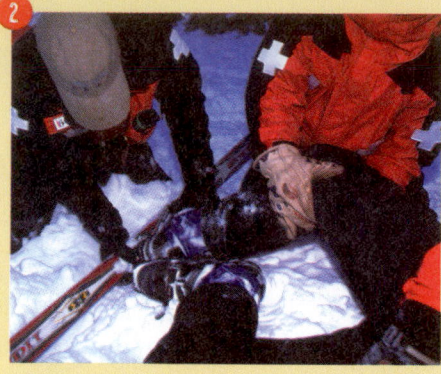

2. After the fracture has been stabilized, another rescuer(s) removes the ski or snowboard and assesses the CMS status of the extremity.

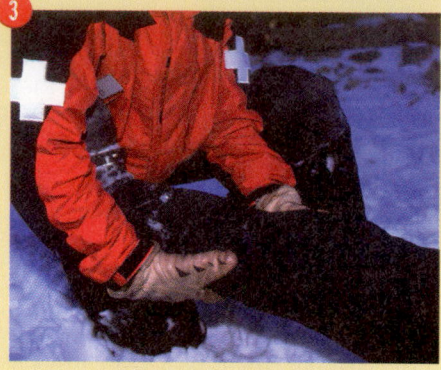

3. The first rescuer firmly grasps the injured leg below the knee and realigns the fracture by manual, longitudinal (axial) traction. The boot can be removed and CMS status assessed at this time as needed.

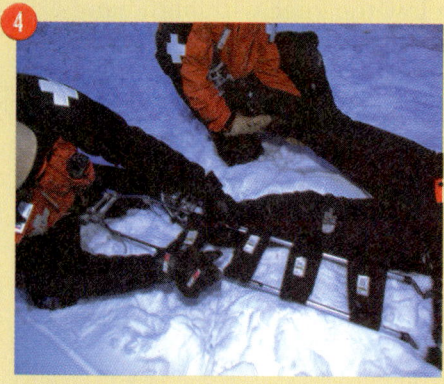

4. The second rescuer sizes and prepares the splint. The ankle hitch should be applied at this time and can be used to maintain manual traction.

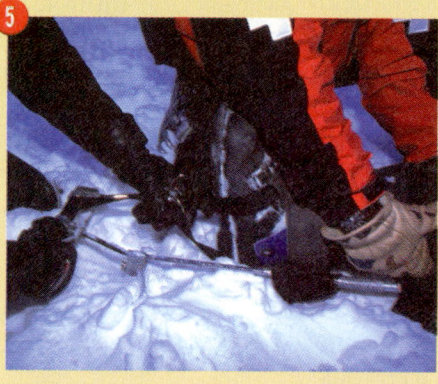

5. The leg is placed in the splint, secured to the upper thigh, and mechanical traction is evenly substituted for manual traction.

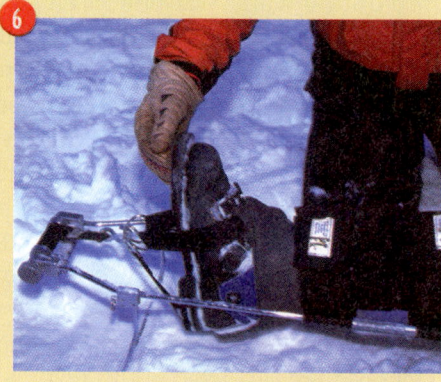

6. Reassess the CMS status of the injured extremity after all straps have been applied.

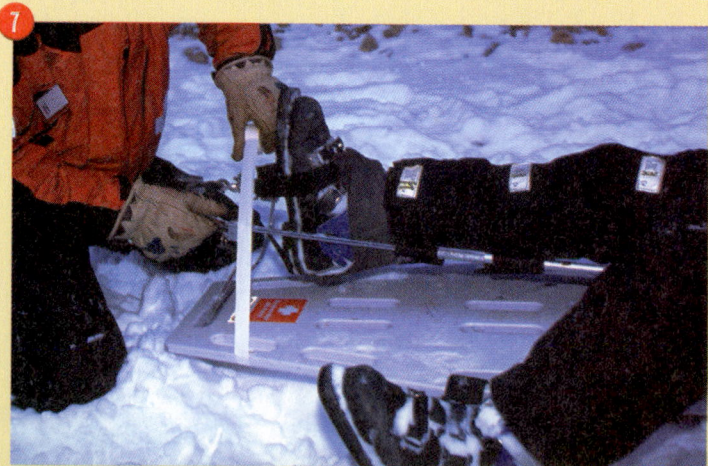

7. Log roll the patient onto his or her uninjured side and place the patient on a long backboard. Secure the splint to the backboard to prevent movement.

APPLICATION OF THE THOMAS HALF RING TRACTION SPLINT. The basic Thomas splint is a rigid, longitudinal metal frame about 4' long, notched at the narrow end and attached at the wide end to a padded half-ring to which is fastened a strap with a buckle. The half-ring is angled to fit comfortably behind the upper thigh against the ischial tuberosity, and hinged so it can be used for either the right or the left lower extremity. The strap is buckled in front of the thigh to keep the half-ring in place.

Expose the injury site (▶ **Figure 24-29A**). Care for any wounds discovered as described previously. If the Thomas splint is an adjustable model, measure it against the patient's uninjured side and adjust it so that the end of the splint extends 6" to 12" beyond the patient's foot or boot. Place the splint beside the injured extremity so that the long side will be on the outside of the extremity. Prepare four cravats (or Velcro support straps) and lay them on the splint, spaced so that two will lie above the knee and two below the knee (▶ **Figure 24-29B**). Prepare the traction pulley system by tying a 50" piece of $\frac{1}{8}$" or $\frac{1}{4}$" braided nylon cord to the end of the splint with two half-hitches (▶ **Figure 24-29C**).

The ankle hitch for a Thomas splint can be a sprained-ankle bandage made from a cravat (▶ **Figure 24-29D**), a hitch made from two cravats (▶ **Figure 24-29E**), or a commercial hitch made of nylon webbing. Unfortunately, many commercial hitches are too small to go around a ski or snowboard boot.

To tie a sprained-ankle bandage, place the middle part of a 2" cravat in the instep of the boot of the injured extremity, forming a stirrup. Cross the ends behind the ankle, bring them around in front of the ankle, and cross them again. Run each end under the first part of the cravat on that side of the foot, then pull it medially around the ankle. Use a square knot to tie the two ends together in front of the ankle, making sure that the cravat is free of wrinkles and snug but not tight.

After the femur angulation has been realigned and the ankle hitch is in place (as described above), rescuer 1 continues to apply manual longitudinal traction through the hitch. Rescuer 2 now moves to support/stabilize the injured thigh, and both rescuers raise the extremity several inches off the ground. Rescuer 2 slides the traction splint (which has been previously prepared) under the extremity until the half-ring is snugly in place against the ischial tuberosity (▶ **Figure 24-29G**).

An aid pack is placed under the distal end of the splint to keep it elevated a few inches off the ground (prevents the patient's heel from touching the ground when the splint is in place). Manual axial traction is continued while the extremity is lowered onto the splint. Rescuer 2 secures the strap in front of the upper thigh to hold the half-ring in place, then threads the end of the 50" nylon line through the stirrup of the ankle hitch, back over the end of the splint, back through the stirrup again, and back to the end of the splint. A pulley system with a 4:1 mechanical advantage is thus created (▶ **Figure 24-29F**).

As rescuer 2 pulls the nylon line tight, rescuer 1 gradually releases manual traction, transferring it to mechanical traction. The traction line is tightened until the pain is reduced, then tied off to the end of the splint with two half-hitches. The loose ends of each of the four cravats lying across the splint are reversed, brought under and around the opposite sides of the splint, over and around the extremity, and tied together at the side of the splint, forming a series of cradle hitches (▶ **Figure 24-29H**). If you are using Velcro straps instead, put them in place firmly around the limb. Do not place a cravat or strap directly over the knee or over a fracture site.

Commercially available modifications of the Thomas splint, such as the Hare splint (▶ **Figure 24-30**), use Velcro straps instead of cradle hitches and a ratchet at the end of the splint for mechanical traction. There are special conversion kits that give an ordinary Thomas splint some of the features of a Hare splint. Rescuers who choose a splint that has ratchet traction should be trained to use it properly. If applied too tightly, such devices are uncomfortable and can cause pressure damage to the buttock, or even loss of pulses in the foot.

APPLICATION OF THE HARE TRACTION SPLINT.

1. Place the splint beside the patient's uninjured leg, and adjust it to the proper length, with the padded support at the ischial tuberosity and the splint extending 6" to 12" beyond the foot. Open and adjust the four Velcro support straps, which should be positioned at the midthigh, above the knee, below the knee, and above the ankle.

2. Follow the protocol as outlined above for *alignment of the fractured femur and application of the ankle hitch.*

3. Next, while rescuer 1 continues to apply longitudinal traction, rescuer 2 now moves back to support/stabilize the injury site, and both rescuers raise the extremity off the ground. Rescuer 2 slides the Hare splint into position under the patient's injured limb, making certain that the pad is seated well on the ischial tuberosity. The

Figure 24-29 Application of a modified Thomas splint.

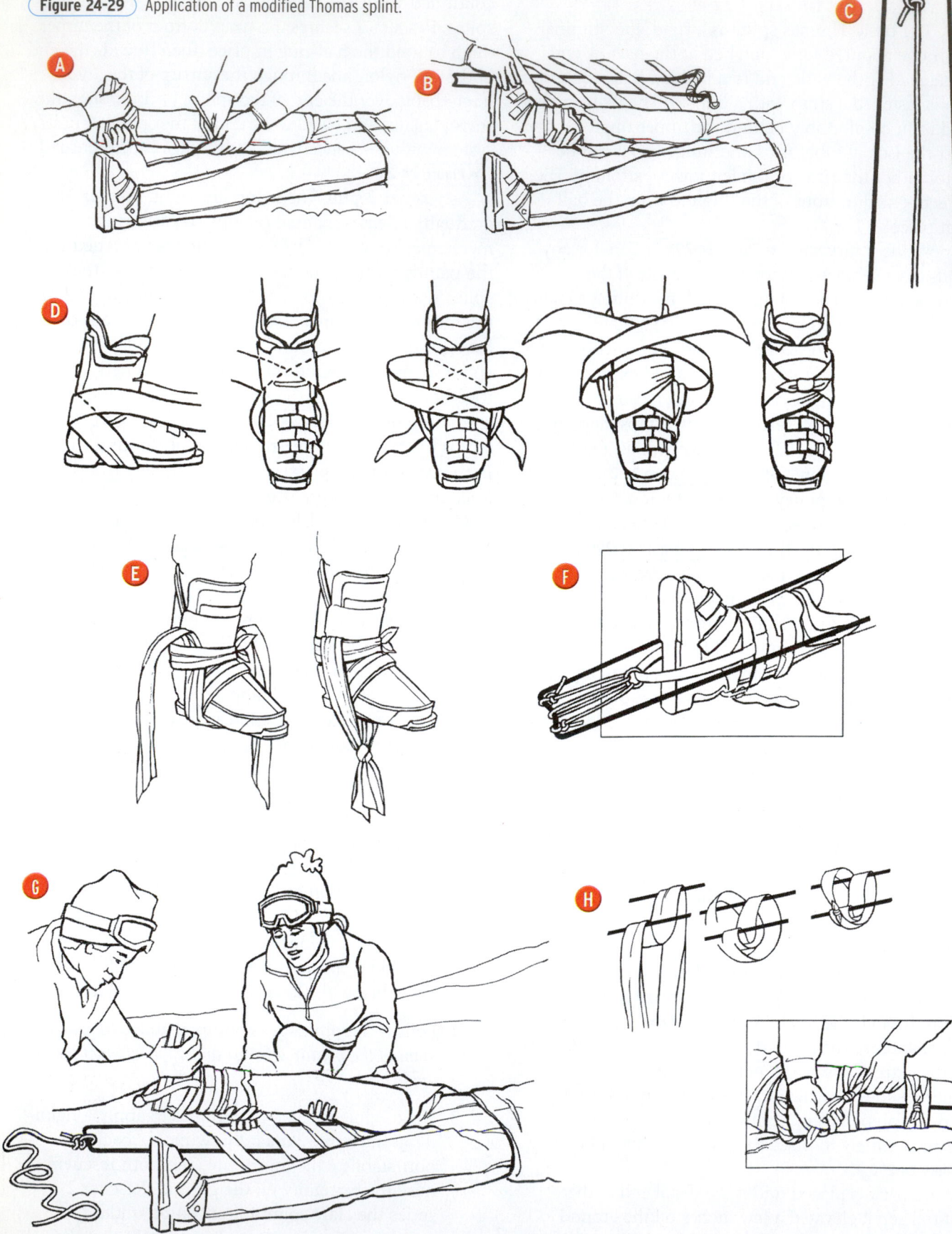

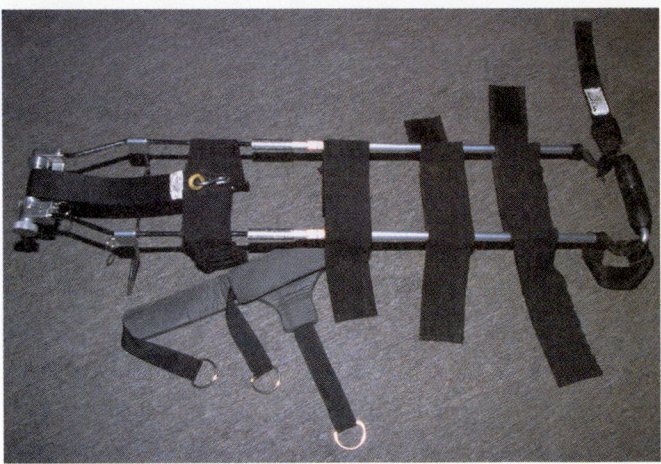

Figure 24-30   Hare traction splint.

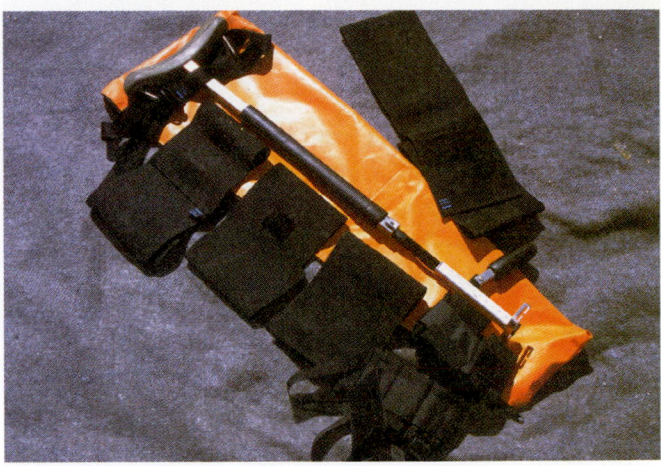

Figure 24-31   Sager splint.

rescuer pads the groin area and applies the ischial strap.

4. Rescuer 1 maintains longitudinal traction through the ankle hitch, and rescuer 2 connects the loops of the ankle hitch to the end of the splint. The ratchet is slowly tightened. Gentle mechanical traction on the injured leg is thereby established through the connecting strap, between the ankle hitch and the splint, just strongly enough to maintain limb alignment. Use caution! This splint comes with a ratchet mechanism to tighten the strap, which can overstretch the limb and further injure the patient. Adequate traction has been applied when the leg is the same length as the other leg and/or the patient feels relief.

5. Once proper traction has been applied, fasten the Velcro support straps so that the limb is securely held in the splint. Check all proximal and distal support straps to make sure they are snug.

6. At this point, reassess the CMS status.

7. Log roll the patient onto the uninjured side, and place the patient securely on a long backboard for transport to the aid room. In the absence of a suspected spinal injury, a cervical collar is unnecessary.

Commercially available ankle hitches are more comfortable and simpler to apply, but, again, some are too small to fit over ski boots, heavy mountaineering boots, or snowboard boots.

When purchasing a traction splint for patients who will be wearing boots, make sure the harness or hitch supplied with the splint is large enough to fit over ski

boots and other large boots. In some cases you may have to order a larger harness separately; it should be the type labeled as "suitable for climbing, ski, or snowboard boots," and should be tried out before being used in the field. You can also improvise a traction hitch from one or two cravats.

It is generally safe to apply traction to a booted foot for up to an hour, but longer periods of time are uncomfortable and introduce the danger of interference with circulation and pressure damage to the tissues of the foot (this is one reason that many patrols are now removing the boot on the hill before applying traction). Question the patient periodically about his or her ability to wiggle the toes and whether there is any new numbness or pain in the toes or foot. If there is any doubt, replace the mechanical traction with manual traction, remove the boot, assess the foot and ankle, and reapply mechanical traction on the unbooted foot.

Several newer devices for traction are portable, lightweight, readily adjustable, and compact enough so that a splinted patient will usually fit into a helicopter. The Sager splint (▲ **Figure 24-31**), which many prefer to Thomas or Hare splints, weighs less than 4$\frac{1}{2}$ lb and breaks down to fit into a tapering package that measures 32" × 64". It has a single longitudinal support that can be positioned either on the inside or outside of the lower extremity. This splint has a great advantage over other traction splints in that the unstable injured thigh *does not have to be lifted off the supporting snow at any time during splint application.* One version of the Sager splint allows traction to be applied to both lower extremities at the same time.

APPLICATION OF THE SAGER TRACTION SPLINT. The following summarizes the application of a Sager splint for a midshaft fractured femur. Also be sure to consult the manufacturer's directions before applying the splint ▶ **Skill Drill 24-7**.

1. Remove the splint from its case and attach the foam-covered, T-shaped groin piece to the top of the splint. **Adjust the plastic buckle so that, when closed, it will be on the front of the patient's thigh** (Step 1).

2. Hold the splint next to the uninjured lower extremity and **adjust it so that the calibrated wheel is just below the patient's heel** (Step 2). Follow the protocol as outlined above for *alignment of the fractured femur and application of the ankle hitch*. Before application of the Sager ankle hitch, estimate the size of the patient's ankle (boot on or boot off), and fold in or out the number of pads on the ankle hitch needed to provide adequate padding and contact around the ankle. Apply the hitch snugly above the malleoli. Check foot pulses before and afterward (if the boot has been removed).

3. After the ankle hitch has been applied, and while one rescuer continues to apply manual longitudinal traction, with the injured thigh supported by the snow, burrow in the snow and slide the thigh strap under the injured thigh so that the groin piece is snug against the patient's crotch and ischial tuberosity. Patients wearing tight underclothing or jeans, especially men, may find this position uncomfortable unless the tight clothing is adjusted.

4. **Close the buckle and tighten the thigh strap** (Step 3) so that the groin piece is drawn sideways into the patient's crotch. Be sure to pad in the crotch and under the strap.

5. Shorten the loop of the ankle hitch harness by pulling on the strap threaded through the square D-buckle. **Connect the ankle hitch latch-hook** to the cable ring of the calibrated wheel at the end of the splint. Make sure the cable ring is snug against the bottom of the foot (Step 4).

6. **Extend the splint** by pressing down on the thumb piece and sliding the inner part out until the desired amount of traction is noted on the calibrated wheel. A rough guide is 10% of the patient's body weight, up to a maximum of 25 lb, with *15 to 20 lb* being average traction for an adult (Step 5).

7. **Fasten the splint to the extremity** by applying the three 6"-wide elastic straps. Place the two shorter straps (1) around the patient's midthigh *over the fracture site* (to tamponade [compress] internal hemorrhage) and (2) at the midcalf level. The third longer strap is applied just above the ankle and around the other leg, to hold the extremities together (Step 6).

8. **Check CMS** in the foot after splint application. Log roll the patient onto the uninjured side to place the patient on a backboard, then transport the patient by sled to the aid room (Step 7).

The Kendrick Traction Device (KTD) is similar to the Sager splint, and uses an aluminum pole much like a tent pole to provide longitudinal support. It weighs 20 oz and breaks down to form a package about 10" × 5½" × 3" ▼ **Figure 24-32**. Because of its simplicity, smaller size, and weight, the KTD is probably the best choice for backcountry rescue groups, while the Sager splint is replacing the Thomas and Hare splints in many ski patrols and urban EMS groups.

Again, when purchasing the splints described above, be sure that the traction harness included is large enough to fit over a ski, snowboard, or climbing boot. Over-snow rescue groups have the option of improvising traction splints from ski poles, described later in this chapter.

Because all the traction splints described previously immobilize the limb by producing countertraction on

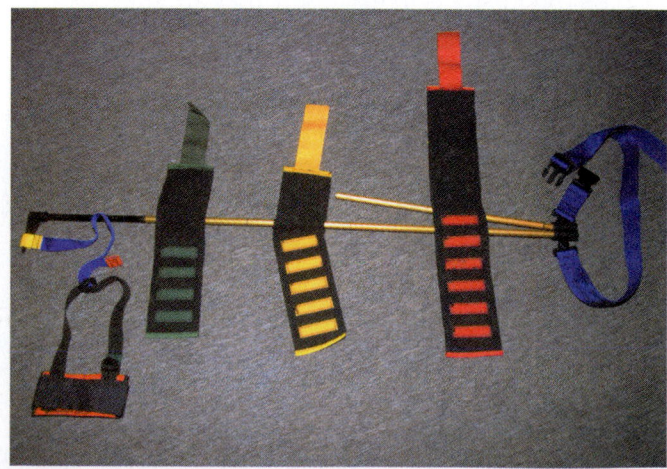

Figure 24-32 KTD splint.

SkillDrill 24-7   Applying a Sager Traction Splint

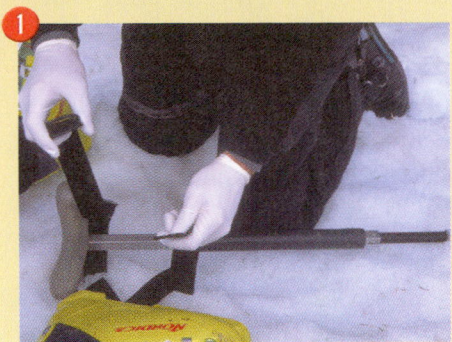

1 Adjust the thigh strap so that it lies anteriorly when secured.

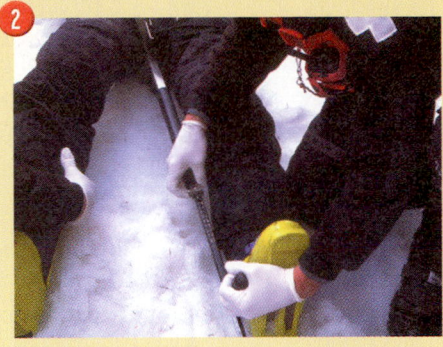

2 Estimate the proper length of the splint by placing it next to the uninjured limb.
Fit the ankle pads to the ankle.

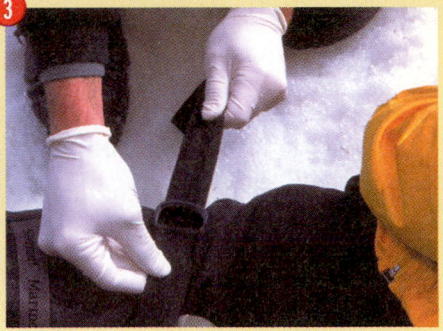

3 Place the splint at the inner thigh, apply the thigh strap at the upper thigh, and secure snugly.

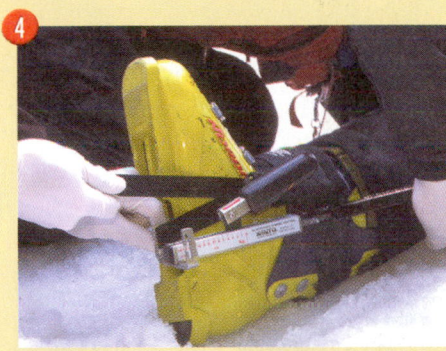

4 Tighten the ankle harness just above the malleoli.
Snug the cable ring against the bottom of the foot.

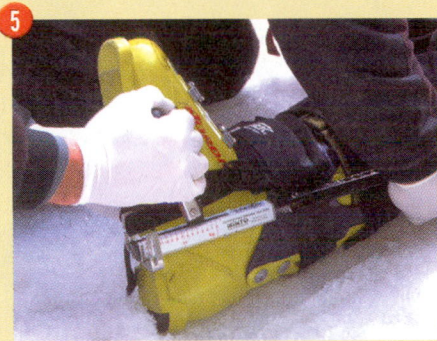

5 Extend the splint's inner shaft to apply traction of about 10% of body weight.

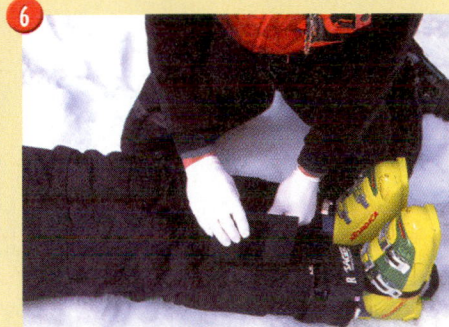

6 Secure the splint with elasticized cravats.

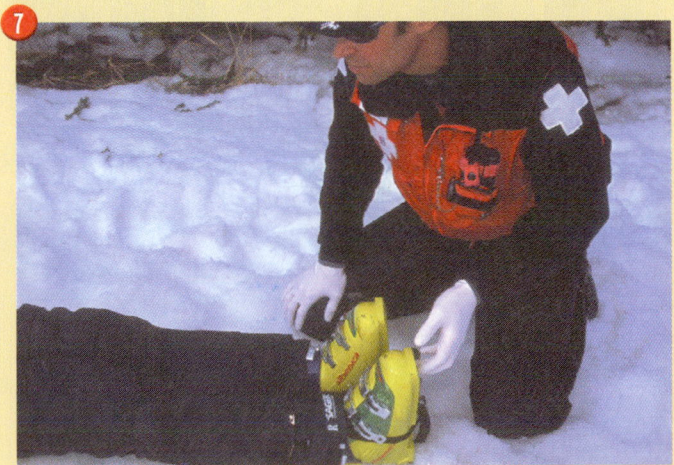

7 Check CMS functions.
Secure the patient to a long backboard.

the ischium and in the groin, use care to pad these areas well. You must avoid excessive pressure on the external genitalia. If at all possible, always use commercially available padded ankle hitches rather than pieces of rope, cord, or tape. Such improvised hitches can sometimes be painful and can potentially obstruct circulation in the foot.

Hazards of Improper Splinting

You must be aware of the hazards associated with the improper application of splints, including the following:

- Compression of nerves, tissues, and blood vessels

- Delay in transport of a patient with a life-threatening injury

- Reduction of distal circulation if the splint is too tight

- Aggravation of the injury

- Injury to tissue, nerves, blood vessels, or muscles as a result of excessive movement of the bone or joint

Once an injured limb is adequately splinted, the patient is ready to be transferred to a backboard and/or sled, and be transported. Very few musculoskeletal injuries justify the use of excessive speed during transport. The limb will be stable once a dressing and splint have been applied. However, the patient with a pulseless limb must be given a higher priority. Still, if the aid room, and subsequently the hospital, are only a few minutes away, haste to the emergency department will make little or no difference in the patient's eventual outcome. However, if the treatment facility is more than an hour away, the patient with a pulseless limb should be transported by helicopter or immediate ground transportation. If circulation in the distal limb is impaired, always alert the rescue squad to notify medical control so that proper steps can be taken quickly once the patient arrives in the emergency department.

IMPROVISED TRACTION SPLINTS. If standard traction equipment is not available, you can improvise a Thomas type of traction splint from a single ski or two ski poles (▼ **Figure 24-33**).

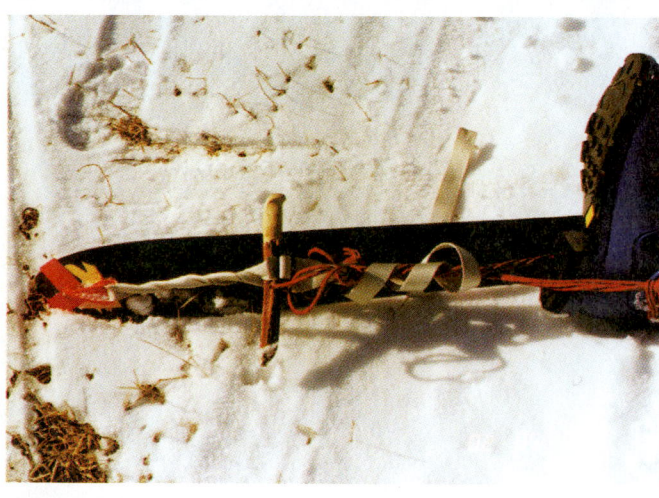

Figure 24-33 Improvised traction splint using a single ski.

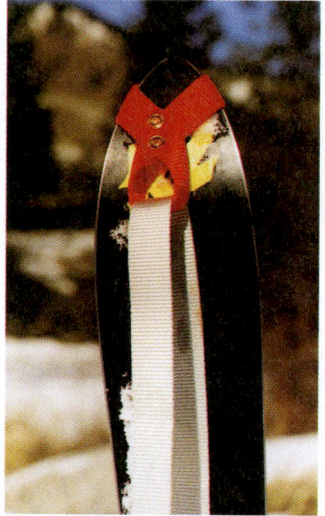 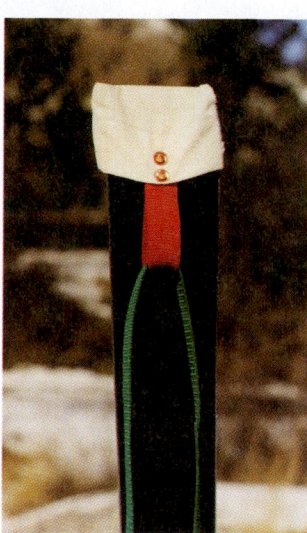

For the single-ski technique, purchase or prepare in advance two canvas pockets—one to slip over each end of the ski. Each pocket should have a grommet on one side of the base. Cravats can substitute for the pockets. To construct the splint, slip the pockets in place, with the tail of the ski toward the patient's armpit, the tip turned out, and the grommets facing the patient.

One rescuer applies continuous manual traction to the patient's foot and calf until splinting is completed. Run a cravat around the patient's upper thigh and pull it snugly up into the patient's groin. Tie the tails of the cravat through the grommet of the tail pocket. Then apply an ankle bandage or hitch to the boot, and apply traction to the boot in the manner previously described for the Thomas half-ring splint, using a nylon cord run in pulley fashion through the grommet of the tip pocket and the stirrup of the ankle hitch.

Pad any areas where the lower extremity touches the ski. Wrap several wide cravats around the patient's limb and ski from ankle to lower thigh. Support the tip of the ski to keep the patient's heel off the ground. After securing traction, stabilize the splint by wrapping cravats around the upper end of the ski and the trunk, and by tying the uninjured leg to the splint.

Another acceptable traction splint can be made from two ski poles or two canoe paddles provided they are long enough. The two ski-pole technique makes a useful, improvised emergency traction splint for ski tourers and over-snow wilderness rescue groups ▼ Figure 24-34 .

This technique requires a length of rope for a pulley and a minimum of six cravats (five if a commercial ankle hitch is available). Interlace or tie the pole straps together to form a half-ring no greater than half of the patient's thigh circumference. Join the baskets with a spreader such as an 8″ length of ski pole with two holes drilled in it the proper distance apart (prepared beforehand and carried in the emergency care kit). Lay four cravats to use as cradle hitches across the two poles, apply an ankle bandage or ankle hitch to the boot, and attach the nylon cord to the spreader.

Use manual axial traction in the same manner as described for the Thomas splint. Slip the splint under the extremity so that the padded pole straps ride up under the patient's buttock. Secure the splint at the patient's groin by tying the handles of the poles together in front of the hip with a cravat. Set up the pulley device to furnish traction, and finally, tighten the cradle hitches in place.

If no traction splint is available, you can apply traction to the lower extremity of a patient on a scoop stretcher (described in Chapter 25) by using the metal bar that forms the end of the stretcher as an anchor for the pulley. However, you must first immobilize the patient's torso on the stretcher to keep the traction from pulling the patient toward the end of the stretcher. Use two cravats to immobilize the torso; loop one around each thigh at the groin and tie them off to the side bar through a handhold.

Figure 24-34   Improvised traction splint using two ski poles.

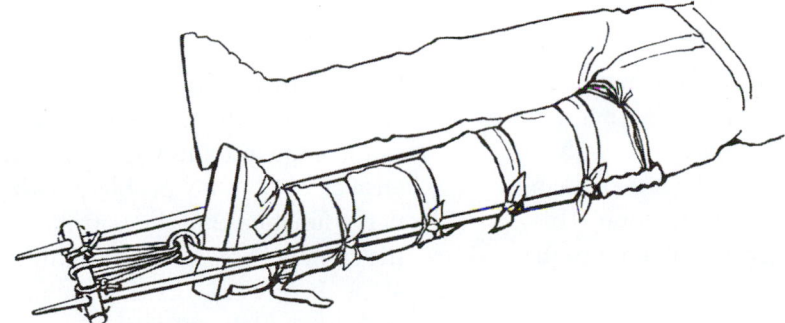

Boot Removal

In a case involving a skier or snowboarder with a lower extremity injury, deciding whether the boot should be removed at the area (whether on the hill or in the aid room) has been and remains the subject of considerable discussion. An important factor to consider is whether the type of injury requires use of a fixation or traction splint. Advantages and disadvantages of boot removal are outlined in (▼ **Table 24-2**) and (▼ **Table 24-3**).

With the advice of its patrol medical advisor, each area should develop a local protocol for boot removal (▶ **Skill Drill 24-8**), taking into consideration environmental conditions at the time of the incident, such as temperature, snow, rain, and wind; transport times from the incident site to the aid room and from the aid room to the hospital; type of injury; type of splint needed; probable or actual CMS status in the extremity distal to the injury; the patient's comfort; and local EMS and emergency department protocols.

The NSP National Medical Committee recommends that, as a rule, the boot should be off before the patient arrives at the hospital.

Table 24-2 Advantages and Disadvantages of Boot Removal in the Aid Room

Advantages:	Disadvantages:
CMS and nerve supply to the foot cannot be assessed directly with the boot in place.	Transport is delayed.
Many local EMS protocols require boot removal for assessment of CMS before transporting the patient.	
The boot has to come off at some point. Because of their experience and training, patrollers are sufficiently prepared to handle boot removal.	

Table 24-3 Advantages and Disadvantages of Boot Removal on the Slope*

This situation applies mainly to femur fractures that require traction splints.

Advantages:	Disadvantages:
Applying traction to a booted foot may be more painful than applying it to a shoeless foot.	Removing the boot on the slope exposes the foot to the cold.
For a patient in a traction splint, removing the boot in the aid room is a complicated process that requires releasing mechanical traction, replacing it with manual traction, taking the boot off, and assessing CMS before reapplying mechanical traction. This process introduces additional manipulation of the fractured limb.	On the slope, CMS can usually be satisfactorily assessed by asking the patient whether he or she can feel the feet and wiggle the toes. Even if the answer is "no," any problem with circulation or nerve function that the patroller can improve on the slope will respond to alignment and splinting alone. In any case, getting the patient off the hill becomes a high priority.
	Removing the boot on the hill takes time perhaps better spent in transport.

* *To make the patient more comfortable while you are deciding whether to remove the boot, slightly loosen both boots by unbuckling and rebuckling them at a looser setting.*

Skill Drill 24-8 Boot Removal

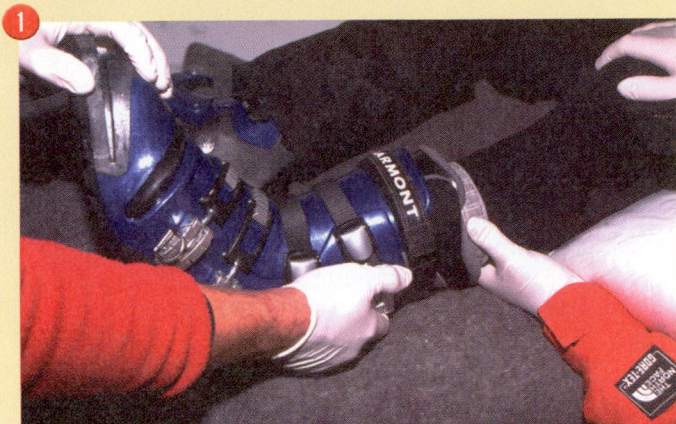

Stabilize the lower leg and the boot.

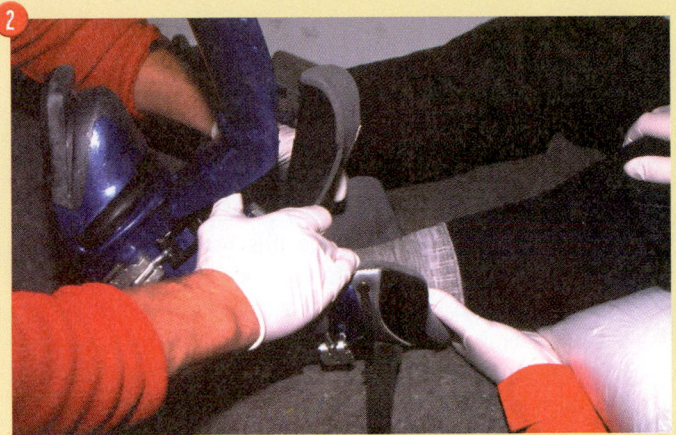

While maintaining manual stabilization, spread the boot shell, pulling the tongue out or opening a rear entry boot as wide as possible. Loosen all devices and provide instructions to the assisting rescuer.

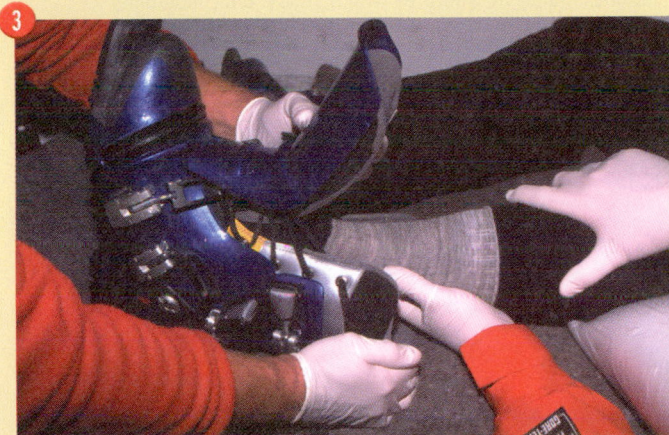

With the boot shell held open and the leg stabilized, apply tension to the boot. Firmly and smoothly pull and rotate the boot off the foot, while using your shoulder as counterpressure against the boot toe.

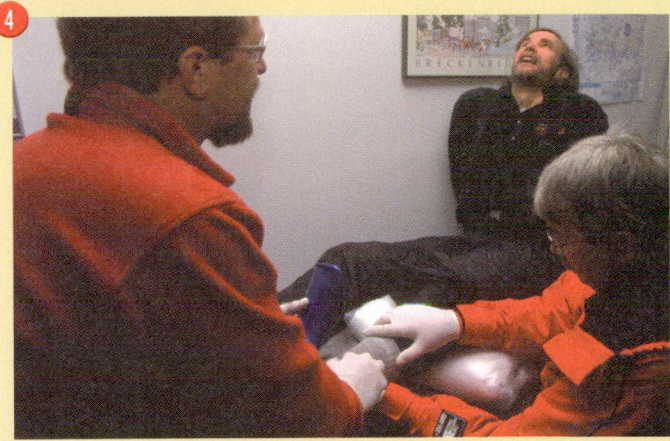

Monitor the patient for indications of excessive pain or resistance. Stop or modify the procedure as appropriate.

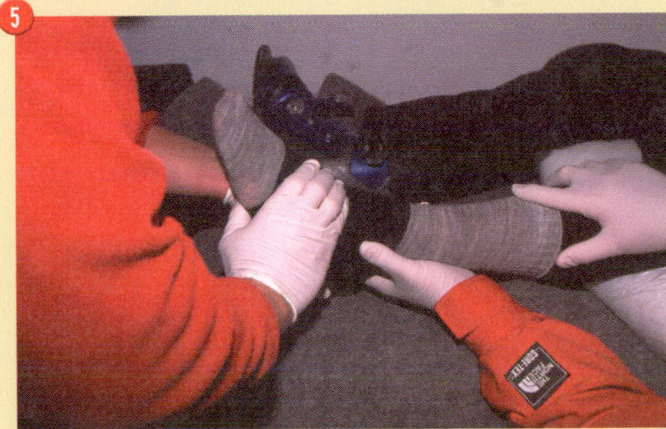

Assess distal circulation and neurologic function, swelling, displacement, or bruising (remove clothing).

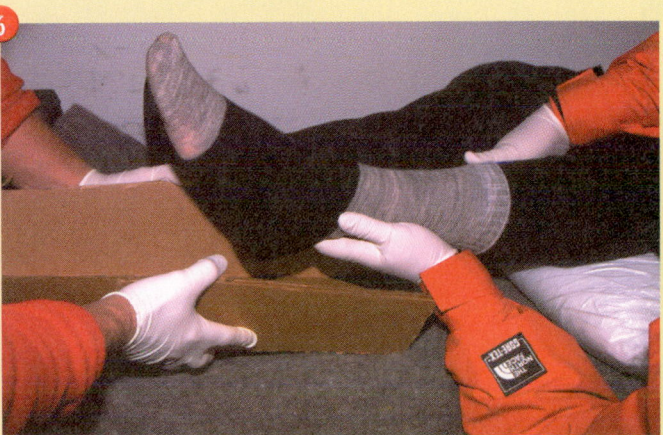

Prepare to splint the lower extremity.

Chapter *Sweep*

Ready for Review

Skeletal or voluntary muscle, which attaches to bone and forms the major muscle mass of the body, is supplied with arteries, veins, and nerves. The 206 bones of the skeleton are living tissue that, when fractured, can bleed and cause severe pain. Wherever two bones come into contact, a joint is formed, strengthened in key areas by ligaments. A fracture is a broken bone; a dislocation is a disruption of a joint; a sprain is a joint injury that involves partial or temporary dislocation of bone ends and partial or complete stretching or tearing of ligaments; and a strain is a muscle pull. Depending on the amount of kinetic energy absorbed by the tissues, the zone of injury may extend to a distant point, so you must always check for associated injuries beyond the obvious ones. Fractures are either open or closed, complete or incomplete, displaced or nondisplaced. Signs of fracture and dislocation include pain, deformity, point tenderness, guarding, swelling, crepitus, and false motion. Signs of sprain include point tenderness, swelling, ecchymosis, and instability of the joint.

Your approach to patients with multiple painful, swollen, deformed extremities should include a rapid initial assessment, stabilization of vital functions and control of serious bleeding, focused physical exam of the injured body part, assessment of neurovascular function in the affected limbs, splinting to immobilize the affected parts, and prompt transport to the aid room. For each limb injured, your neurovascular examination should include pulse, sensation, and motor function. Repeat this exam every 5 to 10 minutes as part of your detailed physical exam.

The principles of splinting include the following: if you suspect a fracture of the shaft of any bone, make sure the splint immobilizes the joints above and below the fracture; with injuries in and around a joint, make sure the splint immobilizes the bones above and below the injured joint; where fracture of a long bone shaft has resulted in severe deformity, use constant, gentle, longitudinal traction to align the limb so that it can be splinted, unless this is too painful. There are three types of splints: rigid fixation splints, soft fixation splints, and traction splints.

Provide immediate transport to any patient if you are unable to restore a pulse to a pulseless limb by applying traction. The only life-threatening musculoskeletal injuries are multiple fractures, fractures with arterial injuries, severe open fractures, limb amputations, and pelvic fractures with hemodynamic instability.

Vital Vocabulary

articular cartilage A pearly layer of specialized cartilage covering the articular surfaces (contact surfaces on the ends) of bones in synovial joints.

closed fracture A fracture in which the overlying skin is not broken.

crepitus A grating or grinding sensation that occurs when fractured bone ends rub together.

dislocation Disruption of a joint in which ligaments are damaged and the bone ends are no longer in normal contact.

displaced fracture A fracture in which bone fragments are separated from one another and not in anatomic alignment.

fracture A break in the continuity of a bone.

involuntary muscle A muscle whose contractions are not under conscious control.

joint The place where two bones come into contact.

ligament A band of fibrous tissue that connects bones to bones, and supports and strengthens a joint.

nondisplaced fracture A simple crack in the bone that has not caused the bone to move from its normal anatomic position; also called a hairline fracture.

open fracture Any break in a bone in which the overlying skin has been violated.

patella The kneecap.

point tenderness Tenderness that is sharply localized at the site of the injury, found by gently palpating along the bone with the tip of one finger.

reduce To return a dislocated joint or fractured bone to its normal position; set.

skeletal muscle Striated muscles that are attached to bones and usually cross at least one joint.

smooth muscle A muscle that is not under voluntary control, found in the respiratory, circulatory, digestive, urinary, and reproductive systems. Smooth muscles help carry out much of the body's automatic internal work. They are called "smooth" because they lack the striations found in skeletal muscle.

splint A flexible or rigid appliance used to protect and maintain the position of an injured extremity.

sprain A joint injury involving damage to supporting ligaments, and partial or complete temporary dislocation of bone ends.

strain Stretching or tearing of a muscle; also called a muscle pull.

tendon A tough, ropelike cord of fibrous tissue that attaches a skeletal muscle to a bone.

traction The act of exerting a pulling force on a structure.

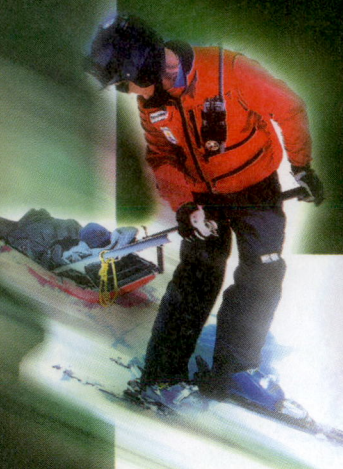

Assessment in Action

You are dispatched to a double black-diamond slope. A skier has jumped from a cornice and landed on rocks below. On arrival you find a 25-year-old man lying on his left side. He is alert and oriented to time, person, and place, but complaining of severe pain in his left thigh, hip, and upper arm. His skin is warm and moist. Vital signs include a pulse of 120 beats/min and full, and respirations of 22 breaths/min and deep. An obvious bone end, from his midthigh, protrudes through the ski pants on his left leg.

1. What is the most accurate description of the mechanism of injury?
   A. Direct force only
   B. Twisting and direct force
   C. Twisting force only
   D. High-energy force

2. Which type of splint is the best choice for the patient's upper left leg fracture?
   A. Ladder
   B. Pillow
   C. Traction
   D. Cardboard

3. Appropriate assessment of this patient's fractured limb includes:
   A. a complete set of vital signs.
   B. assessing pulses, motor, and sensory function.
   C. determining the zone of injury.
   D. palpation of the chest or abdomen.

4. When you are assessing an extremity, it is best to:
   A. compare your findings to your own extremities.
   B. compare the findings to the patient's other extremity.
   C. compare the lower extremities to the upper extremities.
   D. assess each extremity separately and on its own.

5. When you assess your patient's distal pulse, you note that it is noticeably weaker than his pulse in his other foot. Appropriate action would be to:
   A. try gentle longitudinal traction.
   B. use the ladder splint instead.
   C. apply a groin-to-ankle quick splint.
   D. secure the extremity to a backboard.

6. Appropriate care of the open wound on his left thigh would be to:
   A. leave it alone.
   B. cover it with a moist dressing.
   C. cover it with an occlusive dressing.
   D. cover it with a dry, sterile dressing.

7. His injured left arm is unstable, with crepitus and swelling in the mid-portion. How would you manage this injury?
   A. Apply a traction splint to the humerus.
   B. Apply a sling and swathe.
   C. Have him straighten his arm for a ladder splint.
   D. Immobilize the left upper extremity with a long-arm ladder splint and a sling and swathe.

Challenging Questions

8. Of all his injuries, which presents the greatest potential for a threat to his life?

9. You must always check CMS before and after splinting a fractured extremity. Why?

10. It is very important that you handle patients with fractures very gently. Besides not wanting to cause more pain, why is this so important?

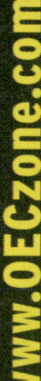

Assessment and Care of Bone and Joint Injuries

Objectives

Cognitive

🌲 **1.** List the assessment and emergency care for injuries of the upper extremities (p 614).

🌲 **2.** List the assessment and emergency care for injuries of the lower extremities (p 624).

Affective

🌲 **3.** Explain the rationale for stabilization of specific injuries to the upper extremities (p 616).

🌲 **4.** Explain the rationale for stabilization of specific injuries to the lower extremities (p 625).

Psychomotor

🌲 **5.** Demonstrate the assessment and emergency care for injuries of the clavicle and scapula (p 615).

🌲 **6.** Demonstrate the assessment and emergency care for injuries of the shoulder (p 616).

🌲 **7.** Demonstrate the assessment and emergency care for musculoskeletal injuries of the humerus (p 617).

🌲 **8.** Demonstrate the assessment and emergency care for musculoskeletal injuries of the elbow (p 619).

🌲 **9.** Demonstrate the assessment and emergency care for musculoskeletal injuries of the forearm and wrist (p 621).

🌲 **10.** Demonstrate the assessment and emergency care for musculoskeletal injuries of the wrist joint and hand (p 621).

🌲 **11.** Demonstrate the assessment and emergency care for musculoskeletal injuries of the pelvis (p 624).

🌲 **12.** Demonstrate the assessment and emergency care for musculoskeletal injuries of the hip (p 625).

🌲 **13.** Demonstrate the assessment and emergency care for musculoskeletal injuries of the femur (p 626).

🌲 **14.** Demonstrate the assessment and emergency care for musculoskeletal injuries of the knee (p 629).

🌲 **15.** Demonstrate the assessment and emergency care for musculoskeletal injuries of the tibia and fibula (p 634).

🌲 **16.** Demonstrate the assessment and emergency care for musculoskeletal injuries of the ankle (p 637).

🌲 **17.** Demonstrate the assessment and emergency care for musculoskeletal injuries of the foot (p 640).

🌲 These are core concepts in initial patrol training.

Points to Ponder

You respond to your resort cafeteria to find a snowboarder with a dislocated shoulder. She is complaining of pain and asks you to "pop it back in." The patient explains that the shoulder has dislocated a couple times before, but she has always been able to "get it back into joint." She has good circulation and neurologic function in the arm. The boarder explains how to pull gently and rotate the arm to get it to pop back in. The patient refuses to go to the hospital. Would you assist the patient in reducing the dislocated shoulder? Should the patient be seen by a care provider? Why or why not?

Issues Scene Management, Risk Management, Equipment and Transport Decisions, Interface with EMS

Online Outlook

Because musculoskeletal injuries occur so often, you must be able to evaluate them properly. Injury to the bones and joints is often associated with injury to the surrounding soft tissue. To improve your knowledge of injuries to the skeletal system, complete Exercise 24 at www.OECzone.com.

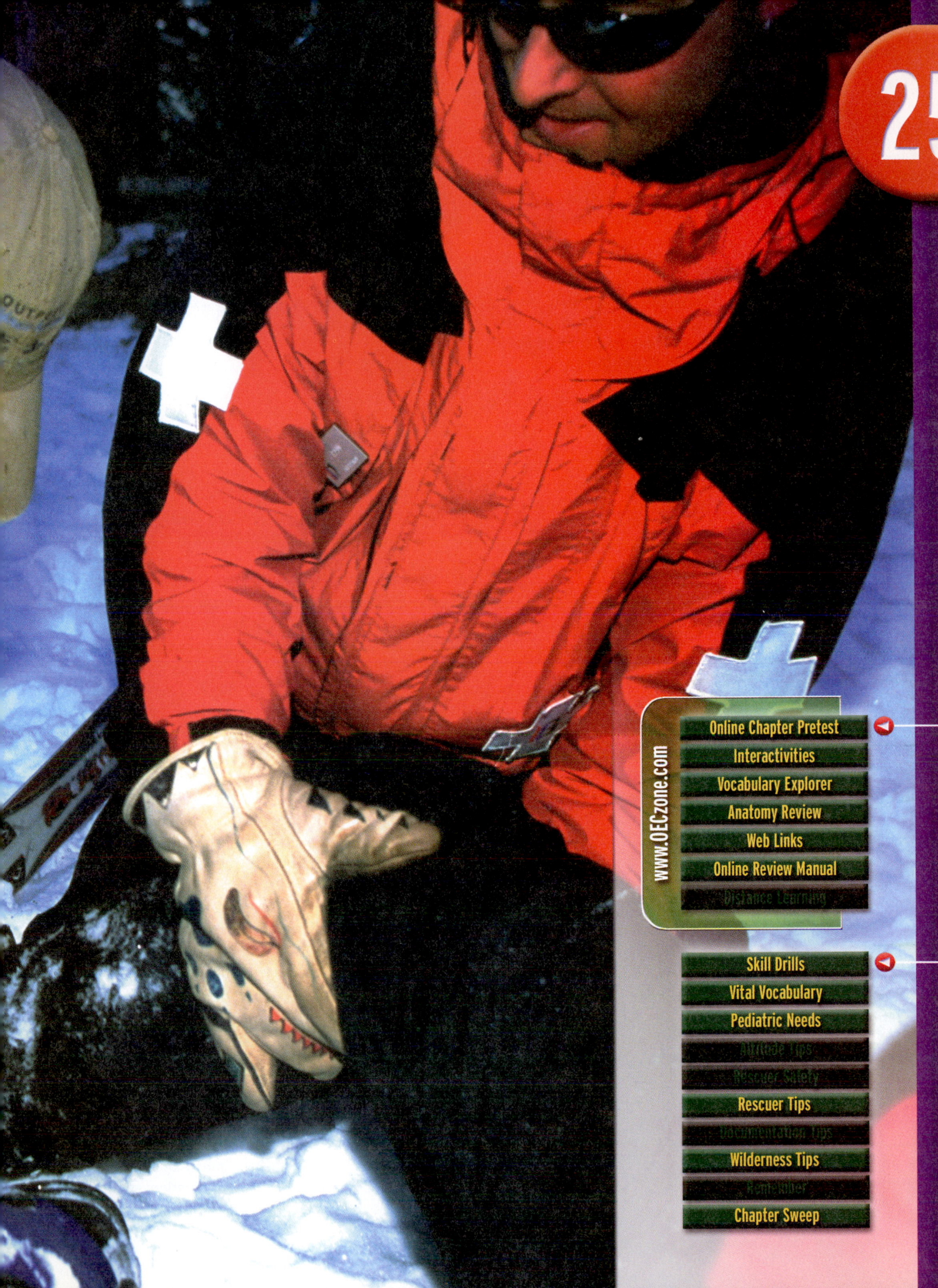

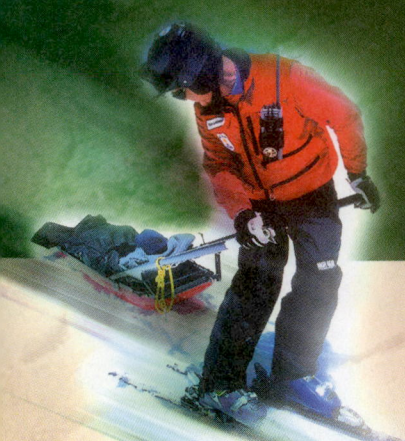

A call comes over the radio that a snowboarder is down in the terrain park and appears to have an injured wrist. You grab a toboggan and respond to the scene quickly.

With the appearance of terrain parks at most snowsports areas across the country, a new emphasis has been placed on extremity injuries. This chapter will present the fundamental of assessment and care relative to musculoskeletal injuries, in addition to helping you answer the following questions.

1. What is the difference on the hill between caring for a suspected fracture and a dislocation?

2. Why is an open fracture more complicated to care for than a closed fracture?

Assessment and Care of Bone and Joint Injuries

This chapter describes the care of specific sprains, fractures, and dislocations of the upper and lower extremities. The general care of soft-tissue injuries is discussed in Chapter 19, and the general principles of bone and joint injury care are discussed in Chapter 24. Before reading this chapter, review Chapters 19 and 24 and be familiar with the appropriate sections on anatomy, physiology, and surface anatomy.

Specific Injuries to the Upper Extremities

In the outdoors, upper extremity injuries usually result from a fall onto an outstretched hand or shoulder, although skiers and snowboarders can also sustain these injuries during collisions with each other or fixed objects such as trees. Fractures, dislocations, and soft-tissue injuries such as lacerations, contusions, and sprains occur frequently. The extent and type of injury depends on the age of the patient, the characteristics of any equipment used, the type, direction, and magnitude of the forces involved, the position of the upper extremity at the time of impact, and the characteristics of the ground, snow, or other surface. A fall onto an outstretched hand can sprain the shoulder, elbow, wrist, or hand; dislocate the shoulder, elbow, wrist, or fingers; or fracture the clavicle, humerus, or bones of the forearm or hand.

When the arm is adducted, ie, drawn toward the body, the head of the humerus moves upward against the arch formed by the distal end of the clavicle and the acromion of the scapula. A person who falls with an arm in this position is more likely to sprain the shoulder joint or the acromioclavicular joint, or fracture the upper humerus, than to injure other parts of the shoulder girdle.

If a person falls with the arm partially abducted, ie, held away from the body, force is transmitted directly to the clavicle, which is likely to be fractured. If the arm is fully abducted and externally rotated (a common position when holding a ski pole or ice ax), the force of the fall is transmitted to the joint capsule. In young people with strong bones, this frequently produces an anterior dislocation of the shoulder. In skeletally immature children and elderly people, whose bones are more fragile than the tendons and ligaments of the shoulder capsule, a fracture of the upper end of the humerus is more common than a shoulder dislocation. An anterior shoulder dislocation may also result from other maneuvers involving abduction and external rotation, such as a high brace in kayaking when the person thrusts his or her arms over the shoulders to regain balance and the paddle catches on the water or an obstacle.

In many types of upper extremity injuries, pain increased by movement causes the patient to self-splint the injured extremity in a characteristic manner. The patient internally rotates the upper arm, flexes the elbow, and holds the extremity against or near the chest wall while supporting the forearm with the opposite hand ▶ Figure 25-1 .

When assessing any injury of the extremities in a conscious patient, if physically possible, always ask the patient to "point with one finger to the area that hurts the most." Only the patient can know the point of maximal tenderness!

When providing emergency care to a patient with an

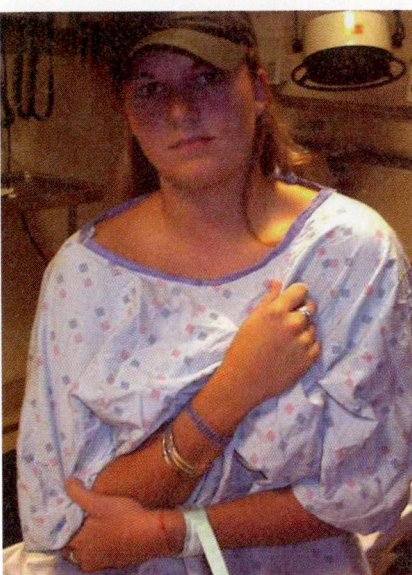

Figure 25-1 Self-splinting an upper extremity injury.

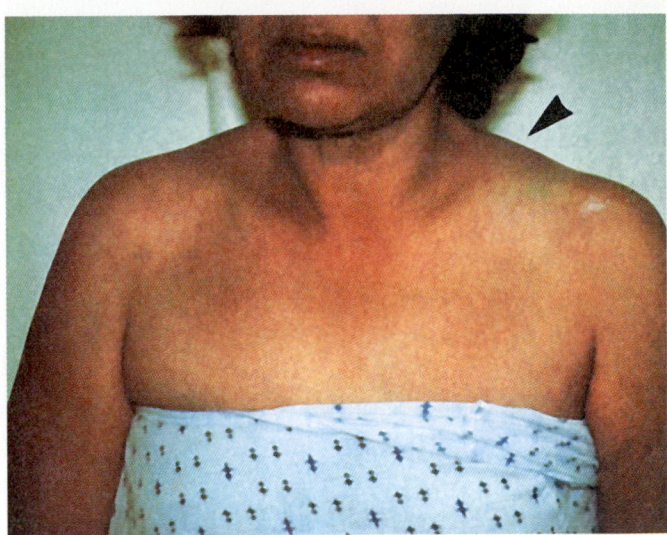

Figure 25-2 A clavicle injury is characterized by swelling, point tenderness, and "tenting" over the fracture fragment.

injured upper extremity, be sure to remove rings, bracelets, and any other jewelry before swelling occurs and before you splint the extremity.

Injuries of the Clavicle and Scapula

The **clavicle**, or collarbone, is one of the most commonly fractured bones in the body. Fractures of the clavicle occur most often in snowsliders when they fall on an outstretched hand. They can also occur with crushing injuries of the chest. A patient with a fracture of the clavicle will report pain in the shoulder and will usually attempt to self-splint the injury. A young child often reports pain throughout the entire arm and is unwilling to use any part of that limb. These complaints may make it difficult to localize the point of injury, but, generally, swelling and point tenderness to palpation will occur over the clavicle injury site. Also, the injured shoulder is usually held lower than the uninjured shoulder. Because the clavicle is subcutaneous (just beneath the skin), the skin will occasionally "tent" over the fracture fragment ▲ Figure 25-2 . The clavicle lies directly over major arteries, veins, and nerves; therefore, fracture of the clavicle may lead to neurovascular compromise.

Fractures of the **scapula**, or shoulder blade, occur much less frequently because this bone is well protected by many large muscles. Fractures of the scapula are almost always the result of a forceful, direct blow to the back, directly over the scapula, which may also injure the adjacent spine and underlying thoracic cage, lungs, and heart. For this reason, you must carefully

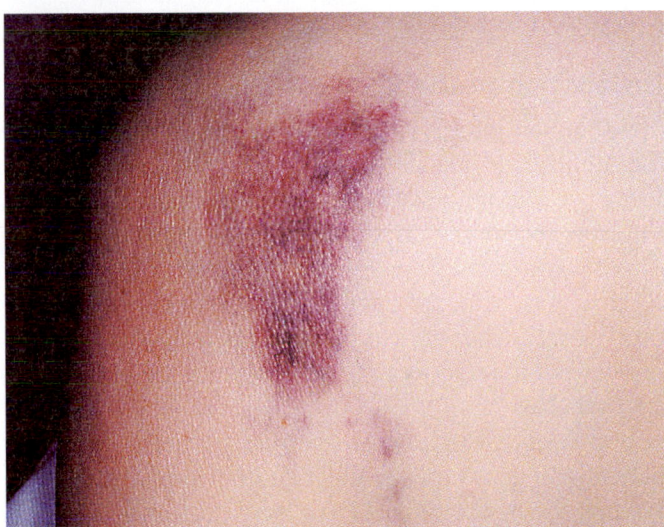

Figure 25-3 Contusions or abrasions over the scapular area may indicate a fracture.

assess the patient for signs of spinal injury or breathing problems. Provide supplemental oxygen and prompt transport for patients who are having difficulty breathing. Remember, it is the associated chest or spinal injuries, not the fractured scapula, that pose the greatest threat of long-term disability.

Abrasions, contusions, and significant swelling may also occur posteriorly over a scapula fracture, and the patient will often limit use of the arm because of pain at the fracture site ▲ Figure 25-3 . The scapula also has bony projections that may be fractured with a lesser degree of force.

The joint between the outer end of the clavicle and the acromion process of the scapula is called the acromioclavicular (A/C) joint. This joint is frequently sprained in snowsports when the skier experiences a forward (outside edge) fall and lands on the point of the shoulder, driving the acromion downward from the outer end of the clavicle. The common term applied to this "true dislocation" is a separated shoulder. If the injury force is significant, a "third-degree injury" occurs, and the distal end of the clavicle will protrude upward. When compared to the opposite shoulder, the injured shoulder cap will have an obvious shelf-like deformity. This deformity is often confused with a severely displaced clavicle fracture. However, the patient will exhibit point tenderness over the A/C joint (▶ Figure 25-4).

Fractures of the clavicle and scapula and A/C separations can all be splinted effectively with a sling and swathe, the application of which is described in Chapter 24.

Dislocation of the Shoulder

The shoulder joint is where the head of the humerus, the supporting bone of the upper arm, meets the glenoid fossa of the scapula forming the glenohumeral joint. It is the most commonly dislocated large joint in the body. Almost always, the humeral head will dislocate anteriorly, coming to lie in front of and inferior to the coracoid process of the scapula as a result of forced abduction (away from the midline) and external rotation of the arm (▶ Figure 25-5).

Shoulder dislocations are extremely painful. The patient will guard the shoulder and try to protect it by holding the dislocated arm in a fixed position away from the chest wall (abducted), with the forearm externally rotated (▶ Figure 25-6). The shoulder joint will usually be locked, and the cap will appear squared off and flattened. The humeral head will protrude anteriorly or inferiorly underneath the pectoralis major muscle on the anterior chest wall.

Because of the humeral head position just described, the injured patient is physically unable to bring his or her hand across the abdomen or chest. Skiers or riders who have clavicle, scapula, and proximal humerus fractures or A/C joint sprains almost always support their injured forearm in front of them. Therefore, on the hill, to differentiate one of the latter injuries from an anteriorly dislocated shoulder, ask (and gently assist) the patient to touch the opposite shoulder cap with their injury-side fingertip. If the patient is able to do this, the shoulder is not dislocated.

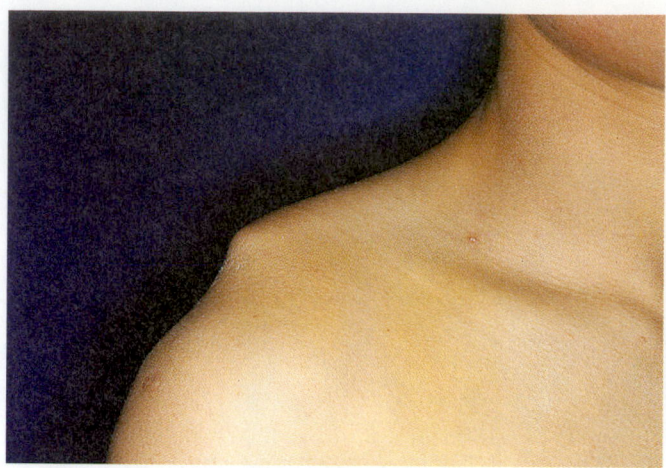

Figure 25-4   With A/C separations, the distal end of the clavicle usually sticks out.

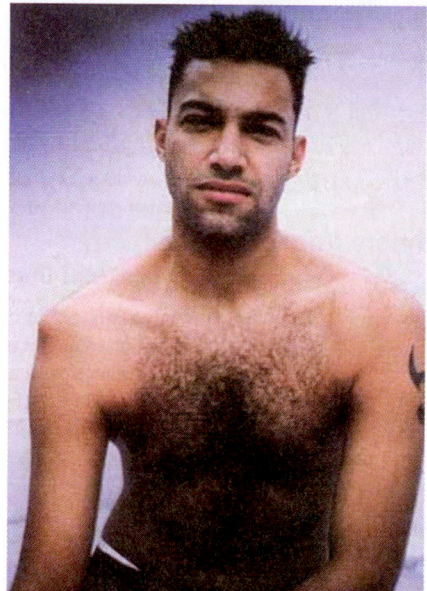

Figure 25-5   The shoulder almost always dislocates anteriorly. Note the absence of the normal rounded appearance of the patient's right shoulder.

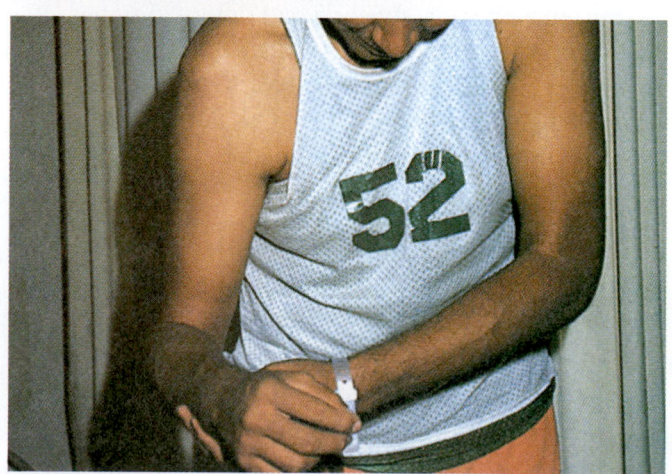

Figure 25-6   A patient with a dislocated shoulder will guard the shoulder, trying to protect it by holding the arm in a fixed position away from the chest wall.

Some patients with dislocated shoulders occasionally report numbness in the hand or skin over the deltoid muscle because of nerve or circulation compromise.

Immobilizing an anterior shoulder dislocation is difficult, because any attempt to bring the arm in toward the chest will produce pain. You must splint the joint in whatever position is most comfortable for the patient. On the hill, it is best to use the blanket roll splint (see Chapter 24). Once the arm is stabilized with a blanket roll splint, the elbow can usually be flexed to 90° without causing further pain. At this point, you can apply a sling and swathe to the forearm and hand to support the weight of the arm (▶ **Figure 25-7**), apply a blanket roll, or have the patient stabilize the forearm. Transport the patient in a sitting or semiseated position in the toboggan, with another rescuer seated behind the patient to help stabilize the injured arm.

Dislocation of the shoulder disrupts the supporting ligaments of the anterior aspect of the shoulder. Often, these ligaments are attenuated by the injury and fail to heal properly, so dislocation recurs, each time causing further neurovascular compromise and joint capsule injury. In most cases, when the shoulder dislocates more than twice, surgical repair is required to prevent further dislocations. Some patients are able to reduce their own dislocated shoulders. Generally, however, this maneuver must be done in a hospital setting and only after X-rays have been obtained. Sometimes, wilderness protocols allow for dislocated shoulder reduction in the field.

A shoulder will dislocate posteriorly instead of anteriorly about once in every 20 occurrences. Football players, especially linemen, and skiers or riders landing on outstretched arms are susceptible to this type of injury. The arm will often be locked in adduction (toward the midline), so it cannot be rotated externally.

Fracture of the Humerus

Fractures of the humerus occur either proximally, in the midshaft, or distally at the elbow (▶ **Table 25-1**). Fractures of the proximal humerus (anatomic or surgical neck) resulting from falls are common in children through the weak proximal growth plate (epiphysis), and among the elderly (▶ **Figure 25-8**). Fractures of the midshaft humerus occur more often in young patients, usually as the result of a violent direct blow (▶ **Figure 25-9**).

Fractures of the distal humerus are discussed with fractures about the elbow. For complete midshaft fractures or any severely angulated humeral fracture, you

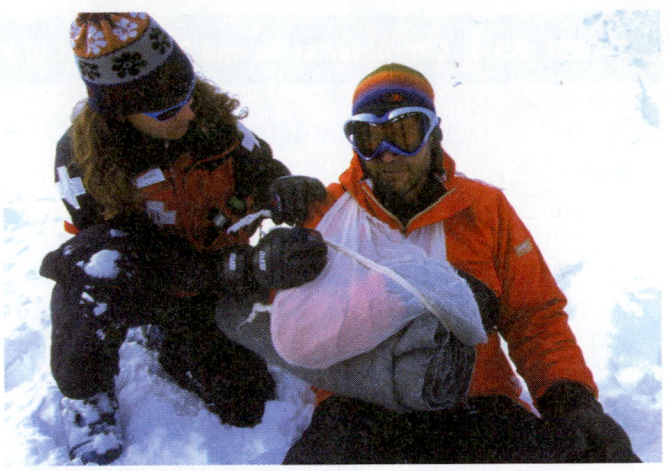

Figure 25-7   Blanket roll splint in place with an additional sling and swathe to support the forearm.

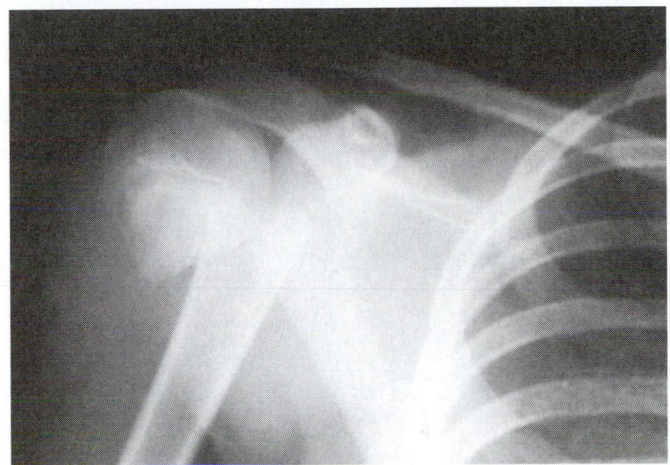

Figure 25-8   Displaced fracture of the proximal humerus.

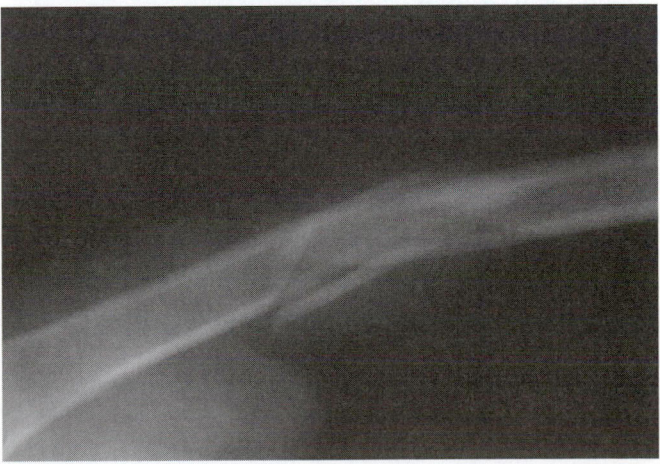

Figure 25-9   X-ray of a closed, midshaft fracture of the humerus.

TABLE 25-1 Characteristics and Treatment of Fractures of the Humerus

Type	Characteristics	Treatment
Proximal Humeral Fractures	• Significant swelling, but no major deformity, of the upper arm • Occasional neurovascular compromise • Any or all of the brachial plexus affected, depending on the degree of displacement • Concurrent soft-tissue injuries • Possible rotator cuff injury (if X-rays show no fracture, a tear of the rotator cuff is possible, especially if the patient cannot move the arm toward the medial plane)	• Immobilize in a sling and swathe or a shoulder immobilizer. • Use the chest wall as a splint, and secure the injured arm to the chest wall. • Place a short, padded board splint on the lateral side of the arm under the sling and swathe for additional support.
Midshaft Fractures	• Gross angulation of the arm • Marked instability and crepitus of fracture fragments • Possible neurovascular compromise • Possible entrapment of the radial nerve (The patient cannot extend or dorsiflex the wrist or fingers and may report numbness on the dorsum of the thumb; classic "wrist drop")	• If the CMS functions in the hand are normal, apply a padded long-arm wire ladder splint and a sling and swathe. • If the CMS functions are abnormal, see the paragraph below.
Distal Humeral Fractures	• Significant swelling at the elbow • Probable neurovascular compromise • Possible injury to the ulnar or median nerves (document nerve status before and after any attempt to immobilize the fracture)	• Immobilize in a padded long-arm wire ladder splint, SAM splint, or similar device, bent to conform to the angle of the elbow; supplement with a sling and swathe. • If CMS is abnormal, follow midshaft fracture information above.

should consider applying gentle longitudinal traction to realign the fracture fragments before splinting them. Check your local area protocol before proceeding with the alignment technique that is described next. Support the site of the fracture posteriorly with one hand, and with the other hand, grasp the two humeral condyles (the lateral and medial protrusions) just above the elbow. Pull gently in line with the normal axis of the limb ▶ **Figure 25-10** . Once you achieve gross realignment and restore length to the limb, have another patroller splint the arm with a padded long-arm wire ladder splint and a sling and swathe ▶ **Figure 25-11** or padded board splints on the medial and lateral aspects of the arm, again with a sling and swathe. If the patient reports a significant increase in pain or resists the gentle traction and realignment attempt, splint the fracture in the deformed position found with either a padded wire ladder or padded board splint.

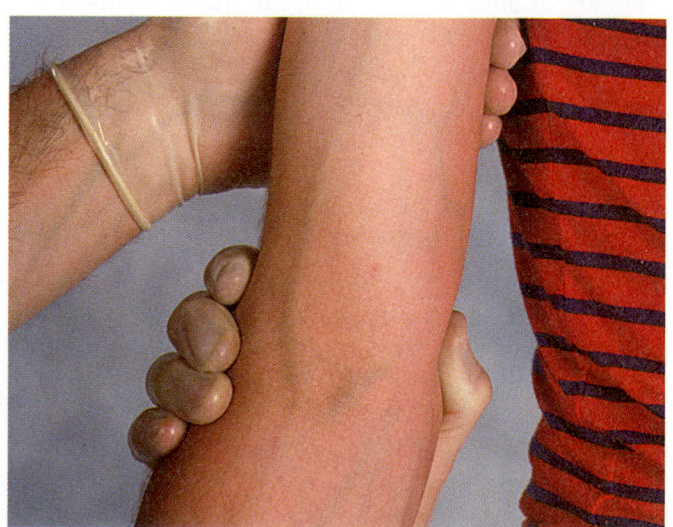

Figure 25-10 To align a severe deformity associated with a humeral shaft fracture, apply gentle axial tension to the humeral condyles, as shown in this uninjured arm.

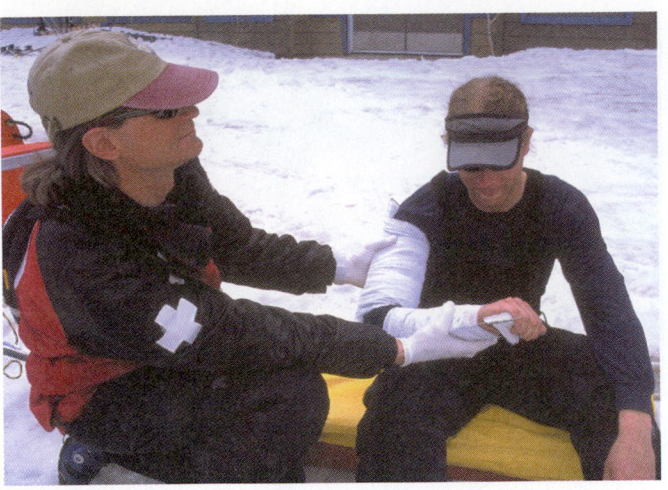
Figure 25-11 Splint a humeral shaft fracture with a padded moldable splint supplemented by a sling and swathe.

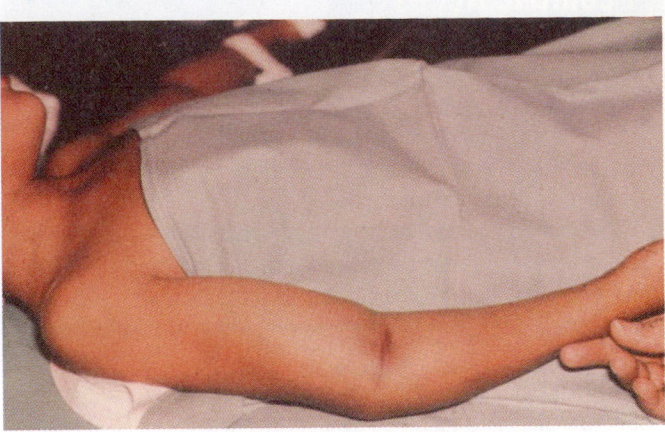
Figure 25-12 Supracondylar fracture of the humerus in a child.

Elbow Injuries

Fractures and dislocations often occur around the elbow, and the different types of injuries are difficult to distinguish without X-rays. However, they all produce similar limb deformities and require the same emergency care. Injuries to nerves and blood vessels that cross the elbow are quite common in this region. Such injuries can be caused or worsened by inappropriate emergency care, particularly by excessive manipulation of the injured joint.

SUPRACONDYLAR FRACTURE OF THE HUMERUS. Fractures just above the elbow are common in children ▶ Figure 25-12 .

These fractures are frequently complicated by nerve and blood vessel injury from the jagged bone fragments at the fracture site ▶ Figure 25-13 . Assessment usually reveals marked swelling and deformity of the elbow area, with tenderness, pain, and ecchymosis. The point of the elbow is often displaced backward. Assessment of the circulation, motor, and sensory (CMS) functions in the hand is crucial.

Emergency care consists of splinting the injury in the position found. A good method is to bend a moldable splint (eg, SAM or ladder) to conform to the angle of the elbow, and place it on the back and underside of the extremity. The splint is held in place with a self-adhering roller bandage or cravats, with the extremity supported by a sling and swathe ▶ Figure 25-14 .

DISLOCATION OF THE ELBOW. This type of injury typically occurs occasionally in adults, but is not seen in young children. A fall on the outstretched hand with the elbow partially flexed produces the injury. The ulna and radius are usually displaced posteriorly. The ulna,

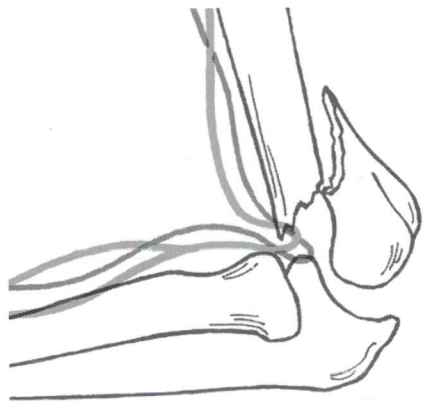
Figure 25-13 Nerves and vessels are occasionally impaled in the fracture site.

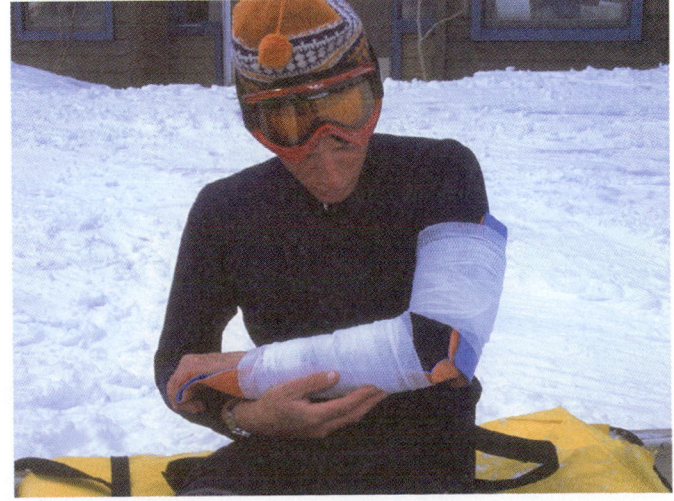
Figure 25-14 Apply a SAM splint to stabilize an elbow fracture in the position found.

Pediatric Needs

Growth plate injuries in children are common, especially around the wrist, elbow, knee, and ankle. Injuries tend to occur through these cartilaginous growth centers because they are inherently weaker than the surrounding bone. Since longitudinal growth of the limb is dependent upon the function of the growth plate, it is extremely important to recognize the possibility of growth plate injuries, stabilize the injured limb, and transport the patient in timely fashion to an appropriate center with pediatric orthopaedic and surgical coverage. Proper functioning of the injured growth plate throughout the remainder of skeletal growth is dependent upon urgent anatomic reduction of the fracture and close follow-up by an orthopaedist.

Any deformity in close proximity to a joint in children younger than 16 years should be assumed to be a growth plate injury and transported and treated appropriately.

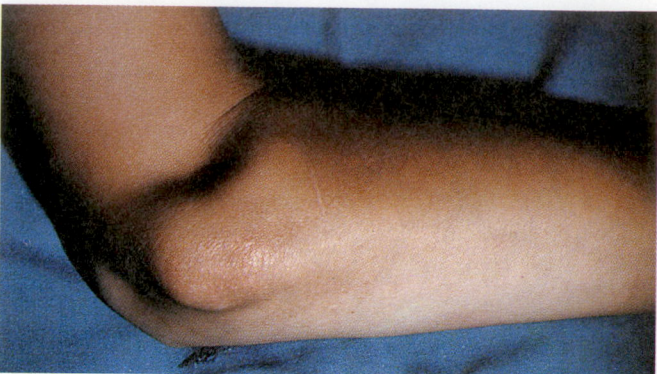

Figure 25-15 Posterior dislocation of the elbow makes the olecranon process of the ulna much more prominent.

the bone on the small finger side of the forearm, and the **radius**, the bone on the thumb side of the forearm, both join the distal humerus. The posterior displacement makes the olecranon process of the ulna much more prominent (▶ **Figure 25-15**). The joint is usually locked, with the elbow in partial flexion; this position makes any attempt at motion extremely painful. As with a fracture of the distal humerus, there is swelling and significant potential for vessel or nerve injury.

ELBOW JOINT SPRAIN. This injury is rare and is usually diagnosed by X-ray. Often, the real problem is a hard-to-detect fracture.

FRACTURE OF THE OLECRANON PROCESS OF THE ULNA. This fracture is usually the result of a direct blow, such as a fall onto the point of the elbow, and therefore is often accompanied by overlying lacerations or abrasions. The patient will be unable to extend the elbow. Almost always, the fracture requires surgical internal fixation for treatment (▶ **Figure 25-16**).

FRACTURE OF THE RADIAL HEAD. Occasionally missed even in the emergency department, this fracture generally occurs as a result of a fall on an outstretched arm or a direct blow to the lateral aspect of the forearm. Attempts to rotate the forearm or wrist are very uncomfortable. Again, surgery is usually required if the fracture is displaced (▶ **Figure 25-17**).

Care of Elbow Injuries

All elbow injuries are serious and require careful management. Always assess distal neurovascular functions periodically in patients with elbow injuries. If you find

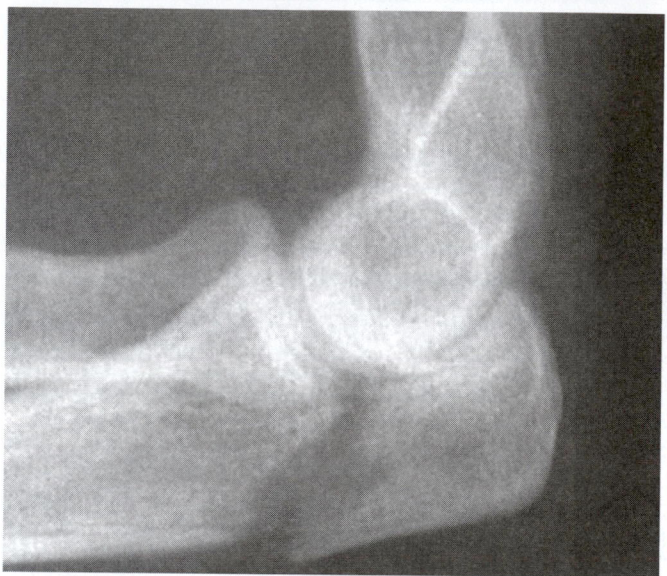

Figure 25-16 X-ray of a displaced olecranon fracture.

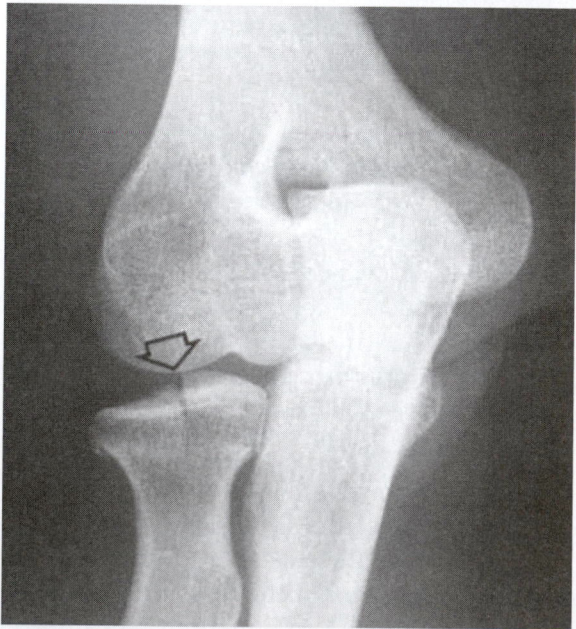

Figure 25-17 Displaced radial head fracture.

strong distal pulses and normal sensation in the hand, then splint the elbow injury in the position in which you found it. A padded long-arm wire ladder splint or SAM splint bent to conform to the angle of the elbow, or two padded board splints, applied to each side of the limb and secured with soft roller bandages or cravats, usually are enough to stabilize the arm. Make sure the board splints extend from the midupper arm to the midforearm, immobilizing the entire bone above and below the injured joint. Supplement both types of splints with a sling and swathe.

A cold, pale hand or a weak or absent distal pulse indicates that the blood vessels have likely been injured at the fracture site. Further care of this patient must be dictated by a physician. Notify the aid room immediately. If you are within 60 minutes of the hospital, splint the limb in the position in which you found it and ask your rescue squad to provide prompt transport.

If the limb is pulseless and significantly deformed at the elbow and total transport time from the ski hill to the hospital will take more than 60 minutes, apply gentle manual traction in line with the long axis of the limb to decrease the deformity. This maneuver may restore the pulse. Be careful, as excessive manipulation will only worsen the vascular problem. If no pulse returns after one attempt, splint the limb in the most comfortable position for the patient. If the pulse is restored by gentle longitudinal traction, splint the limb in whatever position allows the strongest pulse. Provide prompt transport for all patients with impaired distal circulation, even if circulation is restored.

Fractures of the Forearm and Wrist

Fractures of the shaft of the radius and ulna are common in snowboarders. Both bones may break at the same time when the injury is the result of a fall on an outstretched hand (▶ **Figure 25-18**). An isolated fracture of the shaft of the ulna may occur as the result of a direct blow to it; this is known as a nightstick fracture.

Fractures of the distal radius are the most common upper extremity injury in snowboarders and are known as Colles fractures. The term "silver fork deformity" is used to describe the distinctive appearance of the patient's wrist (▼ **Figure 25-19**). In children, this fracture often occurs through the distal radial growth plate (epiphysis) and can have long-term consequences if the growth plate is damaged.

To immobilize fractures of the forearm use a padded long-arm wire ladder or moldable splint, supplemented by a sling and swathe. Splinting of the elbow joint is not essential with fractures near the wrist. A padded forearm splint can be used, placing the hand in the position of function, ie, with the fingers cupped over a gauze roll held in the palm, as if holding a ball. The patient will be more comfortable if you add a sling and swathe.

Injuries of the Wrist Joint and Hand

Injuries to the wrist joint, including both fractures and dislocations, are especially common in snowboarders. True sprains of the wrist are uncommon. Dislocations are usually associated with a fracture, resulting in a fracture-dislocation. The second most common wrist

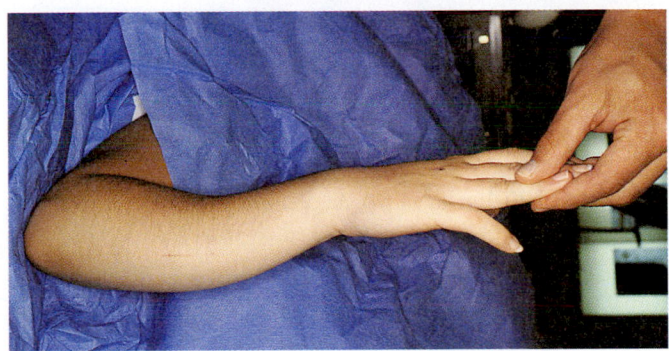

Figure 25-18   Fractures of the mid-forearm often occur in snowboarders as a result of a fall on an outstretched hand.

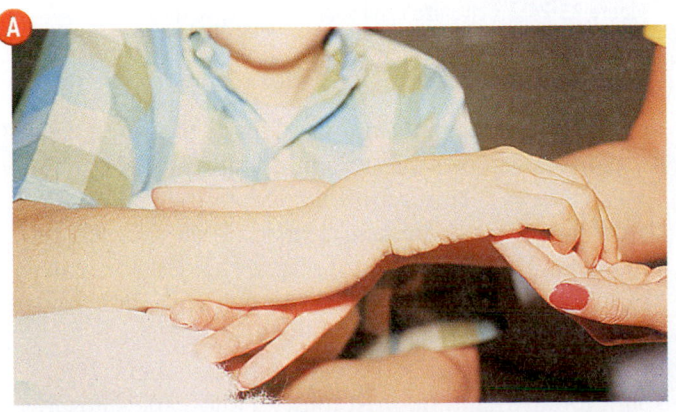
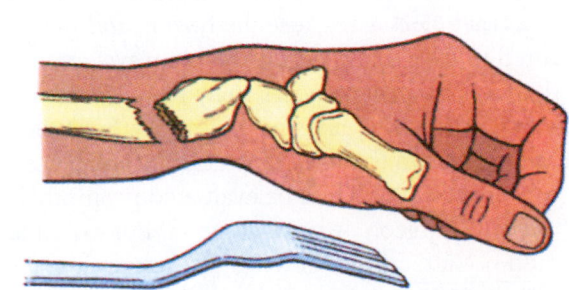

A   B

Figure 25-19   **A.** Fractures of the distal radius produce a characteristic silver fork deformity.   **B.** An artist's illustration of same.

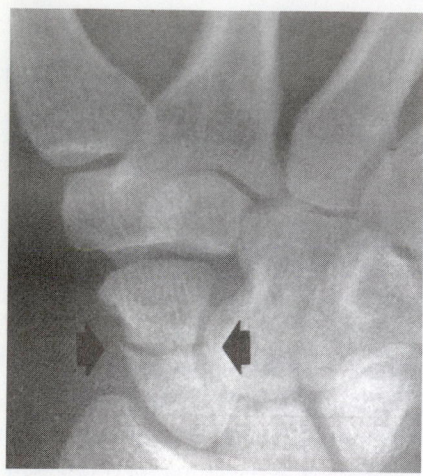

Figure 25-20 Carpal scaphoid fracture.

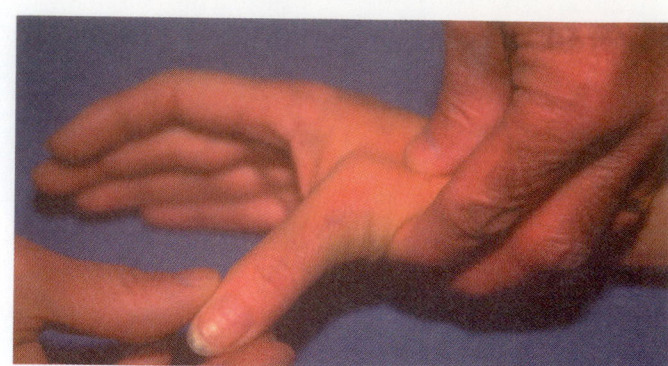

Figure 25-21 Severe ulnar collateral ligament sprain of the right thumb.

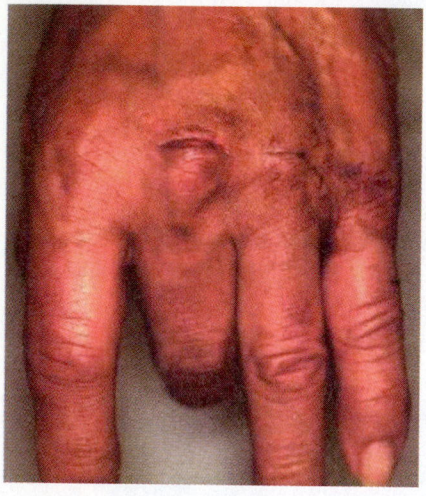

Figure 25-22 Small transverse laceration over the third metacarpal head, with an underlying extensor tendon laceration and resultant "dropped finger."

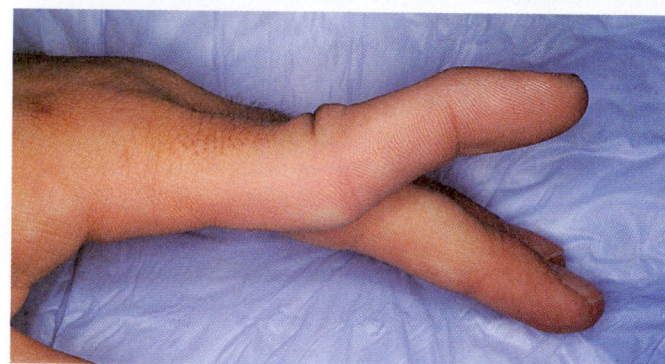

Figure 25-23 Dislocation of an index finger middle joint. Do not be tempted to try to "pop" the joint back into place.

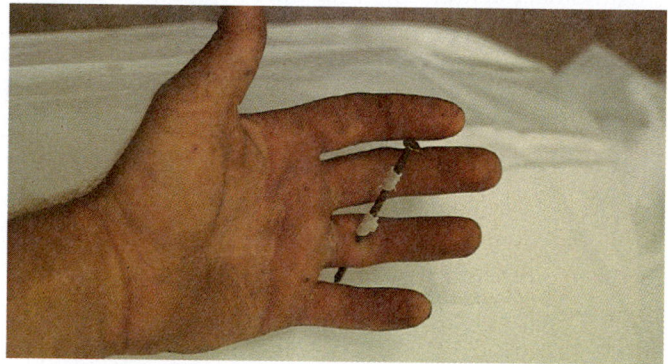

Figure 25-24 Galvanized nail impaled through a finger.

joint fracture is the isolated carpal scaphoid fracture (▲ **Figure 25-20**), and is produced by a fall on the outstretched hand. Any wrist injury should be splinted in a short arm splint and evaluated in the emergency department.

There is a great variety of hand injuries, many with potentially serious consequences. Snowsport accidents often result in sprains, dislocations, fractures, and lacerations of the hand. The most common upper extremity injury in skiing is a sprain of the thumb ulnar collateral ligament, also known as gamekeeper's thumb or skier's thumb (▲ **Figure 25-21**). Because the fingers and hands are required to function in such intricate ways, any injury that is not treated properly may result in permanent disability, as well as a visible deformity. For this reason, all injuries to the hand, including simple lacerations (▲ **Figure 25-22**), should be evaluated promptly by an orthopaedic surgeon or hand surgeon. For example, you should not attempt to reduce a dislocated finger joint (▶ **Figure 25-23**). As with other areas of the body, do not attempt to remove impaled objects in the hand or fingers (▶ **Figure 25-24**). In cases of traumatic amputa-

tions, always bring any amputated parts to the aid room so that they can be sent to the hospital with the patient (▶ **Figure 25-25**). Be sure to wrap the amputated part in a dry or moist sterile dressing depending on your local protocol and place it in a dry plastic bag. Put the sealed bag in a cooled container of water; do not directly soak the part in water or allow it to freeze.

A bulky forearm/hand dressing makes an effective splint for any hand or wrist injury. Follow the steps in (▶ **Skill Drill 25-1**):

SkillDrill 25-1   Splinting the Hand and Wrist

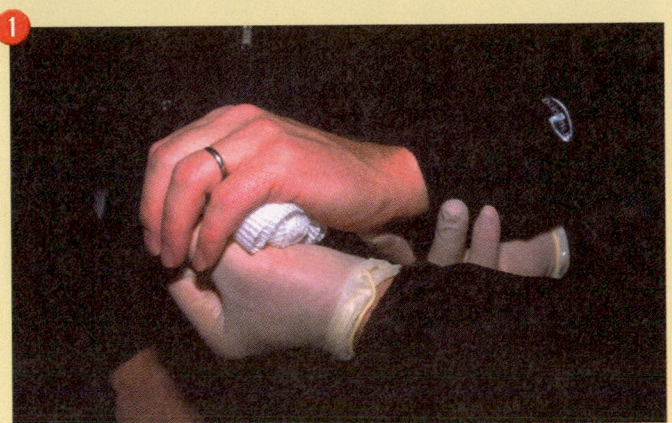

Move the hand into the position of function.
Place a soft roller bandage in the palm.

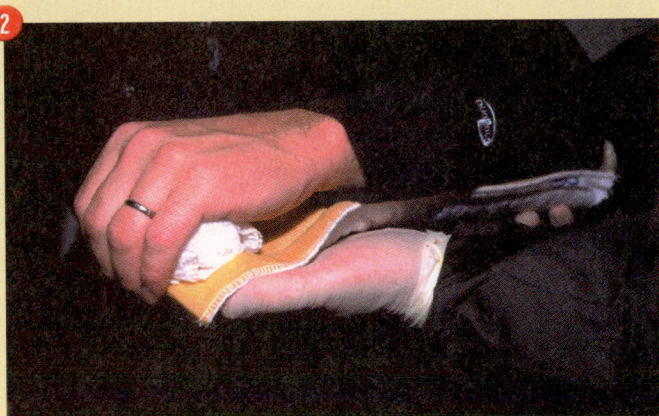

Apply a padded board splint on the palmar side with fingertips exposed.

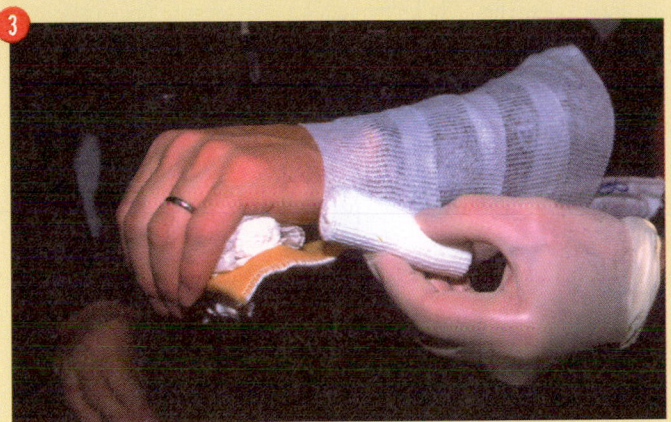

Secure the splint with a roller bandage.

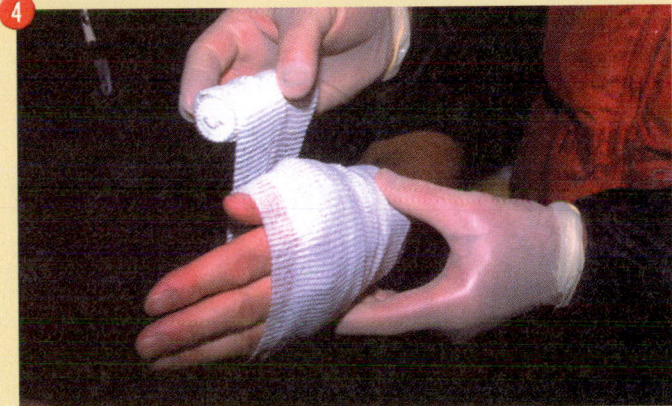

Stabilize a thumb ulnar collateral ligament sprain to the hand with a roller gauze.

1. **Follow BSI precautions.**
2. **Cover all wounds** with a dry, sterile dressing.
3. Supporting the injured limb, **form the injured hand into the** **position of function**, placing a soft roller bandage into the palm of the hand **(Step 1)**. Check CMS function.
4. **Apply a padded board splint to the palmar side of the wrist,** leaving the fingertips exposed **(Step 2)**.
5. **Secure the entire length of the splint** with a soft roller bandage **(Step 3)**.
6. For thumb ulnar collateral ligament spains, **stabilize the injured thumb to the hand with a roller gauze (Step 4)**.
7. **Apply a sling and swathe.** Check CMS function.

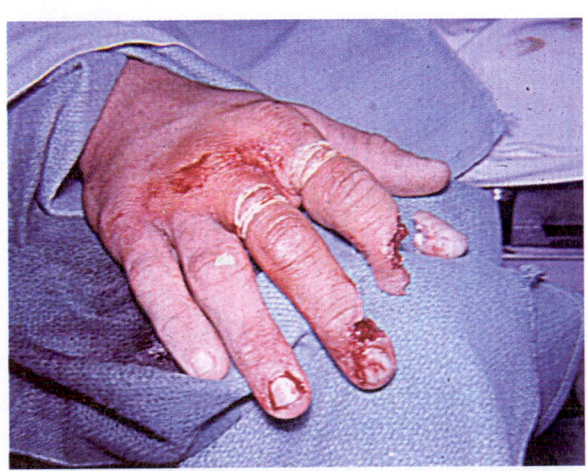

Figure 25-25 Amputated index fingertip transported with the patient was later used as a full-thickness skin graft to the long finger laceration.

Specific Injuries of the Lower Extremity
Fractures of the Pelvis

Fractures of the pelvis most often result from direct compression in the form of a heavy blow that literally cracks or crushes the pelvis. In snowsports, the injury force is usually a moving skier against a tree, or a fall from a height—such as a snowboarder jumping from a cornice onto concealed rocks below. Injuries to the pelvis can also be caused by indirect forces. For example, when the knee strikes the dashboard in a snowmobile crash, the impact of the force is transmitted along the line of the femur, the thigh bone, which is the longest and largest bone in the body. The head of the femur is driven into the pelvis, causing the rim of the hip socket (acetabulum) to fracture. Frequently, posterior dislocation of the hip accompanies this type of pelvis fracture.

Fractures of the pelvis may be accompanied by life-threatening loss of blood produced by the fracture itself and from the laceration of blood vessels affixed to the pelvis at certain key points. Up to several liters of blood may drain into the pelvic space (▶ **Figure 25-26**). The result is significant hypotension, shock, and sometimes death. For this reason, you first must anticipate, then be prepared to take immediate steps to treat shock, even if there is only minimal swelling. Often, there are no visible signs of bleeding until severe blood loss caused by internal bleeding has occurred. You should be prepared to resuscitate the patient rapidly if this becomes necessary.

The bladder, urethra, and rectum lie very close to the anterior ring of the pelvis, as does the uterus and vagina in females (▶ **Figure 25-27**). Because the pelvis is surrounded by heavy muscle, open fractures of the pelvis are quite uncommon. However, pelvis fracture fragments can lacerate the rectum and vagina, creating an open fracture that is often overlooked. Once the protective pelvic ring is broken, the structures it is designed to protect, including the urinary bladder, are open to injury. The bladder may also be lacerated by pelvic bone fragments (▶ **Figure 25-28**), but more often, it tears or ruptures as a result of tension on either the bladder or the urethra. Subsequent complications may include peritonitis (inflammation of the abdominal cavity's membranous wall) and/or sepsis (infection of the abdominal cavity).

You should suspect a fracture of the pelvis in any skier or snowboarder who has sustained a high-velocity injury and complains of discomfort in the lower back, lower abdomen, or pelvic area. On your approach, you will probably find the person either lying supine, with their knees partially flexed, or in the fetal position on the side opposite the injury. Because the pelvis is covered by

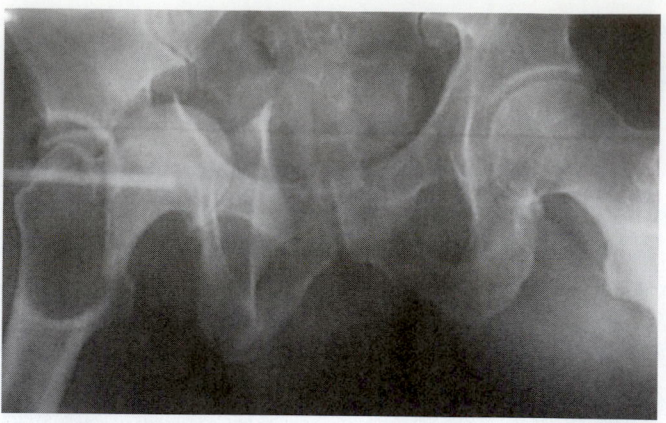
Figure 25-26 Displaced central acetabular fracture of the pelvis that produced severe blood loss.

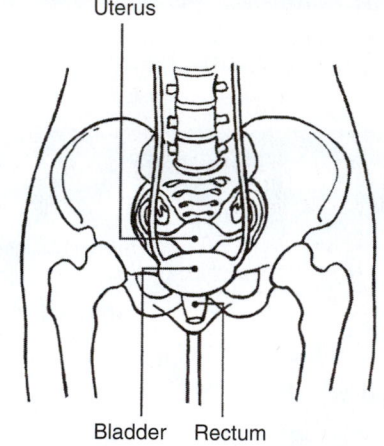
Figure 25-27 Pelvic organs adjacent to the anterior ring of the pelvis.

Uterus

Bladder   Rectum

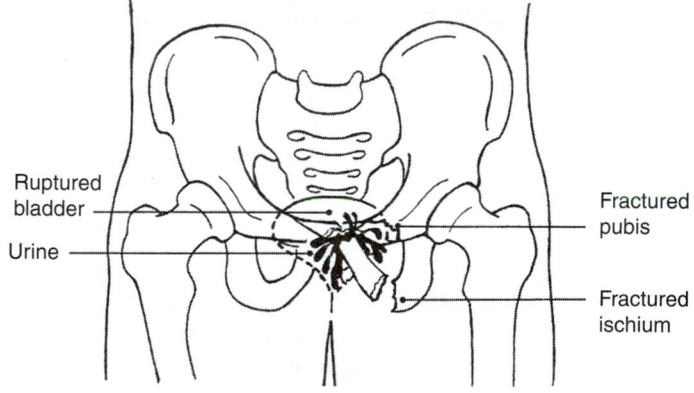
Figure 25-28 Fracture fragments of a pelvic fracture can lacerate the bladder.

Ruptured bladder

Urine

Fractured pubis

Fractured ischium

muscle and soft tissue, deformity or swelling may be very difficult to see. If the pelvis fracture line is located near the center of the anterior pelvic ring, the patient may feel a strong urge to void. Therefore, you should immediately suspect that an injured person who complains of pain in the lower abdomen or pelvis and a

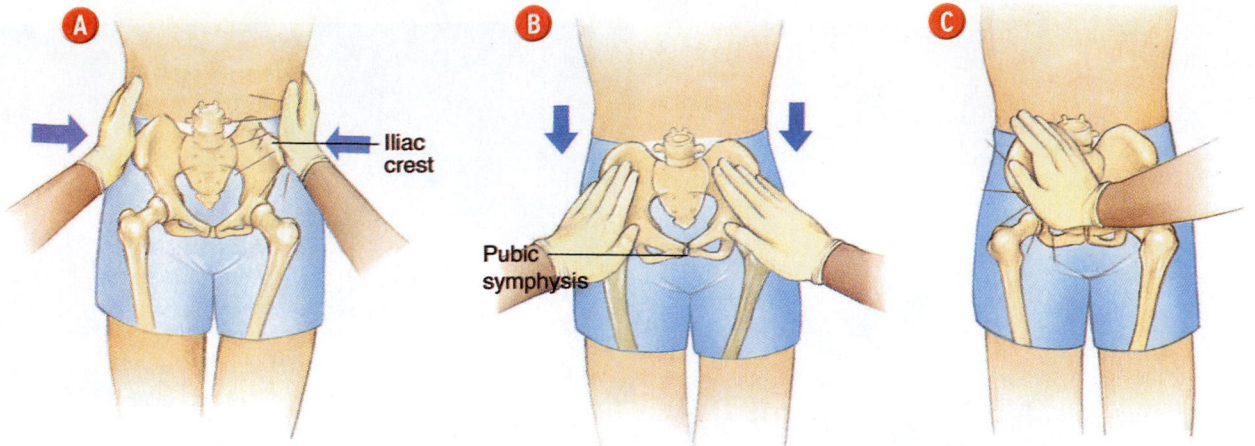

Figure 25-29 **A.** To assess for tenderness in the pelvic region, place your hands over the lateral aspect of each iliac crest, and gently compress the pelvis. **B.** With the patient in a supine position, place your palms over the anterior aspect of each iliac crest, and gently rock the pelvis anteriorly and posteriorly. **C.** Firmly palpate the pubic symphysis with the palm of your hand.

need to urinate may have a fractured pelvis.

The most reliable sign of fracture of the pelvis is simple tenderness on firm compression and palpation. To proceed with assessment (▲ **Figure 25-29**), compress the lateral sides of the pelvis with your open palm. This maneuver will usually produce pain if there is a fracture. If no sign of discomfort is elicited, carefully rock the pelvis back and forth (anteriorly and posteriorly), again with your palm on the lateral pelvis. If the patient still registers no pain, firmly palpate the anterior pubis with your palm. Pain or tenderness caused by any of these maneuvers indicates the possibility of a pelvic fracture. You should therefore avoid further examination of the area, because more manipulation will produce unnecessary discomfort for the patient.

If there has been injury to the bladder or the urethra, the patient will have lower abdominal tenderness and may also have evidence of hematuria (blood in the urine) or blood at the urethral opening.

Perform an initial assessment, and carefully monitor the general condition of any patient who you suspect has a pelvic fracture, because he or she is at high risk for hypovolemic shock. Administer high-flow oxygen by facemask. Transfer the patient to a backboard, using a bridge lift in either the supine or side-lying position, keeping the knees partially flexed. Do not give the patient anything to eat or drink. Treat the patient for shock. Anticipate vomiting and have suction available. Rapidly transport the patient to the aid room, and on to a medical facility, especially if there is evidence of hypovolemic shock.

Dislocation of the Hip

The hip joint is a very stable ball-and-socket joint that dislocates only after significant injury. Almost all dislo-

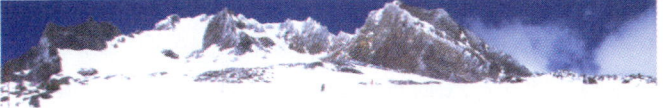

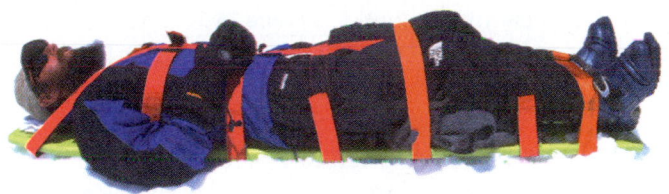

Figure 25-30 Transport a patient with a fractured pelvis on a backboard with the knees partially flexed.

cations of the hip are posterior. The femoral head is displaced posteriorly to lie in the muscles of the buttock. The injury is rare in snowsports because the mechanism of injury—a sudden, severe inward twisting force on the thigh while the hip is partially flexed—does not usually occur. This is not to say, however, that the injury never occurs. Posterior hip dislocation, which is frequently associated with a "rim fracture" of the hip socket as mentioned earlier, can occur among skiers in deep snow when the ski is suddenly caught by a hidden object, such as a tree limb or rock, or the ski releases prematurely while the skier is initiating a turn. In either of these cases, the internal rotational force must be great. Posterior dislocation of the hip more commonly occurs during a motor vehicle crash in which the knee meets with a direct force, such as the dashboard, and the entire femur is driven poste-

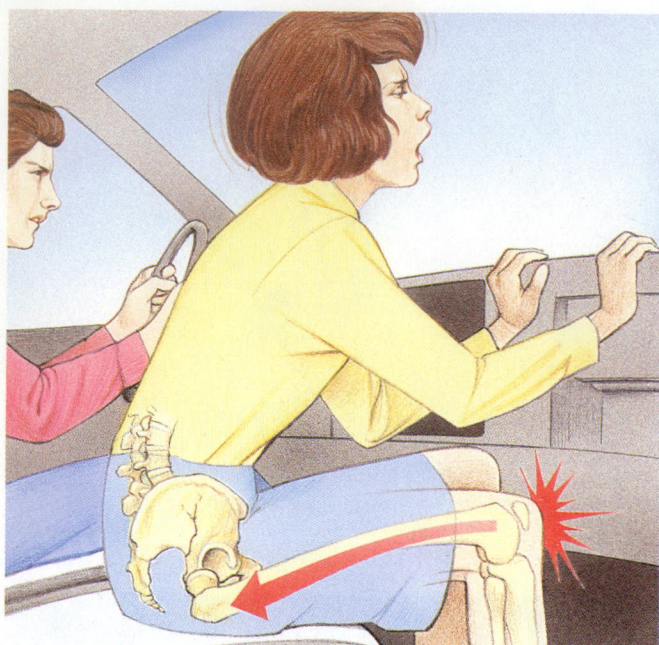

Figure 25-31 Posterior dislocation of the hip can occur as a result of the knee hitting the dashboard in a motor vehicle crash. The impact drives the femur posteriorly (see arrow), dislocating the joint.

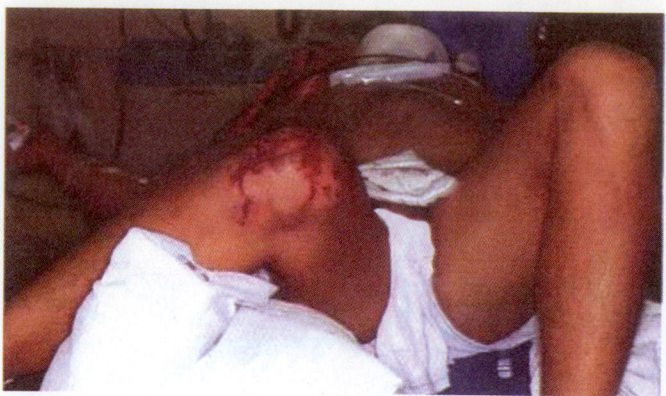

Figure 25-32 The usual position of a patient with a posterior dislocation of the hip. The hip joint is flexed, and the thigh is rotated inward and adducted across the midline of the body.

riorly, dislocating the joint (▲ **Figure 25-31**). Thus, you should suspect a hip dislocation in any patient who has been in an automobile crash and has a contusion, laceration, or obvious fracture in the knee region. Very rarely does the femoral head dislocate anteriorly; in this circumstance, the legs are suddenly and forcibly spread wide apart and locked in this position.

Posterior dislocation of the hip is frequently complicated by injury to the sciatic nerve, which is located directly behind the hip joint. The **sciatic nerve** is the major nerve in the lower extremity; it controls muscle activity in the posterior thigh and below the knee, as well as sensation in most of the leg and foot. When the head of the femur is forced out of the hip socket posteriorly, it may compress or stretch the sciatic nerve, leading to partial or complete paralysis of the nerve. The result is decreased sensation and muscle weakness in the leg and foot and frequently weakness in the foot muscles. Generally, only the dorsiflexors, the muscles that raise the toes or foot, are involved, causing the "foot drop" that is characteristic of damage to the peroneal portion of the sciatic nerve.

Another possible complication of posterior hip dislocation is circulatory in origin. Because the blood supply to the head of the femur runs within the capsule of the hip joint, stretching or tearing of this capsule (as can

occur with dislocation) may interrupt the blood supply to the femoral head. If there is a lack of blood flow to the bone for an extended time, the femoral head will undergo cell death, or osteonecrosis.

Skiers or boarders with a dislocated hip will commonly be found lying supine or on the side opposite the injury, with the injured hip partially flexed, internally rotated, and adducted across the opposite thigh. Also, the affected knee is usually flexed, and the hip appears as though it is "locked" in position. Any attempts you make to move the hip will be met with great resistance and cries of pain (▲ **Figure 25-32**). Check for sciatic nerve injury by carefully assessing sensation and motor function in the foot. Occasionally, sciatic nerve function will be normal at first and then slowly diminish.

As with any other extremity injury, you should make no attempt to reduce the dislocated hip in the field. Splint the dislocation in the position of the deformity and place the patient supine on a long backboard. Support the affected limb with pillows and rolled blankets, particularly under the flexed knee. Then secure the patient to the backboard with long straps so that the hip region will not move. Because of the severe pain and the possibility of circulatory compromise to the femoral head, be sure to provide prompt transport off the hill, and arrange for rapid transfer to a medical facility.

Fractures of the Proximal Femur

Fractures of the proximal femur are also relatively uncommon in snowsports. Although they are usually called hip fractures, they rarely involve the hip joint itself. Instead, the break goes through the neck of the femur (high), the intertrochanteric region (middle), or across the proximal, subtrochanteric shaft of the

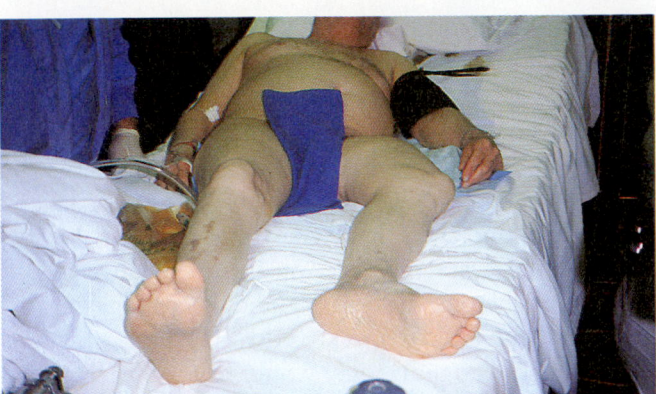

Figure 25-33   A patient with a fracture of the proximal femur will typically present with the extremity externally rotated and the injured leg shorter than the opposite leg.

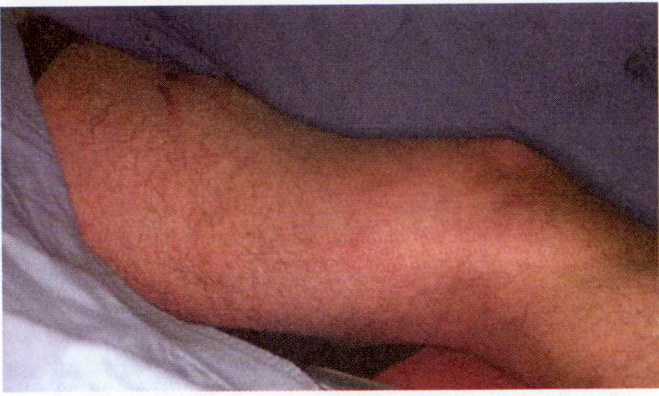

Figure 25-34   Fracture of the right femur with significant swelling.

femur (low). Although these three fracture types occur most often in older patients, particularly patients with osteoporosis, they may also be seen as a result of high-energy injuries in young adults. When a skier or snow-boarder does sustain this injury, most often it results from a collision or fall directly on the lateral aspect of the hip. Injury to adjacent structures—thigh soft-tissue damage or muscle hemorrhaging—is frequent.

All patients with displaced fractures of the proximal femur display a very characteristic deformity. They lie with the leg externally rotated, and the injured leg is usually shorter than the opposite, uninjured limb

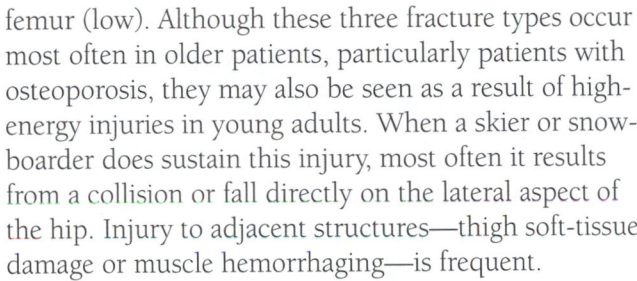

▲ Figure 25-33). When the fracture is not displaced, this deformity is not present. With any kind of hip fracture, patients typically are unable to walk or move the leg because of pain in the hip region or in the groin or inner aspect of the thigh. The hip region is usually tender on palpation, and gentle rotation of the leg will cause severe pain. On occasion, the pain is referred to the knee. Therefore, it is not uncommon for a patient with a traumatic hip fracture to complain of knee pain after a fall. You should stabilize the lower extremity of an elderly patient who has fallen and complains of pain in either the hip or the knee, even if there is no deformity.

The emergency care for a patient with a suspected hip fracture consists of the following:

1. Administer high-flow oxygen by face mask.
2. Gently splint the injured extremity to the uninjured leg by tying the patient's thighs and lower legs together with broad, folded cravats.
3. Log roll the patient toward the uninjured lower extremity, then transfer him or her onto a back-

board. Next, secure the individual to the back-board and place a folded blanket under the knee of the uninjured extremity to keep it partially flexed (which tends to decrease muscle-tension pain in the injured hip).

4. Do not give the patient anything to eat or drink.
5. Monitor the patient's vital signs frequently; be alert for signs of shock.
6. Rapidly transport the patient to a medical facility.

Femoral Shaft Fractures

The term femoral shaft fracture is used to describe fractures of the middle half to three fourths of the femur. These fractures occur as the result of a direct blow to the femur, such as from a fall onto the thigh from a height, or secondary to a violent twisting injury to the thigh, such as an excessive external rotation injury to the leg where the tibia and knee remain stable, and the femur fractures obliquely. Assessment usually discloses an externally rotated and shortened limb with a tender bulge in the thigh. If the patient is seen early, this bulge which represents hematoma and tissue edema may not have had time to develop. The fracture is often angulated. The patient is usually in severe pain, has thigh muscle spasms, and is unable to move the extremity

▲ Figure 25-34).

If the general condition of the patient allows, a fracture of the femoral shaft should be stabilized with a traction splint. Traction splinting counteracts the spasm and pull of the large, powerful thigh muscles. In addition, traction splinting prevents the bone ends from overriding more, causing further shortening of the limb, reduces the potential for damage from sharp bone frag-

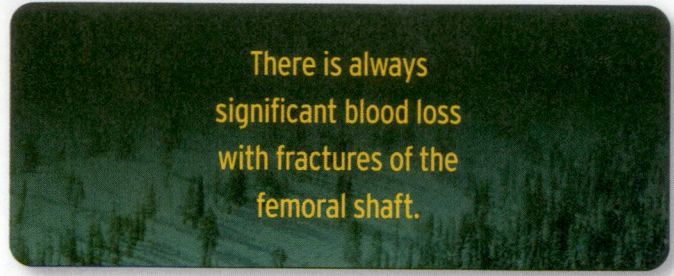

There is always significant blood loss with fractures of the femoral shaft.

ments, decreases pain by stabilizing the fracture site, and minimizes blood loss into the thigh musculature. The purpose of traction is not to pull the bone ends apart or to realign the fracture anatomically. If there is major deformity of the thigh, the injured leg must be realigned before application of the splint.

Bleeding at the fracture site is decreased with use of the traction splint because traction stretches and tightens the musculofascial "envelope" surrounding the fracture, keeping it cylindrical rather than allowing it to shorten and assume a spherical shape. This tends to stop the bleeding by increasing the pressure inside the periosteal (fibrous bone cover) envelope. A fixation splint stabilizes the fracture without tightening the envelope, thereby allowing continued bleeding into the loose envelope. Without a traction splint, considerable time may therefore elapse before enough pressure builds up in the envelope to control the bleeding.

Because the skier or boarder may lose 1,500 to 2,000 mL of blood into a closed femoral fracture site, you should anticipate that mild to moderate shock will develop, accompanied by a pulse rate of more than 100 beats/min. The blood pressure may be relatively normal as long as the patient is recumbent. Because nerves and blood vessels crossing the fracture site may be damaged by the bone ends, check CMS function in the foot during the urgent survey, before and after splinting, and at frequent intervals during the ongoing survey. Traction splinting may improve impaired circulation, motion, and sensation.

If it is unclear whether a traction splint is required, the following assessment strategy may prove helpful: place the heel of one hand on the patient's iliac crest, with your fingers on the greater trochanter. If pressing on this hand with your other hand causes the patient pain, the injury is in the hip area and a traction splint is not indicated. If no pain results, place the heel of one hand on the patient's pubic bone with your fingers pointing down the thigh, and place the heel of the other hand on the patient's patella with your fingers pointing up the thigh. If the pain from a suspected fracture is

between the fingertips of your two hands, a traction splint is indicated.

In the past, emergency care providers were encouraged to place a cravat under the upper thigh before a traction splint was applied, in case a tourniquet was needed to stop severe bleeding. This practice has fallen out of favor and should be avoided because it is now deemed unnecessary, ineffective, and even dangerous. In an open femoral fracture, significant bleeding can be managed with a direct pressure dressing alone. In a closed fracture, a tourniquet would have no effect on the main source of bleeding, ie, broken bone ends tearing into the soft tissues of the thigh. Traction splinting is the proper care for this type of bleeding.

Under most circumstances, a traction splint should not be removed except in a hospital. However, in patrol operations, special circumstances may arise in which a traction splint applied to a fractured femur in the field might reasonably be removed in the aid room and traction reapplied. Such special circumstances might include the following:

1. When a makeshift splint has been applied in preparation for transport from a wilderness accident or off-area rescue, or any other instance where the splint is clearly not doing an adequate job

2. When a patient with traction applied over the boot is unable to wiggle his or her toes or feel the foot, transport to the nearest hospital will take more than an hour, and it is desirable to remove the boot so that CMS function can be checked directly

3. When helicopter transport is necessary and the splint is too long to fit in the helicopter

4. When the patient is in great pain and adjusting traction does not help

5. In the case of traction applied over the boot, when local EMS protocol will not permit patient transport unless the boot is removed to check CMS function. In some places, EMS protocol requires checking CMS function regardless of the signs and symptoms.

Each patrol, with the aid of medical personnel, should develop a local protocol that covers the circumstances in which a traction splint can be removed. Many patrols are now removing the boot on the hill at the accident scene, so that pain from the boot and the uncertainty of traction release at a later time does not occur. If the traction splint is removed or the traction decreased, the injured extremity must be manually stabilized until the new splint is in place and traction is reapplied.

Depending on the general condition of the patient, fractures of the femoral shaft should be stabilized with a traction splint, such as a Sager splint, Hare splint, or Thomas half-ring splint (see Chapter 24).

Injuries of Knee Ligaments

The knee is very vulnerable to injury; therefore, many different types of injuries occur in this region. Ligament injuries, for example, range from mild sprains to complete dislocation of the joint. The patella can also dislocate. In addition, all the bony elements of the knee (distal femur, upper tibia, and patella) can fracture.

The knee is especially susceptible to ligament injuries, which occur when abnormal bending or twisting forces are applied to the joint. Knee sprains are common among people who participate in most outdoor sports, and are the most common injury in skiing. Because of the frequency of knee injuries, you should be thoroughly familiar with its anatomy and function.

The knee is a modified hinge joint. Although its motion is mainly in the single plane of flexion-extension, some degree of rotation of the tibia on the femur occurs going from full flexion of the knee to full extension.

The bones of the knee joint are the femur proximally, the tibia distally, and the patella anteriorly ▼ **Figure 25-35 A and B** . The fibula is only indirectly involved with the knee joint.

The weight-bearing surfaces of the knee are the convex condyles of the femur, which are semicircular and covered with articular cartilage, and the concave tibial plateau on which the femoral condyles sit. The tibial plateau is also covered with articular cartilage. The C-shaped medial cartilage and the O-shaped lateral cartilage (menisci) sit atop the tibial plateau ▼ **Figure 25-35 C and D** , deepen its concavities, cushion the joint, and help align the femur as it sits on the tibia. The patella, whose posterior surface is also covered with cartilage, is located in front of the knee joint in the groove between the femoral condyles.

The knee joint is enclosed by a fibrous joint capsule and lined by a synovial membrane that secretes lubricating synovial fluid ▼ **Figure 25-35 E** . The medial and lateral parts of the knee joint capsule are thicker and stronger than the rest of the capsule, forming the medial and lateral ligaments of the knee, also called "collateral" ligaments. The front and back of the capsule are loose, permitting flexion and extension of the joint.

There are two other important ligaments of the knee joint: the anterior and posterior cruciate ligaments, or ACL and PCL. These originate in the groove between the femoral condyles, cross each other front to back in an X, and insert into the tibial plateau. The ACL crosses in front of the PCL. Because the concavities of the tibial plateau are shallow, the knee joint would be easy to dislocate if not for these four powerful ligaments, the menisci, and the muscles and tendons around the knee. The lateral and medial ligaments are probably the most important in preventing medial and lateral dislocation of the knee—the ACL in preventing forward dislocation and the PCL in preventing backward dislocation. Hyperextension is prevented by both cruciates (mainly the anterior cruciate) and also by the posterior part of the joint capsule.

The major muscles associated with the knee joint are the quadriceps femoris ("quad") anteriorly, which

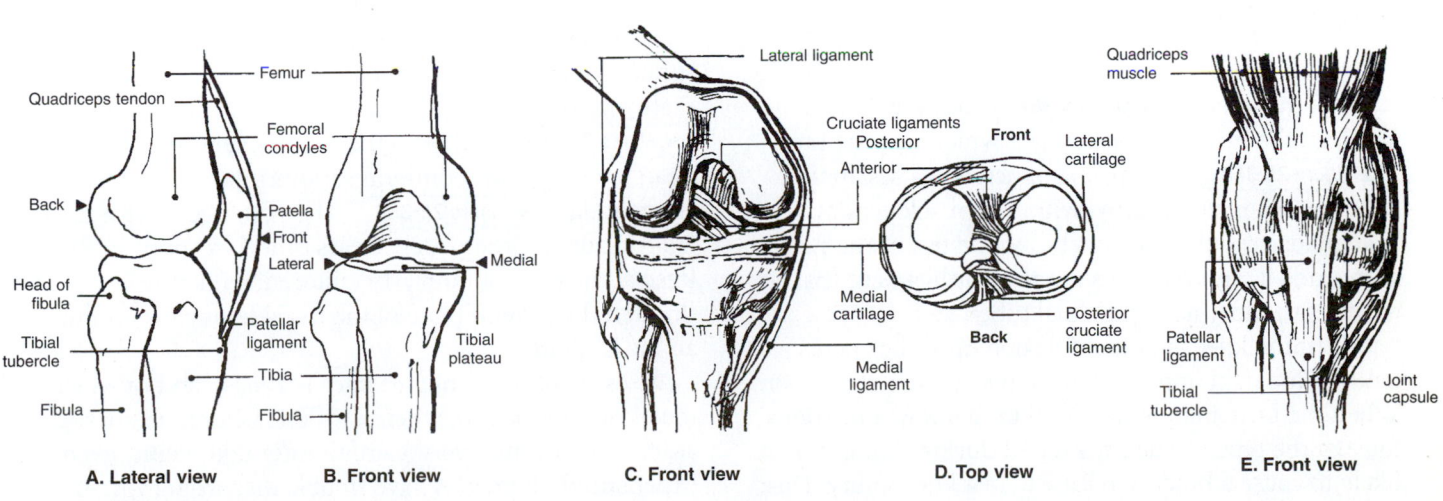

A. Lateral view   B. Front view   C. Front view   D. Top view   E. Front view

Figure 25-35 Anatomy of the knee.

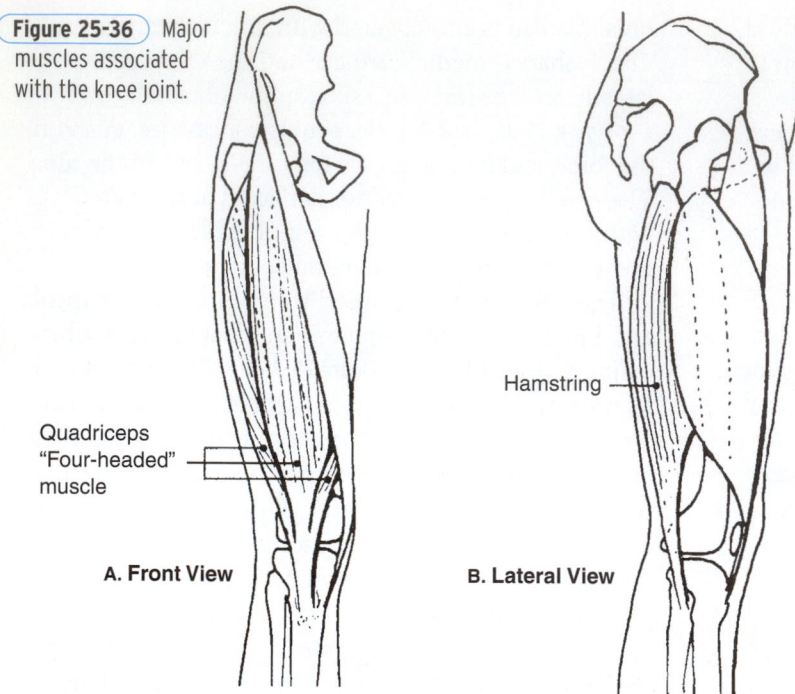

Figure 25-36 Major muscles associated with the knee joint.

Quadriceps "Four-headed" muscle

A. Front View

Hamstring

B. Lateral View

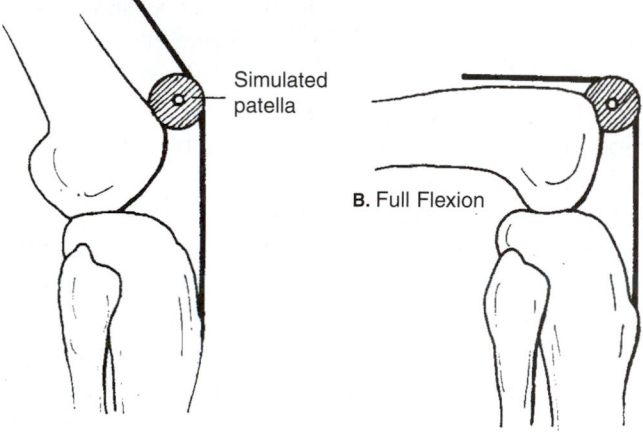

A. Partial Extension

Simulated patella

B. Full Flexion

Figure 25-37 Mechanics of the patellar system.

extends the knee (▲ Figure 25-36A), and the medial and lateral hamstrings posteriorly, which flex the knee (▲ Figure 25-36B). The patella is actually a sesamoid bone, ie, a bone that forms within a muscle tendon. The quadriceps tendon attaches to the top of the patella, surrounds it, and becomes the patellar ligament that attaches to the tibia at the tibial tubercle.

When the knee is in slight flexion, most ligaments and tendons are tight and the joint is in its strongest position. When the knee joint is stabilized in this way, a rotational force of the type frequently exerted during skiing is more likely to cause a binding release than a knee injury. This is why novice skiers are encouraged to keep their knees

bent to maintain better control and prevent knee injuries.

The medial cartilage (meniscus), which is partly fixed by its attachment to the medial collateral ligament, is torn more often than the lateral cartilage, which can move to some extent within the joint.

Prolonged flexion of the knee at close to a 90° angle, which can occur when "sitting back" while skiing bumps, puts a severe strain on the patella. If done frequently, this eventually injures the cartilage that covers the posterior surface of the patella, producing a painful condition called chondromalacia patella. Chondromalacia causes pain in the knee during prolonged sitting with the knees bent 90°, and when ascending or (especially) descending stairs or hills. The knee is also less stable in the 90° flexed position, and the ACL is more prone to injury in this position.

The patella improves knee extension when the knee is partly extended, since it lies on the lower end of the femur just above the condyles, holds the quadriceps tendon away from the joint, and lengthens the lever arm (◄ Figure 25-37A). However, in full flexion, the mechanical advantage of the patellar system is lost because the patella moves downward, sinks between the femoral condyles, and allows the quadriceps tendon to move closer to the joint (◄ Figure 25-37B). Since ski boots with built-in forward lean put considerable stress on the patella, skiers who wear these boots are advised to loosen them and stand up straight when they are not skiing.

Knee injuries make up more than one third of all ski injuries among alpine and nordic skiers and are the most common injury in skiing. Most knee injuries are sprains, many of which involve more than one ligament. Eighty percent of knee sprains involve the MCL joint (► Figure 25-38A) and 40% the ACL. Severe ACL sprains (tears) are the most common serious injuries in alpine skiing today (► Figure 25-38B). They can occur without a fall. Frequently, the patient hears or feels a "pop" in the knee at the time of injury. In children, a fracture through the growth plate of the distal femur may mimic an MCL sprain.

Assessment of an injured knee is easiest, and provides the most information, when it is done before the knee swells and becomes very painful. After this occurs, even experienced physicians have trouble diagnosing specific knee injuries by physical examination alone. Successful

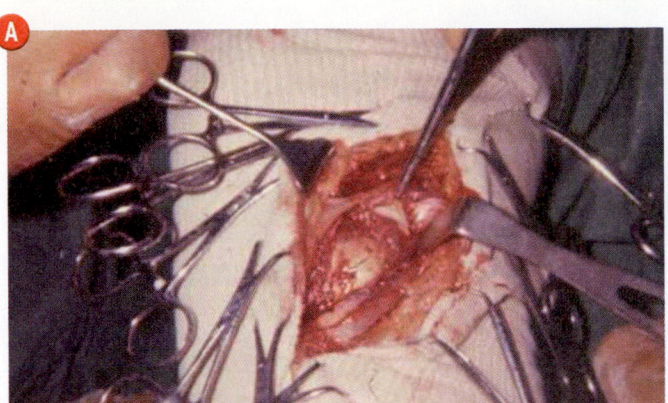

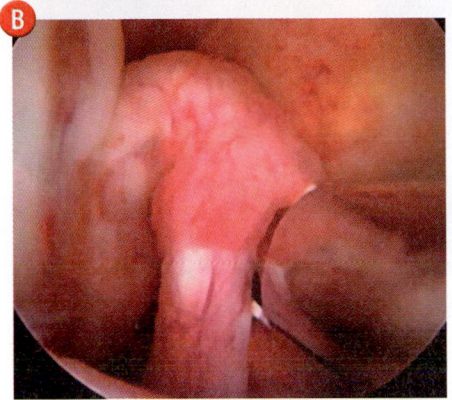

Figure 25-38 **A.** Intraoperative photo showing the surgeon's forceps grasping the torn end of a medial collateral ligament. **B.** Intraoperative arthroscopic photo of a torn anterior cruciate ligament.

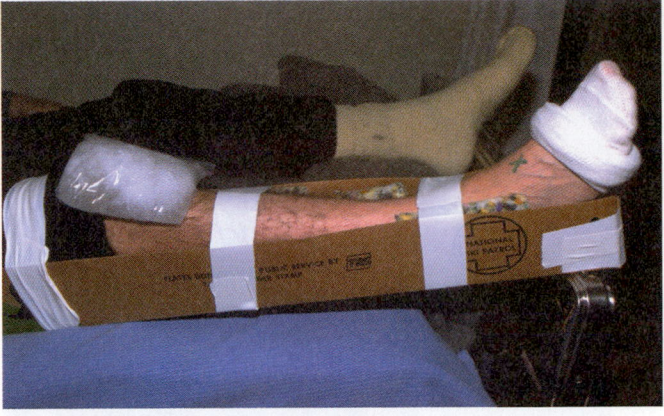

Figure 25-39 With a cardboard splint on an injured knee, the skier is ready for discharge from the aid room.

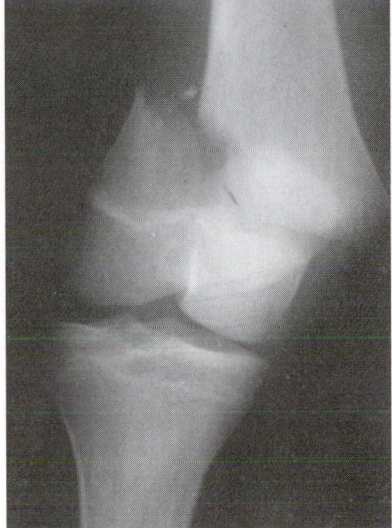

Figure 25-40 X-ray of a displaced fracture through the distal femoral growth line (epiphysis), the overall appearance mimicking severe joint laxity produced by major ligamentous tears of the knee joint.

treatment of many knee injuries depends on prompt diagnosis, which may require examining the interior of the joint with an arthroscope, and possible reconstructive surgery within a week or two. Therefore, advise every patient with a knee injury to promptly see a physician, preferably an orthopaedic surgeon, especially if symptoms are not significantly better within 24 hours.

The knee is best assessed in a warm aid room. You can frequently get a good idea of which parts of the knee have been injured by noting the circumstances of the injury and the areas of tenderness. First, ask the patient to describe the events immediately preceding the injury—including the exact way in which a fall, if any, occurred—and try to reconstruct the probable mechanisms involved. Ask if a "pop" was heard or felt, which indicates a possible ACL injury. Ask the patient to point with one finger to where the knee hurts, then assess the rest of the knee. Look for swelling and deformity, and gently feel for tenderness of the medial and lateral ligaments, the ligaments attached to the patella, the posterior part of the joint capsule, and the hamstring tendons.

Emergency care of a knee sprain on the hill consists of applying a rigid fixation splint (quick splint), and transport to the aid room in a sled. After evaluation in the aid room, a suitable fixation splint is reapplied (usually a cardboard splint), and ice bags are placed over the knee ▲ **Figure 25-39** . It is best to let a physician decide when the patient can remove the splint and bear weight on the injured extremity.

Fractures About the Knee

Fractures in the area of the knee joint may occur at the distal end of the femur, at the proximal end of the tibia, or in the patella. Because of local tenderness and swelling, it is easy to confuse a nondisplaced or minimally displaced fracture near the knee with a ligament injury. Likewise, a displaced fracture close to the knee joint may produce significant deformity that makes it look like a dislocation, or a severe ligament injury ▲ **Figure 25-40** .

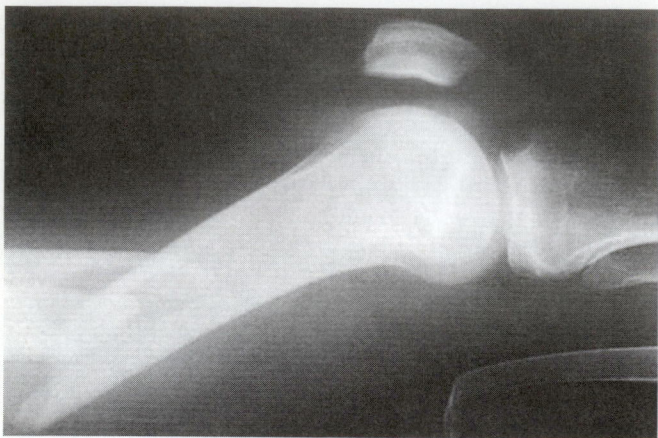

Figure 25-41   X-ray of a patient with a posteriorly angulated supra-condylar fracture of the femur.

A fracture of the femur just above the knee (supra-condylar fracture) is a serious injury. The pull of the thigh muscles tips the lower fragment so that its jagged upper end lies against the nerves and blood vessels running down the back of the thigh, putting them at risk of injury.

Assessment reveals a large, tender swelling in the lower thigh just above the knee, with deformity, pain, and inability to move the knee **▲ Figure 25-41**. CMS function below the injury should be assessed during the urgent survey, before and after splinting (or alignment, if this becomes necessary because circulation or nerve supply is impaired), and at regular intervals during the ongoing survey.

Emergency care consists of stabilizing the fracture with a rigid fixation splint (quick splint) that extends from just below the groin to the foot, as described in Chapter 24, or with a padded board splint applied on each side of the joint in a technique similar to that used to stabilize a fracture above the elbow **▶ Figure 25-42**. Do not use a traction splint.

The patient must be taken to a hospital as soon as possible. However, a single, gentle attempt at fracture alignment is indicated if transport to a definitive care facility will take longer than an hour and the following signs are present:

1. interrupted nerve supply, such as weakness of ankle, foot, or toe movement or loss of sensation below the fracture

2. impaired circulation, such as a cold, pale foot; pain in the foot and leg; or absence or weakness of the posterior tibial and dorsalis pedis pulses

The single attempt at alignment should be done with the patient's knee bent. Grasp the leg just below the

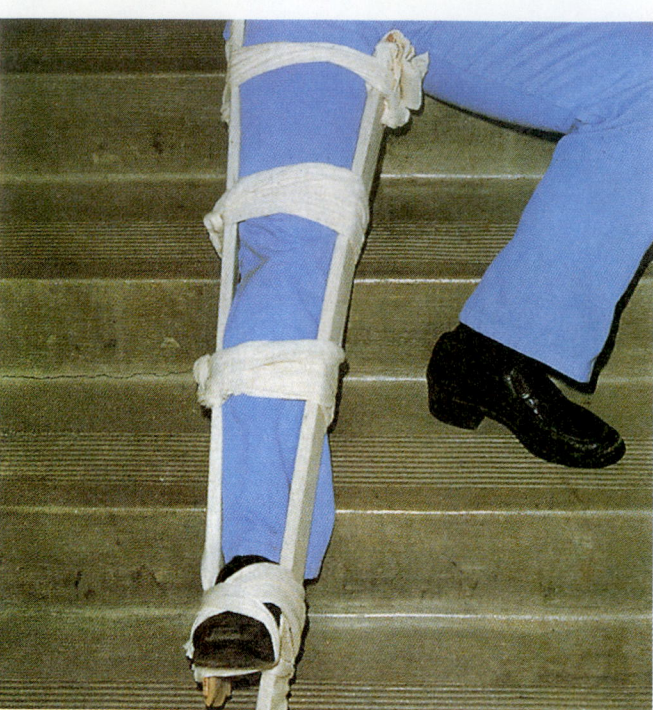

Figure 25-42   Patient immobilized with double-padded board splints.

knee while a second rescuer steadies the upper thigh. Exert longitudinal traction to reduce the posterior angulation of the fracture site. If realignment produces a return of pulses, a decrease in pain, or improvement in color, splint the extremity in the position that produces the strongest pulses. If the attempted realignment is unsuccessful, or causes major resistance or severe pain, splint the injury in the most comfortable position and rapidly transport the patient to a hospital.

Fractures of the proximal tibia in snowsports are caused by the same medial/lateral forces that trigger a collateral ligament sprain and an epiphyseal supra-condylar femur fracture or result from a jump/fall from a height.

These forces usually produce a lateral stress to the knee, and in terms of the proximal tibia, result in an intra-articular compression fracture of the lateral tibial condyle. On assessment, the appearance of the leg will be similar to that described for a supracondylar femur fracture, often with lateral angulation of the lower leg.

Dislocation of the Knee

Complete disruption of the ligaments supporting the knee may result in dislocation of the joint. When this happens, the proximal end of the tibia completely displaces from its articulation with the lower end of the femur, usually producing a significant deformity **▶ Figure 25-43**. Although severe ligament damage always occurs with a knee dislocation, the more urgent

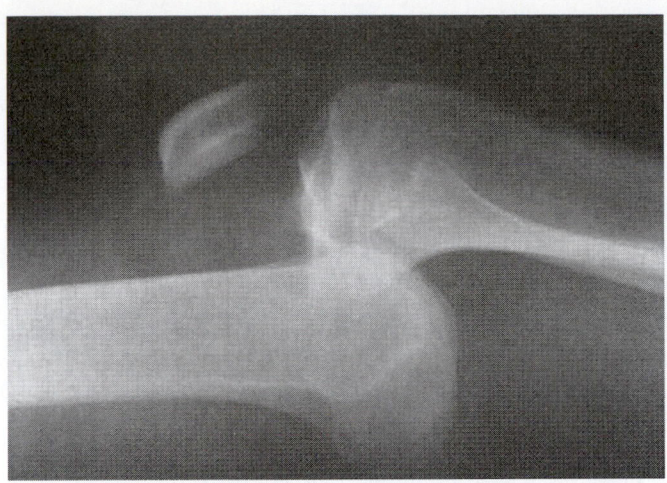

Figure 25-43 Knee x-ray of a patient with a complete dislocation of the knee.

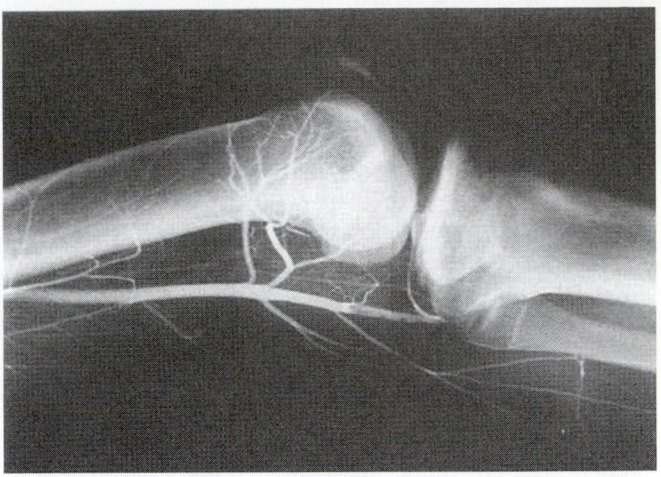

Figure 25-44 Arteriogram x-ray of a blocked popliteal artery secondary to a recent fracture-dislocation of the knee. This injury resulted in amputation of the lower leg.

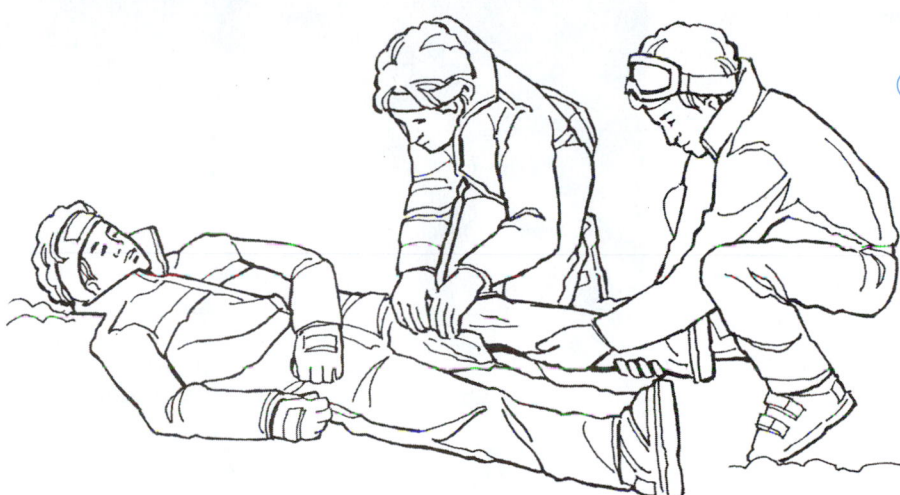

Figure 25-45 Axial traction to improve circulation in a dislocated knee.

injury is to the popliteal artery, which is almost always lacerated or compressed by the posteriorly displaced proximal tibia (▲ **Figure 25-44**).

When gross deformity, severe pain, and an inability to move the joint cause you to suspect a dislocation of the knee, always check the distal circulation carefully before taking any other step. If the distal pulses are absent, and transport time from the ski hill to the hospital is less than an hour, splint the leg with a quick splint in the position found, and rapidly transport the skier to the aid room. Ask your rescue squad to stand by for immediate transport to an emergency department.

If adequate distal pulses are present, also splint the knee in the position in which you found it, and transport the patient promptly. Do not attempt to manipulate any severe knee injury if there are good distal pulses. If the limb is straight, apply a quick splint. If the knee is bent and the foot has a good pulse, splint the joint in the bent

position, using a reversed (upside down) quick splint or parallel padded board splints secured at the hip and ankle joint to provide a stable A-frame. Secure the patient to a backboard with folded blankets and straps to eliminate any motion of the knee during transport.

If there are signs of impairment of circulation or nerve function in the foot distal to the injury and transport to a hospital will take more than an hour, try to improve matters by using gentle longitudinal traction to change the angle of dislocation. Grasp the patient's ankle with one hand and the patient's calf with the other hand while a second rescuer steadies the lower thigh. Then exert gentle traction while flexing the knee slightly (▲ **Figure 25-45**). Test the pulses in the foot with the knee in the new position. If the maneuver is successful, splint the limb in the position that produces the strongest pulses. Make only one attempt; if it is unsuccessful, or elicits severe pain or major resistance, splint the limb in the most comfortable position and rapidly transport the patient to a hospital.

Fractures of the Patella

Patellar fractures are usually caused by a severe blow to the patella or a fall onto the flexed knee. Assessment reveals swelling, tenderness, and ecchymosis around the patella (▶ **Figure 25-46**), and the patient is unable to extend the knee because of pain. Emergency care is the same as that for a fracture just above the knee.

Dislocation of the Patella

A dislocated patella most commonly occurs in teenagers and young adults who are engaged in athletic activities, and snowsports are no exception. Some patients have recurrent dislocations of the patella. As with recurrent dislocation of the shoulder, a minor twisting may be enough to produce the problem. Almost always, the dislocated patella displaces to the lateral side of the joint, causing the knee joint to assume a partially flexed position. The deformity is significant, and quite characteristic (▶ **Figure 25-47**).

Splint the knee in the position in which you found it. To immobilize the knee, apply a "reversed" quick splint or padded board splints to the medial and lateral aspects of the joint, extending from the hip to the ankle. Use folded blankets to support the limb in the sled.

Occasionally, as you apply the splint, the patella will return to its normal position spontaneously. When this occurs, immobilize the knee in extension in a quick splint. The patient still needs rescue squad transport to the emergency department. Report the spontaneous reduction of the patellar dislocation to the rescue personnel so that they can make the hospital staff aware of the severity of the injury.

Injuries of the Tibia and Fibula

The <u>tibia</u> (shinbone) is the larger of the two leg bones and is responsible for supporting the major weight-bearing surfaces of the knee and ankle. The <u>fibula</u> is the smaller bone in the lower leg and functions mainly to provide sites for muscle origin, and distally, as part of the ankle joint mortise. Fracture of the shaft of the tibia or the fibula may occur at any place between the knee joint and the ankle joint. Common skiing fractures are "boot-top fractures," in which a forward fall causes a transverse fracture of the tibia and fibula at the level of the boot top (▶ **Figure 25-48A**), and spiral fractures, in which a twisting fall causes oblique fractures of both bone shafts (▶ **Figure 25-48B**).

When both the tibia and fibula are fractured, the extremity distal to the fracture is usually angulated or

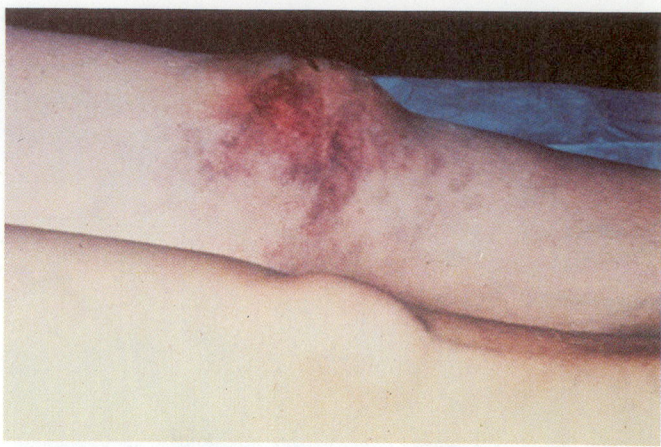

(**Figure 25-46**)   Patellar fracture with ecchymosis.

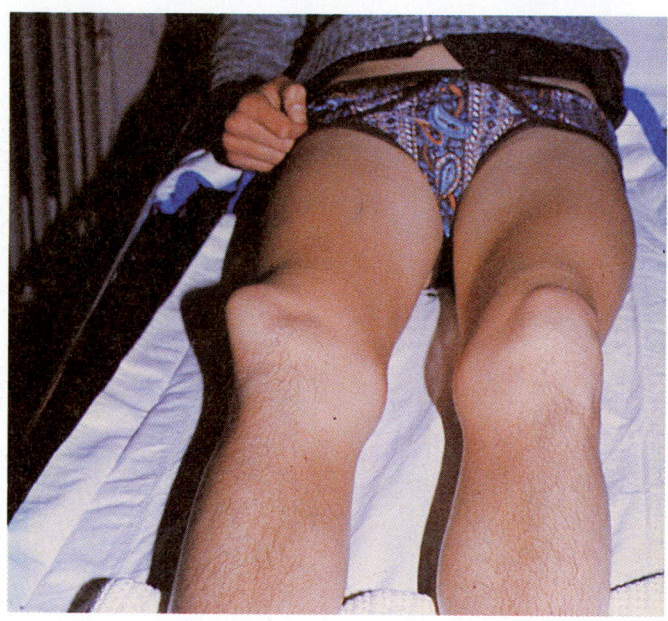

(**Figure 25-47**)   A dislocated patella will typically appear with the patella displaced lateral to the knee and with the knee moderately flexed.

rotated, occasionally as much as 180°. The patient complains of severe pain and resists movement of the leg. Assessment shows swelling and tenderness at the fracture site. Ecchymosis will develop later. Most of the length of the tibia is subcutaneous (just beneath the skin); therefore, open fractures of this bone are common (▶ **Figure 25-49**). Because of the potential tamponade (pressure) effect of the boot on hemorrhage from the open fracture, unless there is excessive bleeding of the lower leg above the boot, do *not* expose the injury site until the boot is removed in the aid room.

Emergency care of a patient with a lower leg fracture consists of applying a quick splint, as described in Chapter 24. Before applying the splint, you frequently must realign the fracture to bring the leg into its proper

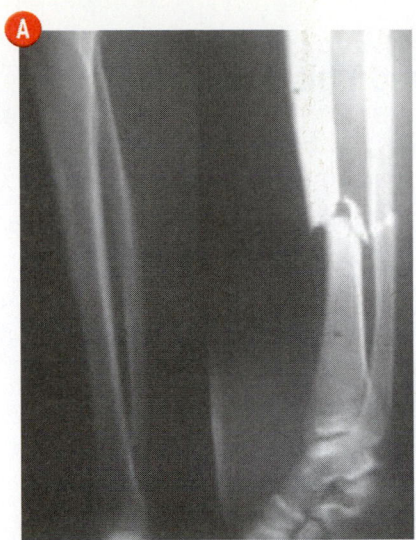

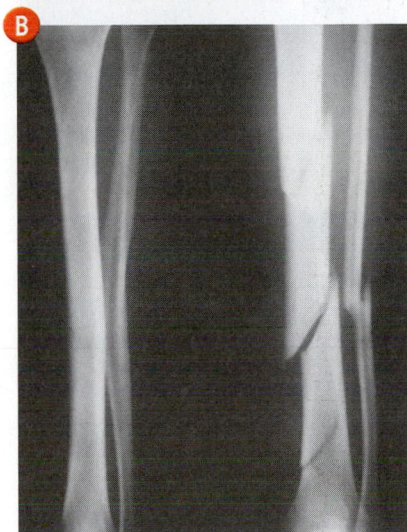

Figure 25-48
A. Lateral X-ray of a boot top fracture of the tibia and fibula, with a normal tibial X-ray on the left.
B. X-ray of a spiral fracture of the tibia secondary to skiing, with a normal tibial X-ray on the left.

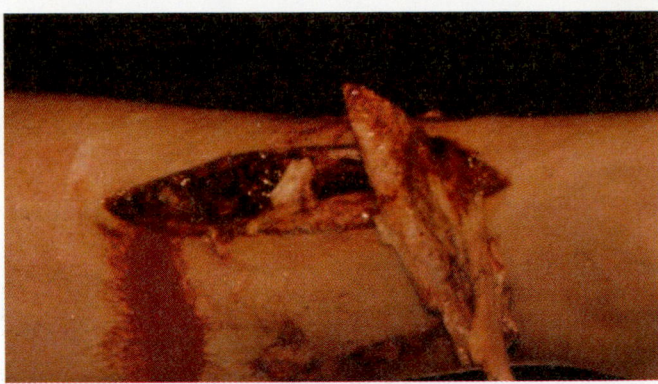

Figure 25-49 Because the tibia is so close to the skin, open fractures are quite common.

stabilize the leg from the groin to the foot. Rescuer 1 lowers the leg into the splint **(Step 3)**.

4. **Rescuer 2 closes the splint** and then tightens the straps. Rescuer 1 slides his or her upper hand out from behind the upper calf as the splint is closed, but does not release control of the foot, and therefore the fracture site, until both straps of the quick splint are snugly secured **(Step 4)**.

5. Rescuer 1 slides his or her hand from around the heel and **checks CMS function (Step 5)**.

This fracture realignment will cause significant pain, and will be met with some resistance from the patient. However, both rescuers must be positive about the benefits of splinting, and once initiated, the maneuver should be carried out to completion without hesitation. The earlier realignment is attempted after the injury, the easier it is to perform. Assess CMS function in the foot during the urgent survey, before and after alignment and splinting, at frequent intervals during toboggan transport to the aid room, and in the aid room.

When both the tibia and the femur in the same limb have been assessed to be fractured ("floating knee fracture"), do not apply a traction splint to the injured leg. Instead, apply gentle longitudinal tension to the extremity to realign the lower leg, and then place the leg in a quick splint from the groin to the foot. The goal here is to restore a position that will allow the use of a standard splint; it is not necessary to attempt realignment of the fracture fragments into their anatomic position.

Fractures of the tibia and fibula are often associated with vascular injury as a result of the distorted position of the limb following injury. Realigning the limb frequently may restore adequate blood supply to the foot. In any incidence, transport the patient promptly to the aid room and have staff summon your rescue squad while you are en route.

anatomic relationship with the foot **▶ Skill Drill 25-2** . To be effective, two rescuers are required to execute this procedure properly. The boot is left in place until the injured skier or boarder has been transported to the aid room.

1. Rescuer 1 kneels at the patient's foot on the same side as the injury, **firmly grasps the boot heel** with one hand, and places his or her hand under the leg just below the knee but above the fracture site **(Step 1)**. Rescuer 2 opens and readies the quick splint.

2. When all is ready, **rescuer 1 applies gentle longitudinal traction** to the lower leg and with both hands lifts, straightens, and derotates the deformed extremity all in one continuous motion **(Step 2)**.

3. **Rescuer 2 slides the splint under the leg** from the medial and below, positioning the splint to

Skill Drill 25-2   Realignment of Angulated, Rotated, Fractured Tibia/Fibula with Application of a Quick Splint

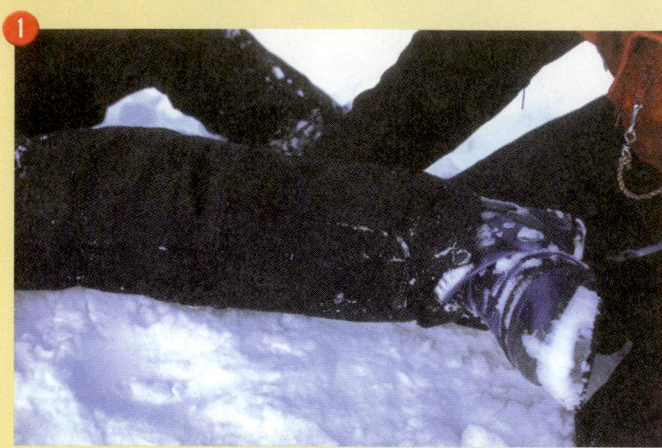

1 Rescuer 1 grasps the boot heel of the injured leg with one hand, while the other hand is placed under the calf just below the knee.

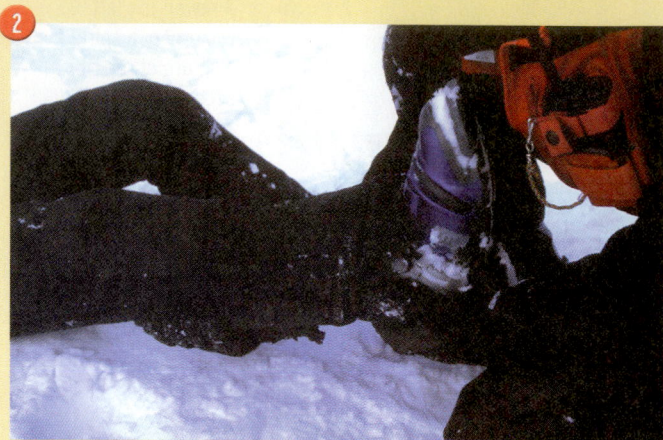

2 When the splint is ready, rescuer 1 applies gentle longitudinal traction, and with both hands, lifts, straightens, and derotates the deformed tibia all in one continuous motion.

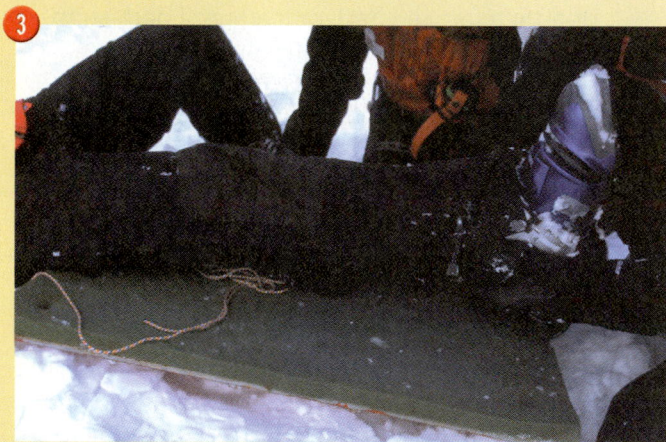

3 Rescuer 2 slides the splint under the leg from medial and below, then rescuer 1 lowers the leg into the splint.

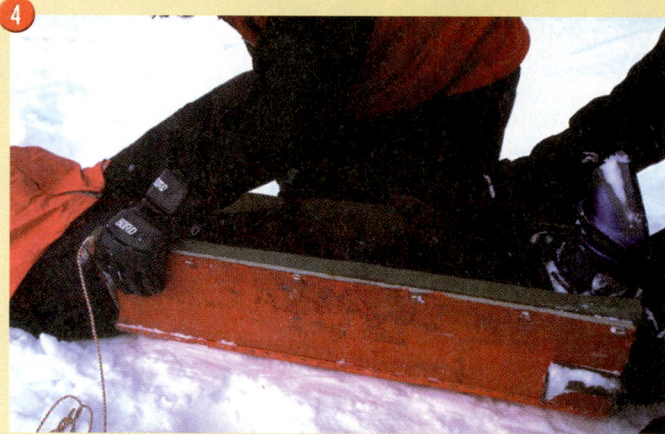

4 Rescuer 2 closes the splint and secures the straps, while rescuer 1 removes his or her upper hand.

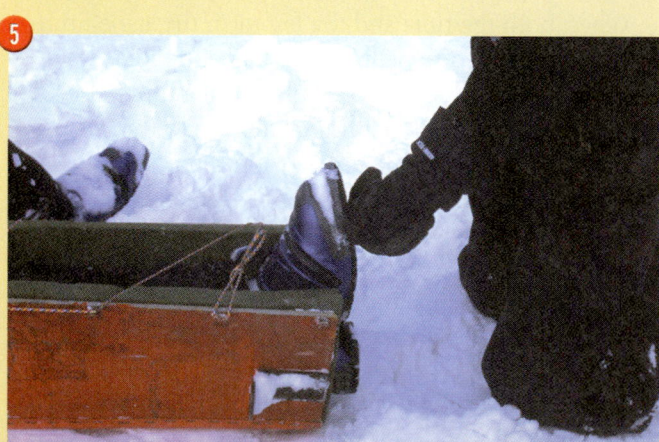

5 Rescuer 1 slides his or her hand out from around the heel, and then checks the CMS function in the foot.

Ankle Injuries

The ankle is the most commonly injured joint. Ankle injuries occur in individuals of all ages and range in severity from a simple sprain, which heals after a few days' rest, to severe fracture-dislocations. Ankle sprains are a hazard for outdoor travelers walking on uneven ground, and for nordic skiers and snowboarders. Although modern hiking and alpine skiing boots tend to protect the ankle, ankle sprains are common among nordic skiers because their bindings do not release and they generally wear low-top boots, and among snowboarders because they often wear soft boots. As the use of higher, stiffer telemark boots, and stiffer snowboarding boots increase, the number of ankle sprains among nordic skiers and snowboarders will probably decrease.

The most frequent mechanism of ankle injury is abruptly "turning the foot under" or "twisting the foot in," which incompletely or completely tears the supporting ankle ligaments. Depending on the severity and particularly the specific ligaments injured, assessment of an injured ankle will reveal tenderness, swelling, and ecchymosis usually around the lateral malleolus (bony projection from the fibula, on the outside of the ankle) and over the top of the foot (▶ **Figure 25-50**).

Emergency care of mild sprains consists of applying cold packs and supporting the ankle with a cravat ankle bandage or a figure-of-8 made from an elastic bandage (▶ **Figures 25-51**). The patient should use a cane or crutches to avoid putting full weight on the injured ankle. Severe ankle sprains are hard to distinguish from fractures and should be treated with a fixation splint designed for the lower leg (quick splint on the hill, and cardboard splint in the aid room). All patients with moderate or severe ankle sprains, or mild sprains that do not improve within a day or two, should see a physician.

In wilderness conditions, a patient with a mild to moderate ankle sprain may have to self-evacuate. An adhesive-tape boot may stabilize the sprain enough to allow the patient to walk or ski out (▶ **Figure 25-52**). Monitor the patient's sensation and movement in the toes because the tape encircling the foot and ankle may produce a tourniquet-like effect.

A "fractured ankle" usually refers to a fracture of the lower end of the tibia and/or fibula. The ankle joint has two "shear pins," the lateral and medial malleoli, which usually break first when a rotational force is applied to the ankle joint, thus preventing a more extensive fracture of the shafts of these bones. Ankle fractures are

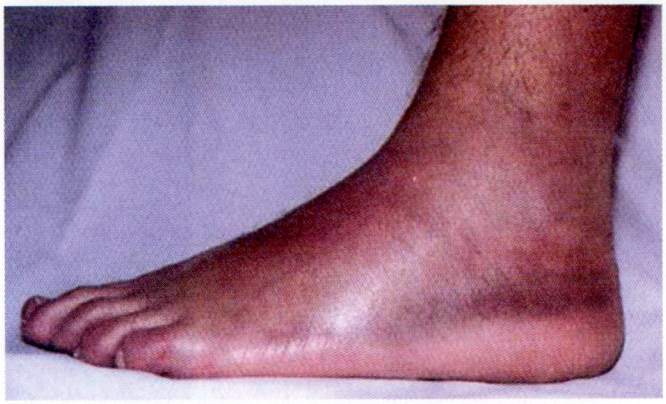

Figure 25-50 Typical appearance of a sprained ankle.

caused by twisting falls and falls from heights. Such fractures are now relatively rare among alpine skiers because of improved boot and binding designs, but they continue to be seen in nordic skiers and snowboarders. An ankle fracture may be hard to distinguish from a severe sprain (▶ **Figure 25-53**).

Assessment reveals swelling, tenderness when the ankle bone is palpated, and sometimes deformity of the ankle. Ecchymosis will develop later. The patient may or may not be able to move the joint. If a malleolus is fractured, gentle pressure over its tip is painful. Any ankle injury that produces pain, swelling, localized tenderness, or the inability to bear weight should be evaluated by a physician (▶ **Figure 25-54**). Surgery with screw fixation is usually necessary to realign and secure the malleoli back in their normal anatomic alignment.

As discussed in the segment on lower leg fractures, the ski or snowboard boot is usually not removed until the patient is in the aid room. Emergency care on the hill consists of applying a fixation splint designed for the lower leg, as described in Chapter 24. In an indoor environment, an improvised splint made of a folded pillow, a tightly rolled blanket, or cardboard, is satisfactory (▶ **Figure 25-55**).

Snowboarders sometimes incur a unique type of ankle fracture that mimics a sprain. This is a fracture of a small, bony projection of the talus (the tarsal bone that lies within the ankle mortise) caused when the toe edge of the snowboard catches and causes a sudden, severe dorsiflexion of the ankle during a forward fall. Suspect this in any snowboarder complaining of pain and tenderness in the anterolateral ankle area, and advise the patient to consult an orthopaedic surgeon.

Ankle dislocations are usually associated with fractures of the lower ends of both the tibia and fibula,

Figure 25-51 Support for sprained ankle.

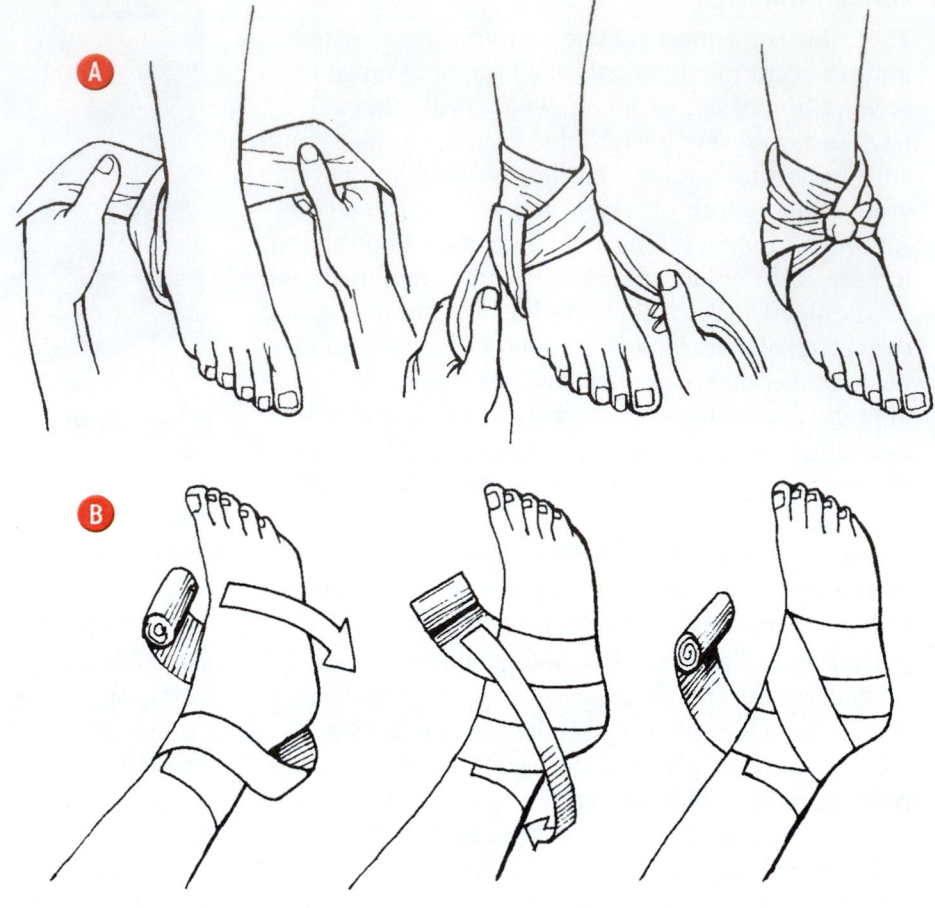

Figure 25-52 Adhesive tape boot for a sprained ankle.

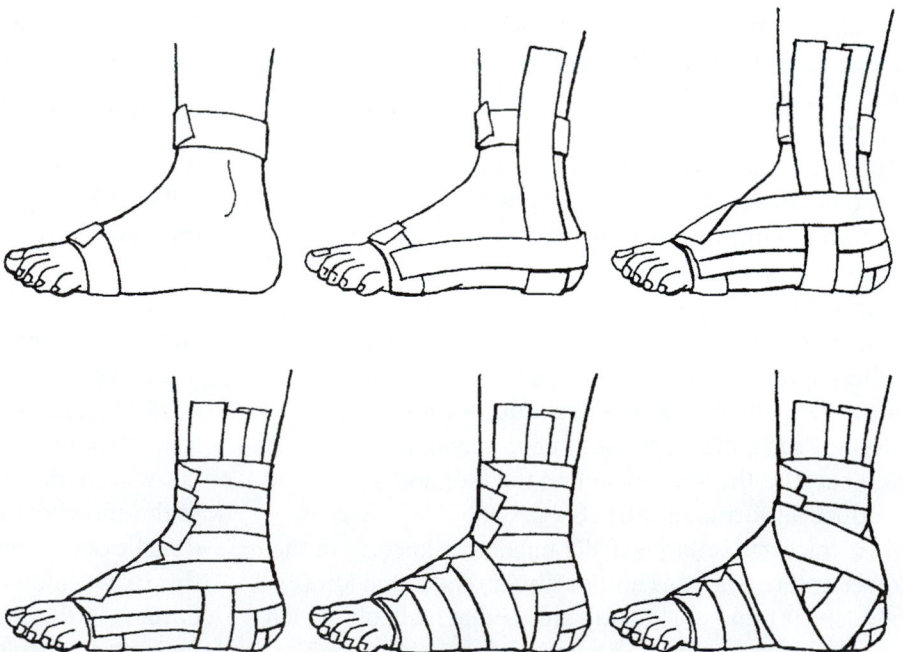

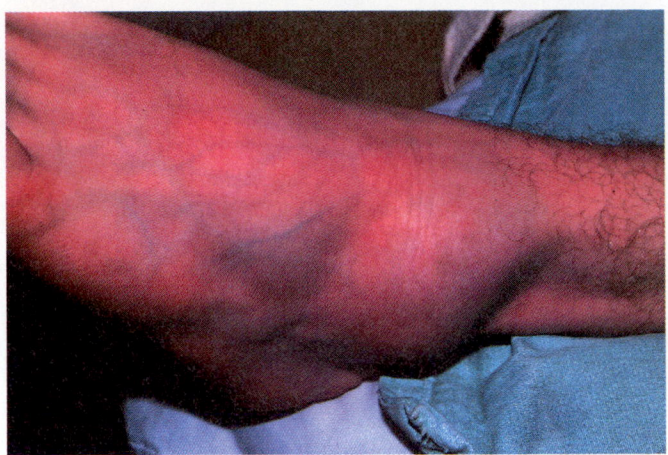

Figure 25-53 Swelling about the ankle is characteristic of sprains, fractures, and dislocations.

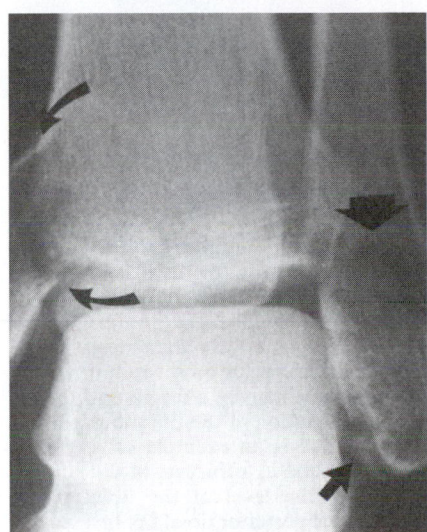

Figure 25-54 X-ray of a fracture of the medial and lateral ankle malleoli.

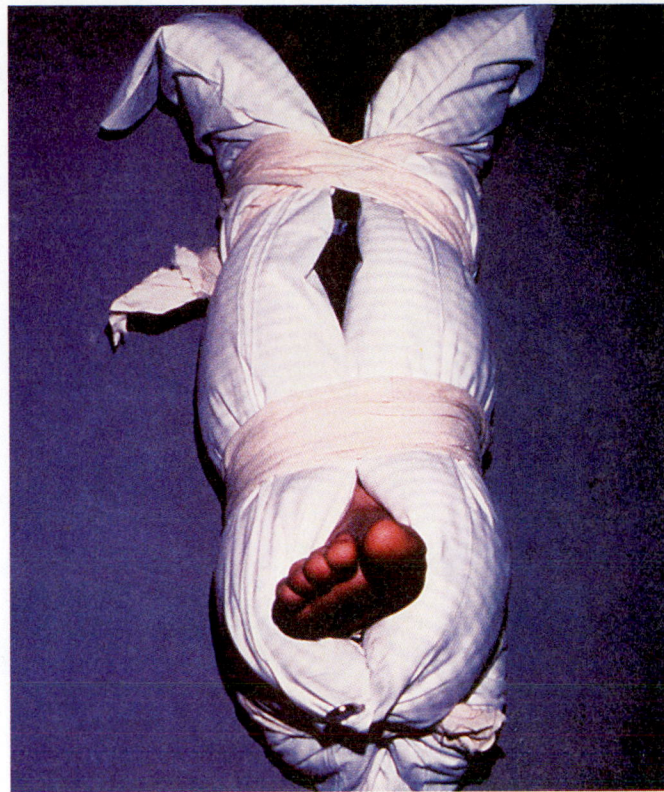

Figure 25-55 A pillow splint for ankle injuries.

and are very often hard to distinguish from displaced fractures ► **Figure 25-56**. Assessment again reveals tenderness, swelling, and deformity of the ankle joint (usually severe), with pain on any attempted movement. A major injury can produce a flail (excessively loose) ankle.

Emergency care on the hill involves applying a rigid fixation splint that includes the knee and the foot. Once in the aid room, remove the boot and assess the circulation and nerve supply below the injury by feeling for the dorsalis pedis pulse, testing sensation over the foot, and having the patient move his or her toes. (The posterior tibial pulse is generally undetectable due to local swelling.) Splint the ankle in the position found. The best splint is probably a pillow, rolled blanket, or well-padded cardboard splint, secured with cravats or tape. Ask your rescue squad to transport the patient to a hospital without delay.

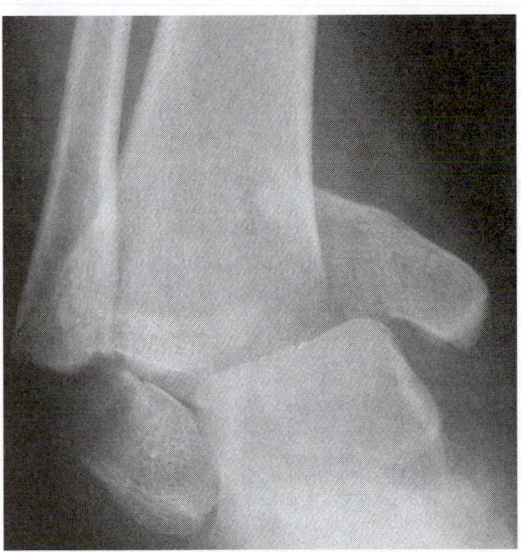

Figure 25-56 Anteroposterior X-ray of a fracture-dislocation of the ankle.

If the foot circulation and nerve supply are impaired and it will take more than an hour to reach the hospital, a single attempt to realign the injury in the position that gives the strongest pulse is justified. Use gentle longitudinal traction, grasping the forefoot with one hand and the heel with the other while a second rescuer steadies the

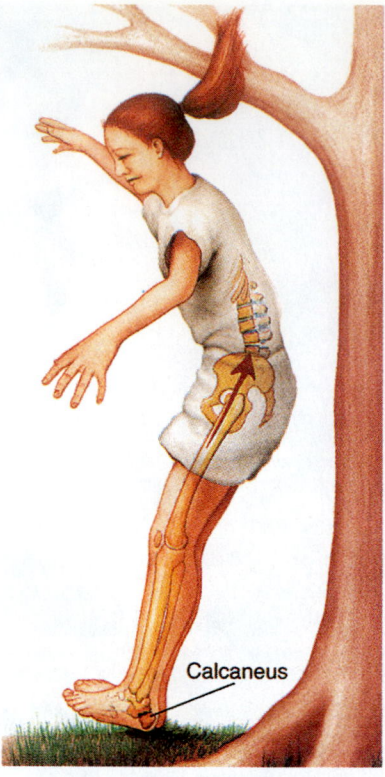

Calcaneus

Figure 25-57 The force of injury is transmitted up the legs to the spine, often resulting in a fracture of the lumbar spine.

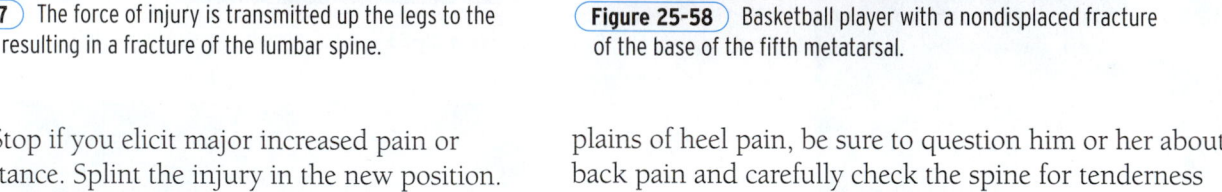
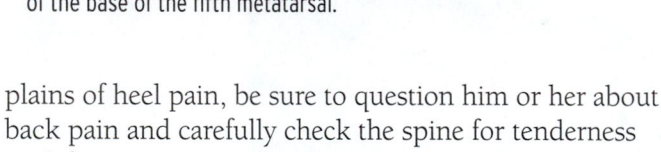

Figure 25-58 Basketball player with a nondisplaced fracture of the base of the fifth metatarsal.

lower leg. Stop if you elicit major increased pain or severe resistance. Splint the injury in the new position.

Foot Injuries

While uncommon in snowsports, recreational injuries to the foot frequently result in the fracture of one or more of the tarsals, metatarsals, or phalanges of the toes. Toe fractures are especially common. Sprains of the midfoot, and of the great toe metatarsophalangeal joint are also common in athletes.

Of the tarsal bones, the **calcaneus**, the heel bone, is the most commonly fractured. Injury usually occurs when the patient falls or jumps from a height and lands directly on the heel. The force of injury compresses the calcaneus, producing immediate severe pain, swelling, and ecchymosis. If the force of impact is great enough, as from a fall from a height, there may be associated fractures in other areas of the body as well.

Frequently, the force of injury is transmitted up the legs to the spine, producing a fracture of the lumbar spine, usually the L2 vertebra (▲ **Figure 25-57**). When a patient who has jumped or fallen from a height com-

plains of heel pain, be sure to question him or her about back pain and carefully check the spine for tenderness or deformity.

Fractures at the base of the fifth metatarsal in the foot occur regularly in those who participate in "jumping sports" such as basketball. The foot-inversion mechanism seen in ankle sprains is the culprit in this injury. In addition, the force is centered more on the midfoot than at the ankle (▲ **Figure 25-58**).

Fatigue fractures, also known as "stress fractures," of the metatarsals occur in long-distance runners, joggers, and hikers who carry heavy packs (▶ **Figure 25-59**).

Traumatic injuries of the foot are usually associated with pain, tenderness, and swelling, but rarely with gross deformity. Ecchymosis may develop later. In the case of a fatigue fracture, the only symptom may be pain in the forefoot increased by walking or running, and the only sign may be tenderness over the fracture site, most commonly the third or fourth metatarsal neck.

Vascular injuries in the foot are not common. However, as in the hand, lacerations about the ankle and foot may damage important underlying nerves and

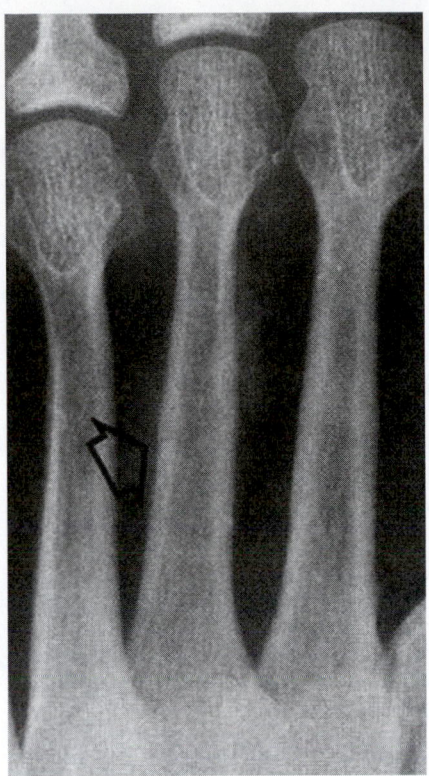

Figure 25-59 Healing stress fracture of the fourth metatarsal neck.

tendons. Puncture wounds of the foot are common and may cause serious infection if not treated early. All of these injuries must be evaluated by a physician.

A patient with a fractured foot should use a cane or crutches to avoid placing weight on the injured foot. If there is little swelling, the patient's boot or shoe can be used to protect and splint the injury. Suspected fractures should be splinted with a folded pillow, tightly rolled blanket, or, if the patient is on the hill, with a quick splint. When the patient is transported in a toboggan, elevate the foot approximately 6″ to minimize swelling. All patients with significant lower extremity injuries should be transported in the supine position with the injury facing uphill to allow for elevation of the limb, unless there are other medical reasons to place the injury downhill. If a patient has fallen from a height and complains of heel pain, use a long backboard to stabilize any possible spinal injury in addition to splinting the foot.

Chapter *Sweep*

Ready for Review

It is mainly falls, collisions, and direct blows that cause extremity injuries. The extent and type of injury depend on the age of the patient; the type, direction, and magnitude of the forces involved; the position of the extremity at the time of injury; the condition of the ground surface; and whether the equipment introducing a lever arm is involved. In the outdoors, upper extremity injuries typically result from a fall onto the outstretched hand, although skiers and snowboarders can also sustain these injuries during collisions. Because of their size and requirement to support weight, the bones of the lower extremity can potentially sustain greater adverse forces without injury. However, this usually means that when the bones and joints of the lower extremity are injured, the causative forces are more violent, and the accompanying tissue damage extensive. Therefore, in lower extremity injuries, rescuers must be especially vigilant to assess adjacent anatomic areas for damage. Thumb ligament injury is one of the most common upper extremity injuries in skiing. In snowboarders, wrist fracture or dislocation is one of the more frequently assessed upper extremity injuries. The most common injury in snowsports continues to be the knee ligament sprain. In outdoor sports, isolated sprains of the elbow and wrist are not typical and usually represent hard-to-detect fractures.

Extremity injuries that occur close to a joint may be particularly serious because of possible injury to adjacent neurovascular structures that cross these areas. This is significant in the upper extremity where vessels/nerves key to hand function come in close contact with both the elbow and wrist joints. All outdoor sport injuries of the hand should be evaluated promptly by a physician (preferably an orthopaedist or hand surgeon).

Accurate assessment and efficient emergency care of extremity injuries allow prompt transport. If definitive medical care is available within 60 minutes of the occurrence of any extremity injury complicated by neurovascular compromise, immobilization in the position found and rapid transport is preferable to injury manipulation with the risk of further traumatic damage.

Extremity injuries are often associated with shock. When assessing any injury of the extremities in a conscious patient, if physically possible, always ask the patient to point with one finger to the area that hurts the most. Evidence of impaired circulation or nerve injury justifies an attempt to realign the extremity using gentle but firm traction.

In many types of upper extremity injuries, pain increased by movement causes the patient to self-splint the injured extremity in a characteristic manner. The patient internally rotates the upper arm, flexes the elbow, and holds the extremity against or near the chest wall while supporting the forearm with the opposite hand. On the hill, the sling and swathe is the useful stabilization device for upper extremity injuries, as is the quick splint for lower extremity injuries. The rescuer should splint an upper extremity injury to the thorax and a lower extremity injury to the opposite uninjured leg.

Injuries to the lower extremity and pelvis are not rare among outdoor enthusiasts. Lower extremity fractures are even more serious than sprains. Whether they impact the pelvis, hip, or bones of the leg, knee, ankle, or foot, these injuries can be debilitating. Emergency care for pelvic and hip fractures require immobilizing the patient on a long backboard. Femoral shaft fractures are best treated using a traction splint. Emergency care for above-the-knee femur, patellar, lower leg, and ankle fractures consists of immobilizing the facture with a fixation splint. Foot fractures may suffice with improvised splinting materials. CMS function in the extremity below the injury should be assessed during the initial assessment, before and after splinting (or alignment, if this becomes necessary because circulation or nerve supply is impaired), and at regular intervals during the ongoing assessment.

Dislocations of the lower extremity are generally very painful and can be quite serious if they jeopardize circulation and nerve supply. Treat these situations as a serious emergency and rapidly transport the patient to the hospital.

Rescuer ingenuity is very important in the emergency care of difficult to manage extremity injuries. Every patient with an extremity injury should be advised to promptly see a physician, especially if symptoms do not clear up within 24 hours.

Vital Vocabulary

acromioclavicular (A/C) joint   A simple joint where the bony projections of the scapula and the clavicle meet at the top of the shoulder.

calcaneus   The heel bone.

clavicle   The collarbone.

fibula   The outer and smaller bone of the two bones of the lower leg.

glenoid fossa   The part of the scapula that joins with the humeral head to form the glenohumeral joint.

humerus   The supporting bone of the upper arm that joins with the scapula (glenoid) to form the shoulder joint and with the ulna and radius to form the elbow joint.

position of function   A hand position in which the wrist is slightly dorsiflexed and all finger joints are moderately flexed.

radius   The bone on the thumb side of the forearm; most important in wrist function.

scapula   Shoulder blade.

sciatic nerve   The major nerve in the lower extremity; controls much of muscle function in the leg and sensation in the entire leg and foot.

tibia   The larger of the two lower leg bones responsible for supporting the major weight-bearing surface of the knee and the ankle; the shinbone.

ulna   The bone on the small finger side of the forearm.

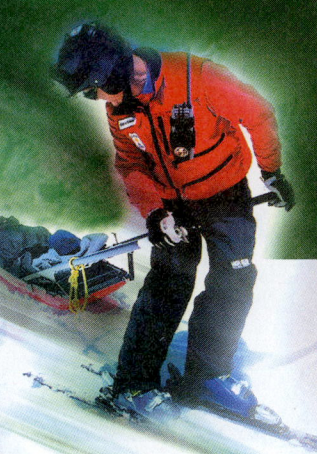

Assessment in Action

You are summoned to a "trails merge" intersection where you find that an 8-year-old snowboarder and an adolescent skier have collided. The rider is lying on her side supporting her right arm. Her elbow is deformed and held in about 40° of flexion. The skier is lying on the snow, sobbing in pain, with an angulated injury to his left thigh just above the knee.

1. The rider's upper extremity injury would be best splinted using a:
   A. sling and swathe.
   B. two board splints and a sling and swathe.
   C. long arm wire ladder splint and a sling and swathe.
   D. long arm cardboard splint.

2. Extremity fractures near a joint in children may be complicated by:
   A. injury to the growth plate (epiphysis) and bone growth retardation.
   B. injury to a major artery that crosses the affected joint.
   C. contusion of nerves that cross the fracture site.
   D. all of the above.

3. In an emergency situation, a fracture injury of the lower extremity can always be splinted:
   A. with a traction splint.
   B. with a ski pole.
   C. to the opposite uninjured extremity.
   D. with a rolled blanket.

4. Immobilization of displaced, angulated long bone extremity fractures often requires:
   A. two padded board splints.
   B. gentle in-line traction to realign the extremity before splinting.
   C. a reversed quick splint.
   D. splinting the injury "where it lies."

5. The most efficient way to determine where a person is injured is to:
   A. look for ecchymosis and swelling.
   B. palpate the zone of injury for the most tender spot.
   C. have the injured patient tell you where it hurts the most.
   D. ask the patient to point with one finger to the area that hurts the most.

Challenging Questions

6. Which of the two injuries described above is potentially more serious? Why?

Points to Ponder

You are on the slope caring for a middle-aged skier who has incurred an open fracture of his right tibia just above the boot. While attempting to place a pressure dressing on the open wound, your glove tears, and a small healing laceration of your index finger touches his blood. During the SAMPLE history, the skier relates that he is a carrier of hepatitis B. What precautions must you follow now? What is your area protocol for body substance exposure?

Issues Well-Being of the Rescuer, Safety, Patient Respect, Reporting Channels

Online Outlook

Because musculoskeletal injuries occur so often, you must be able to evaluate them properly. To improve your knowledge of assessment and emergency care of musculoskeletal injuries, complete Exercise 25 at www.OECzone.com.

www.OECzone.com

Head and Spine Injuries

Objectives

Cognitive

1. State the components of the nervous system (p 646).
♣ 2. List the functions of the central nervous system (p 647).
♣ 3. Define the structure of the skeletal system as it relates to the nervous system (p 649).
♣ 4. Relate mechanism of injury to potential injuries of the head and spine (p 650).
5. Describe the implications of not properly caring for potential spinal injuries (p 651).
♣ 6. State the signs and symptoms of a potential spinal injury (p 652).
♣ 7. Describe the method of determining if a responsive patient may have a spinal injury (p 651).
♣ 8. Relate the airway emergency medical care techniques to the patient with a suspected spinal injury (p 652).
♣ 9. Describe how to stabilize the cervical spine (p 653).
10. Discuss indications for sizing and using a cervical spine immobilization device (p 653).
11. Establish the relationship between airway management and the patient with head and spinal injuries (p 652).
12. Describe a method for sizing a cervical spine immobilization device (p 665).
13. Describe how to log roll a patient with a suspected spinal injury (p 654).
14. Describe how to secure a patient to a long spine board (p 654).
15. List instances when a short spine board should be used (p 656).
16. Describe how to immobilize a patient using a short spine board (p 657).
17. Describe the indications for the use of rapid extrication (p 657).
18. State the circumstances when a helmet should be left on the patient (p 668).
19. Discuss the circumstances when a helmet should be removed (p 668).
20. Explain the preferred methods to remove a helmet (p 668).
21. Describe how the patient's head is stabilized to remove the helmet (p 668).

Affective

♣ 22. Explain the rationale for immobilizing of the entire spine when a cervical spine injury is suspected (p 653).
23. Explain the rationale for utilizing a short spine immobilization device when moving a patient from the sitting to the supine position (p 656).
♣ 24. Explain the rationale for utilizing rapid extrication approaches only when they indeed will make the difference between life and death (p 657).
25. Defend the reasons for leaving a helmet in place while transporting a patient (p 668).
26. Defend the reasons for removing a helmet before transporting a patient (p 668).

Psychomotor

♣ 27. Demonstrate opening the airway in a patient with a suspected spinal cord injury (p 652).
♣ 28. Demonstrate evaluating a responsive patient with a suspected spinal cord injury (p 651).
♣ 29. Demonstrate stabilization of the cervical spine (p 653).
♣ 30. Demonstrate the four-person log roll for a patient with a suspected spinal cord injury (p 654).
♣ 31. Demonstrate securing a patient to a long backboard (p 654).
32. Demonstrate using the short board immobilization technique (p 656).
33. Demonstrate preferred methods for stabilizing a helmet (p 668).
♣ 34. Demonstrate helmet removal techniques (p 668).

♣ These are core concepts in initial patrol training.

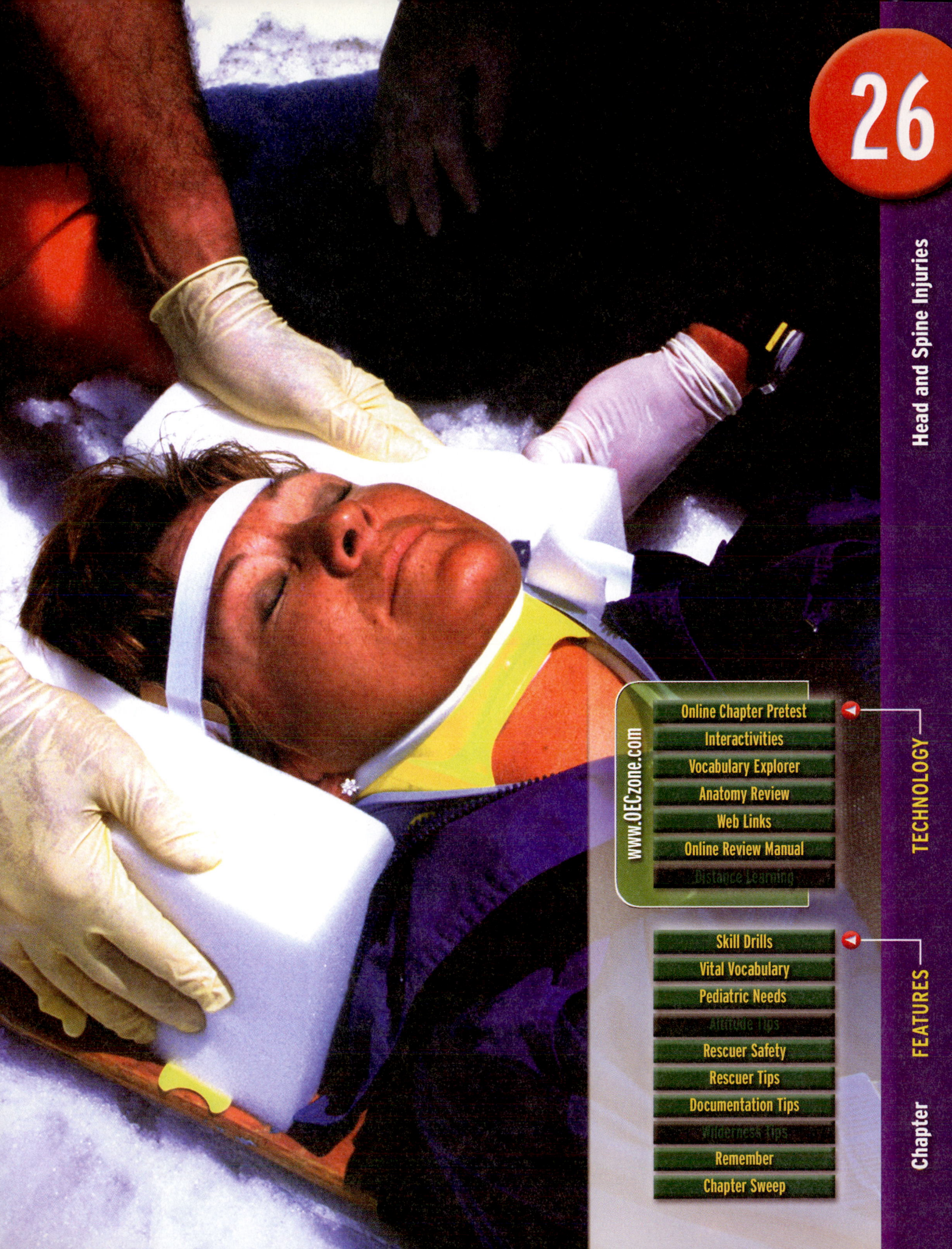

www.OECzone.com

Chapter

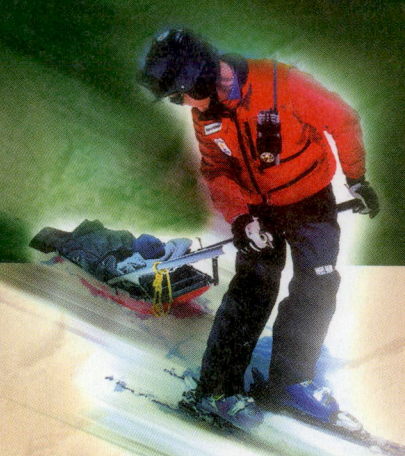

You are patrolling in the backcountry when you are requested to respond for a snowboarder who has inadvertently ridden off a 30' cliff. Upon your arrival, he tells you his chief complaint, along with neck pain, is that he "can't feel his legs."

Spinal cord injuries are among the most devastating types of trauma. This chapter covers the principles of good spinal care —assessment and stabilization—along with care for head and brain injuries. It will also help you answer the following questions:

1. Why is it important to take spinal motion restriction precautions for a trauma patient with a significant mechanism of injury but who has no neurologic deficits?

2. Describe the physical findings and complaints that might make you suspect that your patient has a brain injury.

Head and Spine Injuries

The nervous system is a complex network of nerve cells that enables a person to interpret the environment (sensation) and react (motion) to it. It includes the brain, the spinal cord, and several billion nerve fibers that carry information to and from all parts of the body. Because the nervous system is so vital, it is well protected. The brain lies within the skull, and the spinal cord is inside the bony spinal canal. Despite this protection, serious blows can damage the nervous system.

This chapter first briefly reviews the anatomy and function of the central and peripheral nervous systems and of the protective skeletal system—knowledge that

you will need to make an accurate assessment of injuries to these systems. It then discusses specific head and spinal injuries, including signs, symptoms, and treatment. Extrication of patients with possible spinal injuries and removal of helmets are also described.

Anatomy and Physiology of the Nervous System

The nervous system is divided into two anatomic parts: the central nervous system and the peripheral nervous system ▼ Figure 26-1 . The **central nervous system (CNS)** consists of the brain and spinal cord. The skull and vertebrae cover the brain and spinal cord for

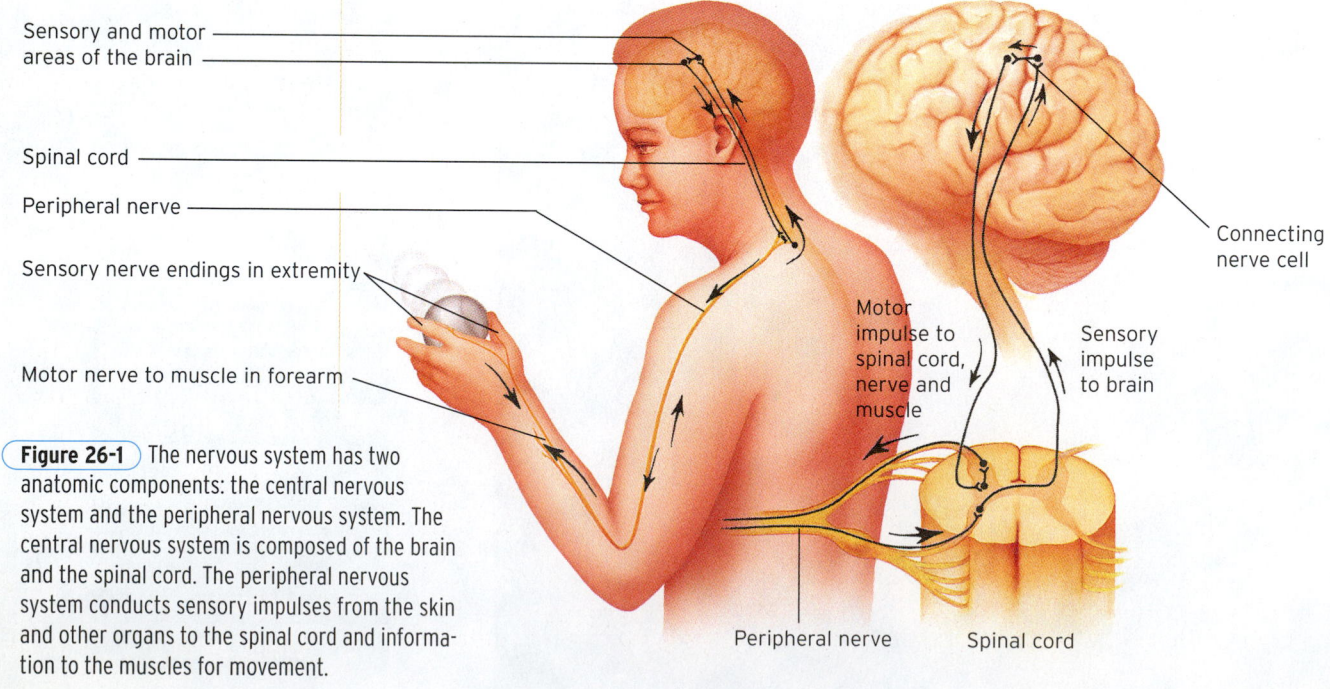

Sensory and motor areas of the brain

Spinal cord

Peripheral nerve

Sensory nerve endings in extremity

Motor nerve to muscle in forearm

Connecting nerve cell

Motor impulse to spinal cord, nerve and muscle

Sensory impulse to brain

Peripheral nerve

Spinal cord

Figure 26-1 The nervous system has two anatomic components: the central nervous system and the peripheral nervous system. The central nervous system is composed of the brain and the spinal cord. The peripheral nervous system conducts sensory impulses from the skin and other organs to the spinal cord and information to the muscles for movement.

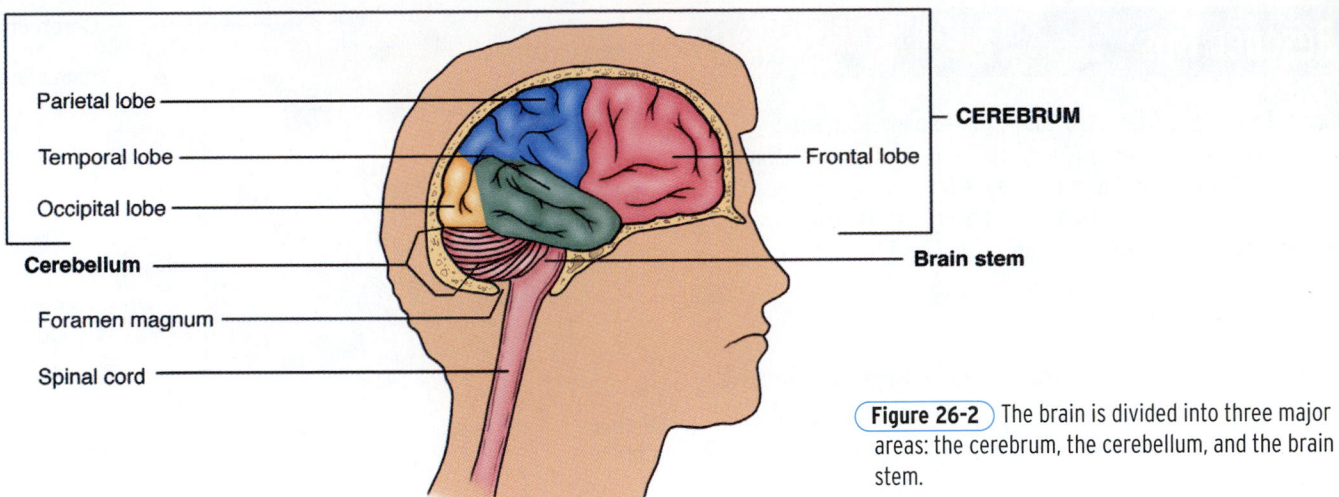

Figure 26-2 The brain is divided into three major areas: the cerebrum, the cerebellum, and the brain stem.

protection. Once the nerves exit the bony protection, they combine to form nerves that make up the **peripheral nervous system**. Long fibers of a neuron, or **axons** link the brain to the body's various organs, carrying information to the brain and reactions from the brain to the organs.

Central Nervous System

The CNS is composed of the brain and spinal cord. The brain is the organ that controls the body, the center of awareness. It is divided into three major areas: the cerebrum, the cerebellum, and the brain stem (▲ **Figure 26-2**).

The **cerebrum**, which contains about 75% of the brain's total volume, controls a wide variety of activities. Underneath the cerebrum lies the **cerebellum**, which coordinates smooth body movements. The most primitive part of the central nervous system, the **brain stem**, controls automatic functions that are necessary for life, including the cardiac and respiratory systems. Deep within the cranium, the brain stem is the best-protected part of the central nervous system.

The spinal cord, the other major portion of the CNS, is mostly made of fibers that extend from the brain's nerve cells. The spinal cord carries messages between the brain and the body.

Protective Coverings of the Brain

The cells of the brain and spinal cord are soft and easily injured. Once damaged, they cannot be regenerated or reproduced. Therefore, the entire CNS is contained within a protective framework.

The thick, bony structures of the skull and spinal canal withstand injury very well. The skull is covered by a layer of muscle fascia and scalp, skin, and galea—

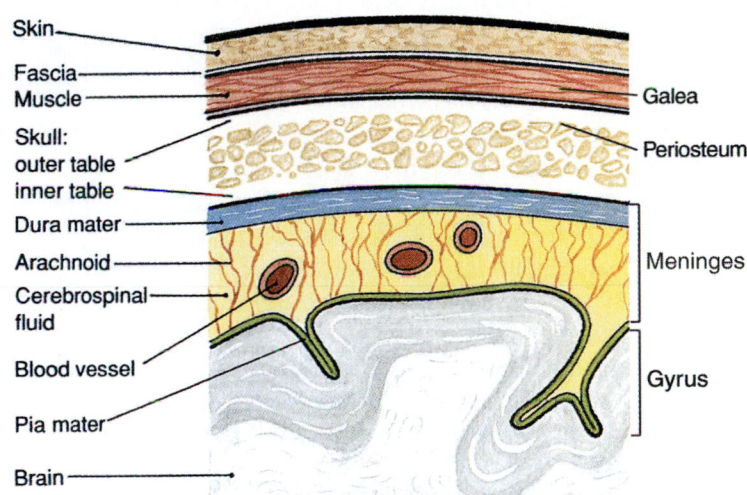

Figure 26-3 The central nervous system has several layers of protective coverings: the skin, bone, and the meninges. The three layers of the meninges include the dura mater, the arachnoid, and the pia mater.

a specialized fascia that allows the skin to lightly glide over the skull. The spinal canal, too, is surrounded by a thick layer of skin and muscles.

The central nervous system is further protected by the **meninges**, three distinct layers of tissue inside the skull that suspend the brain and the spinal cord within the skull and the spinal canal (▲ **Figure 26-3**). The outer layer, the dura mater, is a tough, fibrous layer that closely resembles leather. This layer forms a watertight sac that contains the spinal fluid in the central nervous system, with small openings through which the peripheral nerves exit.

The inner two layers of the meninges, called the arachnoid and the pia mater, are much thinner than the dura mater. They contain the blood vessels that nourish the brain and spinal cord. Cerebrospinal fluid (CSF) produced by the choroid plexus in the brain's fluid-filled sacs called the ventricles acts as an excellent shock absorber. The brain and spinal cord essentially float in this fluid, buffered from injury.

When an injury does penetrate all these protective layers, clear, watery CSF may leak from the nose, the ears, or an open skull fracture. Therefore, if a patient with a head injury has what looks like a runny nose or complains of a salty taste at the back of the throat, you should assume that the fluid is CSF.

Ironically, the very layers of tissue that isolate and protect the central nervous system can contribute to serious problems in brain injuries. Severe injury may cause bleeding of the vessels under the dura mater. This, in turn, causes blood to collect in this space (a subdural hematoma), increasing the pressure inside the skull and compressing softer brain tissue. In many cases, only prompt surgery can prevent permanent brain damage.

Peripheral Nervous System

The peripheral nervous system has two anatomic parts: 31 pairs of spinal nerves and 12 pairs of cranial nerves ▶ **Figure 26-4** .

The 31 pairs of spinal nerves conduct sensory impulses from the skin and other organs to the spinal cord. They also conduct motor impulses from the spinal cord to the muscles. Because the arms and legs have so many muscles, the spinal nerves serving the extremities are arranged in complex networks called plexuses. The brachial plexus, arising from the cervical spinal cord, controls the arms, and the lumbosacral plexus, arising from the lumbar spinal nerve roots, controls the legs.

Cranial nerves are the 12 pairs of nerves that pass through holes in the skull and transmit sensations directly to or from the brain. For the most part, they perform special functions in the head and face, including special senses such as sight, smell, taste, hearing, and movement of muscles for facial expressions.

There are three major types of peripheral nerves. The **sensory nerves**, with endings that can perceive only one type of information each (pain, temperature, and pres-

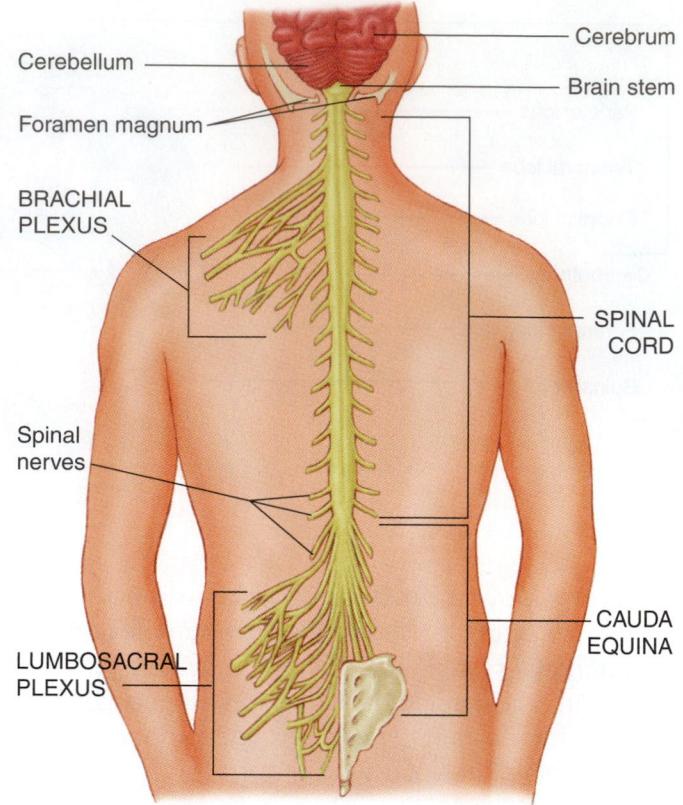

Figure 26-4 The peripheral nervous system is a complex network of motor and sensory nerves. The brachial plexus controls the arms, and the lumbosacral plexus controls the legs.

sure position), carry that information from the body to the brain via the spinal cord. The **motor nerves**, one for each muscle, carry information from the central nervous system to the muscles. The **connecting nerves**, found only in the brain and spinal cord, connect the sensory and motor nerves with short fibers, which allow the cells on either end to exchange messages.

How the Nervous System Works

The nervous system controls virtually all of our body's activities, including reflex, voluntary, and involuntary activities.

In connecting the sensory and motor nerves of the limbs, the connecting nerves in the spinal cord form a reflex arc. If a sensory nerve in this arc detects an irritating stimulus, such as heat, it will bypass the brain and send a message directly to the motor nerve, thus activating muscles to pull away ▶ **Figure 26-5** .

Voluntary activities are the actions that we consciously perform, in which sensory input determines the specific muscular activity—for example, reaching across the table for a salt shaker or to pass a dish. **Involuntary activities** are the actions that are not under the control of our will, such as respirations and heart rate; in most instances, we inhale and exhale without consciously

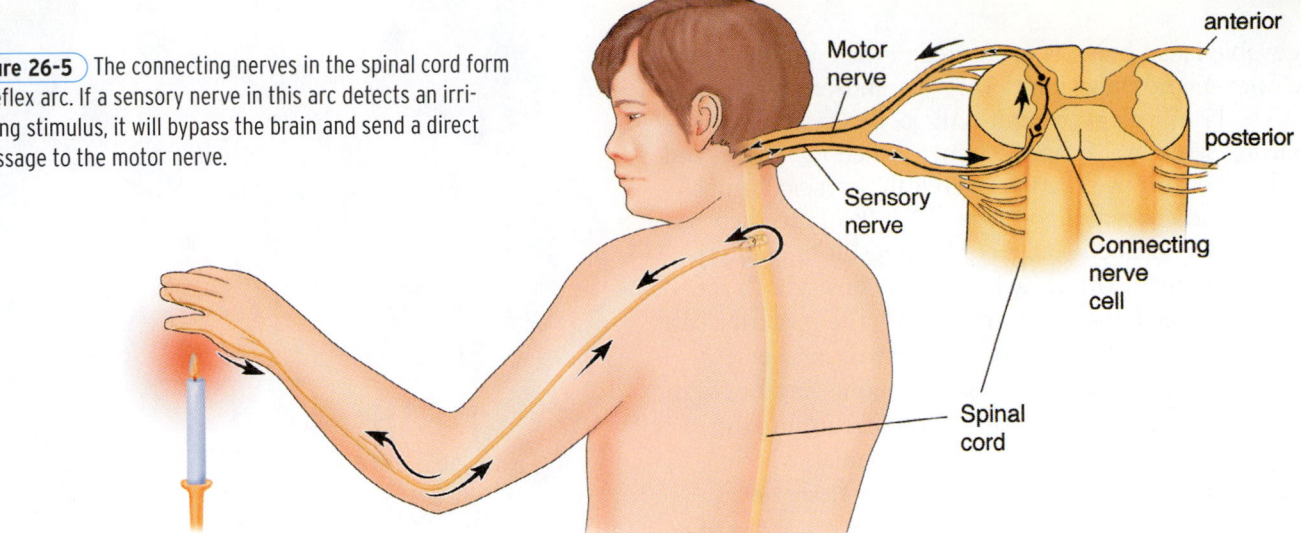

Figure 26-5 The connecting nerves in the spinal cord form a reflex arc. If a sensory nerve in this arc detects an irritating stimulus, it will bypass the brain and send a direct message to the motor nerve.

thinking about it. Many of our body's functions occur independently of thought, or involuntarily.

The part of the nervous system that regulates or controls our voluntary activities, including almost all coordinated muscular activities, is called the **somatic (voluntary) nervous system**. The mechanism of the somatic nervous system is simple. The brain interprets the sensory information that it receives from the peripheral nerves and responds by sending signals to the voluntary muscles.

The body functions that occur without conscious effort are regulated by the much more primitive **autonomic (involuntary) nervous system**. The autonomic nervous system controls the functions of many of the body's vital organs, over which the person has no voluntary control.

The autonomic nervous system, like so much in our nervous system, is composed of two parts: the sympa-

thetic nervous system and the parasympathetic nervous system. Confronted with a threatening situation, the sympathetic nervous system reacts to the stress with the fight-or-flight response. The parasympathetic nervous system has the opposite effect on the body, causing blood vessels to dilate, slowing the heart rate, and increasing digestive activity. These two divisions of the autonomic nervous system tend to balance each other so that basic body functions remain stable and effective.

Anatomy and Physiology of the Skeletal System

The skull has two layers of bone, the outer and inner tables, that protect the brain. It is divided into two large structures: the cranium and the face ▼ **Figure 26-6**. The mandible (lower jaw), the only

Figure 26-6 The skull has two large structures: the cranium and the face.

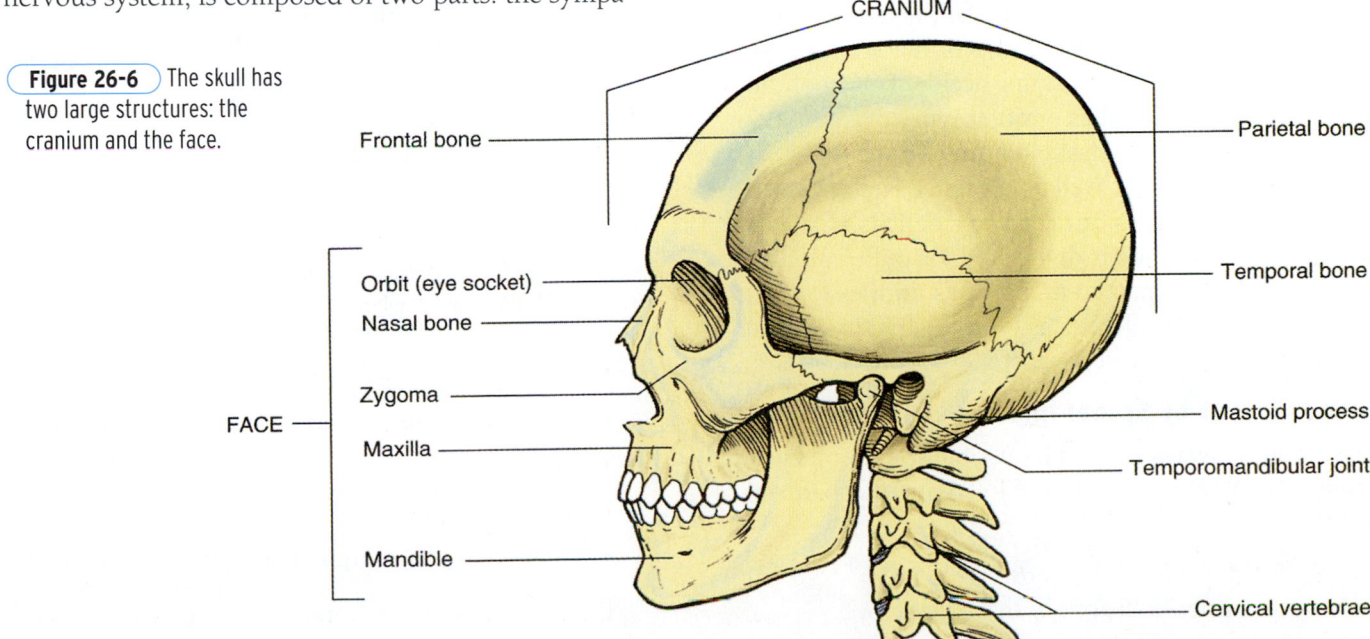

movable facial bone, is connected to the cranium by the temporomandibular joint (TMJ) just in front of each ear.

The bony spinal column is the body's central supporting structure. It has 33 bones, called vertebrae, and is divided into five sections: cervical, thoracic, lumbar, sacral, and coccygeal (▶ **Figure 26-7**). Injury to the vertebrae and associated spinal cord can result in paralysis.

The anterior part of each vertebra consists of a round, solid block of bone called the "body"; the posterior part forms a bony arch consisting of the two transverse processes and spinous process. From one vertebra to the next, the series of arches form a tunnel running the length of the spine. This is the spinal canal, which encases and protects the spinal cord (▶ **Figure 26-8**).

The vertebrae are connected by ligaments and separated by cushions, called **intervertebral disks**. While allowing the trunk to bend forward and back, these ligaments and disks also limit motion so that the spinal cord is not injured. When the vertebra is injured or fractured, the spinal cord and its nerves are left unprotected. Therefore, until the spine is stabilized, you must keep it aligned as best you can to prevent further injury to the spinal cord.

The spinal column itself is almost entirely surrounded by muscles. However, you can palpate the posterior spinous process of each vertebra, which lies just under the skin in the midline of the back. The most prominent and most easily palpable spinous process is at the seventh cervical vertebra at the base of the neck.

Injuries of the Spine

The cervical, thoracic, and lumbar portions of the spine can be injured in a variety of ways. Compression injuries can occur as a result of a fall, regardless of whether the patient landed on his or her feet, coccyx, or, as in some diving and skiing accidents, top of the head. High speed crashes or other types of trauma can extend, flex, or rotate the spine. Any one of these unnatural motions, as well as excessive lateral bending, can result in fractures or neurologic deficits.

Any time the spine is **distracted**, or pulled along its length, you can expect to find serious injuries to the spine. For example, hangings typically fracture the vertebrae high up in the cervical spine.

Assessment of Spinal Injuries

You should always suspect a possible spinal injury any time you encounter one of the following mechanisms of injury:

- Vehicle (snowmobile, car, motorcycle) crashes
- Snowrider collisions with objects
- Falls from heights

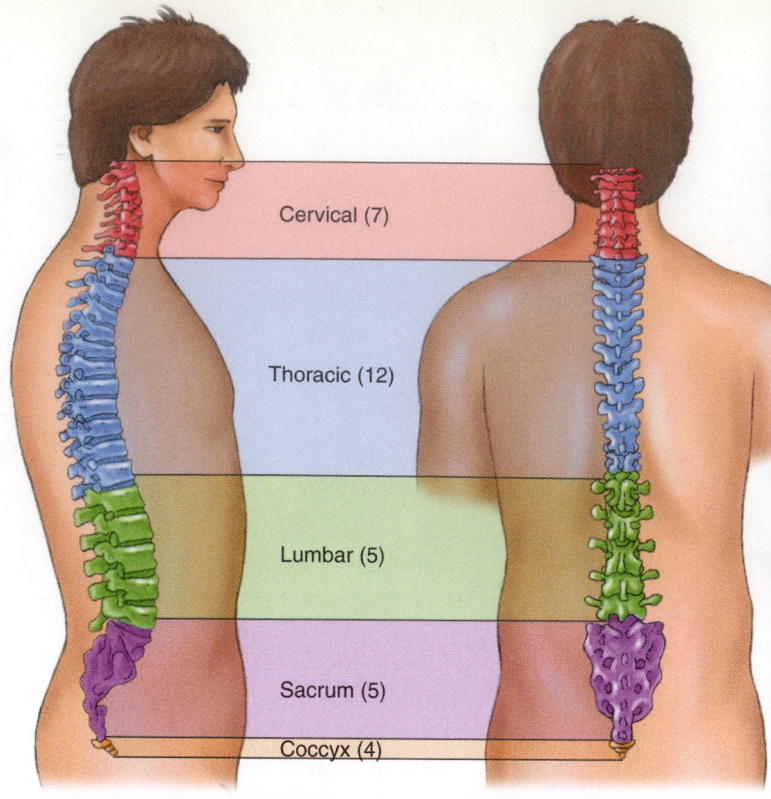

Figure 26-7 The spinal column is the body's central supporting system and consists of 33 bones divided into five sections. Injury to the vertebrae can cause paralysis.

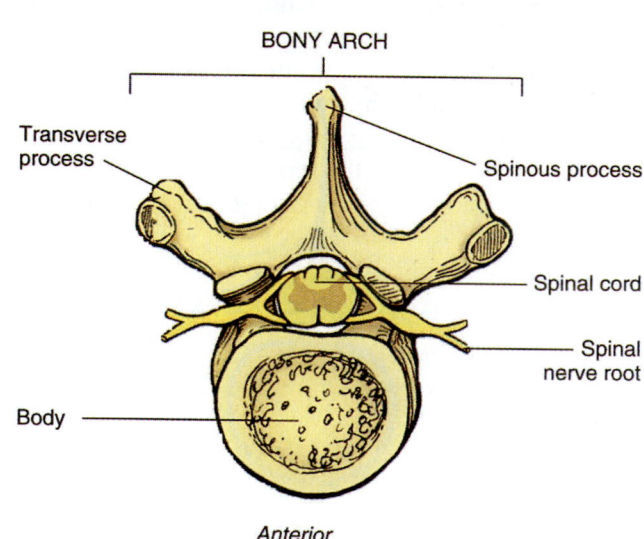

Figure 26-8 The spinal canal is formed by the vertebral body in the front (or anteriorly) and the bony arch in the back (or posteriorly).

- Blunt trauma
- Penetrating trauma to the head, neck, or torso
- Hangings
- Diving injuries
- High-speed recreational and sports accidents

If a trauma patient is unresponsive, you should always assume that he or she has a spinal injury. Take

If a trauma patient
is unresponsive, you should always
assume that he or she
has a spinal injury.

great care to avoid excessive and unnecessary movement that could cause further injury.

In fact, the safest approach to any injured patient, responsive or unresponsive, is to assume that the patient has sustained a vertebral injury that may injure the spinal cord, even if there is no pain or neurologic deficit. The reason is that complications of spinal cord injuries are serious, often leading to death or lifelong disability. Examples include respiratory failure resulting from direct injury to the brain stem or upper spinal cord, and partial or complete paralysis below the point of injury.

When assessing a patient for possible spinal injury, you should begin with an initial assessment, focusing on the ABCs. If the patient is responsive, make sure you ask about the mechanism of injury and about his or her symptoms, starting with these five questions:

1. What happened?
2. Where does it hurt?
3. Does your neck or back hurt?
4. Can you feel me touching your fingers? Your toes?
5. Can you move your hands and feet?

As part of your focused physical exam, inspect the spinal column for DCAP-BTLS: Deformities, Contusions, Abrasions, Punctures/penetrations, Burns, Tenderness, Lacerations, and Swelling. Make sure that you do not move any body parts excessively. Determine whether the strength in each extremity is equal by asking the patient to squeeze your hands and to gently push each foot against your hands ◄ Figure 26-9 . Finally, assess the equality of strength of the extremities by comparing the right limb to the left limb. If no deformities or fractures are detected and the patient is in no pain, ask the patient to lift the legs slightly off the ground. Gentle downward pressure on the limb will determine the strength of that extremity.

With unresponsive patients, you should try to identify the mechanism of injury. As part of your assessment, inspect the patient for DCAP-BTLS. First responders, family members, or bystanders may have helpful information, including when the patient lost responsiveness or what his or her previous level of consciousness was.

Remember that the ability to walk, move the extremities, or feel sensation does not necessarily rule out a spinal cord or vertebral injury. Nor does an absence of pain. Do not ask patients with possible spinal injuries to

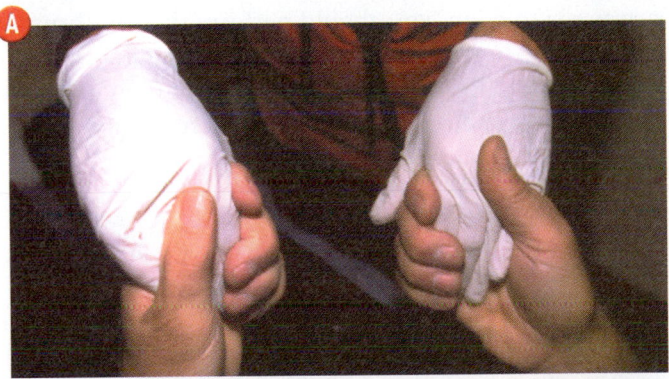

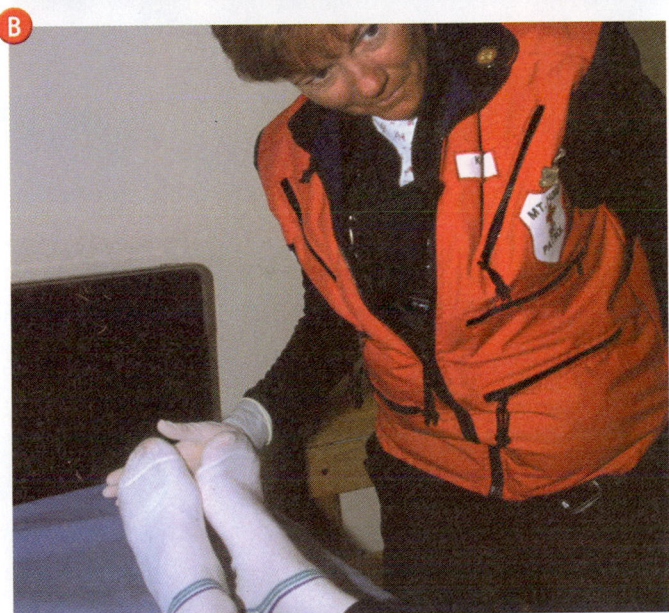

Figure 26-9 **A.** Assess the equality of strength of each extremity by asking the patient to squeeze your hands. **B.** Next, ask the patient to gently push each foot against your hands.

move their torso or spinal column as a test for pain. On the contrary, you should instruct them to be still.

However, pain or tenderness when you palpate the spinal area is certainly a warning sign that a spinal injury may exist. Patients with spinal injuries may complain of constant or intermittent pain along the spinal column or in their extremities. A spinal cord injury may also produce pain independent of movement or palpation.

Other signs and symptoms of spinal injury include an obvious deformity as you palpate the spine; complaint of numbness, weakness, burning or tingling in the extremities; and soft-tissue injuries in the spinal region. Patients with severe spinal injury may lose sensation or experience paralysis below the suspected level of injury or be incontinent (▼ **Figure 26-10**). Obvious injury to the head and neck may indicate injury to the cervical spine. Injury to the shoulders, back, or abdomen may indicate injury to the thoracic or lumbar spine. Injuries of the lower extremities or pelvis may indicate associated injury to the lumbar spine or sacrum.

Emergency Medical Care

Emergency medical care of a patient with a possible spinal injury begins, as does all patient care, with your

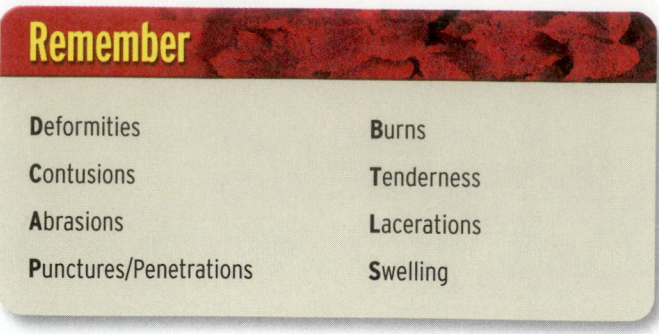

Remember

Deformities	**B**urns
Contusions	**T**enderness
Abrasions	**L**acerations
Punctures/Penetrations	**S**welling

protection; therefore, you must remember to follow BSI precautions. Next, you must maintain the airway in the proper position, assess respirations, and give supplemental oxygen.

MANAGING THE AIRWAY. Knowing that improper handling of a spinal injury can leave a patient permanently paralyzed should not prevent you from establishing an airway. Remember, all patients without an airway will die. If a patient with a suspected spinal injury has an airway obstruction, you should perform the jaw-thrust maneuver to open the airway while maintaining in-line spinal stabilization (▼ **Figure 26-11**). Do not use the head tilt-chin lift maneuver, as it extends the neck and may

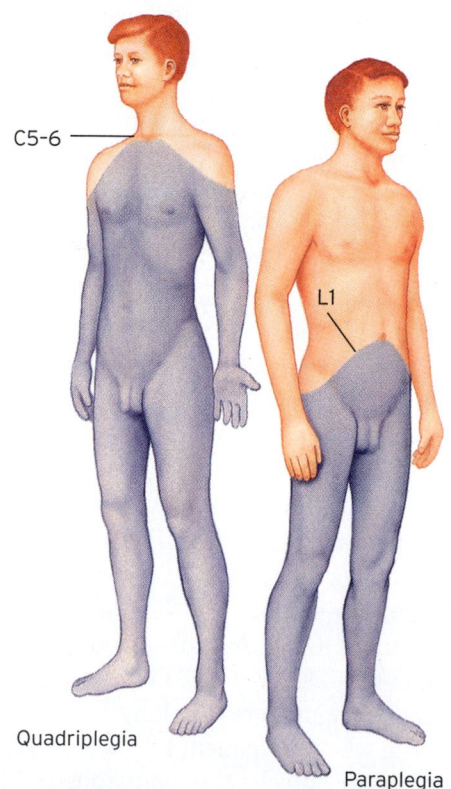

Figure 26-10 With severe spinal injuries, patients may lose sensation or experience paralysis below the suspected level of injury.

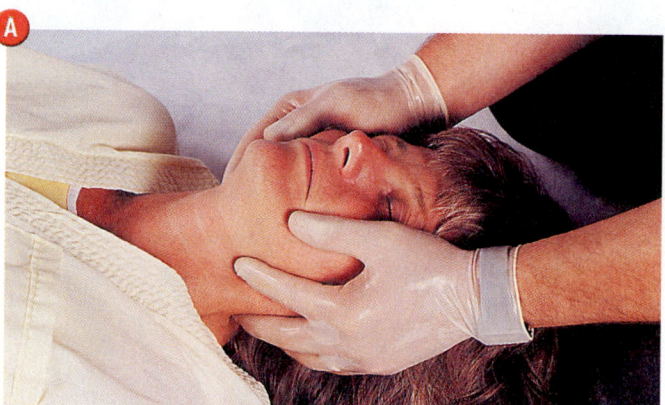

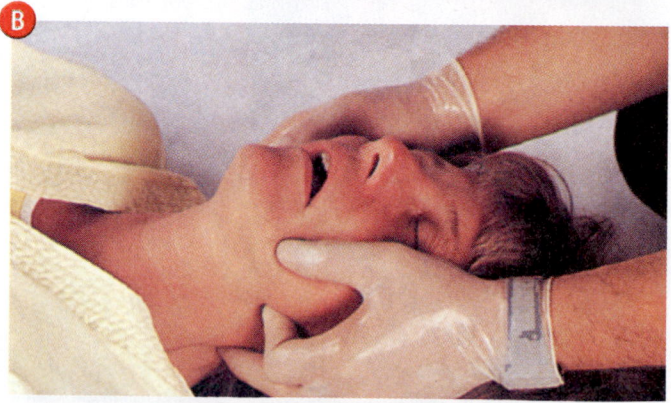

Figure 26-11 Jaw-thrust maneuver. **A.** Stabilize the neck in a neutral, in-line position. **B.** Push the angle of the lower jaw forward.

SkillDrill 26-1   Performing Manual In-Line Stabilization

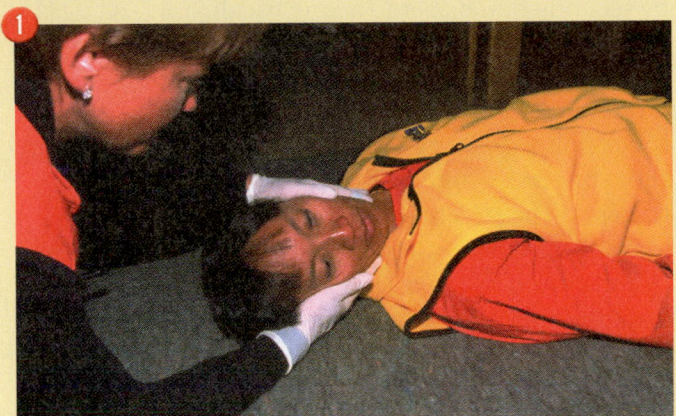

Kneel at the head of the patient and place your hands firmly around the base of the skull on either side.

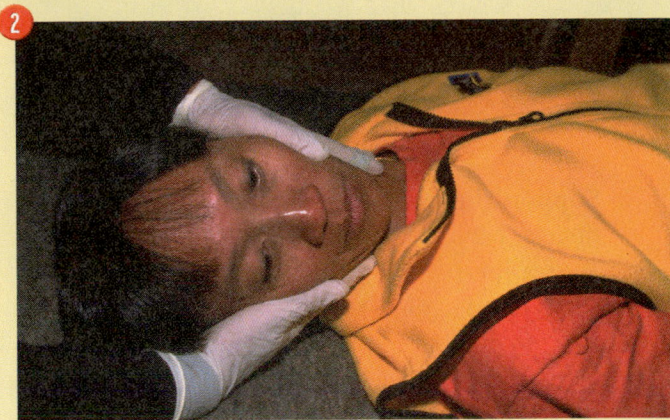

Support the lower jaw with your index and long fingers, and the head with your palms.

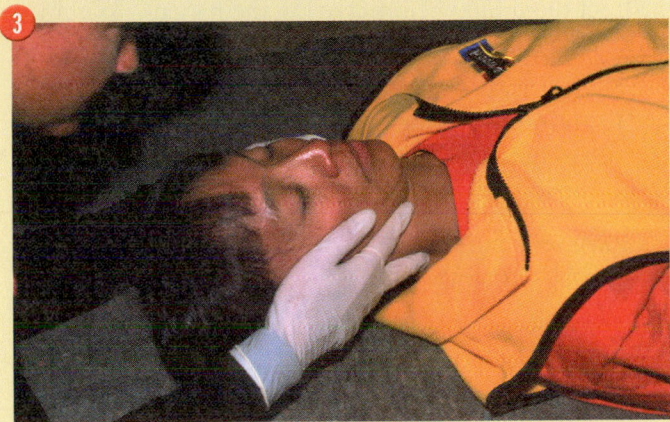

Gently align the head into a neutral, eyes-forward position, aligned with the torso. Do not move the head or neck excessively.

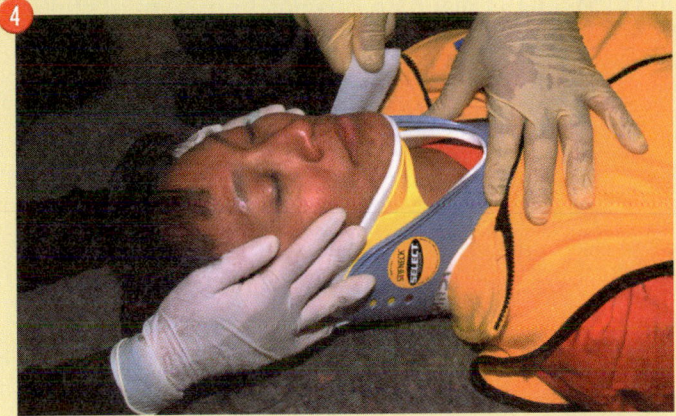

Continue to support the head manually while your partner places a rigid cervical collar around the neck. Maintain manual support until you have the patient secured to a backboard.

further damage the cervical spine. If the patient is unresponsive, you can lift or pull the tongue forward so that you do not have to move the neck. Once the airway is open, hold the head still, in a neutral, in-line position, until it can be fully immobilized.

After you open the airway, consider inserting an oropharyngeal airway. If you do so, be sure to monitor the airway closely and have a suctioning unit available as you will often need to clear away blood, saliva, or vomitus. Give oxygen to any patient who is having trouble breathing.

If you cannot open the airway because of the position of the head, realign the neck. Firmly grasp the patient's head with both hands, pull the head gently and firmly away from the trunk, and turn it to the front. Maintain

the head in this position while you or your partner repeats the jaw-thrust maneuver.

STABILIZATION OF THE CERVICAL SPINE. Stabilizing the airway is your first priority. You must then stabilize the head and trunk and in doing so stabilize the cervical spine so that bone fragments do not do further damage. Even small movements can significantly injure the spinal cord. Follow the steps in ▲ Skill Drill 26-1:

1. **Begin manual in-line stabilization** by holding the head firmly with both hands. Whenever possible, kneel at the head of the patient, and place your hands around the base of the skull on either side **(Step 1)**.

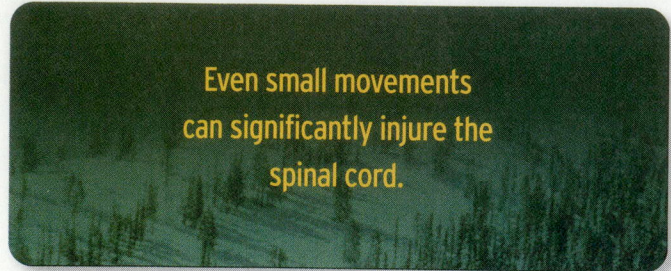

Even small movements can significantly injure the spinal cord.

2. **Support the lower jaw** with your index and long fingers, while you are supporting the head with your palms **(Step 2)**.

3. **Then gently align the head** until the patient's eyes are looking straight ahead and the head and torso are in line. This neutral **eyes-forward position** makes stabilization easier. Align the nose with the navel. Never twist, flex, or extend the head or neck excessively **(Step 3)**.

4. **Manually maintain this position** as you continue to maintain the airway. Have your partner place a rigid cervical collar around the neck to provide more stability. Do not remove your hands from the patient's head until the patient is properly secured to a backboard and the head is immobilized. The patient must remain immobilized until he or she is examined at the hospital **(Step 4)**.

Once the patient's head and neck are manually immobilized, assess the pulse, motor functions, and sensation in all extremities. Then, using observation and gentle palpation, assess the cervical spine area and neck. Keep in mind that the cervical collar is used to provide increased stability to the neck. It is used in addition to, not instead of, manual cervical spine immobilization. An improperly fitting collar can do more harm than good. If you do not have the proper size, place a rolled towel around the top of the head, and tape it to the backboard as you immobilize the patient on the board. In any case, maintain manual support until the patient is fully secured to a backboard.

There are some situations in which you should not force the head into a neutral, in-line position. Do not move the head if any of the following causes the patient to complain of pain:

- Muscle spasms in the neck
- Increased pain
- Numbness, tingling, or weakness
- Compromised airway or ventilations

In these situations, immobilize the patient in the position in which you found him or her.

Preparation for Transport
Supine Patients

A patient who is supine can be effectively immobilized by securing him or her to a long backboard. The ideal procedure for moving a patient from the ground to a backboard is the three- or **four-person log roll**. This procedure is recommended any time you suspect a spinal injury. In other cases, you may choose instead to slide the patient onto a backboard or use a scoop stretcher. The patient's condition, the scene, and the available resources will dictate the method you choose.

You should first take the necessary precautions and then direct the team from a kneeling position by the patient's head so that you can maintain manual in-line immobilization. Your job is to ensure that the head, torso, and pelvis move as a unit, with your teammates controlling the movement of the body. If necessary, you may recruit bystanders to the team, but be sure to instruct them fully before moving the patient. To immobilize a patient on a backboard, follow the steps in ▶ **Skill Drill 26-2** :

1. **Maintain in-line stabilization** from a kneeling position at the patient's head. This rescuer directs the log roll.

2. **Assess pulse, motor, and sensory function** in each extremity **(Step 1)**.

3. **Apply an appropriately sized cervical collar** **(Step 2)**.

4. **The other team members** should position the immobilization device (backboard) and place their hands on the far side of the patient to increase their leverage. Instruct them to use their body weight and their shoulder and back muscles to ensure a smooth, coordinated pull, concentrating their pull on the heavier portions of the patient's body **(Step 3)**.

5. **On command** from the rescuer at the head, the rescuers roll the patient toward themselves. One rescuer quickly examines the back while the patient is rolled on the side, then slides the backboard behind and under the patient. The team rolls the patient back onto the board, avoiding rotating the head, shoulders, or pelvis **(Step 4)**.

6. **Ensure the patient is centered** on the board **(Step 5)**.

7. **Secure the upper torso** to the board once the patient is centered on the backboard **(Step 6)**.

Skill Drill 26-2   Immobilizing a Patient to a Long Backboard

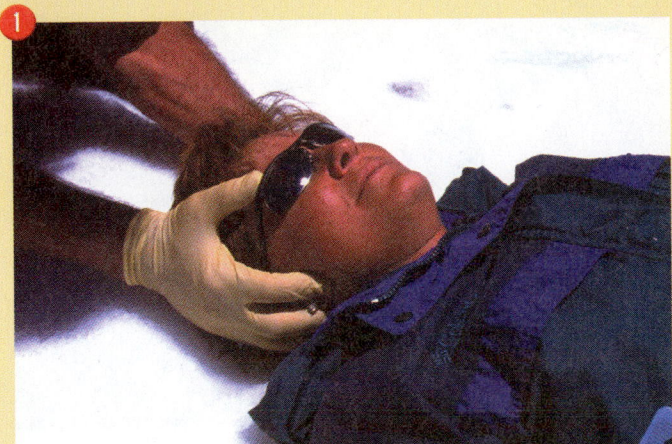

Apply and maintain cervical stabilization.
Assess distal functions in all extremities.

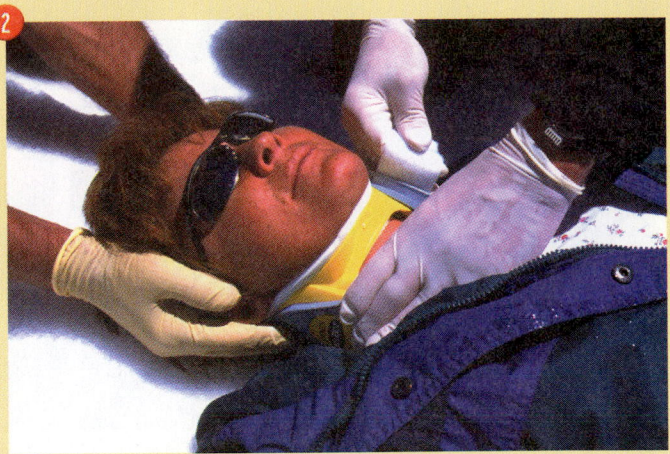

Apply a cervical collar.

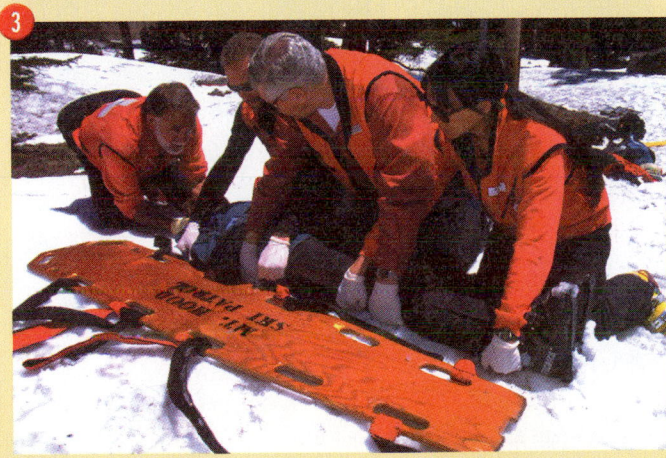

Rescuers kneel on one side of the patient and place hands on the far side of the patient.

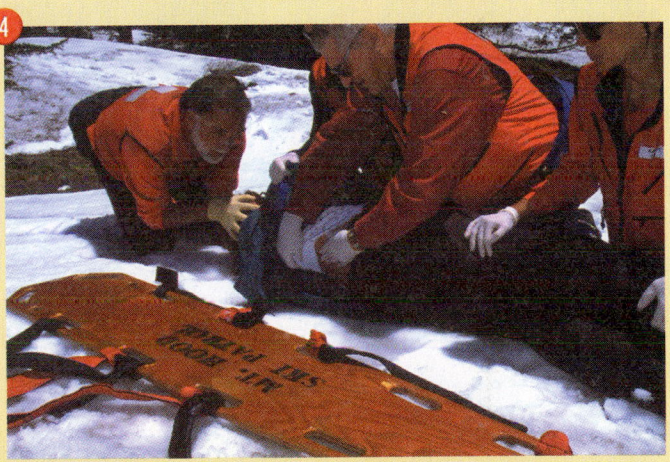

On command, rescuers roll the patient toward themselves, quickly examine the back, slide the backboard under the patient, and roll the patient onto the board.

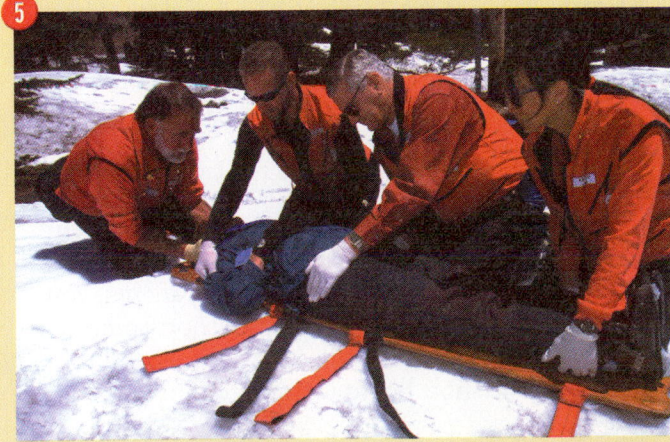

Center the patient on the board.

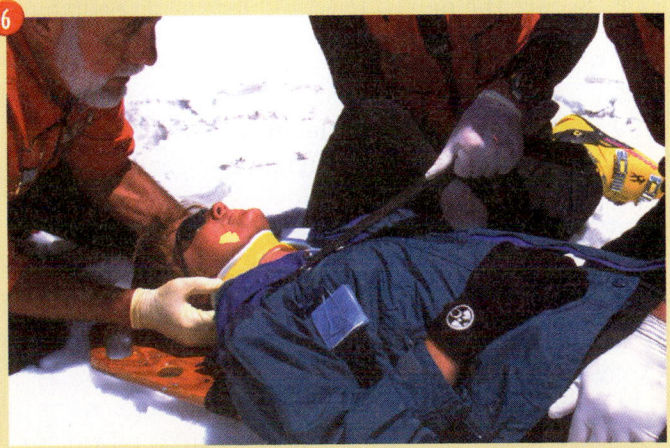

Secure the upper torso first.

Skill Drill 26-2   Immobilizing a Patient to a Long Backboard—continued.

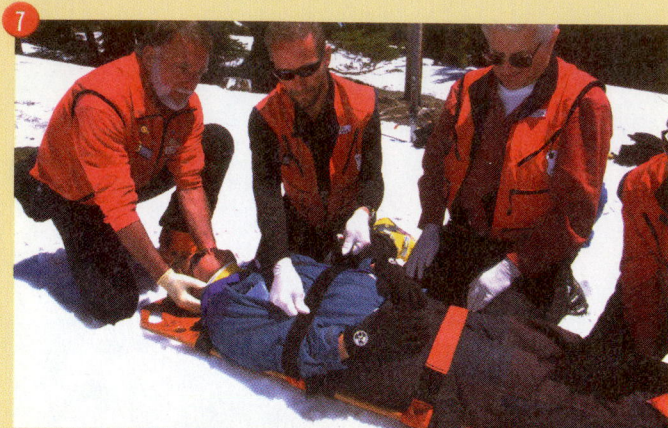

Secure the pelvis, legs, and feet.

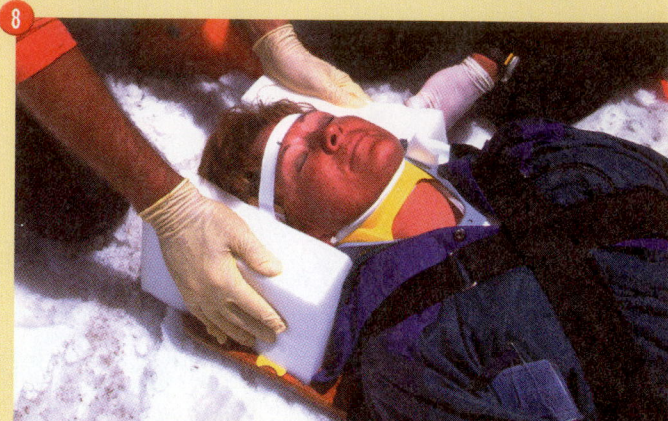

Begin to secure the patient's head using a commercial immobilization device, blanket roll, and/or foam blocks.

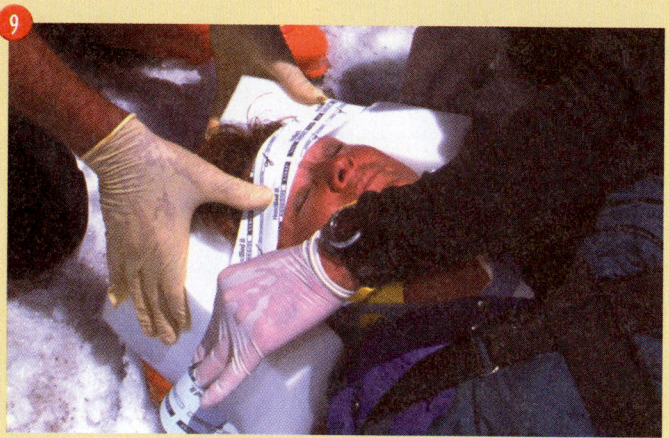

Place tape across the patient's forehead.

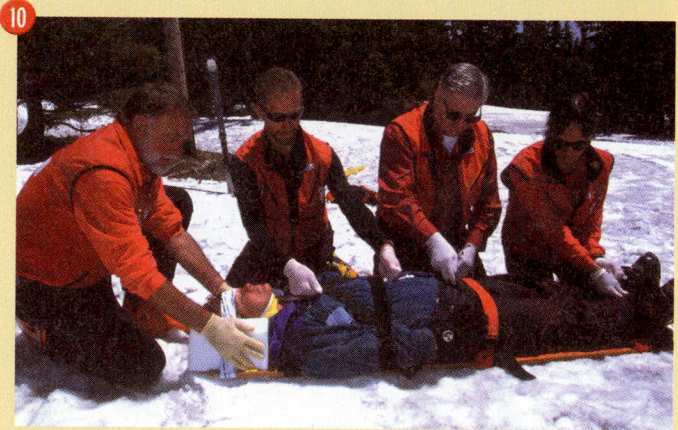

Check all straps and readjust as needed.
Reassess distal functions in all extremities.

8. **Secure the pelvis, legs, and feet** using padding as needed. For the pelvis, use straps over the iliac crests, and/or groin loops **(Step 7)**.

9. **Begin to immobilize the head to the board** by positioning a commercial immobilization device, or towel rolls **(Step 8)**.

10. **Secure the head by taping** the head-immobilization device or towels across the forehead. To prevent airway problems and leave access to the airway, do not tape over the throat or chin **(Step 9)**.

11. **Check and readjust straps** as needed to ensure that the entire body is snugly secured and will not slide during patient movement.

12. **Reassess pulse, motor, and sensory function** in each extremity, and continue to do so periodically **(Step 10)**.

Sitting Patients

Some patients with a possible spinal injury may be in a sitting position, wedged against a tree or rock. Often rescuers will simply come upon patients who have sat down following an accident. With these patients, you should use a short backboard or other short spinal extrication device to immobilize the cervical and thoracic spine. The short board is then secured to the long board.

The exceptions to this rule are situations in which you do not have time to first secure the patient to the short board, including the following situations:

- You or the patient is in danger.
- You need to gain immediate access to other patients.
- The patient's injuries justify urgent removal.

In these situations, your team should lower the patient directly onto a long backboard. Be sure that you provide manual stabilization of the cervical spine as you move the patient. Rapid extrication is indicated only in cases of life-threatening injury or loss of life or limb. In all other cases, follow these steps to immobilize a sitting patient:

1. As with the supine patient, you must **first stabilize the head** and then maintain manual in-line stabilization until the patient is secured to the long backboard.

2. **Assess pulse, motor, and sensory function** in each extremity.

3. **Apply the cervical collar**.

4. **Insert a short spine immobilization device** between the patient's upper back and the seat back.

5. **Open the board's side flaps (if present)**, and position them around the patient's torso and snug to the armpits.

6. Once the board is properly positioned, **secure the upper torso straps first** and then the midtorso straps.

7. **Position and fasten both groin loops** (leg straps). Check all torso straps to make sure they are secure. Make any adjustments necessary without excessive movement of the patient.

8. **Pad any space** between the patient's head and the board as necessary.

9. **Secure the forehead strap**, and then fasten the lower head strap around the cervical collar.

10. **Place the long backboard** next to the patient's buttocks, perpendicular to the trunk.

11. **Turn the patient parallel** to the long board, and slowly lower him or her onto it.

12. **Lift the patient** (without rotating him or her), and slip the long board under the short board.

13. **Secure the short and long boards** together.

14. **Secure the patient's legs and feet** to the longboard.

15. **Reassess the pulse, motor function, and sensation** in all four extremities. Note your findings, and prepare for immediate transport.

Standing Patients

You may arrive at a scene in which you find a patient standing or wandering around after an accident or injury. If you suspect that there may be underlying head, neck, or spinal injuries, you should immobilize the patient to a long backboard before proceeding to assess him or her. This will require three rescuers. Follow the steps in ▶ **Skill Drill 26-3** :

1. **Establish manual, in-line stabilization,** apply a cervical collar, and instruct the patient to remain still.

2. **Position the board upright** directly behind the patient **(Step 1)**.

3. **Two rescuers stand on either side** of the patient and the third is directly behind the patient, maintaining immobilization.

4. **The two rescuers grasp the handholds at shoulder level or slightly above** by reaching under the patient's arms while standing at either side **(Step 2)**.

5. **Prepare to lower** the patient to the ground **(Step 3)**.

6. **Carefully lower the patient** as a unit under the direction of the rescuer at the head. The rescuer at the head will have to make sure the head stays against the board and carefully rotate his or her hands as the patient is being lowered in order to maintain in-line stabilization **(Step 4)**.

Head Injuries

All head injuries are potentially serious. In any significant head injury, trauma to the cervical spine can occur. Stabilization with a cervical collar and backboard is necessary. If not properly treated, those that at first seem minor may end up being life threatening. On the other hand, severe lacerations of the scalp or fractures of the skull may occur with little or no brain injury and may produce minimal or no long-term conditions.

Scalp Lacerations

Scalp lacerations can be minor or very serious. Because both the face and the scalp have unusually rich blood

Skill Drill 26-3   Immobilizing a Patient Found in a Standing Position

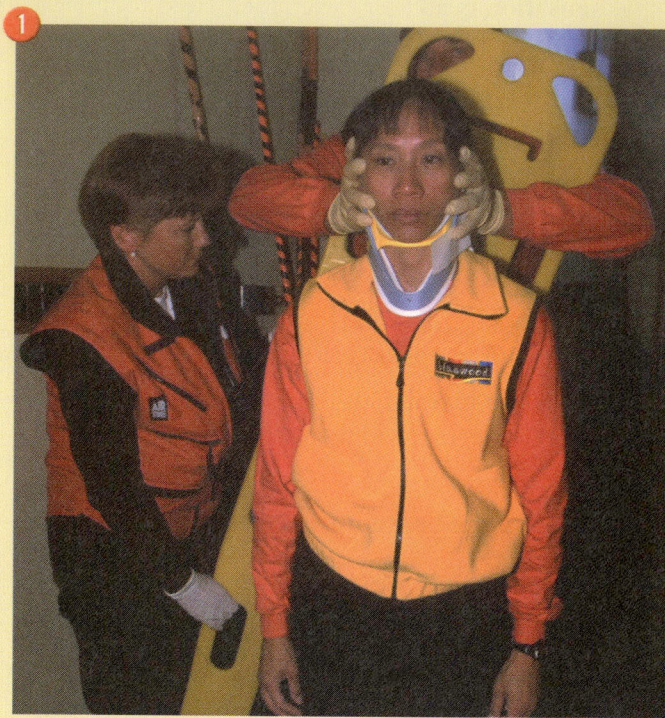

1 After manually stabilizing the head and neck, apply a cervical collar. Position the board behind the patient.

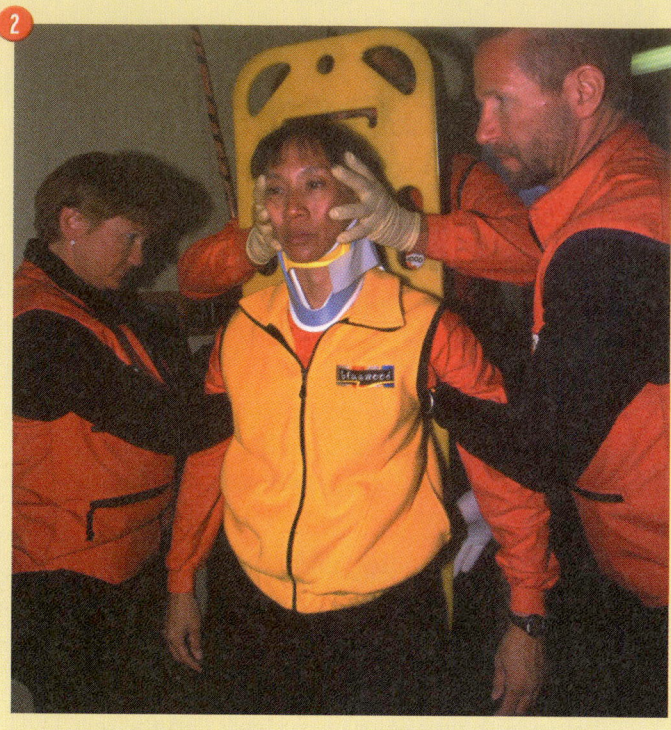

2 Position rescuers at sides and behind the patient.
Side rescuers reach under patient's arms and grasp handholds at or slightly above shoulder level.

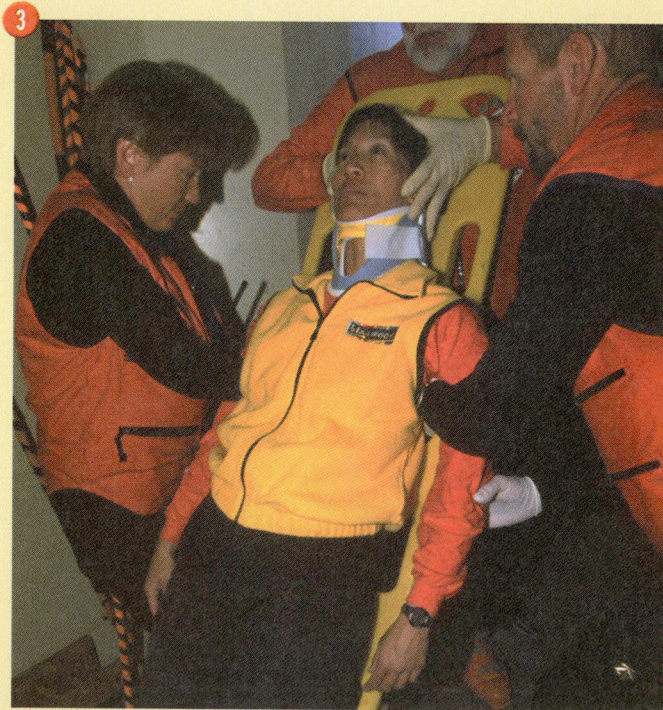

3 Prepare to lower the patient. Rescuers on the sides should be facing the rescuer at the head and wait for his or her direction.

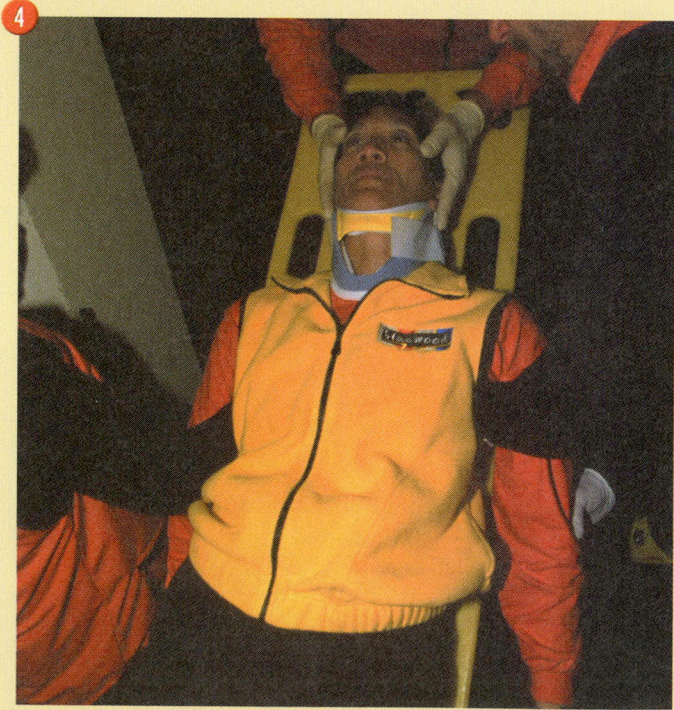

4 On command, lower the backboard to the ground.

supplies, even small lacerations can quickly lead to significant blood loss ▶ **Figure 26-12** . Occasionally, this blood loss may be severe enough to cause hypovolemic shock, particularly in children. In any patient with multiple injuries, bleeding from scalp or facial lacerations contributes to hypovolemia. In addition, since scalp lacerations usually result from direct blows to the head, they often indicate deeper, more serious injuries to the brain.

You can almost always control bleeding from a scalp laceration by applying direct pressure over the wound. Remember to follow BSI techniques. Use a dry, sterile dressing, folding any torn skin flaps back down onto the skin bed before applying pressure ▶ **Figure 26-13A** . In some instances, you will have to apply firm compression for several minutes to control the bleeding ▶ **Figure 26-13B** . If you suspect a skull fracture, do not apply excessive pressure to the open wound. Otherwise, you may increase intracranial pressure or push bone fragments into the brain.

If the dressing becomes soaked, do not remove it. Instead, place a second dressing over the first. Continue applying manual pressure until the bleeding is controlled, then secure the dressing in place with a soft, self-adhering roller bandage ▶ **Figure 26-13C** .

Skull Fracture

Fracture of the skull is an indication that a significant force has been applied to the head. As with any fracture, a skull fracture may be open or closed, depending on whether there is an overlying laceration of the scalp. Injuries from rocks, trees, and tree branches frequently result in fractures of the skull. The diagnosis of a skull fracture is usually made in the hospital by x-ray examination, but you can conclude that a fracture may be present if there is a significant amount of soft-tissue swelling or pain to palpation of the skull or face. A sign of basilar skull fracture that you may see is ecchymosis (bruising) that develops around the eyes (**raccoon eyes**) ▶ **Figure 26-14A** or behind one ear over the mastoid process (**Battle's sign**) ▶ **Figure 26-14B** . Cerebrospinal fluid dripping from the nose or an ear indicates a skull fracture.

Brain Injuries

CONCUSSION. A blow to the head or face may cause **concussion** or minor traumatic brain injury. There is no universal agreement on the exact definition of a concussion, but in general, it means a temporary loss or alteration of part or all of the brain's abilities to function without apparent physical damage to the brain. For

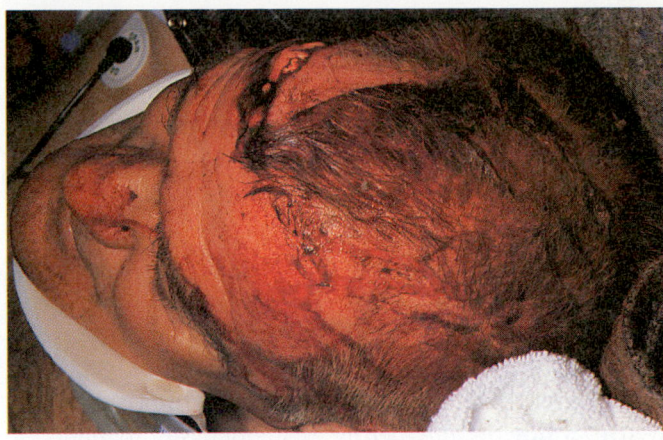

Figure 26-12 The scalp has an unusually rich blood supply; therefore, even small lacerations can result in significant blood loss.

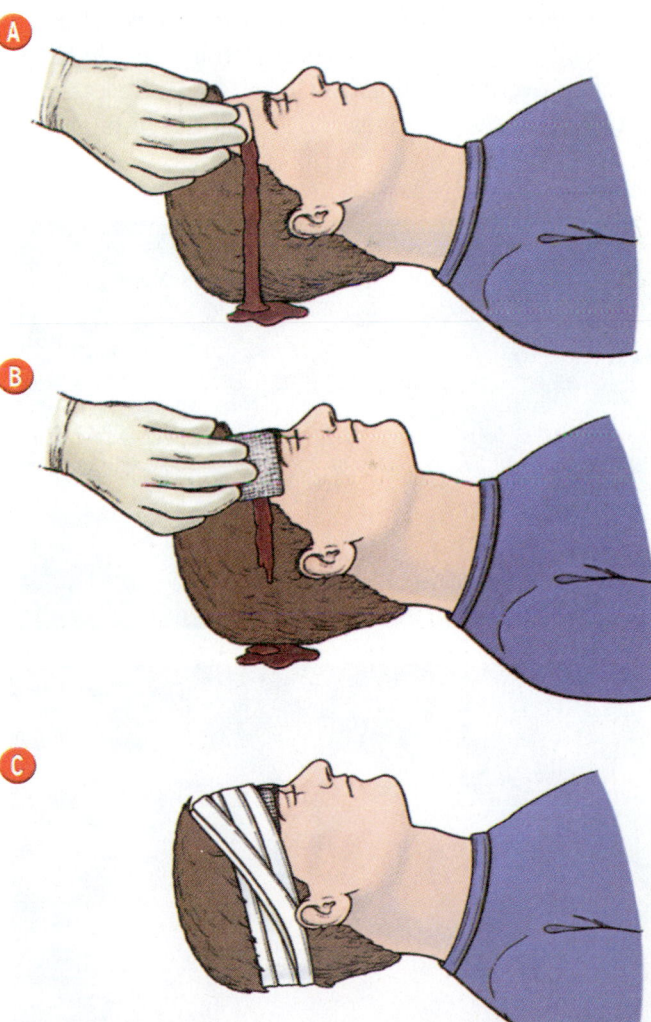

Figure 26-13 **A.** Apply pressure with a sterile dressing for lacerations to the head. **B.** Apply firm compression for several minutes to control the bleeding. **C.** Secure the compression dressing in place with a soft, self-adhering roller bandage. Remember cervical spine precautions.

example, a person who "sees stars" after being struck in the head has had a concussion that affects the occipital portion of the brain. A concussion may result in unresponsiveness and even the inability to breathe for short periods of time.

A patient with a concussion may be disoriented or have amnesia (loss of memory). Ask questions concerning orientation (person, place, date) that test memory. Occasionally, the patient can remember everything but the events leading up to the injury; this is called **retrograde amnesia**. Inability to remember events after the injury is called **anterograde (posttraumatic) amnesia**. Frequently, postconcussion patients will exhibit repetitive speech patterns. Commonly, the individual will ask "what happened" and shortly thereafter, ask the same question again and again. This can sometimes last for hours. This is called perseveration.

Usually, a concussion lasts only a short time. In fact, it is often over by the time you arrive. Nevertheless, you should assess mental status and ask about symptoms of concussion in any patient who has sustained an injury to the head; these symptoms include dizziness, weakness, headache, nausea, ringing in ears, or visual changes. Following any symptoms of concussion, the rescuer should follow local protocols in releasing a patient to continue their previous, or any, activity.

CONTUSION. Like any other soft tissue in the body, the brain can sustain a contusion, or bruise, when the skull is struck. A contusion is far more serious than a concussion, because it involves physical injury to the brain tissue, which may suffer long-lasting and even permanent damage. As with contusions elsewhere, there is associated bleeding and swelling from injured blood vessels. Injury of brain tissue or bleeding inside the skull can cause an increase of pressure within the skull. A patient who has had a brain contusion may exhibit any or all of the signs of brain injury described later in this chapter.

INTRACRANIAL BLEEDING. Laceration or rupture of a blood vessel inside the brain or in the meninges that cover the brain will produce intracranial bleeding (hematoma) in one of three areas (▼ Figure 26-15):

- Beneath the dura but outside the brain (a subdural hematoma)

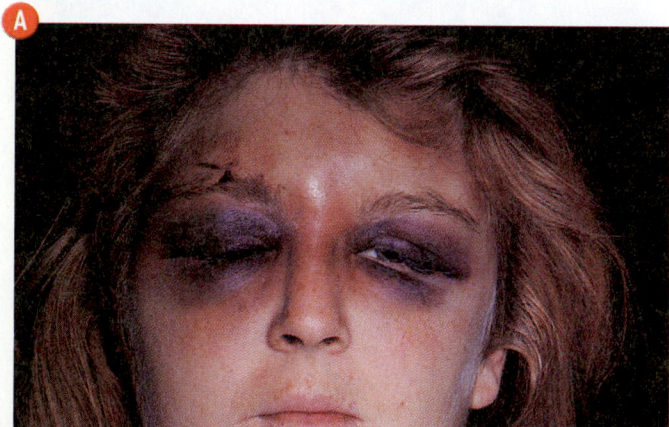
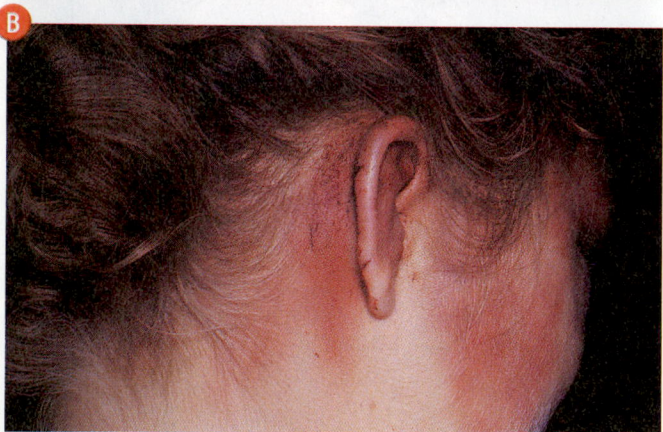

Figure 26-14 Skull fracture is a possibility if a patient has ecchymosis, **A.** Around the eyes (raccoon eyes), or **B.** Behind one ear over the mastoid process (Battle's sign).

TYPES OF INTRACRANIAL HEMATOMAS

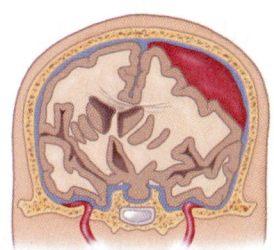
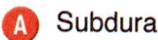

A Subdural

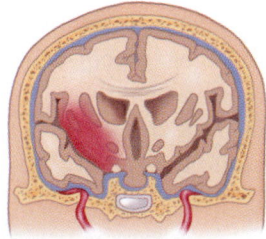
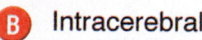

B Intracerebral

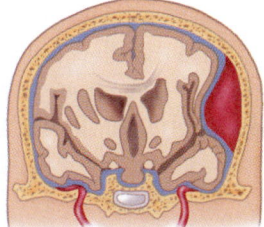

C Epidural

Figure 26-15 Intracranial bleeding can occur in one of three areas. **A.** Beneath the dura but outside the brain (subdural hematoma). **B.** Within the substance of the brain tissue (intracerebral hematoma). **C.** Outside the dura and under the skull (epidural hematoma).

- Within the substance of the brain tissue itself (an intracerebral hematoma)
- Outside the dura and under the skull (an epidural hematoma)

A hematoma may develop rapidly, usually because of arterial injury, as in an epidural hematoma; or it may develop very slowly, as with a subdural hematoma. In any case, because the brain occupies nearly the entire space inside the skull, the result is increased pressure inside the skull, leading to compression of the brain tissue. The expanding hematoma will cause progressive loss of brain function and, if not treated properly, death.

Rapid deterioration of neurologic signs following a head injury is a sign of intracranial hematoma. You must act quickly to evaluate and treat such patients. Maintain an airway in unresponsive patients, provide oxygen, monitor the airway, ensure spinal stabilization during transfer, and provide immediate transport.

Other Brain Injuries

Brain injuries are not always a result of trauma. Certain medical conditions, such as blood clots or hemorrhaging, can also cause brain injuries that produce significant bleeding or swelling. Problems with the blood vessels, high blood pressure, or any number of other causes may lead to spontaneous bleeding in the brain, affecting the patient's level of responsiveness. This is known as altered mental status. The signs and symptoms of nontraumatic injuries are the same as those of traumatic brain injuries, except that there is no obvious mechanism of injury or any evidence of trauma.

Complications of Head Injury

Cerebral edema, or swelling of the brain, is one of the most common complications of any head injury. It is also one of the most serious, because, as we have seen, swelling in the skull compresses the brain tissue, resulting in a loss of brain function.

Cerebral edema is aggravated by low oxygen levels in the blood and improved by high ones. Many patients with altered levels of responsiveness will not be able to maintain their airway. For this reason, you must make sure that the airway is open and that adequate ventilations and high-flow oxygen are given to any patient with a head injury. Do not wait for cyanosis or other obvious signs of hypoxia to develop.

Occasionally the patient with a head injury will have a convulsion, or seizure. This is the result of excessive excitability of the brain, caused by direct injury or the accumulation of fluid within the brain (edema). You should be prepared to manage seizures in all patients who have had a head injury. Another effect of cerebral edema and increased intracranial pressure may be increased blood pressure, decreased pulse, and irregular respirations.

A common response to brain injuries, even among children with very slight head injuries, is vomiting. This is usually the result of increased intracranial pressure. In managing such vomiting, you should pay particular attention to protecting the airway and cervical spine.

As was discussed earlier, the appearance of clear or pink watery CSF from the nose, the ear, or an open scalp wound indicates that the dura and the skull have both been injured. You should make no attempt to pack the wound, ear, or nose in this situation. Cover the scalp wound, if there is one, with sterile gauze to prevent further contamination, but do not bandage it tightly.

Assessing Head Injuries

Skier-skier collisions, skier-snow collisions, skier-tree collisions, and falls from heights are common causes of head injury. A patient who has experienced any of these events should immediately arouse your suspicion and cause you to start looking for specific signs and symptoms of brain injury. A deformed or dented helmet may indicate a major blow to the head, which is likely to have caused injury (▼ **Figure 26-16**). It is

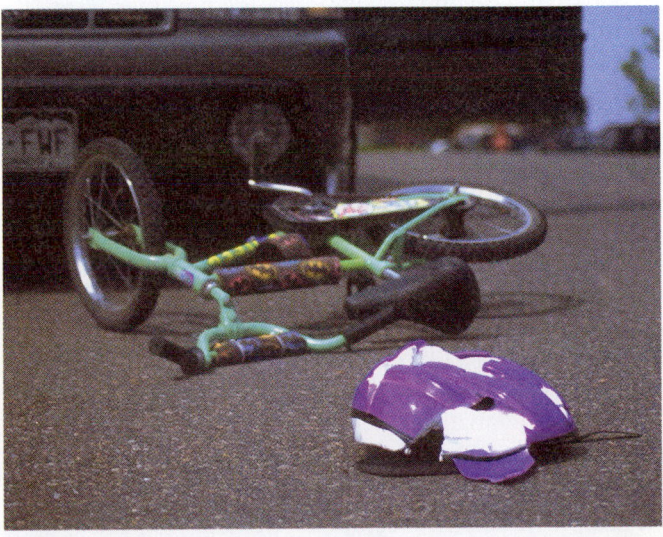

Figure 26-16 Helmet crushing or deformities are direct evidence that significant force has occurred to the head.

Follow local protocols pertaining to continuation of activity when releasing a patient who incurred a concussion.

especially important to evaluate and monitor the level of responsiveness in patients with suspected head injuries, paying particular attention to any changes that may occur.

Types of Brain Injuries

Blunt injuries, usually associated with trauma, are those in which the brain has been injured but the skin has not been broken and there is no obvious bleeding. In assessing a patient with a possible blunt injury, consider the mechanism of injury. Did the patient fall? Did the patient strike his or her head? Was it a high-speed impact? Was there deformity of the helmet? Look for scalp lacerations, contusions, hematomas, or skull deformities suggesting impact of the skull with hard objects. Sometimes, the skull will appear to have been pushed into the brain.

Decreased level of responsiveness is the most reliable sign of this type of injury. Monitor the patient for changes in level of consciousness, including signs of confusion, disorientation, or deteriorating mental status. Is the patient unresponsive or repeating questions? Experiencing seizures? Nauseated or vomiting? Next, assess the patient for decreased movement and/or numbness and tingling in the extremities. Assess the vital signs carefully. People with head injuries may have irregular respirations, depending on which region of the brain is affected. Look for blood or CSF leaking from the ears, nose, or mouth and for bruising around the eyes and behind the ears.

You should also evaluate the patient's pupils, especially if he or she has a decreased level of responsiveness. Often, unequal pupil size after a brain injury signals a serious problem. Developing blood clots may be pressing on the third cranial nerve, causing one pupil to dilate (▶ **Figure 26-17**). Be aware that this condition (anisocoria) occurs naturally in about 5% of the population.

Scalp contusions, lacerations, hematomas, and obvious skull deformities are all signs of **open head injuries**, which are often caused by a penetrating

object. There may be bleeding and exposed brain tissue. Do not probe open scalp lacerations with your gloved finger, as this may push bone fragments into the brain. Do not remove an impaled object. Securely splint it in place and arrange for transport to the hospital.

Signs and Symptoms of Brain Injury

Blunt and penetrating brain injuries have essentially the same signs and symptoms.

Following an injury, any patient who exhibits one or more of these signs or symptoms should be evaluated promptly in the emergency department:

- Lacerations, contusions, or hematomas to the scalp
- Soft area or depression upon palpation
- Visible fractures or deformities of the skull and face
- Ecchymosis about the eyes or behind the ear over the mastoid process
- Clear or pink CSF leakage from a scalp wound, the nose, or the ear
- Failure of the pupils to respond to light
- Unequal pupil size (anisocoria)
- Loss of sensation and/or motor function
- A period of unresponsiveness
- Respiratory distress from swelling or bleeding from the mouth or throat
- Amnesia
- Seizures
- Numbness or tingling in the extremities
- Irregular respirations
- Dizziness

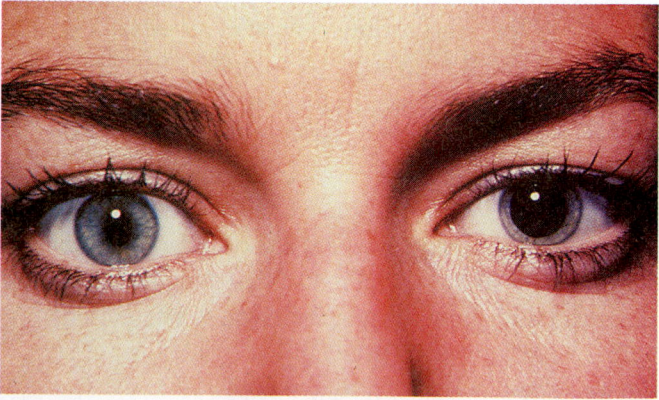

Figure 26-17 Assess pupil size if you suspect a head injury. Unequal pupil size may signal a serious problem.

- Visual complaints
- Combative or other abnormal behavior
- Nausea or vomiting

LEVEL OF RESPONSIVENESS. Change in the level of responsiveness is the single most important observation that you can make in assessing the severity of brain injury. Level of responsiveness usually corresponds to the extent of loss of brain function. As soon as you determine that a brain injury is present, you should perform a baseline assessment using the AVPU scale and record the time. Reevaluate the patient and record your observations every 15 minutes if the patient's condition is stable and at least every 5 minutes if the patient's condition is unstable.

Frequently, the levels will fluctuate, improving, deteriorating, then improving again over time. On other occasions, there is a gradual, progressive deterioration in the patient's response to stimuli; this usually indicates serious brain injury that may need aggressive medical and/or surgical treatment. The physicians who treat the patient will need to know when loss of responsiveness or a diminished level of responsiveness occurred. They will want to compare their neurologic evaluation with the one you performed in the field.

Your organization may choose to use the more detailed **Glasgow Coma Scale** instead of the AVPU scale to a assess a patient's level of responsiveness ▶ **Figure 26-18** . In either case, you should always use simple, easily understood terms when reporting the level of responsiveness, such as "does not remember events immediately preceding injury" or "confused about date and time." Terms such as "semicomatose" or "dazed" have different meanings to different people and should not be used in either written or verbal reports.

CHANGES IN PUPIL SIZE. The nerves that control dilation and constriction of the pupils are very sensitive to pressure within the skull. When you beam a bright light into the eye, the pupil should constrict. Inappropriately large or unresponsive pupils is an early and important sign of increased intracranial pressure. Unequal pupil size may indicate increased pressure on one side of the brain.

As soon as you have assessed the patient's level of responsiveness, determine the reaction of each pupil to light. Sketch the size of both pupils to indicate any difference between the two eyes. Continue to monitor the pupils and document the time and type of pupillary

changes. Any change in their reactions over time may indicate progressive brain damage.

Emergency Medical Care

Patients with head injuries occasionally have injuries to the cervical spine as well. Because cervical spine injuries can be devastating, keep in mind the need to protect and stabilize the cervical spine at all times when treating a patient with a head injury. Keep the patient lying down. Avoid moving the neck unnecessarily until the complete spine can be appropriately stabilized. An initial assessment with spinal immobilization should be done on scene with a complete, detailed physical examination done inside.

Beyond this, you should treat the patient with a brain injury according to three general principles, which are

GLASGOW COMA SCALE

Eye Opening

Spontaneous	4
To Voice	3
To Pain	2
None	1

Verbal Response

Oriented	5
Confused	4
Inappropriate Words	3
Incomprehensible Words	2
None	1

Motor Response

Obeys Command	6
Localizes Pain	5
Withdraws (pain)	4
Flexion (pain)	3
Extension (pain)	2
None	1

Glasgow Coma Score Total	**15**

Figure 26-18 The Glasgow Coma Scale is one method of evaluating level of responsiveness. Note that the lower the score, the more severe the extent of brain injury.

> Change in the level of responsiveness is the single most important observation you can make in assessing the severity of brain injury.

designed to protect and maintain the critical functions of the central nervous system:

1. **Establish an adequate airway.** Remember that unresponsive patients cannot maintain their own airway. Transport of these patients requires continuous and constant monitoring while riding in a toboggan or other evacuation device. If necessary, begin and maintain ventilation and always provide high-flow supplemental oxygen.

2. **Control bleeding**, and provide adequate circulation to maintain cerebral perfusion. Begin CPR, if necessary. Be sure to follow BSI precautions.

3. **Assess the patient's baseline** level of responsiveness, and continuously monitor it.

As you continue to treat the patient, do not apply pressure to an open or depressed skull injury. In addition, you must assess and treat other injuries, prevent hypothermia, dress and bandage open wounds as indicated in the treatment of soft-tissue injuries, splint fractures, anticipate and deal with vomiting to prevent aspiration, be prepared for seizures and changes in the patient's condition, and transport the patient promptly and with extreme care.

MANAGING THE AIRWAY. The most important step in the treatment of patients with head injury, regardless of the severity, is to establish an adequate airway. If the patient has an airway obstruction, you should perform the jaw-thrust maneuver to open the airway. Once the airway is open, maintain the head and cervical spine in a neutral, in-line position until the patient can be fully immobilized with a cervical collar ▶ **Figure 26-19** . Remove any foreign bodies, secretions, or vomitus from the airway. Make sure a suctioning unit is available, because you will often need to clear blood, saliva, or vomitus from the airway.

Once you have cleared the airway, check for oxygenation and ventilation. If the respiratory control center of the brain has been injured, the rate and/or

depth of breathing may be ineffective. Ventilation may also be limited by chest injuries or, if the spinal cord is injured, by paralysis of some or all of the muscles of respiration. Give high-flow oxygen to any patient who is having trouble breathing. This reduces hypoxia and possible cerebral edema. An injured brain is even less tolerant of hypoxia than a healthy brain, and studies have shown that supplemental oxygen can reduce brain damage. However, to be effective, it must be started as soon as possible. *Do not wait until the patient becomes cyanotic.* Continue to assist ventilations and administer supplemental oxygen until the patient reaches definitive care.

CIRCULATION. If the heart is not beating, providing airway maintenance, ventilation, and oxygen accomplishes nothing. You must also begin CPR if the patient is in cardiac arrest, and, if available, call for an AED.

Active blood loss aggravates hypoxia by reducing the available number of oxygen-carrying red blood cells. Although they rarely cause shock except in infants and

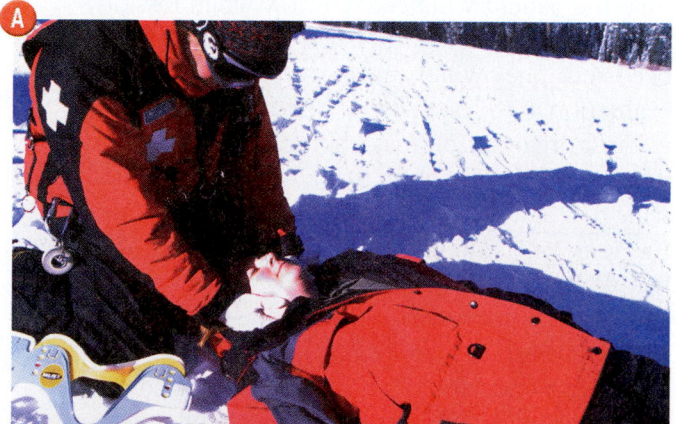

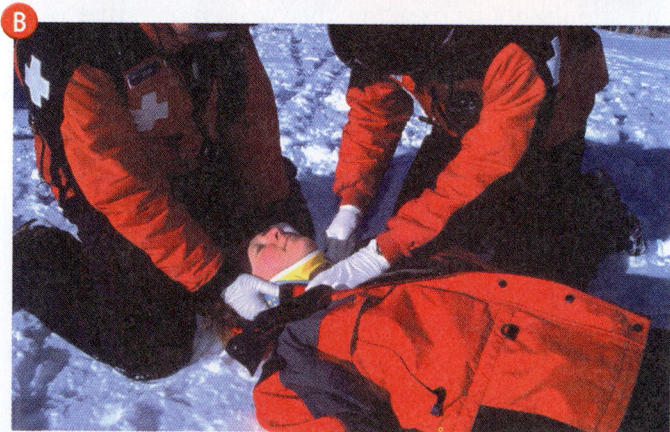

Figure 26-19 **A.** Maintain the head and cervical spine in a neutral in-line position. **B.** Apply a cervical collar as you finish the initial assessment.

Rescuer Safety

Many mechanisms that cause head and spine injuries for the patient can also entail risk to emergency responders. Before you approach the patient, get the "big picture" of scene safety and take any actions necessary to ensure your own well-being.

children, scalp lacerations often cause the loss of large volumes of blood, which must be controlled. Bleeding inside the skull may cause intracranial pressure to rise to life-threatening levels, even though the actual volume of blood lost inside the skull is relatively small.

Shock that develops in a patient with a head injury is usually due to hypovolemia caused by bleeding from other injuries. As with other trauma patients, shock in these cases indicates that the situation is critical. Such patients must be transported immediately to a trauma center. Maintain the airway while you protect the patient's cervical spine, ensure adequate ventilation, administer 100% oxygen, control obvious sites of bleeding with direct pressure, place the patient supine on a spine board, keep the patient warm, and provide immediate transport.

If the patient has a medical condition or nontraumatic injury along with the head injury, place him or her on the left side to prevent aspiration if the patient happens to vomit. *Be sure to maintain the head in the in-line neutral position, with the cervical collar in place.* You should also have a suctioning unit available. When the patient is appropriately and securely strapped to a backboard, it is possible to tip the backboard sideways if the patient vomits.

Immobilization Devices

An injured spine is often very difficult to evaluate in a patient with a head injury. Sometimes, there is no neurologic loss. Pain in the spine may be missed because of shock, because the patient's attention is directed to more painful injuries, or because the patient is unresponsive. Because any manipulation of the unstable cervical spine may cause permanent damage to the spinal cord, you must assume the presence of spinal injury in *all* patients who have sustained head injuries. Use manual in-line immobilization or a cervical collar and long backboard.

CERVICAL COLLARS. Rigid cervical immobilization devices, often called cervical collars, c-collars, rigid collars, or extrication collars, provide preliminary, partial support. A cervical collar should be applied to every patient who has a possible spinal injury based on mechanism of injury, history, or signs and symptoms. Keep in mind, however, that cervical collars do not fully immobilize the cervical spine. Therefore, you must maintain manual support until the patient is completely secured to a spinal immobilization device, such as a long or a short backboard. A scoop stretcher does not provide adequate immobilization to prevent excessive spine motion while on a toboggan or stretcher.

To be effective, a rigid cervical collar must be the correct size for the patient. It should rest on the shoulder girdle and provide firm support under both sides of the mandible, without obstructing the airway or ventilation efforts in any way (▼ **Figure 26-20**). Follow the steps in (▶ **Skill Drill 26-4**) to apply a cervical collar:

1. **One rescuer** provides continuous manual in-line support of the head while the other prepares the collar **(Step 1)**.

2. **Measure the proper size collar** according to manufacturer's specifications. It is essential that the cervical collar fits properly. An improperly sized immobilization device has a potential for further injury. If you do not have the correct size, use a rolled towel; tape it to the backboard

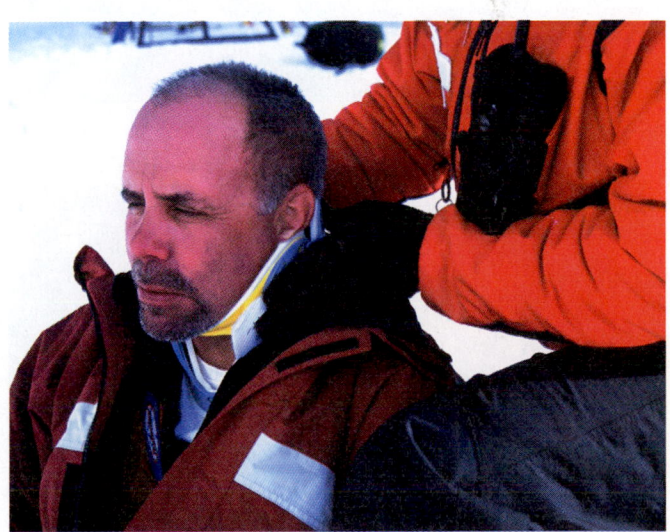

Figure 26-20 Proper fit is essential in applying a cervical collar. The collar should rest on the shoulder girdle and provide firm support under both sides of the mandible without obstructing the airway or any ventilation efforts.

SkillDrill 26-4 Application of a Cervical Collar

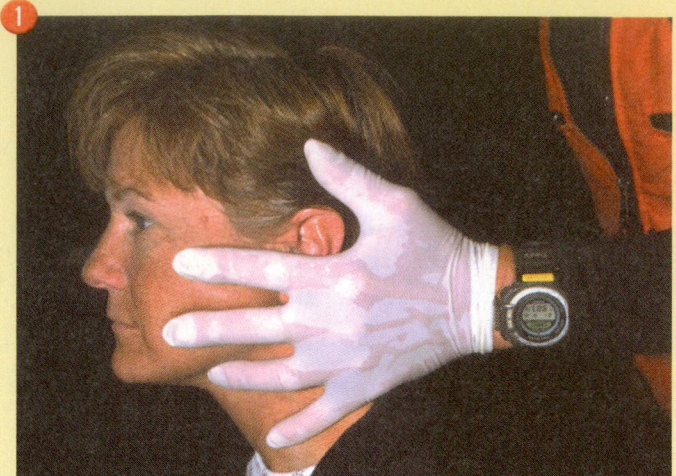

1. Apply in-line stabilization.

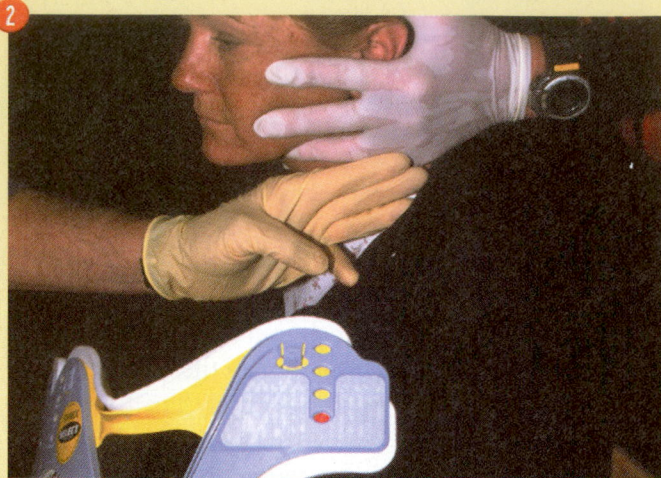

2. Measure the proper collar size.

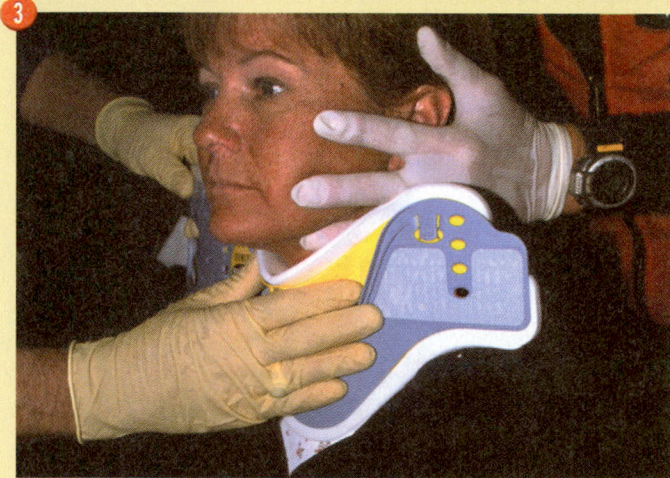

3. Place the chin support first.

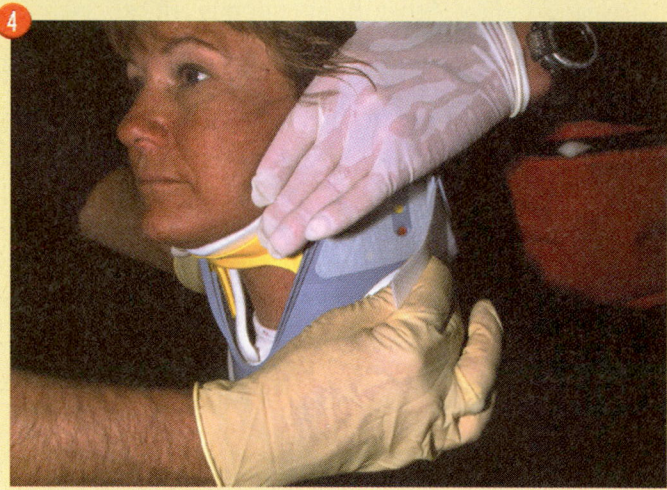

4. Wrap the collar around the neck and secure the collar.

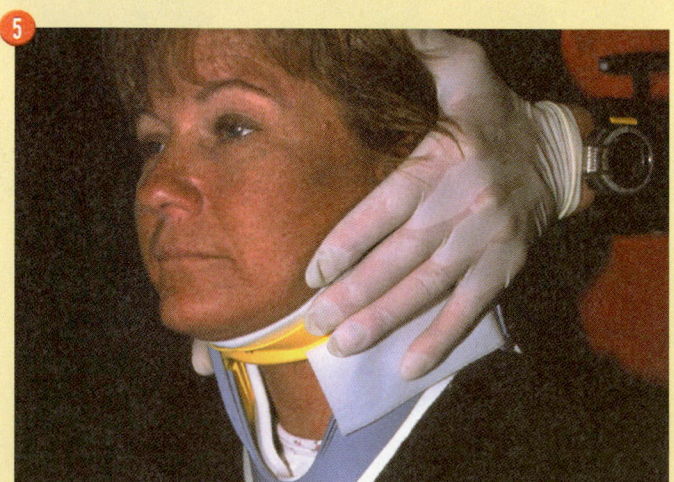

5. Ensure proper fit and maintain neutral, in-line stabilization.

around the patient's head, and provide continuous manual support (► **Figure 26-21**) **(Step 2)**.

3. **Begin by placing the chin support** snugly underneath the chin **(Step 3)**.

4. **Maintaining head stabilization** and neutral neck alignment, wrap the collar around the neck and secure the collar to the far side of the chin support **(Step 4)**.

5. **Ensure that the collar fits properly** and recheck that the patient is in a neutral, in-line position. Maintain in-line stabilization until the patient is completely secured to the board **(Step 5)**.

SHORT BACKBOARDS. There are several types of short-board immobilization devices. The most common are the vest-type device and the rigid short board (► **Figure 26-22**). These devices are for extrication only. They are designed to stabilize and immobilize the head, neck, and torso. They are used to immobilize noncritically injured patients who are found in a sitting position and have possible spinal injuries. The patient should be transferred to a long backboard as soon as possible, with the short board still in place.

As was described earlier in this chapter, the first step in securing a patient to a short board or device is to provide manual, in-line support of the cervical spine. Assess the pulse, motor function, and sensation in all extremities, and then assess the cervical area. Then apply an appropriately sized cervical collar.

Position the device behind the patient, and secure it to the torso. Evaluate how well the torso and groin are secured, and make adjustments as necessary. Avoid excessive movement of the patient. Next, evaluate the position of the patient's head. Pad behind the head as needed to maintain neutral, in-line stabilization.

Now secure the patient's head to the device. Once you have done that, you may release manual support of the head. Rotate or lift the patient to the long backboard. At this point, you must reassess the pulses, motor function, and sensation in all four extremities to determine whether the change in position has affected the patient's vital signs or neurologic status. Finally you should immobilize the patient to the long backboard.

LONG BACKBOARDS. There are several types of long backboard immobilization devices that provide full body spinal immobilization (► **Figure 26-23**). They also provide stabilization and immobilization to the head, neck and torso, pelvis, and extremities. Long back-

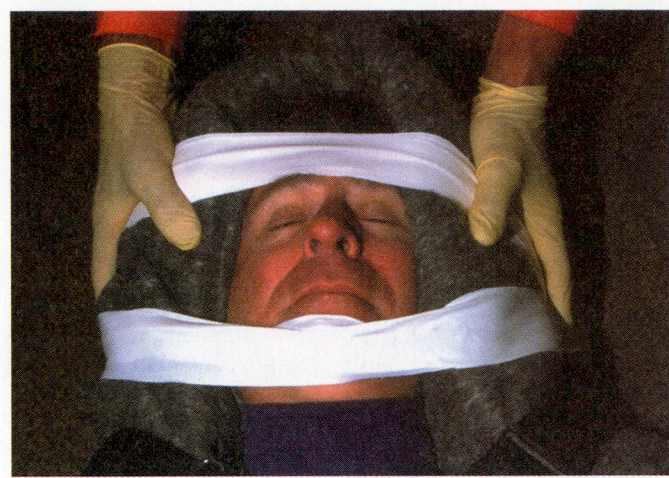

Figure 26-21 If you do not have an appropriately sized cervical collar, you may use a rolled towel. Tape it to the backboard around the patient's head, and provide continuous manual support.

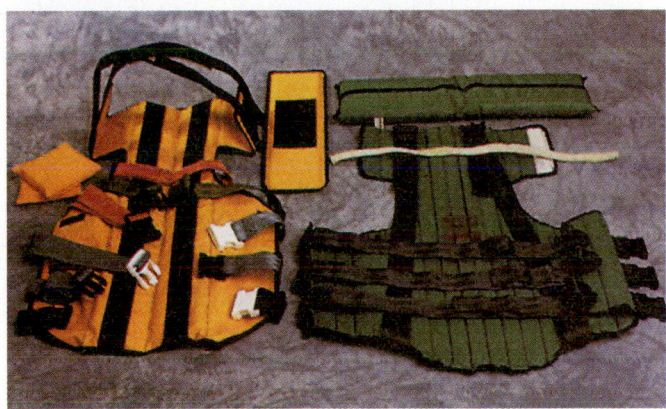

Figure 26-22 The most common types of short-board immobilization devices are vest-type devices.

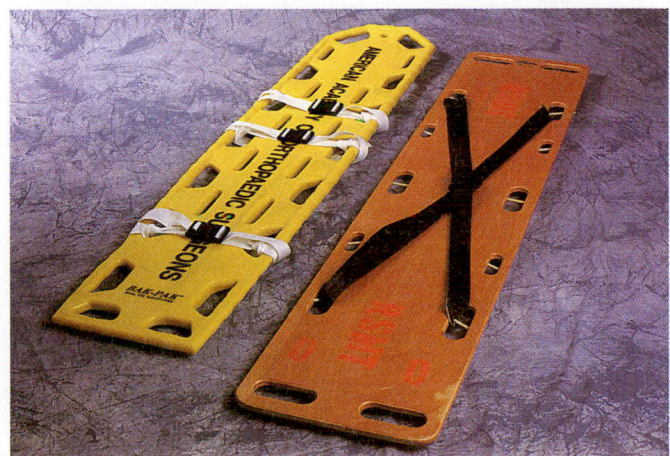

Figure 26-23 Long-board immobilization devices provide full body spinal immobilization, including stabilization of the head, neck and torso, pelvis, and extremities.

boards are used to immobilize patients who are found in any position (standing, sitting, supine), sometimes in conjunction with short backboards. Make certain your local transportation equipment safely accommodates your immobilization devices.

Securing a patient to a long board was described in detail earlier in this chapter. Briefly, you should begin by providing manual, in-line support of the head. Assess pulse, motor function, and sensation in all extremities, and assess the cervical area. Then apply an appropriately sized cervical collar, and proceed as follows:

1. **Position the device.**

2. **Log roll the patient onto the device.** You may also move the patient onto the device by suitable lift or slide or by scoop stretcher. Remember that a scoop stretcher by itself may not provide adequate spinal stabilization. As you maintain in-line support, your partner should kneel by the patient's head and direct the other one or two rescuers as you roll the patient. Your partner's job is to make sure that the head, torso, and pelvis move as a unit. As the patient's back comes into view, quickly assess its condition if you did not do so during initial assessment. One rescuer should position the device under the patient. Then, at your partner's command, roll the patient onto the board.

3. **If there are spaces** between the patient's head and torso and the board, fill them with padding. In an adult, these spaces are usually under the head and torso. In a child, place padding from the shoulders to the toes to establish a neutral position.

4. **Secure the torso to the device** by applying straps across the chest, pelvis, and legs. Adjust these straps as needed. *Then* secure the patient's head to the board.

5. **Reassess pulse,** motor function, and sensation in all extremities.

6. **When the patient is properly secured,** you can safely lift the board or turn it on its side, if necessary.

Helmet Removal

As you plan your care of a patient wearing a helmet, ask yourself the following questions:

- Is the patient's airway clear?
- Is the patient breathing adequately?
- Can you maintain the airway and assist ventilations if the helmet remains in place?
- How well does the helmet fit?
- Can the patient move within the helmet?
- Can the spine be immobilized in a neutral position with the helmet on?

A helmet that fits well prevents the patient's head from moving and should be left on, as long as (1) there are no impending airway or breathing problems, (2) it does not interfere with assessment and treatment of airway or ventilation problems, and (3) you can properly immobilize the spine. You should also leave the helmet on if there is any chance that removing it will further injure the patient.

Remove a helmet if (1) it makes assessing or managing airway problems difficult, (2) it prevents you from properly immobilizing the spine, or (3) it allows excessive head movement. Finally, always remove a helmet from a patient who is in cardiac arrest.

Sports helmets are typically open in the front and may or may not include an attached face mask. The mask sometimes can be removed without affecting helmet position or function by simply removing or cutting the straps that hold it to the helmet. In this way, sports helmets allow easy access to the airway. Motorcycle and snowmobile helmets often have a shield covering the face. This, too, can be unbuckled to allow access to the airway (▶ **Figure 26-24**). If a shield cannot be removed, then the helmet must be removed, as immediate access to the airway is mandatory.

Preferred Method

Removing a helmet is at least a two-person job; however, the technique for helmet removal depends on the actual type of helmet worn by the patient. One rescuer provides constant in-line support as the other moves; you and another rescuer should not move at the same time. You should first consult with medical control, if possible, about your decision to remove a helmet. When you decide to do so, follow the steps in (▶ **Skill Drill 26-5**):

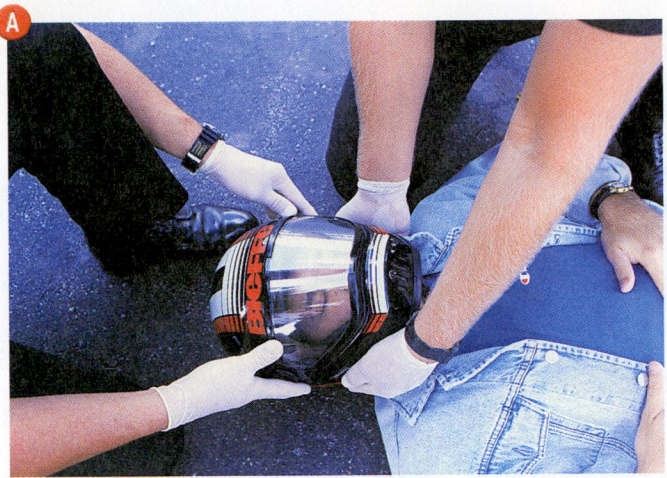
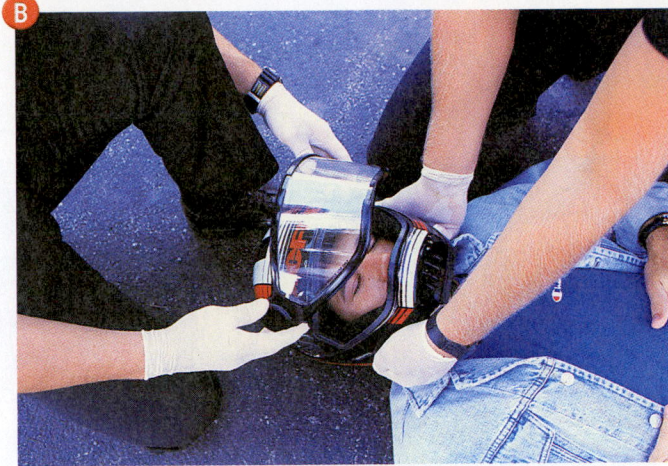

Figure 26-24 Snowmobile and motorcycle helmets often have a face shield that can be removed. **A.** Stabilize the neck in a neutral, in-line position. **B.** Unbuckle or snap off the face shield to access the airway.

1. **Begin by kneeling down** at the patient's head. Another rescuer should kneel on one side of the patient, at the shoulder area.

2. **Open the face shield,** if there is one, and assess the patient's airway and breathing. Remove eyeglasses or goggles if the patient is wearing them **(Step 1)**.

3. **Stabilize the helmet** by placing your hands on either side of it, with your fingers on the patient's lower jaw to prevent movement of the head. Once your hands are in position, another rescuer can loosen the chin strap **(Step 2)**.

4. **Once the strap is loosened,** the other rescuer should place one hand on the patient's lower jaw at the angle of the jaw and the other behind the head at the junction of the head and cervical spine. Once the other rescuer's hands are in position, you may pull the sides of the helmet away from the patient's head **(Step 3)**.

5. **Gently slip the helmet** halfway off the patient's head, stopping when the helmet reaches the halfway point **(Step 4)**.

6. **The other rescuer then slides** his or her hand from the junction of the head and cervical spine to the back of the head. This will prevent the head from snapping back once the helmet is completely removed **(Step 5)**.

7. With the other rescuer's hand in place, **remove the helmet,** and immobilize the cervical spine.

8. **Apply the cervical collar,** and then secure the patient to the backboard.

9. **With large helmets** or small patients, you may need to pad under the shoulders. This will prevent flexion of the neck. If shoulder pads or a heavy jacket is in place, you may need to pad behind the patient's head to prevent extension of the neck **(Step 6)**.

Remember, you do not need to remove a helmet if you can access the patient's airway, if the head is snug inside the helmet, and if the helmet can be secured to an immobilization device.

Pediatric Considerations

Remember that small children may require additional padding to maintain the in-line neutral position. Children are not small adults. They have smaller airways, so padding is important to maintain the airway. Pad under the shoulders to the toes, as needed, to avoid excessive neck flexion (▶ **Figure 26-26**). In addition, place blanket rolls between the child and the sides of an adult-sized board to prevent the child from slipping to one side or the other (▶ **Figure 26-27**). Appropriately sized backboards are available for children.

Removing a Helmet

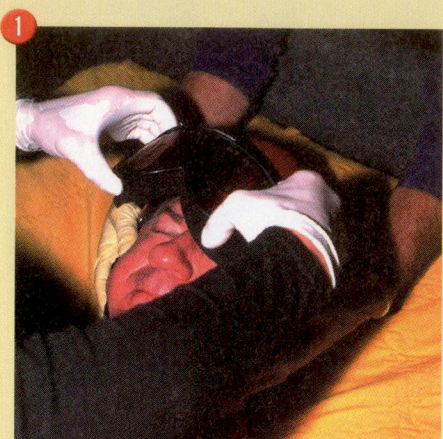

Kneel down at the patient's head with another rescuer at one side.

Open the face shield to assess airway and breathing. Remove eyeglasses or goggles if present.

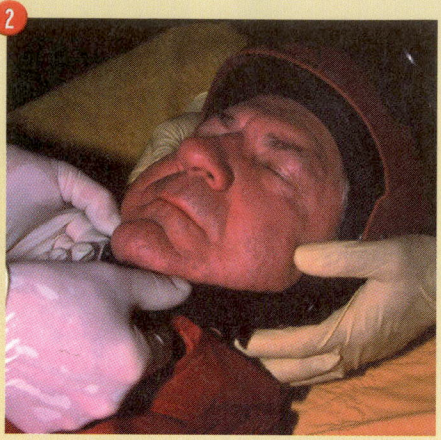

Prevent head movement by placing your hands on either side of the helmet and fingers on the lower jaw. Have another rescuer loosen the strap.

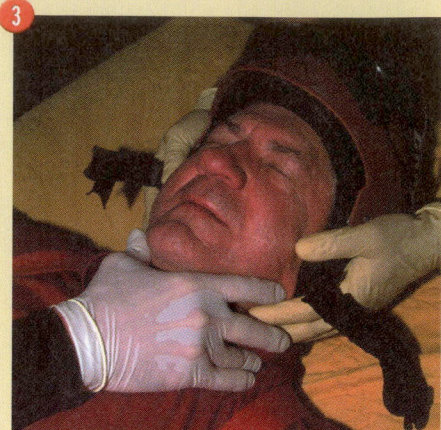

Have another rescuer place one hand at the angle of the lower jaw and the other at the junction of the head and cervical spine.

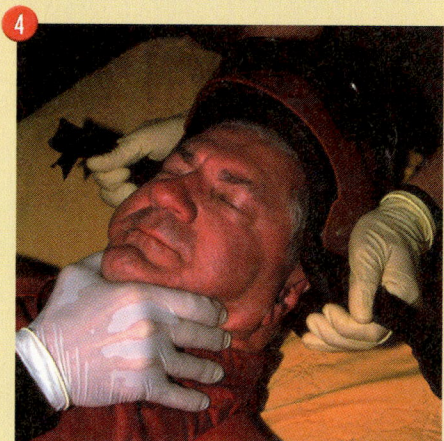

Gently slip the helmet about halfway off, then stop.

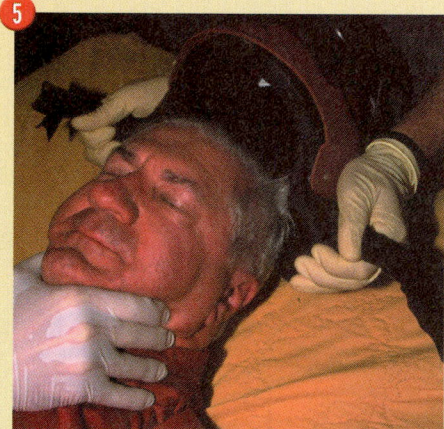

Have another rescuer slide his or her hand from the junction of the patient's head and cervical spine to the back of the head to prevent it from snapping back.

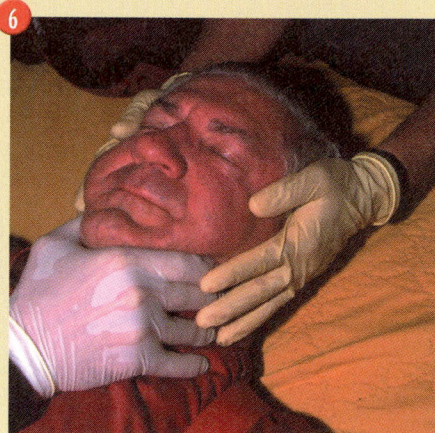

Remove the helmet and stabilize the cervical spine.

Apply a cervical collar and secure the patient to a long backboard.

Pad as needed to prevent neck flexion or extension.

Pediatric Needs

You are likely to find infants and children who have been in automobile crashes still in their car seats. Your best course of action is to immobilize the child in the car seat if possible. Whenever you apply a cervical collar, make sure it is properly sized. If a properly fitting collar is not available, use a rolled towel and tape it to the car seat. Pad the sides of the car seat, if necessary, to prevent lateral movement ▼ **Figure 26-25**, and place additional padding in any spaces between the patient and the car seat. If the child is not in a car seat or was removed before your arrival, use an appropriately sized immobilization device. If the cervical immobilization device does not fit, use a rolled towel, and tape it to the board and manually support the head.

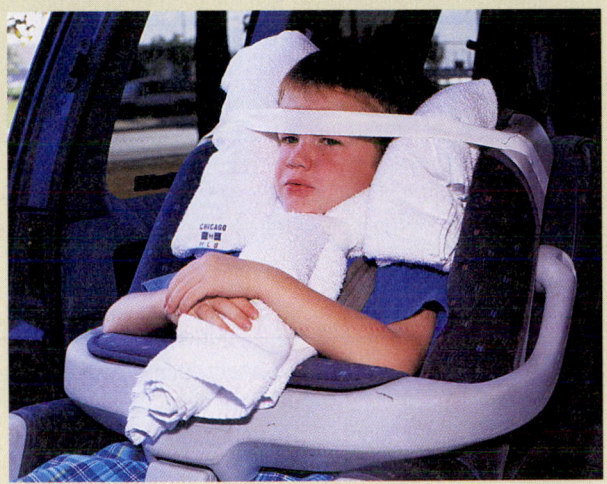

Figure 26-25 If you do not have an appropriately sized cervical collar for a child, you may use a rolled towel and tape it to the car seat. Pad the sides of the car seat, if needed, to prevent lateral movement.

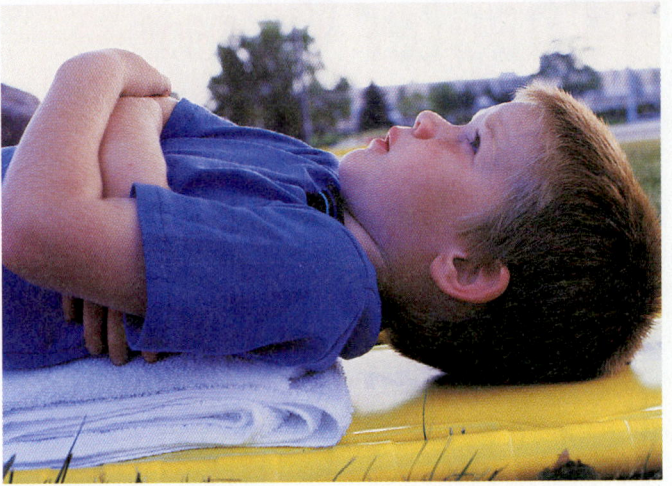

Figure 26-26 Children have proportionately larger heads than adults, so you may need to place padding under the shoulders to avoid excessive flexion of the neck.

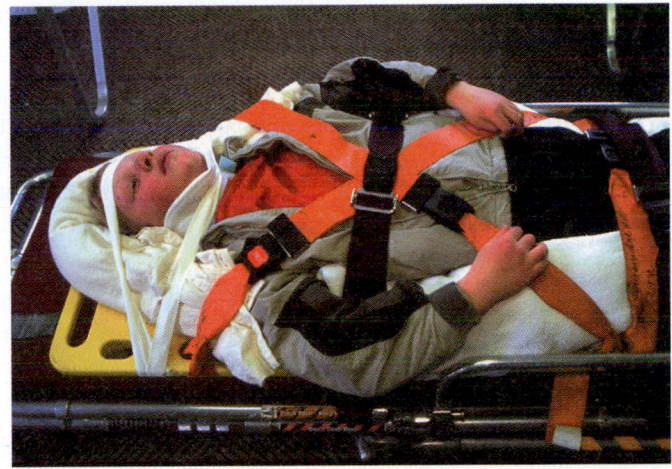

Figure 26-27 Place blanket rolls between the child and the sides of an adult-sized board to prevent the child from slipping to one side or the other.

Chapter *Sweep*

Ready for Review

The nervous system is divided into two parts: the central nervous system and the peripheral nervous system. The central nervous system consists of the brain and the spinal cord. The cables of nerve fibers linking nerve cells in the brain and spinal cord to the body's organs make up the peripheral nervous system. In addition to the skull and spinal canal, the central nervous system is protected by the meninges, three layers of tissue called the dura mater, arachnoid, and pia mater. The peripheral nervous system consists of 31 pairs of spinal nerves, which conduct sensory impulses from the skin and other organs to the spinal cord and conduct motor impulses from the spinal cord to the muscles, and 12 pairs of cranial nerves, which transmit sensations relating to sight, smell, taste, and hearing directly to the brain. The three major types of peripheral nerves are sensory nerves, motor nerves, and connecting nerves.

The part of the nervous system that regulates our voluntary activities is called the somatic or voluntary nervous system. The much more primitive autonomic or involuntary nervous system regulates involuntary body functions. The autonomic nervous system is composed of the sympathetic and parasympathetic nervous systems, which balance each other.

The skull is divided into two large bony structures that protect the brain: the cranium and the face. The spinal column has 33 bones, called vertebrae, in five sections: cervical, thoracic, lumbar, sacral, and coccygeal.

The cervical, thoracic, and lumbar portions of the spine can be injured through compression resulting from a fall; through unnatural motions such as overextension caused by motor vehicle crashes and other types of trauma; and through distraction (pulling) along the length of the spine, as in hanging. Start your assessment of a patient with a possible spinal injury by focusing on the ABCs and, if he or she is responsive, by asking five questions: What happened? Where does it hurt? Does your neck or back hurt? Can you feel me touching your fingers and toes? Can you move your hands and feet? Look for contusions, punctures, or skull deformities; test for strength in the extremities; ask about pain; and check for numbness, weakness, or tingling in the extremities. Patients with severe spinal injury may lose sensation or be paralyzed below the suspected injury.

Keep the head in a neutral, in-line position while you open and maintain the airway, assess respirations, and give supplemental oxygen. Provide manual immobilization until the patient is properly secured to a backboard. A patient who is supine can be immobilized with a long backboard, using the four-person log roll. With sitting patients, you should use a short backboard, then secure the short board to a long board. If the patient is standing, immobilize him or her to a long backboard before starting your assessment; this requires three rescuers.

Common head injuries include skull wounds (scalp lacerations and skull fracture) and brain injuries (concussion, contusion, intracranial bleeding), typically caused by direct blows, collisions, falls from heights, and sports injuries. Cerebral edema, seizures, vomiting, and leakage of cerebrospinal fluid are common complications of both open and closed head injuries. Common signs and symptoms of head injuries include lacerations, visible deformities of the skull, ecchymosis about the eyes or behind the ear, unequal pupil size and failure of the pupils to respond to light, loss of sensation and/or motor function, visual complaints, and irregular respirations.

The single most important observation that you can make in assessing a brain injury is of change in the level of responsiveness. Use the AVPU scale or the Glasgow Coma Scale to assess consciousness immediately and every 15 minutes for a stable patient and every 5 minutes for an unstable patient, recording scores and times as you do so. Also monitor and document pupil size and reactions.

Patients with head injuries occasionally have injuries to the cervical spine as well. Therefore, when treating a patient with a head injury, you must protect and stabilize the cervical spine at all times. Three principles govern treatment of head injuries: airway, ventilation, and high-flow supplemental oxygen; bleeding and circulation; and assessing/monitoring level of responsiveness.

Immobilization devices include cervical collars, which must be the correct size; short backboards, including vest-type devices and rigid short boards; and long backboards.

A helmet that fits well prevents the patient's head from moving and should be left on, as long as it does not interfere with assessment/treatment of airway or ventilation problems and you can properly immobilize the spine. Remove a helmet if it makes assessing or managing airway problems difficult, prevents you from immobilizing the spine, or allows excessive head movement. Never remove a helmet if doing so will further injure the patient. Always remove a helmet if the patient is in cardiac arrest.

www.OECzone.com

Vital Vocabulary

anterograde (posttraumatic) amnesia Inability to remember events after an injury.

autonomic (involuntary) nervous system The part of the nervous system that regulates functions that are not controlled by conscious will, such as digestion and sweating.

axon The long process of a neuron.

Battle's sign Bruising behind an ear over the mastoid process that may indicate skull fracture.

blunt injury Injury to the head in which the brain has been injured but the skin is unbroken.

brain stem The part of the central nervous system that controls virtually all functions that are necessary for life, including the cardiac and respiratory systems.

central nervous system (CNS) The brain and spinal cord.

cerebellum The part of the brain that coordinates body movements.

cerebral edema Swelling of the brain.

cerebrum The largest part of the brain, containing about 75% of the brain's total volume.

concussion A temporary loss or alteration of part or all of the brain's abilities to function without actual physical damage to the brain.

connecting nerves Nerves in the brain and spinal cord that connect the motor and sensory nerves.

distracted The action of pulling the spine along its length.

eyes-forward position A head position in which the patient's eyes are looking straight ahead and the head and torso are in line.

four-person log roll The recommended procedure for moving a patient with a suspected spinal injury from the ground to a long spine board.

Glasgow Coma Scale A method of evaluating level of consciousness that uses a scoring system for neurologic responses to specific stimuli.

intervertebral disk The cushion that lies between two vertebrae.

involuntary activities The actions that we do not consciously control.

meninges Three distinct layers of tissue that surround and protect the brain and the spinal cord within the skull and the spinal canal.

motor nerves Nerves that carry information from the central nervous system to the muscles.

open head injuries Injury to the head in which a penetrating object has caused scalp lacerations, contusions, hematomas, and obvious skull deformities.

peripheral nervous system The 31 pairs of spinal nerves and 12 pairs of cranial nerves that link the body's other organs to the central nervous system.

raccoon eyes Bruising under the eyes that may indicate skull fracture.

retrograde amnesia The inability to remember events leading up to a brain injury.

sensory nerves Nerves that transmit sensory input, such as touch, taste, heat, cold, and pain, from the body to the central nervous system.

somatic (voluntary) nervous system The part of the nervous system that regulates our voluntary activities, such as walking, talking, and writing.

voluntary activities Actions that we consciously perform, in which sensory input determines the specific muscular activity.

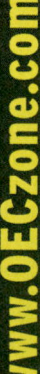

Assessment in Action

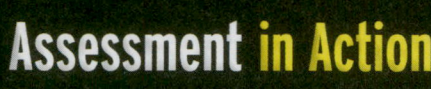

On the first nice weekend of April, two young men take their mountain bikes to the Elk Ridge Trails. With taunts as to who is "King of the Mountain," they race off down the trail. One of the cyclists loses control of his bike and crashes into the underbrush. He is launched over the handlebars and lands on the ground, shaken and disoriented.

His friend quickly rides back to the ranger station to call 9-1-1. You and your partner arrive to find a 23-year-old man still down on the trail. He is wearing shorts, sandals, and sunglasses but no helmet. The patient responds to pain by withdrawing when you pinch his arms or legs. Vital signs include a pulse of 60 beats/min, respirations of 28 breaths/min and irregular, and a blood pressure of 166/98 mm Hg. Additional examination shows multiple abrasions over his entire body and an angulated fracture of his left tibia.

1. Based on the patient's presenting signs and symptoms, which presents the most likely threat to his life?
   A. Fractured tibia
   B. Multiple abrasions
   C. Possible spinal cord injury
   D. Brain injury

2. Whenever possible, in what position should you immobilize a patient's head and cervical spine?
   A. Slight flexion
   B. Moderate extension
   C. Moderate flexion
   D. Neutral

3. Just as you adequately secure the patient to the long spine board, he starts to retch in preparation for vomiting. You should immediately:
   A. leave him supine but prepare to suction the airway.
   B. remove all the straps and roll him over onto his stomach.
   C. keep the patient strapped to the board and turn the board on its side.
   D. remove the head strap and turn the patient's head to the side.

4. En route, you notice a watery, blood-tinged fluid leaking from the patient's nose. You should:
   A. document this finding and bring it to the attention of the receiving physician.
   B. apply direct pressure with sterile dressings.
   C. pack the nostrils and apply direct pressure.
   D. pack the nostrils with tight, sterile dressings.

5. The presence of irregular respirations in this patient indicates which part of the brain is injured?
   A. Cerebrum
   B. Cerebellum
   C. Brain stem
   D. Meninges

6. In this case, with the altered level of responsiveness, irregular respirations, and watery, bloody fluid from the nose, this patient is at risk for which of the following problems?
   A. Aspiration
   B. Seizures
   C. Uncontrollable speech
   D. Tachycardia and low blood pressure

7. Which of the following is the best way to administer oxygen in this patient, provided that the patient accepted any method you chose?
   A. Nonrebreathing mask at 12 to 15 L/min
   B. BVM at a rate of 24 to 30/min
   C. Nonrebreathing mask at 6 to 10 L/min
   D. BVM at a rate of 12 to 16/min

Challenging Questions

8. Patients with neck injuries causing paralysis are at risk for developing breathing problems. Why?

9. If a patient is talking, alert, and oriented, the presence of unequal pupils does not necessarily mean a serious head injury is present. Why?

10. A more detailed method of assessing the level of responsiveness in a patient is called the Glasgow Coma Scale. What three parameters does it measure?

Points to Ponder

You find a victim of an avalanche in the debris field curled under a tree. The patient is conscious and complaining of pain in his abdomen, neck, and left ankle. He also explains that every time he moves his head, a burning pain shoots down his back. The patient is able to move his fingers and toes, except right after the shooting pain. The patient now begins to complain of nausea. Within a couple of minutes of complaining of nausea, the patient begins to vomit. Would you move this patient? Why or why not? When would you move the patient? How would you move him?

Issues Scene Management, Total Patient Care, Decision-Making Skills

Online Outlook

Review cutting edge scientific information pertaining to the grades of concussions, their evaluation in sports medicine, and the effect of this information on emergency care in Exercise 26 at www.OECzone.com.

www.OECzone.com

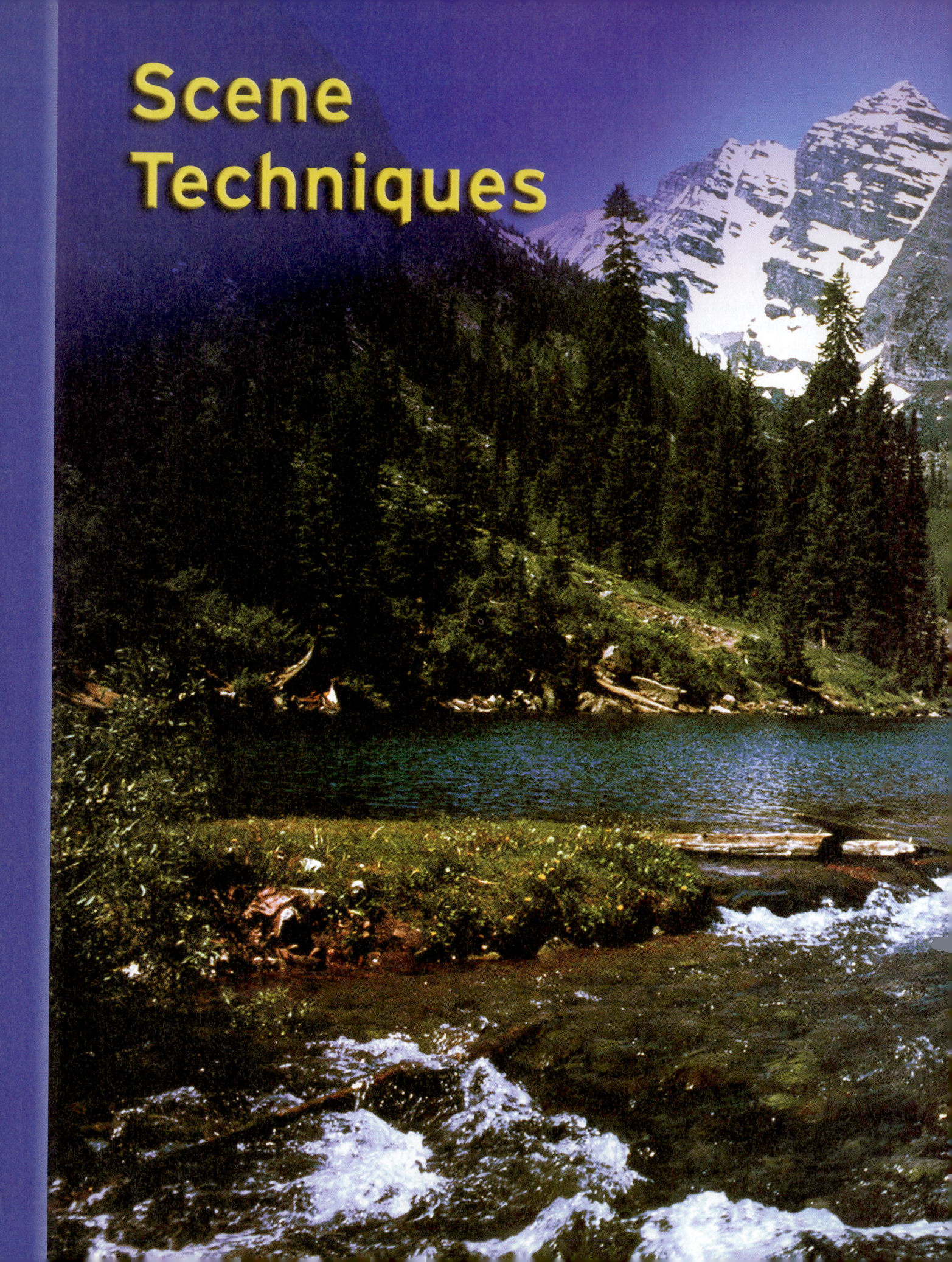

Scene Techniques

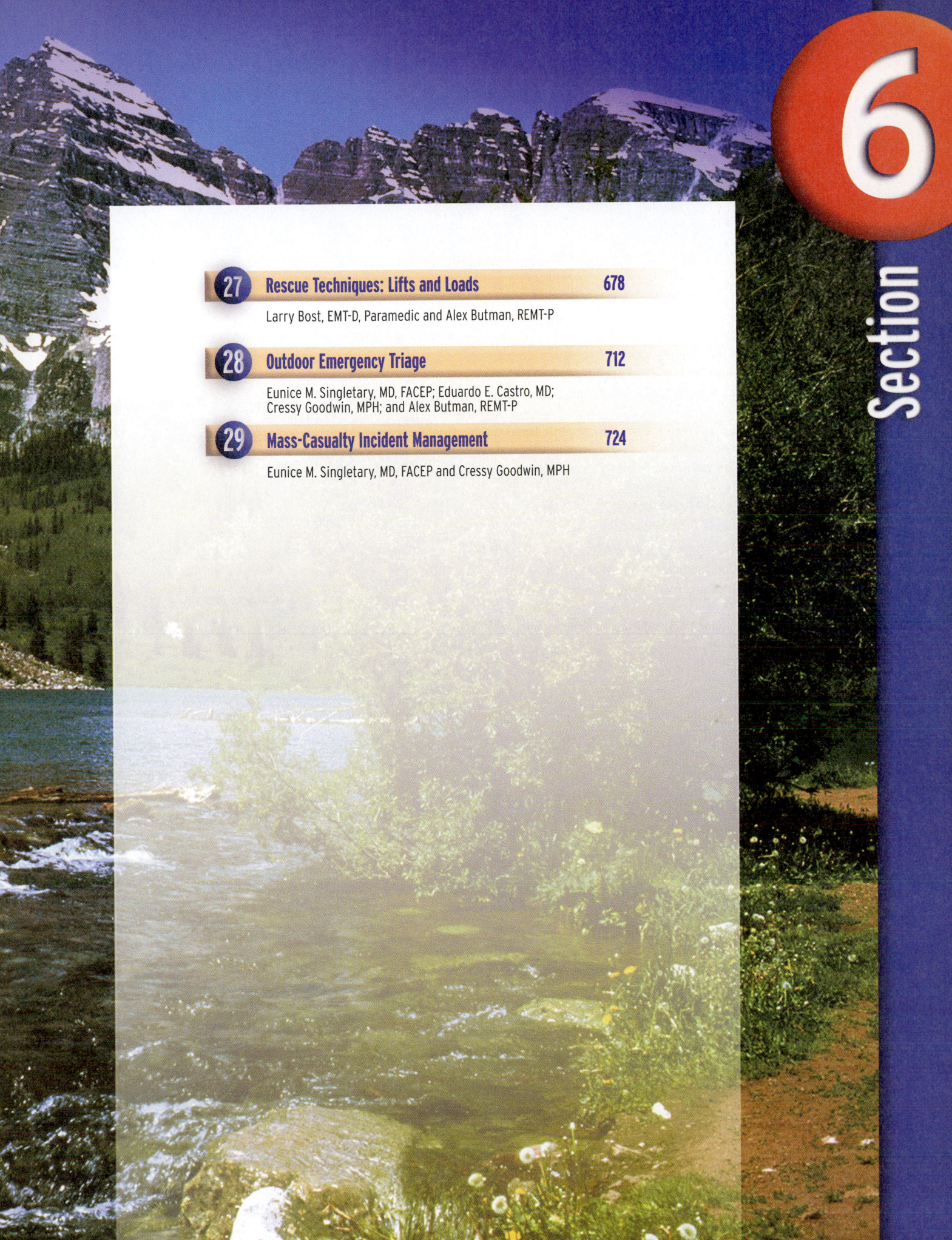

Section

6

Rescue Techniques: Lifts and Loads

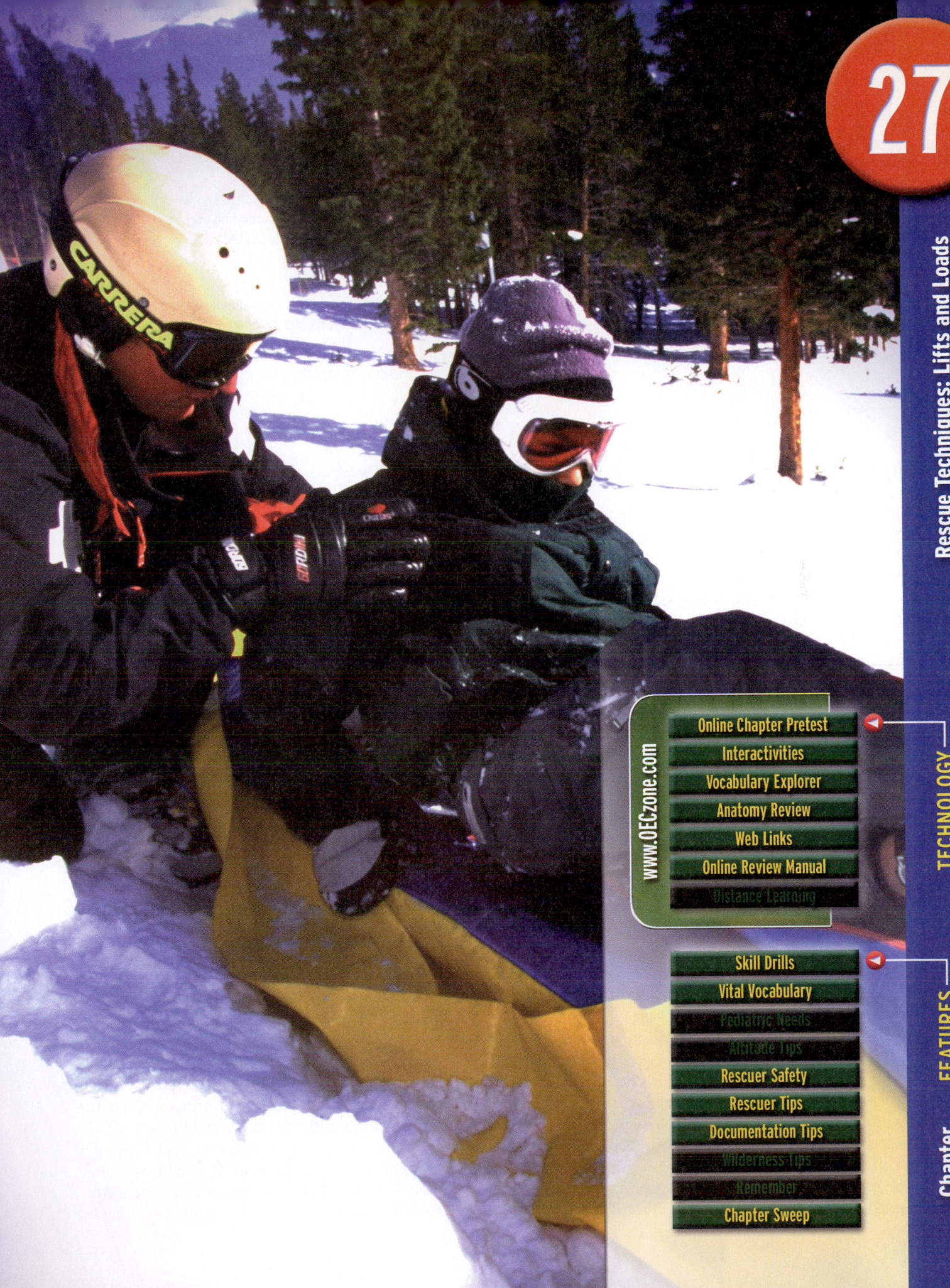

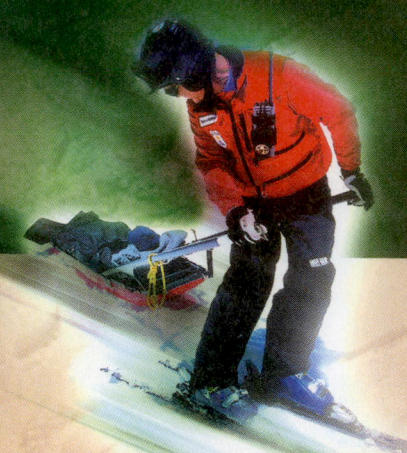

During your morning patrol briefing you are informed that Jason, another patroller, was injured and taken to the clinic the previous day. When you ask for details, you find out that Jason hurt his back while loading a patient into a toboggan and is expected to be off for the next few days.

Most patients encountered in the field will require some combination of lifting and moving. This chapter will cover the principles and key concepts that you should follow when performing these activities, as well as help you answer the following questions:

1. Why are proper body mechanics and clear communications key elements of safe lifting and moving activities?

2. What's the reason for every rescue group having such a wide variety of devices for lifting and moving patients?

Overview of the Rescue Process

When you first see the patient, you should note the location and position compared to your own and determine the fastest and most efficient way to reach him or her with all necessary equipment. Also note hazardous aspects of the scene that may endanger the patient or rescuers. Specific hazards include potential rockfall, steep slopes, heavily traveled ski runs, technical terrain, snow avalanches, slippery rocks in the middle of rivers, whitewater, flash floods, approaching storms, forest fires, weakening structures, moving machinery, and heavy vehicular traffic. Always wear head protection such as a hard hat or helmet in situations where falls or injuries from falling objects such as rocks or parts of buildings could occur.

As a general rule, do not approach a patient from directly above or directly below unless there is no alternative. The safest route of access may be difficult to determine. Whenever possible, remove the obstacle from the patient, not the patient from the obstacle. Also, move the patient from the incident site only after the patient has been stabilized and an exit route prepared.

After the patient has been located and given initial emergency care, often the patient must be removed from the original location to a place where it is more conducive to continue emergency care and package him or her for tranport. This process, called **extrication**, involves delicate techniques designed to move the patient without causing further injury to the patient or endangering the rescuers. After extrication, the patient is transferred, first to a backboard or other device, if necessary, then to a transportation device such as a litter or toboggan.

Following the transfer, packaging requires the patient to be properly positioned in the transportation device, padded, strapped in securely, and protected from the elements and hazards, such as falling rocks, by various types of insulation and shielding. After being packaged, the patient is transported to definitive medical care.

Despite your altruistic intentions, you must first protect yourself and your fellow rescuers before you can attend to the patient's safety. To avoid injury to the patient, yourself, or your fellow rescuers, you also will have to learn how to lift and carry the patient properly, using proper body mechanics and a power grip. You will have to learn to be able to move a patient safely and properly in the various situations that you will encounter in the outdoor environment. At times, you and your team will need to move a patient who weighs more than 300 lb or carry a patient over snow, ice, or rocks, on a trail, or across rugged terrain. You will need to know the special techniques for extricating, lifting, loading into a transfer or carrying device, and transferring the patient from the transfer device to a transportation device, then to a cot or bed in the aid room, medical clinic, or emergency care center, and potentially to an ambulance, helicopter, or other vehicle.

Lifting and carrying are dynamic processes. To ensure that no individual suddenly bears unexpected, dangerous weight and to reduce the risk of injury to a rescuer or the patient, you must know where rescuers should be positioned and how to give and receive lifting commands so that all parties act simultaneously. You will also need to know how to prepare immobilization, transfer, and transportation devices and when and how to use them. This chapter will cover principles of extrication and transfer, carrying, and searching techniques as well as principles of moving patients, including emergency, urgent, and nonurgent moves. In addition, different types of equipment and patient positioning will be discussed in detail.

Principles of Extrication and Transfer
Basic Anatomic Positions

There are six basic <u>anatomic positions</u> in which a patient may be found (▼ **Figure 27-1**): three main positions and three variations. Originally taught by Peter Goth, MD, and his colleagues at Wilderness Medical Associates, the technique of aligning and extricating patients found in these positions is often referred to as "<u>jams and pretzels</u>."

Position 1: The patient is supine, in the neutral, anatomic position with the back straight, the eyes facing forward, and extremities straight with the palms against the sides of the thighs. This is the position that the patient must be aligned into before being immobilized on a long backboard.

Position 1a: The patient is supine, but the head, neck, back, and extremities may be rotated, bent, or in any position other than the anatomic one.

Position 2: The patient is on his or her side, but in the neutral, anatomic position with the back straight, the eyes facing forward, and the extremities straight with the palms against the sides of the thighs. In the log roll, this is the position that the patient must be in when rolled to one side.

Position 2a: The patient is on his or her side but with the head, neck, back, and extremities in any position except the anatomic position.

Position 3: The patient is prone but in the neutral, anatomic position, except that the head is usually turned to the side.

Position 3a: The patient is prone, with the head, neck, back, and extremities in any position except the neutral, anatomic position.

The ultimate goal of extrication is to place an injured patient, especially one with a suspected neck or back

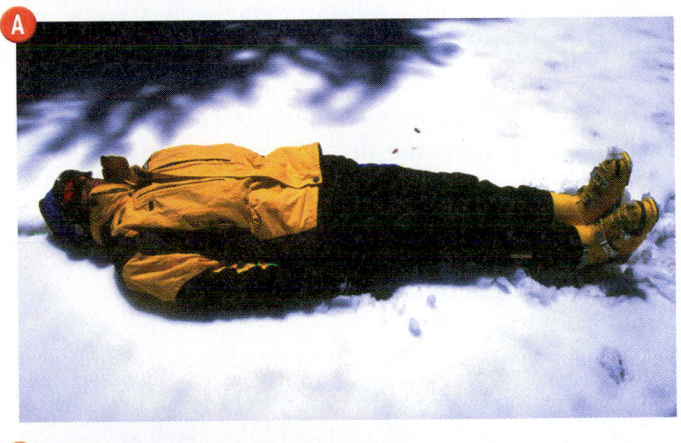
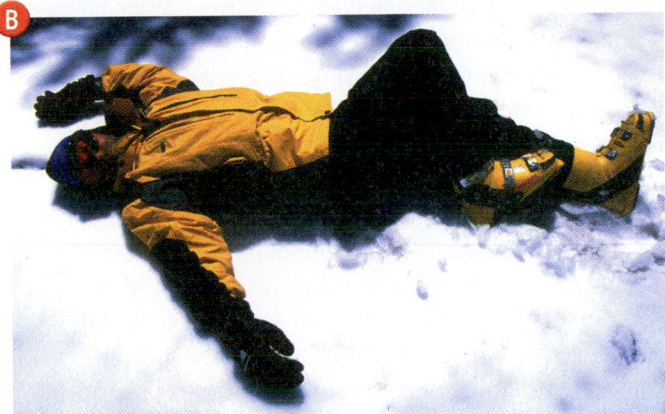
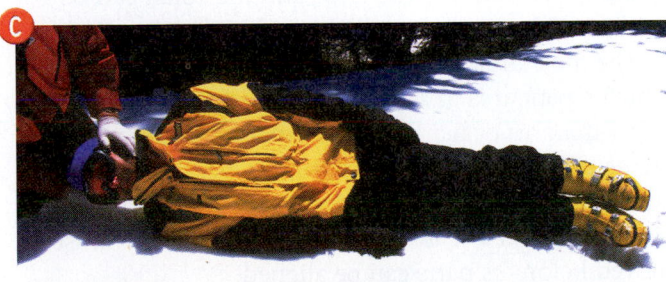
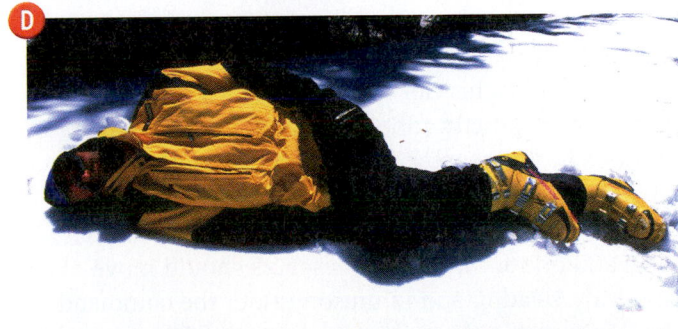
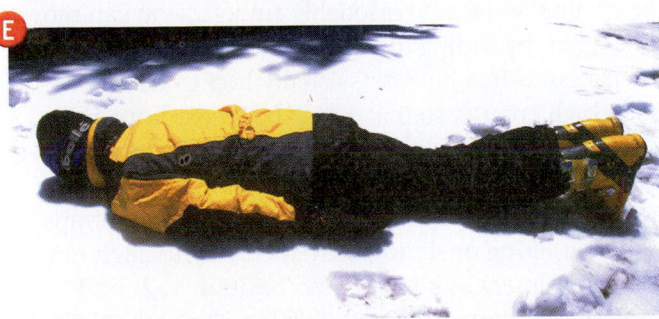
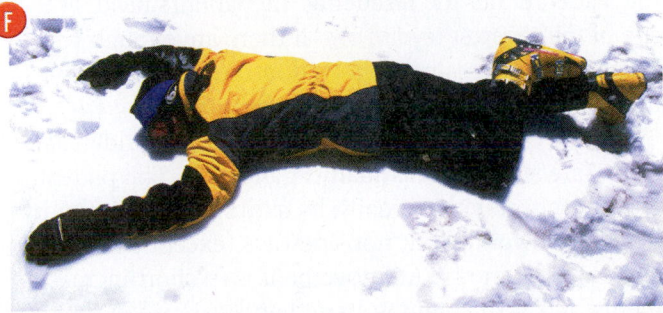

Figure 27-1 Basic anatomic positions in which a patient may be found. **A.** Position 1; **B.** Position 1a; **C.** Position 2; **D.** Position 2a; **E.** Position 3; **F.** Position 3a.

injury, in position 1 on the ground or on a long back-board.

The spine can be visualized as two long bones and three joints. The bones are the cervical and thoraco-lumbar segments of the spine; the joints are the joint between the skull and the first cervical vertebra, the joint between the seventh cervical and first thoracic vertebrae, and the joint between the fifth lumbar vertebra and the sacrum. Proper immobilization of an injured spine requires that all three of these joints be immobilized.

Think of a flat surface on which a patient lies as a flat spinal plane. As the patient lies supine in the anatomic position on the flat surface, the occiput, shoulders, upper back, buttocks, sacrum, calves, and heels are in contact with this plane. Three important reference points to keep in mind are the head, shoulders, and hips. The goal is to align the patient so that these three points are in line with each other, at right angles to the spine, and related to each other as though the patient were lying on this spinal plane in the neutral, anatomic position: they should remain so during any movement of the patient.

If this can be accomplished, the three joints of the spine will be stabilized and there will be little or no motion of the areas of the spine between the joints. When moving the patient, keep the concept of the spinal plane in mind at all times so that the three reference points are kept in proper relationship to each other.

Aligning the spine of an injured patient is a delicate procedure. Ideally, four to six rescuers are needed to smoothly align and stabilize the patient. However, in some situations this can be accomplished with fewer rescuers who strictly adhere to the alignment principles outlined in this chapter. To align the patient, one rescuer should be at the patient's head, one at the shoulders (or at each shoulder), one at the hips (or at each hip), and one at the legs. All rescuers should move smoothly, steadily, and in unison under the command of the leader, either the rescuer at the patient's head, at the site of the severest injury, or—if there are enough rescuers—one who is not involved in the patient movement but can observe the entire scene.

The three reference points—the head, shoulders, and hips—are stabilized manually at all times. The patient's body is moved either axially, by sliding, or vertically, by lifting or lowering, but not sideways (except occasionally on steep snow). All movement is in short increments of 6″ to 12″ and is started and stopped at the leader's command.

When the limbs or the head and neck must be straightened, only one joint at a time is moved in one plane at a time while the three reference points are manually stabilized. Align all body parts into position 1, 2, or 3 as early as possible, unless pain or resistance occurs. The head and neck are usually aligned first to protect the airway. Parts that cannot be brought into anatomic position at first because of the patient's position or location are manually stabilized in the position found during all movement of the patient and until the patient reaches a place where there is room for the rescuers to work.

Perform the maneuvers rapidly but not hastily. The number of positions should be kept to a minimum, and generally should progress from higher- to lower-numbered positions. For example, a patient in position 2a is aligned into position 2 and then log rolled into position 1. A patient in position 1a is aligned into position 1. A patient in position 1 is lifted a few inches off the ground by the bridge lift (or log rolled into position 2) to be placed on a long backboard.

Alignment of a patient in position 3a with the head turned to the side is more complicated. In this case, the body and extremities are aligned into position 3, but the head and neck are stabilized in place. The patient is then log rolled into position 2a with the head maintained in position before the head and neck are aligned so that the patient is in position 2. Finally, the patient is log rolled into position 1.

Apply a rigid collar as soon as possible, for example, when the head has been moved into a neutral, aligned position in relation to the torso and the collar can be applied with minimal movement of the head and neck.

The most difficult extrication problems are those in which a patient is in a closely confined area not much larger than his or her body or located so that body parts are held in nonanatomic positions by being jammed against other objects, such as a foot or head against a tree (▶ **Figure 27-2**). In this case, the entire body must be moved before its parts can be aligned.

If you can access enough of the patient's body and the ground surface is reasonably smooth, you can move the patient by sliding the body axially. Otherwise, or if the patient is in a hole, it is usually best to raise the body high enough so that a long backboard or similar rigid object can be slid underneath. This is done by adapting the multiple-rescuer bridge lift, if necessary using belts, cravats, or nylon webbing as lifting straps.

Before lifting or sliding the patient, try to align him or her as closely as possible into position 1, 2, or 3. Parts that cannot be aligned must be stabilized in place. While moving the patient, maintain stabilization of the

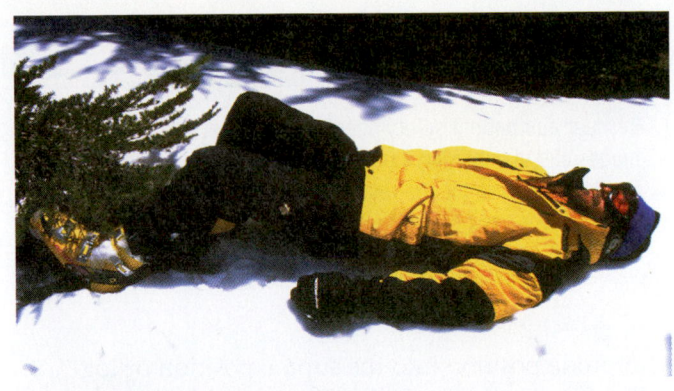

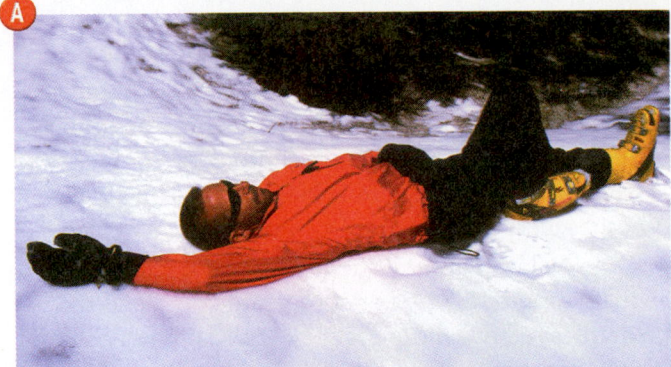

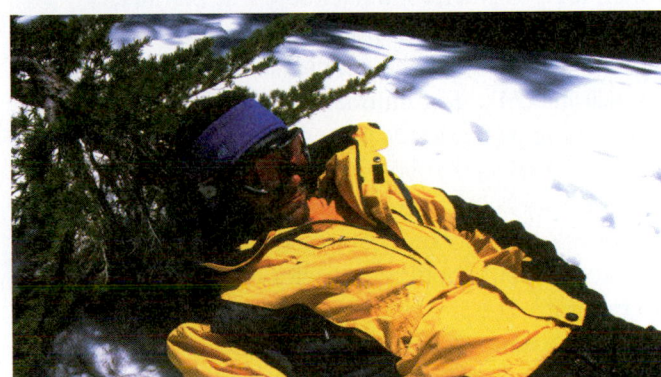

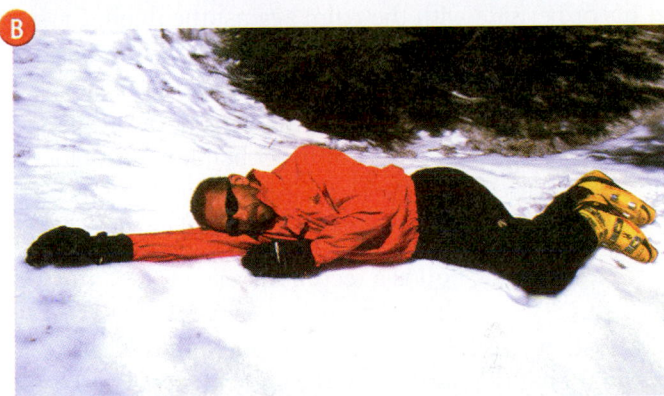

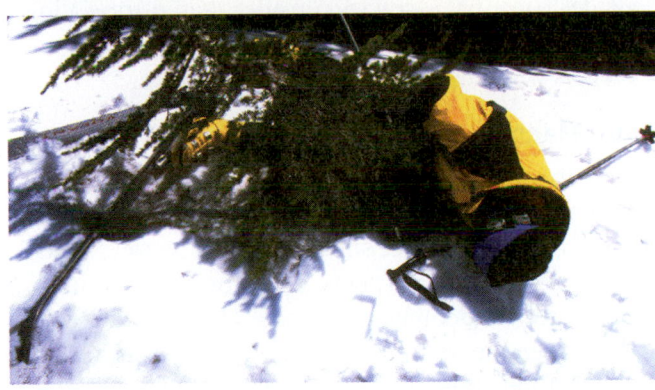

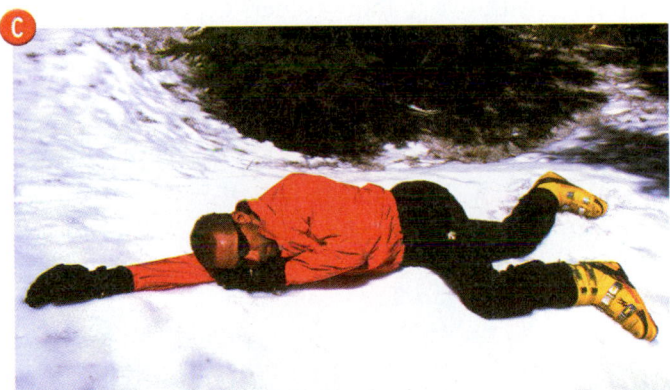

Figure 27-2 A person may be jammed in a confined space in a nonanatomic position.

Figure 27-3 Placing a patient in the recovery position. **A.** and **B.** Roll the patient onto the left side so that the head, shoulders, and torso move at the same time without twisting. **C.** The patient's left arm should be extended and the right hand placed under the cheek.

three reference points and maintain all other body parts in either their aligned or original positions. After the patient is on the backboard, complete alignment into the neutral, anatomic position (position 1).

The same principles apply when removing a seated patient from a vehicle.

It is important to pay attention to footing and balance, especially on slippery rocks, icy stairs, and wet or snowy inclines. Make movements smoothly and in unison with fellow rescuers. During all multiple-rescuer lifts and carries, one rescuer should be designated as the leader. All movements should be made on agreed-upon signals from the leader.

RECOVERY POSITION. After completing the rapid body survey, if the patient does not require rescue breathing or assisted breathing and trauma is unlikely, place him or her in the **recovery position**, also called the stable side, semiprone, rescue, or NATO position (▲ Figure 27-3). This position protects the airway by making it less likely that the tongue will fall back and block the pharynx or that the patient will inhale any vomit or accumulated secretions.

Even after putting the patient in this position, continue to monitor the individual closely.

ONE-RESCUER SIDEROLL. Always remember that an injured or ill patient may vomit. If you are alone, use the one-rescuer sideroll (turning technique) to immediately roll the patient to the side, protecting the neck as well as possible if the patient is injured. Also, this is a reasonably satisfactory alternative when there are no other rescuers to help you (▼ Figure 27-4).

Quickly kneel at the patient's side, far enough away so that you can roll the patient toward you. Bend the patient's far elbow and place his or her far hand behind the head. Straighten the patient's near arm and place it at his or her side with the palm against the thigh. Cross the patient's far ankle over the near ankle. With one hand behind the patient's far shoulder and the other behind the far hip, quickly roll the person toward you onto his or her side. A minimum of bending or rotation of the spine may occur with this maneuver, but it is preferable to having the patient vomit and aspirate.

LOG ROLL. A **log roll** is a technique used to roll a patient 180° (usually from prone to supine) or to the side so that a backboard can be slipped underneath without bending or twisting the spine. It is generally performed with two to four rescuers depending on whether the patient is being log rolled from a prone or

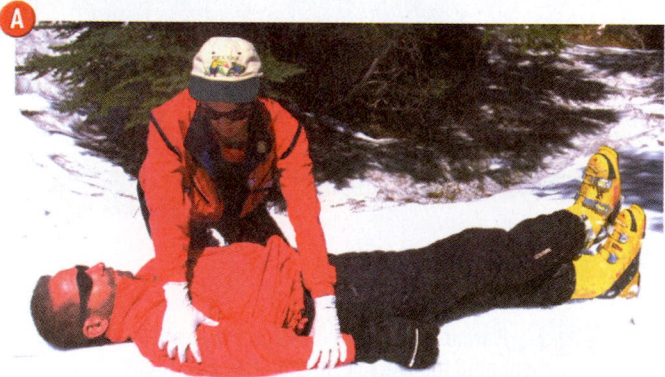

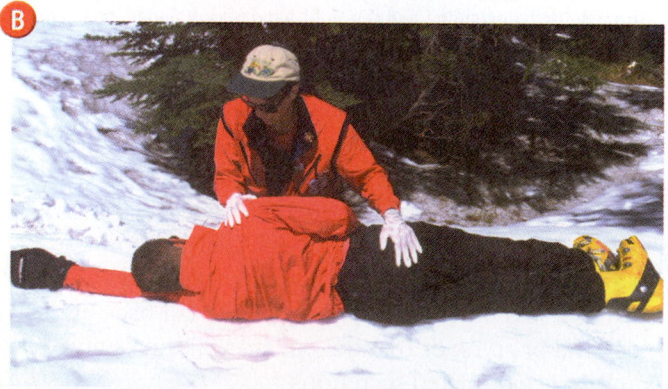

Figure 27-4 One-rescuer sideroll. **A.** Kneel at the patient's side and **B.** quickly roll the patient toward you.

Rescuer Tips

Rescuer and patient safety depends on proper lifting techniques and maintaining a proper hold while lifting and carrying. Loss of grasp by one rescuer may cause injury to another team member as well as the patient.

semiprone position into the supine position or log rolled for placement of a backboard or blanket.

Generally, when log rolling a patient onto his or her side, you will initially have to reach farther than 18" (▶ Skill Drill 27-1). To minimize this distance, kneel as close to the patient's side as possible, leaving only enough room so that your knees will not prevent the patient from being rolled. When you lean forward, keep your back straight, and lean solely from the hips. Be sure to use your shoulder muscles to help with the roll. To minimize the amount of time you are extended like this and to support the patient's weight, roll the patient without stopping until the patient is resting on his or her side. Some EMS experts consider that, during a log roll, you should pull rather than push the patient. Local protocols will guide your training in this area.

Body Mechanics

The safety of the rescuers is an important consideration in any move. To avoid injuring the back or another body part, every rescuer should know how to lift and carry heavy loads. It is unwise to lift or carry too heavy a load without adequate assistance. The back is especially vulnerable to injury during common mistakes such as lifting while twisted to the side or while bending forward with the knees straight (as when moving a cooler from the trunk of a car).

Therefore, lift with the hips and legs rather than the back. Keep the back straight; don't twist or bend forward or to the side. Hold the load as close to your body as possible, and avoid sudden jerky movements.

Anatomy Review

The shoulder girdle rests on the rib cage and is supported by the vertebrae that lie inferior to it. The arms are connected to and hang from the shoulder girdle. When the person is standing upright, the individual weight-bearing vertebrae are stacked on top of each other and aligned over the sacrum. The sacrum is both the mechanical weight-bearing base of the spinal column and the fused central posterior section of the pelvic girdle.

SkillDrill 27-1   Log Roll

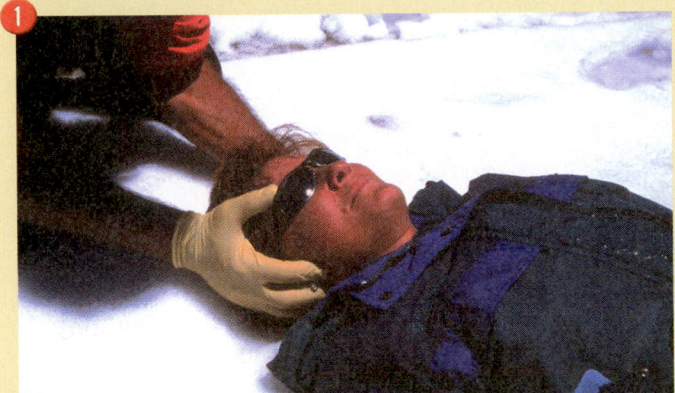

① Manually stabilize the head and neck.

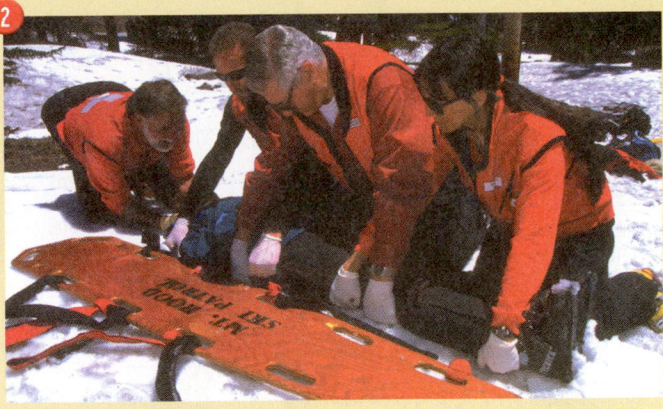

② Position sufficient rescuers on the same side of the patient, kneeling as close to the patient's side as possible.

Position hands on the far side, taking body mass into consideration. Keep your back straight and lean solely from the hips. Overlap hands if possible.

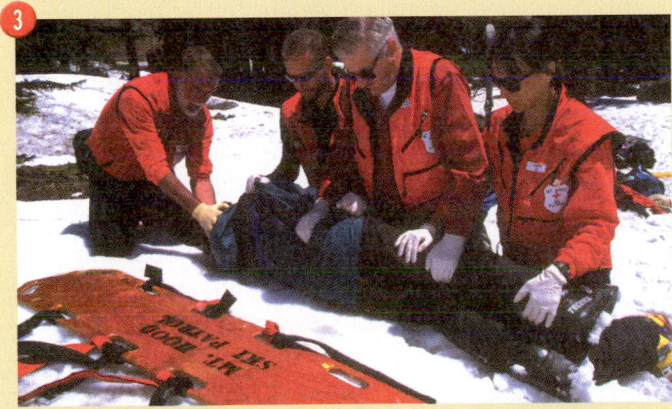

③ Roll the patient as a unit toward the rescuers on command from the leader (at the head), keeping the body in line and while monitoring vital signs. The patient's arm may be alongside the body or elevated, depending on local protocols.

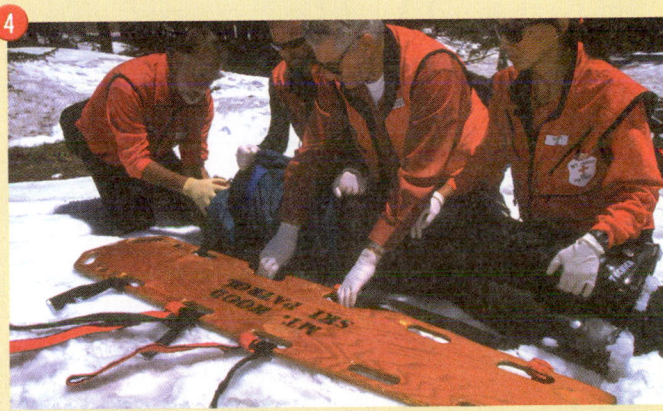

④ Place the backboard, blanket, or stretcher alongside the patient and underneath as far as possible without excessive movement.

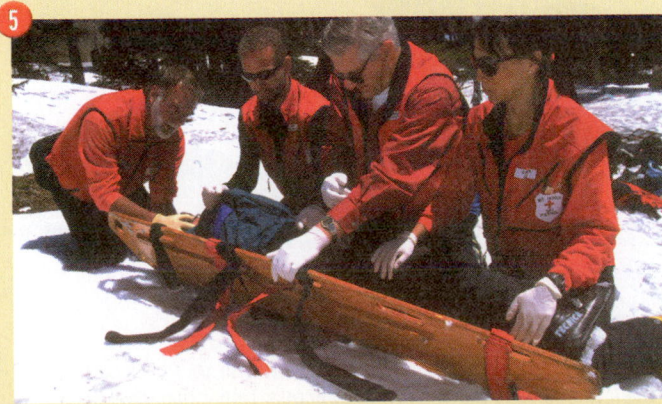

⑤ When using a backboard, bring the device as close as practical to the patient's back.

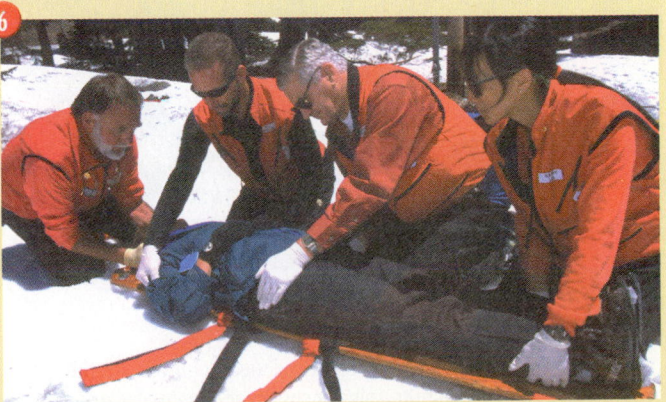

⑥ Roll the patient onto the device on command from the leader, keeping the body in line.

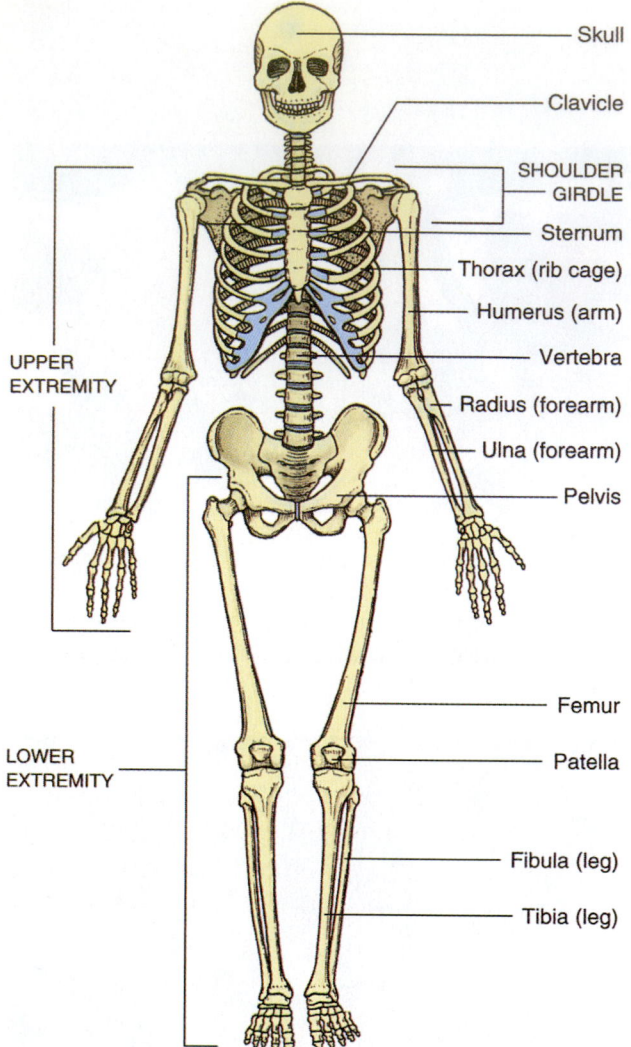

Figure 27-5 When you are standing upright, the weight of anything that you lift and carry in your hands is borne by the shoulder girdle, the spinal column, the pelvis, and the legs.

Labels on skeleton:
- Skull
- Clavicle
- SHOULDER GIRDLE
- Sternum
- Thorax (rib cage)
- Humerus (arm)
- Vertebra
- Radius (forearm)
- Ulna (forearm)
- Pelvis
- Femur
- Patella
- Fibula (leg)
- Tibia (leg)
- UPPER EXTREMITY
- LOWER EXTREMITY

When a person is standing upright, the weight of anything being lifted and carried in the hands is reflected onto the shoulder girdle, the spinal column inferior to it, the pelvis, and then the legs (◄ Figure 27-5). In lifting, if the shoulder girdle is aligned over the pelvis and the hands are held close to the legs, the force that is exerted against the spine occurs in an essentially straight line down the strong, stacked vertebrae in the spinal column. Therefore, with the back properly maintained in an upright position, very little strain occurs against the muscles and ligaments that keep the spinal column in alignment, and significant weight can be lifted and carried without injury to the back (◄ Figure 27-6). However, you may injure your back if you lift with your back curved or, even if straight, bent significantly forward at the hips (▼ Figure 27-7). With the back in either of these positions, the shoulder girdle lies significantly anterior to the pelvis, and the force of lifting is exerted primarily across, rather than down, the spinal column. When this occurs, the weight is supported by the muscles of the back and ligaments that run from the base of the skull to the pelvis (keeping the spinal column in alignment) rather than by each vertebral body and disk resting on those aligned below it. In

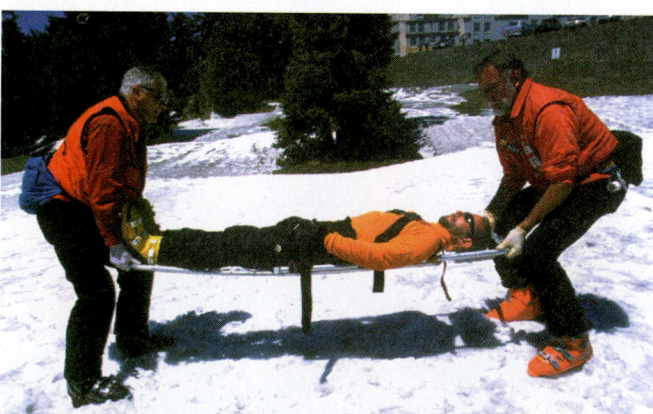

Figure 27-6 If your body is properly aligned when you lift, the line of force exerted against the spine occurs in an essentially straight line down the vertebrae. In this way, the strong, stacked vertebrae support the lift.

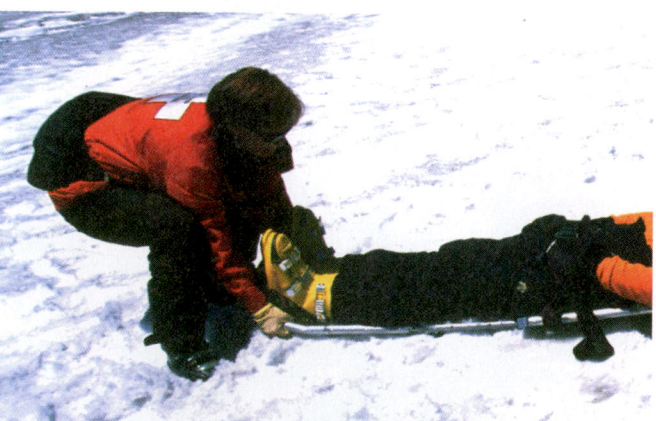

Figure 27-7 You may be injured if you lift with your back curved, as the lifting force is exerted primarily across, rather than down, the spinal column. When this occurs, the muscles of the back, not the vertebrae, are supporting the lift.

addition, the upper spine and torso serve as a lever so that the force that is exerted against the muscles and ligaments in the lumbar and sacral regions, as a result of the mechanical advantage produced, is many times that of the combined weight of your upper body and the object you are lifting. Therefore, the first key rule of lifting is to always keep the back upright (vertical) in a slightly inward curve, and to lift without twisting.

When lifting, you should spread your legs about 15″ apart (shoulder width) and place your feet so that your center of gravity is properly balanced between them. Then, with the back held upright, bring your upper body down by bending the legs. Once you have properly grasped the patient or cot and made any necessary adjustments in the location of your feet, lift the patient by raising your upper body and arms and by straightening your legs until you are again standing. Because the leg muscles are exercised by walking, climbing stairs, or running, they are well developed and extremely strong. Therefore, as well as being the safest way to lift, lifting by extending the properly placed flexed legs is also the most powerful way to lift. This method is appropriately called a **power lift**. The power lift position is also useful for individuals who have weak knees or thighs.

Even if the back is held properly upright, the same adverse force across the spinal column and leverage against the lower back will occur if you lift a heavy object with your arms outstretched so that your hands are significantly anterior to the plane described by the front of the torso. Therefore, you should *never* lift a patient or other heavy object while reaching any significant distance in front of your torso or face. Whenever you are lifting or carrying a patient, be sure to hold your arms so that your hands are almost immediately adjacent to the plane described by your anterior torso (the anterior torso and imaginary lines extended vertically above and below it). Always keep the weight that you are lifting as close to your body as possible.

Lateral force across the spine and sideways leverage against the lower back must also be avoided. If you lift with only one arm or with the arms extended more to one side than the other, more force will be exerted against one side of the shoulder girdle than the other, causing lateral force to be exerted across the spinal column. To prevent this, keep your arms approximately the same distance apart as when hanging at each side of the body, with the weight distributed equally and properly centered between them. If the weight is not balanced between both arms or properly centered between the shoulders when you are preparing to lift, turn your

body and/or move to the left or right until the weight is properly balanced and centered. To lift safely and produce the maximal power lift, you should take the following steps ▶**Skill Drill 27-2** :

1. **Tighten your back in its normal upright position** and use your abdominal muscles to lock it in a slight inward curve.

2. **Spread your legs apart about 15″**, and bend your legs to lower your torso and arms.

3. **With arms extended down each side of the body,** grasp the cot or backboard with your hands held palm up and just in front of the plane described by the anterior torso and imaginary lines extending vertically from it to the ground.

4. **Adjust your orientation and position** until the weight is balanced and centered between both arms **(Step 1)**.

5. **Reposition your feet** as necessary so that they are about 15″ apart with one slightly farther forward and rotated so that you and your center of gravity will be properly balanced between them. In the outdoor environment, make sure you have established a firm footing. Be sure to straddle the object, keep your feet flat, and distribute your weight to the balls of the feet or just behind them **(Step 2)**.

6. **With the arms extended downward,** lift by straightening your legs until you are fully standing. Make sure your back is locked in and that your upper body comes up before your hips **(Step 3)**.

Reverse these steps whenever you are lowering the backboard or stretcher. Always remember to avoid bending at the waist.

Your safety, as well as that of the other rescuers and the patient, depends on the use of proper lifting techniques and having and maintaining a proper hold when lifting or carrying a patient. If you do not have proper hold of the transfer or carrying device, or of the patient in a body lift, you will not be able to bear a proper share of the weight, and there is an increased chance that you can suddenly lose your grasp with one or both hands. If you temporarily lose your grasp with one or both hands, the position and weight distribution of the transfer or carrying device changes suddenly, and the other members of the team must quickly reach beyond a safe distance to avoid dropping the patient. As a result, sudden excessive force

Skill Drill 27-2 Performing the Power Lift

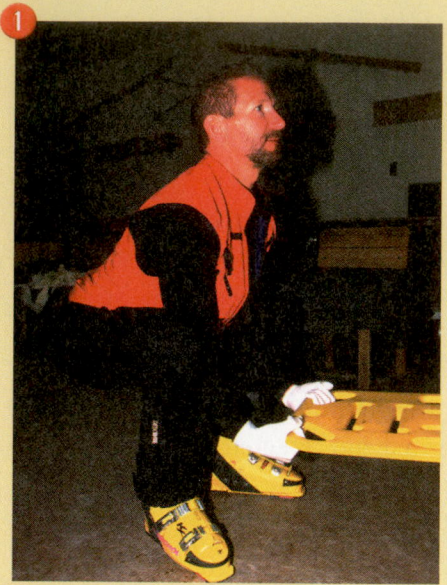

Lock your back into an upright, slightly inward curve.

Spread and bend your legs.

Grasp the backboard, palms up and just in front of you.

Balance and center the weight between your arms.

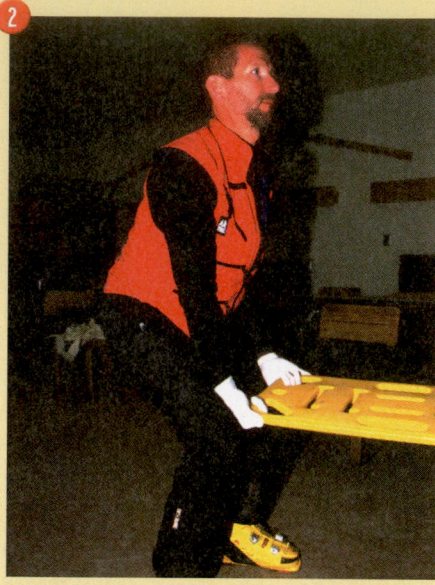

Position your feet, straddle the object, and distribute weight.

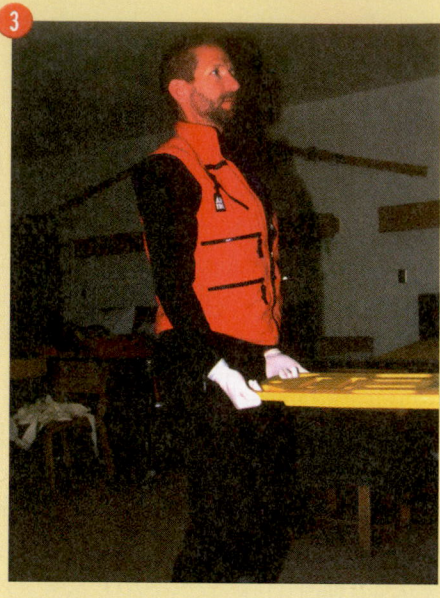

Straighten your legs and lift, keeping your back locked in.

---

may be placed across each one's spine, causing lower back injury.

You should use the **power grip** to get the maximum force from your hands whenever you are lifting a patient ▶ Figure 27-8 . The arm and hand have their greatest lifting strength when facing palm up. Whenever you grasp a transfer or carrying device, your hands should be at least 10″ apart. Each hand should be inserted under the handle with the palm facing up and the thumb extended upward. You should then advance the hand until the thumb prevents further insertion and the cylindrical handle lies firmly in the crease of the curved palm. Curl your fingers and thumb tightly over the top of the handle. All your fingers should be at the same angle. To have the proper power grip, make sure that the underside of the handle is fully supported on your curved palm with only the fingers and thumb preventing it from being pulled sideways or upward out of the palm.

If you must lift the object higher once you have lifted by extending your legs, you will be able to "curl" the object higher by using your biceps to flex the arms while maintaining the power grip and weight supported in the palms.

When directly lifting a patient, you should tightly grip the patient in a place and manner that will ensure that you will not lose your grasp on the patient.

Working in ski and snowboard boots can offer additional challenges when lifting. While designed to main-

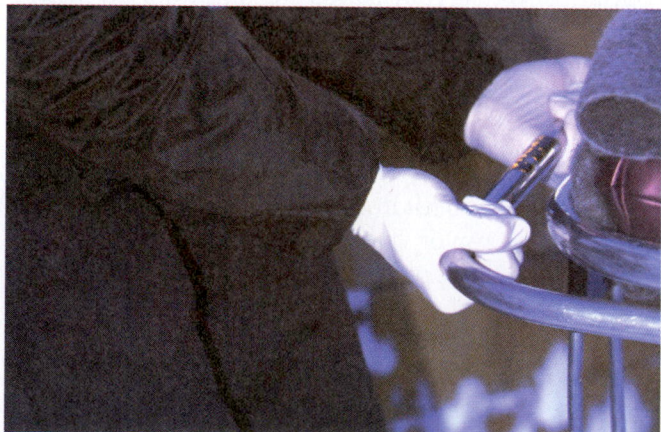

Figure 27-8 To perform the power grip, grasp the handle of the litter with your palms up and your thumb extending up. Make sure your hands are about 10″ apart and that your fingers are all at the same angle. The underside of the handle should be fully supported by the palm of your hand.

tain the foot in an efficient snow riding position, these types of footwear can affect the ergonomics of lifting. Ski boots are especially challenging because the foot is not allowed to bend at the ball and can put undue strain on the toes. Additionally, most boots fix the ankle to some degree and affect the lower leg position used for correct lifting techniques. Be aware of the limits that your boots place on lifting techniques and practice safe lifting while wearing your snow-riding boots.

Weight and Distribution

You must make sure that you understand and follow certain guidelines for carrying a patient on immobilization, transfer or carrying, and transportation devices. (▼ Table 27-1) shows the guidelines.

If a patient is supine on an immobilization or transfer device or is lying or in a semisitting position on a transportation device, his or her weight is not equally distributed between the two ends of the device. Between 68% and 78% of the body weight of a patient in a horizontal position is in the torso. Therefore, more of the patient's weight rests on the head half of the device than on the foot half.

A patient on an immobilization or transfer device should be carried feet first to place the lightest load on the rescuer at the patient's feet, who, to walk forward, must turn and grasp the handles with his or her back to the device. Carrying the patient feet first will also allow a conscious patient to see in the direction of movement.

It is important that you and your team use the correct lifting techniques to lift the backboard or stretcher. You must also make sure that your team members are positioned to take advantage of similar height and strength.

When you must carry a patient on rough terrain, a flight of stairs, or other significant incline, use the most appropriate equipment available. When you use a backboard, stretcher, or stair chair, be sure that the patient is

anatomically secured to the device in such a way that he or she cannot slide significantly when the stretcher is at an angle.

Whenever possible, you should use the patient's armpits as similar anatomic anchors and support points when you use a direct body lift or drag to move the patient or when assisting a patient who can stand.

Directions and Commands

To safely lift and carry a patient, you and your team must anticipate and understand every move, and each move must be executed in a coordinated manner. The team leader should indicate where each team member is to be located and rapidly describe the sequence of steps that will be performed to ensure that the team knows what is expected of it before any lifting is initiated. If you must lift and move the patient through a number of separate stages, the team leader should first give an abbreviated overview of the stages, followed by a more detailed explanation of each stage just before it will occur.

Orders that will initiate the actual lifting or moving or any significant changes in movement should be given in two parts: a preparatory command and a command of execution. For example, if the team leader says "All ready to stop. STOP!," the "All ready to stop" will get your attention, identify who should act, and prepare them to act; the declarative "STOP!" will indicate the exact moment for execution. Commands of execution should be delivered in a louder voice. Often, a countdown is helpful when you need to lift a patient. To avoid confusion in using a countdown, always clarify whether "three" is to be a part of the preparatory command or whether it is to serve as the order to execute. You can say "We're going to lift on three. One-two-THREE!" or "I'm going to count to three and then we're going to lift. One-two-three-LIFT!"

TABLE 27-1 Guidelines for Carrying a Patient on an Immobilization or Transfer Device

- Be sure that you know or can find out the weight to be lifted and the limitations of the team's abilities.
- Coordinate your movements with those of the other team members while constantly communicating with them.
- Do not twist your body as you are carrying the patient.
- Keep the weight that you are carrying as close to your body as possible while keeping your back in a locked-in position.
- Be sure to flex at the hips, not at the waist, and bend at the knees, while making sure that you do not hyperextend your back by leaning back from your waist.

Additional Lifting and Carrying Guidelines

You should estimate how much the patient weighs before attempting to lift him or her. Commonly, adult patients weigh between 100 and 210 lb. If you use the correct technique, you and one other rescuer should be able to safely lift this weight. Depending on your individual strength, you and another rescuer may be able to safely lift an even heavier patient. However, because it is quite a bit safer to have four rescuers lift, you should try to use four rescuers whenever the available resources allow. *You should know how much you can comfortably and safely lift and should not attempt to lift a proportional weight (the share of the weight that you will bear) that exceeds this amount.* If you find that lifting the patient places strain on you, call for the lifting to be stopped and the patient to be lowered. You should then obtain additional help before again attempting to lift the patient. Be sure to communicate clearly and frequently with your partner and other rescuers whenever you are lifting a patient.

You should not attempt to lift a patient who weighs more than 250 lb with fewer than four rescuers, regardless of individual strength. Protocols should include a method to rapidly summon additional help to lift and carry such a patient or, as in the case of a cardiac arrest, provide and maintain the necessary care in the field and when moving and transporting the patient. In addition, you must know, or be able to find out, the weight limitations of the equipment you are using and how to handle patients who exceed the weight limitations.

Because more than half of a patient's weight is distributed to the head end of the backboard or stretcher, the strongest of the available rescuers should be located at the head end of the device. Even with four or more rescuers carrying the patient, the strain on the rescuer carrying the head end of the device will be increased when you must negotiate rough or slippery terrain, a narrow area, or flight of stairs. In carrying a patient up or down trails or rugged terrain, proportionally greater weight will also be distributed to the rescuer who is carrying the foot end when the backboard or stretcher becomes angled because of the incline. You should anticipate this and, in such cases, make sure the two strongest rescuers are positioned at the head and foot ends of the board. Because of the incline of the stairway, if one of the two rescuers is considerably taller than the other, it will be easier if the shorter of the two is at the head end and the taller is at the foot end.

The dynamics that are involved in carrying a patient for any significant distance will not allow you to carry as much proportional weight as you can to safely lift or support the patient during a move onto a nearby backboard or cot. Therefore, if you feel that you are approaching your maximum lifting capacity as you are moving the patient onto a backboard or other transportation device, you should not attempt to lift and carry the patient for any significant distance. You can again attempt to lift and carry the patient after you have decreased the amount of proportional weight you will be carrying by changing your position on the device or that of the others on the team or have obtained additional help.

Always remember to keep your back in a locked-in position and to flex at the hips, not the waist. You should also bend at the knees and keep the patient's weight and your arms as close to your body as possible. Try to avoid any unnecessary lifting and carrying of the patient. If an assist, log roll, bridge lift, or long-axis drag will not harm or jeopardize the patient, use one to move the patient onto the backboard, stretcher, or other transporting device.

Principles of Safe Reaching and Pulling

When you use a long-axis drag to move a patient over snow or other smooth terrain, the same basic body mechanics and principles apply as when lifting and carrying. Your back should always be locked and straight, not curved or bent laterally, and you should avoid any twisting so that the vertebrae remain in normal alignment. When you are reaching overhead, avoid hyperextending your back. When you are pulling a patient who is on the ground, you should always kneel to minimize the distance that you will have to lean over ▶ **Figure 27-9A**). To keep your reach within the recommended distance, reach forward and grasp the patient so that your elbows are just beyond the anterior torso ▶ **Figure 27-9B**). When you are pulling a patient who is at a different height from you, bend your knees until your hips are just below the height of the plane across which you will be pulling the patient ▶ **Figure 27-9C**). During pulling, you should extend your arms no more

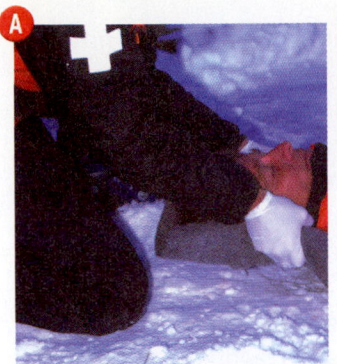 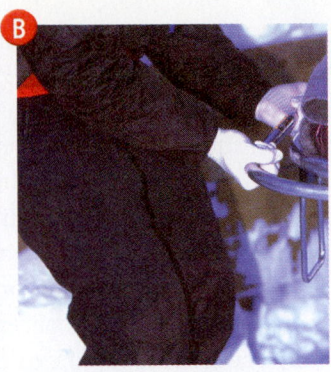 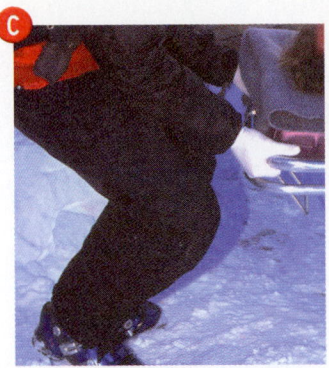 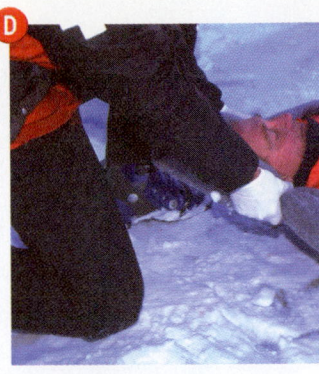

Figure 27-9 Reaching and pulling safely. **A.** Kneel to pull a patient who is on the ground. **B.** When pulling, your elbows should only extend just beyond the anterior torso. **C.** Bend your knees to pull a patient who is at a different height than you are. **D.** Position your feet or knees to balance the force of pull.

than about 15″ to 20″ in front of your torso. Reposition your feet (or knees, if kneeling) so that the force of pull will be balanced equally between both arms and the line of pull will be centered between them
▲ Figure 27-9D. Pull the patient by slowly flexing your arms. When you can pull no farther because your hands have reached the front of your torso, stop and move back another 15″ to 20″. Then, when properly positioned, repeat the steps. You should alternate between pulling the patient by flexing your arms and then repositioning yourself so that your arms are again extended with your hands about 15″ in front of your torso. By not moving yourself and the patient simultaneously, you will prevent undesirable jostling of the patient and the chance that sudden unscheduled force will occur across your spine. You should also try to prevent injury to yourself by avoiding situations that involve strenuous effort lasting more than 1 minute.

LONG-AXIS DRAG Sometimes a **long-axis drag** is necessary for a patient when not an emergency move. This maneuver is performed by sliding the patient headward or footward in the direction of the long axis of the body. The patient should be supine and aligned into the neutral, anatomic position, with a rigid collar in place. *Do not move the patient sideways* because this may bend the spine. Rescuers must maintain manual stabilization of the head and neck, but avoid accidentally applying traction or compression to the head and neck. They must not slide a patient with suspected shoulder or clavical injuries headward, or a patient with suspected lower-extremity or pelvic injuries footward.

The long-axis drag requires at least three rescuers. For a headward drag, the first rescuer, who is in charge, is at the patient's head, stabilizing the head and neck. The second and third rescuers are on either side of the patient, with one hand in the patient's armpit and the

other hand grasping the patient's belt or clothing at the waist **▼ Figure 27-10**.

On command, the rescuers drag the patient a previously specified distance, usually about 12″. The rescuers then reposition themselves and repeat the drag until reaching the desired location.

For a footward drag, the process is the same except the second and third rescuers are positioned on each side of the patient's legs, with one hand grasping the ankle and the other the belt or clothing at the waist. The patient's wrists should be tied together in front of the body.

General Considerations

Moving a patient should normally be done in an orderly, planned, and unhurried fashion. This approach will protect both you and the patient from further injury and reduce the risk of worsening the patient's condition when he or she is moved.

At a minimum, on most ski area and other outdoor rescue calls you will have to lift the patient onto a

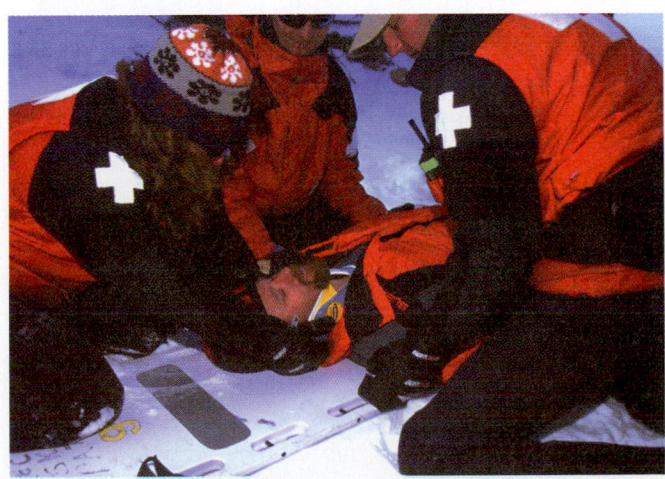

Figure 27-10 Long-axis drag.

transfer device, and then move the patient onto a transportation device. An additional move would occur when the patient reaches more definitive care—such as to a gurney or cot in an aid room or loading the patient into an automobile, ambulance, or helicopter.

You should carefully plan ahead and select the methods and equipment that will involve the least lifting and carrying. Remember to always consider whether there is an option that will cause less strain to you and the other rescuers.

Emergency Moves

You should use an **emergency move** to move a patient before initial assessment and care are provided when there is some potential danger, and you and the patient must move to a safe place to avoid possible serious harm or death. The presence of snowslides, rockslides, fire, explosives, or hazardous materials and your inability to protect the patient from other hazards or gain access to others who need lifesaving care are all situations in which you should use an emergency move.

The only other time you should use an emergency move is if you cannot properly assess the patient or provide immediate, potentially critical emergency care because of the patient's location or position.

Rapid extrication techniques are used only when there is a true emergency (less than 1 minute) and no time to get help or to use the standard immobilization devices. (▼ Table 27-2) describes the situations in which you should use rapid extrication techniques.

In such cases, the delay that occurs in applying an extrication-type vest or half-board is contraindicated. However, the manual support and immobilization that you provide when using rapid extrication techniques produce a greater risk of spine movement. You

TABLE 27-2 Situations in Which to Use Rapid Extrication Techniques

- The scene or vehicle is unsafe.
- The patient cannot be properly assessed before being removed from the scene.
- The patient needs immediate intervention that requires a supine position.
- The patient's condition requires immediate transport to the hospital.
- The patient blocks the rescuer's access to another seriously injured patient.

should not use rapid extrication techniques if no urgency exists.

The steps of rapid extrication techniques must be considered a general procedure to be adapted as needed. Every situation will be different—varied terrain, different obstacles, a different car, a different patient, and a different crew. You will handle a large, heavy adult differently than a small adult or child. Your resourcefulness and ability to adapt are necessary elements to successfully perform the rapid extrication technique.

If you are alone and danger at the scene makes it necessary for you to use an emergency move, regardless of a patient's injuries, you should use a drag to pull the patient along the long axis of the body. This will help to keep the spinal column in line as much as possible. When performing an emergency move, one of your primary concerns is the danger of aggravating an existing spinal injury. Remember that it is impossible to remove a patient quickly from a vehicle while providing as much protection to the spine as you would give by using an immobilization device. However, if you follow certain guidelines during the move, you can usually move a patient from a life-threatening situation without causing further injury to the patient.

You can move a patient on his or her back along the floor or ground by using one of the following methods.

- **Emergency clothes drag.** Pull on the patient's clothing in the neck and shoulder area (► Figure 27-11A).
- **Blanket drag.** lace the patient onto a blanket, coat, or other item that can be pulled (► Figure 27-11B).
- **Arm drag.** Rotate the patient's arms so that they are extended straight on the ground beyond his or her head, grasp the wrists, and, with the arms elevated above the ground, drag the patient (► Figure 27-11C).
- **Arm-to-arm drag.** Place your arms under the patient's shoulders and through the armpits, and, while grasping the patient's arms, drag the patient backward (► Figure 27-11D).

If you are alone and must remove an unconscious patient or to move patients over snow or other smooth terrain, make certain to maintain manual stabilization of the head and neck throughout the maneuver. Roll the patient into the supine position. This movement is difficult for the single rescuer because the patient must be rolled without twisting the neck or back (► Figure 27-12).

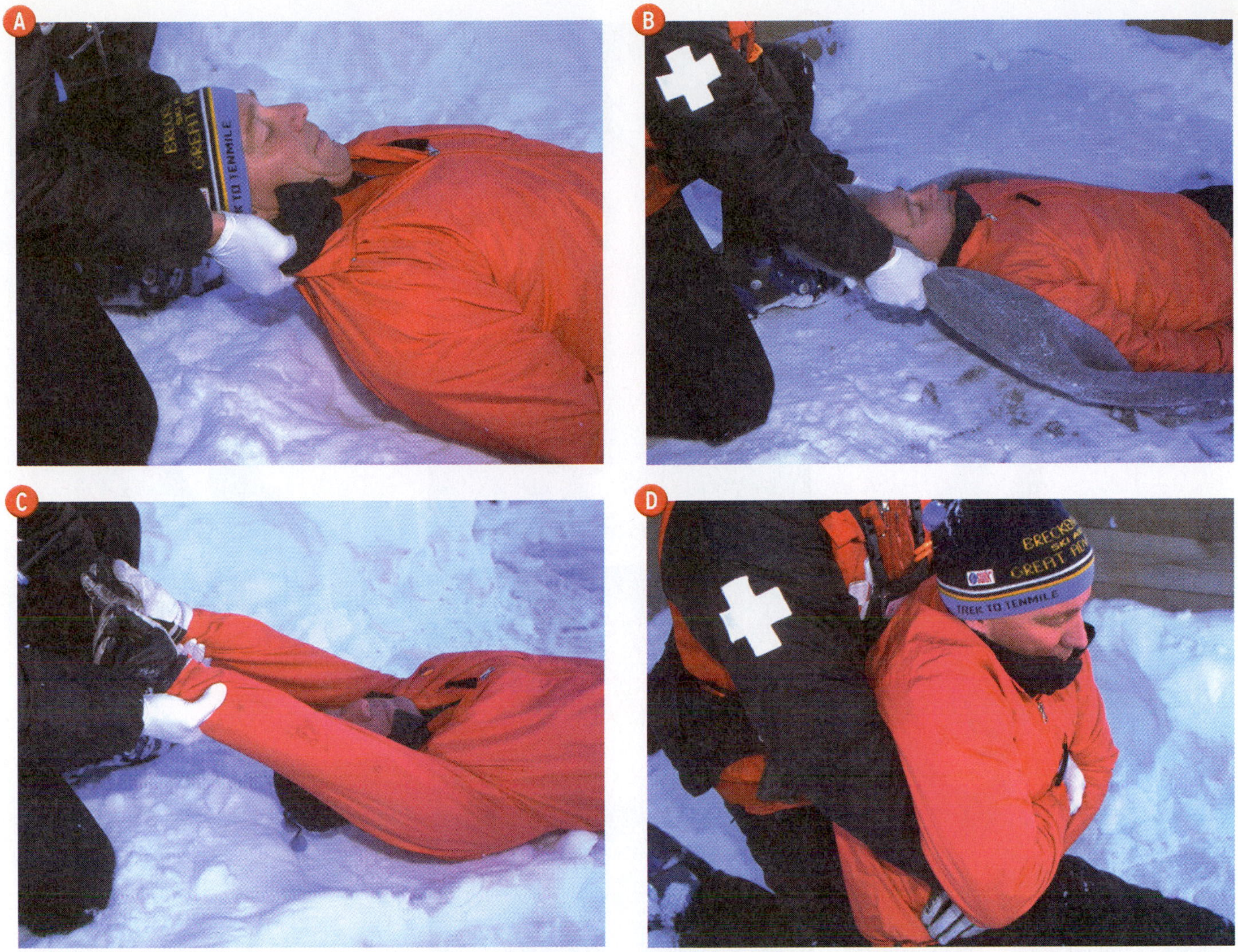

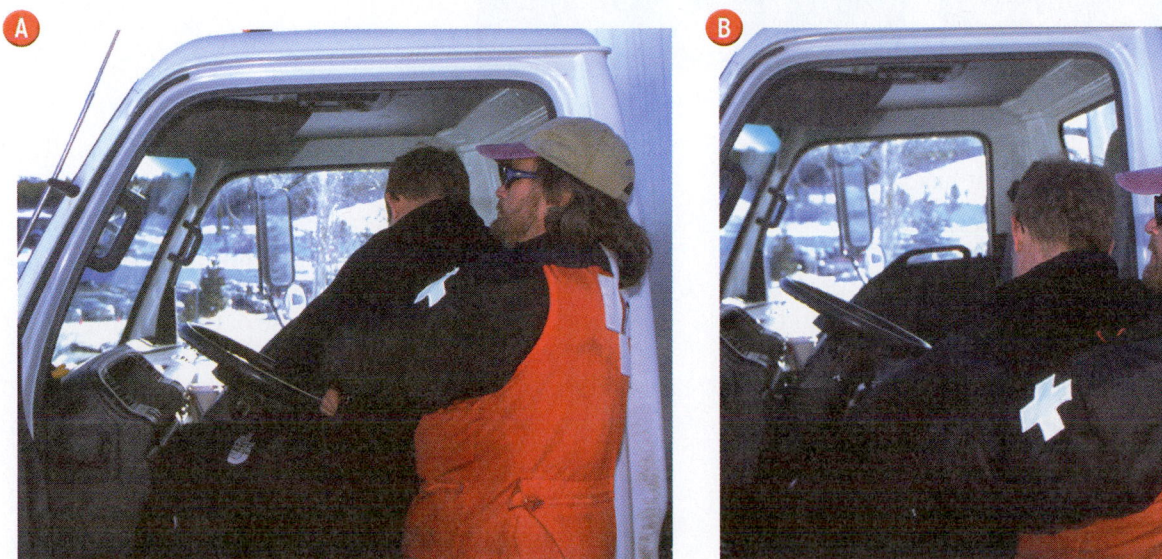

Figure 27-11 Long-axis dragging methods. **A.** Emergency clothes drag. **B.** Blanket drag. **C.** Arm drag. **D.** Arm-to-arm drag.

Figure 27-12 One-person technique for moving an unconscious patient. **A.** Grasp the patient under the arm. **B.** Pull the patient slowly into a supine position.

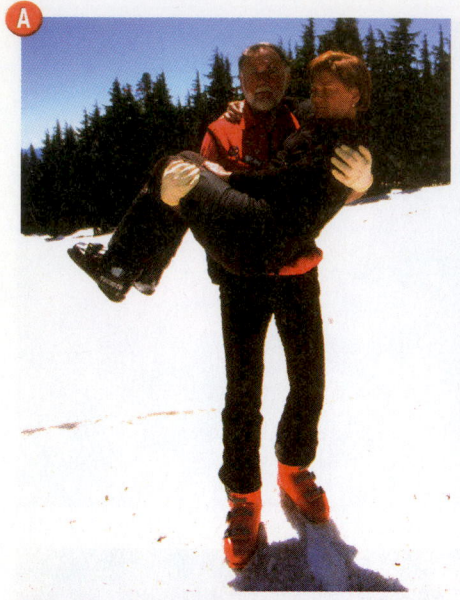

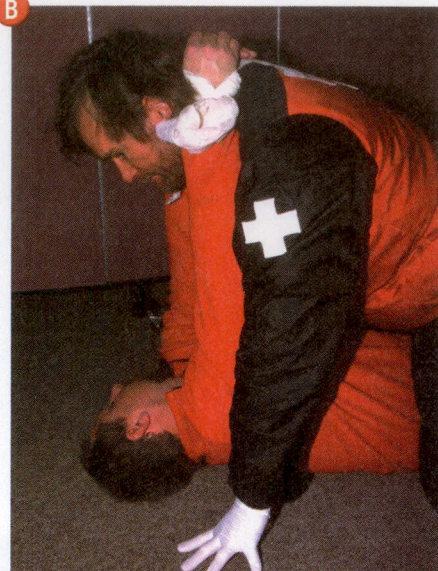

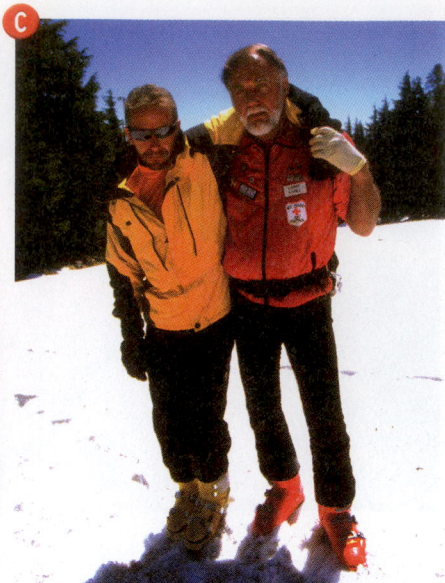

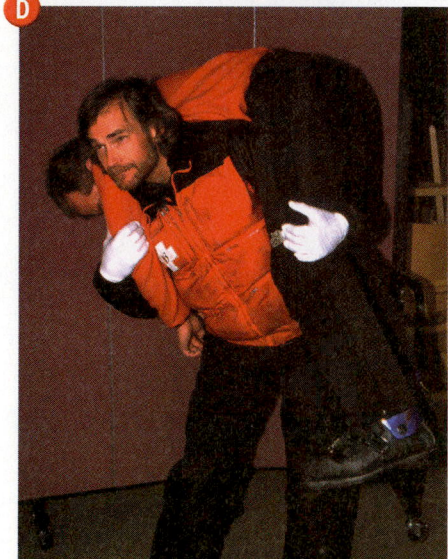

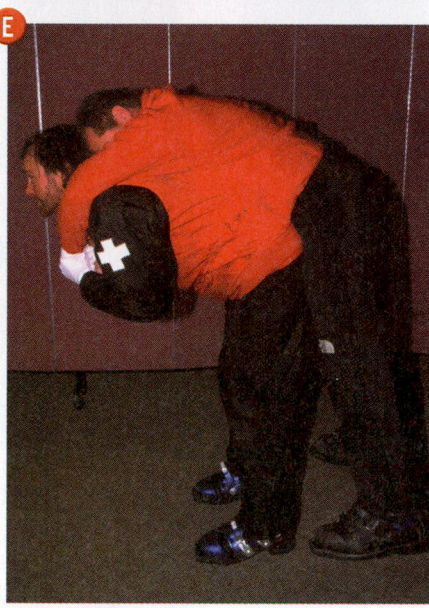

Figure 27-13 One-rescuer drags, carries, and lifts. **A.** Front cradle. **B.** Firefighter's drag. **C.** One-person walking assist. **D.** Firefighter's carry. **E.** Pack strap.

The patient can be pulled by the feet or trousers and dragged feet first. To drag a patient head first, extend the patient's arms above his or her head, cradle the patient's head in the neutral position between his or her arms, and pull the patient by the wrists. Move in a crouched position, pulling the patient slowly and smoothly about 12″ at a time. Reposition and repeat the drag until you reach the desired location.

It is preferable to pull the patient on a sheet of material such as a poncho or space blanket, if available. Roll the patient (if found nonsupine) onto the material or place the material under the patient by first pleating or tightly rolling it lengthwise, leaving one third flat. Place the rolled side of the material alongside the patient and push it under the patient's body, then pull it from the opposite side so that it unrolls under the individual. If done properly, it unrolls so that the patient ends up at its center.

You should use one-person techniques to move a patient only if a potentially life-threatening danger exists and you are alone or, because of the pressing nature of the danger, another rescuer is moving a second patient simultaneously. Additional one-rescuer drags, carries, and lifts are shown in ▲**Figure 27-13**.

Urgent Moves

An urgent move may be necessary for moving a patient with an altered level of consciousness, inadequate ventilation, or shock (hypoperfusion). An extreme weather condition may also make an urgent move necessary. In some cases, patients must be urgently moved from the location or position in which they are found. When a patient who is sitting in a car or truck must be urgently moved, you should use the rapid extrication technique.

Nonurgent Moves

When both the scene and the patient are stable, you should carefully plan how to move the patient. If your patient move is rushed or not well planned, it may result in discomfort or injury to the patient, you, and your team. Before you attempt any move, the team leader must be sure that there are enough personnel, any obstacles have been identified or removed, the proper equipment is available, and the procedure and path to be followed have been clearly identified and discussed.

In nonurgent situations, you and your team may choose one of several methods for lifting and carrying a patient. Some general methods are presented here, which may serve as a basis for your plan. You may adapt these procedures to meet your needs on a case-by-case basis.

BRIDGE LIFT The **bridge lift** is a nonemergency move for a patient with no spinal injury that requires at least three rescuers. With a possible spine injury, this same maneuver would require at least four but preferably six rescuers. This bridge lift maneuver requires the rescuers to form a bridge by bracing their heads against the shoulders of opposite rescuers or a stationary object such as a tree. All rescuers should have a mental image of the spinal plane whenever moving the patient so that during movement, the patient's head, shoulders, and hips are maintained in line with each other, at right angles to the spine, and parallel to the spinal plane.

The bridge lift is preferred to the direct ground lift because it allows rescuers to lift the patient with their arms and shoulders instead of their backs. It is also a more stable lift because rescuers are in better balance, lifting requires less effort, and it is easier to stabilize the patient's spine.

One rescuer is designated as the leader preferably one who is positioned so that he or she can easily see the entire scene. In addition to the other rescuers involved in the actual lift, an extra person is required to slide the long backboard in place under the patient. Before getting into position for the lift, the rescuers should agree on the height they wish to raise the patient, usually 6″ to 12″. ▶ **Skill Drill 27-3** shows how to do the bridge lift.

1. **The first rescuer is at the patient's head, maintaining manual stabilization of the patient's head and neck (Step 1).** A rigid collar should be in place.

2. **Rescuers 2 and 3 are on one side of the patient, faced by rescuers 4 and 5, respectively, on the opposite side.** The rescuers kneel close to the patient's body, with their knees 8″ to 12″ apart **(Step 2)**.

3. **Each rescuer butts his or her head against the shoulder of the rescuer kneeling opposite of him or her,** ie, rescuers 2 and 4 brace against each other and rescuers 3 and 5 brace against each other. The rescuer's arms should hang freely **(Step 3)**.

4. Rescuers 2 and 4 then place their hands at the level of the patient's shoulders and lower chest; rescuers 3 and 5 place their hands at the level of the patient's lower abdomen or upper thighs and legs. Each hand is placed under the patient's body directly below the rescuer's shoulder so that lifting can be straight and up.

5. At a word from the leader, the four rescuers at the patient's sides brace their heads against their opposite partner's shoulders and prepare to lift. On command, the rescuers smoothly lift the patient to the height previously agreed on. An assistant then slides the long backboard beneath the patient **(Step 4)**.

In some cases, cramped quarters or other constraints prevent the rescuers from bringing the backboard close to the patient, so the patient must be moved a short distance. This can be done by means of a long-axis drag or by the direct ground lift-and-carry procedure.

DIRECT GROUND LIFT. The **direct ground lift** is used for patients with no suspected spinal injury who are found lying supine in a neutral, anatomic position. You should use this lift when you have to lift and carry the patient some distance to be placed on the cot. If you find the patient semiprone or lying on his or her side, you should first roll the patient onto his or her back. Ideally, the direct ground lift should be performed by three or more rescuers; however, it can be done with only two. It is difficult to perform with small rescuers or a heavy patient, and the chance of injury to the rescuers' backs is greater than with the bridge lift. The direct ground lift is performed as follows ▶ **Skill Drill 27-4** :

1. **Line up on one side of the patient** with rescuer 1 at the patient's head, rescuer 2 at the patient's waist, and rescuer 3 at the patient's knees. All rescuers kneel on one knee, preferably the same knee **(Step 1)**.

2. **The patient's arms should be placed on his or her chest, if possible (Step 2)**.

3. **Rescuer 1 places one arm under the patient's neck and shoulders** and cradles the patient's head, then places the other arm under the patient's lower back **(Step 3)**.

Skill Drill 27-3 The Bridge Lift

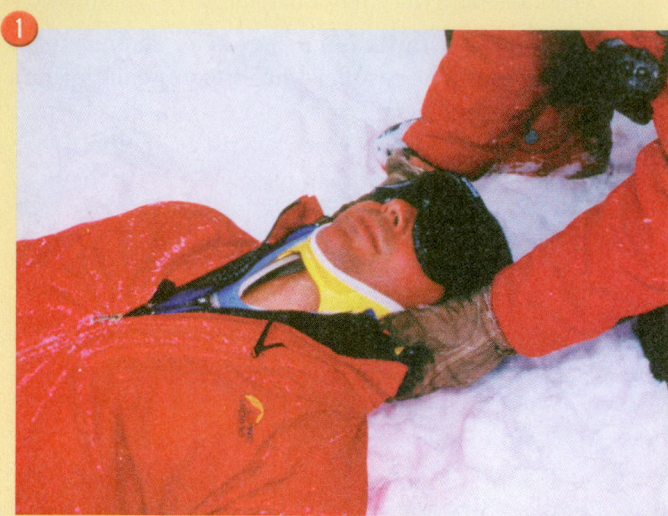

Manually stabilize the head and neck.

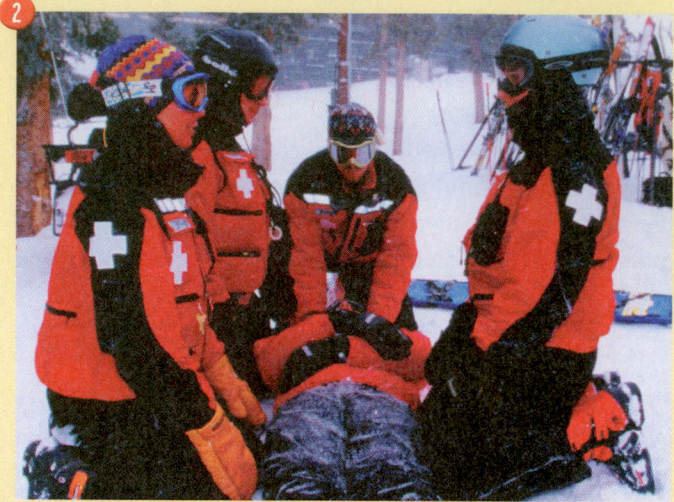

With five rescuers, the first rescuer is at the head, rescuers 2 and 3 are at one side, and rescuers 4 and 5 are at the other side.

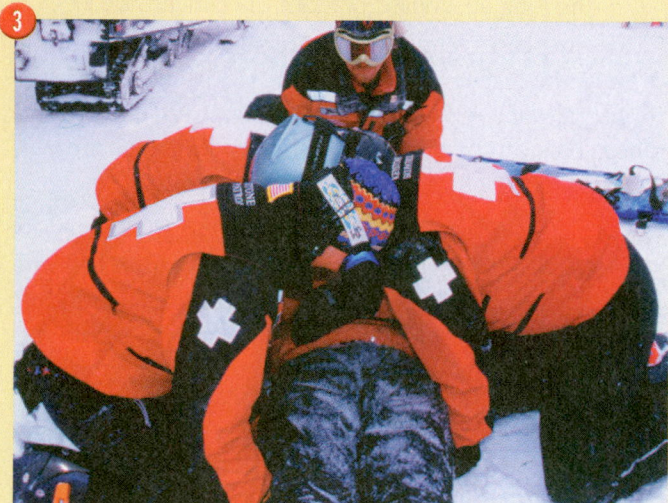

Position the rescuers and have them form a bridge over the patient, head-to-shoulder or shoulder-to-shoulder. All rescuers must use the same configuration.

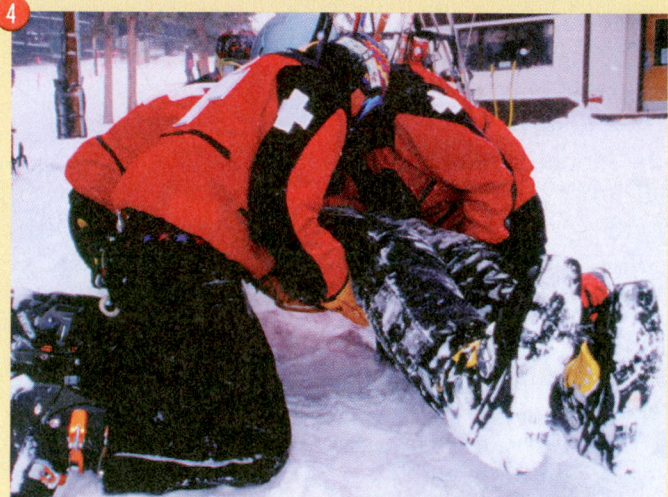

Position hands underneath the patient to lift at points of body mass and ensure the rescuer's commitment and distribution across the bridge.

Lift the patient just enough to place a backboard underneath.

SkillDrill 27-4 Direct Ground Lift

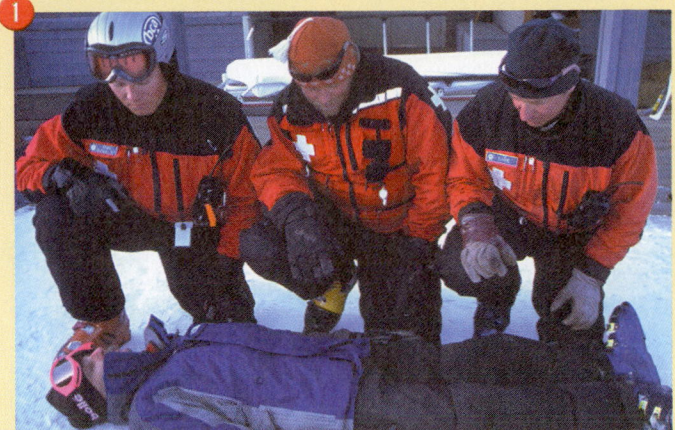

Line up on one side of the patient with rescuer 1 at the patient's head, rescuer 2 at the patient's waist, and rescuer 3 at the patient's knees. All rescuers kneel on one knee, preferably the same knee.

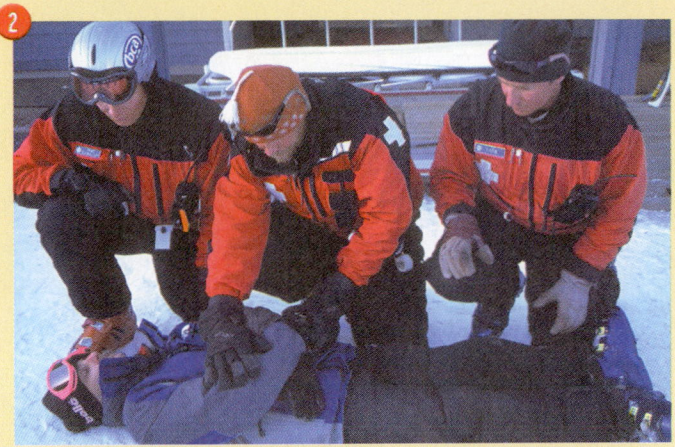

The patient's arms should be placed on his or her chest, if possible.

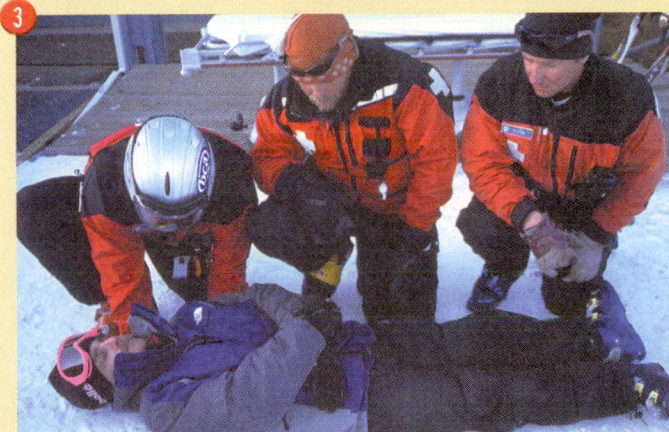

Rescuer 1 then places the other arm under the patient's shoulder.

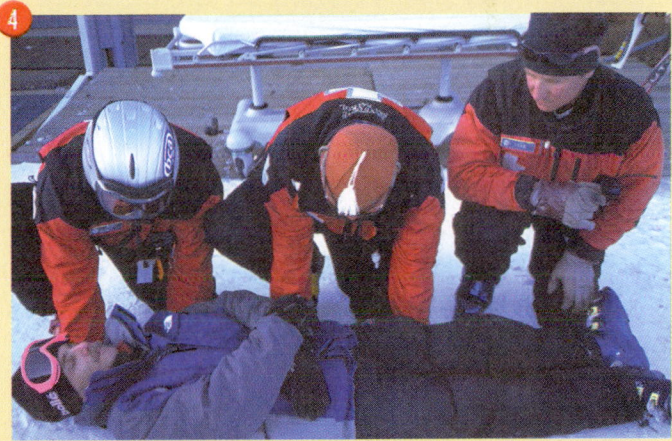

Rescuer 2 places both arms under the patient's lower back and buttocks.

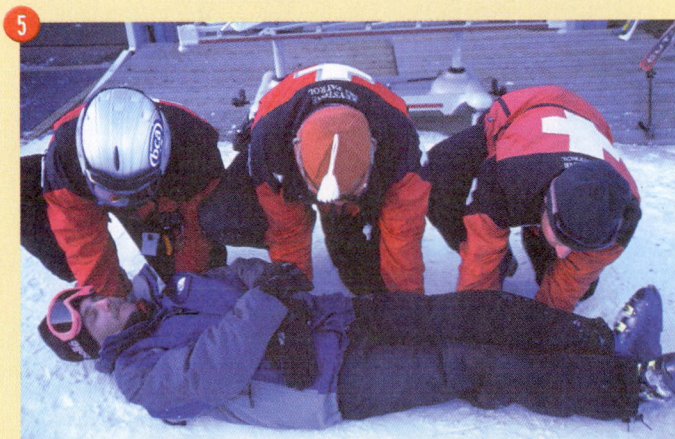

Rescuer 3 places both arms under the patient's legs.

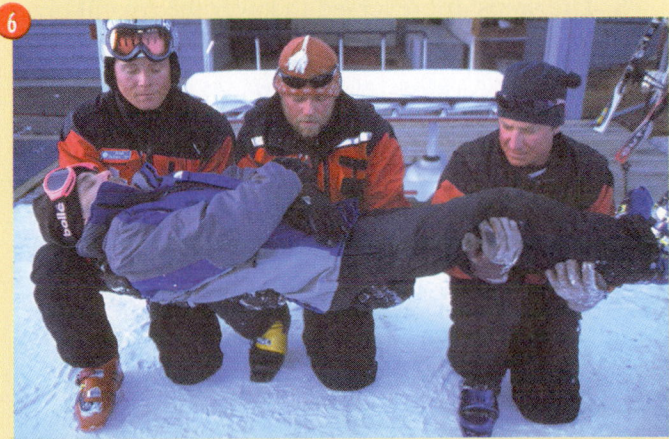

On command, the team lifts the patient up to knee level as each rescuer rests an arm on his or her knee.

Continued.

Skill Drill 27-4   Direct Ground Lift—continued.

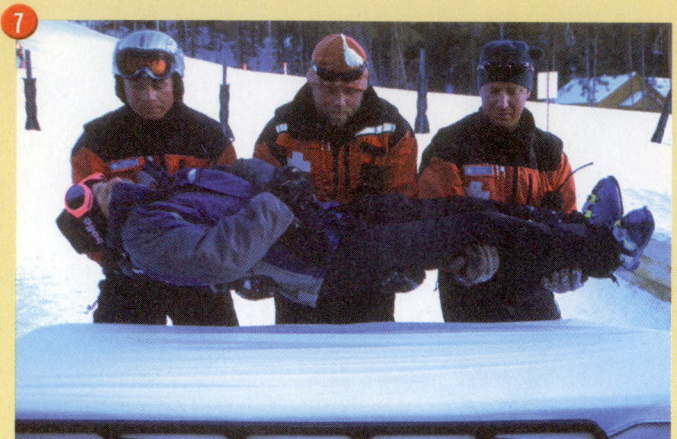

As a team and on signal, each rescuer rolls the patient in toward his or her chest. Again on signal, the team stands and carries the patient to the carrying or transportation device.

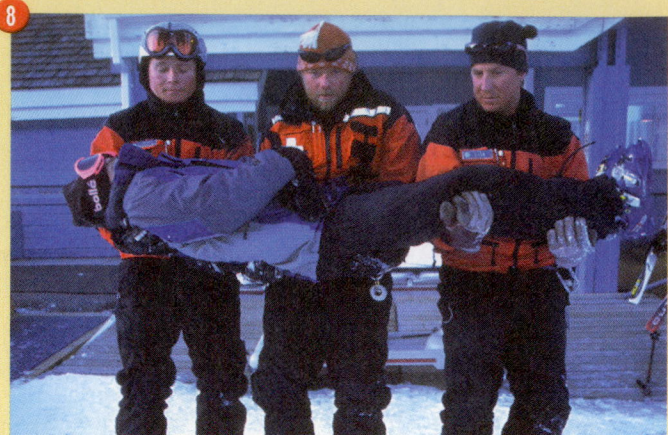

The steps are reversed to lower the patient onto the carrying or transportation device.

4. **Rescuer 2 places both arms under the lower back and buttocks,** and rescuers 1 and 3 slide their arms either up to the midback or down to the buttocks as appropriate **(Step 4)**.

5. **Rescuer 3 places one arm under the patient's knees** and the other above the buttocks **(Step 5)**.

6. **On command, the team lifts the patient** up to knee level as each rescuer rests an arm on his or her knee **(Step 6)**.

7. **As a team and on signal,** each rescuer rolls the patient in toward his or her chest. Again on signal, the team stands and carries the patient to the carrying or transportation device **(Step 7)**.

8. **The steps are reversed** to lower the patient onto the carrying or transportation device **(Step 8)**.

EXTREMITY LIFT. The **extremity lift** may also be used for patients with no suspected extremity or spinal injuries who are supine or in a sitting position on the ground. The extremity lift may be especially helpful when the patient is in a very narrow space or there is not enough room for the patient and a team of rescuers to stand side by side.

Communication is the key to success with this lift. You and your partner must coordinate your movements through direct verbal commands.

The first rescuer kneels behind the patient's head as the second rescuer kneels at the patient's feet. The two rescuers are facing each other. The patient's hands should be crossed over his or her chest. The first rescuer places one hand under each of the patient's armpits. The second rescuer grasps the patient's wrists. The two rescuers pull and lift the upper torso until the patient is in a sitting position. The first rescuer reaches his or her arms through the patient's armpits and grasps the patient's forearms, or his or her own wrists. The second rescuer moves to a position between the patient's legs, facing in the same direction as the patient, and slips his or her hands under the patient's knees. Both rescuers move up to a crouching standing position and make sure they are balanced with a good grip on the patient. As the rescuer at the head gives the command, both stand fully upright and move the patient to the carrying device ▶ **Figure 27-14**.

You will be less likely to injure yourself if you bend at the hips and knees and use your legs for lifting. However, this lift and carry method increases pressure on the patient's chest, so the patient may be uncomfortable in this position.

Transfer Moves

There are several ways to transfer the patient from an immobilization or transfer device onto a transportation device.

DIRECT CARRY. Transfer a supine patient from the ground or a bed to the toboggan or other transportation device using the direct carry method ▶ **Figure 27-15**. Position the transportation device parallel to the patient. Be sure that you prepare the transportation device by

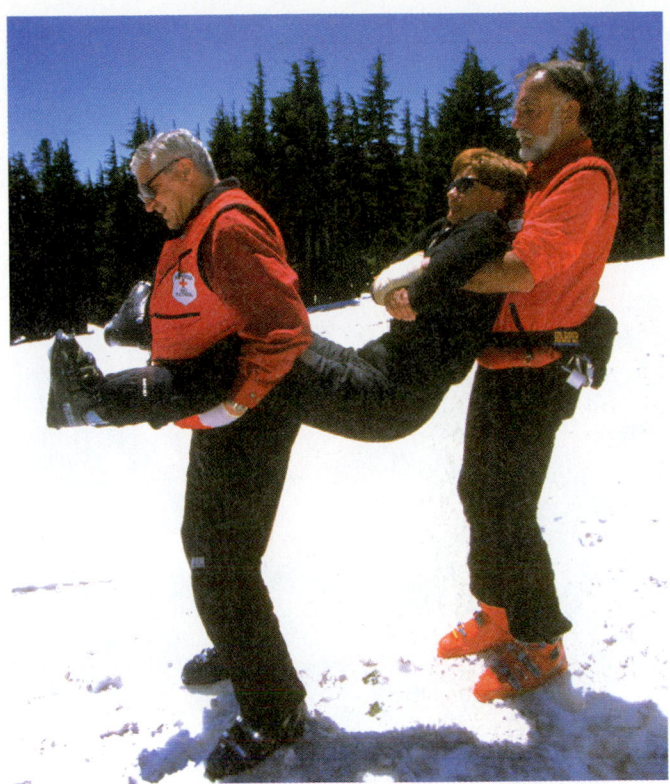

Figure 27-14 When performing the extremity lift, stand upright and move the patient to the carrying device when the rescuer at the head gives the command.

unbuckling the straps and removing any other items from it and firmly securing it on the terrain. You should slide one arm under the patient's neck and cup the patient's shoulder. Another rescuer should slide his or her hand under the patient's hip and lift slightly. You should then slide your other arm under the patient's back, and the other rescuer should place both arms underneath the patient's hips and calves. If a third rescuer is available, he or she can place his or her hands under the patient as well. Slide the patient to the edge of the transportation device without compromising the injury, lift and curl the patient toward your chests, and gently place the patient onto it.

BLANKET LIFT. To move the patient lying on a sheet or blanket to a bed, use the blanket lift, (often referred to as the direct sheet method) ▼ **Figure 27-16** . If necessary, roll the patient onto the sheet or blanket. Place the transportation device next to the bed, making sure it is at the same height as the bed and rails are lowered and straps are unbuckled. Be sure to hold the device to keep it from moving.

Roll the sides of the blanket underneath the patient to provide a better grip. Reach across the device and grasp the sheet or blanket firmly at the patient's head, chest, hips, and knees. Gently slide the patient onto the device.

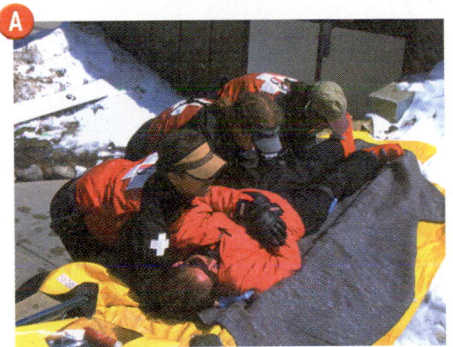
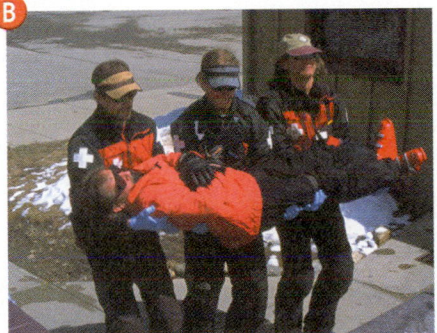
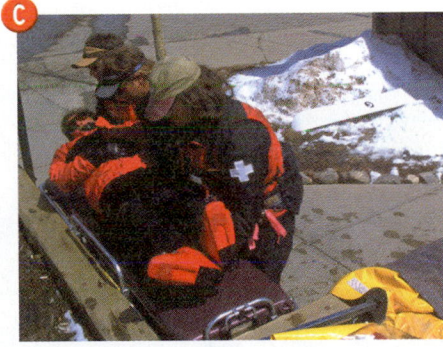

Figure 27-15 The direct carry method. **A.** Position the cot nearby and line up next to the patient. **B.** Lift the patient in a smooth, coordinated fashion. Slowly position him or her over the cot. **C.** Slowly and gently lower the patient onto the cot.

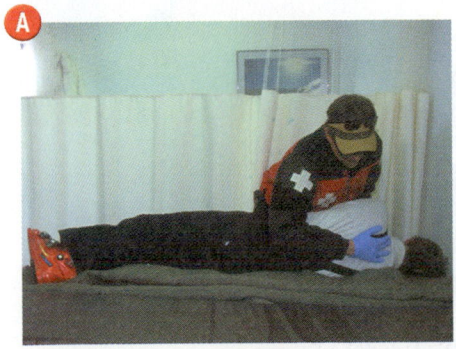
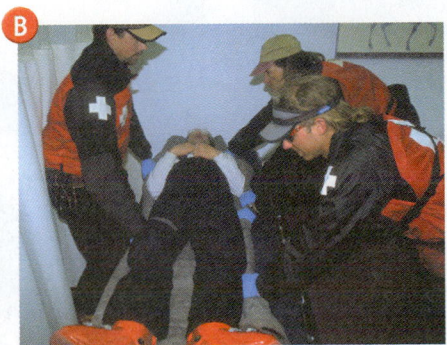
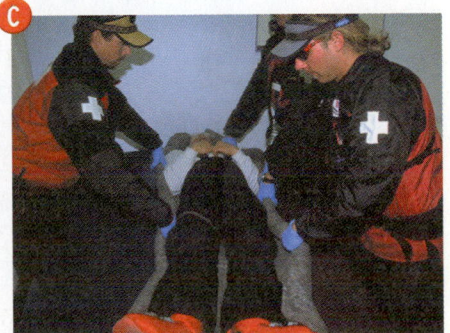

Figure 27-16 The blanket lift method. **A.** Roll the patient onto a blanket or sheet. **B.** Bring the cot in parallel to the bed. Gently pull the patient to the edge of the bed. **C.** Transfer the patient to the cot.

Skill Drill 27-5 Using a Scoop Stretcher

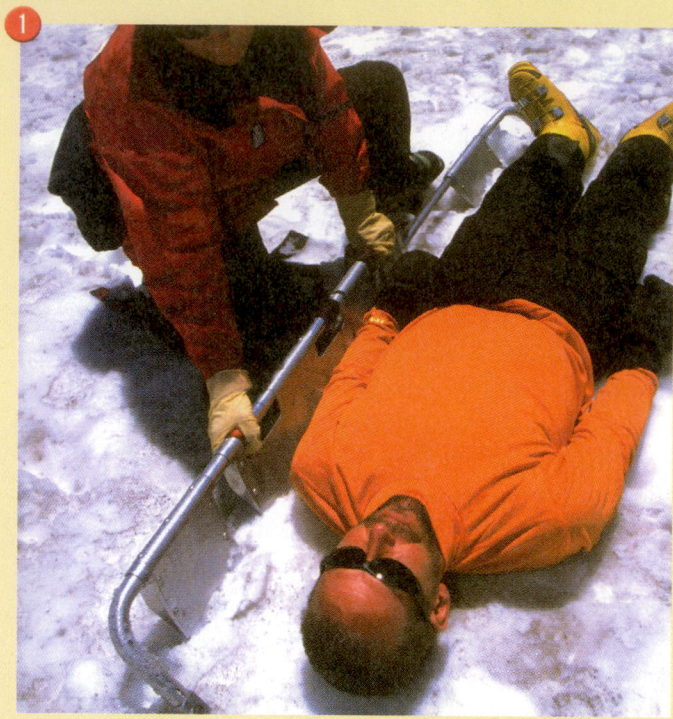

1 Adjust stretcher length.

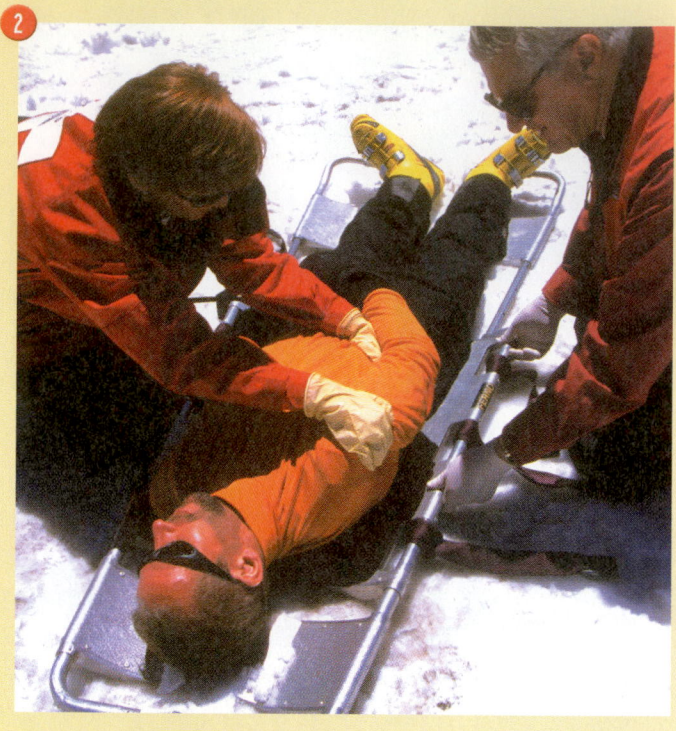

2 Lift patient slightly and slide stretcher into place, one side at a time.

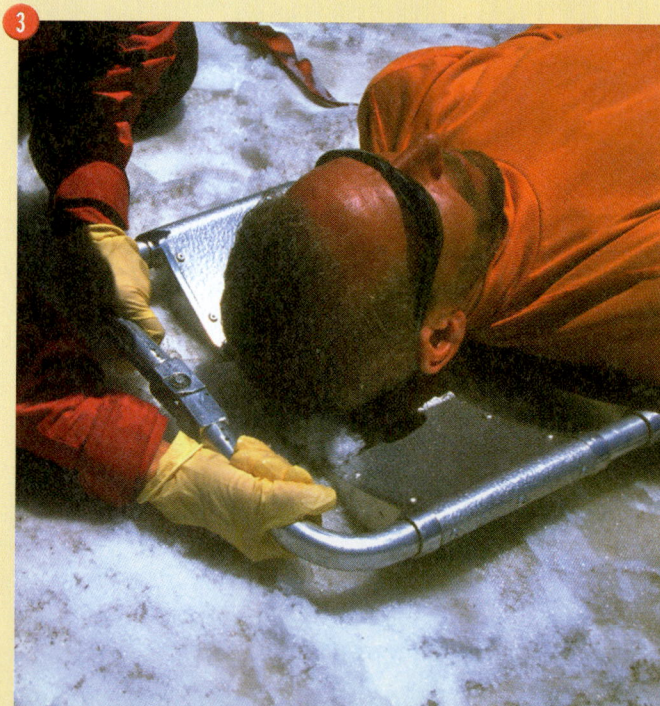

3 Lock the stretcher ends together, avoiding pinching.

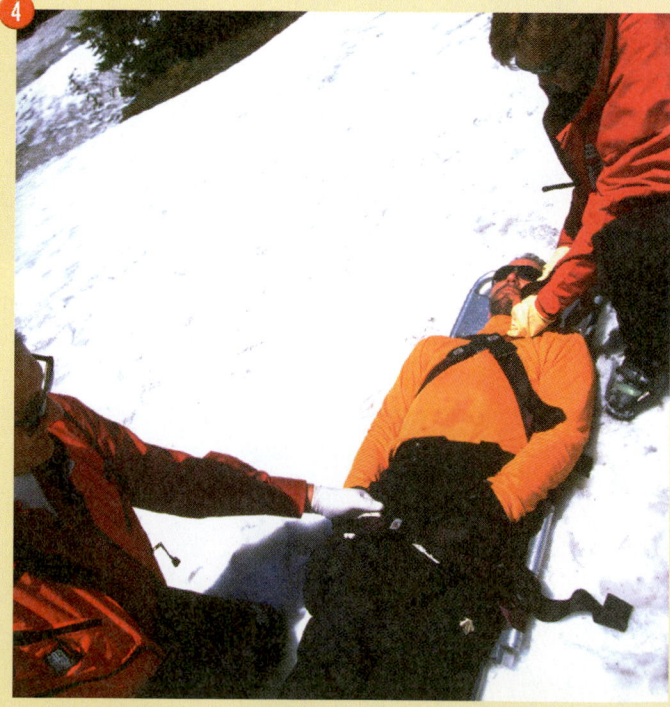

4 Secure the patient and transfer to the cot.

OTHER CARRIES. Other carries are performed in the following manner:

- Place a backboard or blanket next to the patient and, after using a log roll or slide to move the patient onto the backboard, secure the patient and lift and carry the backboard to the nearby prepared bed.

- Insert the halves of a scoop stretcher under each side of the patient, and fasten the two sides together. Lift and carry the patient to the nearby prepared bed. Follow the steps in ◀ **Skill Drill 27-5** . (Note that you can also log roll a patient onto a scoop stretcher that is already locked together.)

1. **With the scoop stretcher separated,** measure the length of the scoop and adjust to the proper length **(Step 1)**.

2. **Position the stretcher,** one side at a time. One rescuer lifts the patient's side slightly by pulling on the far hip and upper arm, while the other rescuer slides the stretcher into place **(Step 2)**.

3. **Lock the stretcher ends together** by engaging their locking mechanisms one at a time and continuing to lift the patient slightly as needed to avoid pinching **(Step 3)**.

4. **Apply and tighten straps** to secure the patient to the scoop stretcher before transferring to the cot **(Step 4)**.

- Assist an able patient to the edge of the bed, and, placing the patient's legs over the side, help the patient to sit up. Move the cot so that its foot end touches the bed near the patient. Help the patient to stand and rotate so that he or she can sit down on the center of the cot. Lift the patient's legs, and rotate them onto the cot while your partner lowers the torso onto the cot.

To avoid the strain of unnecessary lifting and carrying, you should use the draw sheet method or assist an able patient to the cot whenever possible.

To move a patient from the ground or the floor onto the cot you should use one of the following methods:

- Lift and carry the patient to the nearby prepared cot using a direct body carry.

- Use a log roll or long-axis drag to place the patient onto a backboard, and then lift and carry the backboard to the cot. Place both the backboard and the patient onto the cot.

- Insert the halves of a scoop stretcher under the patient and, after securing the halves together, lift and carry the stretcher to the prepared cot. You can also log roll the patient onto the scoop stretcher. Separate and remove the scoop stretcher once the patient has been placed on the cot.

- Log roll the patient onto a blanket, centering the patient on the blanket and rolling up the excess material on each side. Lift the patient by the blanket, and carry him or her to the nearby cot.

With minor lower-extremity injuries, two rescuers can help the patient stand and provide support from either side to move a patient from the aid room to a nearby vehicle. The patient balances on the uninjured foot and puts one arm around each rescuer's neck. The rescuer on the side of the injury supports the splinted extremity. The patient, supported and partially carried by the rescuers, then hops to the waiting vehicle ▼ **Figure 27-17A** . The patient should be oriented so that the splinted leg rests along the back of the seat. To load a patient into the backseat of a four-door vehicle, open both rear doors so a third rescuer can enter the far door to help pull the patient onto the seat ▼ **Figure 27-17B** .

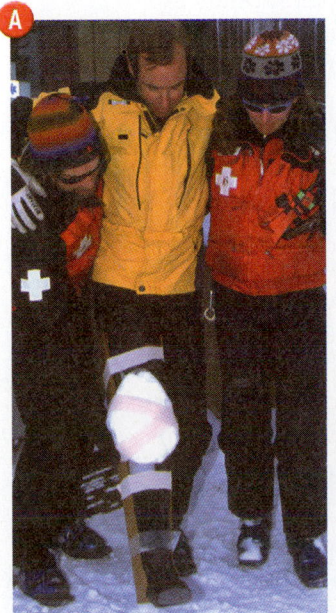
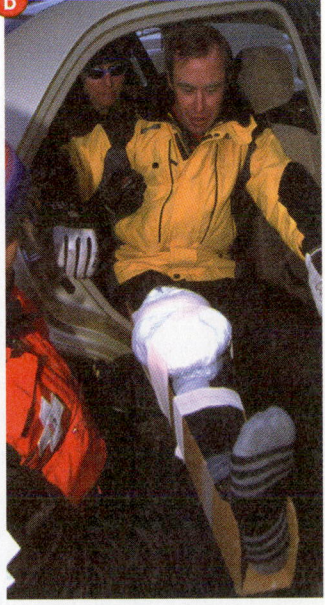

Figure 27-17 **A.** Assisting a patient from the aid room. **B.** Positioning a patient in a vehicle.

Transfer Devices

BACKBOARDS. Backboards are long, flat boards made of rigid, rectangular material ▶ Figure 27-18 . Backboards were originally made of wood but are now made of other materials as well, mostly plastic. They are used to carry patients and to immobilize supine patients with suspected spinal injury or other multiple trauma. Plastic backboards can be slippery on snow and ice. Rescuers should make accommodations for this so that the patient won't "slip away." Backboards can also be used to move patients out of awkward places. They are 6' to 7' long and are commonly used for patients who are found lying down. Parallel to the sides and ends of the backboard are a number of long holes that are about ½" to 1" from the outer edge. These holes form handles and handholds so that the board can be easily grasped, lifted, and carried. The handles and adjacent holes also allow straps used to secure and immobilize the patient to the backboard to be secured to each side and end of the backboard at any needed location.

For many years, backboards were made of thick marine plywood whose surface was sealed with polyurethane or another marine varnish. Wooden backboards are still used in some places. If wooden backboards are used, you must follow infectious control procedures before you can reuse the backboards. Where wooden backboards are no longer used, they have generally been stored so that they will be available in the event of a multiple-casualty situation. Newer backboards are made of plastic materials that will not absorb blood or other infectious substances.

You can use a short backboard, also called a half-board, or an extrication vest to immobilize the torso, head, and neck of a seated patient with a suspected spinal injury until you can immobilize the patient on a backboard. Short backboards are 3' to 4' long. The original short wooden backboard has generally been replaced with a vest-type device that is specifically designed to immobilize the patient until he or she is moved from a sitting position to supine on a backboard ▶ Figure 27-19 . The vest-type devices are easier to use than the wooden backboard. They are made of fabric strengthened with fiberglass or rods. These are designed to temporarily immobilize a patient in a confined area such as a tree well or an automobile seat when a long backboard cannot be used.

STRETCHERS. Several types of commercial flexible stretchers, such as the SKED, Reeves, or Navy stretcher, are available and can be rolled up across either the stretcher's width or, in the case of the SKED, its length, so that the stretcher becomes a smaller tubular package for storage and carrying ▶ Figure 27-20 . When you must carry the equipment a considerable distance from

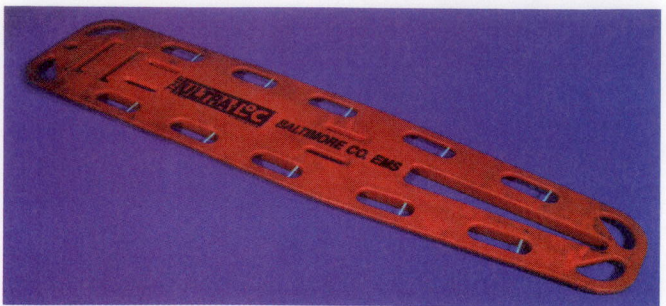

Figure 27-18 A long backboard.

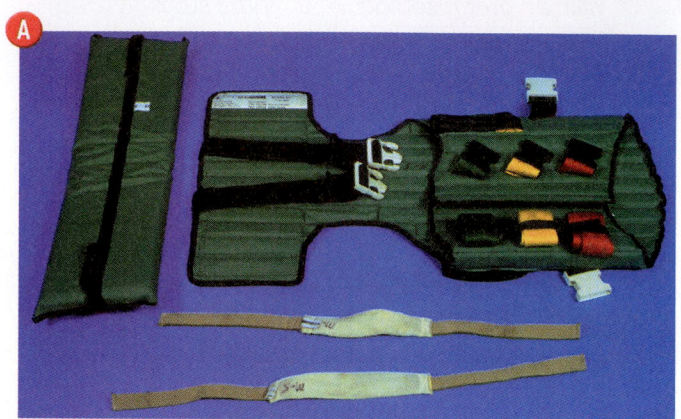

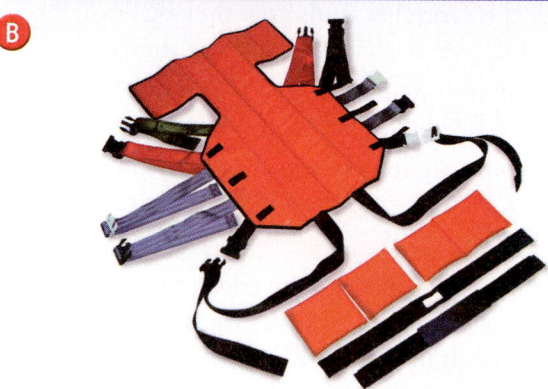

Figure 27-19 Vest-type short immobilization devices. **A.** KED. **B.** Oregon-type backboard.

Figure 27-20 A flexible stretcher.

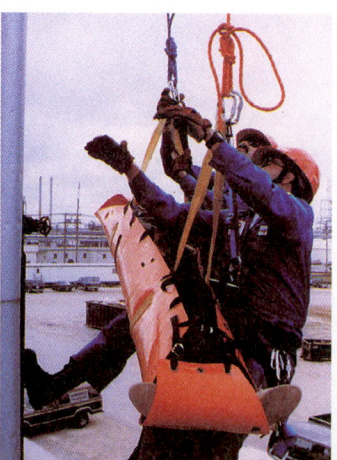

the nearest place that the ambulance can be located, this is an important consideration. A flexible stretcher forms a rigid stretcher that conforms around the patient's sides and does not extend beyond them. When these stretchers are extended, they are particularly useful when you must remove a patient from or through a confined space. The SKED stretcher can also be used if the patient must be belayed or rappelled by ropes.

The flexible stretcher is the most uncomfortable of all the various devices; however, it provides excellent support and immobilization. When the stretcher is wrapped around the patient and the straps are secured, the patient is completely immobilized. The stretcher can then be lowered by rope or slid down a flight of stairs by resting it on the front edge of each step.

SCOOP STRETCHERS. The **scoop stretcher**, or split litter, is designed to be split into two or four pieces (▼ **Figure 27-21**). These sections are fitted around a patient who is lying on the ground or another relatively flat surface. The parts are reconnected, and the patient is lifted and placed on a long backboard or stretcher. There are metal and more lightweight molded plastic models.

A scoop stretcher is efficient; however, both sides of the patient must be accessible. You must also pay special attention to the closure area beneath the patient so that clothing, skin, or other objects are not trapped. As with the long backboard, you must fully stabilize and secure the patient before moving him or her; however, you cannot slip a scoop stretcher under the long axis of the patient's body. Scoop stretchers are narrow, well constructed, and compact and have excellent body support features but are not adequate when used alone for standard immobilization of a spinal injury and are generally not recommended. Scoop stretchers can be excellent devices for extrication; however, the limitations of this piece of equipment should be taken into account when used. Good training is the key to the successful use of a scoop stretcher.

If a scoop stretcher is used to help stabilize and extricate a patient with a suspected spinal injury, a rigid cervical collar should be used and the patient should be placed on a backboard as soon as possible. You must be particularly careful to strap the patient securely to the

stretcher so it can be safely tipped to the side if the patient vomits. Further, the metal scoop interferes with X-rays and scans, can be cold for the patient and for rescuers' hands unless padded, tends to gape in the middle when loaded with a heavy patient, and has latches that can fill with snow and freeze.

STOKES (RIGID BASKET STRETCHERS). You should use a rigid **basket stretcher**, often called a Stokes litter, to carry a patient across uneven terrain from a remote location that is inaccessible by ambulance or other vehicle (▼ **Figure 27-22**). If you suspect that the patient has a spinal injury, you should first immobilize him or her on a backboard and then place the backboard into the basket stretcher. Once you have reached the ambulance, you can remove the patient and backboard from the basket stretcher and place them on the cot.

Basket stretchers either are made of plastic with an aluminum frame or have a full steel frame that is connected by a woven wire mesh. The wire basket is very uncomfortable for the patient unless the wire is padded. Either type can be used to carry a patient across fields, rough terrain, or trails or on a toboggan, boat, or all-terrain vehicle. Basket stretchers surround and support the patient, yet their design allows water to drain through holes in the bottom. Basket stretchers are also used for

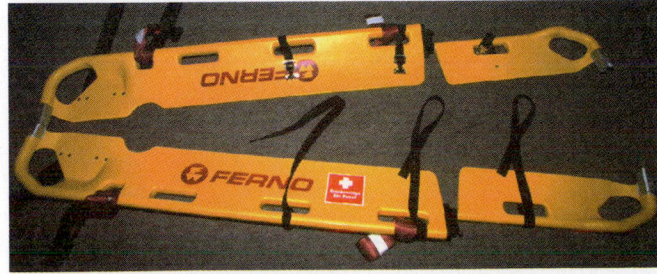

Figure 27-21 A scoop stretcher.

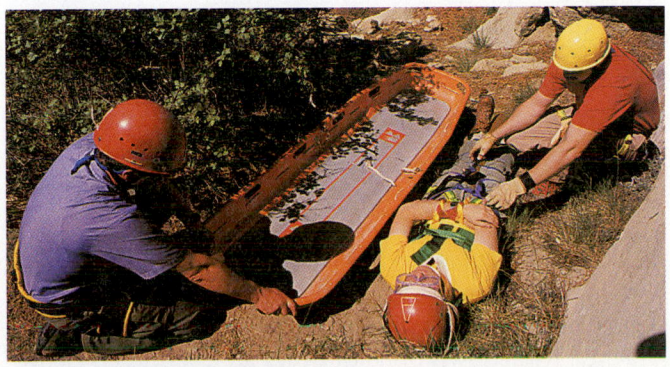

Figure 27-22 A basket stretcher.

technical rope rescues and some water rescues. Not all basket stretchers are rated or appropriate for each of these specialized rescue uses. The types of basket stretchers that are acceptable for specialized rescue must be determined by individuals with additional special training.

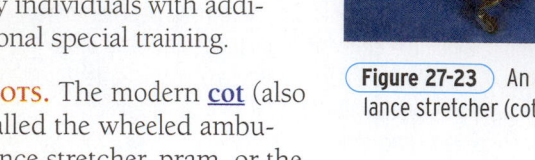

Figure 27-23   An ambulance stretcher (cot).

Cots. The modern <u>cot</u> (also called the wheeled ambulance stretcher, pram, or the clinic gurney) is available in a number of different models, which may include different features **▲ Figure 27-23**. Before using this equipment, you should be fully familiar with the specific features of the device used by your aid room or rescue service. You must know where the controls to adjust and lock each feature are located and how each works.

The cot has a specific head end and foot end. The cot has a strong horizontal rectangular tubular metal main frame to which all of its other parts are attached. The cot should be pulled, pushed, and lifted only by its main frame or handles, which are attached to the main frame specifically for this purpose.

In most instances, it is best if you pull the foot end of the cot while your partner guides it from the head end. When the cot must be carried, it is best if four rescuers are available to carry it. There is more stability with a four-person carry, and the carry requires less strength. One rescuer should be positioned at each corner of the cot to provide an even lift. A four-person carry is much safer if the cot must be moved over rough ground. If only two rescuers are available, or if limited space will allow room for only two rescuers to carry the cot, there is risk that the cot will become unbalanced. In a two-person carry, the two rescuers should stand facing each other, with one person at the head end of the cot and the other at the foot end. With this type of carry, one rescuer will have to walk backward.

Transportation Devices

Toboggans. The <u>toboggan</u> is the most commonly used device to move and transport patients in the winter environment **▶ Figure 27-24**. They are ultra-maneuverable rescue devices found on almost all ski slopes. Features will vary based on geographic and terrain criteria. They come with two or four handles, most with locking handle capabilities for easier maneuverability with a patient aboard. The toboggan may be attached to a snowmobile or other all terrain vehicle for transport over flatter terrain and to support the

toboggan handler. Information on various toboggan types and their handling capabilities can be found in NSP's toboggan transportation text.

After splinting and providing other emergency care, lift the patient into the toboggan **▶ Skill Drill 27-6**, being careful not to aggravate injuries. When placing a patient in a toboggan, the general rule is to position the injury uphill to decrease swelling, slow bleeding, and keep the patient's weight from jamming the injured extremity against the end of the toboggan during a downhill ride. With dislocated upper extremities, the patient is usually more comfortable in a sitting position rather than lying down **▼ Figure 27-25**.

However, no rule is absolute, and the patient's comfort should be a strong guide in deciding how to position him or her in the toboggan **▶ Table 27-3**.

When a patient has multiple, serious injuries, a head or chest injury may indicate a head-uphill position, but the presence of shock may indicate a head-downhill position. Your decision must be based on your estimate of the most life-threatening conditon, even though some requirements may conflict with others.

Placing the patient directly on a canvas litter or tarp will make removal from the toboggan easier. Wrap the patient in a blanket or sleeping bag covered with a tarp or other snowproof and windproof cover, and strap him or her in securely. Toboggan straps should not put pressure on the site of injury. A jacket or emergency care belt can be used as a pillow, if necessary.

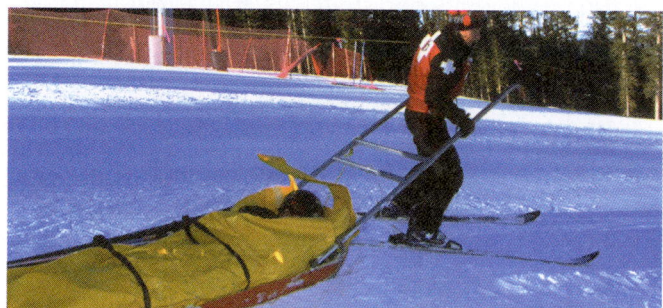

Figure 27-24   Toboggan rescue equipment.

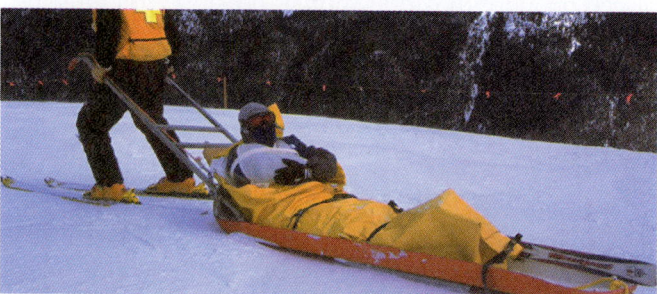

Figure 27-25   The patient with a dislocated shoulder will need to be supported by another rescuer or improvised device during toboggan transport.

If the patient is on a long backboard, make sure the board is positioned and secured so that the patient's head or feet do not jam against the toboggan ends.

You should also give forethought as to how to manage vomiting in the patient. Either the backboard or the entire toboggan will have to be tipped to the side. In the former case, the backboard cannot be strapped in place in the toboggan.

Take the toboggan down the hill to the aid room by the safest, smoothest, and shortest route, and try to avoid jostling and bumping. Strap the patient's equipment to the side of the toboggan opposite the injury with any tips pointing toward the patient's feet, or have another rescuer carry them. Never leave a loaded toboggan unattended.

You should take the following steps when transferring a patient into a transportation device:

1. Assess the factors:
   - Position of the patient in the toboggan
   - Nature and extent of the injury
   - Patient responsive/unresponsive
   - Patient mobility—ability to assist
   - Number of people able to assist
   - Terrain (steep or flat)
   - Conditions (hard/soft; poor footing)
   - Type of transportation device (with/without basket; height of edges)

2. Position the toboggan and all of the other equipment

3. Ensure all rescuers are in the appropriate position

4. Perform the lift smoothly without compromising the injury

5. Ensure that the patient clears the side of the device

BACKCOUNTRY RESCUE EQUIPMENT When cross-country skiers and ski mountaineers become sick or injured in difficult or isolated terrain, patrols and other winter rescue groups should be familiar with the techniques of backcountry over-snow rescue and toboggan handling.

If the site is accessible by snowmobile or helicopter, the best practice is often to stabilize the patient and send for such help. Otherwise, the patient will have to be moved by a toboggan that can be brought to the site or built from available materials (▼ **Figure 27-26**).

A toboggan loaded with a heavy patient can be very difficult to pull uphill or handle in deep snow with an insufficient number of rescuers. When transporting a patient, attach one or more ropes to the front of the toboggan so additional rescuers can help pull. Other rescuers should guide the toboggan from the rear, using the rear handles or a tail rope. This is especially important on sidehills, in difficult snow, or on steep downhill stretches. Toboggans should be belayed on steep terrain and dangerous sidehills.

Improvised toboggans are made from one or more pairs of skis held together by a frame that forms a platform to which the patient can be strapped. Improvised

Table 27-3 Toboggan Positioning Guidelines

Head Downhill
Cardiac arrest

Shock

Hypothermia

Lower extremity and pelvic injuries

Abdominal injuries (unless the patient is short of breath)

Head Uphill
Injury to the head, eye, face, neck, and upper extremity

Shortness of breath

Unresponsiveness

Suspected heart attack

Very steep terrain

Position of Comfort (Usually Head Uphill)
Chest injury

Recovery Position
Nausea and vomiting

Unresponsiveness not caused by trauma

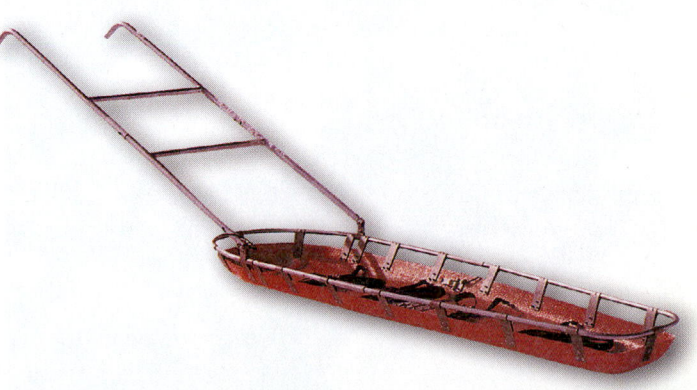

Figure 27-26 Commercial backcountry toboggans are lighter and smaller than those used by alpine patrols.

Skill Drill 27-6   Lifting a Patient into a Toboggan or other Transportation Device

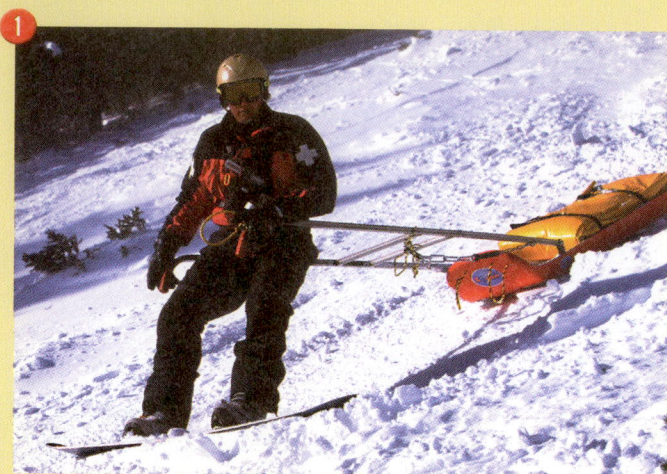

Assess the factors:
  a. Position of the patient in the toboggan
  b. Nature and extent of the injury
  c. Patient responsive/unresponsive
  d. Patient mobility—ability to assist
  e. Number of people able to assist
  f. Terrain (steep or flat)
  g. Conditions (hard/soft; poor footing)
  h. Type of transportation device (with/without basket; height of edges)

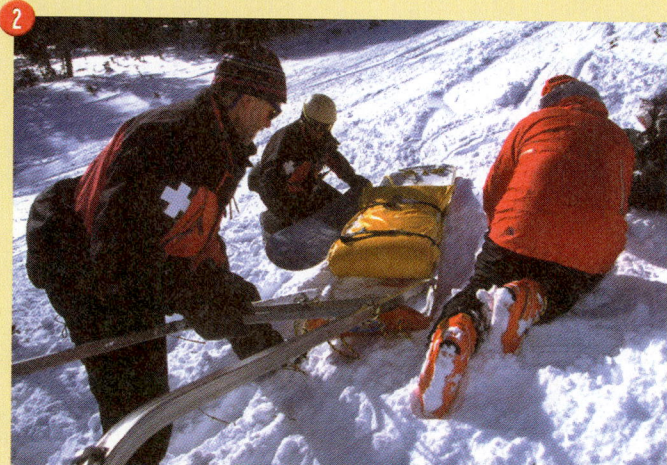

Position the toboggan and all of the other equipment.

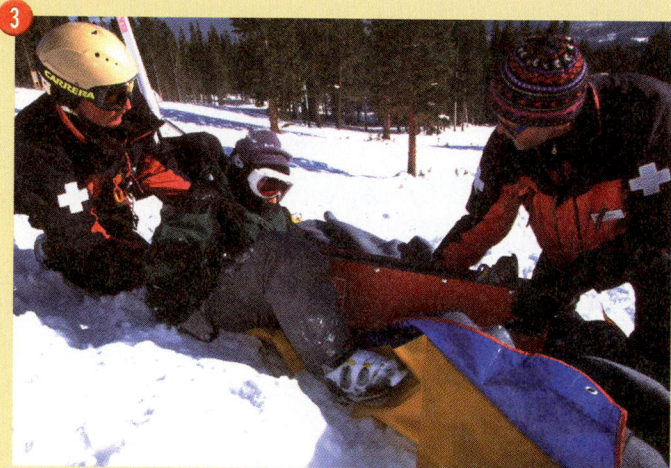

Ensure all rescuers are in appropriate position.

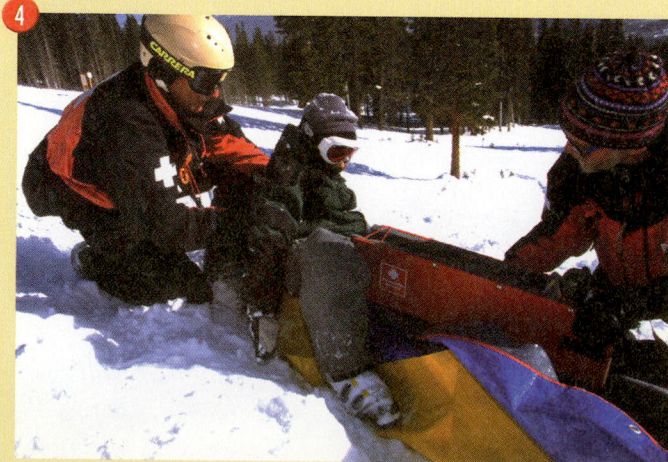

Perform the lift smoothly without compromising the injury.

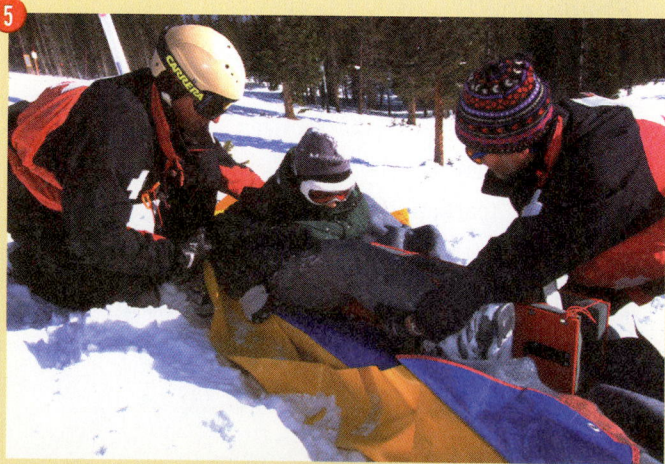

Ensure that the patient clears the side of the device.

toboggans are usually weaker, more difficult to handle in snow, and more difficult to pull over long distances than commercially available toboggans. However, improvised toboggans can be handled much like commercial toboggans.

OVERLAND WHEELED STRETCHERS. The <u>overland wheeled stretcher</u> (▼ **Figure 27-27**), or cot, is the most commonly used device to move and transport patients in the outdoor environment.

Most patients are placed directly on the overland wheeled stretcher. However, you will need to place and secure patients with a possible spinal injury or multiple system trauma onto a backboard. Patients who may need CPR or must be carried down (or up) a trail while supine should also be placed on a backboard. The backboard and patient are then secured onto the wheeled stretcher.

PORTABLE/FOLDING STRETCHERS. A <u>portable stretcher</u> is a stretcher with a strong rectangular tubular metal frame and rigid fabric stretched across it (▶ **Figure 27-28**). Portable stretchers do not have a second multipositioning frame or adjustable undercarriage. Some models have two wheels that fold down about 4" underneath the foot end of the frame and legs of a similar length that fold down from the head end at each side. The wheels make it easier to move the loaded stretcher. The legs should not be used as handles.

Some portable stretchers can be folded in half across the center of each side so that the stretcher is only half its usual length during storage. Many ambulances carry a portable stretcher to use if a patient is in an area that is difficult to reach with a wheeled ambulance stretcher or a second patient must be transported on the squad bench of the ambulance.

A portable stretcher weighs much less than a wheeled stretcher and does not have a bulky undercarriage. However, because most models do not have wheels, you and your team must support all of the patient's weight and any equipment along with the weight of the stretcher.

STAIR CHAIRS. <u>Stair chairs</u> are folding aluminum frame chairs with fabric stretched across them to form a seat and seat back (▼ **Figure 27-29**). They have fold-out handles to help you carry their head and foot ends up or down a flight of stairs, and most have rubber wheels at their back with casters in front so that they can be rolled along the floor and make turns. Stair chairs serve as an adjunct for moving a conscious patient up or down stairs to the ground floor, where the prepared wheeled ambulance stretcher is waiting. You can roll the stair chair on the floor until you reach the stairwell, then carry it (rather than roll and bump it) up or down the stairs. Once you reach the ground floor, you can roll it to the waiting cot and assist or lift the patient onto the cot.

Be sure to follow manufacturer's directions for maintenance, inspection, repair, and upkeep for any device that you use as patient-handling equipment.

IMPROVISED STRETCHERS. Improvised litters and stretchers tend to be uncomfortable and are usually insufficiently rigid for patients with spine injuries. They should be limited to short-distance transport.

An emergency soft stretcher can be improvised from two long poles and a blanket or several jackets or parkas. If you are using parkas, make sure they are all about the same size. Leave the arms as is or turn them inside out so that they remain inside the body of

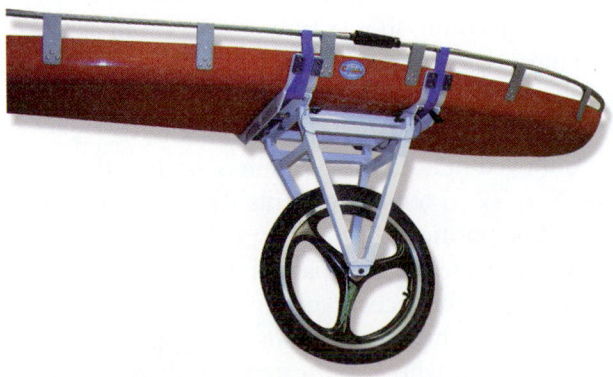

Figure 27-27 The overland wheeled stretcher is ideal for evacuation from mountain trails.

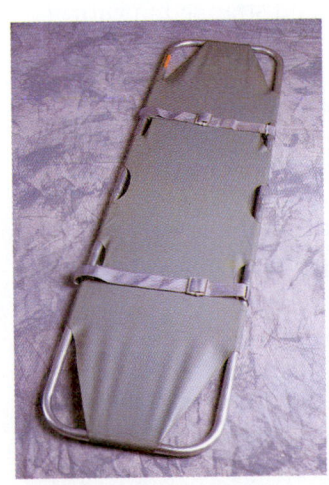

Figure 27-28 A portable stretcher.

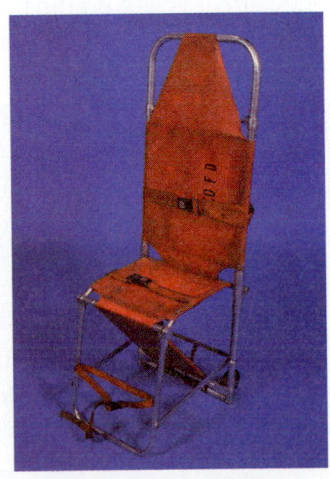

Figure 27-29 A stair chair.

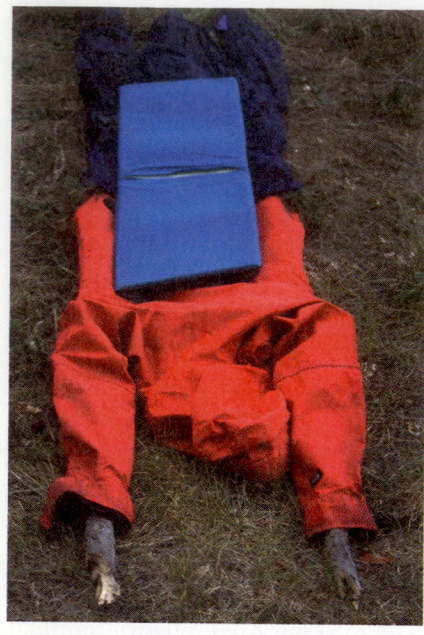

Figure 27-30 Improvised stretcher made from two parkas.

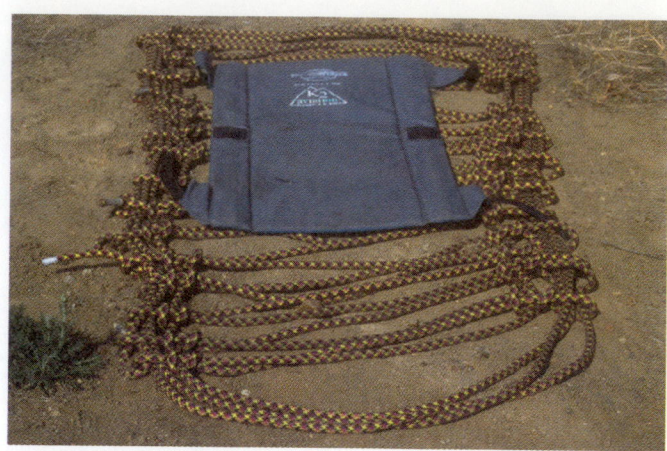

Figure 27-31 Rope stretcher.

the parka. Zip the parkas closed and insert the poles, one on each side, inside the parkas and through their arms ▲ **Figure 27-30** . The poles are carried by one or two rescuers at each end and other rescuers at the sides.

Stretchers can also be made from external pack frames or climbing ropes. Two external pack frames can be tied end to end, and strengthened by one or two additional frames. This type of litter can be carried by itself or by tying it to two poles. It should be cushioned with foam pads, sleeping bags, or clothing.

A rope stretcher can be improvised from a 150′ climbing rope ▶ **Figure 27-31** . The rope stretcher can serve as an improvised long backboard if rigid objects such as skis, snowshoes, canoe paddles, or poles are laid on it. These are padded with multiple foam pads, and the patient is laid on the pads and strapped in with cravats, straps, or a continuous sling or rope.

Moving and Positioning the Patient

Every time you have to move a patient, you must take special care that neither you, your team, nor the patient is injured. Patient packaging and handling are technical skills that you will learn and perfect through practice and training.

Training and practice are required to use all the equipment that is described in this chapter. You must master the skills necessary for their use and understand the advantages and limitations of each device. Practice each technique with your team often so that when you must move a patient, you can perform the move quickly, safely, and efficiently. After each patient transfer, you and

your team should evaluate the appropriateness of the technique that you used, as well as your technical skill in completing the transfer. You must also be sure to maintain your equipment according to the manufacturer's instructions. Using clean, well-maintained equipment is but one part of providing high-quality patient care.

Delivering a patient to definitive care may involve several moves and transfers. After this is accomplished, you and your team must begin preparing for your next call. Review the positive points about the transport. Discuss changes that would improve the next run. This process of review and evaluation identifies the following:

- Procedures that need more practice
- Equipment that needs to be cleaned or repaired
- Skills that you need to review or acquire

Most important, a critical review helps you and your team to become more confident and better-skilled rescuers.

Certain patient conditions, such as head injury, shock, spinal injury, and pregnancy, call for special lifting and moving techniques. Patients with chest pain or difficulty breathing should sit in a position of comfort, as long as they are not hypotensive. Patients with suspected spinal injuries must be immobilized on a long backboard. Patients who are in shock should be packaged and moved in a supine position or with their legs elevated 6″ to 12″. Pregnant patients who are hypotensive should be positioned and transported on their left sides. Move an unresponsive patient with no suspected spinal injury into the recovery position by rolling the patient onto his or her side without twisting the body. Transport a patient who is nauseated or vomiting in a position of comfort, but be sure that you are positioned appropriately to manage the airway.

Chapter *Sweep*

Ready for Review

The first key rule of lifting is to always keep your back in an upright position and lift without twisting. You can lift and carry significant weight without injury as long as your back is in the proper upright position.

The power lift is the safest and most powerful way to lift. The safety of you, your team, and the patient depends on the use of proper lifting techniques and maintaining a proper hold when lifting or carrying a patient. If you do not have a proper hold, you will not be able to bear your share of the weight, or you may lose your grasp with one or both hands and possibly cause a lower back injury to one or more rescuers.

Regardless of the devices used, you must constantly coordinate your movements with those of the other team members and make sure that you communicate with them.

When lifting a patient or a cot, you must make sure that you and your team use correct lifting techniques. If you must carry a loaded backboard or cot in rough or slippery terrain up or down stairs or other inclines, be sure that the patient is tightly secured to the device to prevent sliding. Be sure to carry the backboard or cot foot end first so that the patient's head is elevated higher than the feet.

Directions and commands are an important part of safe lifting and carrying. You and your team must anticipate and understand every move and execute it in a coordinated manner. The team leader is responsible for coordinating the moves.

You should try to use four rescuers whenever resources allow. You should also know how much you can comfortably and safely lift and not attempt to lift more than this amount. Rapidly summon additional help to lift and carry a weight that is greater than you are able to lift.

The same basic body mechanics apply for safe reaching and pulling as for lifting and carrying. Keep your back locked and straight, and avoid twisting. Do not hyperextend your back when reaching overhead.

You should normally move a patient with nonurgent moves, in an orderly, planned, and unhurried fashion, selecting methods that involve the least amount of lifting and carrying. At times, you may have to use an emergency move to move a patient before providing initial assessment and care. You should perform an urgent move if a patient has an altered level of consciousness, inadequate ventilation or shock, or in extreme weather conditions.

The toboggan is the most commonly used device to move and transport patients in the outdoor winter environment. Other devices that are used to lift and carry patients include portable stretchers, flexible stretchers, backboards, basket stretchers (Stokes litters), scoop stretchers, overland wheeled stretchers and stair chairs.

Whenever you are moving a patient, you must take special care so that neither you, your team, nor the patient is injured. You will learn the technical skills of patient packaging and handling through practice and training. Training and practice are also required to use all the equipment that is available to you. You must practice each technique with your team often so that you are able to perform the move quickly, safely, and efficiently.

Chapter *Sweep*

Vital Vocabulary

anatomic position In the outdoor rescue setting, the six positions in which a patient may be found.

backboard A device that is used to immobilize a patient who is suspected of having a hip, pelvic, spinal, or lower extremity injury. Also called a spineboard, trauma board, or long board.

basket stretcher A rigid stretcher commonly used in technical and water rescues that surrounds and supports the patient yet allows water to drain through holes in the bottom. Also called a Stokes litter.

bridge lift A lift performed by four or more rescuers. Each rescuer braces his or her head against the shoulder of an opposite rescuer, allowing lifting to occur with the arms instead of the back.

cot (wheeled ambulance stretcher) A specially designed stretcher that can be rolled along the ground. A collapsible undercarriage allows it to be loaded into the ambulance. Also called an ambulance cot, gurney, or pram.

direct ground lift A lifting technique that is used for patients who are found lying supine on the ground with no suspected spinal injury.

emergency move A move in which the patient is dragged or pulled from a dangerous scene before initial assessment and care are provided.

extremity lift A lifting technique that is used for patients who are supine or in a sitting position with no suspected extremity or spinal injuries.

extrication The process of freeing or removing a patient from an awkward, confined, or poorly accessible situation or position.

extrication vest A vest-shaped device made of fabric strengthened with lightweight materials to form a lightweight and collapsible short backboard; designed to temporarily immobilize the trunk, head, and neck of a patient in a confined area such as an automobile seat or tree well when a long backboard cannot be used. Common types are the Kendrick extrication device (KED) and Oregon Spine splint.

flexible stretcher A stretcher that can become smaller for carrying and storage but when in use will wrap around the patient to provide support and stabilization.

jams and pretzels Techniques for aligning and extricating a patient found in an awkward position or confined location.

log roll A technique used to roll a patient 180° (usually from prone to supine) or to the side so that a backboard or blanket can be slipped underneath without bending or twisting the spine.

long-axis drag (axial slide) A technique of moving a patient by sliding him or her in the direction of the long axis of the patient's body.

overland wheeled stretcher A stretcher on a wheel assembly for use in outdoor conditions. The most commonly used device in outdoor rescue.

portable stretcher A stretcher with a strong rectangular tubular metal frame and rigid fabric stretched across it.

power grip A technique in which the litter or backboard is gripped by inserting each hand under the handle with the palm facing up and the thumb extended, fully supporting the underside of the handle on the curved palm with the fingers and thumb.

power lift A lifting technique in which the rescuer's back is held upright, with legs bent, and the patient is lifted when the rescuer straightens the legs to raise the upper body and arms.

recovery position The preferred body position for an unconscious patient with no suspected spine injury. The patient lies on his or her side with the opposite knee flexed and the head cushioned on the hand. Also called the semiprone, rescue, stable side, or NATO position.

scoop stretcher A stretcher that is designed to be split into two or four sections that can be fitted around a patient who is lying on the ground or other relatively flat surface; also called a split litter.

stair chair A lightweight folding device that is used to carry a conscious, seated patient up or down stairs.

toboggan A rescue sled found on most ski slopes. Construction and features vary to accommodate a variety of terrain and snow conditions. Comes with two or four handles. Rescuer steers the toboggan from within or outside the front handles. On steep or difficult terrain a second rescuer uses a tail rope or the second set of handles for better stability in the rear.

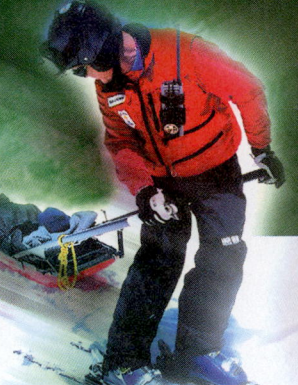

Assessment in Action

As you are carrying a patient from the aid room to an ambulance, the patient's weight suddenly shifts as you descend a small step.

To prevent the patient from falling, you are forced to bend forward to restrain the patient. After loading the patient, your back feels stiff. The following questions refer to this situation.

1. Which of the following methods would be best to prevent the patient from slipping while moving?
   A. Keep the stretcher level at all times.
   B. Have more people help you carry the stretcher.
   C. Secure the patient with straps at the armpits and groin.
   D. Take the patient down head first.

2. In this situation, the center of gravity was not properly balanced when lifting. How can you ensure a proper position for the center of gravity?
   A. Place your legs about 15" apart with your pelvis centered.
   B. Place your legs about 15" apart with your pelvis slightly to the left.
   C. Place your legs 30" apart with your pelvis and right leg slightly ahead.
   D. Place your legs 30" apart with your pelvis and right leg slightly behind.

3. When the back is maintained in an upright position while lifting, where is most of the force transmitted?
   A. To the muscles and ligaments of the spine
   B. Along the stacked vertebrae
   C. Against the pelvic ring
   D. To the parallel arms

4. What are possible alternatives for moving the patient that would help to avoid this situation?
   A. Emergency one-person technique
   B. Wheeled chair
   C. Backboard
   D. Rapid extrication technique

5. Once you have lifted a stretcher using good body mechanics, if you need to lean to either side to compensate for a weight imbalance, you have probably:
   A. exceeded your weight limit.
   B. assumed the heavier end of the stretcher.
   C. exceeded your height limit.
   D. exceeded your arm length.

6. The safest and most powerful method of lifting is the:
   A. body twist.
   B. power lift.
   C. power grip.
   D. clean and jerk.

7. To obtain the maximum force from your hands when lifting a patient, you should grasp the litter with your hands at least:
   A. 10" apart, palms down.
   B. 10" apart, palms up.
   C. 15" apart, with one palm up, one down.
   D. 15" apart, with palms up.

8. One of the best ways to move a patient from a bed to the cot is to use:
   A. an emergency move.
   B. the extremity lift.
   C. the direct sheet method.
   D. the scoop stretcher.

Challenging Questions

9. In this situation, your back felt stiff after the lifting incident. Why?

10. Why is the sacrum considered the mechanical weight-bearing base of the spinal column?

11. Twisting while pulling or lifting is one of the most frequent causes of back injury for rescuers. Why does this so frequently occur?

Points to Ponder

A visitor at your resort begins having breathing difficulties while eating lunch on the second floor at the lodge. Upon arrival, you find a 55-year-old man who appears to weigh more than 400 lbs. Protocols are very clear that this patient should be transported (not walked) to the aid room on a stretcher. It appears to you that the patient is too large to move down the steps on a stretcher but that given enough time and assistance he could walk down the stairs. No other patrollers are available. How would you deal with this situation? Would you go against protocol? Why or why not? How long would you wait for assistance?

Issues Best Care for Patients, Making and Admitting Mistakes, Preventing Accidents, Personal Injuries

Online Outlook

Seven patient-carrying devices were discussed in this chapter. To improve your knowledge of this equipment, complete Exercise 27 at www.OECzone.com.

www.OECzone.com

Triage

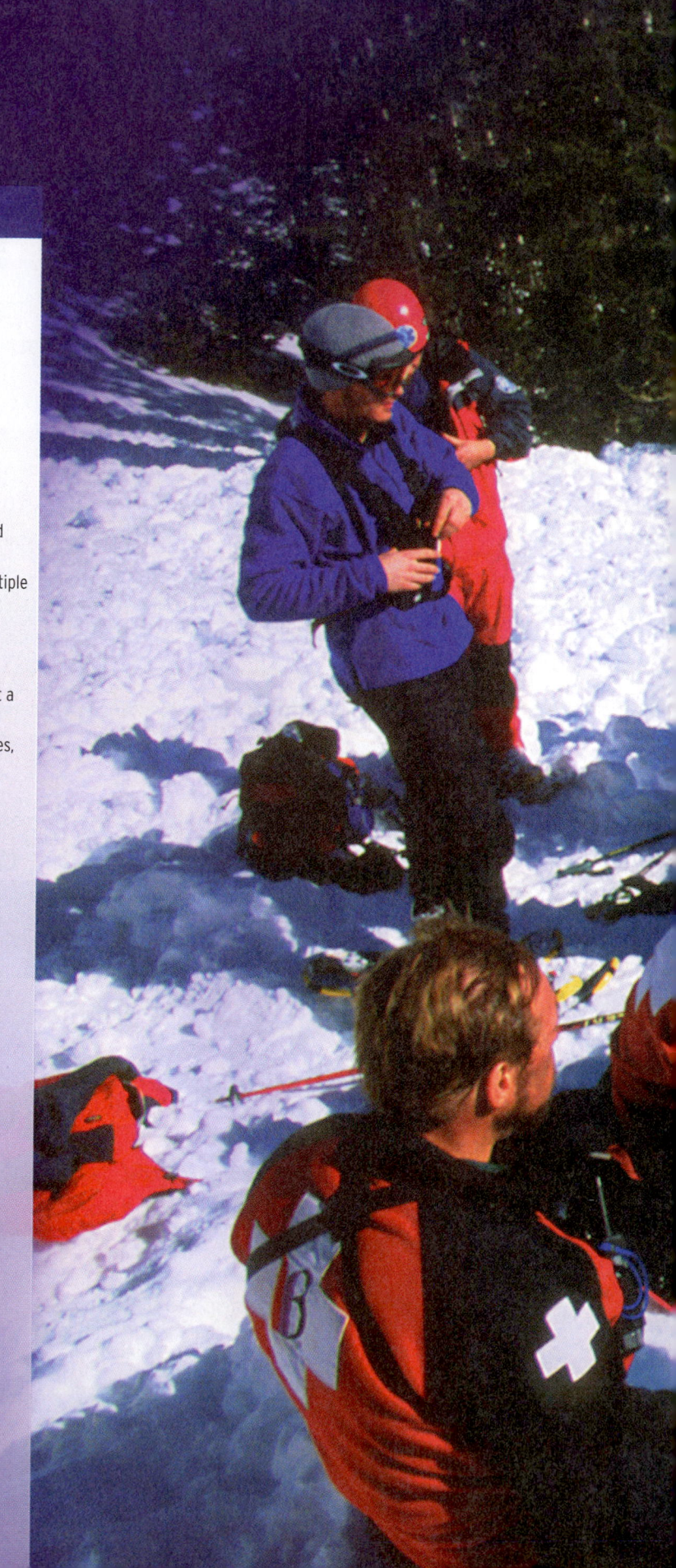

Objectives

Cognitive

🌲 **1.** Explain the purpose, use, and benefits of the triage process (p 714).

2. Describe components of an ideal triage system (p 715).

🌲 **3.** Describe the four-colored categories used in primary triage (p 715).

4. Describe a simple, five-step approach to the triage process (p 715).

🌲 **5.** Summarize the four steps of the START system for triage (p 717).

6. Explain what special situations can change triage priorities (p 719).

🌲 **7.** Describe methods of identifying triage categories (p 715).

8. Define primary and secondary triage and explain when they are applied (p 714).

🌲 **9.** Describe the sequence of emergency care for a single patient with multiple injuries (p 720).

Affective

10. Discuss the psychological impact of wanting to act but recognizing that a scene is not safe to enter (p 714).

11. Discuss the psychological impact of triaging a patient with lethal injuries, but who has not yet expired, as lowest (black) priority (p 717).

Psychomotor

🌲 **12.** Given a scenario of a mass-casualty incident, perform triage correctly using the START algorithm (p 718).

🌲 These are core concepts in initial patrol training.

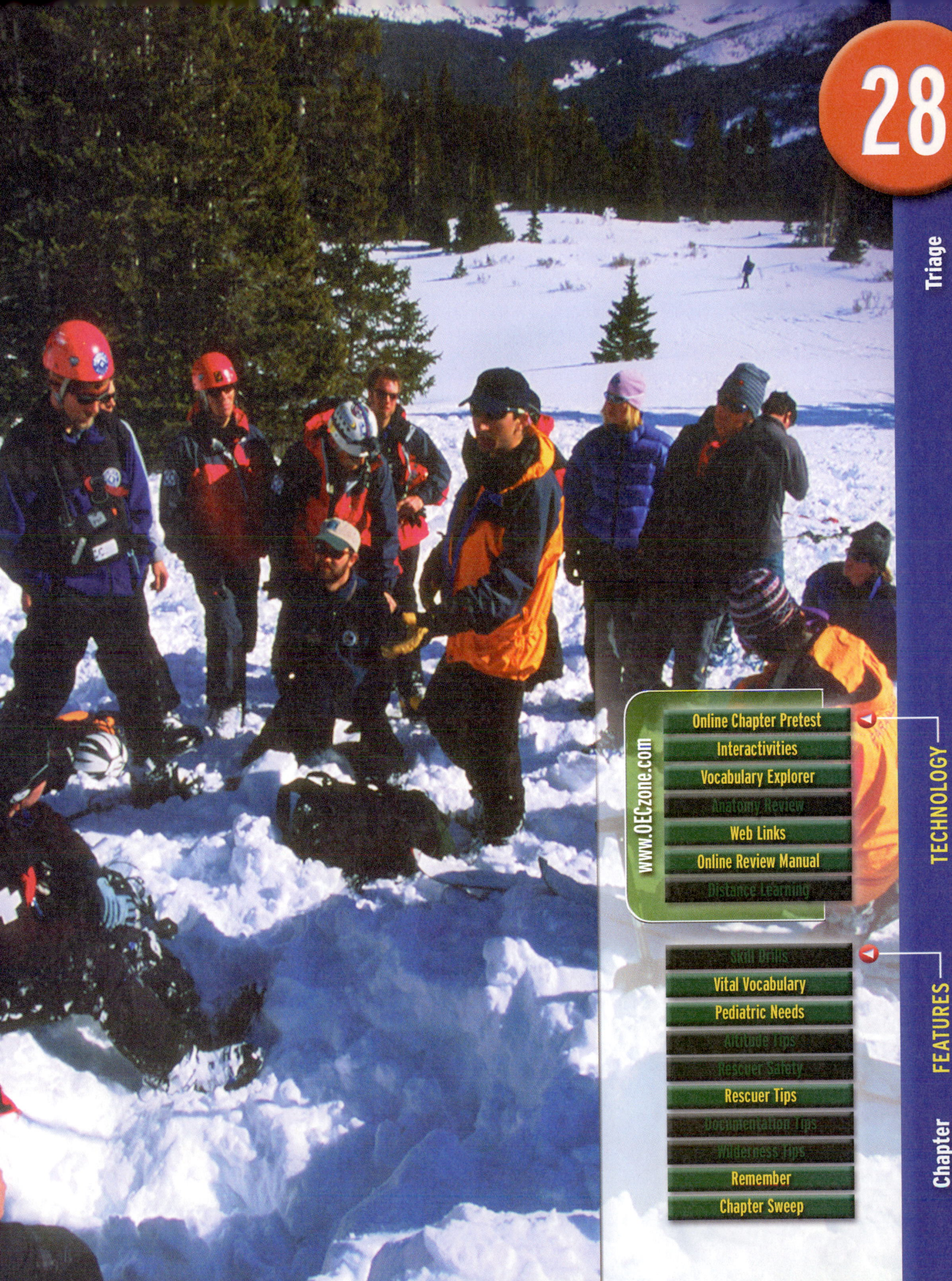

www.OECzone.com

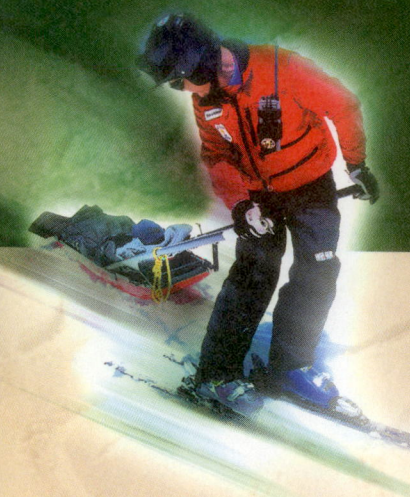

You are the rescuer

It is a cold, starlit night at Snowflake Ski Area, a small resort served by four fixed-grip triple chairlifts and one double chairlift. You are working the 3- to 11-pm patrol shift when you hear on the radio that the main bull wheel of chairlift 3 has collapsed and there has been a derailment. You are first to arrive at the top of the lift. Because the slope beneath the lift is well lit for night skiing, you are able to see approximately 12 victims lying on the slope where they have been thrown. Other skiers remain in chairs above, hanging from a derailed haul cable that in many places sags close to the ground.

The outdoor environment is an unpredictable and often uncontrolled place to work. Some types of responses will require much more from you than patient care. Managing scenes that you find in disarray, avoiding risks at those scenes and helping others avoid them, and calling for and coordinating the arrival of additional resources—all of these can be your responsibility. You also may be called on to assist with complex scenes already being managed by other agencies. This chapter introduces the concept of triage in the outdoor environment. It will help you answer the following questions:

1. What are the general procedures for initial responses to a mass-casualty incident in the outdoor environment?

2. How is triage performed at a mass-casualty incident, especially a large-scale incident?

3. How does triage in the outdoor environment differ from triage in the urban setting?

4. How is an individual patient with multiple injuries triaged?

Triage

As an outdoor emergency care rescuer, you will typically care for one or two injured patients at a time. The potential for multiple simultaneously injured patients, however, is substantial and requires a different approach to assessment.

When you respond to a **mass-casualty incident (MCI)**, you cannot rush in to provide patient care. Rather, you must take time to assess the scene accurately by identifying the size of the hazard area, find a safe and sheltered location to which patients can be removed, and take self-protective measures. *Safety is your prime consideration.* The assessment of multiple-injured patients is performed through a process known as triage (▶ Figure 28-1). A simplified approach to the triage process for OEC providers is presented in this chapter.

It is important to note that in this text, a mass-casualty incident refers to any call that involves more than one patient, as well as any situation that places such a great demand on available equipment and personnel that the system is stretched to its limit or beyond. Examples include fires, lift roll backs, tower collapses, avalanches, terrorist attacks, or bus and airplane crashes.

Primary Triage

Most emergencies encountered by OEC rescuers involve a single injured person. Nevertheless, the potential for multiple simultaneously injured persons in the outdoor recreational environment is considerable, particularly with chairlift or tram accidents, bus accidents, structural

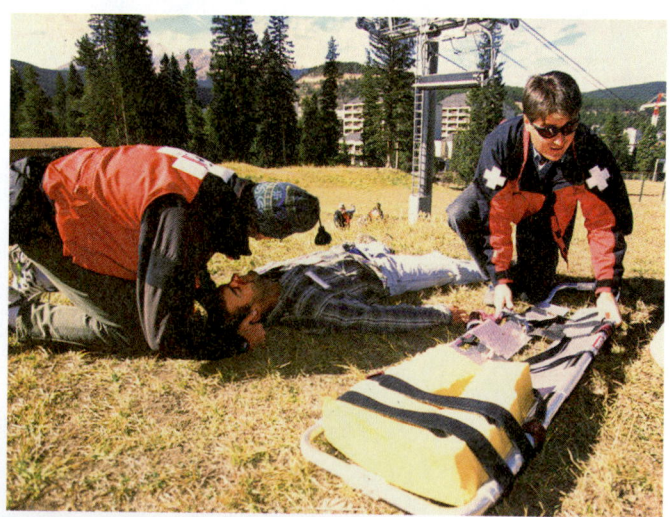

Figure 28-1 Triage is an essential component of operations at a mass-casualty incident.

collapses, avalanches, and river raft accidents. These mass-casualty incidents present a unique challenge to patrols and area resources.

Triage is essential at all mass-casualty incidents. Triage is the sorting of two or more patients based on the severity of their conditions to establish priorities for care based on available resources. If the scene is safe, or as soon as it is, the triage process is begun and patients are ranked in order of severity. When additional emergency care providers are available and time permits, the patient with the most severe injuries is given priority attention. After counting the number of patients and notifying the dispatcher of additional help that is needed, initial assessment of all patients begins. As more personnel arrive, either the first rescuer on the scene or the most experienced rescuer should assume the job of triage officer. This person should assign crews and equipment to priority patients first. Remember that if you assume the initial duties of the triage officer, you should not become involved in patient care.

Triage in the outdoors follows the same principles as triage under urban conditions except that terrain, weather, equipment, manpower, communication, and distance from definitive medical care often make decisions more difficult and may require modifications of standard triage protocols. For example, a multiple-casualty incident in a remote location during the winter may be complicated by numerous cases of hypothermia, necessitating modification of treatment priorities.

The Triage Process

A simplified approach to triage can be remembered as "The five S's of Triage" (▶ Table 28-1). Before triage is begun, the first arriving rescuer surveys the scene to assess for **S**afety for rescuers. Simultaneously, you **S**ize up the scene to get an initial idea of what type of incident occurred, the estimated number of persons involved, and geographic or weather considerations for rescuers. This information is called (or **S**ent) in to dispatch as soon as possible so that EMS resources can be requested and area hospitals notified. **S**etting up the scene for triage involves identifying triage collection points (keeping in mind access and egress), and quickly locating triage ribbon. The fifth "S" stands for "START" triage.

Triage Priorities

Patients are sorted into four triage levels early. Patients are color-coded according to their triage level to enable visual identification of the severity of the condition and to avoid unnecessary repeat patient assessments (▶ Table 28-2).

Red

Red is the category for first- or high-priority patients. These patients usually have injuries to the circulatory

Table 28-1 The 5 S's of Triage

1. Safety Assessment
   - Assess scene for safety
2. Simultaneous scene size-up
   - Size and severity
     - Type of incident
     - Approximate number of patients
     - Severity of injuries
     - Area involved, access
3. Send information
   - Contact dispatch with your scene size-up information
   - Request assistance and additional resources
4. Setting up the scene
   - Obtain triage ribbon
   - Identify triage areas
   - Consider scene access and egress
5. START triage process
   - Begin where you are
   - Relocate green-tagged patients
   - Move in an orderly pattern
   - Maintain a patient count of casualties
   - Provide minimal treatment

or respiratory systems. Red-priority patients generally include patients in whom:
- Hypoxia or shock is either present or imminent.
- Survival is probable with immediate care and rapid transport to the hospital.
- Stabilization is possible without constant attention.

Note that patients with severe head injuries and major blunt trauma to the chest and abdomen (and who appear stable) usually do not meet these criteria.

Red-priority patients may include those with the following specific conditions:
- Upper airway obstruction
- Shock
- Respiratory distress due to a flail chest, sucking chest wound, closed pneumothorax, tension pneumothorax, or critical burns
- Major external or internal hemorrhage
- Pericardial tamponade
- Head injuries showing progressive deterioration
- Altered mental status
- Medical emergencies such as poisoning, heart attack, diabetic hypoglycemia

Table 28-2 Triage Priorities

Triage Category	Typical Injuries
Red (Highest) Priority Patients who need immediate care and transport. Treat these patients first and transport as soon as possible.	• Airway and breathing difficulties • Uncontrolled or severe bleeding • Decreased level of consciousness • Severe medical problems • Shock (hypoperfusion) • Severe burns
Yellow (Second) Priority Patients whose treatment and transportation can be temporarily delayed	• Burns without airway problems • Major or multiple bone or joint injuries • Back injuries with or without spinal cord damage
Green (Low) Priority Patients whose treatment and transportation can be delayed until last	• Minor fractures • Minor soft-tissue injuries
Black (Lowest) Priority Patients who are already dead or have little chance for survival. If resources are limited, treat salvageable patients before these patients.	• Obvious death • Obviously nonsurvivable injury, such as major open brain trauma • Full cardiac arrest

Yellow

Yellow is the category for second- or delayed-priority patients. These patients are considered serious but not as urgent as red-priority patients. They are more likely to have severe injuries to the musculoskeletal or nervous systems. Yellow-priority patients are typically able to wait longer than red-priority patients before being transported. Yellow-priority patients generally include those who:

- are seriously injured but not yet hypoxic or in shock
- appear able to wait without serious risk for 45 minutes or longer before being transported to a hospital
- need more attention than red-priority patients
- have less chance of survival than red-priority patients

Yellow-priority patients may include those with the following specific conditions:

- severe burns without respiratory distress
- back or spinal cord injuries
- multiple fractures
- pelvic or femur fractures without shock
- open fractures

- stable abdominal injuries, including open abdominal injuries without shock
- eye injuries
- severe head or chest injuries, if stable

Green

Green is the category for patients whose injuries have third or lowest priority. They may be ambulatory or even uninjured and are regarded as able to wait several hours before being transported to a hospital. Green-priority patients generally those who:

- have minor injuries that do not present a risk to life
- can be stabilized with a minimum of emergency care
- are uninjured but whose presence at the MCI scene needs to be noted

Typically referred to as the "walking wounded," green-priority patients may include those with the following specific conditions:

- single, closed fractures
- minor burns
- most psychological problems
- localized soft-tissue injury

Black

Black is the category for nonsalvageable patients. Black-priority patients generally include those who:

- are dead
- will die during emergency care
- have lethal injuries and no chance of survival, even in a hospital

Black-priority patients may include those with the following specific conditions:

- cardiac arrest
- absent respirations not responding to opening the airway
- massive (especially open) injuries of the head, chest, or abdomen
- total body burns (90% or more)
- obvious death

Patients who are tagged red should later be reassessed in the <u>treatment area</u> to determine who should receive limited resources such as paramedic assessment and care. The sorting of multiple red-tagged patients in the treatment area who need to be seen immediately by advanced life support providers will depend on the number of advanced life support providers available at that time. The order in which the patients will be transported is determined after the initial triage and treatment is completed.

If patients are entrapped, <u>extrication</u> is required. If circumstances such as heavy smoke or fear of a hazardous material exposure exist, triage will be difficult if not impossible. The immediate concern is the removal of the patients to a safe area for triage to be done later. The <u>triage area</u> is the name usually given to such a collecting area for patients to be initially triaged and color coded before being sent to the treatment area. The triage officer is located here. For patients located in nonhazardous areas, this initial triage can begin immediately where they are found.

Triage Tags

Triage tags and ribbon are used to rapidly identify a patient's priority for treatment and transportation (▶ Figure 28-2). Triage categories can be marked with specialized color-coded tags that are attached to the patients or to their clothing. In the outdoor environment, however, tags may be damaged by rain or snow, or blown away by wind. A practical and simple way to identify triage categories is through use of colored tape or colored surveyor's ribbon. Rolls of red, green, yellow and black tape or ribbon can be easily stored on a "D" ring and carried to the incident scene. If tags are not available, write the initial of the appropriate color (R, Y, G, or B) on a piece of adhesive tape and attach it to the patient's forehead. Once a patient is transported to a

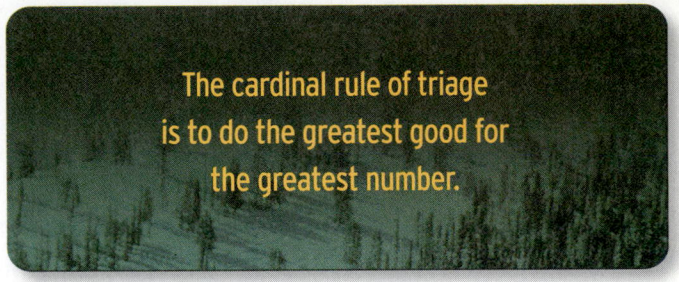

The cardinal rule of triage is to do the greatest good for the greatest number.

treatment area and reassessed, triage ribbon is replaced by a triage tag on which one can write additional information about the patient's injuries.

Triage Techniques

Triage identifies patients who require rapid medical care to save life and limb. It provides rational distribution of casualties and by separating out minor injuries, reducing the urgent burden on each hospital. A number of different approaches to triage rely on specific injuries and physical findings in order to categorize and prioritize patients. An in-depth assessment requires more time than may be available. Thus, the ideal triage system should be simple, does not require advanced assessment skills, does not rely on specific diagnoses, provides for rapid and simple lifesaving interventions, and is easy to teach and learn.

The <u>Simple Triage And Rapid Treatment (START)</u> system meets these requirements. Developed at California's Hoag Memorial Hospital, the START protocol is an effective method of <u>primary (initial) triage</u> based on the patient's respirations, pulse, and mental status.

The START System

The START process (▶ Figure 28-3) begins by making a clear announcement to all injured that those who can walk should get up and proceed to an easily designated recognized point, away from immediate danger and outside the initial triage area. As these (green) patients

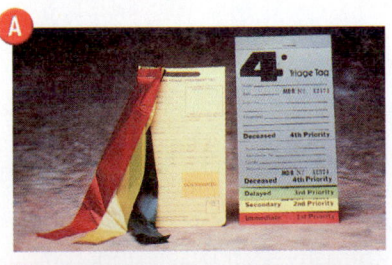

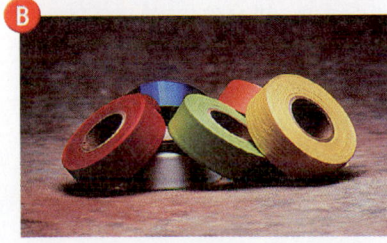

Figure 28-2
A. Triage tags.
B. Triage tape.

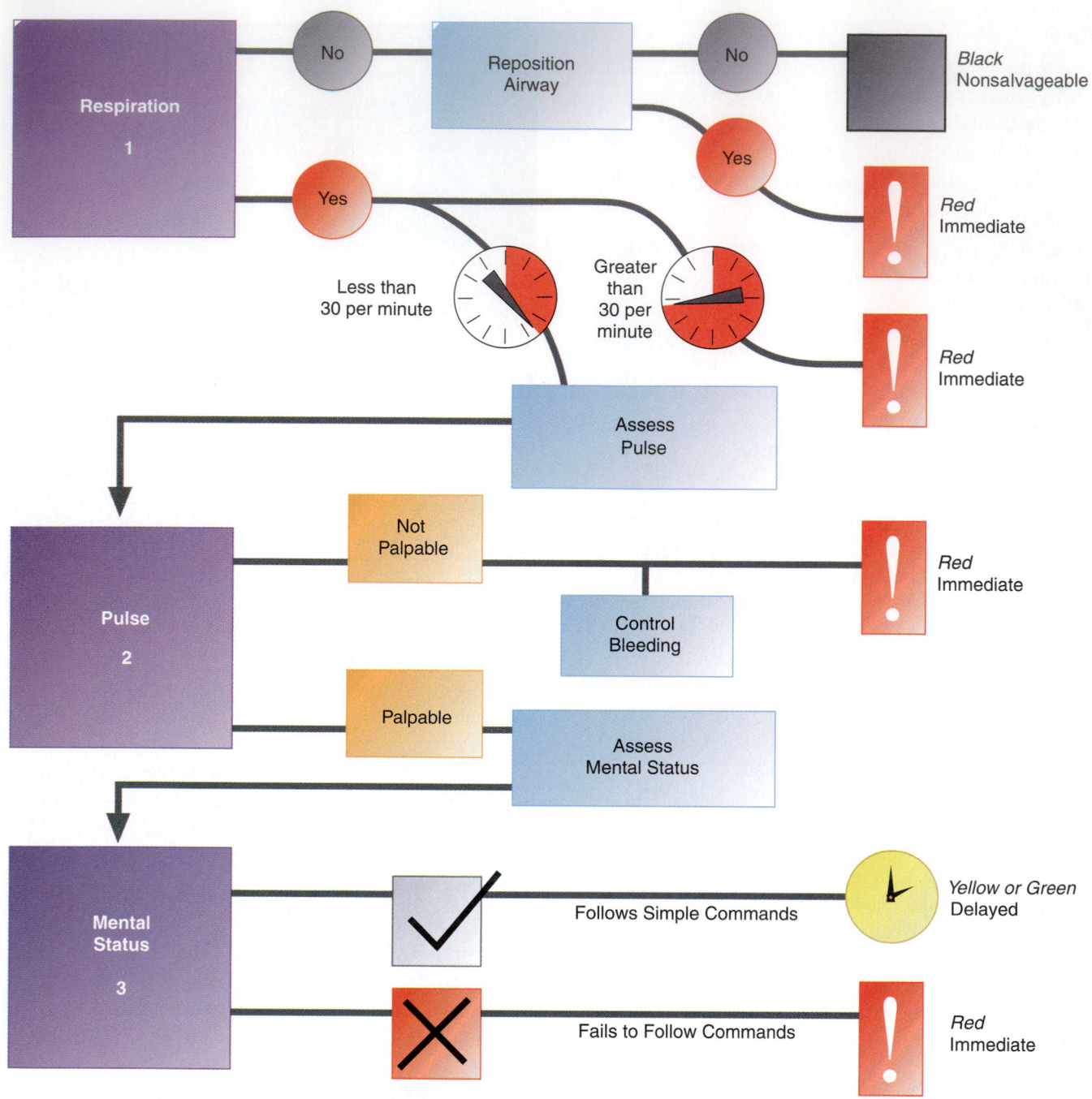

Figure 28-3 START algorithm.

are relocating, move through the remaining patients in an orderly pattern. Begin with the patient nearest to you, assessing each casualty you come upon and marking the category with easily seen triage ribbon or tape affixed to the patients' *body* (clothing may be removed). Maintain a count of the casualties. This can be easily accomplished by marking on a 2″ to 3″ piece of tape on your thigh, or by saving a small piece of triage ribbon from each person you have triaged.

Provide only minimal treatment. Use only two inter-

ventions: (1) open the airway and (2) stop excessive bleeding. Heroic resuscitative efforts are not appropriate as they take too much time, require equipment that can be used for salvageable patients, and are staffing intensive. In a normal response, four or more providers may work on a single patient; in mass casualties, this ratio is reversed.

It is important to keep moving! START assessments should last only 15 to 30 seconds per patient.

Remember

Heroic resuscitative efforts are not appropriate as they take too much time, require equipment that can be used for salvageable patients, and are staffing intensive. In a normal response, four or more providers may work on a single patient; in mass casualties, this ratio is reversed.

Remember

To help you remember the sequence of assessment for triage, think "RPM" for respirations, pulse, and mental status.

STEP 1—GET UP AND WALK. The first step in the assessment was when you directed the patients to get up and walk—they sorted themselves out. These patients are tagged green.

STEP 2—RESPIRATION. Step 2 is a check for respiratory compromise. If the airway is closed, open the airway. If there are still no respirations, the patient is marked with black ribbon (lowest priority). If respirations are more than 30 breaths/min, the patient is marked with red ribbon (immediate/highest category). If a patient is breathing more than 30 times a minutes, that means the patient is breathing once every other second. This rate is so fast, it can be recognized without actually having to count respirations. If respirations are less than 30 breaths/min, further evaluation is required and you should proceed to step 3 (Perfusion).

STEP 3—PERFUSION. Step 3 is a radial pulse check. Some EMS systems use capillary refill, but this is an unreliable indicator in cold weather. If the radial pulse is not palpable, the patient is marked with red ribbon (immediate). Severe bleeding may be controlled by direct pressure using a bystander with protective gloves. If the radial pulse is palpable, then further evaluation is required and you should proceed to Step 4 (Mental Status).

STEP 4—MENTAL STATUS. Step 4 is a check for compromise of mental status. Asking the patient to follow simple commands is an easy way to assess mental status. Ask the patient to open or close his or her eyes or to squeeze your hand. This step may have been accomplished simultaneously with assessments of respirations and perfusion. If mental status is altered, mark the patient with red ribbon (immediate). If mental status is appropriate, mark the patient with yellow ribbon (delayed) or green (minor) ribbon according to other findings, such as obvious injuries or illnesses.

Secondary Triage

Priorities may change as the condition of each patient changes and as more help arrives so that more attention can be given to those with less chance of survival.

Thus, setting priorities is an ongoing process. After you complete an initial evaluation of all patients and as additional rescuers and necessary equipment arrive, patients assigned to the red priority are transported to a designated treatment area. This may be a rental shop, a nearby warehouse, or similar structure. Patients in the red group who are awaiting transportation from the incident scene as well as yellow priority patients can be monitored and given more extensive assessment and care. Patients whose conditions have deteriorated are moved to a higher priority category. For smaller scale incidents, a treatment area may be located nearby.

Once patients are transported to the treatment area, they undergo **secondary triage**. This is an in-depth reassessment and allows for the patient's triage category to be changed. Standard **triage tags**, such as the METTAG ▼ **Figure 28-4** are used at this stage to indicate the triage category and specific injuries or vital signs. Further triage can also be performed in the ambulance on the way to the hospital and again on arrival at the hospital.

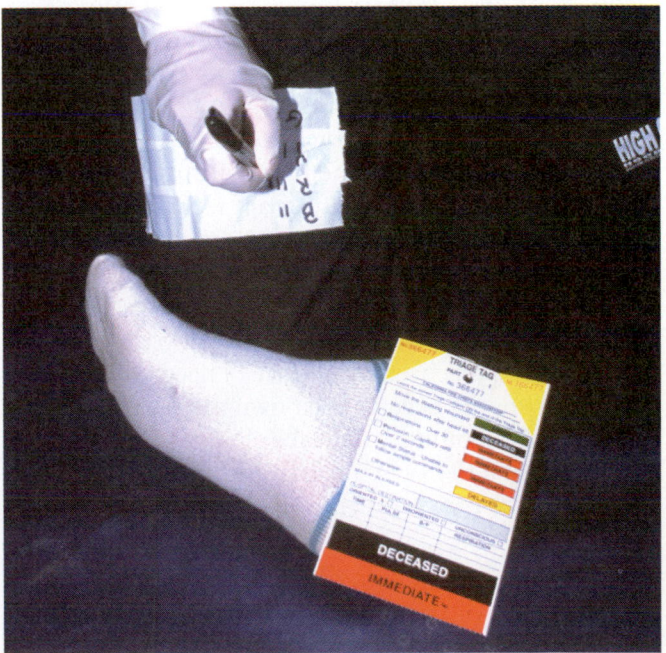

Figure 28-4   METTAG triage tag

Special Triage Situations

In some cases, factors other than respirations, pulse, mental status, or type of injury may influence the category to which a patient is assigned. An injured rescuer or relative of a rescuer is automatically assigned to the red category regardless of the severity of injuries. This is done to minimize distraction and maintain rescuer morale. A disruptive or hysterical patient, or patient with a hysterical relative, also should be assigned a higher priority than the injury might otherwise warrant. Alternatively, another ambulatory patient might be asked to stay and comfort a hysterical patient or unaccompanied child. Children, likewise, are assigned a higher category. When possible, rescuers should transport children with a parent. Because of their excellent cardiovascular reserve, children tend to maintain a fairly normal pulse rate and blood pressure even in the face of shock, until their blood pressure begins a precipitous decline. For this reason, it may be wise to check capillary refill in children, particularly once they have been removed from a cold environment. Capillary refill is checked by applying pressure to the nailbeds or fingertips until they blanch. Once pressure is released, a normal pink color should return within 2 seconds. Shock, as well as cold temperatures, may prolong capillary refill time.

Hypothermia is a significant risk for persons injured in a mass-casualty incident in the outdoor environment. This risk needs to be anticipated when responding to such incidents during inclement weather. A patient who becomes hypothermic could be changed to a higher priority.

A lack of light may hamper efforts at triage, particularly when the geographic area of an incident is substantial. Consider using supplemental lighting from headlamps, or headlights from snowmobiles, all-terrain vehicles, snow groomers, and other off-road vehicles.

It is not enough to know the triage techniques that your organization or EMS system uses to identify patients for transport to specialized treatment facilities. As with the other skills you are learning, you must practice these techniques as well. Mass-casualty incident plans must be developed and practiced in advance of need. Ski areas and resorts should develop their own triage and MCI protocols and coordinate annual drills with the participation of the local EMS system. The mass confusion of an MCI is no time to experiment with organization.

Triage of the Patient with Multiple Injuries

The proper sequencing of emergency care for a single patient with multiple injuries involves a form of triage. To some extent, the sequencing depends on how much

Pediatric Needs

Children, because of their excellent cardiovascular reserve, tend to maintain a fairly normal pulse rate and blood pressure even in the face of shock, until their blood pressure begins a precipitous decline. Therefore, check capillary refill in children, particularly once they have been removed from a cold environment.

Rescuer Tips

Definitions of mass-casualty incidents vary from one place to another, and training on such specialized topics may not be frequent. As a new rescuer, you may have to do some research and studying on your own to be sure that you understand and can apply local policy and procedure for large-scale incidents.

help is immediately available. If transportation is ready and waiting, rescuers should remain in the field only long enough to stabilize the patient.

Remember the **Golden Hour**, the average amount of time that elapses before a patient with serious or multiple injuries starts to deteriorate rapidly. For every 30-minute period after the Golden Hour, the patient's chances of survival are *cut in half*. To improve the patient's odds, rescuers must be knowledgeable, experienced, able to work quickly and efficiently, and capable of establishing priorities and improvising when necessary. Rescuers should also remember that their job is to buy time for the patient until a hospital is reached or an ambulance or helicopter arrives. A seamless interface with local EMS advanced life support (ALS) providers is essential to rapidly transfer the multiple-injured patient to the nearest trauma center.

Life-threatening injuries usually involve the circulatory, respiratory, or nervous systems. Fortunately, the assessment techniques you have already learned are designed to discover and care for these injuries immediately. You do not have to learn anything new; you basically need to practice your assessment techniques until you automatically do the right things in the right order right away.

No matter how much blood is on the ground, your first and most important considerations are always the airway and assessment of breathing and circulation. To open the airway, use the jaw-thrust maneuver rather than the head tilt-chin lift maneuver. Then use the finger sweep method or suction (as soon as it is available) to remove any obstructing material such as snow, vomit, or blood. If necessary, perform the Heimlich maneuver to remove a foreign body from the airway. If the patient is unresponsive and has no gag reflex, insert an oral or nasopharyngeal airway. Provide rescue breathing or assist ineffective breathing by using a pocket mask or bag-valve-mask (BVM) device. Add high-flow oxygen as soon as it is available. Meanwhile, stabilize the head and neck as the number of personnel on hand permits. It is not necessary to perform CPR on a patient who has experienced cardiac arrest due to severe trauma.

If the airway cannot be maintained by using the techniques listed above, particularly if there is an injury to the patient's neck or face, it will probably be necessary to combine advanced airway maintenance techniques with BVM ventilation. These methods include endotracheal intubation, in which a tube is introduced through the mouth or nose into the trachea, by laryngeal mask airway (LMA) ventilation and cricothyroidotomy, in which a tube is introduced into the trachea through the membrane between the cricoid and thyroid cartilage. These techniques are performed by ALS providers, again emphasizing the need to rapidly interface with the local EMS system.

A simple pneumothorax, sucking chest wound, or flail chest can be treated in the field with techniques described in previous chapters. A tension pneumothorax and cardiac tamponade, however, require advanced techniques such as the introduction of needles and tubes into the chest. Again, if no one at the scene is trained to perform these procedures, the patient may die unless you can rapidly transport him or her to a trained individual who is capable of administering this treatment.

As soon as the patient's airway and breathing are stable or being managed by another rescuer, assess the cause of any bleeding. For the moment, ignore nonbleeding or slowly bleeding wounds, regardless of their size. Control active bleeding by applying direct pressure. A pressure bandage is useful when not enough help is available to keep manual pressure on the wound.

A diminished level of responsiveness suggests a head injury, hypoxia, or lack of brain perfusion caused by shock. Assessing the ABCs helps you discover any life-threatening conditions that need to be cared for immediately. Although the rapid body survey is largely a search for threats to limb, it also reveals other potentially fatal injuries, such as those to the musculoskeletal and nervous systems, which can cause shock. Therefore, if an injured patient in shock has no obvious external bleeding, suspect a fractured femur, fractured pelvis, multiple extremity fractures, or a spinal cord injury.

In the field, a rescuer can do little more to treat shock than control external bleeding, give oxygen, support ineffective ventilations, elevate the patient's legs, and arrange for rapid transport.

Assess and monitor the patient's level of responsiveness, state of the pupils, peripheral pulses, ability to move, and perception of pain and touch. Use the AVPU scale to record and monitor the level of responsiveness, which can be altered by hypoxia. Also keep in mind that hypoxic patients may be agitated or belligerent rather than dull and listless. Always administer high-flow oxygen to any patient with multiple injuries.

Use judgment in exposing the patient, especially in inclement weather, and always cover the patient afterward. Although major injuries, especially bleeding injuries, should be detected as soon as possible, you should often delay a detailed, clothes-off body assessment until the patient reaches shelter. At an alpine ski area, full exposure usually takes place only in the aid room. However, this detailed physical exam should not delay transport to a hospital.

Because of the need for rapid transport, it is almost always preferable to immobilize the multiple-trauma patient on a long backboard or whole body vacuum splint rather than to treat individual fractures and other extremity injuries separately. This saves time, is the best care for spine and spinal cord injuries, and is effective for managing most fractures or other injuries that may be present. An exception is a femur fracture. Because of the need to control bleeding into the fracture site, the femur fracture should be treated separately with a traction splint if time, other injuries, and the patient's general condition allow.

Chapter *Sweep*

Ready for Review

Triage in the outdoor environment is unique in that terrain, weather, lighting, communication difficulties, and distance from definitive medical care can be challenging and require modification of standard treatment protocols. In a mass-casualty incident, the most highly trained medical person on the scene directs triage. This means assigning treatment and transport priorities according to the severity and survivability of patients' injuries. There are four triage categories. Highest (red) priority is given to patients whose injuries are critical but probably survivable with prompt treatment. The cardinal rule of triage is to do the greatest good for the greatest number. Treatment and triage continue until all patients have been transported.

The START system of triage prioritizes patients based on their respirations, perfusion as indicated by radial pulse, and mental status. Initial or primary triage categories may be easily marked in the outdoor environment using four-colored surveyor's tape. Secondary triage occurs as patients are moved to treatment areas and allows for changes in a patient's condition.

Patients with multiple injuries are also "triaged" to allow proper sequencing of emergency care and rapid transfer to the nearest trauma center. Prompt use of advanced airway techniques and treatment for shock by Advanced Life Support providers may be critical for survival, emphasizing the need for a seamless interface with local EMS systems.

Vital Vocabulary

extrication Removal of a patient from entrapment or a dangerous situation or position, such as from a rock slide, avalanche, wrecked vehicle, industrial accident, or building collapse.

Golden Hour The average amount of time before a patient with multiple injuries starts to deteriorate rapidly; for every half hour after the first hour, the patient's chances of survival are cut in half.

mass-casualty incident (MCI) An emergency situation involving more than one patient that can place such a great demand on equipment or personnel that the system is stretched to its limit or beyond.

primary triage The initial triage performed on the scene of a mass-casualty incident.

secondary triage An in-depth reassessment of a patient's condition that allows for a change in triage category.

START Simple Triage And Rapid Treatment system of initial (primary) triage.

treatment area Location in a mass-casualty incident where patients are brought after being triaged and assigned a priority, where they are reassessed, treated, and monitored until transport to the hospital.

triage The process of sorting patients based on the severity of injury and medical need, to establish treatment and transportation priorities.

triage area Designated area in a mass-casualty incident where the triage officer is located and patients are initially triaged before being taken to the treatment center.

triage officer The individual in charge of the incident command triage area, who directs the sorting of patients into triage categories in a mass-casualty incident.

triage tag A tag attached to a patient in a mass-casualty incident that indicates the person's triage category and specific injuries or vital signs. The triage tag is typically used once patients undergo secondary triage at a treatment area.

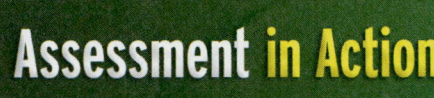

Assessment in Action

A van carrying a church group loses control on a snow- and ice-covered road approaching a ski area. You are the first to arrive on the scene while driving to work. The van is found off road lying on its side, on a heavily treed, snow-covered bank.

1. What is your priority when you arrive at the scene?
   A. Request that dispatch contact the news media.
   B. Extricate any survivors that you can find in the wreckage.
   C. Begin to triage victims.
   D. Ensure that the scene is safe for you and your partner to enter.

2. A survey of the scene shows six passengers inside the vehicle and two young men climbing out. The two ambulatory passengers tell you they they are "OK" except for some scrapes and bruises, but that there are two persons in the van who are not talking or moving, two others complaining of neck pain, one with severe leg pain and one with a cut on the forehead that is "gushing blood." The two passengers who have crawled out of the van would be triage priority:
   A. Red
   B. Yellow
   C. Green
   D. Black

3. You are able to reach in the side door of the van and find an 8-year-old girl crying that her leg hurts. She has an obvious deformity of the thigh, respirations of 26 breaths/min, a strong radial pulse, and intact mental status. This child's triage priority is:
   A. Red
   B. Yellow
   C. Green
   D. Black

4. A special consideration in transporting this child would be:
   A. transporting the child with a parent, if possible.
   B. checking capillary refill in addition to radial pulse.
   C. raising the priority level, since this is a child.
   D. all of the above.

5. The driver of the vehicle has gasping respirations at a rate of 8 breaths/min, no palpable pulse, and is unresponsive with obvious massive head injury. This individual's triage priority would be:
   A. Red
   B. Yellow
   C. Green
   D. Black

Points to Ponder

You arrive at the scene of a gondola accident in which three cars, each carrying four passengers, have fallen between 20' and 30' to the ground. After calling in to dispatch, you begin triage at the first car and find four individuals have been injured. One patient appears dead with obvious head injury and no respirations or pulse. A second patient is conscious with bilateral femur deformities, respirations of 28 breaths/min, and a weak but palpable radial pulse. A third patient is a 70-year-old man, conscious and alert, in respiratory distress with a sucking chest wound and respirations of more than 30 breaths/min. The fourth patient is a 30-year-old man you recognize as a fellow patroller. He is unresponsive with massive head and chest injuries. His respirations are approximately 8 breaths/min, shallow and irregular, and his radial pulse is not palpable. Additional help has not yet arrived. There are two more gondola cabins containing injured persons in need of triage.

How would you prioritize the injured patroller? How might this change with additional help? Since you did not have an opportunity to grab triage ribbon, what could you do to identify each patient's triage category?

Issues Scene Safety, Determining Risk, Delaying Patient Care, Critical Incident Stress Debriefing (CISD)

Online Outlook

Learn more about triage techniques used in outdoor emergency care to identify patients for transport to specialized treatment facilities. To learn more about triage systems, complete Exercise 28 at www.OECzone.com.

Mass-Casualty Incident Management

Objectives

Cognitive

1. Explain the rescuer's role during a call involving hazardous materials. (p 727)

♠ **2.** Discuss the various environmental hazards that affect the rescuer. (p 726)

3. Describe the criteria for a multiple-casualty incident. (p 727)

♠ **4.** Evaluate the role of the OEC technician in the multiple-casualty incident. (p 726)

5. Summarize the components of basic triage. (p 730)

6. Define the role of the rescuer in a disaster operation. (p 731)

7. Describe basic concepts of incident management. (p 727)

♠ **8.** Review the local mass-casualty incident plan. (p 727)

♠ **9.** Define incident command system (ICS). (p 727)

♠ **10.** Identify main ICS functions and their responsibilities during a mass-casualty incident. (p 727)

♠ **11.** Describe the advantages of using ICS as an organized approach to the management of mass-casualty incidents. (p 727)

Affective

12. Discuss the psychological impact of wanting to act but recognizing that a scene is not safe to enter. (p 726)

♠ **13.** Explain how the ICS structure expands or contracts to meet the needs of an incident. (p 727)

♠ **14.** Describe where you might be assigned within an ICS structure and list possible job responsibilities. (p 729)

Psychomotor

15. Given a scenario of a mass-casualty incident, perform triage. (p 730)

♠ **16.** Apply the four color-coded categories to a mass-casualty incident. (p 730)

♠ **17.** Apply the sequence of emergency care for a single patient with multiple injuries. (p 727)

♠ These are core concepts in initial patrol training.

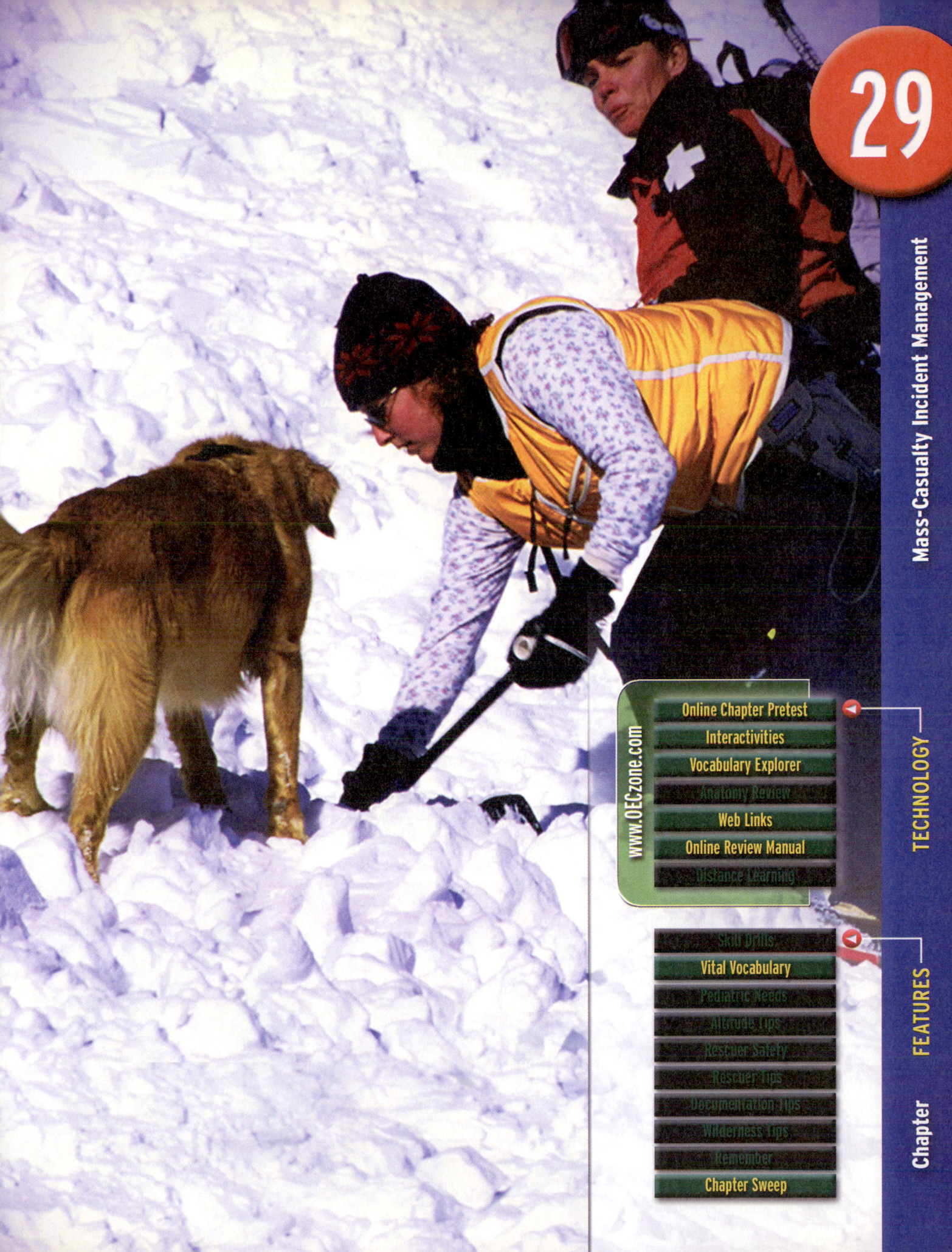

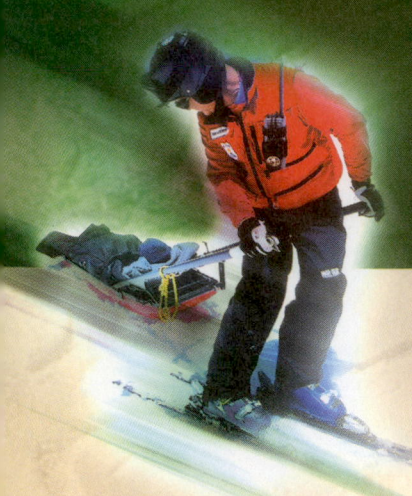

You are the rescuer

You are working as a white-water rafting guide on a three-raft expedition carrying 21 guests, two second-year guides, and one guide trainee. As you approach a narrow bend on the river, you are the last raft through. You come around the bend and encounter one raft broached on a rock and the other raft floating upside down in the current. More than a dozen persons are overboard, some clinging to rocks and tree branches, and at least two persons have been swept downstream ahead of you. Others are clinging to the side of the raft.

As an OEC provider working in the outdoor environment, you typically prepare to encounter extreme weather conditions and, at times, hazardous surroundings. Under the best of circumstances, managing a scene in which the victims outnumber the rescuers is a challenge. When faced with an incident involving multiple victims that takes place in adverse weather or hostile terrain, you may be required to provide much more than emergency medical care. Managing these scenes while avoiding risks to yourself and other rescuers and obtaining additional support are critical responsibilities that you may take on as an OEC provider. This chapter introduces several subjects related to complex and dangerous scenes. It will help you answer the following questions:

1. What are the general procedures for initial responses to a mass-casualty incident in the outdoor environment?

2. What are the different roles in which an OEC provider may be asked to serve within a local incident command system?

Mass-Casualty Incident Management

The first section of the chapter describes multiple-victim, mass-casualty incidents (MCI) as may be encountered in the outdoor environment. This is followed by a very basic introduction to incident command systems (ICS). The purpose of this section is to give you an idea of the larger structure that is at work during complex incidents.

A final section describes the different roles of the rescuer at an MCI. Again, under the ICS, EMS personnel will fulfill one of several identified roles to manage a large number of patients at a single event. The usual EMS response of triaging three or four patients will be difficult when there are 25 or more casualties. To ensure that all patients receive appropriate care and transportation to a hospital consistent with the severity of his or her condition, a more organized operation is required with three major responsibilities assigned: triage, treatment, and transportation.

As described in Chapter 28, this text defines a mass-casualty incident as any call that places such a great demand on available equipment or personnel that the system is stretched to its limit or beyond. Airplane, bus or railroad crashes, and earthquakes are obvious examples of MCIs (▶ **Figure 29-1**). However, other causes of MCIs are far more common than such disasters and are usually much smaller in scope.

In the outdoor environment, mass casualties can be anticipated from incidents involving ski lifts, ice, rock or mountain climbing, river rafts, or avalanches. These technical rescue situations may contain hidden dangers, and special skills often are needed for personnel to enter and move around the scene safely. It is not safe to include in such a response any personnel without the necessary specialized training and experience in situations such as avalanche, mountain, and/or white-water rescue. A **technical rescue team** is made up of individuals from one or more regional groups who are trained and on call for certain types of technical rescue. Many members of a technical rescue team are also trained as OEC technicians or EMT-Bs so that they can provide the necessary immediate care when only they can safely reach the patient. Generally, nothing but essential simple care is provided until the rescuers can bring the patient to the nearest safe, stable location. Mass-casualty incidents that require

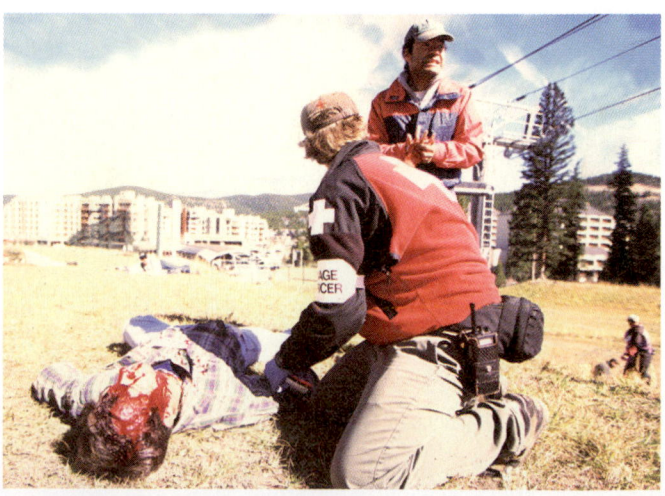

Figure 29-1 Every incident requires cooperation, as each responder has a specific role at the scene.

outdoor technical rescue may not include only physical trauma from the incident, but also environmental exposure and subsequent hypothermia or hyperthermia and dehydration. These injuries are further complicated by the delay in transport to advanced medical care that is inherent with technical rescue situations.

Multiple-victim incidents in the outdoor environment also may be the result of environmental exposure alone. Examples include heat exhaustion or heat stroke that develops in multiple participants and spectators of a mountain biking competition or hypothermia that develops in a group of students on a backcountry hiking trip who become lost during a snowstorm.

When handling an MCI, ask yourself the following questions:

- Does the situation require technical rescue skills and that a team be summoned?
- What equipment will you need to take to the rescue scene to treat, immobilize, and carry out patients?
- What environmental injuries, such as heat or cold injuries, will need to be treated or prevented in both patients and rescuers?
- What happens when you have three or more patients who need treatment?

The Emergency Operations Plan

The key to managing an MCI in the outdoor environment is a well-designed, well-practiced emergency operations action plan. This plan provides you with a systematic way of responding to an emergency situation. The organizational structure that is implemented for an emergency such as an MCI should be as similar as possible to that used for day-to-day operations. At a ski area, a written emergency operations action plan defines the roles of management, emergency responders, including patrollers, lift operators and maintenance personnel, or even ski school personnel, in the event of such specific emergencies as a lift derailment or avalanche. White-water rafting organizations or climbing clubs and other outdoor groups also can benefit from such a plan. Regardless of how many local resources you have within an organization or community, if you have no plan to put them to use, they are of little value.

▼ Table 29-1 lists some basic emergency functions that should be included in a local emergency operations plan. Emergency operations plans work best when coordinated with the local EMS system and integrated into an existing community emergency operations plan and ICS. The plan should be flexible and expandable enough to be used when there is a large-scale incident. To be effective, an emergency operations plan must be well-publicized, realistic, and frequently practiced. Many EMS systems schedule periodic simulation drills in which the fire, rescue, EMS, and police units in the region are alerted and a large number of mock victims are triaged and treated from the onset of the incident to delivery and retriage at the hospital.

The Incident Command System

In recent years, a number of leadership and command systems have been developed to improve the on-scene management of emergency situations. The ICS was developed in the 1970s in response to a series of major wildland fires in California and is a tool for command, control, and coordination of a response to all types of incidents. ICS is designed for use in daily operations and has been adapted and used by many EMS organizations to organize their own operations better. However, the ICS is most effective when used to organize large numbers of personnel at complex incidents such as mass-casualty incidents.

Components and Structure of an Incident Command System

At a large fire, a hazardous materials incident, or a mass-casualty incident, fire, rescue, HazMat, police, and EMS units from many different areas usually will become involved in some way. To ensure clear lines of responsibility and authority, a preestablished system is needed to identify who is in charge of different activities and who reports to whom. Even with a single patient incident and no need for any other services, the implementation of an incident command system is helpful to identify the roles and responsibilities of each rescuer and to ensure an effective response and the efficient, safe use of resources.

The incident command system is structured such that there is a single authority with overall responsibility

Table 29-1 Basic Emergency Functions Included in an Emergency Operations Plan		
• Communications	• Emergency medical care	• Public works/utility repair
• Public information	• Security	• Logistics
• Evacuation	• Fire and rescue	• Direction/control

to manage the incident. This person is identified as the **incident commander**. The incident commander usually remains at a **command post**, the designated field command center. A field command center is typically a vehicle or building at the scene where the incident commander establishes an "office." From here, the commander oversees and coordinates the activities of the various groups and leaders.

Functions normally centered at the command post include information, safety, and liaison with other agencies and groups who are responding. In a typical ICS operation, all information to the public and the news media originates at the command post. The incident commander will usually appoint a **safety officer** who will circulate among responding personnel. It is essential that every rescuer understand that any order or directive issued by a safety officer has the full authority of the incident commander and must be immediately followed. Many times rescuers cannot see a hazard or problem they are walking into, and the safety officer is responsible for protecting all personnel and any victims of the incident. Finally, an officer may be named by the incident commander to coordinate incoming fire, police, and EMS units.

In the initial response, the incident commander may assume direct control over the groups and task forces being set up. In this circumstance, a **medical group supervisor** may be named to coordinate all EMS activity, or a rescue group supervisor may be appointed to deal with people entrapped in the wreckage. In extended operations that may go on

for hours, days, or longer, the typical incident command structure may have multiple sectors including operations, planning, logistics, finance. **▼ Figure 29-2** shows a sample ICS organization chart that includes these sectors. Each of these sections will have a single officer acting as the person in charge, the **sector commander**. Not all positions are used at every incident. The incident commander will select the individual positions and teams and will choose which to use depending on the nature of the incident.

Major incidents often require another level of management, known as **unified command**. With unified command, the incident commander is joined at the command post by one officer who is in charge of all fire operations, one who is in charge of all rescue, one who is in charge of all EMS operations, and one who is in charge of all law enforcement. This group, under the direction of the incident commander, directs the overall operations at the scene. Because the different public safety officers are stationed at the command post, they can be easily found and can collectively advise the incident commander of changes and problems that are communicated to them. The incident commander can also involve them in making the necessary decisions and in rapidly conveying orders to those under their command. In addition to unified command, this system ensures that the actions of each different type of responder are properly coordinated.

How these systems work together depends on the nature of the event. For example, during a large avalanche incident, the leading agency might be the local

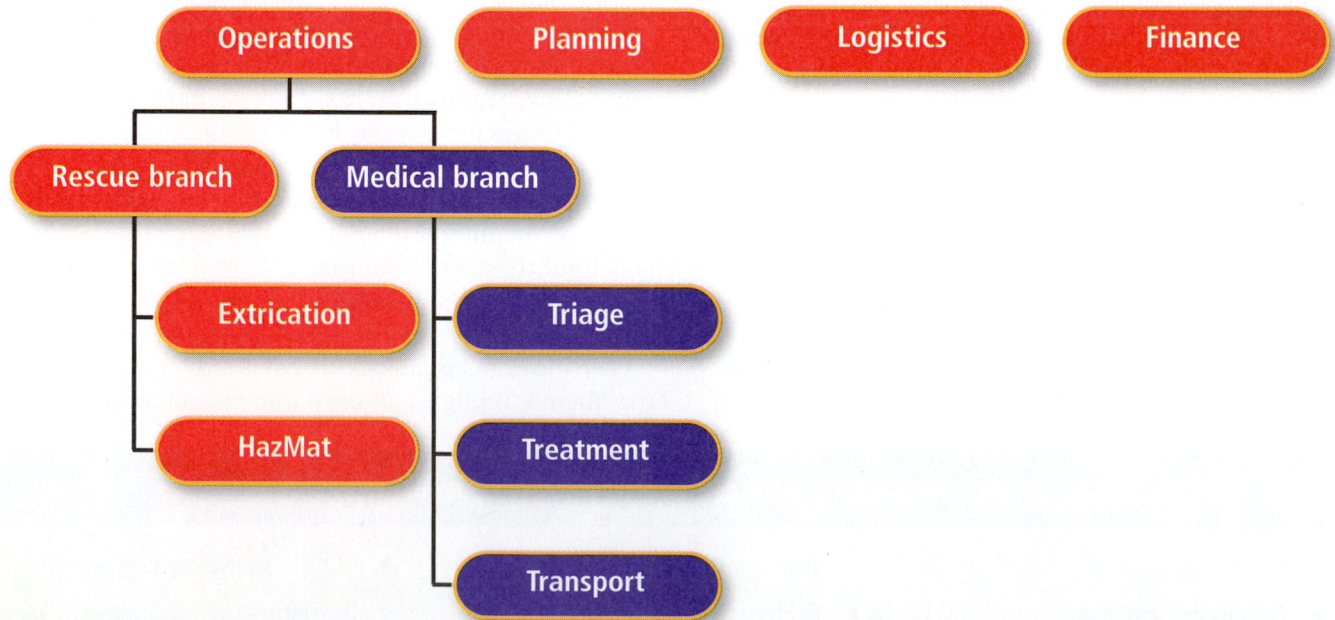

Figure 29-2 Incident command structure. Not all positions will be filled in every incident. However, the incident commander is responsible for all activity until subordinates are appointed to assist in managing the incident. © National Wildlife Coordinating Group

search-and-rescue team. In this situation, ski patrollers could be one aspect of the overall incident command system. Within their own organization, ski patrollers would establish and carry out their tasks. However, ultimate control of the incident would rest with the search-and-rescue incident commander.

Medical Command

As an example of how responsibilities may be assigned at a major EMS incident, consider the following typical assignments (▼ **Table 29-2**). Where might you fit in as an OEC technician?

- **Command center.** This is typically a vehicle or building at the scene where the EMS commander establishes an "office." From here, the commander oversees and coordinates the activities of the various groups and leaders.

- **Staging area.** This is a holding area for arriving ambulances and crews until they can be assigned a particular task. The **staging area manager** is the person who ensures that resources are available, positioned, deployed, and properly allocated. In some incidents, this may include resources such as portable lighting and heating, fans, and generators.

- **Extrication area.** This is where patients are disentangled and removed from a hazardous environment, allowing them to be moved to the triage area. If weather is harsh it should preferably be inside, if a building is close to the scene.

- **Triage area.** The **triage area** is a sorting point where each patient is assessed and tagged, using color-coded tags or tape, according to their injuries. A **triage officer** directs activities in this area. Triaged patients are then directed to specific locations in the treatment area(s), according to

their assigned priority. When patients are spread over a large geographic area, such as a ski slope, initial triage may take place where the patients lie. As toboggans become available, red-priority patients are the first patients transported to the treatment area.

- **Treatment area.** This is where a more thorough assessment is made and on-scene treatment is begun while transport is being arranged. The treatment area is organized and managed under the authority of the **treatment officer**. Patients are given care under the standards of the rescue protocols system in the treatment area before being transported. This means that all fractures should be splinted, and all care normally rendered under a focused assessment should be accomplished before the patient is released for transport (▼ **Figure 29-3**).

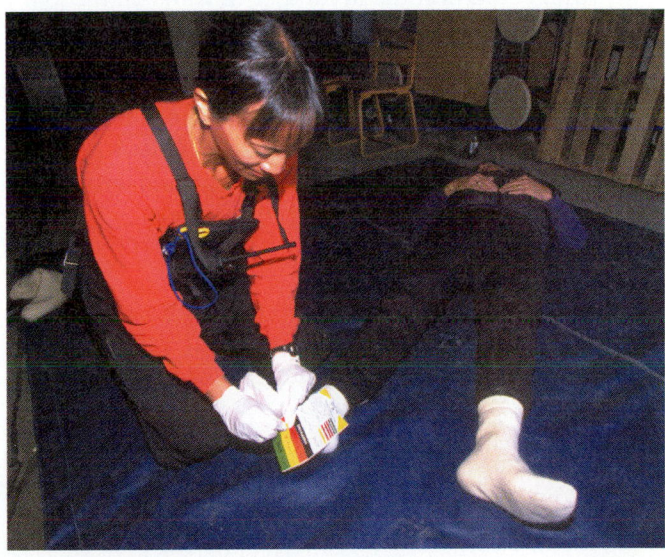

Figure 29-3 Triage area.

Table 29-2 Key Components at a Mass-Casualty Incident

- Incident commander, command post, and incident command system
- On-site communications system
- Adequate supply of long backboards, straps, or ties
- Extrication/retrieval team
- Triage officer and designated triage area
- Staffed patient collection area

- Staffed patient treatment area
- Supply location adjacent to the treatment area
- Transportation officer and transport area
- Staging area to hold resources until they are needed
- Fire and law enforcement personnel
- A secure perimeter

- **Supply area.** This is an area in which to assemble extra equipment and supplies, such as blankets, oxygen cylinders, bandages, and backboards, for dispersal to other areas as needed.

- **Transportation area.** This is where ambulances and crews are organized to transport patients from the treatment sector to area hospitals. The transportation area is managed by the **transportation officer**, who will assign patients to waiting ambulances. The transportation officer also works with area hospitals to determine their capabilities, so that no single hospital is overburdened by large numbers of patients.

- **Rehabilitation area.** This area provides protection and treatment to firefighters and other personnel working at the emergency scene. As workers enter and leave the scene, they are medically monitored and provided any needed care. This helps to ensure the safety and health of emergency workers who could become injured or ill while on the job. It is also an area where personnel may go for rest, nourishment, hydration, and sanitary facilities.

Incident command systems will vary from place to place, and different terms may be used (▼ **Figure 29-4**). You should become familiar with the specific terms and chain of command that are used in your area.

The Medical Response

Medical response at a major emergency incident can be divided into three stages: triage, treatment, and transport. The medical sector supervisor will appoint a triage officer, treatment area officer, transportation officer, and possibly a staging officer.

The first rescuer on the scene performs a scene size-up to determine whether the scene is safe or technical rescue may be necessary. An estimate of the number of patients is made and communicated to dispatch. Triage is begun at the scene, as described in Chapter 28. Triage at a large-scale mass-casualty incident should be done in several steps. Patients who are tagged red should later be reassessed in the treatment area to determine who should receive limited resources such as paramedic assessment and care. The sorting of multiple red-tagged patients in the treatment area who need immediate treatment by paramedics will depend on the number of paramedics available at that time. The order in which the patients will be transported from the treatment area will be determined after the initial triage and treatment is completed.

The following triage steps are accepted by most larger-scale mass-casualty operations:

- Lifesaving care should be rapidly administered to those in need.

- Color coding is provided to indicate priority for treatment and transport at the scene. Red-tagged patients are the highest priority, yellow-tagged patients are the second priority, and green- or black-tagged patients are the lowest priority.

- Red-tagged patients are rapidly removed for treatment in the field and transport as ambulances are available.

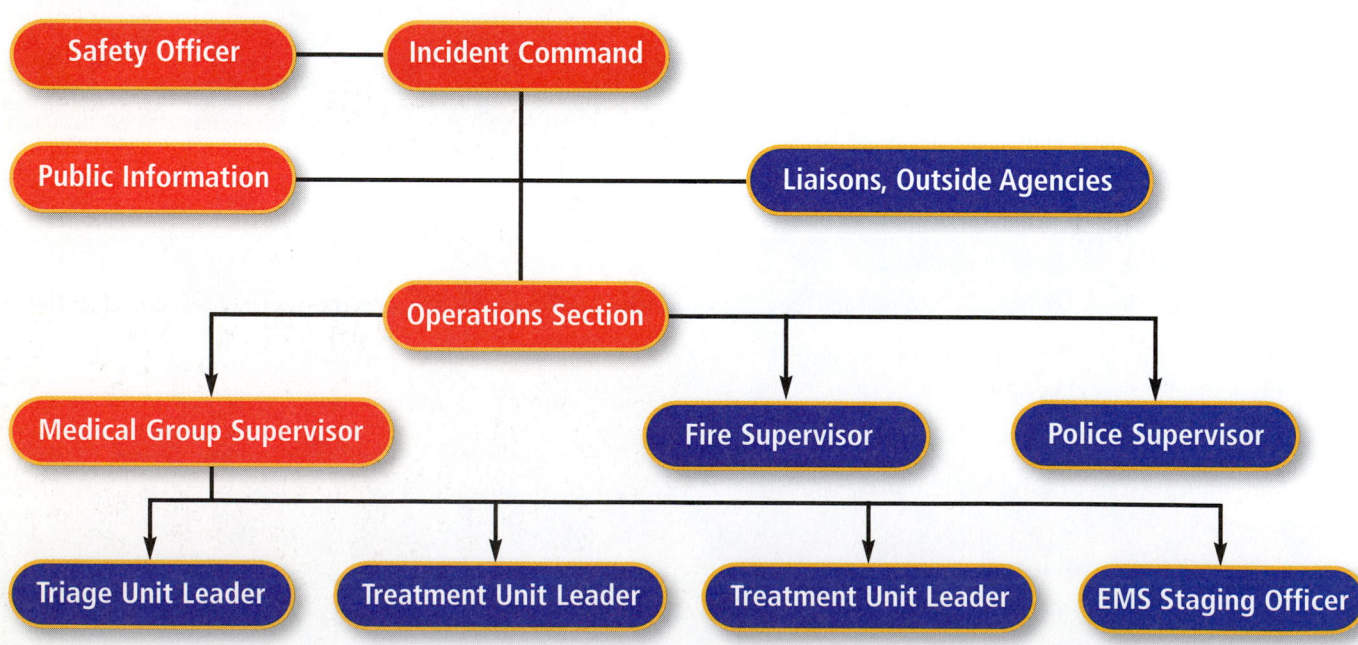

Figure 29-4 A common incident command system used by the EMS community. Copyright © Ski Patrol Magazine, Winter Issue 2000, pg. 29. Reprinted with permission.

- A separate treatment area should be used to care for red-tagged patients if transportation is not immediately available. Yellow-tagged patients also can be monitored and cared for in the treatment area while waiting for transportation.

- When more patients are waiting to be transported than there are ambulances available, the transportation officer decides which patient should be loaded next. The use of specialized transportation resources (air ambulance, paramedic ambulances, etc) requires separate decisions.

The transportation officer is responsible for sending an ambulance to the appropriate hospital or the next hospital in turn. This rotation must occasionally be altered to allow specific patients to be taken to the most appropriate facility, such as a pediatric center, or to another hospital if a hospital has notified the transportation officer that it needs to be skipped for one rotation.

As patients are loaded into an ambulance, the transportation officer or his or her scribe logs their mass-casualty incident number, their overall condition, and the hospital to which they will be taken. As the ambulance leaves the scene, the transportation officer radios or telephones the receiving hospital and briefly describes the patients, the unit transporting them, and the time they left the scene. To minimize radio traffic during such incidents, personnel on individual ambulances do not use their radios except to obtain advice from medical control or to notify the transportation officer that they are leaving the hospital and returning to the field.

After giving a verbal report to hospital staff and transferring the patient, the ambulance returns to the staging area without further delay, helping to keep a continuous flow of ambulances moving between the MCI site and the hospital. Equipment that is collected at the hospital or additional supplies that are needed in the field are brought to the staging area in the next returning ambulance.

If additional ambulances are needed, the transportation officer should radio the command center, which then directs the resources from the staging area. If additional ambulances are not available at the staging area, the EMS chief notifies the dispatcher to obtain them elsewhere. To prevent a lack of ambulances, extra ambulances should be requested as early as possible in a triage situation.

After all the first-priority (red-tagged) patients have been transported, the second-priority (yellow-tagged) patients are transported, followed by the third-priority (green-tagged) patients. After all patients have been transported, several units usually stay at the incident site to protect other rescuers who remain in case others become injured and require emergency care.

Treatment and triage continue until all patients have been treated and transported. After the MCI has ended, all personnel who were involved should be debriefed and evaluated to determine whether they need counseling.

The success of any ICS depends on all personnel performing their assigned tasks and working within the system. For example, suppose a rescuer who is assigned to perform triage decides instead to bypass triage and treatment and evacuates patients from the scene directly to the transport areas. As a result, those patients who were not yet triaged would not receive the initial assessment. Always remember that the cost of "doing your own thing" may include the loss of lives.

Disaster Management

A **disaster** is a widespread event that disrupts functions and resources of a community and threatens lives and property. Many disasters may not involve personal injuries. On the other hand, many disasters such as floods, fires, and avalanches also result in widespread injuries.

The role of the rescuer in a disaster is to respond when requested and to report to the ICS for assigned roles. One such role might be to record baseline vital signs and assessment of other response personnel before they enter the area. Later, the rescuers may provide medical care and support to those who become exhausted or injured and return to the rehabilitation area.

In a disaster with an overwhelming number of casualties, area hospitals may decide that they cannot treat all patients at their facility. In this case, they may mobilize medical and nursing teams with equipment. Using a facility such as a warehouse near the disaster scene, they will set up a **casualty collection area**. The ambulance crew would then be requested to transport patients to this alternative facility instead of to the local emergency department. Once at the casualty collection area, triage can be performed, medical care provided, and patients transported to the hospital on a priority basis.

If a casualty collection area is established, it will be coordinated through the ICS in the same way as all other branches and areas of the operation. This is usually done only in a major disaster such as an earthquake when transportation to a hospital facility is impossible or has prolonged delays. It may take several hours to establish a casualty collection area. This delay can limit the number of events where such an area is an effective method for handling the incident.

Chapter Sweep

Ready for Review

In the outdoor environment, incidents resulting in mass casualties may require rescue by persons trained in specialized technical rescue skills. Delays in extrication combined with environmental weather extremes contribute further to injuries sustained. Rescuers themselves also are at risk from the environmental conditions and need to plan accordingly.

When faced with an incident involving multiple patients, use of an emergency operations action plan will assist rescuers by providing an organized, coordinated approach. Large-scale incidents will require OEC-trained rescuers to interface with the EMS system and other agencies. The ICS allows for coordination of police, fire, and EMS activities in an emergency situation. In major incidents, there is usually a unified command center, which has a single command post where decisions are made by agency leaders. Rescuers may be assigned to the medical group to assist with triage, treatment, or transportation from the scene to the treatment area.

For an emergency operations action plan to be effective, rescuers must be trained in the response and they should practice or drill the plan on a regular basis. All emergency care providers from OEC technicians to medical command officers have an important role to play in the successful management of a mass-casualty incident. The success of any ICS depends on all personnel performing their assigned tasks and working within the system.

Vital Vocabulary

casualty collection area A designated location where victims of a mass-casualty incident may be taken for triage and initial medical care prior to transport to a hospital.

command post A designated center where an incident commander establishes a location to oversee and coordinate the response activities.

disaster A widespread event that disrupts community resources and functions, in turn threatening public safety, citizens' lives, and property.

incident commander The individual who has overall command of the scene in the field.

medical group supervisor The individual named to coordinate the activities of emergency medical personnel.

rehabilitation area The area that provides protection and treatment to firefighters and other personnel working at an emergency. Here, workers are medically monitored and receive any needed care as they enter and leave the scene.

safety officer The individual responsible for protecting mass-casualty incident response personnel and victims from unseen hazards or dangers.

sector commander The individual delegated to oversee and coordinate activity in an incident command sector; works under the incident commander.

staging area manager The individual responsible for ensuring that resources are available, positioned, deployed, and properly allocated.

technical rescue team A team of individuals trained for special or hazardous rescue situations.

transportation area The area in a mass-casualty incident where ambulances and crews are organized to transport patients from the treatment area to receiving hospitals.

transportation officer The individual in charge of the transportation sector in a mass-casualty incident, who assigns patients from the treatment area to waiting ambulances in the transportation area.

treatment officer The individual, usually a physician, who is in charge of and directs EMS personnel at the treatment area in a mass-casualty incident.

triage area Designated area in a mass-casualty incident where the triage officer is located and patients are initially triaged before being taken to the treatment center.

triage officer The individual in charge of the incident command triage sector, who directs the sorting of patients into triage categories in a mass-casualty incident.

unified command Incident command process shared by the various agency area commanders (fire, rescue, EMS, law enforcement).

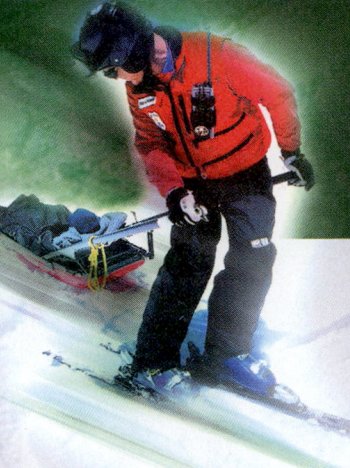

Assessment in Action

A small plane carrying one pilot and three passengers crashes in dense cloud cover at a local ski area. The plane appears to have hit several trees adjacent to a slopeside house, shearing off the wings. The fuselage is twisted and has come to rest on a deck outside the house. You proceed to the scene after hearing the low-flying plane and subsequent impact from the top of the slope where you are patrolling. You are the first rescuer to arrive. Several curious skiers have removed their skis and are approaching the scene from the slope.

1. This is an example of a mass-casualty incident.
   A. True
   B. False

2. Your first action as a rescuer should be to:
   A. attempt to pull out any surviving victims from the wreckage.
   B. warn the occupants of the house to get out before there is an explosion.
   C. determine if the scene is safe to enter.
   D. call the local TV station.

3. Two fire engines and the fire chief arrive on the scene. In the ICS, the fire chief will take the role of:
   A. medical command.
   B. incident command.
   C. transportation officer.
   D. staging officer.

4. An ambulance arrives shortly after with one paramedic and one first responder. Two other patrollers also arrive. The paramedic requests that you assist with initial triage as passengers are removed from the airplane and have the other patrollers carry them to a treatment area next to the ambulance in the driveway. Under the ICS, your role would be defined as the:
   A. treatment officer.
   B. triage officer.
   C. transportation officer.
   D. safety officer.

5. All but one of the passengers are removed from the fuselage. Additional, specialized tools are needed to extricate the last remaining passenger. The incident commander requests this equipment from the:
   A. transportation officer.
   B. staging officer.
   C. logistics officer.
   D. medical command.

6. Which of the command staff positions should the incident commander establish immediately?
   A. Information officer
   B. Media officer
   C. Safety officer
   D. None of the above

Points to Ponder

As part of your local emergency operations plan, you are the designated medical command officer for a mass-casualty incident that has taken place at a private ski area where you work as patrol director. The incident involves a chairlift that derailed near the top of the mountain, throwing an estimated 15 skiers and snowboarders to the slope below. You have appointed a triage officer at the scene and additional patrollers to coordinate transportation from the scene to a designated treatment area in a rental shop, and you have called for assistance from nearby EMS agencies. A paramedic with the first arriving ambulance informs you that he is now assuming the role of medical command. How would you deal with this situation?

Issues Scene Safety, Duty to Act, Risks of Being a Rescuer, Critical Incident Stress Debriefing (CISD), Legal Liability

Online Outlook

Incident command systems allow for coordination of OEC technicians, EMS, search and rescue, and other activities in an emergency situation. In major incidents there is usually a unified command, with a single command post where decisions are made by the designated leader. To learn more about major incident command systems, complete Exercise 29 at www.OECzone.com.

www.OECzone.com

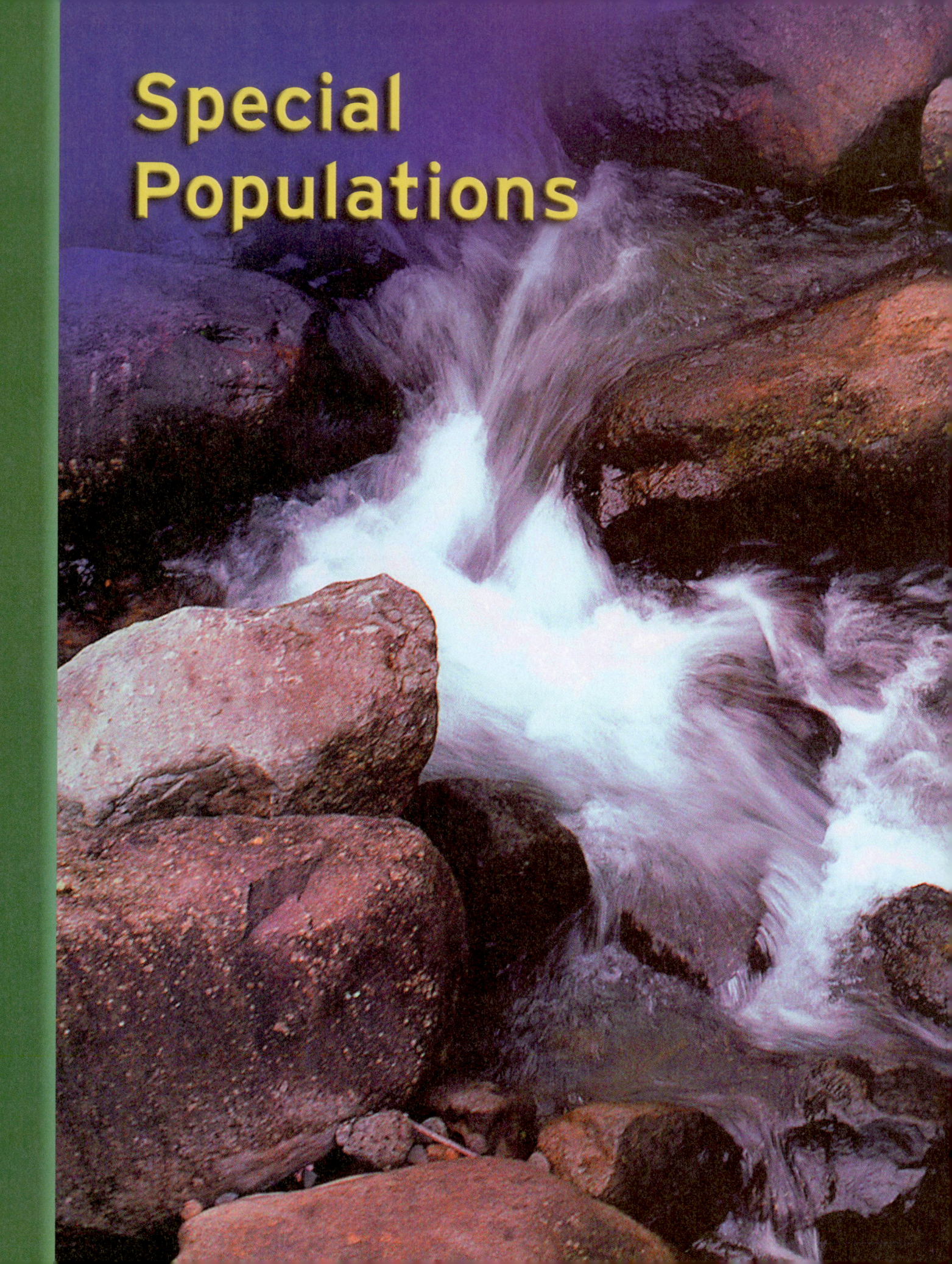

Special Populations

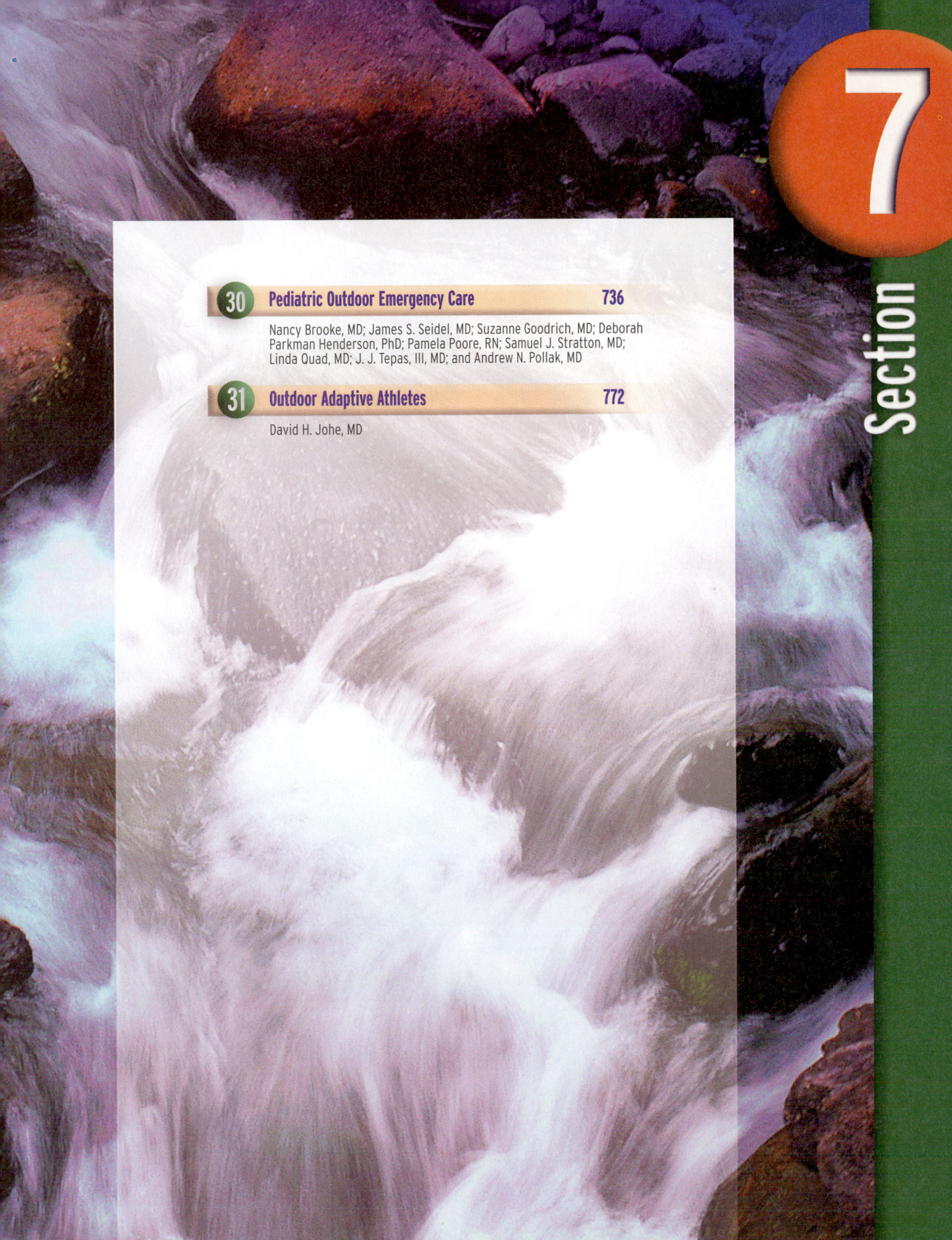

Section

7

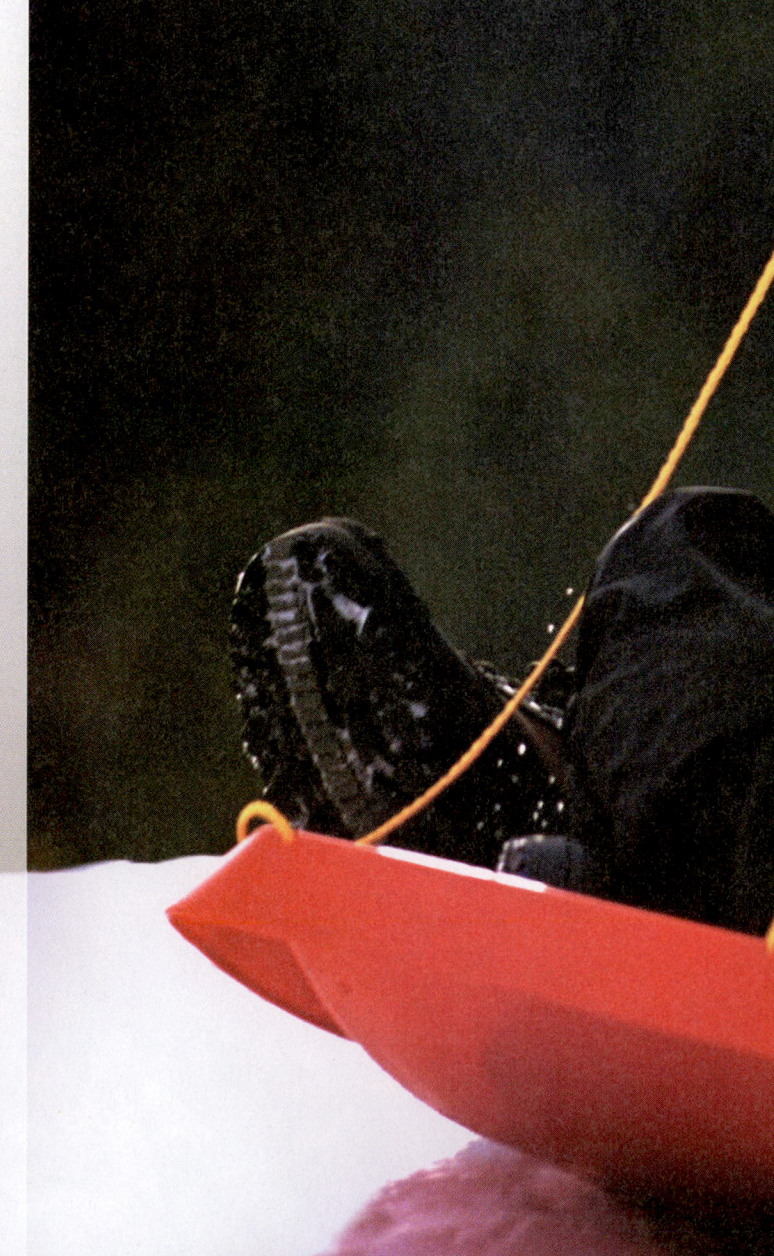

Pediatric Outdoor Emergency Care

🌲 These are core concepts in initial patrol training.

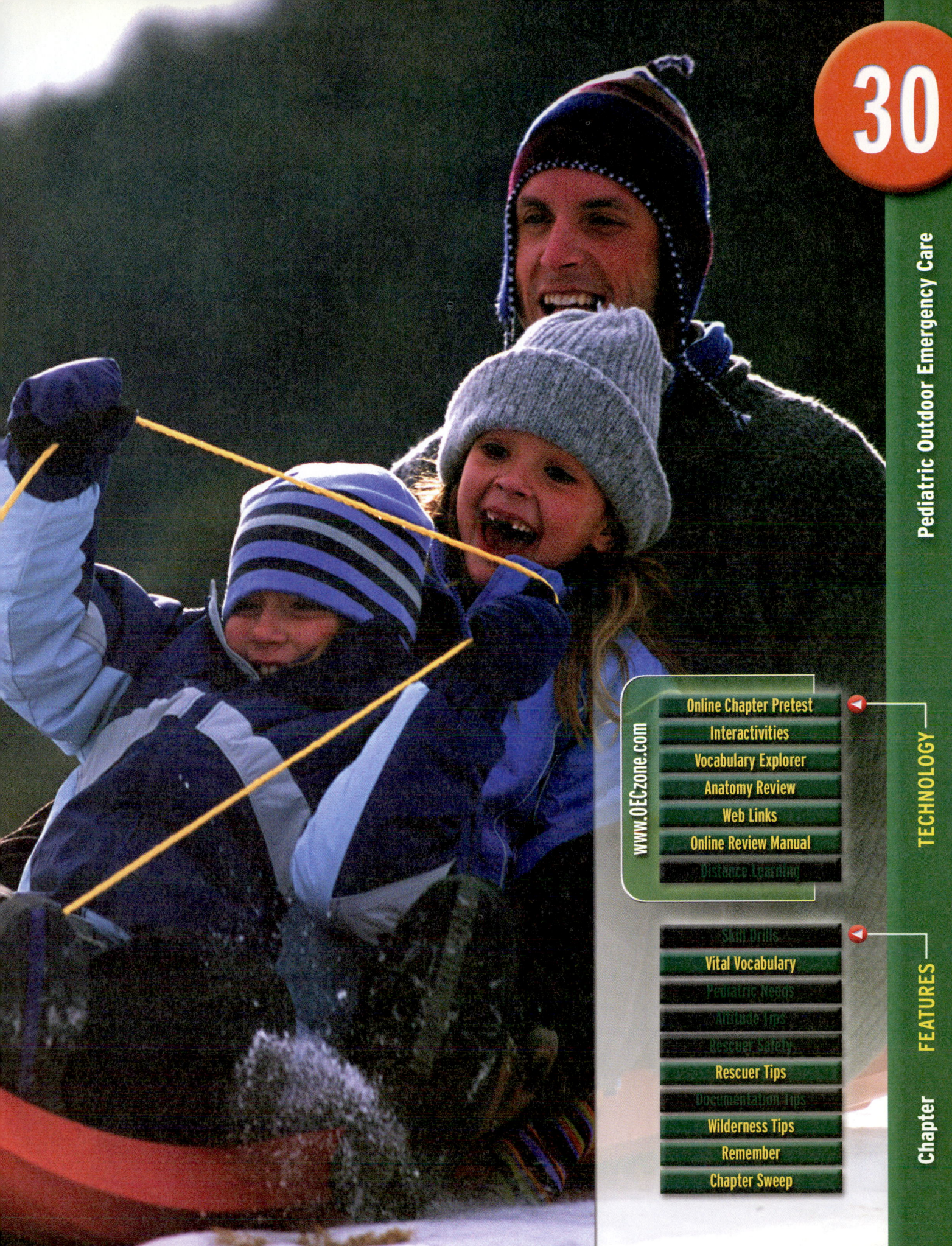

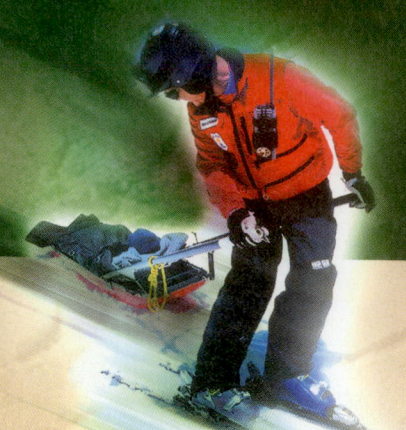

You are alerted at the year-round resort medical clinic that a child has been injured on the alpine slide.

This chapter will focus on pediatric patient assessment along with the most common pediatric emergencies. It will also help you answer the following questions:

1. How does the age of a child affect both your assessment and management? Give two age-specific examples.

2. Are there certain physical characteristics that make children more at risk than adults when they are injured? What are they?

Pediatric Outdoor Emergency Care

This chapter first describes the different developmental stages of childhood and some of the special challenges in caring for sick or injured children.

Children have many unique health problems. Similarly, many problems that are common in adults do not occur in children. Therefore, there is a specialized medical practice devoted to the care of the young, called **pediatrics**. In most situations, handling an infant or child means dealing with the parents as well. Therefore, it is vital that you remain calm and professional when you care for a child ▶ Figure 30-1 .

Working with infants and children has its own nuances. As the rescuer approaches the pediatric patient, certain important considerations in care, both anatomically and physiologically, need to be understood. Patient assessment has its own unique needs. Shock is discussed because it occurs rapidly in children. Specific pediatric medical and traumatic emergencies are discussed. Care for burns, poisoning, submersion injuries, seizures, hypothermia, hyperthermia, sepsis, and dehydration are covered. Child abuse, a topic that all rescuers should understand, is also discussed.

An important part of caring for children is dealing with their parents. In addition to feeling love and concern for their children, parents often become anxious about a child who is injured or ill, and they may express this anxiety by questioning your competence as a rescuer or by appearing agitated or hysterical. They may also feel guilty—rightly or wrongly—if they feel they were a factor in causing the child's injury or contributed to worsening an illness by not bringing the child to care sooner. At times you will be dealing with a caregiver rather than a parent. If the child trusts the caregiver, include this individual in the care as you would a parent. The terms *parents* and *caregivers* may be used interchangeably in this chapter.

As an emergency care provider, you should remain calm, nonjudgmental, and impartial. Explain what is going on, what needs to happen, and that everything necessary is being done as thoroughly and as quickly as possible. In general, allow the parents to remain with the child. When painful procedures are necessary, explain this beforehand and give the parents the option of remaining with the child or leaving temporarily.

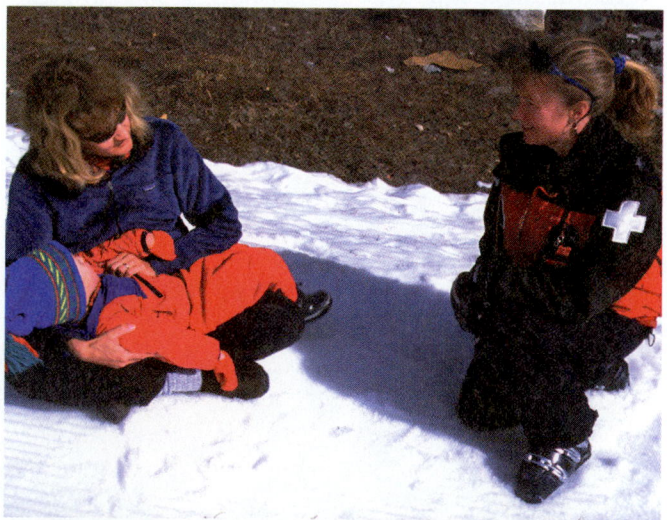

Figure 30-1 Handling a sick or injured child can be extremely challenging. A calm, professional demeanor is of utmost importance as you care for the child and communicate with the parents.

Anatomy and Physiology

There is no other time in our lives that our bodies are growing and changing as fast as during childhood. Infants quickly change once outside the mother's body. Toddlers learn to walk and talk. School-age children explore the world without thought of consequences. These changes can create difficulties with assessment of the child if the rescuer does not expect these differences.

The airway changes greatly during the early years of life. The tongue is larger and more rounded compared with the size of the mandible, or lower jaw, in younger children. This makes the tongue a greater risk for obstruction. The mandible will grow and pull the tongue forward while it flattens with age ▼ **Figure 30-2**.

The soft tissue in the rear of the mouth can also contribute to airway problems in the youngest of children. The tonsils, adenoids, and soft palate in combination with the tongue produce a smaller opening to move air easily. Upper airway colds can make a child work hard just to breathe. Also, the trachea is softer and narrower. The cartilage that makes up the support matures as we grow; however, the trachea can be occluded from compression. Even during the head tilt–chin lift technique, the airway can be occluded if the maneuver is performed too aggressively.

An infant needs to breathe faster than an older child. The child's lungs will grow and develop better abilities to handle the exchange of oxygen as they age. A respiratory rate of 40 to 60 breaths/min is normal for the newborn, while the teenager is expected to have rates closer to the adult range. Breathing also requires the use of the chest muscles and diaphragm. Infants have very little use of their chest muscles to make their chests expand during inspiration. They use their diaphragm. Anything that puts pressure on the abdomen of a young child can block the movement of the diaphragm and cause respiratory compromise.

Rescuer Tips

Pediatric Characteristics

- Smaller body mass
- Thinner skin
- A larger body surface area-to-mass ratio
- A larger, heavier head in relation to body size, supported by a relatively weaker neck
- A relatively larger tongue
- Smaller airway passages
- A more elastic but weaker skeleton (because ligaments may be stronger than their associated bones)
- Faster heart and breathing rates
- Higher metabolic rates and oxygen requirements
- Less effective control of body temperature
- Ability to compensate for developing shock to the extent that a drop in blood pressure occurs later than in adults
- In the young infant, a preference for breathing through the nose rather than the mouth

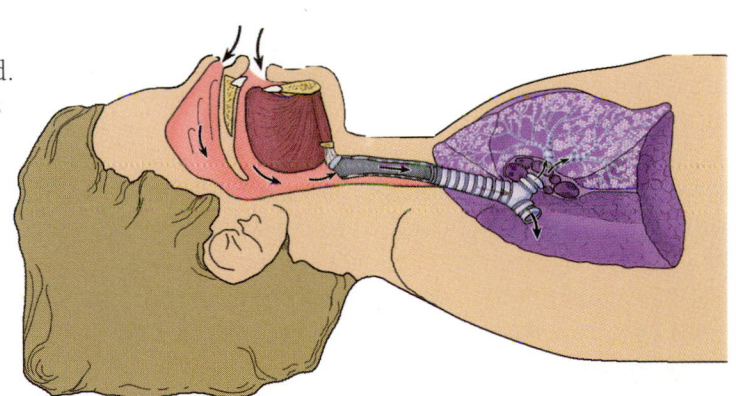

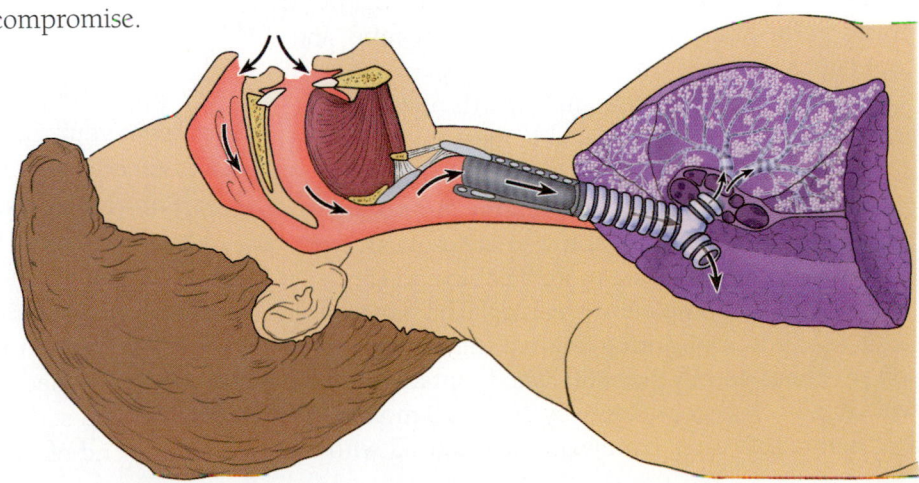

Figure 30-2 The anatomy of a child's airway differs from that of an adult's in several ways. The back of the head is larger in a child, so head positioning requires more care. The tongue is proportionally larger and more anterior in the mouth. The trachea is smaller in diameter and more flexible. The airway itself is lower and narrower.

Common Medical Causes of Respiratory Distress in the Pediatric Patient

Upper Airway
- Above the larynx: severe tonsillitis, abscess of the tonsillar area or back of the throat
- Larynx: croup, epiglottitis
- Below the larynx: foreign body, infection (tracheitis)

Lower Airway
- Asthma
- Bronchiolitis
- Bronchitis
- Pneumonia
- Foreign body

Young children also experience muscle fatigue much more quickly than older ones. This can lead to respiratory failure if a child has had to breathe hard for long periods.

An infant's heart rate can become as high as 200 beats/min or more if the body needs to compensate for injury or illness. This is the primary method for the body to compensate for decreased oxygenation. It is important to know the normal ranges when evaluating children. The ability of children to constrict their blood vessels gives them the ability to keep the vital organs well perfused. Pale skin is an early sign that the child may be compensating for decreased perfusion. Constriction of the vessels can be so profound that blood flow to the extremities can be diminished. Signs of vasoconstriction can include weak distal (eg, radial) pulses in the extremities, delayed capillary refill, and cool hands or feet.

The skeletal system contains growth plates at the ends of long bones, which enable these bones to grow during childhood. Children's fractures commonly occur in the growth plate between the layer of new uncalcified bone cells and the next layer of calcified cells. Children's bones are more flexible and can "bend" without completely breaking. The bones of the skull also grow, but during infancy. Infants have two soft openings within the skull called fontanels. These will usually close completely by about 18 months of age; before that time, handle an infant's head with care.

Growth and Development

There are specific issues that are important to different age groups. However, no two children grow and develop along the same timetable. There are some general guidelines the rescuer should use when caring for a child of any age ▶ Table 30-1 .

Between birth and adulthood (age 21), many physical and emotional changes occur in children. While each child is unique, the thoughts and behaviors of children as a whole are often grouped into stages: infancy, the toddler years, preschool age, school age, and adolescence. Children in each stage grapple with different developmental issues.

How you examine children and how you help them to cope with the emergency depend on several practical considerations, including the child's stability and mental status, the anticipated transport time, the availability of other personnel, and the protocols in your area. However, there are a number of simple techniques that will let you calm and comfort most children during emergency treatment and transport. Here are some suggestions about approaching and caring for the different childhood age groups.

The Infant

Infancy is usually defined as the first year of life; the first month after birth is called the neonatal or newborn period. At first, infants respond mainly to physical stimuli such as light, warmth, cold, hunger, sound, and taste. Crying is one of their main avenues of expression during this period. After the first few months, however, they learn to coo, smile, roll over, and recognize their parents or caregivers. Infants are usually not afraid of strangers, because they become the center of attention in most families. However, by the end of their first year, they may show signs of preferring to be with their caregivers and may cry if they are separated.

Begin your assessment by observing the infant from a distance, preferably in a caregiver's arms. This initial size up can reward the rescuer with valuable information. The work of breathing, skin color, alertness, and level of activity provide a good overall picture of the infant's condition. Older infants, from 6 months to a year, may begin to cry when touched or picked up by a stranger, so let the caregiver continue to hold the baby as you start your examination. Warm your hands and the end of the stethoscope, then begin by listening

TABLE 30-1 Helpful Tips in Caring for Infants and Children

1. **Try to remain calm and appear confident.** Children are used to having other people take charge. They are also easily frightened by noise, so speak with a soft voice whenever possible.

2. **Remember that you are caring for the whole family, not just the child.** Children are quick to pick up on their caregivers' anxiety. It may calm both parties if you can establish good rapport with the caregivers and allow them to help with the child's care. To avoid confusion, avoid using technical terms.

3. **Honesty is the best policy.** Telling a child or a caregiver that a procedure won't hurt (when you know that it will) or that it will be over quickly (when it won't) can boomerang: Once you lose their trust, any additional procedures that you attempt are more likely to meet with resistance.

4. **Tell both the caregivers and the child what is happening as often as you can.** Lack of information is very stressful for everyone; the imagination can run wild in an effort to make sense of what is going on. In children, we call this frightening fantasies; in caregivers, we call it worst-case scenarios.

5. **Keep the family together as much as possible.** This is not always possible, but children and their caregivers generally feel safer when they are together. Parents can sometimes be encouraged to help by holding the child's hand, talking to the child, or telling a story.

6. **Provide hope and reassurance to the caregivers and to the child.** Even when you are very concerned about the child's condition, be careful not to eliminate hope in the patient and family. Children especially need reassurance, rewards, and praise during painful events. Remember that no one can be absolutely certain about the outcome. Children have an amazing ability to bounce back from what looks to be death's door.

> Between birth and adulthood, many physical and emotional changes occur in children.

to the chest and assessing the heart rate. Next, examine the abdomen, then the head, and then the rest of the body. This torso-to-head approach works well because infants see their world centered around their head. Near the end of their first year, an infant's world will increase in size to include their torso as well.

Provide as much sensory comfort as you can: use a soothing voice and a kind, unhurried, parental approach. Keep the infant warm, and offer a pacifier if the caregiver allows it. Have a caregiver hold the infant, if possible, during procedures. Plan to complete any painful procedure in an efficient manner. When splinting a suspected fracture, be sure to have all of the equipment you will need in order to avoid making the procedure take longer than necessary. Always explain to the caregiver what you are doing.

The Toddler

After infancy, until about 3 years of age, a child is called a **toddler**. During this period, children begin to walk and to explore the environment. They are able to open doors, drawers, boxes, and bottles. Ask the parent for permission to render care. Because they are explorers by nature and are not afraid, injuries in this age group are more frequent.

Stranger anxiety develops early in this period. Toddlers may resist separation from caregivers and be afraid to let others come near them. Ask the parent for permission to render care. Because of toddlers' newly found independence, they may also be very unhappy about being restrained or held for procedures ▶ **Figure 30-3** . Two-year-olds in particular have a well-deserved reputation for having their own ideas about almost everything, which is why these years are often called the "terrible twos." Toddlers have a hard time describing or localizing pain. Pain in the abdomen may be "My tummy hurts," and examination may reveal tenderness throughout the body. This is not because the child is trying to be difficult but because he or she cannot tell the difference.

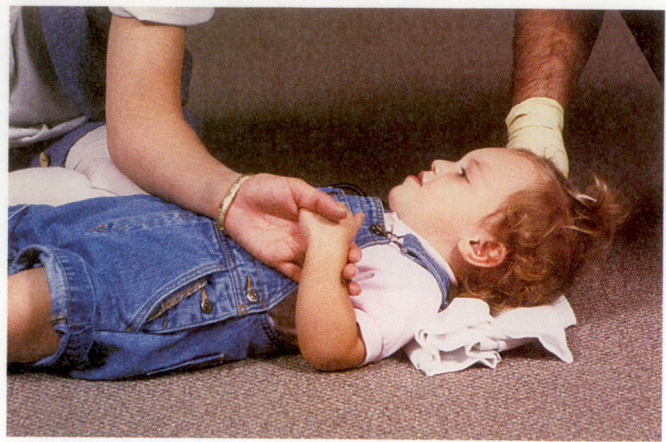

Figure 30-3 Because of their newly found independence, toddlers may be unhappy about being restrained or held for procedures.

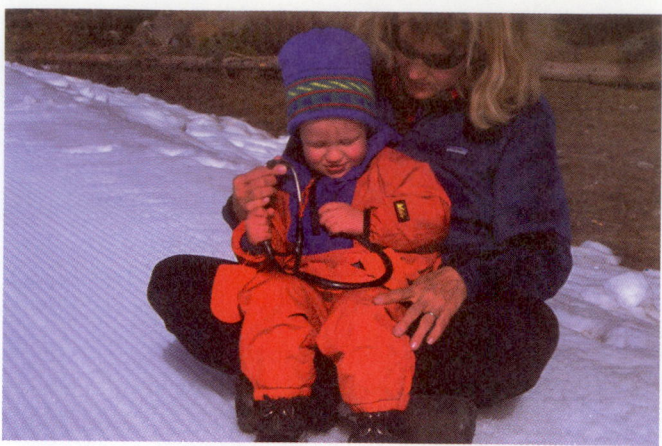

Figure 30-4 Make the exam less threatening by allowing the patient to handle some pieces of equipment.

Make as many observations as you can before touching the child: level of alertness, work of breathing, and skin color. When appropriate, examine the child on the caregiver's lap, and use toys or puppets to distract him or her.

Toddlers can be curious and adventuresome, so you may able to distract them. For example, you might allow the child to play with a tongue depressor. Restrain the child for as short a time as possible, and allow him or her to be comforted immediately after a painful procedure. Begin your palpation assessment *away* from the suspected area of injury or pain. If you go straight to this area, the child may become upset, making the rest of your evaluation difficult.

The Preschool-Age Child

Preschool-age children (age 3 to 6 years) are able to use simple language quite effectively and have lively imaginations. They can understand directions, be much more specific in describing their sensations, and identify painful areas when questioned. They tend to respond positively to a request to "help find out what is wrong," or when the rescuer asks, "Can you show me where it hurts?" Much of their history must still be obtained from caregivers, however. Preschool-age children have a rich fantasy life, which can make them particularly fearful about pain and change involving their bodies. At this age, they often believe that their thoughts or wishes can cause injury or harm to themselves or to others. They can believe that an injury was due to a bad deed they did earlier in the day.

Try to distract the child during the examination with simple conversation and questions, or use a toy, game, or puppet. Make the examination less threatening by allowing the child to handle some pieces

of equipment, such as your stethoscope or a tongue depressor ▲ **Figure 30-4**. Do not use words that suggest invading the child's body, such as "shot," "cut," "poke," or "stick." At this age, children may take your remarks literally, so choose your words carefully.

Tell the child what you are going to do immediately before you do it; this way, the child has no time to develop frightening fantasies. At this age, children are easily distracted with counting games, small toys, or conversation. Be sure to adjust the level of game to the developmental level of the child; health care providers often assume that preschool children understand more than they actually do. Use adhesive bandages to cover the site of an injection or other small wound, because the child might be worried about keeping his or her body together in one piece.

The School-Age Child

School-age children (age 6 to 12 years) are beginning to act more like adults. They can think in concrete terms, respond sensibly to direct questions, and help take care of themselves. Your assessment, therefore, is more like an adult assessment; talk to the child, not just the parent, in taking the medical history.

The school-age child is usually familiar with the process of physical examination. They have been to the doctor for childhood check-ups and immunizations. Whenever possible, give the child appropriate choices: Would you like to sit up or lie down? Would you like to take off your clothes yourself? Only ask questions that you can control the answer. If you ask "Can I take your blood pressure?" and the answer is NO! you will not be able to take it without upsetting the child. Encourage cooperation by allowing the child to listen to his or her own heartbeat through the stethoscope.

School-age children can understand the difference between emotional and physical pain; they have concerns about the meaning of pain. Give them simple explanations about what is causing their pain and what will be done about it. Games and conversation may distract them. Ask them to describe their favorite place, their pets, or their toys. Ask the caregiver's advice in choosing the right distraction. Rewarding the school-age child after a procedure can be very helpful in his or her recovery, but only reward a child for completing the procedure.

The Adolescent

Most **adolescents** (age 12 to 18 years) are able to think abstractly and can participate in decision making. This is a period where the focus of their strength has moved from parents to peers. They are very concerned about body image and how they appear to their peers and to others. They may have very strong feelings about being observed during procedures, even—or especially—by their caregivers. The rescuer should become aware of special problems sometimes associated with this age group, especially substance abuse, sexually transmitted diseases, and pregnancy.

Respect the adolescent's privacy at all times. Remember that adolescents can often understand very complex concepts and treatment options; you should provide them with information when they request it. You will find them more helpful and understanding of necessary procedures.

Adolescents have a clear understanding of the purpose and meaning of pain. Whenever possible, explain any necessary procedures well in advance. Assess their pain by facial and body expression as well as by asking questions; adolescents can be very stoic and may not request relief from pain even when they need it. To distract them, find out what they are interested in, such as sports, books, movies, or friends, and get them talking about this.

Assessing Pediatric Patients
Approach to Assessment

Always approach pediatric patients at their eye level (sit down if possible) ▶ **Figure 30-5** . During the first impression, note whether the child appears injured or ill, critical or not, active or quiet, and what the child is doing, eg, crying, talking, or playing with toys.

When a child becomes sick or injured, the young body begins to compensate for the extra needs of the body. The work-of-breathing (WOB) increases. This is often seen as faster breathing, retractions along the chest wall, or the way the child sits and positions himself or

> Adolescents need to be treated in a matter-of-fact manner and shown consideration for their desire for independence. Nevertheless, they may regress into childlike behavior when ill or injured.

herself. The heart rate increases to allow more oxygenated blood to pass through the body. The skin color may turn pale or cyanotic depending on the problem. The child will become anxious as the oxygen level in the brain decreases. Assessment of the level of responsiveness will give clues to the amount of oxygen reaching the end-organs of the body. Grade responsiveness according to the AVPU scale. In the newborn, infant, or young toddler, response to verbal stimuli consists of actions such as turning in response to a parent's voice, eye opening, crying, nonverbal noises, or calming down. Grade the patient's behavior by comparing it with that of a normal child at this stage of development. It is important to note whether the patient recognizes a parent and responds to his or her voice.

Because pediatric patients have a relatively large head size, a greater body surface area-to-mass ratio, and a less stable system for regulating body temperature, they are more prone to heat loss and therefore more susceptible to hypothermia. Be sure to protect the patient from the elements. In a cold environment, always insulate the head as well as the body. In an extremely hot environment, children are also more susceptible to hyperthermia than adults. If the brain is feeling oxygen starved, other parts of the body will also.

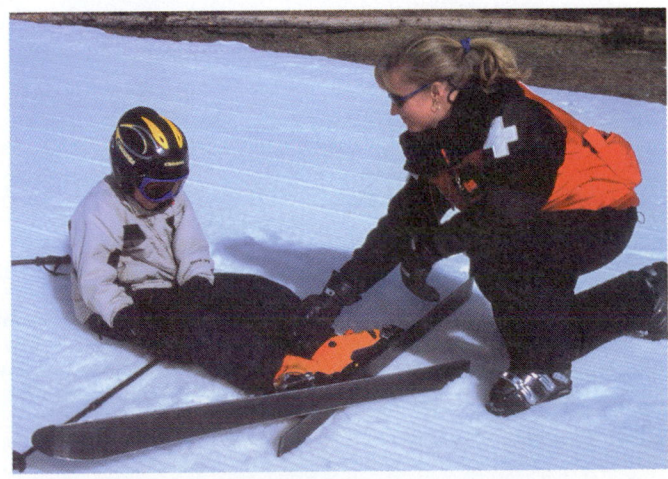

Figure 30-5 Always approach pediatric patients at their eye level.

Patient Assessment

Scene Size-Up

Body Substance Isolation
Scene Safety
Determine Mechanism of Injury/Nature of Illness
Determine Number of Patients
Request Additional Assistance
Consider C-Spine Immobilization

Initial Assessment

Form General Impression of the Patient
Assess Responsiveness
Assess the Airway, Breathing, and Circulation (ABCs)
Stabilize ABCs
Identify Priority Patients
Initiate Transport Decision

Unresponsive Patients

Rapid History and Physical Exam

Rapid Body Survey
Baseline Vital Signs
SAMPLE History
    (from friends, family,
    or bystanders)
Rapid Transport

Responsive Trauma Patients

Focused History and Physical Exam

Reconsider the Mechanism of Injury

Significant MOI	No Significant MOI
Rapid Trauma Assessment (Rapid Body Survey)	Focused Physical Exam Based on Chief Complaint
Baseline Vital Signs and SAMPLE History	Baseline Vital Signs and SAMPLE History
Rapid Transport	Reevaluate Transport

Responsive Medical Patients

Focused History and Physical Exam

History of Illness
SAMPLE History
Focused Physical Exam:
    Based on Chief Complaint
Baseline Vital Signs
Reevaluate Transport

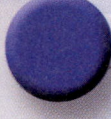

Detailed Physical Exam

Head-to-toe Steps
Systematic Exam Using DCAP-BTLS
Baseline Vital Signs

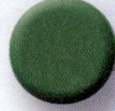

Ongoing Assessment

Repeat the Initial Assessment (ABCs)
Reassess Vital Signs
Repeat Focused Assessment
Check Interventions

Figure 30-6 Base your approach to a child on the same general steps you use for adults.

Although each child and situation is unique, you should follow a few basic guidelines when assessing and caring for infants and children. First, you should follow the same general approach to children that you use for adults ◄ Figure 30-6 . Remember that children most commonly have respiratory arrest, not cardiac arrest. Management of the airway and breathing is paramount. You should consult a pediatric BLS publication such as AHA, ARC, NSC, or ASHI for specifics of pediatric cardiopulmonary resuscitation (CPR).

The Pediatric Airway
Positioning the Airway

Positioning the airway correctly is critical in pediatric emergency care. Always position the airway in a neutral sniffing position ▼ Figure 30-7 . This accomplishes two goals at once: it keeps the trachea from kinking when the neck is bent back (hyperextended) or forward (flexed), and it maintains the proper alignment if you have to immobilize the spine. If the child has been involved in trauma or trauma is suspected, use the jaw-thrust maneuver to open the airway.

Follow these steps to position the airway in a child or infant:

1. **Place the patient on a firm surface** such as a short backboard or pediatric immobilization device.

2. **Fold a small towel to a thickness of approximately 1″, and place it under the patient's shoulders and back.**

3. **Place tape across the child's forehead** to limit rolling of the head during transport.

Airway Adjuncts

In children with inadequate ventilation, whatever the reason, you should use an airway adjunct to maintain an open airway. Airway adjuncts are devices that help to maintain the airway or assist in providing artificial ventilation, including oral and nasal airways, bite blocks, and BVM devices. Placing the adjuncts correctly starts with choosing the appropriately sized equipment.

Assisting Ventilation and Oxygenation

After opening the airway, you should assess the patient's ventilation status. Look, listen, and feel for breathing. Remember to observe chest rise in older children and abdominal rise in younger children and infants. Skin condition indicates the amount of oxygen getting to the organs of the body. Patients with pale, mottled, or blue skin may have inadequate levels of oxygen in their blood. All trauma patients should receive oxygen. If the patient has sustained trauma to the face, assisting ventilations may be difficult.

Airway Obstruction

Children, especially those younger than 5 years, can (and do) obstruct their airway with any object that they can fit into their mouth: hot dogs, balloons, grapes, or coins ▼ Figure 30-8 . In cases of trauma, a child's teeth may have been dislodged into the airway. Blood, vomitus, or other secretions can also cause partial or complete obstruction.

Another source of airway obstructions are infections, including pneumonia, croup, and epiglottitis ► Figure 30-9 . Croup is an infection of the airway below the level of the vocal cords, usually caused by a virus. Epiglottitis is an infection of the soft tissue in the area above the vocal cords. Infection should be

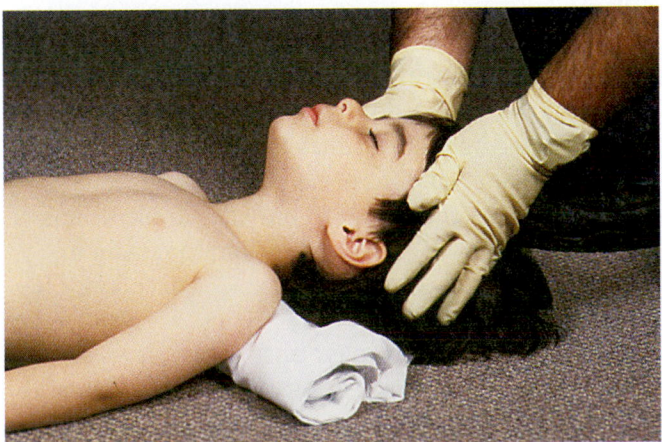

Figure 30-7 The airway should be placed in a neutral sniffing position to keep the trachea from kinking when the neck is flexed or hyperextended.

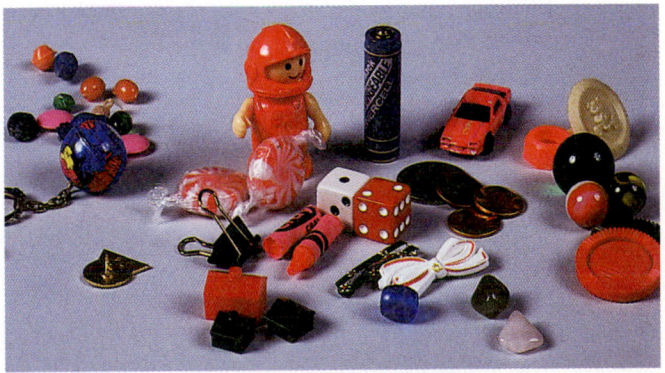

Figure 30-8 Any number of objects can obstruct a child's airway. Some of the more common ones include batteries, coins, toys, buttons, and candy.

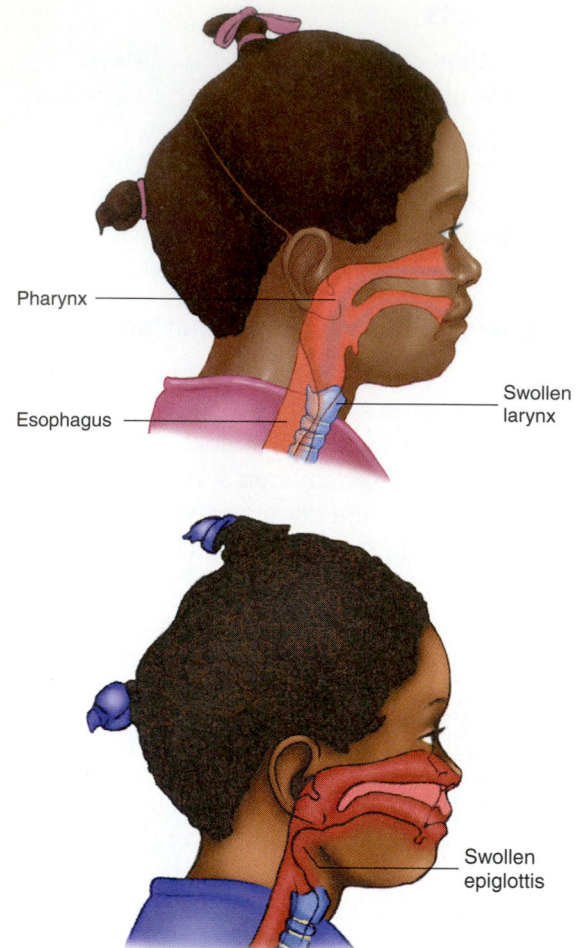

Figure 30-9 Epiglottitis is an infection that can cause airway obstruction in children.

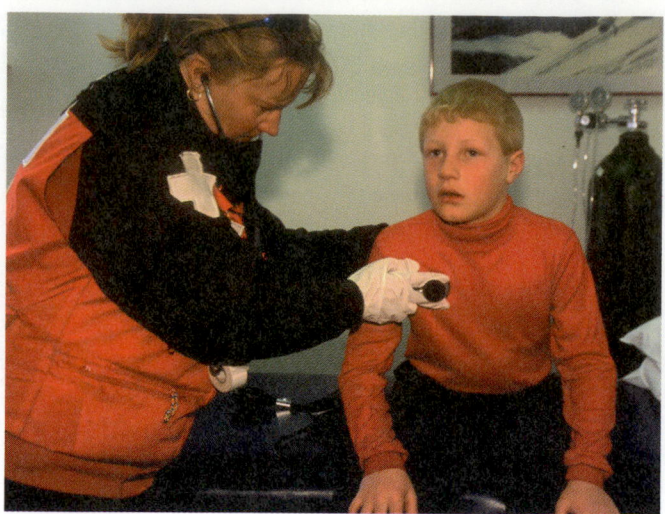

Figure 30-10 Auscultate breath sounds at the level of the armpit.

considered as a possible cause of airway obstruction if a child has congestion, fever, drooling, and cold symptoms. Such children must be taken immediately to the emergency department. Without special equipment and training, attempts to clear an airway that is blocked by infection can worsen the obstruction.

Signs and Symptoms

Obstruction by a foreign object may involve the upper or the lower airway. Signs and symptoms that are frequently associated with an upper airway obstruction include decreased or absent breath sounds and stridor. **Stridor** has been described as a high-pitched noise heard mainly on inspiration and is usually caused by swelling of the area surrounding the vocal cords or upper airway obstruction. In children with croup, it resembles the bark of a seal.

Signs and symptoms of a lower airway obstruction include **wheezing**, a whistling sound caused by air

traveling through narrowed air passages within the bronchioles, and/or rales. **Rales** are caused by the flow of air through liquid, present in the air pouches and smaller airways in the lungs. They produce a crackling sound like that of blowing bubbles through a straw in a glass filled with liquid. The best way to auscultate breath sounds in a child is to listen on both sides of the chest at the level of the armpit (▲ **Figure 30-10**).

Emergency Medical Care

Treatment of the child with an airway obstruction depends on whether or not the patient is unconscious and whether the obstruction is partial or complete.

If the child is conscious and you know for sure that there is a foreign body in the airway—that is, if someone actually saw the object go into the child's mouth—encourage the child to cough to clear the airway. Abdominal thrusts are also recommended to relieve a complete airway obstruction in a child. If the material in the airway does not completely block the flow of air, the obstruction is not complete and the child may be able to breathe adequately on his or her own without any intervention. If the obstruction is only partial, do not intervene except to provide supplemental oxygen (▶ **Figure 30-11**). Allow the child to remain in whatever position is most comfortable, and monitor his or her condition.

If you see signs of complete obstruction, however, you must attempt to clear the airway at once. The signs include the following:

• Ineffective cough (no sound)

• Inability to speak or cry

• Increasing respiratory difficulty, with stridor

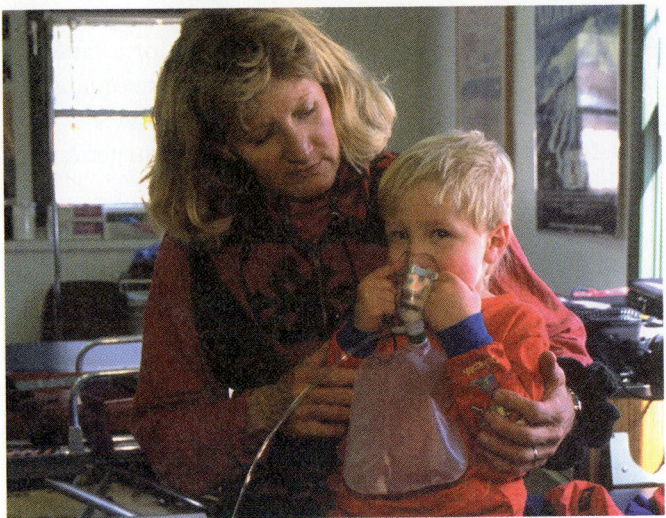

Figure 30-11 If a child has a partial airway obstruction, do not intervene except to give supplemental oxygen and allow the child to remain in whatever position is most comfortable.

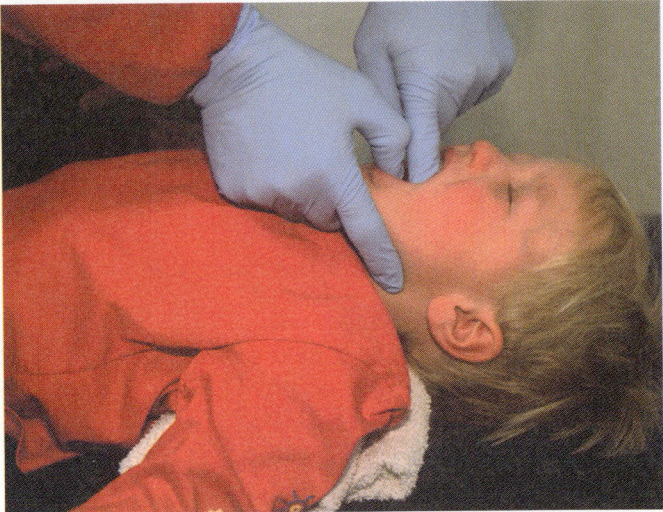

Figure 30-12 Use the tongue-jaw lift to open the mouth in an unconscious child. If the object is visible, try to remove it by using a finger sweep.

- Cyanosis
- Loss of consciousness

MANAGEMENT OF AIRWAY OBSTRUCTION IN A CHILD. If there is reason to believe that an unconscious child has a foreign body obstruction, check the upper airway to see whether the obstructing object is visible. The best way to do this is to grasp the tongue and jaw between your finger and thumb and lift to open the mouth; this is called the tongue-jaw lift (▶ Figure 30-12). If the object is visible, try to remove it using a finger sweep motion. Never use finger sweeps in infants or children if you cannot see the object, as you may push it further into the airway.

Abdominal thrusts are recommended to relieve a complete airway obstruction in a child. These thrusts increase the pressure in the chest, creating an artificial cough that may force a foreign body from the airway.

The following lists the steps for applying abdominal thrusts to the unconscious child who you suspect has a foreign body airway obstruction:

1. **Place the child in a supine position** on a firm, flat surface.

2. **Inspect the upper airway** using the tongue-jaw lift. If you see the foreign object, try to remove it.

3. **Attempt rescue breathing.** If the first try is unsuccessful, reposition the child's head and try again.

4. **If ventilation is still unsuccessful, kneel beside or straddle the child's hips.** Place the

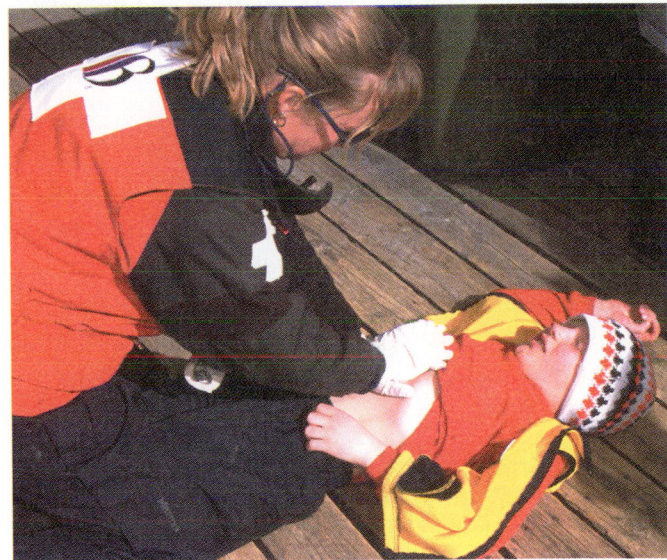

Figure 30-13 If ventilation is unsuccessful, position your hands on the abdomen above the navel and well below the chest cage. Give five abdominal thrusts.

heel of one hand on the front of the child's abdomen just above the navel and well below the rib cage and sternum. Place your other hand on top of the first hand.

5. **Press both hands into the abdomen** in an upward motion, giving five distinct thrusts (▲ Figure 30-13).

6. **Open the airway** using the tongue-jaw lift and visualize the airway.

7. **If you see the foreign body,** remove it. Only attempt to remove objects you can actually see. Blind sweeps may push the object back into the airway.

8. **Attempt rescue breathing.** If the foreign body is not expelled on the first attempt, reposition the child's head and try again.

9. **If the airway remains obstructed,** repeat the abdominal thrusts.

The following steps are used to remove a foreign body obstruction from a conscious child who is in a standing or sitting position (▶ **Figure 30-14**):

1. **Kneel on one knee behind the child,** and circle his or her body with both arms around the patient's chest. Prepare to give abdominal thrusts by placing your fist just above the patient's navel and well below the lower tip of the sternum. Place your other hand over that fist.

2. **Give the child five rapid, distinct abdominal thrusts** in an upward direction. Be careful to avoid applying force to the lower rib cage or sternum.

3. **Repeat this standing technique** until the child expels the foreign body or fully loses consciousness.

4. **If the child becomes unconscious,** inspect the airway using the tongue-jaw lift. If you see the foreign body, try to remove it.

5. **Attempt rescue breathing.** If the first attempt fails, reposition the head and try again.

6. **If the airway remains obstructed,** repeat the abdominal thrusts.

If you manage to clear the airway obstruction in an unconscious child but he or she remains without spontaneous breathing or circulation, perform CPR.

MANAGEMENT OF AIRWAY OBSTRUCTION IN AN INFANT.
Abdominal thrusts are not recommended for infants because of the risk of injury to the immature organs of the abdomen. Instead, use back blows and chest thrusts to try to clear a complete airway obstruction in an infant, as follows (▼ **Figure 30-15**):

1. **Hold the infant face down,** with the body resting on your forearm. Support the infant's jaw and face with your hand, and keep the head lower than the rest of the body.

2. **Deliver five back blows** between the shoulder blades, using the heel of your hand.

3. **Place your free hand behind the infant's head and back,** and bring the infant upright on your thigh, sandwiching the infant's body between your two hands and arms. The infant's head should remain below the level of the body.

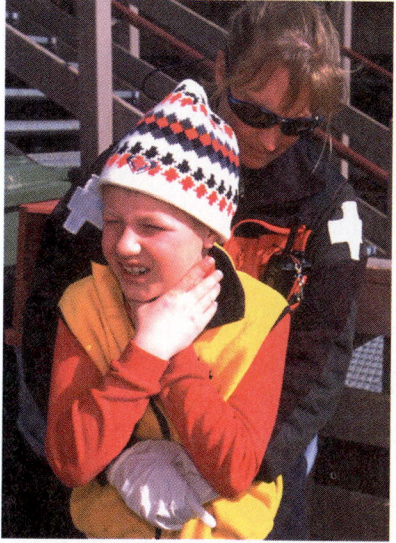

Figure 30-14 Kneel or stand behind the child, wrap your arms around his or her body, and place your fist just above the navel and well below the lower tip of the sternum.

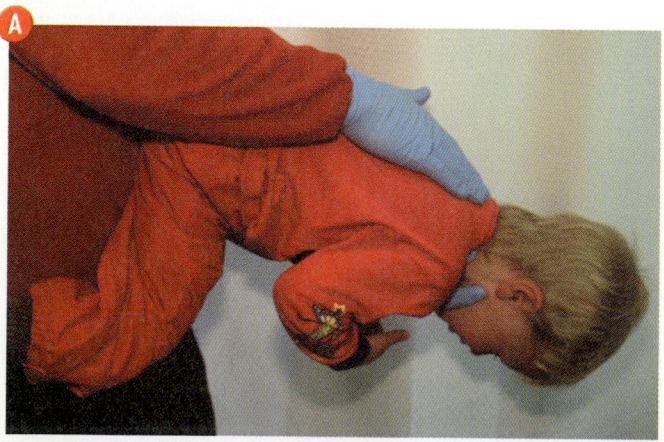

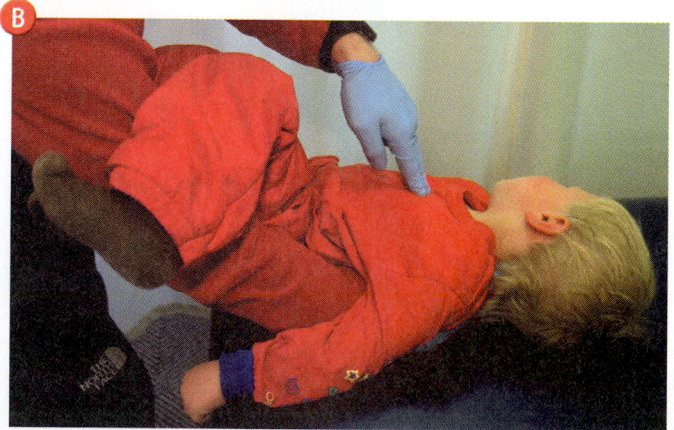

Figure 30-15 **A.** Hold the infant face down with the body resting on your forearm. Support the jaw and face with your hand, and keep the head lower than the rest of the body. Give the infant five back blows between the shoulder blades, using the heel of your hand. **B.** Give the infant five quick chest thrusts, using two fingers placed on the lower half of the sternum.

4. **Give five quick chest thrusts** in the same location and manner as chest compressions, using two fingers placed on the lower half of the sternum. For larger infants, or if you have small hands, you can perform this step by placing the infant in your lap and turning the infant's whole body as a unit between back blows and chest thrusts.

5. **Check the airway.** If you can see the foreign body now, remove it. If not, repeat the cycle as often as necessary.

6. **If the infant is still unconscious** after removal of the object, check for circulation and perform CPR, if necessary.

If the infant regains consciousness, keep him or her in the recovery position during transport.

After your first impression, you should take a child's vital signs early in the field because you are the eyes, ears, and hands of more definitive care. During your assessment, you should obtain a complete set of baseline vital signs, including respirations, pulse, blood pressure (when possible), skin signs, level of activity, muscle tone, and movement. It is always a good idea to inform the base or receiving hospital about the status of a pediatric patient so that the facility can prepare to meet the child's particular needs.

The condition of infants and children may deteriorate rapidly during transport. You should use pediatric resuscitation equipment when necessary. Arrange transport of infants and children to facilities that are capable of providing the appropriate level of care whenever possible. Not all community hospitals offer all higher levels of care

for children. You may have to bypass closer emergency care facilities to reach a pediatric center. When this is not possible, as in many rural areas, a hospital may arrange for secondary transportation after stabilizing the child's condition.

After registering the first impression, assess the patient's level of responsiveness and perform the ABCs. A normal voice or lusty cry indicates a good airway. If the patient has altered responsiveness, is unable to talk, or has stridor, perform the head tilt-chin lift technique (or the jaw-thrust maneuver if trauma is likely). Do *not* hyperextend the neck; this may cause or worsen airway obstruction.

Vital Signs

Note that normal vital signs in pediatric patients vary with the age of the child (▼ Table 30-2). Remember that your approach to taking vital signs also varies with the age of the child. Be gentle, talk to the child, assess respirations and pulse next, and assess blood pressure last (► Figure 30-16). Warm your stethoscope on your hands or a cloth before placing it on the skin. You may also want to let the child hold the equipment or stethoscope before placing it on him or her.

RESPIRATIONS. Abnormal respirations are a common sign of illness or injury in children. Respirations should be counted for at least 30 seconds. However, do not base your evaluation by counting the number of times the chest rises and falls in infants and children younger than 3 years. Rather, count the rise and fall of the abdomen. This is usually easier to do with the child in the caregiver's lap. Note the effort the child makes in breathing, and listen for noises during respiration.

TABLE 30-2 Vital Signs by Age

Age	Respirations (breaths/min)	Pulse (beats/min)	Systolic Blood Pressure (mm Hg)
Newborn: 0 to 1 month	40 to 60	120 to 160	50 to 70
Infant: 1 month to 1 year	30 to 60	100 to 160	70 to 95
Toddler: 1 to 3 years	24 to 40	90 to 150	80 to 100
Preschool-Age: 3 to 6 years	22 to 34	80 to 140	80 to 100
School-Age: 6 to 12 years	18 to 30	70 to 120	80 to 110
Adolescent: 12 to 18 years	12 to 16	60 to 100	90 to 110
Older than 18 years	12 to 20	60 to 100	90 to 140

PULSE. Pulses may be difficult to feel if they are very weak, very fast, or slow (▶ **Figure 30-17**). In infants, feel over the brachial area or in the femoral area. In older children, use the carotid artery. Count the pulse for at least 1 minute. Note the strength of the pulse: is it weak or strong?

BLOOD PRESSURE. Measuring a child's blood pressure in the field can be tricky. To get an accurate reading, you must have a cuff that covers two thirds of the patient's upper arm (▼ **Figure 30-18**). If conditions at the scene make it impossible to measure blood pressure accurately, do not waste a lot of time trying. For patients 3 years of age or younger, technical difficulties reduce the value of a blood pressure in the field. Consider the effects a cold environment has on the skin, as this can change your findings.

SKIN SIGNS. Feel the skin for temperature and moisture at the same time that you measure the other vital

signs. Is the skin warm and dry, or cold and clammy? Estimate capillary refill by squeezing the end of a finger or toe for several seconds and then observing the return of blood to the area (▼ **Figure 30-19**). Color should return in less than 2 seconds after you let go. Again, capillary refill is decreased in cold weather.

Specific Respiratory Emergencies

In the early stages of respiratory distress or failure, respirations may be too slow or too fast for the patient's age. This suggests that gases are not moving effectively

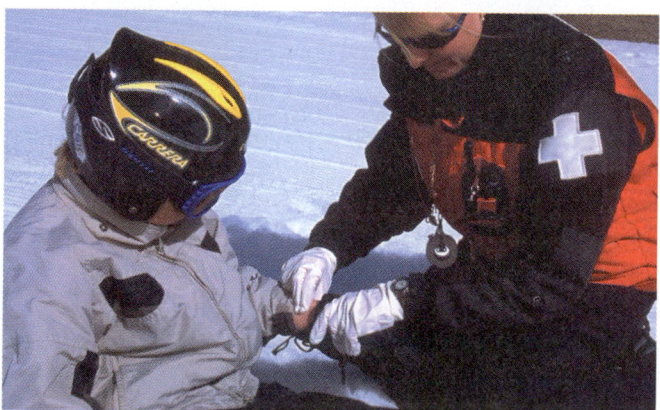

Figure 30-16 Always take vital signs in the field. Begin by talking to the child, then assess respirations and pulse.

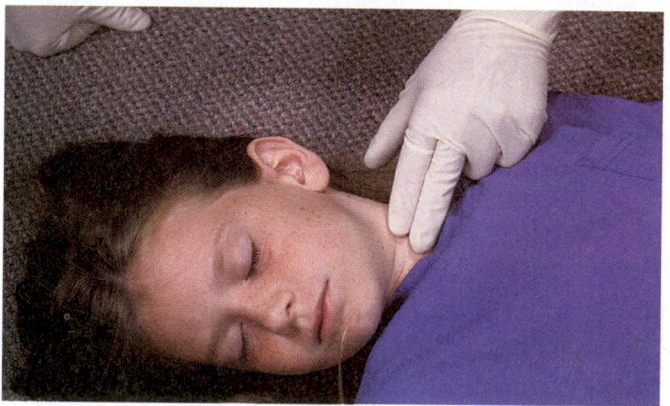

Figure 30-17 In older children, palpate over the carotid artery to assess the pulse.

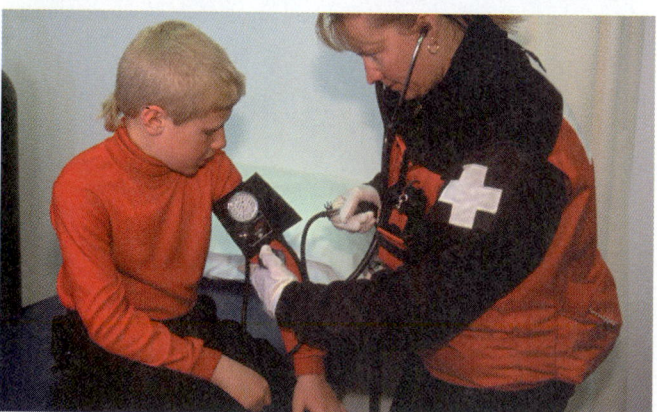

Figure 30-18 When measuring a child's blood pressure, use the proper size cuff, which should cover two thirds of the patient's upper arm.

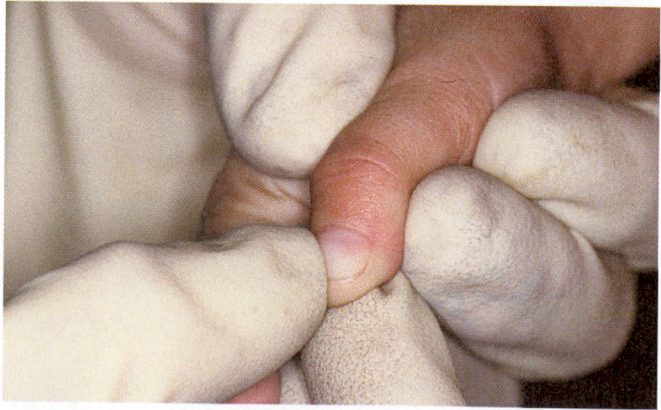

Figure 30-19 Estimate capillary refill by squeezing the end of a finger or toe for several seconds until the fingertip blanches. Normal color should return within 2 seconds after you let go.

into and out of the lungs. If, like most people, you find it hard to memorize normal vital sign ranges for infants and children, keep reference charts handy for this purpose. Respirations of greater than 60 breaths/min are a sign of a problem. In most cases, you should begin to assist ventilation immediately, even if the child appears to be breathing adequately. But remember, you are treating the child, not the numbers. A child breathing 60 breaths/min who is playing happily does not need assisted ventilation; a child breathing 60 breaths/min who is lying unconscious on the floor does.

Signs and Symptoms

In the early stages of respiratory distress, you may note changes in the child's behavior, such as combativeness, restlessness, and anxiety. As the body attempts to maximize the amount of air going into the lungs, the work of breathing (WOB) increases. Signs and symptoms of increased WOB include the following:

- Nasal flaring, as the body tries to increase the size of the airway

- Grunting respirations, as the body attempts to keep the alveoli expanded at the end of expiration

- Wheezing, stridor, or other abnormal airway sounds

- Accessory (intercostal) muscle use; remember that in young children, the diaphragm is the major muscle of ventilation

- Retractions, or movements of the child's flexible rib cage

- The **tripod position** (► **Figure 30-20**); in older children this position will maximize their airway.

As the child progresses to possible respiratory failure, efforts to breathe decrease; the chest rises less with inspiration. A definite diagnosis of respiratory failure is made in the hospital. The body has used up its available energy stores and cannot continue to support the extra WOB under these conditions. At this point, cyanosis, which is a late sign, may develop. Be aware that not all children become cyanotic. You should be just as concerned about a child with pale skin as one with bluish skin.

Changes in behavior will also occur until the child demonstrates an altered level of consciousness. The patient may experience periods of **apnea** (absence of breathing). As the lack of oxygen becomes more serious, the heart muscle itself becomes hypoxic and

slows down. This leads to **bradycardia**, a condition in which the heart rate is less than 60 beats/min in children or less than 80 beats/min in newborns. Bradycardia is almost always related to a lack of oxygen and is an ominous sign in pediatric patients. If the heart rate is fast, you need to investigate the cause. However, if the heart rate is slow or absent, you must intervene immediately. Without aggressive airway management, bradycardia may quickly progress to cardiopulmonary arrest.

Of course, respiratory failure does not always indicate airway obstruction. It may indicate trauma, problems with the nervous system, dehydration (often caused by vomiting and diarrhea), or metabolic disturbances. For example, a child with diabetes might have a blood glucose level that is too high or too low; a child might have a pH imbalance, as can happen with some rare childhood diseases. Regardless of the cause, your first step is always to focus on ensuring adequate oxygenation and ventilation.

Never forget that a child can progress from respiratory distress to respiratory failure at any time. For this reason, you must reassess the child frequently.

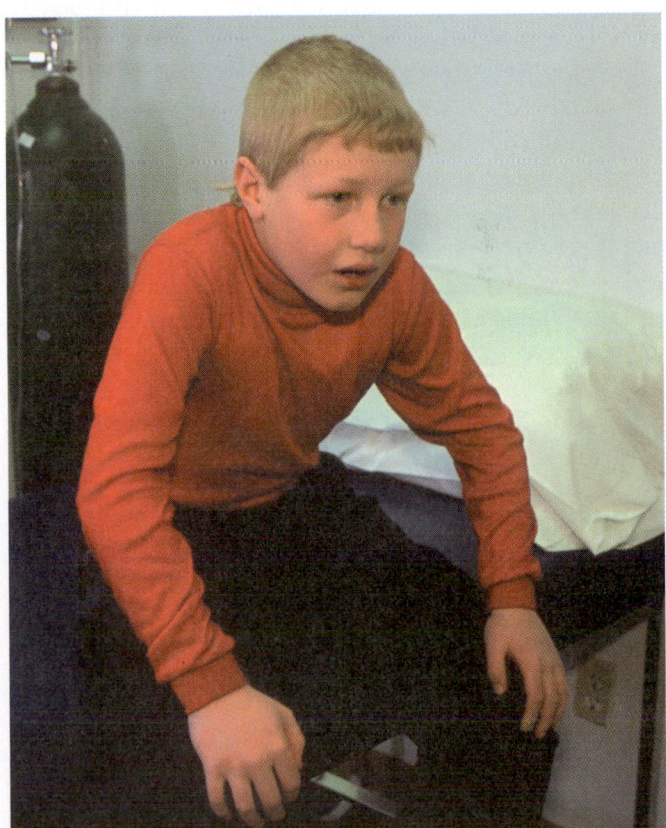

Figure 30-20 The tripod position in older children will maximize their airway.

Croup

Croup, a viral infection of the respiratory tract, is responsible for 90% of stridor noted in pediatric patients and is most common in children age 1 to 3 years. The illness usually begins as an upper respiratory tract infection that is followed by hoarseness, a characteristic barking cough, and a low-grade fever.

Croup almost always responds to hydration (administering fluids by mouth) and by inhaling cool mist generated by a nebulizer. If the patient's condition fails to improve or stridor develops, an evaluation by a physician is necessary.

Epiglottitis

Epiglottitis, a potentially life-threatening infection, is most commonly caused by Haemophilus influenzae and generally affects patients age 18 months to 7 years. It has been seen much less frequently since the HIG vaccine was developed in 1985. The onset is acute, causing fever, difficulty swallowing, a muffled voice, progressive stridor, and increasing respiratory distress. The patient usually sits upright, possibly in the tripod position, breathes through the mouth, and may drool. A patient with epiglottitis has a higher fever and looks more ill than a patient with croup does.

Epiglottitis is a pediatric emergency that can be rapidly fatal because, without treatment, it may quickly progress to complete airway obstruction. During assessment, do not look in the patient's mouth, put a tongue blade in the mouth, or gag the patient—any of which might precipitate airway obstruction. Give all patients with stridor high-flow oxygen unless it frightens them and they fight it, and immediately transport them to medical care.

Asthma

Asthma is common in children and may be evident as early as during the first few weeks of life. Upper respiratory tract infections, allergen exposure, exercise, and cold air may precipitate asthma attacks, and in infants and young children, asthma attacks may occur without wheezing and be mistaken for attacks of bronchitis.

The emergency care of a pediatric patient who is having an acute asthma attack includes high-flow oxygen using a nonrebreathing mask, and rapid transport. If the child's inhaler is available, allow self-administration—usually under the direction of the parent or caregiver—of the appropriate number of "puffs." In rare cases, the child's parent may have an Epi-Pen, and self-administration (or administration by a parent) is appropriate.

Bronchiolitis, Bronchitis, and Pneumonia

Bronchiolitis is an infection, usually viral, of the smaller air passages of the lung. It resembles asthma and is most common in patients younger than 2 years. Signs and symptoms include respiratory distress, wheezing, and cough.

Bronchitis is an infection of the large and small air passages, and pneumonia is an infection of the alveoli (the smallest air sacs of the lungs) and the spaces between them. Bronchitis and pneumonia are common lung infections that can occur at any age and are caused by either viruses or bacteria. Signs and symptoms include fever, respiratory distress, and cough.

In very young infants, the first sign of these three diseases may be complete cessation of breathing (apnea).

Emergency care of all three diseases includes administering high-flow oxygen, suctioning the nostrils as

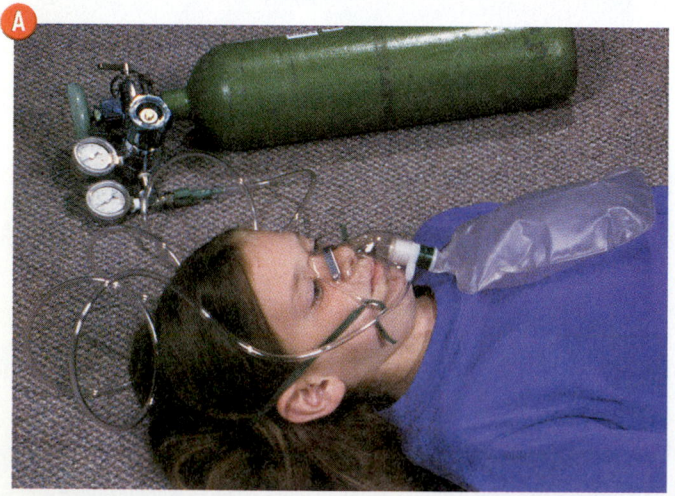
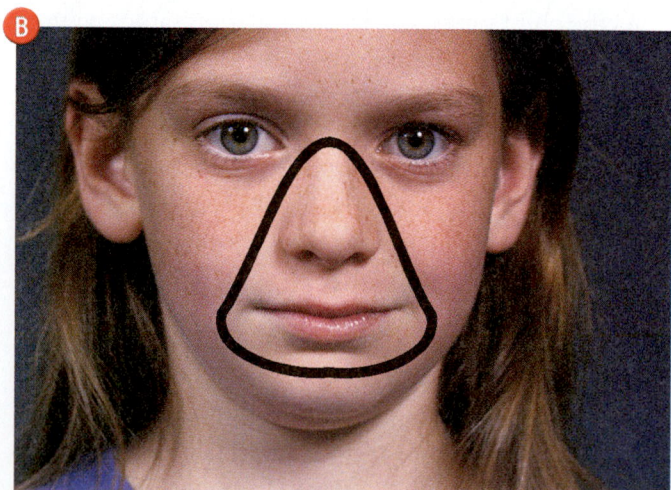

Figure 30-21 **A.** Use a properly fitting nonrebreathing mask to deliver supplemental oxygen. **B.** Area covered on a child's face with a properly fitting mask.

needed, supporting breathing as necessary, and immediately transporting the patient to medical care.

Emergency Medical Care

A child or infant in respiratory distress or possible respiratory failure needs supplemental oxygen. Remember, anxiety, agitation, or crying may increase the effort or work of breathing, so use whichever method seems least upsetting to the child: mask, blow-by, or nasal cannula (◄ Figure 30-21). You may need to get creative by distracting the child with games, a toy, or talking.

Allow the child to remain in a comfortable position. For a small child, this may mean sitting on the caregiver's lap. Give nothing by mouth, in case the child's condition deteriorates suddenly.

If the patient has progressed to respiratory failure, you must begin assisted ventilation immediately and continue to provide supplemental oxygen.

Other Emergencies

The reasons for cardiopulmonary arrest differ in children and adults. In adults, cardiac arrest is usually the result of an abnormal cardiac rhythm, which is itself caused by underlying cardiac disease. Because most children have healthy hearts, sudden cardiac arrest is rare. More commonly, children have cardiopulmonary arrest because of respiratory or circulatory failure from illness or injury. For this reason, the airway and breathing are the focus of pediatric basic life support (BLS) (▼ Table 30-3).

The procedure for performing infant chest compressions is shown in (► Figure 30-22).

Respiratory problems leading to cardiopulmonary arrest in children can have a number of different causes, including the following:

- Injury, both blunt and penetrating
- Infections of the respiratory tract or another organ system
- A foreign body in the airway
- Near drowning
- Electrocution
- Poisoning or drug overdose
- Sudden infant death syndrome (SIDS)

TABLE 30-3 Review of Pediatric BLS

Action	Infants Younger Than 1 Year	Children Between Age 1 and 8 Years
Airway	Head tilt-chin lift; jaw-thrust if spine injury is suspected	Head tilt-chin lift; jaw-thrust if spine injury is suspected
Breathing		
Initial	2 breaths at a rate of 1 to 1½ seconds/breath (Use a BVM device with oxygen connected if available.)	2 breaths at a rate of 1 to 1½ seconds/breath (Use a BVM device with oxygen connected if available.)
Subsequent	20 breaths/min	20 breaths/min
Circulation		
Pulse check	Brachial/femoral arteries	Carotid artery
Compression area	Lower half of sternum	Lower half of sternum
Compression width	2 or 3 fingers or 2 thumb encircled hands	Heel of hand
Compression depth	½" to 1"	1" to 1½"
Compression rate	At least 100/min	100/min
Ratio of Compressions to Ventilations	5:1 (pause for ventilation)	5:1 (pause for ventilation)
Foreign Body Obstruction	Back blows and chest thrusts	Abdominal thrusts

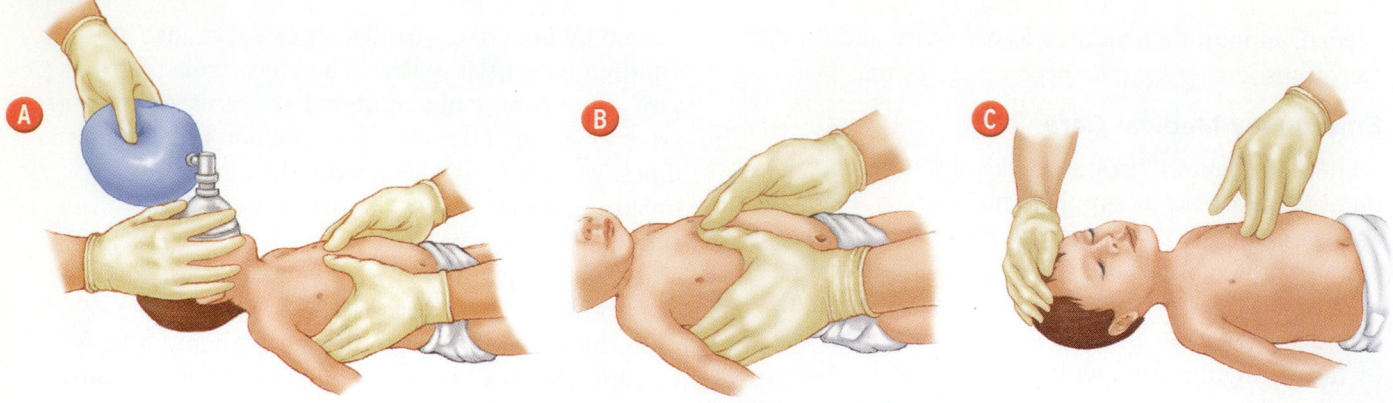

Figure 30-22 **A.** Chest compressions should be given with the hands encircling the infant and thumbs side by side. **B.** In very small infants, you may need to overlap the thumbs. **C.** In larger infants, you may use the two-finger technique, using the middle and ring fingers.

Seizures

A seizure is the result of disorganized electrical activity in the brain. It can be very frightening to people around the patient. Therefore, it is important to reassure the family and to approach assessment and management in a calm, step-by-step manner.

SIGNS AND SYMPTOMS. Seizures in children may appear in several different ways, including shaking of the whole body or movement in just a single arm or leg. Seizures can also appear as lip smacking, eyes blinking, or staring off into space. In a true seizure, movements cannot be stopped on command or by holding an extremity. The duration of movement varies from patient to patient.

There are several general categories of seizures. In the course of an epileptic episode, a patient may experience one or more of these types of seizures:

- **Generalized (grand mal) seizures** appear as back-and-forth motions of both upper and lower extremities. The patient is unresponsive to verbal commands or painful stimulation.

- **Partial seizures** may appear as movement in one limb, lip smacking, or eye deviation only (eyes turned to either side or up or down).

- **Absence (petit mal) seizures** appear as an unresponsiveness with or without any movement and may last seconds to minutes.

Altered mental status and the inability of others to stop a movement or range of movements in the affected limb are common to all seizures. Some patients may feel pins and needles, hear sounds, and see hallucinations. In all but absence seizures, there is a **postictal period** of extreme fatigue or unresponsiveness after the seizure for anywhere from a few minutes to several hours. During this time, the patient may appear sleepy and/or confused and is not able to interact appropriately. A short period of seizure activity (less than 30 minutes) is not in itself harmful to the patient. After 30 to 45 minutes, however, the brain may run low on energy stores, and continued activity can be harmful. **Status epilepticus** is a continuous seizure, or multiple seizures without a return to consciousness, for 30 minutes or more.

If you can identify the cause of the seizure, you will be better able to monitor the patient for any potential complications associated with the underlying problem ▼ **Table 30-4** . In particular, be alert to the presence of

TABLE 30-4 Common Causes of Seizures

- Electrolyte imbalance
- Fever
- Hypoglycemia (low blood glucose level)
- Idiopathic (no cause can be found)
- Infection
- Ingestion
- Lack of oxygen
- Medications
- Poisoning
- Previous seizure disorder
- Recreational drug use
- Trauma
- Child abuse

medications, possible poisons, and indications of abuse or neglect.

FEBRILE SEIZURES. Febrile seizures are common in children between the ages of 6 months and 6 years. Most pediatric seizures are due to fever alone, which is why they are called febrile seizures. These seizures typically occur on the first day of a febrile illness, are characterized by generalized tonic-clonic seizure activity, and last less than 15 minutes with a short postictal phase or none at all. They may be a sign of a more serious problem, such as meningitis. Obtain a history from the caregivers, as these children may have had a prior febrile seizure.

If you are called to care for a child who has had a febrile seizure, you often will find that the patient is awake, alert, and fully interactive when you arrive. Keep in mind that a persistent fever can lead to another seizure. Carefully assess the ABCs, begin cooling measures with tepid water (not cold), and provide prompt transport; all children with febrile seizures need to be seen in the hospital setting (▼ **Figure 30-23**).

EMERGENCY MEDICAL CARE. Although medical management of seizures in the hospital setting may vary according to cause, your assessment and management of these patients remain essentially the same from patient to patient. First, ensure that the scene is safe for you and

for the patient. Next, perform an initial assessment, focusing on the ABCs. If possible, obtain a brief history from the caregivers about previous serious illnesses or seizures and current medication or trauma.

Securing and protecting the airway are your priorities. To avoid obstruction from the tongue falling back into the airway, place a child who is having a seizure or who is postictal in the recovery position if you can do so without having to use extreme force against the seizure activity (▼ **Figure 30-24**). In the case of trauma, place the head in a neutral in-line position and ensure that the cervical spine is protected with spinal precautions. Be ready to use suction to prevent aspiration of stomach contents, blood, or vomitus. Do not place your fingers in the mouth of a patient who is having a seizure.

A patient who is having a seizure or is in a postictal period may not be breathing adequately. Assessing the rate and depth of respirations in this situation can be difficult but is essential. Patients may have shallow, rapid breathing or may have occasional deep respirations. Signs that a patient is not breathing adequately include the following:

- Very slow respirations
- Very shallow breaths
- Bluish tint to lips or pale lips
- Snoring respirations caused by the tongue blocking the airway

Deliver oxygen by mask or nasal cannula. If there are no signs of improvement, begin BVM ventilation with appropriately sized equipment.

Patients who are experiencing a seizure usually maintain adequate blood pressure and pulse rate

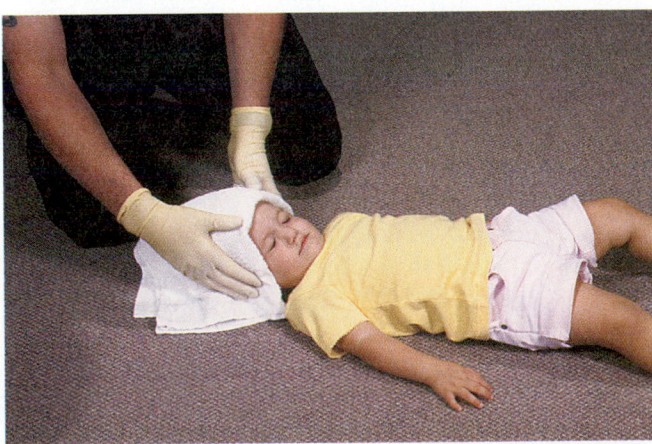

Figure 30-23 Following a febrile seizure, carefully assess the child's ABCs. Then begin cooling measures, and prepare the child for transport.

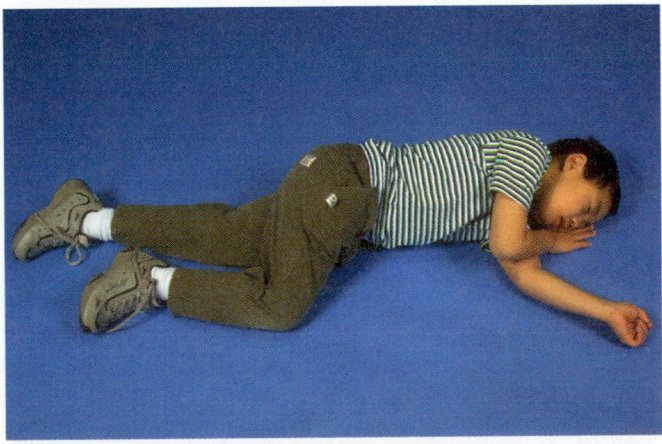

Figure 30-24 A child in the postictal state following a seizure should be placed in the recovery position.

unless the seizure is caused by an underlying circulatory or neurologic problem or trauma, including bleeding, heart problems, or brain injury. Nevertheless, you must evaluate the pulse and blood pressure and reevaluate them. Once the ABCs have been addressed, assessment and management should proceed as follows. If the patient is having an active seizure, note the type of movement and position of the eyes, as this information may be very helpful for hospital staff in making a diagnosis. If there is a fever, begin cooling measures such as removing clothing and placing towels moistened with tepid water on the child. A child with febrile seizures can have another seizure if the body temperature remains high. Do not use alcohol or cold water to cool a patient. Make sure the patient is protected from hitting the sides of the stretcher or nearby equipment. Give any medications or possible poisons at the scene to the EMS team during transfer.

Altered Level of Consciousness

People who are aware of themselves and their surroundings are said to be conscious. Nonverbal infants may demonstrate consciousness by following a person's face or an object (tracking), by babbling and cooing, or by crying. Infants and children may exhibit an **altered level of consciousness** (also called altered mental status) in many ways, including lack of response to vocal commands and pain, combative behavior, confusion, thrashing about, drifting into and out of an alert state, or a change in the pitch and nature of their cry.

Common causes of altered level of consciousness in a pediatric patient can be found in the mnemonic AEIOU-TIPS:

- **A**lcohol
- **E**pilepsy, endocrine, or electrolyte abnormalities
- **I**nsulin or low blood glucose levels
- **O**piates or other drugs
- **U**remia
- **T**rauma or temperature
- **I**nfection
- **P**sychogenic or poison
- **S**hock, stroke, or shunt obstruction

Your first step in caring for a patient with an altered level of consciousness is to assess the ABCs and provide appropriate care as necessary. As you determine responsiveness, remember to use the AVPU scale. Then obtain a brief history from the patient's caregivers, focusing on the following points:

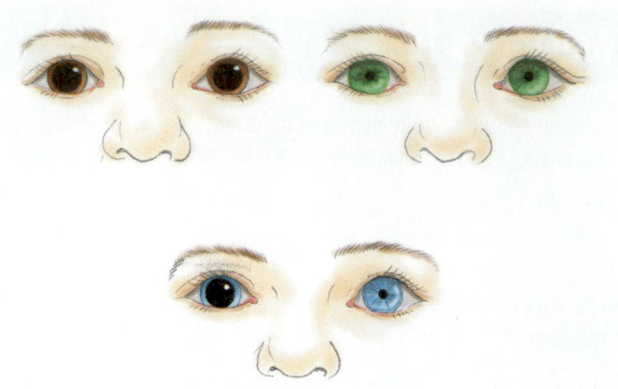

Figure 30-25 Observe a child's eyes for changes in pupillary size.

- Does the patient have any illnesses?
- Does the patient take any medications? When was the last dose?
- Did the patient ingest any substances (eg, poisons, drugs, or plant material)?
- Has the patient been ill?
- Has the patient had any behavior problems?

Next, observe the patient's pupils: Are they dilated or pinpoint? Do they react to a light by constricting ▲ **Figure 30-25** ? Are the eyes turned to the right, left, up, or down? Is the patient staring without moving his or her eyes? Is the patient posturing ▶ **Figure 30-26** ?

Once you have completed your initial assessment, immediately secure the airway. If respirations are inadequate, provide assisted ventilation with a BVM device. If you suspect trauma, log roll the child onto a backboard, and apply a cervical collar. Give supplemental oxygen by mask or nasal cannula. If the child is having an active seizure, follow the care described earlier in this chapter on seizures. Remember to call for ALS backup as necessary. No matter what the cause, you should support the patient's vital functions and provide prompt transport.

Poisoning

Poisoning is common among children. It can occur by ingesting, inhaling, injecting, or absorbing a toxic substance ▶ **Figure 30-27** . The signs and symptoms of poisoning vary widely, depending on the substance and the age and weight of the child ▶ **Table 30-5** . The child may appear normal at first, even in serious cases, or he or she may be confused, sleepy, or unconscious.

Infants may be poisoned as a result of being fed a harmful substance by a sibling or a caregiver or as a result of child abuse. Infants can be exposed to drugs

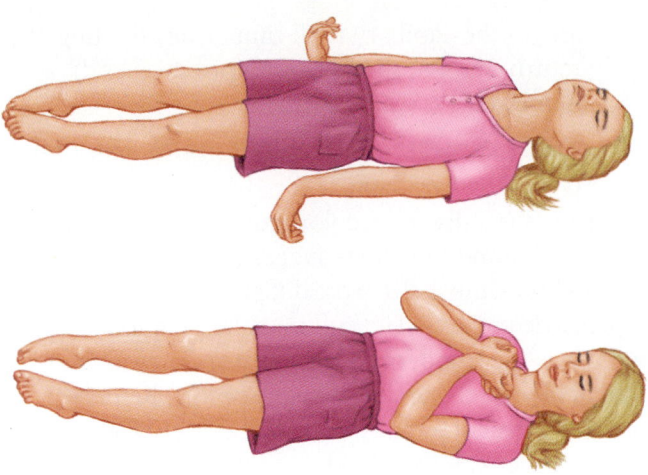

Figure 30-26 Observe a child for posturing.

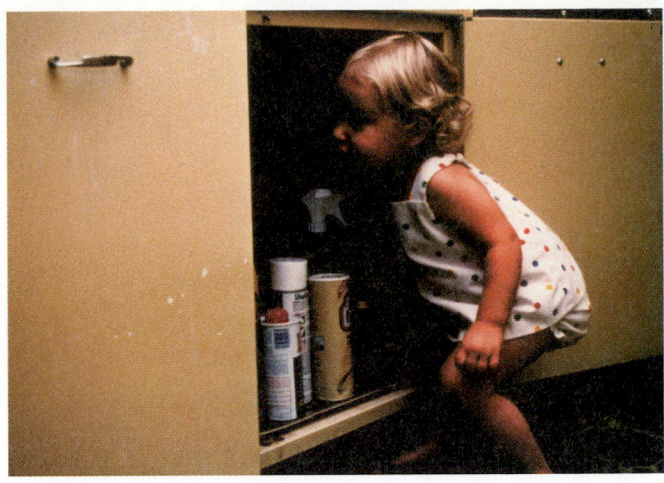

Figure 30-27 A curious child will try to taste or swallow almost any substance. A common victim of accidental ingestion of dangerous compounds is the unsupervised toddler.

and poisons left on floors and carpeting. They can also be exposed in a room or automobile in which harmful drugs, such as crack, cocaine, or PCP, are being smoked. Toddlers are curious and often ingest poisons when they find them in the home or garage. For example, some people store petroleum products in soda bottles. Toddlers may believe the substance to be soda. Adolescents are more likely to have ingested alcohol and street drugs while "partying" or in a suicide attempt.

After you have completed your initial assessment and have notified EMS, you should ask the caregiver the following questions:

- What is the substance(s) involved?

- Approximately how much of the substance was ingested or involved in the exposure (eg, number of pills, amount of liquid)?

- What time did the incident occur?

- Are there any changes in behavior or level of consciousness?

- Was there any choking or coughing after the exposure? (These can be signs of airway involvement.)

Because a child's level of consciousness may be affected by the poison, your care will be guided by how awake and alert the child appears. For a child who is responsive, your protocols may dictate that you contact medical control and your local poison control center to report the situation. Focus on the ABCs, keeping in mind that the child's condition may change over time. Assess the patient's level of consciousness, and support the vital functions as necessary, including giving supplemental

oxygen. If the patient is combative and/or agitated, protect yourself from injury. Do not administer syrup of ipecac (if this is still used in your system) unless directed to do so by medical control. Call for an ALS transport if the patient's condition becomes unstable. As you prepare the patient for transport, try to find the container that held the suspected poison, collect any vomitus from the child and place it in a plastic bag, and give both to EMS personnel and take to the emergency department.

If the child is unresponsive, make sure that you focus immediately on the ABCs, and be prepared to provide artificial ventilation if necessary. Give supplemental oxygen, and then call medical control to report the situation. Arrange for prompt transport to the emergency department, keeping in mind that the child's condition could change at any time.

TABLE 30-5 Common Sources of Poisoning in Children

- Alcohol
- Aspirin and acetaminophen
- Household cleaning products such as bleach and furniture polish
- Houseplants
- Iron
- Prescription medications of family members
- Street drugs
- Vitamins

Shock

Shock is a condition that develops when the circulatory system is unable to deliver a sufficient amount of blood to the organs of the body. This results in organ failure and eventually cardiopulmonary arrest. In children, shock is rarely due to a primary cardiac event, such as a heart attack. Shock may be due to many things; the most common causes include the following:

- Traumatic injury with blood loss (especially abdominal)
- Dehydration from diarrhea and vomiting
- Severe infection
- Neurologic injury such as severe head trauma
- A severe allergic reaction to an insect bite or allergen (anaphylaxis)
- Diseases of the heart
- A collapsed lung (pneumothorax)
- Blood or fluid around the heart (cardiac tamponade or pericarditis)

Infants and children have less blood circulating in their bodies than adults do, so the loss of even a small volume of fluid or blood may lead to shock. Pediatric patients also respond differently than adults to fluid loss. They may respond by increasing their heart rate, increasing their respirations and showing signs of pale or blue skin. You must be able to recognize the signs of shock in infants and children.

Begin by assessing the ABCs, intervening immediately as required; do not wait until you have completed a detailed assessment to take action. Children in shock often have increased respirations but do not demonstrate a fall in blood pressure until shock is severe.

In assessing circulation, you should pay particular attention to the following:

- **Pulse.** Assess both the rate and the quality of the pulse. A weak, "thready" pulse is a sign that there is a problem. The appropriate rate depends on age; anything greater than 160 beats/min suggests shock.
- **Skin signs.** Assess the temperature and moisture on the hands and feet. How does this compare with the temperature of the skin on the trunk of the body? Is the skin dry and warm, or cold and clammy?
- **Capillary refill.** Squeeze a finger or toe for several seconds until the skin blanches, then release it. The time it takes for the blood to return to the

area is the capillary refill time. Does the fingertip return to its normal color within 2 seconds, or is it delayed?

- **Color.** Assess the patient's skin color. Is it pink, pale, ashen, or blue?

Changes in pulse rate, color, skin signs, and capillary refill are all important clues suggesting shock.

Blood pressure is the most difficult vital sign to take in pediatric patients. The cuff must be the proper size: two thirds the length of the upper arm. The value for normal blood pressure is also age-specific. Remember that blood pressure may be normal; this is called compensated shock. If the blood pressure is low, this is a sign of decompensated shock, a serious condition that requires care that an ALS team can provide.

Part of your assessment should also include talking with the caregivers to determine when the signs and symptoms first appeared and whether any of the following has occurred:

- Decrease in urine output (with infants, are there fewer than 6 to 10 wet diapers?)
- Absence of tears, even when the child is crying
- Changes in level of consciousness and behavior

Shock is a serious condition; limit your care to the following steps:

1. **Ensure that the airway is open.**
2. **Be prepared to provide artificial ventilation** if necessary.
3. **Control bleeding** if present.
4. **Give supplemental oxygen** by mask or nasal cannula as tolerated. Continue to monitor airway and breathing.
5. **Position the patient** with the head lower than the feet by elevating the feet with blankets.
6. **Keep the patient warm** with blankets.
7. **Arrange for immediate transport** to the nearest appropriate facility.
8. **Continue monitoring vital signs.**
9. **Contact ALS** backup as needed.
10. **Make sure that EMS personnel are aware of the presence of a caregiver** so that he or she is able to accompany the child whenever possible.

Be sure to activate EMS early in the process and limit your management to these simple interventions. Time should not be wasted in field procedures. Immediate transport is of utmost importance.

Dehydration

Dehydration occurs when fluid losses are greater than fluid intake. The most common cause of dehydration in children is vomiting and diarrhea. If left untreated, dehydration can lead to shock and eventually death. Infants and children are at greater risk than adults for dehydration because their fluid reserves are smaller than those in adults. Life-threatening dehydration can overcome an infant in a matter of hours. Again, your ability to recognize a child with this condition is a critical part of your job.

Dehydration can be described as mild, moderate, or severe. The severity of the dehydration can be gauged by looking at several clues (▼ **Table 30-6**). For example, an infant with mild dehydration may have dry lips and gums, decreased saliva, and fewer wet diapers throughout the day. As the dehydration grows more severe, the lips and gums may become very dry, the eyes may look sunken, and the infant may be sleepy and/or irritable, refusing bottles. The skin may be loose and have no elasticity (tenting); this is called poor skin turgor (▶ **Figure 30-28**). Also, infants may have sunken fontanels.

Young children can compensate for fluid losses by decreasing blood flow to the extremities and directing it to vital organs such as the brain and heart. Children who are moderately to severely dehydrated may have mottled, cool, clammy skin and delayed capillary refill. Respirations will usually be increased. Be aware that blood pressure may remain normal until the child is in shock.

After activating EMS, emergency medical care should include careful attention assessing the ABCs and obtaining baseline vital signs. However, if the dehydration is severe, ALS backup may be necessary

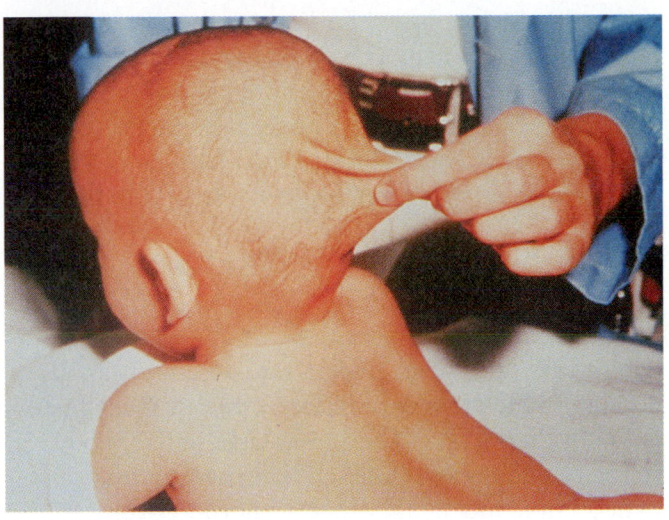

(**Figure 30-28**) An infant with mild dehydration may exhibit "tenting" or poor skin turgor.

TABLE 30-6 Vital Signs and Symptoms of Dehydration

	Mild Dehydration	Moderate Dehydration	Severe Dehydration
Pulse	Normal	Increased	Increased; 160+ is sign of impending shock.
Level of Activity	Normal or slowed	Slowed	Variable, weak to unresponsive
Urine Output	Decreased	Decreased	No output
Skin	Normal	Cool, mottled; poor turgor	Cool, clammy; poor turgor; delayed capillary refill time
Mouth	Saliva may have drooling, bubbles	Dry mucous membranes	Dry mucous membranes
Eyes	Normal	Tears	Sunken eyes
Anterior Fontanel	Normal to sunken	Sunken	Very sunken
Level of Consciousness	Normal	Altered	Altered; lethargic
Blood Pressure	Normal	Normal	Normal to low when shock sets in

so that IV access can be obtained and rehydration can begin. All children with signs and symptoms of moderate to severe dehydration should be transported to the emergency department.

Hyperthermia

Pediatric patients produce more heat for their size than adults and are less effective at regulating their temperature. They also acclimatize more slowly. Because an infant's body temperature rises higher than an older child's does before he or she starts to perspire, avoid overdressing an infant in hot weather. Exertional heat stroke may develop in older children and adolescents.

The principal emergency care measure for this condition is to rapidly cool the patient by whatever means are available and arrange for immediate transport to medical care.

Hypothermia

Pediatric patients—especially newborns and premature babies with little subcutaneous fat—lose heat rapidly because of their large heads, lower proportions of body fat, poor thermal regulation, and large ratio of body surface area to mass. Older children also become hypothermic much faster than adults do.

To prevent hypothermia, it is important to dress the child properly in cold weather (especially by providing a warm hat) and keep him or her dry. Moreover, it is crucial that you pay close attention to insulating and warming an injured or ill pediatric patient in a cold environment. Put a blanket under and over the patient who is lying on the snow.

The emergency care of the pediatric population for drowning, seizures, hypothermia, and hyperthermia is the same as that for an adult and is found in other parts of this book.

Severe Infection (Sepsis)

An infant or child with sepsis looks ill, is usually either irritable or lethargic, and may fail to recognize his or her parents. The patient's skin is commonly pale, ashen, or cyanotic, and may be hot or cool. Capillary refill may be abnormal and the blood pressure low; the heart and respiratory rates are usually high until the patient is terminal, when they fall.

There is almost always a history of an upper respiratory tract infection, fever, vomiting, diarrhea, lethargy, irritability, or feeding problems. Ask whether the child was recently exposed to sick people. It is important to take the patient's temperature, which is usually high but may also be lower than normal.

A patient with sepsis should be given high-flow oxygen and transported immediately to medical care. Do not attempt to cool a patient with sepsis, but remove any excess layers of clothing.

Sports Activities

Children, especially those who are older or adolescents, are often injured in organized sports activities. Head and neck injuries can occur after high-speed collisions in contact sports such as skiing, snowboarding, roller blading, skateboarding, bicycling, football, wrestling, ice hockey, field hockey, soccer, or lacrosse. Remember to immobilize the cervical spine when caring for children with sports-related injuries. You should also be familiar with your local protocols related to helmet removal.

Injuries to Specific Body Systems
Head Injuries

Head injuries are common in children. This is due, in part, to the fact that the size of a child's head, in relation to the body, is larger than that of an adult. The signs and symptoms of head injury in a child are similar to those in an adult, but there are some important differences. Nausea and vomiting are common signs and symptoms of head injury in children; however, it is easy to mistake these for an abdominal injury or illness. You should suspect a serious head injury in any child who experiences nausea and vomiting after a traumatic event.

Your single most important step in caring for a child with a head injury is to ensure that the airway is open. Whenever you suspect trauma, you should immobilize the cervical spine and use the jaw-thrust maneuver to open the airway, as the child's tongue may have relaxed back into the throat, blocking the airway. As you immobilize the child onto a backboard, avoid using sandbags to immobilize the head (▼ **Figure 30-29**). If the child begins to vomit and the board has to be turned to the

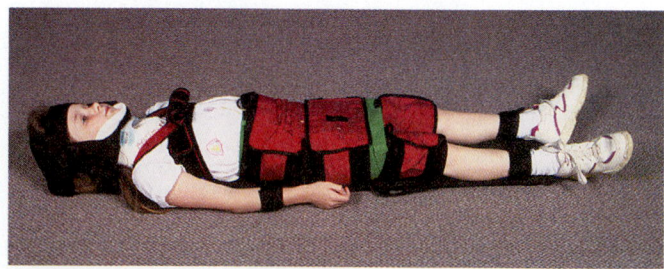

Figure 30-29 Use a proper pediatric immobilization device rather than sandbags to immobilize a child's head. If you need to turn the board to the side in the event of vomiting, sandbags could shift and cause further injury.

side, the weight of the sandbags on the head could cause additional injury. <u>Hyperventilation</u> (rapid ventilation) of the child with a head injury should not be attempted until normal ventilations have been established with a bag-valve-mask device for several minutes.

Respiratory arrest can also occur as a result of head injuries in children. You should be prepared to assist ventilations or provide rescue breaths in any child who has evidence of severe head injury.

Chest Injuries

Chest injuries in children are usually the result of blunt trauma rather than penetrating objects. Remember that children have very soft, flexible ribs that can be compressed a great deal without breaking. Keep this in mind as you assess a child who has sustained high-energy blunt trauma to the chest. Even though there may be no external sign of injury, such as broken ribs, contusions, or bleeding, there may be significant injuries within the chest.

Abdominal Injuries

Abdominal injuries are very common in children. Remember, though, that children can compensate for significant blood loss better than adults without signs or symptoms of shock developing. They can also have a serious injury without early external evidence of a problem. All children with abdominal injuries should be monitored for signs and symptoms of shock, including a weak, rapid pulse; cold, clammy skin; decreased capillary refill (an early sign); confusion, and decreased systolic blood pressure (a late sign). Even in the absence of signs and symptoms of shock, or with only very few signs and symptoms, you should remain cautious about the possibility of internal injuries.

Children can lose a greater proportion of their blood volume than adults can before signs or symptoms of shock develop. What makes this situation dangerous is that infants and children have less blood circulating in their bodies than adults do, so the loss of even a small volume of fluid or blood may lead to shock ▼ **Figure 30-30**.

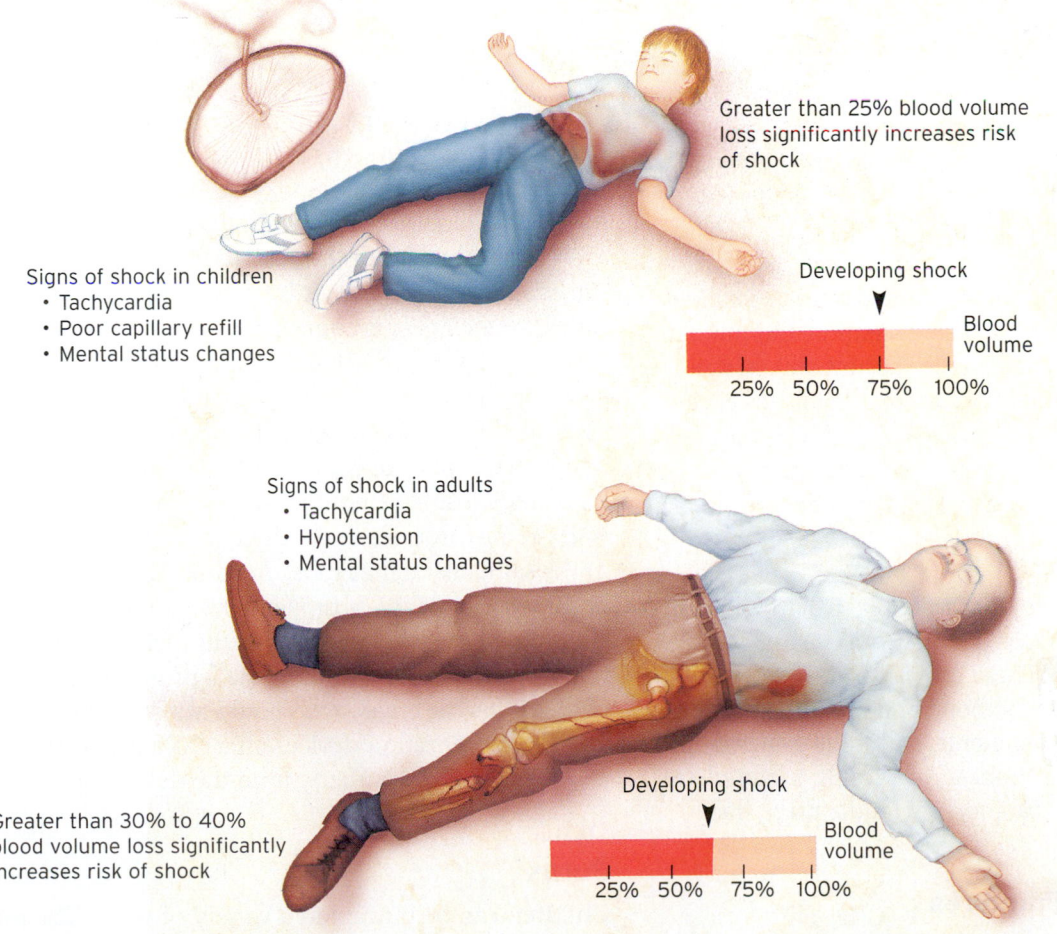

Figure 30-30 Children can lose a greater proportion of their blood volume than adults can before signs or symptoms of shock develop.

Greater than 25% blood volume loss significantly increases the risk of shock in children.

Signs of shock in children include the following:

- tachycardia
- poor capillary refill
- mental status changes

Signs of shock in adults include the following:

- tachycardia
- hypotension
- mental status changes

Greater than 30% to 40% blood volume loss significantly increases risk of shock in adults.

You should always suspect hidden internal injuries in children after a high-energy trauma. One of the problems associated with abdominal injuries in children is the presence of air in the stomach. Children, especially those who have had a traumatic injury, tend to swallow air. Air in the stomach can cause distention and interfere with your assessment. Air can also accumulate in the stomach with artificial ventilation, making it less effective. This is one of the reasons to use the jaw-thrust maneuver to position the airway, as it decreases the amount of air accumulating in the stomach.

Injuries of the Extremities

Children have immature bones with active growth centers. Growth of long bones occurs from the ends at specialized growth plates. These growth plates are potential weak spots in the bone and are often injured as a result of trauma. In general, children's bones bend more easily than adults' bones. As a result, incomplete or greenstick fractures can occur. Handle these fractures with care.

Specific Common Fractures

The clavicle is the most commonly fractured bone in the pediatric population. Children rarely dislocate a shoulder or separate the acromioclavicular (AC) joint in the shoulder until they become teenagers.

In the arm, wrist fractures are common and can be severely displaced causing neurologic or vascular compromise. Also common are midshaft forearm fractures that may be grossly angulated, and difficult to splint straight. Generally, the rescuer should splint deformed limbs in children as they are found. The exception to this is if there is no pulse distally: one attempt at anatomic realignment is allowed. The rescuer should palpate the extremity where the pulse is located, slowly straighten the extremity, and stop when the pulse returns (even if some deformity is still present), and splint in that position.

Elbow fractures in the pediatric population are common and usually true emergencies. Rapid transport after splinting is recommended. The brachial artery can be damaged easily in children, and large nerves cross the elbow close to the bone. Splint as found if a pulse is present, as moving the arm could damage the brachial artery. If no pulse is present and the transport time to definitive medical care is more than 1 hour, try to gently anatomically realign the arm once; and, if there is still no pulse, splint and make sure the child is transported. Time is very important in pulseless children's extremities ▶ **Figure 30-31**.

Femur and tibia fractures occur with less force in children. Older children's fractures may displace, while toddlers and preschoolers may be "bent" (greenstick fracture). Ankle fractures are less common in children than adults, but when they occur, they are usually on the outside of the ankle. A fracture of the central bone (talus) of the ankle is commonly seen in children who snowboard when they land flat after jumping. The ankle hurts on the outside. Treat femur, tibia, and ankle fractures in children as you would in an adult, with an appropriate splint or stabilization device. This reduces bleeding, most importantly, and also reduces pain.

Extremity injuries in children are generally managed in the same manner as those in adults. Painful deformed limbs with evidence of broken bones should be splinted. Specialized splinting equipment, such as a traction splint for fractures of the femur, should be used only if it fits the child. You should not attempt to use adult immobilization devices on a child unless the child is large enough to properly fit in the device.

Other Considerations
Burns

Children can be burned in a variety of ways. The most common involve exposure to hot substances such as scalding water in a bathtub, hot items on a stove, or

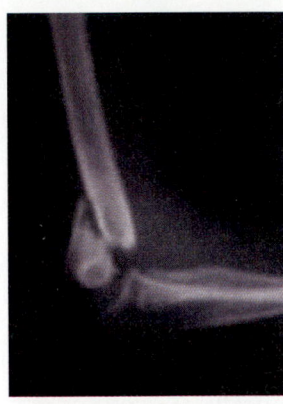

Figure 30-31 Supracondylar elbow fracture in a pediatric patient. This injury is a true emergency when distal circulation and nerve function is impaired.

TABLE 30-7 Severity of Burns in Children	
Severity of Burn	**Body Area Involved**
Minor	Partial-thickness burns involving less than 10% of the body surface
Moderate	Partial-thickness burns involving 10% to 20% of the body surface
Critical	Any full-thickness burn
	Any partial-thickness burn involving more than 20% of the body surface
	Any burn involving the hands, feet, face, airway, or genitalia

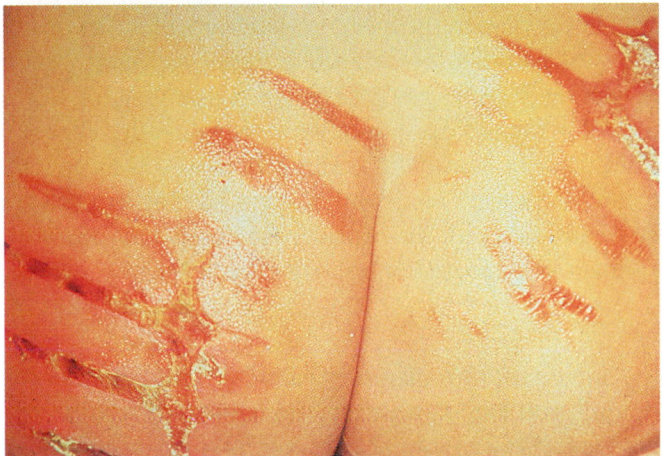

Figure 30-32 The most common burns in children involve exposure to hot surfaces. This child's buttocks were placed against a hot heating grate.

exposure to caustic substances such as cleaning solvents or paint thinners ▲ **Figure 30-32** . You should suspect possible internal injuries from chemical ingestion when you see a child who has burns, particularly around the face and mouth.

One common problem following burn injuries in children is infection. Burned skin cannot resist infection as effectively as normal skin can. For this reason, sterile techniques should be used in handling the skin of children with burn wounds.

As when you are caring for adults, you should first remove all clothing from the burned skin as part of a complete exposure of the patient. Leaving charred clothing in place prevents you from clearly assessing the patient. In addition, the clothing may still be hot and continue to burn the underlying skin if it is not removed. After chemical burns, it is particularly important to remove the clothing rapidly, since chemical materials that are retained within the clothing may also cause damage to the underlying skin. After the skin has been

exposed, you should place dry, sterile dressings on the skin as soon as possible to decrease the risk of infection.

You must learn your local protocols regarding the immediate referral of children to burn centers. ▲ **Table 30-7** provides some general guidelines to follow in assessing a child who has been burned. These guidelines may help you to determine which children should be treated primarily at specialized burn centers. Also note that you should consider the possibility of child abuse in any burn situation. Make sure you report any information about your suspicions to EMS personnel so they can notify hospital staff.

Submersion Injury

Submersion injuries include near drowning and drowning. In submersion situations, you must always take steps to ensure your own safety when retrieving the patient from the water.

Drowning is the second most common cause of unintentional death among children in the United States; children younger than age 5 years are at particular risk. At this age, children often fall into swimming pools and lakes, but many drown in bathtubs and even buckets. Older adolescents, who account for the most drownings after toddlers, drown when swimming or boating; alcohol is frequently a factor.

The principal injury from submersion is lack of oxygen. Even a few minutes (or less) without oxygen affect the heart, lungs, and brain, causing life-threatening

Wilderness Tips

Painful musculoskeletal injuries are a potential complication of wilderness activities. Pain medication for children should be included in the medical kit (see Appendix C).

problems such as cardiac arrest, respiratory difficulty, and coma. Submersion in icy water can rob the body of heat, causing hypothermia. While a very few, very cold victims of submersion hypothermia have survived long periods in cardiac arrest in icy water, most people in this situation die. Diving into the water, of course, increases the risk of neck and spinal cord injuries.

Assessment and reassessment of the ABCs are critical in submersion injuries. First assess breathing and pulse, because the patient may be in cardiac or respiratory arrest. Immediately check breathing effort, skin color, and capillary refill in addition to vital signs. Always immobilize the cervical spine of patients who were diving. Lung injuries may progress, causing breathing difficulty over time, so be sure to reassess the patient frequently while waiting for the ambulance to arrive.

If you cannot effectively ventilate the patient, consider the possibility of a foreign body airway obstruction; water alone does not obstruct the airway. If you can see the object, be sure to use removal techniques that are appropriate to the patient's age.

If it is within your scope of practice, consider using a nasogastric tube to protect the airway in unresponsive patients, as they will usually vomit. Always have a suction device ready in case of vomiting or water in the airway.

Remove wet clothing so that the patient does not get colder. Keep the patient warm and monitor vital functions during transport.

A child may appear completely normal after being submersed, and then problems may develop minutes or hours later. This is called secondary drowning and happens when the lungs are filled with fluid from within the lung (pulmonary edema).

Emergency Care of the Injured Pediatric Patient

Emergency care of the injured pediatric patient includes administering high-flow oxygen, suctioning the nostrils as needed, supporting ineffective respirations, caring for fractures and other specific injuries, and arranging for rapid transport to definitive medical care as indicated.

A pediatric patient with actual or suspected spine trauma must be stabilized on a long backboard designed so the number and location of strap holes will accommodate his or her size.

Because of the relatively large head size in a pediatric patient, place padding (such as a blanket folded to a thickness of 2" to 3") under the trunk of a patient younger than 8 years so that the head and neck are in the neutral, anatomic position. Always use a pediatric cervical collar when stabilizing the spine. If a rigid collar of the proper size is not available, you can improvise one with a SAM splint or a blanket roll.

When transporting children on toboggans or other carrying devices in the outdoor environment, do not allow the parent to hold the child during transport. Always take special precautions when strapping the patient in the toboggan or other carrying device. The child may not fit into this equipment as well as an adult would, so slower speeds and cautious turning will provide extra safety for the pediatric patient. Do not allow your emotions to get control of the situation.

Family Matters

It is important to remember that when children are injured, you may have several patients to treat rather than just one ▼ Figure 30-33 . Family members, especially the primary caregiver, often need help or support when medical emergencies or problems develop. A calm parent usually helps to contribute to a calm child. An agitated parent usually means that the child will act the same way. Make sure that you are calm, efficient,

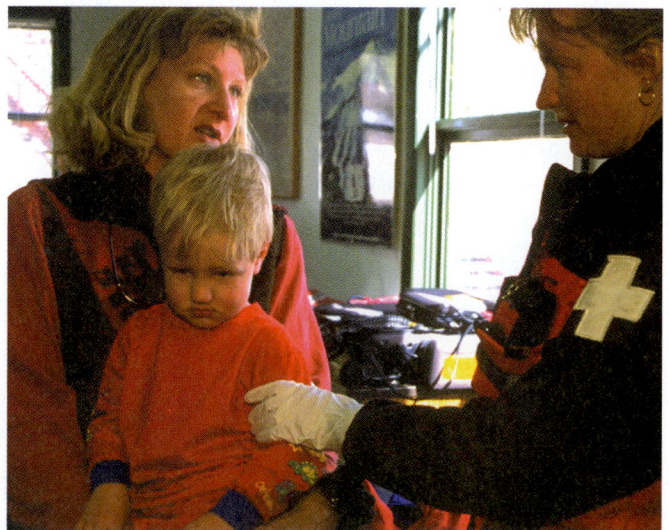

Figure 30-33 Remember that you are caring for at least two patients: the infant or child, and the parent or caregiver.

professional, and sensitive as you deal with children and their families.

Child Abuse

The term <u>child abuse</u> means any improper or excessive action that injures or otherwise harms a child or infant; it includes physical abuse, sexual abuse, neglect, and emotional abuse. The intentional injury of a child, whether physical or emotional, is not rare in our society. More than 2 million cases of child abuse are reported to child protection agencies annually. Many of these children suffer life-threatening injuries, and some die. If suspected child abuse is not reported, the child is likely to be abused again and again, perhaps suffering permanent injuries or even dying. Therefore, you must be aware of the signs of child abuse and neglect, and of your responsibility to report suspected abuse to law enforcement or child protection agencies.

Signs of Abuse

If you suspect that physical or sexual abuse is involved, you should ask yourself the following questions:

- Is the injury typical for the developmental level of the child?

- Is the method of injury reported by the parent or caregiver consistent with the child's injuries?

- Is the caregiver behaving appropriately (concerned about the child's well-being)?

- Is there evidence of drinking or drug use at the scene?

- Was there a delay in seeking care for the child?

- Is there a good relationship between the child and the caregiver?

- Does the child have multiple injuries at different stages of healing?

- Does the child have any unusual marks or bruises that may have been caused by cigarettes, grids, or branding injuries?

- Does the child have several types of injuries, such as burns, fractures, and bruises?

- Does the child have any burns on the hands or feet that involve a glove distribution (marks that encircle a hand or foot in a pattern that looks like a glove)?

- Is there an unexplained decreased level of consciousness?

- Is the child clean and an appropriate weight for his or her age?

Table 30-8   CHILD ABUSE Mnemonic for Assessing Possible Child Abuse
Consistency of the injury with the child's developmental age
History inconsistent with injury
Inappropriate parental concerns
Lack of supervision
Delay in seeking care
Affect
Bruises of varying ages
Unusual injury patterns
Suspicious circumstances
Environmental clues

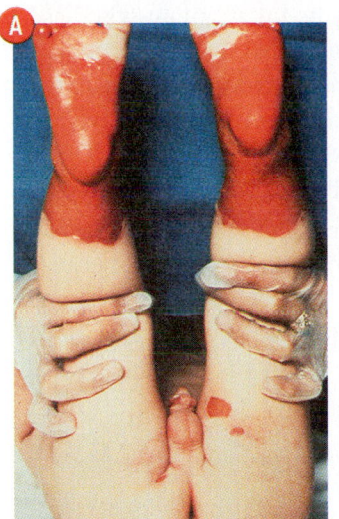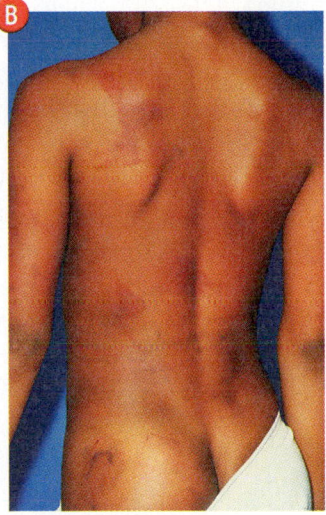

Figure 30-34 Signs of child abuse. **A.** Scald. **B.** Multiple injuries at different stages of healing.

- Is there any rectal or vaginal bleeding?

- What does the home look like? Clean or dirty? Is it warm or cold? Is there food?

Your assessment in the field will allow a better assessment by the medical staff later. An easy way to remember these is the mnemonic CHILD ABUSE shown in ▲ **Table 30-8** .

As you assess the child, look for and pay particular attention to the following signs ▲ **Figure 30-34** .

BRUISES. Observe the color and location of any bruises. New bruises are pink or red. Over time, bruises turn blue, then green, then yellow-brown and faded. Note the location. Bruises to the back, buttocks, or face are suspicious and are usually inflicted by a person.

BURNS. Burns to the penis, testicles, vagina, or buttocks are usually inflicted by someone else, as are burns that encircle a hand or foot to look like a glove. You should suspect abuse if the child has cigarette burns or grid pattern burns.

FRACTURES. Fractures of the humerus or femur do not normally occur without major trauma, such as a fall from a high place or a motor vehicle crash. Falls from bed are not usually associated with fractures.

SHAKEN BABY SYNDROME. Infants may sustain life-threatening head trauma by being shaken or struck on the head, a life-threatening condition called **shaken baby syndrome**. With this condition, there is bleeding within the head and damage to the cervical spine as a result of intentional, forceful shaking. The infant will be found unconscious, often without evidence of external trauma. The call for help may be for an infant who has stopped breathing or is unresponsive. The infant may appear to be in cardiopulmonary arrest, but what has likely occurred is that the shaking tore blood vessels in the brain, resulting in bleeding around the brain. The pressure from the blood results in a coma.

NEGLECT. Children who are neglected are often dirty or too thin or appear developmentally delayed because of lack of stimulation. You may observe such children when you are treating other problems. Report all cases of suspicious neglect.

Symptoms and Other Indicators of Abuse

An abused child may appear withdrawn, fearful, or hostile. You should be particularly concerned if the child refuses to discuss how an injury occurred. Occasionally, the parent or caregiver will reveal a history of several "accidents." Be alert for conflicting stories or a marked lack of concern from the parents or caregiver. Remember, the abuser may be a parent, caregiver, relative, or friend of the family. Sometimes the abuser is an acquaintance of a single parent.

Emergency Medical Care

Your priority is to care for ABCs, as in all other instances. Care for all wounds, splint fractures, and keep the infant or child warm and comfortable. Arrange for transport in all instances in which you suspect abuse has occurred. You are not there to solve the problem or to accuse a parent or caregiver. In fact, you need their cooperation, as a child cannot be transported without consent from the parent or guardian. You do not have to prove that there has been abuse. Law enforcement and child protection agencies are mandated to investigate all reported cases.

Response to Pediatric Emergencies

After care and transport of a sick or injured child, you may experience a wide range of powerful emotions. These emotions result from the call itself or from your previous experience (or inexperience) in caring for infants and children. You may feel anxious if you have not had much experience in dealing with infants and children. You may also think of your own children or the children of a loved one.

As a result, you must be prepared to care for children. Practice with children and pediatric equipment is necessary. As you know, children are not simply small adults. However, many of the skills and principles you use to care for adults can be applied to children. You must simply remember there are differences in anatomy and emotions.

After difficult incidents involving children, debriefing is helpful in working through the stress and trauma. It is also a means to help you in the future if you are faced with similar situations. The ability to seek help after difficult episodes is a sign of maturity and confidence.

Chapter *Sweep*

Ready for Review

Child anatomy contributes to some special challenges in assessment and care. The tongue is large relative to other structures, so it poses a higher risk of airway obstruction than in an adult. Tonsils and other tissue more posterior can also pose this problem, as does a relatively soft and narrow trachea. Head size and shape also make airway positioning a specialized task in children. Newborns and infants have high respiratory rates, and breathe primarily with their diaphragms.

There are five development stages in childhood: infancy, the toddler years, preschool age, school age, and adolescence. Each stage requires a slightly different approach to assessment and pain management. General rules for dealing with children of all ages include appearing confident, being honest, and keeping caregivers together with the patient as much as possible.

Always take the patient's vital signs in the field and use pediatric resuscitation equipment. To measure respirations in children younger than 3 years, count the rise and fall of the abdomen rather than the chest. Feel for a pulse in the brachial or femoral artery in infants and small children, and in the carotid artery in older children.

In treating possible respiratory failure in a child, always position the airway in a neutral position. Use an airway adjunct to maintain an open airway.

Use a BVM device with a child whose breathing and tidal volume are inadequate and who has an altered level of consciousness. There are three keys to successful use of the BVM device in a child: (1) Have the appropriate equipment in the right size, (2) maintain a good face to mask seal, and (3) ventilate at the appropriate rate and volume: 20 breaths/min for an infant or child, 30 for a neonate, 1 to 1$\frac{1}{2}$ seconds per ventilation. Squeeze gently, and stop squeezing as the chest wall begins to rise.

Children younger than 5 years often obstruct their upper and lower airway with a variety of foreign objects. If the child is conscious, encourage him or her to cough to clear the airway. If the child is unconscious, you should first use the tongue-jaw lift and finger sweeps to try to remove an object that you can see. In treating an unconscious child with complete airway obstruction, use abdominal thrusts (in a series of five), alternating with attempts at artificial breathing; in infants, substitute back blows and chest thrusts. In a conscious child who is sitting or standing, apply abdominal thrusts from behind.

A child who is in early respiratory distress may be breathing too slowly or too fast. Rates greater than 60 breaths/min are a sign of a problem requiring assisted ventilation in most cases. Look for signs of extra effort to breathe, including nasal flaring and grunting respirations; these may give way to cyanosis. You must intervene immediately if bradycardia develops in a child in respiratory distress. Use the least upsetting method to administer supplemental oxygen, adding assisted ventilations if these become necessary; use a BVM device without an artificial airway.

Seizures in children may appear as a shaking of the whole body (generalized), a movement in a single arm or leg or eye (partial), or a momentary unresponsiveness (absence seizure). Complications of seizures are due to injury from seizure motion, airway obstruction, or poor breathing effort. Do not put anything into the mouth of a child who is having a seizure. Do position the child so that the tongue is not an obstruction, and be prepared to suction secretions or vomitus. Febrile seizures, typically occurring on the first day of a fever, may be a sign of a more serious problem such as meningitis. Begin cooling measures, and arrange for transport to the hospital.

Other childhood conditions that require immediate transport include altered level of consciousness, which you may assess using the AVPU scale; severe dehydration; and poisoning. The best way to cool a child with a fever is with wet towels that are at room temperature, not cold.

Infants and children can go into shock after the loss of even a small volume of fluid or blood, which may be caused by an injury, dehydration, severe infection or allergic reaction, heart disease, or a collapsed lung. Children who are in shock often have increased respirations but normal blood pressure until the condition is severe. Changes in skin color and capillary refill are important signs of shock.

The most common cause of dehydration in children is vomiting and diarrhea. Life-threatening diarrhea can develop in an infant in hours. You can determine whether a child's dehydration is mild, moderate, or severe by assessing the child's urine output, level of activity, mental status, skin tone, and pulse. For severe dehydration, EMS should arrange for ALS backup so that IV fluids can be given.

When you care for a seriously ill or injured child, remember also that attending to the stress of others involved will help calm the patient. Try to keep the child with—or at least near—a parent or caregiver during transport.

For several reasons, you face special challenges when you are called on to care for children who have traumatic injuries. Children are not only smaller than adults and more vulnerable; they are also anatomically, physiologically, and psychologically different from adults in some important ways. You must understand these differences to provide the best possible care for children who have been injured.

You should remember that children's bones are more flexible and bend more with injury and that the ends of the long bones, where growth occurs, are weaker and may be injured more easily. Children's heads are proportionately larger and are more likely to be injured in automobile mishaps. Children's internal organs are not as insulated by fat and may be injured more severely, and children have less circulating blood, so that, although children exhibit the signs of shock more slowly, they go into shock faster. Children are not always as cautious as adults and tend to have more accidental poisoning, diving, and bicycle injuries.

If you cannot effectively ventilate a victim of submersion, consider the possibility of a foreign body airway obstruction, as water alone does not obstruct the airway.

There is rarely anything more satisfying than helping or saving the life of an injured child, but injured children who are unconscious or in pain can be difficult. Therefore, you must always be prepared emotionally to care for children who have been injured and seek counseling or debriefing if necessary after caring for a traumatically injured child.

Vital Vocabulary

adolescents Children between 12 to 18 years of age.

altered level of consciousnes A mental state in which infants and children may be unresponsive, combative, or confused, may thrash about, or may drift into and out of an alert state; also called altered mental status.

apnea Absence of breathing.

bradycardia A heart rate of less than 60 beats/min in children or less than 80 beats/min in infants.

child abuse Any improper or excessive action that injures or otherwise harms a child or infant; includes neglect and physical, sexual, and emotional abuse.

croup Infection of the airway below the level of the vocal cords, usually caused by a virus.

dehydration A state in which fluid losses are greater than fluid intake into the body, leading to shock and death if untreated.

epiglottitis An infection of the soft tissue in the area above the vocal cords.

febrile seizure Seizure relating to a fever.

hyperventilation Rapid or deep breathing that lowers blood carbon dioxide levels below normal.

infancy The first year of life.

neonatal The first month after birth.

pediatrics A specialized medical practice devoted to the care of the young.

postictal period The period immediately following a seizure, characterized by extreme tiredness or listlessness.

preschool-age Children between 3 to 6 years of age.

rales A crackling breath sound caused by the flow of air through liquid in the lungs; a sign of lower airway obstruction.

school-age Children between 6 to 12 years of age.

shaken baby syndrome Bleeding within the head and damage to the cervical spine of an infant who has been intentionally and forcibly shaken; a form of child abuse.

shock A condition that develops when the circulatory system is not able to deliver sufficient blood to body organs, resulting in organ failure and eventual death if untreated.

status epilepticus The term used to describe a continuous seizure, or multiple seizures without a return to consciousness, for 30 minutes or more.

stridor A high-pitched breath sound heard mainly on inspiration that is a sign of upper airway obstruction.

toddler The period following infancy until 3 years of age.

tonic-clonic seizure A seizure that features rhythmic back-and-forth motion of an extremity and body stiffness.

tripod position An abnormal position to keep the airway open; it involves leaning forward onto two arms stretched forward.

wheezing A whistling breath sound caused by air traveling through narrowed air passages within the bronchioles; a sign of lower airway obstruction.

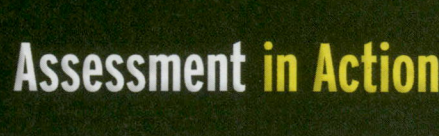

Assessment in Action

While patrolling at a cross-country ski area, you are called to the chalet halfway around the 6-mile course. There is a 12-year-old girl sitting with her hands on her knees having difficulty breathing, who says, "I can't get enough air." It is 0°F outside. Her mother says she has exercise-induced asthma.

The patient tried the inhaler twice with minimal results and the mother was reluctant to try it again. The family doctor did not return a page, so they called the patrol. Your patient appears slightly pale. She does not pay attention to you or your partner and does not respond when you say her name. Her gaze is vacant and she appears tired. The mother states that the patient is receiving no other medication other than her albuterol inhaler. She has no other medical problem.

1. Which of the following signs should be used to determine whether this child is sick or well during your initial assessment?
   A. Body position and skin color
   B. Skin color and pupil size
   C. Pupil size and attention to you
   D. Attention to you and body position

2. In this patient, which of the following observations of respiratory distress can only be observed if her shirt is removed?
   A. Nasal flaring
   B. Sternal retraction
   C. Audible wheezing
   D. Grunting

3. Tripoding is significant because it suggests:
   A. severe abdominal pain.
   B. accessory muscle use.
   C. abnormal circulation.
   D. impending seizures.

4. As you are conducting your assessment, you find that this child has sternal retractions, intercostal retractions, and nasal flaring. Vital signs include a pulse of 150 beats/min, respirations of 46 breaths/min, and a blood pressure of 96/68 mm Hg. Lung sounds have wheezes in all lobes. Assuming that local protocols would allow, which of the following treatments is appropriate for this patient?
   A. Administering oxygen by nasal cannula and rapid transport to definitive care
   B. Rewarming in the aid room, then transport
   C. Administering metered dose inhaler and oxygen, then transport
   D. Administering aspirin and oxygen by mask, then rapid transport

5. Given all her assessment signs, which of the following statements is accurate for this child? She is in:
   A. respiratory failure.
   B. respiratory arrest.
   C. no acute distress.
   D. the recovery phase.

6. Your partner states that this patient is tachypneic. What does that mean?
   A. Her heart rate is too fast.
   B. Her respiratory rate is too fast.
   C. She has poor perfusion.
   D. She has poor attention.

7. As your partner is administering treatment, you complete the assessment and note that her legs are mottled. You know this indicates:
   A. fever.
   B. infection.
   C. poor perfusion.
   D. a cold environment.

8. You complete your detailed physical assessment and note the presence of petechiae, which is:
   A. bruising.
   B. cerebrospinal fluid.
   C. hematoma.
   D. a fine red or maroon rash.

Challenging Questions

9. Why may blood pressure be inaccurate as an indicator of perfusion in a child?
   A. The blood pressure becomes more accurate as the child grows because of the total blood volume.
   B. The blood pressure is only accurate when compared to the pulse of a child who is awake and alert.
   C. Blood pressure cuffs do not come properly sized for the pediatric patient.
   D. A child with poor perfusion frequently has a normal blood pressure because of compensation.

10. What would the appropriate description of this child's AVPU scale be?
    A. She is alert.
    B. She is unresponsive.
    C. She does not respond to her name.
    D. She responds to painful stimuli.

Points to Ponder

You arrive at the scene of a collision involving a 5-year-old girl and an adult. The adult appears to be fine physically but is very stressed and anxious about the condition of the child. Your assessment finds the child to be unresponsive, with multiple small wounds and abrasions. You suspect a spinal injury. You do not have any pediatric spinal stabilization equipment in the top dispatch nor is there any on either of the toboggans coming to the scene. You feel this situation warrants a load and go. What are the risks of using equipment that is too large? What are the risks of waiting for proper equipment to come from the base medical clinic?

Issues Decision-Making Skills, Problems Without Clear Answers, Alternative Resources, Calming Excited Participants, Duty to Transport, Scene Investigation/Risk Management

Online Outlook

Children are not simply small adults; they come in a wide variety of sizes with anatomy and physiology that are different from those of adults. However, the treatment priorities in children who sustain serious trauma are similar to those in adults. To learn more about pediatric medical and trauma emergencies, complete Exercise 30 at www.OECzone.com.

www.OECzone.com

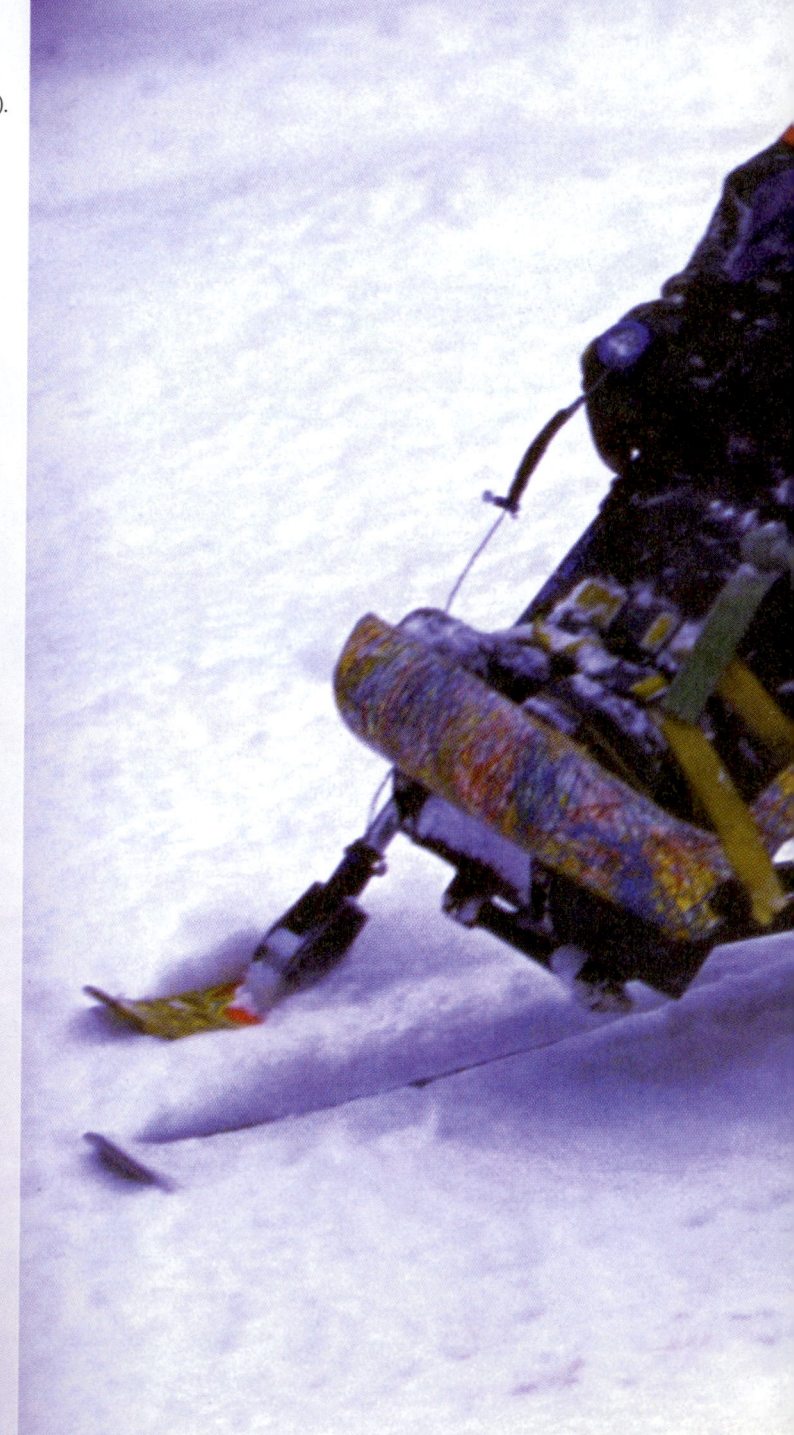

Outdoor Adaptive Athletes

Objectives

Cognitive

1. Identify the outdoor adaptive population (p 775).

Affective

🌲 **2.** Determine special needs of patients who are mentally challenged (p 775).

🌲 **3.** Determine special needs of patients who are physically challenged (p 777).

Psychomotor

🌲 **4.** Demonstrate the special care needs required when treating adaptive patients (p 775).

🌲 These are core concepts in initial patrol training.

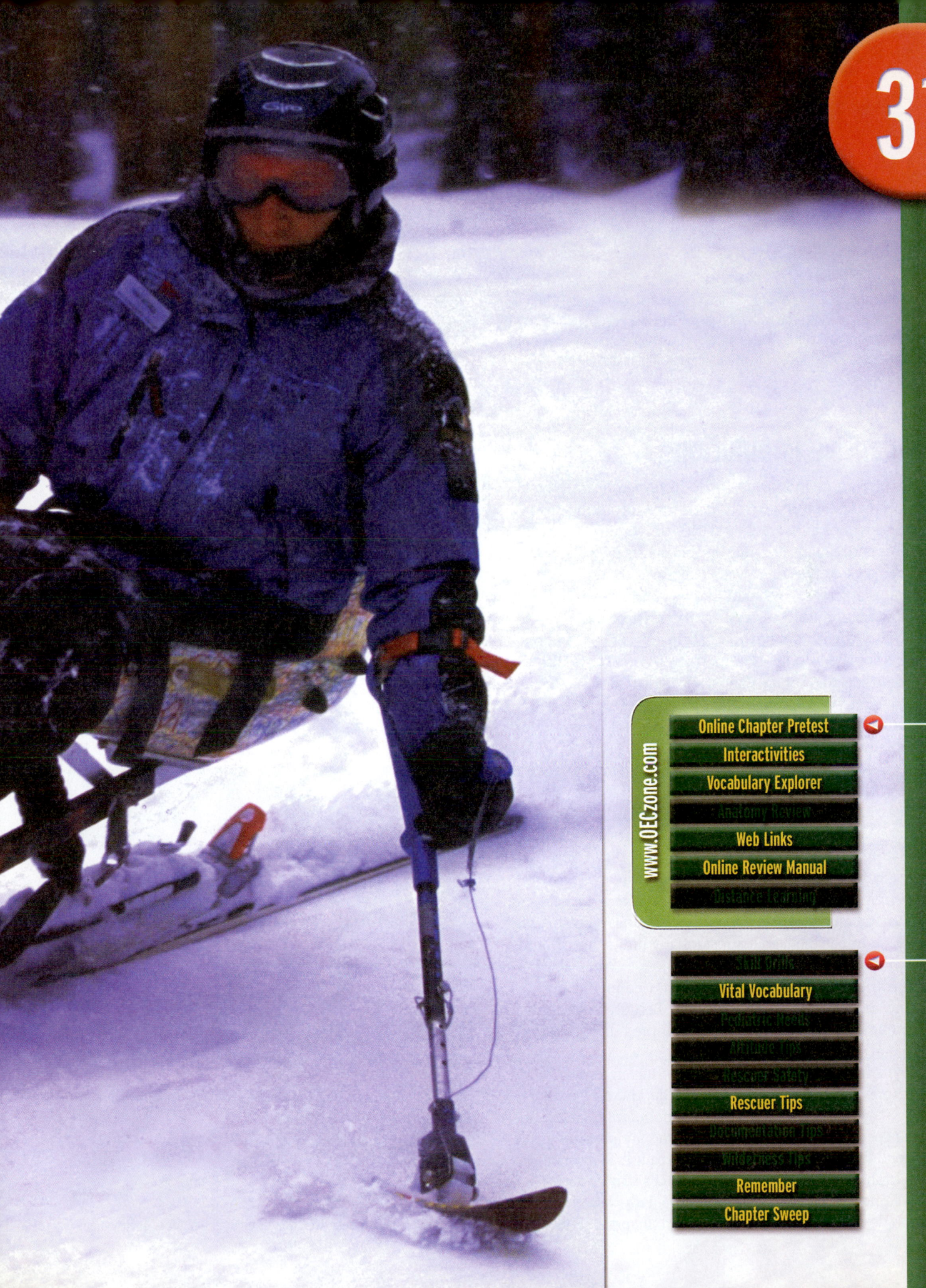

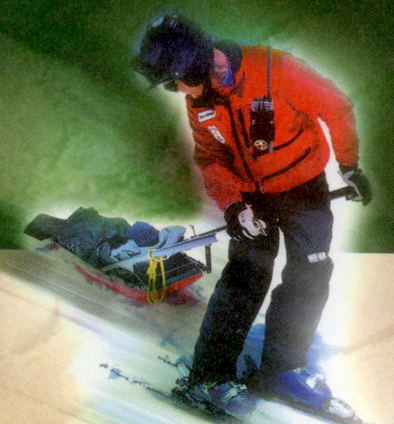

You are the rescuer

It's a very cold mid-January day. On Judy's Run there is a three-tracker over the bank about 20' down over the edge. His guide is with him. Radio control says, "Possible head and shoulder injuries."

Adaptive athletes have special needs and can be a challenge to evaluate and treat. You will discover what these needs are and how the care for these individuals differs. This chapter will introduce you to the outdoor adaptive athlete and his or her special needs and treatment.

1. Who are adaptive athletes?

2. What unique conditions and treatment should the rescuer learn in order to care for these individuals?

Adaptive Populations

No longer are individuals who have significant physical, mental, or emotional handicaps forced to sit on the sidelines and watch athletic competition. Many of these individuals are outdoor enthusiasts ▼ Figure 31-1 . Even so, when injured, they have special needs. Communication, evacuation, and treatment may need modification to fit the conditions of these individuals.

The **Americans with Disabilities Act (ADA)** of 1990 opened up new frontiers for persons with disabilities in regard to employment, programs, and services provided by the government, and access to most publicly used facilities. Participation in the sports world for the disabled is now common.

The terms *impairment, disability,* and *handicap* need to be understood. According to the World Health Organization's guidelines, an **impairment** is defined as any loss or abnormality of psychological, physiologic, or anatomic structure or function. A **disability** is any restriction in or lack of ability to perform an activity in the manner or within the range considered normal for a human being. The US government defines a person who has an impairment that substantially limits one or more of life's activities as **handicapped**.

Although these terms have been used interchangeably, they have separate meanings. Because these terms can be demeaning, the NSP has adopted the term **adaptive athlete** to describe an individual who is physically or mentally challenged and participates in a sport. This chapter will discuss the origin of adaptive athletic programs, define the adaptive sports population, determine the special needs of participants who are physically and mentally challenged, and show the outdoor rescuer how to evaluate and treat these individuals appropriately.

Long before the 1990 Americans with Disabilities Act, people with disabilities participated in sports. Following World War II, Sir Ludwig Guttman in England started wheelchair competition for rehabilitation and as "recreation to prevent boredom." In 1960, the first Paralympic Games were held in Rome following the Olympics. Slowly, athletes with other impairments (including visual problems, hearing problems, paralysis, cerebral palsy, amputation, polio, muscular dystrophy, arthrogryposis, dwarfism, Down syndrome, brain injury, and many other post-traumatic injuries to the musculoskeletal or nervous system) began to participate in athletics.

The summer Paralympics has now become a regular post-Olympic event and includes many sports such as archery, basketball, cycling, equestrian, fencing, judo, running, rugby, soccer, swimming, table tennis, and vol-

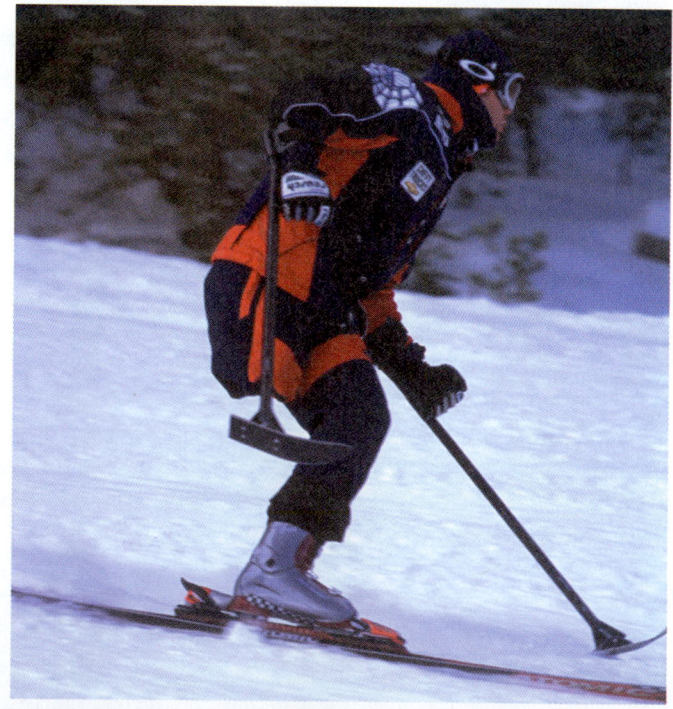

Figure 31-1 Many adaptive athletes enjoy the outdoor environment.

leyball. Winter Paralympic Events include both nordic and alpine skiers with many of the disability conditions previously listed.

The adaptive outdoor athlete seems to have originated in Europe before WW II. The Swiss amputees used crutches instead of poles for nordic skiing. Following a WW II injury, Franc Wendel, a German, entered a ski competition as an amputee, putting a second set of short skis on the end of his crutches, the first known outriggers. Austria created a ski school for amputees in the 1950s.

The United States had several smaller programs for the winter skiing athlete in the 1960s. Then in 1967, disabled war veterans from the Tenth Mountain Division began teaching adaptive skiing techniques in the Sierra Mountains of northern Colorado. Winter Park ski area in Colorado developed the first comprehensive adaptive ski program in the 1970s. The first gold medal for the adaptive snowsports athlete was presented in 1992 at the Winter Olympics.

With the advent of many adaptive snowsports programs in the United States, you now have probably seen many types of adaptive populations gracefully descending the slopes. Because of increased numbers of adaptive snowsports athletes, the Professional Ski Instructors of America (PSIA) now has adaptive snowsports schools at many ski areas in the United States. The outdoor rescuer must now be able to care for these adaptive athletes both during mountain sports activities (winter and summer) and when asked to assist at sporting events such as cycling or wheelchair races.

In order to understand the special needs of these athletes, it is important to know about their various mental and physical medical conditions.

Mentally Challenged Individuals

Individuals who are mentally challenged may have several different conditions. Included are learning disabilities, mental retardation, cognitive disabilities (both congenital and acquired), autism, and individuals who have psychological disorders such as psychosis. The rescuer needs to understand the psychological characteristics of each condition in order to care for these people.

People with **learning disorders** who are not mentally retarded usually have either attention-deficit disorder or dyslexia. **Attention-deficit disorder (ADD)** is often an inherited neurologic disorder characterized by short attention span, distractibility, impulsiveness, hyperactivity, and restlessness. Medications can help these individuals cope with activities of daily living. A person with ADD may also have **dyslexia**. Processing information is

difficult (sometimes backwards) or mixed up. These individuals have normal or above-normal intelligence; however, there is usually a significant delay in learning ability. This delay can be social, academic, emotional, physical, or a combination of these.

Mental retardation (MR) refers to below-average intellectual capacity from birth or childhood associated with difficulties in learning and socialization. Most individuals who can participate in sports demonstrate only mild MR (IQ between 51 to 70). There are many causes or types of MR. More common prenatal types or causes include genetic (predominantly Down syndrome and Fragile X syndrome), fetal alcohol syndrome, microencephaly, and drugs that affect an embryo. Postnatal brain infections, poisoning (lead or mercury), asphyxia, and head trauma all can cause MR. Developmental social categories of MR include lack of mental stimulation and physical abuse.

The rescuer must try to understand the individual's level of intelligence and social development while giving care. These patients may exhibit hyperactivity, anxiety, impulsiveness, bad judgment, apathy, or be easily distracted as their normal behavior. Communicating with a person who is mentally retarded is therefore not the same as communicating with someone who has normal cognitive abilities.

Down syndrome is a more common genetic condition resulting in mental and physical anomalies. The easygoing personality of many of these individuals could confuse the rescuer into thinking they are not injured or ill. Mental retardation makes it difficult for the rescuer to assess their condition ▼ Figure 31-2 .

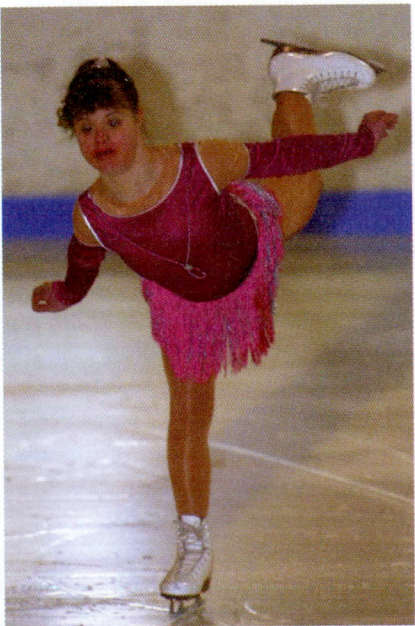

Figure 31-2 Athlete with Down syndrome.

Physical congenital defects in persons with Down syndrome can affect their athletic performance. Congenital cervical spine conditions (instability of C1 or C2) make neck injuries a concern. There are many athletic programs for the disabled that require medical clearance of the C-spine in persons with Down syndrome prior to competition. Laxity of ligaments can make the joints in their extremities more susceptible to injury.

Autism is a developmental neurologic disorder that includes severe problems with communication and behavior. These individuals shun normal human interaction. They have learning and language disorders and thus cannot communicate effectively. They have inappropriate social responses, sleep disturbances, feel isolated, and at times are very aggressive. They can be hyperactive and demonstrate repetitive actions. Therapy and medication may help people with autism. Working with these individuals may be challenging because communication can be very limited, you may not understand their behavior, and your encounter may be frustrating.

Acquired brain injury as a child or an adult can decrease cognition. A **cognitive disability** is from damage or deterioration on any portion of the brain that affects the ability to process information, coordinate and control the body, and/or move in space. Most snow-sports athletes who independently ski or snowboard have reasonable control over motor movements; however, some may sit to ski and have mental and physical problems. Many individuals who have had brain injury can experience seizures; keep this in mind when caring for these patients and be prepared to treat a potential seizure (see Chapter 13).

Individuals who have **psychosis** may function reasonably well if they take appropriate medications. At times, however, their mental status is not in reality, and they may experience hallucinations and hear voices. **Schizophrenia** and **manic-depressive** disorders are the two most common psychotic conditions. Individuals with psychosis, when medicated, can work and participate in athletics. Because these individuals have very different thinking processes, their care may be challenging. Being patient and calm is most important when caring for patients with psychosis.

Special Needs of the Mentally Challenged

Athletes who are mentally challenged can be very hard to assess. Cognitive, social, emotional, and behavioral aspects of the patient's preexisting problem make evaluation and treatment difficult. Generally, a patient who is mentally challenged will have a supervising adult with him or her. This person can usually "read" the patient. The rescuer should heed his or her interpretation of what is wrong. Just as a parent knows when a child is ill, this adult will probably know what is wrong with the person in his or her care.

When you approach such a patient, do so with a gentle, calm, caring attitude. Try to understand the underlying mental condition: Does the patient understand basic questions? Can the patient comprehend a more complex statement? Does the underlying mental problem allow short-term memory capability? Does the patient know the time, place, person, and situation? Will the patient allow you to touch him or her to assess? Is he or she confused or distracted because of the underlying mental condition? Only after you can answer these questions can you provide care.

A dilemma in assessing the mental status of a patient who is mentally challenged is determining whether the cause of the behavior is the underlying mental or psychological problem, or a new problem due to head trauma or another medical condition. If you are not sure, always consider the altered mental status to be a new problem, and treat the patient appropriately.

Table 31-1 Chart of Adaptive Snowsports Terms	
Outriggers	Forearm crutches that have short skis built onto the bottom, to help with balance.
Three tracker	A person who has lost a leg and skis without a prosthesis, on one ski, and uses outriggers on both arms.
Four tracker	A person who uses two skis on both legs (one or both could be artificial) and outriggers on both arms.
Mono skier	A person who sits in a "bucket" or seat that is mounted onto one ski or snowboard under the bucket. Most use outriggers.
Bi-skier	A person who sits in a bucket that is mounted to two skis. Most use outriggers.

Physically Challenged Individuals

Patients who are physically challenged can also make assessment difficult, although communicating with the injured athlete is usually easier. Physical conditions include amputations, ataxia, cerebral palsy, deafness, epilepsy, multiple sclerosis, muscular dystrophy, post-polio syndrome, spina bifida, spinal cord injuries, stroke and brain trauma, and visual difficulties.

Special Needs of the Amputee Patient

A large group of adaptive snow athletes have amputations. Today's adaptive equipment makes it possible for these athletes to participate in many sports. Amputations can be traumatic or surgical, or an individual can be born without one or more limbs. Generally, the athlete who has more of his or her amputated extremity remaining has a higher level of function. The person may be missing part or all of the foot, have a below-knee (through the tibia) amputation, or above-knee (through the femur) amputation, or a hemipelvectomy (through part of the pelvis). An amputation at a joint is called a disarticulation, ie, an amputation between the tibia and femur is called a knee-disarticulation. Athletes with amputations of an arm generally participate in outdoor sports no differently than athletes with arms, except they may use only one pole when skiing.

Some single-legged athletes wear a prosthesis (artificial limb) and use two skis, while others without a prosthesis use one ski (▶ Figure 31-3). When you are examining an amputee with a decreased level of consciousness who has a prosthesis, the artificial limb will have no sensitivity and can make assessment difficult. Also, swelling, infection, and ulceration can occur at the stump site.

A broken femur on the same side as a below-knee amputation poses an interesting dilemma for the rescuer. Applying traction to the ankle of the prosthesis usually will only pull the artificial leg off. If the fracture is just above the knee, remove the prosthesis gently, as it acts as a weight across the fracture site. Cover up the stump to keep it warm, and apply a rigid fixation splint such as a quick-splint. For a midshaft fracture, do the same, as there is not a good way to apply traction to the stump. Tighten the straps on the quick splint as needed to make the patient comfortable. Immobilization at the fracture site to stop bleeding and decrease pain is key. A hip fracture is treated by "good leg splinting," ie, bandage the broken hip on the below-knee amputated leg to the other normal leg.

If the fractured leg on the below-knee amputee is the leg without the amputation, treat it the same way you would treat a person with two legs—apply a traction splint.

More upper extremity injuries occur to adaptive athletes who use outriggers. When the individual falls down with force on the outrigger, axial pressure is exerted through the wrist, the elbow, and then to the shoulder. This can cause significant upper extremity injury, including a dislocated shoulder, fracture of a long bone, or elbow injury.

In the arm with an amputation, the rescuer should modify a sling and swathe with or without a malleable rigid splint (cardboard, ladder, SAM). Use body or chest splinting on a humerus fracture. A fractured elbow in a below-elbow amputee is best treated either as found or in a slightly more than 90° angle in anatomic position.

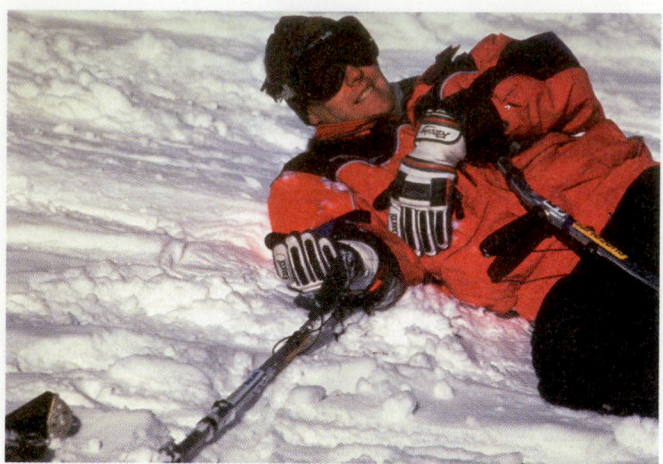

Figure 31-3 Take care of the patient's extra gear, such as outriggers.

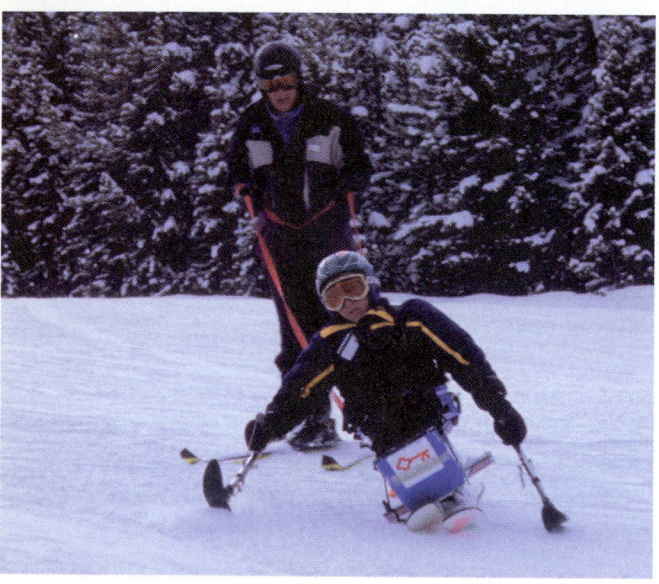

Figure 31-4 Many adaptive athletes need a skiing helper.

Do what is most comfortable for the injured patient.

Individuals with **ataxia**, or inability to walk, must sit to ski. Ataxia can be caused by balance or muscular problems. Since balance is a problem, most individuals with ataxia are sitting bi-skiers, with a skiing helper and a tether (▲ **Figure 31-4**). They have the same injuries and are cared for the same way as other sit-skiers.

Special Needs of the Patient with Cerebral Palsy

Cerebral palsy (CP) is a disability resulting from brain injury before, during, or shortly after birth, which is usually caused by anoxia or insufficient oxygen to brain cells. Depending on what part of the brain is destroyed or damaged, different patterns of CP can be seen. Although

> ### Rescuer Tips
>
> Traction is not an appropriate method of care for all patients. It can worsen spasticity in patients with cerebral palsy and is ineffective in patients with a prosthesis.

mental status can be affected, usually the person with CP has normal mentation. The body and its voluntary muscular coordination are impaired. This can be very mild, as in an individual who has very slight dysfunction in only one extremity, to a wheelchair bound person with no voluntary control of all extremities. Three basic patterns are seen: spastic, athetoid, and dystonic.

Spastic CP is the most common and characterized by constant involuntary muscle contraction, which can occur in one or more extremities. Individuals with very mild spastic CP may be able to ski or snowboard, while the more severely affected will sit (mono or bi-ski) to participate. Body movements in these individuals tend to be jerky, and at times the body is contorted. Balance is a problem. These individuals may not have the ability to relax their limbs when they fall, increasing the severity of the injury.

Athetoid CP is characterized by constant slow, writhing movements. These individuals generally sit to participate, even though some can ambulate with braces and supports.

Dystonic CP is seen in individuals with extreme rigidity of the body muscles. It is difficult for them to participate, although modified buckets or seats in a sit-ski device may allow them to participate, with a guide steering them down the slope.

It can be extremely difficult to apply splints, cravats, a sling and swathe, or traction in patients with CP. Individuals with spastic or dystonic CP are often the hardest to treat. Traction can make spasticity worsen. If traction increases muscle spasm, releasing the traction is appropriate. Remember the principle of fracture care: immobilization is the best possible way to prevent further damage and slow bleeding from the fracture site. Immobilize the injury in the way that is most comfortable for the patient.

Special Needs of the Patient with Multiple Sclerosis

Multiple sclerosis (MS) is a neurologic condition that causes weakness or paralysis of the extremities, loss of stamina, and balance difficulties. Cranial nerves tend to be affected. Visual problems, mood changes, and possibly slurred speech can occur.

Many individuals with MS have cycles of disease exacerbation and remission. During a remission, a person may be able to function reasonably well and could ski, probably as a three-tracker (sitting) if there are balance difficulties.

Individuals with MS may take a longer time to assimilate information and respond to your questions, and several seconds may lapse before they are able to answer.

Special Needs of the Patient with Muscular Dystrophy

Progressive and irreversible muscle wasting is the hallmark of **muscular dystrophy (MD)**. There are several different types affecting different muscle groups. Most are hereditary.

Weak muscles and easy fatigability are seen in persons with MD. Because of their weak muscles, their joints may be hypermobile and are injured more easily. Nearly all snowsports athletes with MD sit to ski. Mental status and pain response are normal. The rescuer must handle these individuals gently to prevent further injury.

Special Needs of the Patient with Postpolio Syndrome

Poliomyelitis in the western world is a disease of the past. However, there are still people who were infected with this virus nearly 50 years ago who experience residual effects. The Sabin and Salk vaccines have eradicated this disease in North America.

Individuals with **postpolio syndrome** who participate in outdoor athletic activities can have one or more extremities "wasted," generally with a shortened atrophied arm or leg. The limb can have some function or be paralyzed. Years after the disease has caused initial paralysis, effects on breathing muscles and balance can recur. Because an extremity is not fully developed, circulation is not normal and cold weather injury can be a problem.

Special Needs of the Patient with Spina Bifida and Spinal Cord Injury

There is a large population of mono- and bi- (sitting) skiers who fall into these two categories. Athletes with spina bifida and spinal cord injury may seem to have the same physical problems with paralysis below the level of the lesion of the spinal cord, but each condition has special characteristics.

> **Remember**
>
> Patients with spina bifida also are allergic to latex. If the allergy is unrecognized, the patient may experience anaphylactic shock and die. Always use latex-free gloves when caring for a patient with SB.

A congenital malformation of the spinal cord (usually the bony spine in the same area) in which segments of the spine fail to fuse results in an anomaly called **spina bifida (SB)**. The spinal cord can be damaged anywhere from the neck down, but nearly all athletes with this have damage in the lumbar region. Thus, they generally have paralysis and sensory alteration below the spinal level affected.

Individuals with SB can have abnormal circulation of cerebrospinal fluid (CSF). Because of this, they can develop hydrocephalus (an enlarged head with too much spinal fluid around the brain). When hydrocephalus exists, a shunt or tube is surgically placed from the base of the skull into the chest area. This tube allows cerebrospinal fluid to drain to release pressure. If this tube becomes clogged, kinked, or has pressure on it (from a helmet), pressure can build up, causing the patient's mental status to change. This situation should be considered when you are assessing the mental status of an athlete with SB.

The area where the spine was open at birth that was repaired shortly afterward is susceptible to injury. The skin in this area is thin. If the rescuer places a patient with SB on a backboard, padding (donut shaped pad) around this area is necessary to prevent skin breakdown and discomfort. Remember, the individual is neurologically compromised only *below* the level of congenital anomaly. A spinal injury can occur *above* this level, necessitating a backboard.

Patients with SB also are allergic to latex. If the allergy is unrecognized, the patient may experience anaphylactic shock and die. Always use latex-free gloves when caring for a patient with SB.

The spinal cord is in some ways similar to a telephone cable with many wires in it. Thousands and thousands of nerves are in the spinal cord. Each nerve has a special function: some are motor neurons for muscular function, some are for sensation, and others serve other functions.

Trauma to the spinal column (vertebral bones stacked on each other) can damage the spinal cord and result in

Hypothermia is especially a concern in an injured paraplegic with a long toboggan transport time.

a **spinal cord injury (SCI)**. Full or partial loss of function can occur below the level of the injury to the cord. If damage is in the cervical or neck region, quadriplegia can result. Injuries to the thoracic or lumbar spine can cause paraplegia. Generally, patients with paraplegia, not quadriplegia, can sit to ski, and usually only if the injury is at T5 level or below. Following injury, most of these athletes have had their spine stabilized with metal rods so they can sit better, but this does not return neurologic function below the injury.

Autonomic dysreflexia (AD) is a condition in which the body below the spine injury level does not have ability to sense and react normally to certain stimuli. AD occurs in individuals with spinal cord injuries. This condition can be life threatening, producing extreme hypertension, stroke, and death. A pressure point on the sacrum or lateral hip, bowel or bladder distention, severe hyperthermia or hypothermia, or trauma can be the inciting irritation to the central nervous system. At first, the patient with an SCI may be unaware of the occurrence of AD. Be aware of this in these patients.

Signs and symptoms occur as the condition worsens. These include a panicky feeling of impending doom, flushed skin, sweating, headache, blurred vision, or mental status changes. Eliminating the cause usually corrects the impending life-threatening extremely high blood pressure. Bowel or bladder evacuation (a bladder catheter may be obstructed) can be lifesaving.

It may be necessary to relieve a pressure point or remove a sharp object sticking into the skin below the level of the spinal cord injury. Remember, the individual cannot feel pain in the same way an unimpaired person would, and therefore does not recognize stimulation.

Patients with SCI have abnormal autonomic temperature regulating systems. Because the individuals cannot sense hot or cold below their spinal cord level, frostbite can occur unknowingly to the toes or feet of the adaptive athlete. Hypothermia and hyperthermia are also causes for concern, especially in an injured

paraplegic with hypothermia and a long toboggan transport time.

The insensate and paralyzed extremities in athletes with SB and SCI have several important considerations. A fracture can occur without pain. You should treat trauma or injury to a paralyzed leg the same as you would in a person without paraplegia. However, too much traction causing a pressure point from a splint can cause AD in the patient with an SCI. Monitor blood pressure frequently after applying a splint or traction.

Because these individuals are sitting in a hard plastic bucket with their legs strapped to the sit-ski, lower extremity injuries are infrequent. However, because of the outriggers and exposure of the arms to increased forces when the outrigger ski is on the ground or snow, there is an increase in the incidence of upper extremity injuries. Dislocated shoulders, fractures of the upper extremity and clavicle, and rotator cuff shoulder injuries are common.

Removal of the injured person from a sit-ski usually requires several people. Be gentle and remember to assess and palpate both legs completely, looking for a painless deformity (a broken leg).

Special Needs of the Patient with Stroke and Brain Trauma

Individuals who have experienced **stroke and brain trauma** have special needs. A stroke occurs when part of the brain becomes **anoxic** from loss of blood supply. Nerves in the brain are damaged or die from penetrating or nonpenetrating trauma. Depending on the portion and how much of the brain is damaged, the individual can be minimally or profoundly disabled.

Athletes with stroke and brain trauma can have emotional or psychological problems as well. Also, **aphasia** can occur. Expressive aphasia occurs when the person cannot verbalize, and receptive aphasia occurs when the person cannot understand the words he or she hears.

Brain-injured people are also predisposed to seizures. Look for a medical alert bracelet, and treat seizures appropriately.

Special Needs of the Visually Impaired Patient

The number of **visually impaired** outdoor athletes is increasing. Instead of a guide dog, these athletes ski or snowboard with a guide buddy who gives continuous verbal directions to the person ▶ Figure 31-5 . Statistically, blind athletes have a higher incidence of injury than do athletes with normal vision; however, they experience the same types of injuries. Talk with these patients while you are caring for them so that they know what you are doing to help them.

Special Needs of the Hearing Impaired Patient

Most athletes who are hearing impaired or underline deaf can read lips and communicate very well. Although knowing sign language can help the rescuer evaluate the patient, simply looking directly at the individual and speaking clearly and normally may be all that is needed for lip reading. Remember, the person cannot hear you and does not know you are communicating unless you have his or her attention. Also, many people who are hearing impaired have some speech difficulties but can usually vocalize their thoughts.

Special Needs of the Patient with Epilepsy

Many different medical, post brain trauma, or congenital conditions cause epilepsy. Treatment of epilepsy is found in Chapter 13. Always look for a medic alert bracelet on a person who is an outdoor enthusiast. Be ready to care for a seizure.

Other Treatment Concerns for the Adaptive Athlete

Adaptive athletes also use braces, appliances, and other equipment. The rescuer may encounter situations in which it is necessary to understand the devices and appliances that the individual uses and how to deal with them.

Ostomy bags are appliances that attach by special adhesive to abdominal wall ports of some individuals who have had abdominal surgery (▼ **Figure 31-6**). The two most common surgically created ports on the abdominal wall are for urine and feces. Generally, following abdominal or pelvic surgery, if the bowel or urinary tract cannot be reconnected immediately, a pink stoma or port is created on the abdominal wall to facilitate excretion. A urinary port is called a urostomy, a small bowel port an ileostomy, and a large bowel or colon port, a colostomy. The plastic bag on the abdominal wall collects the excreted substance. The individual then empties or replaces the bag as needed. Bags are sometimes used for other purposes as well. For example, a patient could have a tube exiting the abdominal cavity in order to drain bile resulting from complications of a gallbladder surgery.

If the patient has one of these appliances, placing straps (when backboarding) or pressure on the bag can make it leak. If it is full, it may be necessary to help the patient empty it.

Generally, these appliances go unnoticed in most individuals. However, if a patient has an ostomy bag, you should inspect the bag for blood during your initial assessment. A tube (Foley catheter) may have been placed up the urethra into the bladder to drain urine. Again, the tube can become kinked in an individual with an SCI, causing autonomic dysreflexia. If the collection bag has bloody urine, this could indicate kidney damage.

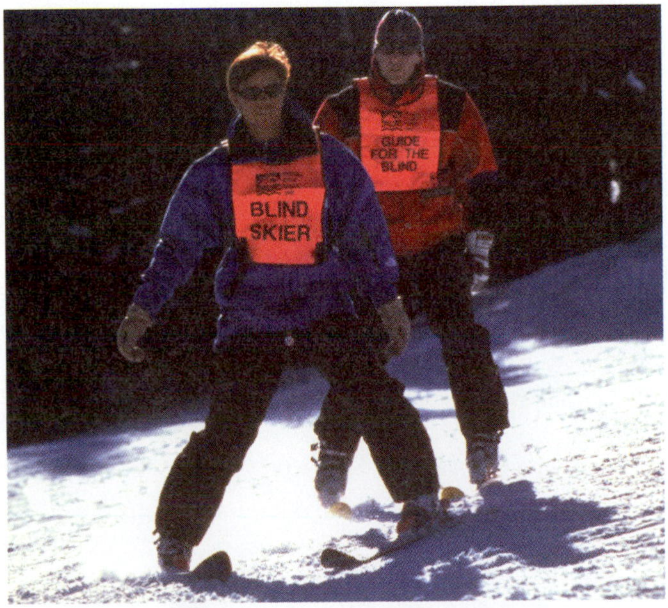

Figure 31-5 Skiers who are visually impaired are usually followed by their guide buddies.

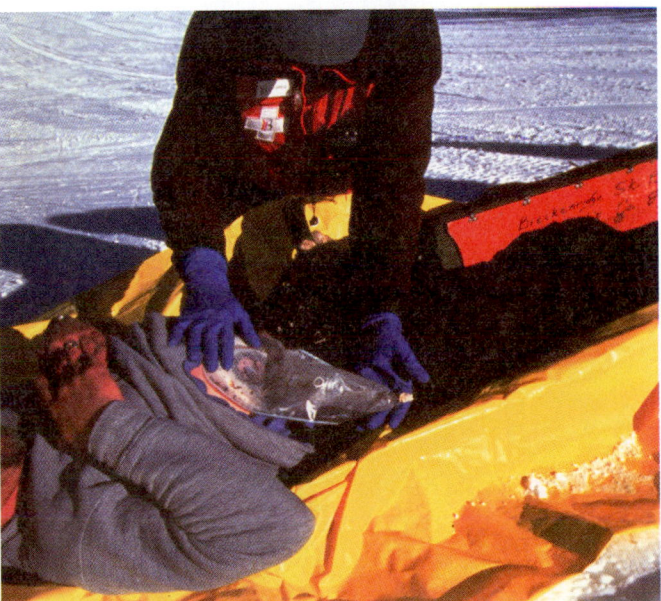

Figure 31-6 If the patient has an ostomy bag, make sure you inspect the bag for any signs of bleeding.

Today, individuals with kidney failure receive dialysis while waiting for a transplant. There are two methods of dialysis. Abdominal peritoneal dialysis involves a tube that goes into the abdominal cavity. Specialized fluid is put into the peritoneal space, absorbs waste products and then is drained out. The person usually does this on an alternating day routine, clamping the tube when not using it. These individuals are susceptible to infection in the abdominal cavity.

Abdominal peritoneal dialysis treatment can be cumbersome; therefore, many people undergo hemodialysis with an artificial kidney machine instead. Hemodialysis occurs every other day, so these individuals may participate in outdoor activities on alternate days. While hooked up to a dialysis machine for 6 to 8 hours, their blood is cleansed of impurities. The access for hemodialysis is by a needle put into a shunt under the skin. These shunts can be confusing to the rescuer, as a buzzing sensation can be felt through the skin over the location of the shunt. Surgically, an artery is directly connected to a vein, permitting rapid flow of blood through a shunt, causing the buzzing sensation.

Dialysis patients can have electrolyte problems, hypotension or hypertension, and can become nauseated easily. When a dialysis patient experiences signs or symptoms of these conditions, a physician should be consulted.

Rescuer Tips

Removing the patient from an overstimulating or threatening environment can bring about behavior change or calmness. Examples of negative environmental stimuli are noisy, crowded buildings, loud snowmaking guns, or the presence of an overprotective caregiver.

The equipment that many adaptive outdoor athletes use is expensive. Artificial arms and legs cost thousands of dollars. If it is necessary for you to remove a limb, care for it appropriately. Wheelchairs, three tracks, and four tracks have become extremely sophisticated and are also expensive. An outrigger can break if it is thrown out of the way at an emergency scene. Remember, if you remove a brace, artificial limb, or device from an adaptive athlete, it compromises the ability to function and should only be removed if necessary.

Many adaptive athletes take medications. Seizure, blood pressure, and psychiatric medications are common. Ask patients what medications they are taking, and if you do not know what it is for—ask. This will give you important information about the person's medical problems.

Lift Evacuation and Transportation Problems

Understanding the handicap or disability of an adaptive athlete is the first step in providing outdoor emergency care. Using common sense and applying the principles of care presented in this chapter will make your job much easier in the outdoor environment.

Certain problems can arise with lift evacuation of adaptive snowsports athletes. Problems primarily occur with sit-skiers (mono and bi) and blind skiers. Sit-skiers should always have tucked in their bucket a leash device that clips onto the bucket at three points. This then attaches to the rope thrown over the chair lift cable, and affords easy descent from the chair. The rescuer must make certain that all three leashes are connected to the bucket before having the skier push out of the chair lift seat (▶ Figure 31-7).

Skiers who are visually impaired may be very frightened when being evacuated from a chair. Talk with the individual even more than you would with an individual who can see. The guide who serves as the skier's eyes will be on the chair with him or her. The skier should always go before the guide. When the skier is on the ground, hold or touch him or her to convey a feeling of safety. Do not let go of the person until the guide has evacuated the lift and can aid the individual.

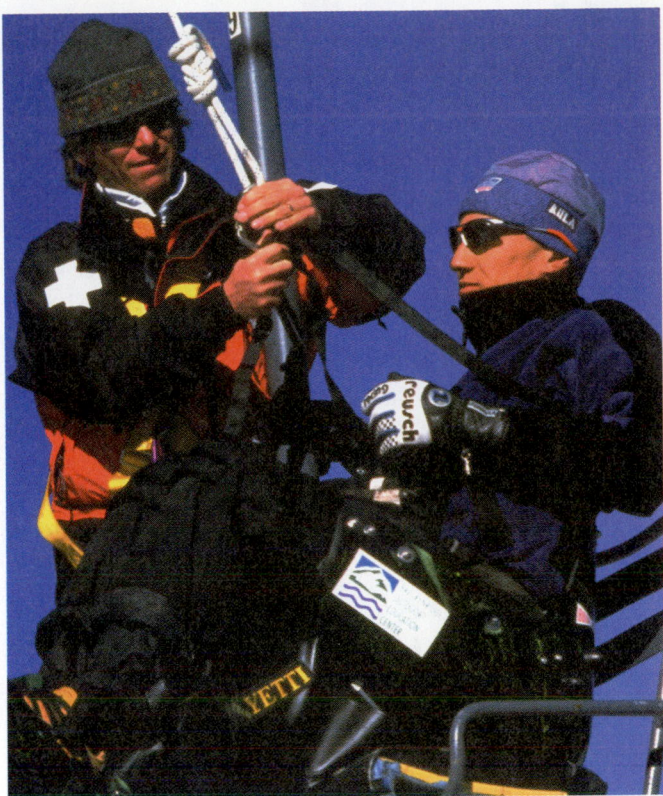

Figure 31-7 Adaptive skiing equipment is equipped with a safety-rated harness permanently attached to the device that provides a point interface with the area's evacuation equipment.

Chapter *Sweep*

Ready for Review

Outdoor adaptive athletes have special needs in relation to their disability or disabilities, in the equipment that they use because of their disability, and within the environment in which they choose to recreate or compete. It is important for the rescuer to understand the patient's disability or disabilities and how to handle emergency care situations. Likewise, the rescuer must become familiar with the specific equipment or devices that have been modified for use and are being used in his or her local areas. Lifting, moving, and transporting adaptive athletes is another key element of emergency care.

Vital Vocabulary

adaptive athlete An individual who is physically or mentally challenged and participates in a sport.

Americans with Disabilities Act (ADA) Comprehensive legislation that is designed to protect individuals with disabilities against discrimination.

amputation A complete separation from the body by cutting or tearing.

anoxic Diminished oxygen in the arterial blood despite normal ability of the blood to contain and carry oxygen. May be due to reduced oxygen supply, respiratory obstruction, reduced surface area in lungs for exchange of gases, or inadequate respiratory movements.

aphasia The inability to communicate verbally.

ataxia Loss of muscle coordination leading to difficulty in maintaining balance and inability to walk.

athetoid cerebral palsy A disorder in which a person makes constant, slow writhing movements.

attention deficit disorder (ADD) Neurologic syndrome that is usually hereditary. Symptoms include distractibility, short attention span, impulsiveness, hyperactivity, and restlessness that interfere with everyday function.

autism A developmental neurologic disorder that includes severe problems with communication and behavior.

autonomic dysreflexia (AD) A condition in which the body below the spine injury level does not have ability to sense and react normally to certain stimuli.

cerebral palsy (CP) A disability resulting from brain injury before, during, or shortly after birth.

cognitive disability Damage or deterioration in any portion of the brain that affects the ability to process information, coordinate and control the body, and/or move in space.

deaf Partially or completely incapable of hearing.

disability Any restriction in or lack of ability to perform an activity in the manner or within the range considered normal for a human being.

disarticulation An amputation that occurs at a joint.

Down syndrome A common genetic condition resulting in mental and physical anomalies.

dyslexia Condition characterized by a significant delay in one or more areas of learning.

dystonic cerebral palsy A condition in which an individual's muscles are extremely rigid.

epilepsy Recurrent episodes of seizures caused by an abnormal focus of electrical activity within the brain that may cause impaired responsiveness, abnormal movements, or psychic, sensory, or autonomic disturbances.

handicapped A term used to describe a person with an impairment that substantially limits one or more of life's activities.

impairment Any loss or abnormality of psychological, physiologic, or anatomic structure or function.

learning disorders A lack of order or impairment with learning skills.

manic-depressive A mentally ill person with a cyclic affective psychosis in which there are alternating moods of depression and mania (madness, characterized by excessive excitement).

mental retardation (MR) A below average intellectual capacity from birth or childhood associated with difficulties in learning and socialization.

multiple sclerosis (MS) A neurologic condition that causes weakness or paralysis of the extremities, loss of stamina, and balance difficulties.

muscular dystrophy (MD) Progressive and irreversible muscle wasting.

ostomy bag An appliance that attaches by special adhesive to the abdominal wall of some people who have had abdominal surgery.

postpolio syndrome After-effects of poliomyelitis, a viral infection of the spinal cord which may cause either broadly distributed or local paralysis. Years after the initial paralysis, the person may exhibit fatigue, shortness of breath, and balance problems.

psychosis Any severe mental disorder characterized by deterioration of normal intellectual and social functioning and by partial or complete withdrawal from reality.

schizophrenia A group of mental disorders characterized by disturbances of thinking, mood, and behavior. With schizophrenia, there is an altered concept of reality and in some cases delusions and hallucinations. Mood changes include inappropriate emotional responses and loss of empathy. Withdrawn, regressive, and bizarre behavior may be noted.

spastic cerebral palsy A condition in which there is constant involuntary contraction of an individual's muscles.

spina bifida (SB) A congenital malformation of the spinal column (usually the bony spine in the same area) in which segments of the spine fail to fuse, allowing the spinal cord to protrude.

spinal cord injury (SCI) Damage to the spinal cord resulting from trauma.

stoma A port created on the abdominal wall to facilitate excrement. This term is also used to describe an opening in the neck that connects the trachea directly to the skin.

stroke and brain trauma A condition that results when part of the brain becomes anoxic from loss of blood supply.

visual impairment Disability involving reduction or loss of vision, usually described in terms of acuity or range. Classifications include legal blindness, partial sightedness, or total blindness.

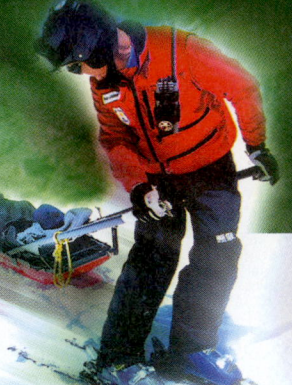

Assessment in Action

An expert skier on a mono-ski was taking a bump run, caught an edge, and tipped over on the hard edge of a bump. He also put out his hand while holding an outrigger to break the fall, and felt his shoulder jolt as he hit. The temperature is about 32º F. The skier is affixed to the mono-ski so that any movements the skier makes will be transmitted through the seat to the ski.

The skier's vital signs are stable. You suspect a fractured wrist and dislocated shoulder. The skier's lower body is strapped to the mono-ski while the patient's upper body is on the snow.

1. Given the mechanism of injury and his special equipment, how serious is this patient's problem?
   A. Not serious; he is alert and oriented
   B. Serious; he is alert and oriented
   C. Serious; he has a fracture and dislocation
   D. Not serious; he has a fracture and dislocation

2. As part of the history taking, which question may indicate the presence of another immediate problem?
   A. When did you eat last?
   B. Why did you fall?
   C. Are you on any medications?
   D. Are you allergic to anything?

3. To assess the patient's complaints adequately, questions should be phrased as:
   A. simple yes-no questions.
   B. all open-ended questions.
   C. specific questions with choices.
   D. written down—these patients will not understand language.

4. After correctly identifying the patient's condition, what is the appropriate treatment for the dislocated shoulder?
   A. Cervical collar and backboard
   B. Improvised stabilization in a position of least discomfort
   C. Quick splint
   D. Load and go

5. What is the best toboggan placement given the terrain and the injury?
   A. Head uphill
   B. Head downhill
   C. Patient on side with no injuries
   D. Patient sitting up

Challenging Questions

6. If this sit-down skier had ataxia, what other concerns and solutions would you have for your transportation plan?

7. If you had to evacuate this individual out of a back bowl requiring an up-load before coming down on the front side of the mountain, what risk management issues would need to be addressed?

Points to Ponder

A skier who is visually impaired has collided with another skier. The blind skier has severe facial abrasions from hitting the snow and has a lower-leg fracture that hurts if she tries to move it. Otherwise, her vitals are stable. The other skier has stress-induced asthma and is having an attack as the rescuer arrives. The blind skier's guide is trying to ward off approaching traffic.

What steps should you take to verify scene safety? What risk management concerns will need to be reported to area management? What is the appropriate use of rescuers and the guide in the emergency care and transport of these two patients?

Issues Scene Safety, Determining Risk, Decision-Making Skills, Communication, Emotional Well-Being of Patients, Calming Excited Participants

Online Outlook

In order to provide effective treatment to the growing number of outdoor adaptive athletes, all rescuers must have an increased understanding of mentally and physically challenged patients. Learn more about adaptive athletes, the activities they engage in, and the equipment that they use by completing Exercise 31 at **www.OECzone.com**.

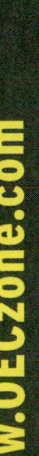

Appendix A

Scenarios

Warren D. Bowman, MD, FACP

Contents

Patient Assessment and Life Support Interventions

Scenario 1

The following scenario is about a patient who responds in a hostile manner toward the rescuer—a situation that is stressful and sometimes difficult to deal with.

You have just brought a toboggan down to a reported incident scene. As you approach the site, you see a young woman lying on the snow crying loudly. One leg and foot, with the ski attached and binding unreleased, is doubled under her other leg at an abnormal angle.

The leg looks broken to you. Several of her friends surround her. You stop the toboggan below her and anchor it with your skis. As you approach the patient, you see a fellow patroller, Mike, come over the rise and head for the site.

You: "Miss, I'm Charlie Dole of the High Range Ski Patrol. Can I help you?" (After putting on a pair of rubber gloves, you reach for her wrist to check her pulse, but she pulls her hand away and continues to cry.) "Miss, I'm here to help you. What's happened?"

Patient: "Don't touch me! My leg is broken—I know it's broken. Get me an orthopaedic surgeon right away. Call a helicopter!"

You: "Miss, if you'll let Mike and me help you, we can take your ski off and look at your leg."

Patient: "Who are you? How do I know you have any training? I'm a nursing student, and I can tell if you know what you're doing."

You: "Miss, I've been trained in Outdoor Emergency Care to take care of ski accidents, and I've been patrolling at High Range Ski Area for 20 years. It looks like you've hurt your leg. We can put a splint on it and take you to the bottom of the mountain in just a few minutes, then get you to a hospital if necessary." (At this, the patient cries louder.) "The first thing we'd better do is to get that ski off. I'm sure it's making your leg hurt worse than it would otherwise."

Patient: "Don't touch me! I want you to call a helicopter right now. My father is a lawyer."

You: "I'm sorry, Miss. We can't land a helicopter here because the slope is too steep and the trees are too close together. Even if we could, it would take 45 minutes to get here. If you'll let us put a splint on your leg, it will feel much better." (At this point, you decide to try calming the patient by distracting her from her injury.) "What's your name?"

Patient: "Sue Happy."

You: "Where do you live, Sue?"

Patient: "Dust Bins, Oklahoma."

You: "Where do you go to nursing school?"

Patient: "The One-Horse Hospital and Health Center."

You: "What year are you?"

Patient: "My first year."

You: "You probably know a lot about anatomy. Show me where your leg hurts."

Patient: "Right there." (The patient points to her leg.)

You: "Can you feel your toes? Can you wiggle them?"

Patient: "Yes."

You: "Let me check your pulse." (This time she lets you palpate her radial pulse, which is normal.) "Have you ever studied first aid?"

Patient: "Not since I was in Girl Scouts."

You: "How did you hurt your leg?"

Patient: "I was skiing over to the side when I lost my balance. I must have twisted my leg when I fell. I heard it snap."

You: "We can carefully straighten your leg and put a splint on it. You know that will help."

Patient: "But that's going to hurt!"

You: "It'll only hurt temporarily while we're straightening it, but it's going to feel better as soon as we get the splint on. Let's get that ski off. Mike, will you steady the boot, please?" (Mike steadies the boot, and you release the binding and remove the ski. Then, you carefully unbuckle the tight boot and rebuckle it at a looser setting.) "That's better, isn't it?"

Patient (reluctantly): "Maybe. What are you going to do next?"

At this point, you take a bit more charge of the situation and ignore her question. Instead, you continue to question her about her condition.

You: "Did you hit your head or hurt your neck or back? Did you hurt yourself anywhere else?"

Patient: "No."

You: "I'm going to check your leg very carefully to see what's going on."

The patient offers no objection, and you gently palpate her leg and thigh through her ski pants. There is no blood on the outer clothing. There is a tender swelling and moderate angulation of the leg just above the top of the boot, and her foot is rotated abnormally inward. When you ask, "Does that bother you?" she says no. You take a quick splint from the toboggan and open it on the snow beside her.

Patient: "What are you doing?"

You: "This is the splint we're going to use. As you can see, it's padded and won't pinch your leg. It will keep your leg from moving and prevent any further damage. It goes on very quickly and fastens with Velcro straps."

Patient: "Do you have to move my leg?"

You: "We'll have to straighten it to get the splint on, but it should be straightened anyway to help the circulation." (The patient starts to cry again.) "We'll show you how we do it, and we'll tell you everything we're going to do before we do it. This is the type of thing you'll need to know how to do as a nurse, too."

You radio the base and tell them that you are putting a splint on an injured leg and request that the physician on call with the doctors' patrol meet you at the base in a few minutes. While you are working, you briefly ask the patient about any allergies, medicines, and chronic illnesses. The answers are all negative and the patient tells you that her most recent meal was the two Twinkies and Coke she had about 3 hours ago.

Patient: "I'm getting cold. I feel dizzy."

You take a blanket from the toboggan, put it around her shoulders, and recheck her pulse, which is still strong with the rate unchanged.

You: "The sooner we get you off the hill, the better you'll feel."

You and Mike are able to straighten her injured leg and apply the quick splint, although the patient continues to cry. However, she clearly feels better with the splint in place, and you are able to lift her into the toboggan and take her down the hill to the aid room.

At the aid room, the patient is seen by Dr. Karen Fixx of the doctors' patrol. She asks to see the doctor's credentials, then refuses to let the doctor examine her because she is not an orthopaedist. The doctor persuades her with some difficulty to have her leg x-rayed and a cast applied at a local hospital rather than to make the 36-hour trip back home in the ski bus, wearing a temporary splint.

Scenario 2

The following scenario provides an example of how to conduct the urgent survey and prepare a patient for transport in a toboggan.

You are answering a radio message from the base about a skier who fell on Big Elk Run just below its juncture with Little Elk Run. As you ski up, you see a teenage girl sitting in the snow, holding her right knee. Both skis are off and she is surrounded by three of her friends. There is no blood on the snow.

You: "Hi, I'm Ben Schussen of the High Range Ski Patrol. Can I help you? What's your name?"

While talking, you take off your skis and approach the girl.

Patient: "Oh, I'm so glad to see you! My name is Eileen Ann Wintz. I fell and really hurt my knee."

You: (Observing her face, noting that the skin is dry and ruddy from the cold): "Excuse me a minute, Eileen. I'm going to put your skis up in the snow to warn uphill skiers to ski around us."

You form an upright X with the patient's skis uphill from the accident. Then, you radio for a toboggan and return to the patient. As you talk to the patient, you grasp her wrist and note that her pulse is strong, regular, and has a normal rate. Her breathing appears normal too.

You: "You hurt your right knee?"

Patient: "Yes. I was trying a turn, and one ski went one way and one went the other. I fell down between them."

You: "Did your bindings release?"

Patient: "Yes, both of them, but my knee twisted when I fell down."

You: "Did you feel a pop in your knee when you fell?"

Patient: "No."

By this time, you have established that Eileen's airway, breathing, circulation, and level of responsiveness are normal. As you expected, there is no obvious severe bleeding. You have assessed her facial color and moisture, her pulse, and the temperature, color, and moisture of the skin of her wrist, all of which are normal. The mechanism of injury does not suggest the possibility of a serious injury, but there are two more questions you need to ask.

You: "Did you hurt your head, neck, or back when you fell?"

Patient: "No."

You: "Did you hurt yourself anywhere else?"

Patient: "No."

It is now time for you to assess the site of major complaint.

You: "I've called for a toboggan so we can give you a ride down the hill. Let me put my jacket around you to keep you warm. I'll also loosen your boots. While we're waiting, I'll take a look at your knee. Can you feel your toes okay?" (The patient says yes.) "Can you wiggle them?" (She nods affirmatively.)

You put on a pair of rubber gloves and examine the patient's knee through her ski pants, noting that there is no swelling, torn clothing, or sign of blood. You palpate the major ligaments around the knee.

You: "Does your knee hurt here? How about here? Here?"

Patient: "It's a bit tender here." (The patient indicates the inner [medial] part of the joint).

You: "Here comes the toboggan. We'll put a splint on your leg to stabilize your knee and make you more comfortable while we give you a ride down to the patrol room."

Scenario 3

In this scenario, the urgent survey of a more seriously injured patient unfolds.

You are patrolling the upper part of High Range Mountain when you intercept a radio message that a skier is down in the trees on the left side of upper Big Elk Run. You notify the base that you can handle the call.

As you approach the scene, you see several skiers gathered at the side of the run. A skier is lying on his side with his chest and left arm against a large tree about 10′ off the run. A set of ski tracks leads from the edge of the run to the skier; both skis are off. As you approach, you see that the patient's eyes are closed and his breathing is fast and shallow. You quickly get out of your bindings and approach the patient.

You: "Hi, I'm Justin Thyme of the High Range Ski Patrol. Do you need some help?"

Patient (opening his eyes): "Yes, thanks, I'm hurting bad…" (panting) "…in my right side and…can't breathe."

You reach over and perform a one-handed jaw thrust to open the airway, but the patient's breathing doesn't improve. You ask the patient what happened as you grasp his wrist and feel the radial pulse, which is strong and regular but faster than normal. The patient's face is pale and there are beads of perspiration on his forehead.

Patient (panting): "Not sure…was skiing the powder…along the side and lost it….Went in the woods and hit this tree."

You: "What's your name?"

Patient: "Mark Sitz."

You: "Mark, did you hit your head, neck, or back, or knock yourself out?"

Patient: "No, just hit my side."

By this time, you've determined that the patient's airway is open, he's breathing, and he has a pulse and normal level of responsiveness. However, his breathing is labored and his pulse is rapid, and you suspect that the patient may have a serious injury.

You: "Excuse me a minute. I'll call for a toboggan to get you off the hill."

You key in to base on the radio.

You: "Thyme to Summit, copy?"(Summit replies.) "I have an accident at location M-5 on upper Big Elk run. I need a toboggan, oxygen, a trauma kit, a long backboard, and some help."

You then ask one of the onlookers to set up the patient's skis in an upright X at the side of the run.

Patient (panting): "Tell them to hurry….I'm feeling worse."

You: "Hold still right as you are, Mark. I need to check you some more and ask you some questions."

You put on a pair of rubber gloves and assess the patient's head. There are no abnormalities of the scalp, both pupils are equal, there is no discharge from the nose or ears, and the mouth appears normal. You then assess his neck. There are no areas of tenderness, particularly over the spinous processes, and no crepitation, swelling, or other abnormalities. The trachea is in the midline.

Moving quickly, you open the patient's jacket and pull up his turtleneck and longjohn shirt. Assessing the chest from the top down, you note that the right side of his chest is not moving as well as the left. There is a bruise over the lower right ribs laterally, extending down onto the upper right lateral abdomen. Palpation reveals a crackling sensation in the skin over several ribs.

You then pull the patient's clothing back down over his chest and expose his upper abdomen. He is quite tender in the right upper quadrant. There is no pain from pressure on the iliac crests.

While you do this, you ask him about any allergies,

medicines, or drugs he's taken, and any history of significant illness. All answers are negative.

You now have a good idea of what has happened. The patient must have been traveling quite fast and collided with a tree, hitting his right chest and abdomen. As a result, several ribs are broken and there is some crepitation, indicating injury to the underlying lung. He also has tenderness in the right upper quadrant, raising the possibility of liver injury. He is in respiratory distress and has signs of early shock, possibly from internal bleeding since there is no obvious external bleeding. He is seriously injured and needs to be taken to a hospital as soon as possible.

You: "Thyme to hill chief, copy?" (The hill chief replies.) "We need an ALS ambulance to meet us at the aid room. Would you please page Dr. Caduceus of the doctors' patrol and ask him to meet us there also?" (The hill chief affirms, and you turn back to the patient.) "Mark, do you hurt anywhere else besides your chest and right side?"

Patient: "No."

You quickly palpate the patient's extremities and find nothing abnormal.

You: "Can you move your legs and feet and wiggle your toes?"

Patient: "Yes."

You: "Do your hands or feet feel numb or tingly?"

Patient: "No."

You ask the patient to move his arms, which he is able to do, and to squeeze your hands, which he is also able to do. As you gently pinch the skin of his anterior thighs through his ski pants, you ask him whether he can feel it. The patient responds that he can, so you gently pinch the skin on the backs of both of his hands. The patient indicates that he can feel that, too, and that both sides feel the same.

Next, you palpate his back, paying particular attention to the spinous processes. There is no deformity and no tenderness except in the right flank.

You have now established that, despite the serious nature of the accident, there appear to be no additional injuries, particularly to the head, neck, or back. Ideally, the patient should be strapped to a long backboard because of the mechanism of injury; however, it is unlikely that he will be able to breathe well enough in that position.

You: "I'll loosen your boots so you'll be more comfortable. Here comes the toboggan. We'll give you some

oxygen so you can breathe easier, and we'll be on our way down in a few minutes."

Scenario 4

The following scenario describes how to assess a responsive patient with a common medical illness.

You and three climbing friends have just finished a 2-day trip on skis from the trailhead to Diorite Peak (13,000'), the highest summit in the Granite range. You plan to spend the night in a snow cave at about 11,000' and do a winter climb of the 1,500' south face the next day.

Your alarm watch goes off at 4 a.m. and you awake to hear your friend Lucky coughing. You reach for a match to light a candle. The light reveals that he is flushed and appears ill.

You: "Hey, are you feeling okay?"

Patient: "Not really."

You: "What's the matter?"

Patient: "My throat was starting to feel scratchy after we ate last night. I've been hurting all over and feeling hot and cold. I didn't sleep at all. Now my throat is so sore I can hardly swallow, my head hurts, my chest hurts, and I'm coughing up some awful stuff."

You: "Have you had an earache, stuffy nose, or drainage down the back of your throat?" (While talking, you place your hand on his forehead; the skin is hot.)

Patient: "No."

You next check the patient's pulse, which is strong, regular, and somewhat faster than normal, which is consistent with both fever and the altitude.

You: "Any nausea, diarrhea, or painful urination?"

Patient: "No, I feel bad enough without anything else."

You note that the patient is breathing at a normal rate and without difficulty.

You: "Where does your chest hurt?"

Patient: "Right in the middle." (The patient points to his sternum.)

You get the emergency care kit and a flashlight out of your pack and ask Lucky to open his eyes wide and look straight ahead. His pupils are round, regular, and equal, and both respond to light.

You then ask him to open his mouth and say "ah." Aiming the flashlight, you use a spoon from the cook kit as a tongue blade so you can inspect his mouth and throat. You can see that his throat is red, his tonsils are swollen and red with white spots on them, and his uvula is swollen. When you take his temperature, the thermometer registers 100.5°F.

You: "You have a fever, Lucky."

Patient: "Yeah, well, I feel hot."

You feel under both sides of the patient's jaw and down both sides of his neck. There is a tender, almond-sized enlargement under the right jaw angle.

You: "Does this feel sore anywhere?"

Patient: "Yes, on that right side."

You ask the patient to put his chin on his chest. He is able to do so easily, indicating that his neck is not stiff.

You tell the patient you want to listen to his chest, and you unzip his shirt and pull up his undershirt, laying your ear on the upper and lower parts of the anterior chest, then the posterior chest. You hear a few scattered rattles on both sides as he breathes in and out. He coughs and the rattles clear.

It is now evident that Lucky has a significant infection—probably tonsillitis and bronchitis. There is no indication of gastroenteritis or a urinary tract infection, which are other possible causes of fever on backcountry trips. You're worried that the altitude might aggravate his condition. Fortunately, his pulse, respirations, and level of responsiveness are normal.

There will be no climbing for him today. He needs to stay in base camp in his sleeping bag, with one of the other party members to watch him. He will need water, simple food, and some mild pain medicine such as aspirin, acetaminophen, or ibuprofen. If his physician has prescribed an antibiotic for his emergency care kit, he should probably take it.

With good luck, the patient will be better tomorrow and able to ski back out, although part of his pack may have to be distributed among the other party members. With bad luck, he will be worse, and two party members will have to ski out to get help since the party is too small to pull him the 12 miles out on an improvised toboggan. The group also should consider moving the camp to a lower altitude if that would be logistically feasible.

Scenario 5

This scenario illustrates the assessment of a patient with a more serious medical condition.

You are having a cup of hot tea in the patrol room after bringing down a patient with an injured knee. The telephone rings; it is the cafeteria manager. "Ski Patrol? We need someone up here in the cafeteria to help a man who has passed out."

You grab your radio and patrol belt and jog outside, across the snow to the nearby cafeteria. Inside, a crowd of onlookers is gathered around a portly, elderly man lying on his side on the floor. A distraught woman is kneeling at his side. There's a tray on the floor with overturned dishes, a large cinnamon bun, and spilled soup nearby.

The patient is obviously breathing, with deep, slow, and noisy respirations. He breathes through his mouth, and as he exhales, his right cheek puffs out more than his left. His eyes are closed and his face is flushed. You notice that the right side of his face seems smoother than the left.

You: "Hi, I'm Connie Serned of the High Range Ski Patrol. What's happened here?"

Woman: "It's my husband. He was eating lunch and he just slumped down in his chair and slid onto the floor. I can't get him to say anything."

You: "Did he hit his head, neck, or back when he fell?"

Woman: "I don't think so."

You put on a pair of gloves, and as you steady the patient's forehead with one hand and shake his shoulder gently with the other, you ask him whether he is okay. The patient moans weakly. You note that the skin of his forehead is dry and warm and his color is normal. You perform the jaw-thrust maneuver with the one-handed technique. The patient's respirations become noticeably less noisy.

You: "Has anything like this happened to him before?"

Woman: "No."

As you remove your hand from the patient's jaw, you notice that his respirations remain easier and quieter. You radio the patrol room, requesting a stretcher, oxygen, suction, some help, and an ambulance to meet you at the aid room.

You: "What's your husband's name?"

Woman: "Sid Enterry."

As you assess the patient's carotid pulse, you note that it is strong and regular at a rate that appears slightly faster than normal.

You: "How old is he?"

Woman: "He's 62."

You: "Was he having any type of trouble before this happened—headache, dizziness, chest pain, or anything?"

Woman: "He didn't say anything about that."

You: "Does he have any medical conditions that I should know about?"

Woman: "He's had high blood pressure for years, but he takes medicine for it. I believe it's called lisinopril."

You: "Any heart disease, diabetes, or stroke?"

Woman: "He has some mild diabetes, but he controls it with diet."

You: "Is he taking any other medicines or drugs?"

Woman: "No."

As you assess the patient's pupils with a flashlight you note that they are both round, equal in size, and react to light.

You: "Does he have any allergies?"

Woman: "No."

You: "I'm going to check his arms and legs to see if he moves them normally."

Taking each of his hands in one of your own, you ask the patient to squeeze your hands. Nothing happens. You then pinch the index finger of each hand between your thumb and forefinger. The patient withdraws his left arm but not his right. Next, you pinch the skin of each leg. He withdraws his left leg but not his right.

You can now sum up the situation: An elderly man with a history of high blood pressure and mild diabetes collapses suddenly while eating. He is partly responsive, with a V rating on the AVPU scale. His airway is open, so this isn't a case of food aspiration. His circulation is good. He appears to move less well in response to pain on the right side than the left. He probably has had a stroke and has a paralyzed right side (right hemiplegia).

You hesitate to put an oral airway in place, since he probably has a gag reflex and you don't have anything with you to suction him if he vomits. Anyway, he is moving air well and is already on his side in the recovery position.

You: "Is there anything else about your husband that I should know?"

Woman: "No, I can't think of anything. He's always been so healthy."

You: "Here come some of our people with a stretcher. We're going to give him some oxygen and take him down to the aid room. I've called an ambulance and we'll get him to the hospital as soon as possible."

Woman: "What do you think has happened?"

You: "I'm not sure, Ma'am, but we'll take good care of him until the ambulance gets here."

Bleeding and Shock
Scenario 6

This scenario illustrates the assessment and emergency care of an injured skier in shock.

You're about to get on the upper lift at High Range Ski Area when you hear a transmission that a skier is down on Mad Dog, a black diamond run on the lower mountain. You duck under the rope and ski to the trail, which is 100 yards away off the east cat track. You stop and look down; there's an X in the center of the run about two thirds of the way to the bottom, with a small group of skiers nearby.

A minute later you're close enough to see a skier lying on her side below a large mogul. You don't see any blood on the snow. You remove your skis and approach the downed skier. Her face looks pale, her eyes are closed, and her respirations are easy but fast. You grasp her wrist and note that her radial pulse is strong and fast.

You: "Miss, are you okay?"

Patient: "No, something's wrong. My left side is hurt."

You: "I'm Bonnie Waydell of the High Range Ski Patrol. Can I help you?"

Patient: "Yes, please."

You: "What happened?"

Patient: "I lost an edge on the ice on the downside of that bump and hit my left side hard. It hurts to breathe."

You: "Were you feeling okay before that happened?"

Patient: "Yes."

You: "Did you hit your head?"

Patient: "I may have—I don't know."

You: "Were you knocked out at all?"

Patient: "No."

You: "Did you hurt your neck or back?"

Patient: "No."

You: "Do you hurt anywhere else?"

Patient: "No."

You reach for your radio and call base.

You: "Waydell to Midway, copy?" (Midway replies.) "I need a toboggan, oxygen, suction, and at least two more patrollers to help. I'm on Mad Dog, two thirds of the way to the bottom." (Midway confirms.)

Turning to the patient, you put your hand on her forehead; it's cool and clammy.

You: "What's your name?"

Patient: "Helen Wheels."

You: "Where are you from, Helen?"

Patient: "Dallas."

You: "Do you know today's date and what day it is?"

Patient: "It's Friday, March 13."

You: "I need to check a few things, if it's all right with you."

The patient nods in assent, so you put on a pair of gloves, pull down the neck of her turtleneck and note that her neck looks normal: there are no wounds, tenderness, lumps, or bleeding, and in particular, no tenderness of the spinous processes. The trachea is in the midline, and there are no obvious abnormalities to palpation of the upper chest.

You pull up her turtleneck and longjohn top. Her lower chest also looks normal and both sides are moving equally. Quickly, you feel the ribs on both sides one by one, finding no lumps or tenderness.

You pull her clothes back down and unfasten the belt of her jeans. The upper abdomen looks normal. Slipping your hand under her clothing, you carefully palpate her abdomen, starting in the right upper quadrant and moving clockwise. She's very tender in the left upper quadrant and the muscles are tight in this area. At this point, she starts to retch and vomits in the snow. The vomit appears to be the contents of a recent meal; there is no sign of blood.

You stop a moment and think. The patient is alert and oriented, but her pulse is fast and her breathing is fast, although not labored. Her radial pulse is strong, so her blood pressure is at least 80 mm Hg. Her chest appears normal, but she's very tender in her left upper abdomen, where she hit when she fell.

You recheck the pulse again, counting it this time. Pulse is 130 beats/min and seems weaker than before. Something is going on; possibly internal bleeding that is causing early shock.

You radio the hill chief and request an ambulance.

You: "The toboggan will be coming soon and we'll take you down to the aid room."

Patient: "I'm feeling really weak and dizzy."

You: "I'm going to check some other areas and ask you some more questions while we're waiting, if you don't mind."

Patient: "Okay."

You assess the patient's head. There are no signs of wounds or bleeding on her face and no swelling, tenderness, or lumps on her scalp. You tell the patient that you are going to shine a light in her eyes to check her pupils; you find that her pupils are round, regular, and equal. There is no bleeding or discharge from her ears. You ask her to open her mouth; there is no bleeding and her teeth look regular.

You: "Have you had any chronic medical conditions such as diabetes, epilepsy, or heart trouble?"

Patient: "No."

You move on to the patient's pelvis, pressing on the iliac crests from side to side and the pelvis from back to front.

You: "Does this hurt?"

Patient: "No."

You: "Did you hurt your arms or legs when you fell?"

Patient: "No, just my side."

You palpate her lower extremities through her clothing and find nothing abnormal. You then palpate her upper extremities through her clothing and again find nothing abnormal. As you are doing this, you continue to ask the patient questions.

You: "Are you taking any drugs or medicines regularly?"

Patient: "No."

You: "Any allergies?"

Patient: "No."

You: "Is there anything else about you I should know?"

Patient: "Well, I'm just getting over a case of mono. You know, the doctor told me my spleen was enlarged and I shouldn't ski or play any contact sports."

You: "Oh?"

Patient: "I already had my tickets for here and they aren't refundable. It's spring break, so I decided to come anyway. Maybe I shouldn't have."

You: "Maybe not."

You palpate her spinous processes through her jacket, from the base of the head to the sacrum, finding no tenderness or deformities. As you are doing this, the toboggan arrives.

You: "Here's the toboggan. We'll lift you into it and be on our way. We're going to put you in with your head at the front end so you won't feel so weak and dizzy. We'll give you some oxygen to help your breathing."

Shortly afterward, the patient was examined in the local hospital emergency department and admitted. At surgery, she was found to have a ruptured spleen with several liters of blood in the peritoneal cavity.

Skin and Soft-Tissue Injuries, Burns, and Bandaging

Scenario 7.

The following scenario illustrates the care of two different types of wounds.

It's a beautiful spring day, and a foot of powder fell the night before. You are getting off the upper lift at High Range Ski Area when you receive a transmission about a skier who is hurt and bleeding in the trees on the left side of Autobahn about two thirds of the way down. You wave to the patroller on duty at the top and radio that you are taking a toboggan down to check it out.

As you arrive at the incident scene, you see a man lying in the snow at the edge of the run. There is obvious blood in the snow near his head; his skis are still on. You park the toboggan below the skier and anchor it with your skis.

As you approach, you can see that his eyes are open and he's breathing. His hat is off and there's blood dripping onto the snow from a large laceration on the left side of his head. There's also a large tear in his left sleeve, and there is blood on his glove.

You: "Hi, I'm Ben Schussen of the High Range Ski Patrol. Can I help you?"

Patient: "Yes."

You put on a pair of rubber gloves, grasp the patient's uninjured forearm, and assess the radial pulse. It is strong and regular; the rate appears normal.

You: "What happened?"

Patient: "I guess I clipped a tree."

You: "Did you just clip it or actually hit it head on?"

Patient: "I think I just got too close to it and one of the branches cut my head. It knocked me down, though."

You: "Skiing the powder along the edge, eh? What's your name?"

Patient: "Otto Control."

You: "Did you hit your head at all?"

Patient: "No."

You: "Were you knocked out?"

Patient: "No."

You: "Does your neck or back hurt?"

Patient: "No."

You: "Do you know where you are and what day it is?"

Patient: "It's Saturday and I'm at High Range."

You: "You're bleeding from a cut on your head. I need to get that stopped."

You take off your emergency care belt, open it, and take out a flashlight, a Swiss Army knife, a packet containing a sterile alcohol pad, three 3″ × 4″ sterile packages of Telfa, a tongue blade, and a roll of 2″ Kling. You assess the patient's head and find a 3″ laceration just above the hairline on the left forehead, bleeding freely. There are three large pieces of bark in the wound. The skin of the patient's forehead is warm and there are a few beads of sweat on it.

You clean the forceps of your knife with alcohol and then use them to remove the three pieces of bark. You then take the compresses out of their packages and place them over the wound. Holding pressure on the wound with one hand, you feel the rest of the scalp carefully; there are no other injuries.

After a minute, you note that the bleeding has stopped. Holding the compresses in place, you retrieve the patient's cap and put it carefully back on his head. The compresses stay in place, and there is no further obvious bleeding.

You then assess the rest of the patient's head, using the flashlight to check both pupils and look in the mouth, ears, and nose. The scalp has no additional abnormalities. The pupils are round and equal, and there is no bleeding or clear drainage coming from the nose or ears. You also examine the patient's mouth with the assistance of the tongue blade; the mouth appears normal.

Moving down, you assess the neck and find no wounds, swelling, tenderness, or other abnormalities. In particular, there is no tenderness over the spinous processes.

You: "Did you hit your chest or abdomen?"

Patient: "No."

You: "I need to take a look at your arm; there's blood on your sleeve and glove, and your sleeve is torn. Does your arm hurt?"

Patient: "Yes. I didn't even notice that."

You: "Do you hurt anywhere else?"

Patient: "No."

You: "Are you feeling cold?"

Patient: "No."

You remove the patient's glove, and with a pair of paramedic shears, you enlarge the tear in the arm of his windshirt and longjohn top to expose the forearm. There's a 1″ puncture wound with a 2″ piece of a tree branch sticking out of it. It's oozing a little blood, and there's blood over most of the distal forearm. The patient's radial pulse is strong and unchanged. After noting the quality of his pulse, you ask him about allergies, medications, preexisting illnesses, and his last meal. The answers are all negative, and he ate 3 hours ago.

At this point, a fellow patroller arrives. You ask her to remove the patient's skis. She places them in an upright X uphill from the accident and loosens the patient's boots.

You: "Can you wiggle your fingers on your left hand?" (The patient does so.) "Make a fist, and then spread your fingers like this." (The patient imitates you.) "Does your hand feel numb or tingly?"

Patient: "No."

You take two more sterile compresses and use them to stabilize the branch in the wound, covering the wound. You take a cravat and a 3″ roll of Kling from your emergency care belt, form the cravat into a donut, and lay it over the compresses. You use the Kling to wrap around the forearm, holding the cravat, the compresses, and the impaled object in place.

You can now pause and review the situation. The patient is alert and oriented, and although he has a scalp laceration, he has no sign of a serious head or neck injury. His breathing and circulation are normal, and there is no airway problem. He had significant bleeding from the scalp wound, although it wasn't enough to produce hypovolemic shock. This bleeding is now controlled. He also has an impalement injury in his forearm that did not bleed significantly. There is no evidence of damage to nerves and blood vessels from the arm injury, which is now stabilized and bandaged.

The other patroller has brought the toboggan closer to the patient. However, because of the mechanism of injury, before the patient is moved you need to finish the rapid body survey to make sure there are no other significant injuries.

You assess the patient's chest and abdomen through his clothing. You find no bleeding, swelling, or tenderness, and both sides of the chest move equally. You then assess the injured extremity and the three uninjured extremities through the patient's clothing. There is no tenderness, swelling, or deformity. As you move from one extremity to the next, you ask the patient whether it hurts, and each time he answers no. As you pinch each arm and leg, you ask whether the patient can feel the pinch. The patient says he can.

You: "Does it feel the same on both sides?"

Patient: "Yes."

You: "Can you feel your fingers and toes?"

Patient: "Yes."

You: "Can you wiggle them?"

Patient: "Yes."

As you begin to assess the patient's back, you ask him whether he has any pain in his back, and he says no. You quickly run your hand down his back to his tailbone, asking as you go whether anything feels tender. There are no tender spots, step-off deformities, or swelling.

It is now time to load the skier into the toboggan and take him to the patrol room, where the nonurgent survey can be carried out.

Emergency Care of Bone and Joint Injuries: General Principles

Scenario 8

The following scenario illustrates the care of two types of injuries to bones.

You have just received a transmission from the hill chief asking you to check out a jump some skiers have made on an ungroomed run just below the summit. As you approach, you see a group of teenage boys gathered at the top of a narrow run leading to a mound of heaped snow. One boy is preparing to push off from the top of the run. To your experienced eye, the landing area below the mound looks like it is very close to a small rock pile.

Before you can get within shouting distance, the skier is on the run and heading swiftly for the jump. His form doesn't look good to you, and as he sails off the top of the mound, his balance is off. When he lands, he bounces off a large rock, falls, and starts to scream. One of his companions waiting below starts sidestepping up to him.

You arrive at the patient's side, kick out of your bindings, and stick your skis in the snow in the form of an upright X. You quickly approach the skier, who is lying on his back, moaning softly, with his left thigh bent at an abnormal angle.

You: "I'm Ben Schussen of the High Range Ski Patrol. Can I help you?"

Patient: "My leg is killing me! Oh, please…it hurts!"

You remove one of the patient's gloves and assess his radial pulse; it's strong, regular, and slightly faster than normal. His breathing appears easy and quiet but faster than normal.

You: "I saw you land. Did you hurt yourself anywhere else besides your thigh?"

Patient (moaning): "My back hurts between my shoulder blades."

You radio for a toboggan, backboard, trauma pack, traction splint, oxygen, suction, and some help.

You: "Did you hit your head?"

Patient: "No."

You: "Did you hurt your neck?"

Patient: "No."

You: "Lie as still as you can until we get some help and can get you down the hill. What's your name?"

Patient: "Dan Jerass."

You: "Where are you from, Dan?"

Patient: "Denver."

You: "Do you know the date and what day it is?"

Patient: "Saturday, March 3rd."

You are satisfied that the patient's airway is normal. He's alert, his breathing is adequate, and his circulation is normal. It's time to examine the areas of complaint: the patient's thigh and back. You put on a pair of latex gloves.

You: "I'm going to examine your thigh, Dan. I'll let you know everything I do before I do it."

You gently palpate the patient's left thigh starting at the groin. He winces when you reach the midthigh and you believe there is a bulge there. You compare it with the same area of the right thigh and see that there is definitely a difference.

You continue down the thigh and palpate the knee and leg. There are no obvious additional abnormalities. You then assess the right lower extremity; it appears normal.

You: "Can you feel your left foot?"

Patient: "Yes."

You: "Can you wiggle your toes?"

Patient: "Yes."

You: "Next, I'm going to run my hand behind your neck and back. Let me know if I hit a tender spot. Try not to move."

You gently palpate each spinous process in turn from the base of the skull to the lower sacrum. There is definite tenderness over two of the midthoracic spinous processes.

So far there is no sign of the toboggan and no other patrollers have arrived yet. Because of the positive mechanism of injury, you proceed with the rest of the rapid body survey.

You: "Dan, were you feeling okay before you wiped out?"

Patient: "Sure."

You: "Are you taking any medicines for anything? Any drugs?"

The patient answers no. You start assessing his scalp, face, eyes, ears, nose, and mouth. There are no signs of wounds, bleeding, tenderness, or swelling. His pupils are equal and respond to light. There is no bleeding or discharge from his nose and ears, and you don't see any obvious abnormalities in his mouth.

You: "Do you have any chronic illnesses or medical problems we should know about?"

Patient: "No, I've always been real healthy."

Moving down to the patient's neck, you find no wounds, bleeding, tenderness, or swelling. The trachea is in the midline.

You: "Any allergies?"

Patient: "No."

By the time you've assessed the patient's chest, abdomen, and pelvis, finding nothing significant, you catch sight of your coworker Joe headed over with the toboggan, accompanied by three other patrollers.

You: "When did you last have anything to eat?"

Patient: "I had lunch 2 hours ago."

You quickly assess the upper extremities as Joe arrives with the toboggan and anchors it with his skis below the patient. You direct your fellow patrollers to assist you. Mike places one hand on each side of the patient's head and stabilizes the head and neck manually. Pete takes out an adjustable Stifneck collar, measures the distance between the patient's shoulder and chin, adjusts the collar, and places it around the patient's neck. Joe takes the Sager splint out of the toboggan and removes the splint from its container.

Meanwhile, you've unbuckled the patient's left boot and rebuckled it slightly looser. While Joe supports the patient's thigh with one hand on each side of the injury, you grasp the toe of the patient's boot with one hand and his upper calf with the other.

You: "Dan, we're going to put this traction splint on your leg, and it'll feel much better as soon as we get it on. First, I have to straighten your leg a little. I'll be as gentle as I can, but it'll hurt for a short time."

You gently straighten the angulated thigh with the aid of slight axial traction. Meanwhile, Joe has assembled the splint and slipped the groin piece between the patient's legs and up against his left ischial tuberosity while Pete supports the patient's leg and thigh. Joe next secures the upper end of the splint by tightening the groin strap, then secures a special ankle harness, large enough to go around the ski boot, to the patient's ankle and attaches it to the end of the splint. He extends the end of the splint slowly until the gauge reads 15 lb, and ties the two ankles together.

You: "Does that feel better?"

Patient: "Yes."

The patient's thigh and leg are secured to the splint with the three 6″ straps. Meanwhile, Haley brings over the long backboard and lays it on the snow. You assess the patient's pulse and breathing again; the pulse is strong and 100 beats/min, and his respirations are 18 breaths/min.

You: "Dan, because you may have hurt your back, we're going to transport you down the hill on this special board. I'm going to straighten your arms and then we'll lift you carefully onto the board."

Patient: "Okay."

Carefully, the patient's arms are arranged by his side and his wrists tied together in front of him. Four of you lift him 6″ off the snow using the bridge lift while the fifth patroller slides the long board under him. You don't detect any twisting or bending of the patient's spine.

The patient is quickly immobilized on the board with straps across his chest just under his axillae, across his pelvis, and across his legs, but not across his thighs. Crisscross straps are put in place over his shoulders and across his lower abdomen. His arms are secured to his sides with an additional strap. Towel rolls are placed on the outside of each leg beneath the leg strap and padding under the small of his back and beneath his head. His head is immobilized with two towel rolls and two straps of adhesive tape, one around the top of the board, over the towel rolls, and across his brow, and the other across the towel rolls and the rigid collar.

You and your four fellow patrollers lift the board with the patient on it into the toboggan with the patient's head toward the front of the toboggan. In a few minutes, the patient is on his way to the warm aid room.

Specific Injuries to the Upper Extremity
Scenario 9

The following scenario illustrates how to manage a typical injury to the upper extremity.

You and three friends are taking a 4-day fishing and backpacking trip through the Moose Flop Wilderness Area. This involves a 20-mile approach by trail to a mountain range that forms the backbone of the area, followed by 3 miles of scrambling and boulder hopping to get across a pass, then 4 miles of travel to a campground where you left a van. The weather forecast is favorable.

The first 2 days go well. You and your companions eat the steaks and heavy fresh food the first night so that the packs are noticeably lighter the next day. By the second night, you start to feel the altitude as you make camp at timberline in a beautiful meadow below a small lake. That night, your friend Lucky takes out his harmonica, and you sing old western songs around a small campfire.

The next morning, after burying the remains of the campfire, you set out, scrambling across boulders at the lake edge until you reach the inlet, then up steep grassy slopes to a small saddle. As you're descending through a large boulder field on the other side of the saddle, you hear a cry behind you. Turning, you see that Lucky has fallen between two large boulders. His pack is over his head and all you can see are his legs. You and the other two party members reach him at about the same time.

You: "Are you okay, Lucky?"

Patient: "I can't move my shoulder. Help me get this damn pack off."

You and the other hikers carefully undo the buckle, remove the pack, and set it aside. Lucky is lying on his side with his feet on one of the boulders, holding his left arm with his right hand.

You: "Where does it hurt?"

Patient: "My shoulder."

You: "Anywhere else?"

Patient: "No."

You: "Did you hit your head or hurt your neck or back?"

Patient: "No."

You: "Can you get up by yourself?"

Patient: "I need some help."

You and the others gently help the patient to a sitting position against a small boulder, being careful to avoid moving his left upper extremity. You tell the patient that you will assess his injury.

You hold his left wrist and assess his radial pulse. It is strong and regular. You carefully palpate the left clavicle, shoulder joint, arm, elbow, and forearm. There is a large, tender bulge in the center of the clavicle. As you scrape the back of his hand and the tips of his index and little fingers with your fingernail, you question the patient.

You: "Can you feel this?"

Patient: "Yes."

When you ask the patient to wiggle his fingers and then make a fist and spread his fingers and thumb, he is able to do both.

You: "Does your arm or hand feel numb or tingly?"

Patient: "No."

You: "Looks like you injured your collarbone."

Patient: "I was afraid of that. I put my hand out to catch myself when I slipped, but I hit too hard."

You: "Well, we can get a sling and swathe on your arm and take your pack. Do you feel up to walking out? It's 4 miles to the van from here. The trail starts about a quarter mile from where we are."

Patient: "I don't know. I'll have to see."

You: "We can give it a try. If it doesn't work we can send out for help. Have you ever ridden a horse?"

Patient: "Sure."

You: "Before I put on the sling, I need to check a few other things."

You open the patient's shirt, pull his undershirt out of the way, and expose the clavicle. There is a large swelling at its midpoint, but no open wound. You note that the chest shows no open wounds, ecchymosis, or swellings. You palpate each rib in turn. The patient winces when you touch the left fourth rib and answers yes when you ask him if it hurts. When you ask the patient to take a deep breath, he winces again.

You: "You may have hurt that rib when you fell."

Patient: "I didn't notice it until you touched it. I guess the collarbone was hurting too much."

You reach in your pack and pull out your emergency care kit. Fortunately, you have two triangular bandages. You make a sling with one, supporting the patient's left forearm but putting all the weight on his

right shoulder. You fold the other into a cravat and bind his left arm to his chest.

You: "How does that feel?"

Patient: "Better."

You then assess the patient's head, neck, abdomen, lower extremities, and back, and ask him about previous illnesses and injuries, medications he's taken, allergies, and any additional problems. The answers are all negative. The patient's pack is emptied and its contents distributed into the other three packs. You strap his empty pack to the outside of your own. With the aid of a walking stick and some steadying help over rough spots, the patient slowly and carefully makes his way through the rest of the boulder field to an area of rolling tundra that leads to the trail at the tree line. The pace picks up as soon as you reach the trail, and it looks as if the patient will be able to self-evacuate.

You: "Lucky, you have to quit doing things like this or the next time we'll leave you at home."

Specific Injuries to the Lower Extremity and Pelvis
Scenario 10

The following scenario illustrates how to manage a typical injury to the lower extremity.

It is after 4 p.m., and the upper lift has closed. The last skier has just gotten off the lift awkwardly, and he has skied down the cat track. You hope he doesn't plan to ski Mad Dog, but your sweep assignment is Autobahn.

You step into your bindings and push off, making slow, wide turns and looking at the remaining skiers far ahead. One of them falls, sending up a huge cloud of snow.

As you approach the scene, you note that the skier is still down. As far as you can tell, he has not moved. Several other skiers have stopped and are looking uphill at their companion. His right ski is off; however, the left ski is still on. You ski to a stop just below the skier.

You: "Hello, I'm Howie Werkitt of the High Range Ski Patrol. Do you need help?"

Patient: "Yes. I think I did a number on my leg."

You: "The one with the ski still on?"

Patient: "Yes."

You take off your skis and approach the patient. You grasp the patient's hand and feel his pulse. It is strong and regular, with a normal rate. You notice that the skier's left foot seems to be rotated out to an abnormal degree.

You: "What's your name?"

Patient: "Will Clyde."

You: "Will, can you feel your toes?"

Patient: "Yes."

You: "Can you wiggle them?"

Patient: "Yes."

You: "Did you hurt yourself anywhere else?"

Patient: "No."

You: "Did you hit your head, or hurt your neck or back?"

Patient: "No."

You call the sweep chief at the summit and ask her to bring down a toboggan. Warning the skier that you will need to take his ski off, you carefully release the heelpiece of the binding without moving his leg or foot, then remove the ski. You plant the skis in the snow, forming an X uphill from the patient.

You: "That will help the toboggan handlers find us. Now I'm going to examine your leg. Where exactly does it hurt?" (The patient points to a place just above the top of the boot.) "Do you remember how you fell?"

Patient: "I caught an edge, one ski went one way and this ski went another. It didn't release, and I twisted my leg when I fell."

You: "Did you feel or hear a 'pop'?"

Patient: "No."

As you palpate the leg and find a swollen, tender area just above the top of the boot, the skier yells "Ouch." At this point, the toboggan arrives, pulled by a veteran patroller, Bea Friendly.

You: "Bea, this is Will Clyde. He injured his left leg above the boot."

Bea parks the toboggan below the patient, anchors it with her skis, and unpacks it. She removes the quick splint, opens it, and lays it on the snow by the skier's injured left lower extremity.

You: "I'll have to expose your injury to make sure there is no open wound. I'll use a seam ripper so that you can repair your jeans and no one will know the difference."

The patient nods his agreement, and after putting on a pair of latex gloves, you take a seam ripper out of your emergency care belt and expertly open the seam of the left pant leg to the knee. Then you open the seam of the left longjohn leg to the knee. There is no sign of blood and no open wound. There is a swelling of the midleg but no ecchymosis yet.

You ask Bea to steady the patient's leg while you loosen his boot. You carefully unbuckle the boot and ask Bea to steady the patient's thigh so you can put some slight traction on his foot.

Bea uses the "pant-leg pinch lift" to steady the thigh and raise it slightly while you grasp the toe and heel of the boot. Using axial traction, you straighten and rotate the leg slightly so that it's back in the anatomic position. The patient grimaces and you notice some pallor and sweat on his forehead.

Bea reaches over with one hand and slides the opened quick splint beneath the patient's extremity. Then, as you lower his extremity into the splint with the knee slightly bent, she folds up the sides and closes the Velcro straps.

You: "We'll lift you into the toboggan and then give you a ride down to the aid room where we can make you more comfortable and take a closer look at your leg."

Patient: "Okay, thanks. It feels a little better since you put the splint on, but I bet I broke it."

Injuries to the Head, Eye, Face, and Soft Tissues of the Neck
Scenario 11

The following scenario illustrates how to provide emergency care for a patient with a head and face injury. Although some of the techniques described are beyond the scope of this book, they are included to provide a comprehensive view of how to properly manage this type of injury in the nonurban environment.

You are the subdistrict ranger in charge of an area of Grandstone National Park that adjoins a national forest where snowmobiling is popular. The park has a mutual aid agreement with the county to help out with medical emergencies. The nearest doctor is 50 miles away; the nearest hospital is 100 miles away.

You are relaxing after your second cup of coffee one Sunday morning in February when the phone rings. It is the manager of a motel in a town several miles away, a community where hundreds of snowmobilers congregate each weekend during the snowy months. A snowmobiler has lost control of his machine and crashed into a tree several miles north of town. One of his friends rode out to get help, while several others stayed with the patient, who is described as unresponsive and having difficulty breathing. One of the friends has had first responder training, but the group has no first aid equipment.

You reach for your radio, alert the communication center at park headquarters, and summon Russ, the other ranger in the compound. Grabbing your jacket and keys, you run outside to the ambulance, which is parked next to a snowmobile trailer loaded with two snowmobiles and a long sled. You back the ambulance up and hitch the trailer to it.

Russ arrives, and the two of you drive up the road to town, where several of the local snowmobile search and rescue people have assembled. It takes only a few minutes to orient all personnel, unload the sled and snowmobiles, and transfer the trauma bag, cardiac monitor/defibrillator, portable suction unit, oxygen backpack, and a long backboard from the ambulance to the sled. Shortly afterward, you are heading up the unplowed road north of town as the injured snowmobiler's friend leads the way.

Twenty minutes later you arrive at the accident scene. An expensive racing snowmobile is lying against a tree, the windshield and front end smashed. Nearby, a middle-aged man is lying supine on a space blanket in the snow; a friend of the injured man is stabilizing his head and neck and keeping his airway open with the jaw-thrust maneuver. The patient's helmet is off and he is breathing deeply and noisily. There is blood on the snow near his head, his face is bruised and covered with blood, and his eyes are swollen partially shut. He is not moving. You lift the trauma bag and suction machine from the sled and approach the patient. As you approach, you put on a pair of rubber gloves from your emergency care kit.

You: "Hi, I'm Ranger Aiden Assyst and this is Ranger Russ Kewer. What's the situation?"

As you speak, you set up the suction machine and attach a Yankauer tip to the tubing.

Friend: "Thanks for coming. I'm Duane Carruthers, and my friend is Will Clyde. He's in a bad way. He's unresponsive and I'm having trouble keeping his airway clear because of the blood and mucus."

You: "Let's try some suction. Just keep maintaining his airway and be sure to keep his head and neck stabilized."

You grasp the patient's wrist and feel the radial pulse. It is strong and slow. You then loudly ask the patient if he is okay. There is no response to your voice. You take out a tongue blade and a small flashlight and gently open the patient's mouth. Several teeth are missing and several more are turned at an abnormal angle, obviously loose. There is so much blood in the mouth, you can't see anything. Blood is coming from both nostrils.

You turn on the suction machine and use the Yankauer tip to remove blood and mucus from the mouth and nose, sucking in 15-second spurts and removing your finger from the side port whenever you move the tip. A lot of material ends up in the jar and the patient's respirations become easier and less noisy. You turn off the machine for a minute.

Russ exposes the patient's arm, assesses the pulse, and takes the blood pressure. You remove the oxygen backpack from the sled, attach a nonrebreathing mask and tube to the outlet nipple, fill the reservoir bag, and turn the flow valve to 15 L/min. You then position the mask on the patient's face.

You: "What did you find when you assessed your buddy?"

Friend: "You know about his airway. His breathing is slow, deep, and regular—10 to 12 breaths per minute. His carotid pulse is strong and I got 80 beats per minute about 10 minutes ago. He isn't responding to my voice. I've been too busy to check his response to pain. He isn't moving spontaneously at all."

Russ: "His pulse is now 60, his blood pressure is 160 over 90."

You: "Did you see the accident happen?"

Friend: "No. I was on the other side of the hill. When he didn't show up, I turned around and came back and found him like this, but face down in the snow. I turned him as carefully as I could so I wouldn't hurt his neck, and he started breathing right away on his own. The way the machine looks, he must have been really moving when he went over that ridge and hit the tree. Looks like he went through the windshield."

You: "Russ, take over with the suction. I'm going to check a few things."

You: "Duane, while I'm checking him, I need to ask you some questions. Was he looking and feeling okay when he got up this morning?"

Friend: "He looked fine to me, and he wasn't complaining of anything. He had a few beers last night. He ate a good breakfast."

You grasp the patient's wrist again and reassess the pulse. It is strong, regular, and measures 56 beats/min. Respirations are deep, regular, and measure 10 breaths/min.

You: "Is Will allergic to anything, such as medicines or drugs?"

Friend: "Not that I know of."

Starting at the patient's head, you carefully assess the scalp. You find no obvious wounds and no bleeding. On his face, there is a large blue swelling over the left forehead and a large laceration above the left eye, which is oozing blood. You take a sterile compress out of the trauma bag and place it on the laceration.

You: "Is he taking any drugs or any medicine for any condition that you know of?"

Friend: "I don't believe so."

Moving down, you note that the area around the left eye is quite swollen and blue; the area around the right eye is swollen but not blue. The left eye is swollen shut, the right eye almost so. There is a lot of swelling around the nose, which is obviously flattened and bent to the right side, with blood flowing slowly from each nostril. The area over each maxilla is swollen, and the skin is blue. There is blood around the mouth and a large swelling at the midpoint of the left jaw. You suspect a broken jaw.

Moving back to the patient's eyes, you open each one with some difficulty, shining a flashlight into each eye in turn. The left pupil is larger than the right and does not react as well to light. Turning to the ears, you find some pinkish fluid draining out of the left ear. To reassess his level of responsiveness, you shout into his ear, "Will, are you okay?" He doesn't respond. You measure the distance from the corner of the patient's mouth to his earlobe, select an oropharyngeal airway, and quickly rotate it into place. The patient does not gag.

You: "Has he eaten anything since breakfast?"

Friend: "No."

You: "Is he seeing a doctor for any chronic condition, like diabetes or high blood pressure?"

Friend: "I don't know of anything."

You: "Is there anything else about his health that we should know?"

Friend: "Nothing that I'm aware of."

Picking up your radio, you contact the communication center, explain the situation, and arrange for a LifeFlight helicopter to meet you at the helipad in town as soon as possible. Next, you reach into the trauma bag and take out the BVM device. You remove the nonrebreathing mask from the patient's face, hook up the oxygen line to the BVM device, and start

assisting the patient's respirations at 15 breaths/min (one breath every 4 seconds). The patient's chest rises well. You recruit Victor, who is an EMT-Basic and a member of the local search and rescue team, to take over head stabilization and managing the face mask.

Russ takes over for you at bag compressions as you proceed downward to assess the patient's neck. The skin is pale, cool, and moist. There are no swelling, wounds, or deformities, and the neck seems to line up normally with the shoulders. The trachea is in the midline. Running your fingers down the spinous processes, you encounter no step-off deformities and no swelling.

You unzip the patient's heavy snowmobile suit and after unbuttoning the shirt and pulling up his undershirt, you palpate each rib in turn. You find no swelling, wounds, or crepitation. Placing a hand on each side of the lower chest, you note that expansion of the chest on each side is equal. Pulling a stethoscope out of your pocket, you listen to the breath sounds on each side of the chest. They are normal. Using the knuckle of your middle finger, you press firmly on his sternum with a slight rotary motion. He winces and moans.

Opening the lower part of the snowmobile suit, you assess the abdomen. There are no obvious wounds, bleeding, bruises, or swelling. You push the two iliac crests together with a rotary motion and then push each crest backward. There is no crepitus and the patient does not wince.

You turn to the lower extremities. Without cutting the suit legs away or removing the boots (which in this case would waste valuable time), you palpate each extremity through the clothing. There is no swelling or deformities, the extremities are the same length, and the feet are in the proper anatomic relation to the legs. You pinch the skin of each lower leg gently but firmly. The patient withdraws the left lower extremity; the right does not move.

Moving to the upper extremities, you again find no swelling or deformities through the clothing. You pinch the skin of the midpoint of each inner arm gently but firmly. The patient withdraws the left upper extremity; the right does not move.

You pause to think. Russ is doing a good job of pumping the bag, and Victor is doing a good job of stabilizing the patient's head and neck and maintaining the mask-to-face seal despite the face and jaw injuries. You suction the patient's nose and mouth again. His airway is open, and his pulse is good although somewhat slow for the severity of his injuries. He is responsive to pain (a P on the AVPU scale) but is moving only the left side of the body. When you retake the blood pressure, you find it is 170/80 mm Hg and the pulse is 48 beats/min.

The patient has a badly injured face and probably has sustained facial bone fractures as well as a fractured jaw. The pinkish fluid draining from the ear indicates a possible skull fracture. There are no other obvious severe injuries, in particular to the chest, abdomen, or pelvis. The rising systolic blood pressure, increasing pulse pressure, slowing pulse, large left pupil, and right-sided weakness make you concerned about a progressive brain injury with increasing intracranial pressure, probably a hematoma or contusion of the left side of the brain. The patient needs to see a neurosurgeon as soon as possible.

At this point, you remove a Stifneck collar from the trauma pack, adjust it to size, snap it into shape, and apply it to the patient's neck.

Friend: "You know, this guy broke his leg last year at High Range Ski area; that's why he took up snowmobiling this year. Maybe he should have stayed with skiing."

You: "If you're not careful, you can get hurt doing anything."

With the assistance of other members of the rescue team, the patient is lifted onto the long backboard, strapped into place, and then lifted into the sled and covered with two blankets. A third blanket is rolled and placed beneath the head end of the backboard to lift his head about 6″. An IV of lactated Ringer's solution, which you have brought along and kept warm inside your parka, is started, using a large bore needle in the patient's right arm and running just fast enough to keep the line open.

With the patient in tow, Victor slowly drives the snowmobile back to town, trying to avoid a bumpy ride. You and Russ ride in the sled with the patient, assisting his breathing and keeping suction ready. The helicopter will be there to meet you when you arrive.

Neck and Back Injuries
Scenario 12

The following scenario describes the care of a patient with a possible neck and back injury, among other problems.

You have just skied off the Midway lift at High Range Ski Area and are tightening your boots when you overhear a transmission from the base. A skier has fallen off the Number 5 lift just above tower 30. Realizing that this is about 200 yards below and to the north of you, you note the time on your watch (11:15 a.m.) and call

to the patroller at the top of the lift: "Joe, I'll check it out. Get the backboard, trauma kit, oxygen, and suction unit loaded on the toboggan, and I'll call you as soon as I get down there. Tell the base that I'm answering the call but will need more help."

In 60 seconds you are at the scene. A young man is spread-eagled face down in the snow, surrounded by a crowd of curious onlookers. You quickly get out of your bindings and hurry to him, noting that he is not moving and there is no blood on the snow. Because of his heavy clothing, you can't tell if he is breathing. You quickly scoop away the snow around his nose and mouth to create a large breathing space, being careful not to cause any movement of his head and neck.

You (speaking loudly): "Sir, are you okay? Don't move! I'm with the ski patrol, and I'm here to help."

You carefully open his airway with the jaw-thrust maneuver as he stirs with a faint groan, and you are relieved to see that he is breathing. Keeping the airway open with one hand, you key your lapel microphone. "Schussen to Midway, copy." (Midway replies.) "I need the toboggan, the equipment I told you about, and lots of help just above Tower 30 on the Number 5 lift."

You relax the jaw thrust and note that the patient's respirations remain strong. His carotid pulse is strong, regular, and slightly faster than normal. You tell yourself that things are now under control as you stabilize the patient's head and neck with both of your hands.

At this moment, an excited skier approaches you.

Skier: "Ski Patrol, how's my brother?"

You: "Okay so far. Were you with him?"

Skier: "Yes."

You: "I'm Ben Schussen of the High Range Ski Patrol. Pardon me for not shaking hands. What's his name?"

Skier: "Barry Careless. I'm his brother Les."

You: "What happened?"

Skier: "We were sitting in the chair when he started to act strange. He grabbed me, mumbled something, and almost pulled me off. The next thing I knew he went headfirst out of the chair and landed face down in the snow. I came down as soon as I could get off the lift. Is he going to be okay?"

You: "It's too early to tell just what's going on. Right now, he's breathing well and has a good pulse. I'm stabilizing his head and neck in case he has a neck injury. I have some help coming. In a minute, we'll turn him over onto his back, put him on a backboard, and get him to a doctor. Do you have any idea why this happened?"

Skier: "He was up pretty late last night drinking with some buddies and had a headache this morning. He didn't feel like eating breakfast; he wanted to go skiing and thought the cold air would help his headache. He fell down several times on the first run and didn't seem to be in his usual form."

You: "Was he feeling okay before he went out last night?"

Skier: "Yes, he looked okay to me."

You: "Is there anything medically wrong with him?"

Skier: "He has diabetes."

You: "Does he take good care of his diabetes?"

Skier: "Most of the time. He tries to eat right and takes his insulin every day, but occasionally he gets fed up with it and really pigs out, like last night."

You: "Did he take his insulin this morning?"

Skier: "I don't know."

You: "Does he take any other medicine besides insulin?"

Skier: "No."

You: "Does he have any allergies?"

Skier: "No."

You: "Has he had anything to eat at all today?"

Skier: "Not that I know of."

You: "Is there anything else we need to know about his health in order to help him?"

Skier: "That's about it. He's always been healthy and active."

At this point, your coworker Joe and several other patrollers arrive with the toboggan. You ask Joe to call the base and hill chief to arrange for an ambulance from town, and ask a patroller named Ann to assess the patient's neck and back. After putting on a pair of rubber gloves, she runs her fingers beneath the patient's jacket, along the spinous processes of the cervical, thoracic, and lumbar vertebrae. There are no prominences, step-off deformities, indications of swelling or obvious tenderness, or evident open wounds. Next, Ann pinches the tip of each index finger firmly but gently between her index finger and thumb. The patient withdraws both upper extremities equally. When she presses her knuckles firmly against each tibia, the patient withdraws both lower extremities equally.

Joe brings the long backboard, oxygen, and portable suction unit from the toboggan. Then, you and three of the other patrollers carefully align the patient's extremities and log roll him into the supine position on the long backboard. Ann places a rigid collar around the patient's neck, while you continue to stabilize the head and neck. The patient is too far to the side and has to be pulled 6″ headward and 6″ footward before he is centered on the board. Ann then starts to administer oxygen using a nonrebreathing mask at 15L/min.

The patient now has his eyes open and is starting to stir. You again ask him if he is okay, and he weakly replies, "No." He is able to tell you that he has pain in his face—where the skin over the cheekbones and around the eyes is red and noticeably swollen—his neck, and his anterior chest. Despite this, his breathing remains regular, deep, and at 16 breaths/min. His pulse is strong and steady at 90 beats/min.

You ask the patient if he took his insulin this morning, and he tells you that he did. After asking him whether he feels nauseated and receiving a negative reply, you ask John to take a tube of Instant Glucose out of your aid belt and squeeze some of it into the patient's mouth for him to swallow.

After doing this, John quickly assesses the patient's head and face while you maintain the manual stabilization and Ann continues to administer oxygen. John determines that the pupils are equal and respond to light. The swollen areas over the cheekbones are tender, but there are no open wounds. The teeth are symmetrical and there are no lumps or tender areas over the sides of the jaw. John quickly performs the remainder of the rapid body survey. He finds no obvious open wounds, bleeding, deformities, or swelling; and no tenderness except over the mid-sternum. Both sides of the patient's chest expand equally during breathing. The patient is able to squeeze both of John's hands and says he can wiggle his toes and feel his feet. He is able to feel a gentle pinch on all four extremities. You and the other patrollers strap the patient securely to the backboard and immobilize his head and neck.

You retrieve a notebook and pencil from your emergency care belt and start making notes. It is 11:35 a.m. You ask yourself whether all this could have happened in only 20 minutes.

As the board and patient are being lifted into the toboggan, the patient starts to gag. Quickly, the four of you lower the board to the snow and tilt it on its side, and Ann snatches the oxygen mask from the patient's face. Joe hands you the V-Vac suction unit while the patient vomits about a cupful of thin, yellow liquid onto the snow. You move the suction tip in and around his mouth and nose, wishing that you'd thought to put

appendix a

on some rubber gloves when you had the chance. When the patient has stopped vomiting, you and the other patrollers lift the backboard into the toboggan, cover the patient with a sleeping bag, and strap him into place, placing the oxygen backpack beside him. Before the toboggan starts to move, you give him another dose of Instant Glucose. Then you put on a pair of latex gloves.

You: "I'll take the V-Vac and ski beside him. If he vomits again we'll have to stop right away and tilt the toboggan on its side. Remember, let's go slow and easy."

You surmise that he must have passed out from low blood sugar and was limp when he hit the snow. The adrenaline surge brought on by the low blood sugar and injury must have raised his blood sugar enough to wake him up. You tell yourself with relief that the patient lucked out. Even though he did a 20' whole-body plant, face first into 3' of snow, the most obvious injury seems to be soft-tissue damage to the face. Even if he has a cervical spine fracture, there is probably no cord damage.

Chest Injuries
Scenario 13

The following scenario illustrates how to manage a patient with an open chest wound.

You and three companions are all students at State University, which is located 100 miles from Grandstone National Park. You have 4 days left of spring break and have decided to use the time to explore the country just north of the park boundary. The plan is to leave two vehicles at a parking area off the main road and take a trail 5 miles north into a range of 10,000' peaks where there should be some good powder skiing.

You will establish a base camp and spend 2 days exploring the high country before heading back after lunch on Sunday. All four of you have your Ortovox transceivers and Lucky has brought Bandit, an avalanche-trained German shepherd with a good nose. You discover that some other skiers have broken trail ahead of you, which means easier trail skiing and more time for the powder.

The party is 2 miles up the trail and going strong through a narrow draw between two meadows. Bandit is out in front. You round a bend and see a huge male bison about 30 yards away. He is standing sideways on the trail; and you hear him snort as he swings his head around to look at you. "Bandit, NO!" cries Lucky, but it is too late. Bandit is heading full tilt for the bison, barking aggressively.

The big animal lowers his head and raises his tail as he turns toward the dog. The party members have all stopped in their tracks and are nervously stepping off the trail—there are steep banks on each side and no place to go to avoid a charge. You recall that male bisons weigh 1 ton and can run 25 mph.

"Bandit, COME!" shouts Lucky. The dog is dancing around in front of the bison, barking furiously. The bison takes a step forward and hooks his head up sharply. The tip of a horn catches the dog and tosses him high up on the bank. He lies there yelping loudly. With a snort, the bison heads for Joe, the nearest skier, who is yelling and frantically sidestepping up the bank. The rest of you stand frozen and watch in horror as the big animal hooks a horn below Joe's armpit and tosses him straight up.

Joe lands screaming in the snow, halfway up the bank. The bison stops, snorts, then turns and walks slowly away up the trail.

Joe is lying on his side. He is moaning with pain, and the moans are interrupted by gasps for breath. As soon as the bison is out of sight, you take off your skis and run over to Joe. Joe's jacket is torn below his left armpit, and there's blood on his clothing and on the snow. You grasp Joe's wrist and feel his pulse.

You: "Joe, are you okay?"

Joe: "He got me in the chest. I can't breathe."

Joe's pulse is strong, regular, and fast. His breathing rate is at least twice normal with obvious respiratory distress. His skin is pale with a cyanotic cast, and there is cold sweat on his forehead.

You: "Joe, did he get you anywhere else? Did you hit your head or hurt your neck or back when you landed?"

Joe (weakly): "No."

By now you know that Joe's airway, breathing, and circulation are adequate but stressed. He clearly has a serious injury to his chest. After retrieving the emergency care kit from your pack and putting on latex gloves, you unzip Joe's jacket, unbutton his shirt, and expose his chest by pulling up his undershirt. Both sides of the chest are moving equally with respirations. There is an open wound the size of a 50-cent piece in the right anterolateral chest. Joe's clothing is blood-soaked, and the wound is bleeding. You hear a sucking noise as he inhales, and when he exhales you can see bloody bubbles in the wound as air comes out of it. You think, *Yikes! A sucking chest wound. I have to get that covered up.*

From the emergency care kit you take a roll of 2″ adhesive tape and a plastic bag filled with sterile compresses of various sizes. You open three of the sterile 4″ × 4″ compresses and stack them over the wound.

You: "Mike, look in the top flap pocket of my pack and get out one of those clean, empty plastic bags. Lucky, tear me off three strips of tape, about 8″ long."

You place a clean Ziploc bag over the top compress and tape three sides of the occlusive dressing firmly to the skin, which you have wiped dry of blood with a fourth compress. You pull down Joe's undershirt, button his shirt, and zip his jacket.

You: "Can you breathe better, Joe?"

Joe: "Yes, a little. I need to sit up."

You: "Don't move yet, let me check your neck and back first. It won't take but a minute."

You quickly run your fingers from the base of Joe's skull down to his coccyx, pressing on each spinous process in turn.

You: "Does this hurt anywhere?"

Joe: "No."

As you help Joe sit up, you note that he appears less anxious and his breathing rate is slower. You time it at 30 breaths/min. You pull up Joe's clothing to look at the wound again; the blood has not soaked through the compresses yet.

You and your buddies agree that Joe must be moved out of this bowling alley in case the bull comes back. The three of you carry Joe slowly and carefully 60 yards out of the gully and into the woods, laying him down on a foam sleeping pad.

You: "Mike, you're the fastest skier. Take your pack and head back to the cars as fast as you can. Here are my keys. Drive to the Alpine Motel in town—the man who runs it is head of the local rescue unit. Ask him to notify the EMTs and bring a snowmobile with a toboggan up here so we can get Joe back to town. The EMTs have some oxygen—have them bring it in along with their trauma gear. Call the LifeFlight helicopter to meet us there. Lucky and I will stay here with Joe."

Lucky has retrieved his dog, who now seems his usual self. Bandit has a superficial laceration on the side where the big horn caught him, but the skin was so loose that he sustained no deeper injuries.

Joe is starting to shiver, so you pull his down parka out of his pack and tuck it over and around him.

As Mike disappears down the trail, Lucky starts to collect wood for a fire and you start the rest of the

urgent survey. Joe has always been healthy, is taking no medications, and has no allergies. There are no abnormalities of his head, face, pupils, ears, nose, mouth, or anterior neck. The trachea is in the midline. There are no abdominal wounds, and you find no tenderness on palpation. There are no deformities, swelling, or indications of tenderness over the extremities. Joe is able to wiggle his toes and squeeze both your hands. You set about making him as comfortable as possible by the fire while waiting for help.

You: "Lucky, you should train that dog not to chase anything bigger than a cat."

Injuries to the Abdomen, Pelvis, and Genitalia

Scenario 14

The following scenario describes how to manage a patient with an abdominal injury.

It's noon on a cold, blustery day in early March. The sky is overcast, and it's beginning to snow. You've just finished your lunch and have dropped into the patrol room when the telephone rings. It's your friend Sheriff Brown. He says there's been an accident at Silver Falls, a popular ice-climbing area about 2 miles inside the Big Bear Wilderness just beyond High Range Ski Area. He needs some experienced ski mountaineers to help the county search and rescue (SAR) team.

Sheriff Brown relays the details provided to him by the victim's companion, Bill, who summoned help. The victim had just finished putting on his crampons at the bottom of the main part of the frozen falls when he slipped on the ice and slid down the frozen rapids below the falls. He had abdominal pain and was unable to stand, so the companion wrapped him in spare clothing and, realizing that he needed medical attention, skied out to the road at the edge of the wilderness area where there was a public campground with a phone. Bill notified the sheriff, then skied back to the falls to do what he could for his friend.

Confirming what you already suspect, the sheriff says emergency care and an over-the-snow evacuation is necessary because the weather is too bad for a helicopter evacuation.

You think about what you need to know as you question the sheriff. There was no sign of bleeding at the accident site. The patient was responsive and coherent, although he was having considerable abdominal pain. Bill saw him slide at full speed into a large log at the side of the frozen stream and believes he hit the log with his abdomen. He also believes his friend may have an abdominal ice-ax wound. The patient grabbed his ice ax as he slipped, but he could not stop himself on the glare ice.

You check the roster. Luckily, four other patrollers with ski mountaineering experience are on duty with you, and there are enough off-duty people available to keep the mountain covered. You clear your plans with the area manager, radio the assistant hill chief to take over your duties, then call the other four patrollers to assemble at the base.

You call the summit and ask the duty patroller to send down the four-handled fiberglass Akja. While waiting, you open the off-area locker and take out five rescue packs, an emergency care kit, and two 150′ coils of climbing rope. You then retrieve an extrication vest and an oxygen backpack from the gear closet. Next, you put a liter bag of physiologic saline solution inside your undershirt against your chest.

By this time, the four other patrollers have arrived. Fortunately, you all have your telemark gear in your vehicles, one of which is a large pickup truck. Within a few minutes, the telemark gear and emergency care equipment is loaded and, after calling the sheriff's office to notify them of your departure, you leave for the trailhead about 10 miles away.

When you arrive, half a dozen members of the local SAR unit are assembling their gear. The rescue party puts climbing skins on their skis and gets into their bindings. Accompanied by several members of the SAR unit, your fellow patrollers set off up the trail with the Akja. Three skiers pull on a length of rope attached to its front end and one skis between the rear handles. You and a member of the SAR team ski ahead with the off-area emergency care kit and oxygen. It is about 18°F, still overcast and snowing lightly, but the wind has died down.

It takes you 45 minutes to ski 2 miles up the narrow trail and ½ mile through deep snow to the accident site. You can see the bright flames and smoke of a fire as you approach. The patient is a few feet from the fire, lying on two daypacks and covered with a parka. An ice ax is planted in the snow nearby. There is blood on the pick but no obvious blood on the snow.

As Bill comes to meet you, you recognize him as an acquaintance you have climbed with in the past. He took the Outdoor Emergency Care course with the patrol candidates 2 years ago. You glance at your watch; it is now 2 p.m.

You: "Bill, how does it look?"

Bill: "I've checked him over as well as I can. We don't have any first aid equipment along. He took a long

slide down the ice of the creek and hit that log. He has a wound in his abdomen—probably landed on the pick of his ice ax. He's bleeding some but not much. His pulse is strong but he's in a lot of pain."

You: "What time did this happen?"

Bill: "About 11 a.m."

You: "What's his name?"

Bill: "Howard Angle."

You grasp the patient's wrist and feel his pulse. The pulse is strong, regular, and faster than normal. As you take the pulse, you introduce yourself to the patient.

You: "Howard, I'm Ben Schussen from the High Range Ski Patrol. Looks like you need some help."

Patient: "Yes, I've met you before. Thanks for coming."

The patient speaks carefully; it obviously hurts to talk. His breathing is rapid and shallow. You glance quickly at his body from head to toe, noting that there is no obvious blood on his clothing.

You: "Exactly what happened?"

Patient: "Slipped and took a fast ride down the ice. Hit that log pretty hard, landed on my ax. Terrible pain in my gut."

You: "Did you hit the log with your abdomen?"

Patient: "Yes."

You: "Do you have any pain anywhere else? How about your neck and back?"

Patient: "No."

You: "Did you hit your chest? You're having trouble breathing."

Patient: "My gut hurts when I breathe."

You: "Did you hit your head?"

Patient: "No."

You: "Are you cold?"

Patient: "Not bad. The fire helps."

You: "Sorry to have to ask you so many questions, but we need to know what happened."

You have now established that his airway is open, he's breathing well, his pulse is strong, and he's alert and able to give a coherent history. It's time to examine the area of chief complaint, the abdomen. As you put on a pair of latex gloves, you explain to the patient that you'll need to open his clothes to examine his abdomen.

The skin of the abdomen is warm. There's a small tear penetrating all the way through his parka, down sweater, pile jacket, and polypropylene undershirt. It matches up with an open wound the size of a quarter in the midabdomen, just to the right of the navel. There's a small amount of blood around the wound and along the track through the clothing. The wound looks free of dirt and other foreign matter, which doesn't surprise you, given the circumstances. Some shiny, yellow material covered with blood—probably fat—is protruding from the wound.

You open the emergency care kit and take out a flashlight, tongue blade, several large, sterile compresses, some 2″ tape, a large package of sterile Vaseline gauze, the V-Vac suction unit, and a set of IV tubing. After removing the IV bag of physiologic saline from inside your undershirt, you carefully inspect and palpate the abdomen, avoiding the area immediately around the wound. The abdomen is slightly distended and generally tender. There are no other open wounds, swelling, or ecchymosis. You press the iliac crests toward each other, and then backward, and none of these maneuvers cause any additional pain.

At this point, the patient starts to retch. You help him turn on his side and he vomits into the snow. You grab the V-Vac and suction his mouth. When he seems to have finished, you put on a new pair of latex gloves, open two large compresses, and place them over the wound. Attaching the IV tubing to the bag, you let enough saline flow onto the compresses to wet them all the way through, then put a large piece of Vaseline gauze over the top. You cover this with a large dry dressing, tape its edges to the skin of the abdomen, and replace the patient's clothing.

You: "Howard, you have an ice-ax wound in your abdomen. The toboggan will be here in a few minutes and we're going to load you into it and take you back to the trailhead. First, if you don't mind, I need to ask you a few more questions and make sure nothing else is wrong. I'll try to phrase the question to keep your answers short. Are you still warm enough?"

Patient: "I'm okay."

You: "Were you feeling all right before you got hurt?"

Patient: "Yes."

You obtain the SAMPLE history, which is negative, and perform the rapid body survey, which does not turn up anything else significant. You take a low-reading thermometer out of the off-area kit, shake it down, and place it under the patient's tongue for 3 minutes. The patient has a temperature of 100.2°F that you suspect is caused by peritonitis. His pulse is 110 beats/min and strong, his respirations are shallow with a rate of 24 breaths/min.

By this time, your companions have arrived with the Akja, maneuvered it beside the patient, and opened the tarp and sleeping bag. You and the other patrollers use the bridge lift to carefully raise the patient, while members of the SAR team shove the Akja underneath him. You lay the patient in the Akja with his knees bent for comfort and cover him up, leaving his head exposed to permit ongoing monitoring. Oxygen is started at 6 L/min, by nasal cannula in case the patient vomits again. You would prefer high-flow oxygen, but this is the best compromise.

One member of the team takes the front handles of the Akja; another takes the rear. You carry the suction unit and ski immediately behind the person at the rear of the Akja. Four skiers are carrying the climbing rope attached to the front of the Akja in case they are needed to pull, and two are in a belay position holding the other rope attached to the back.

Fortunately, it is mostly downhill to the road. One of the other rescuers has radioed ahead so that an ambulance will meet you at the trailhead—about a half hour away with luck and strong legs.

Common Medical Complaints
Scenario 15

The following scenario illustrates how to manage a patient with a respiratory complaint.

You are enjoying a beautiful day of spring patrolling at High Range Ski Area when a transmission from the base announces that a snowboarder is in trouble about halfway down Big Elk run. No details are given. You stop for a moment to reply that you can respond to the call, then continue down.

After a minute, you see several skiers standing around a man in his 30s who is sitting in the snow. As you approach, you see that he is obviously uncomfortable and breathing heavily. His snowboard is off. There are no obvious extremity abnormalities and you see no blood on the snow. You quickly remove your skis and approach him.

You: "Hi, I'm Ben Schussen of the High Range Ski Patrol. Can I help you?"

Patient (panting): "Thanks, I'm having a hard time breathing. I don't know why."

Reaching for the patient's nearest hand, you remove his glove and assess his pulse; it is regular, strong, and faster than normal. His breathing is deep and about twice the normal rate. There are no obvious audible wheezes or other abnormal breathing sounds. His face is pale and his lips are bluish.

You: "Did you fall and hurt yourself?"

Patient: "No. I was cruising along and I felt a sudden pain in my chest and now I can't breathe. I had to stop riding."

You: "Where is the pain?"

The patient points to his upper right anterior chest.

Patient: "It was right here. It's better now though."

You: "How long did it last?"

Patient: "Just a few seconds."

You: "Does it hurt to breathe at all now?"

Patient: "Not really, but the right side of my chest doesn't feel right."

You: "Were you feeling okay before this happened?"

Patient: "Yes."

As you reach for your radio, you tell the patient that you're going to call for a toboggan and give him a ride off the mountain.

You: "Schussen to Summit. I need a toboggan and oxygen pack on Big Elk, halfway down on the left side of the run."

Summit confirms. You use your skis to make an upright X in the snow about 20′ above the patient, then ask the patient his name.

Patient: "Ike Antinhale."

You: "Ike, have you ever had anything like this before?"

Patient: "No."

You: "Do you have any history of heart or lung disease or other serious medical problems?"

Patient: "No."

You: "Have you had a recent cold, cough, or the flu?"

Patient: "No."

You: "Are you taking any medicines or drugs for any condition?"

Patient: "No."

You: "Is there anything else medically important that we should know about you?"

Patient: "Not that I can think of."

You: "Ike, while we're waiting for the toboggan, I'm going to check you over and see if we can figure out what's going on."

The snowboarder nods. After putting on a pair of rubber gloves, you assess his neck and find no abnormal lumps or distended veins. Moving downward, you assess the position of the trachea with your forefinger just above the sternal notch. It is in the midline. You open the snowboarder's jacket and place one hand on each side of his chest. Both sides are moving equally as he breathes. You palpate each rib and interspace in turn on each side of the chest. There are no tender areas or swelling.

A stir in the crowd announces the arrival of another patroller, Pete, who has brought the toboggan and oxygen pack. You unzip the pack, take out the non-rebreathing mask, and attach the tubing to the output nipple of the oxygen regulator. You open the main tank valve and note that the tank is three fourths full as registered on the pressure gauge. Turning the regulator valve to 15 L/min, you fill the reservoir bag, then turn to the patient.

You: "Ike, I'm going to put this mask over your mouth and nose and give you some oxygen. It should make you much less short of breath."

You attach the mask to the patient's head with the elastic strap. The patient's breathing seems to slow somewhat and become less deep after a few minutes.

You: "We're going to help you into the toboggan. I want you to sit up rather than lie down, and keep breathing the oxygen."

You and Pete slowly and carefully take the patient to the bottom of the hill, where he is loaded into a waiting ambulance and taken to the hospital. You later hear that a chest x-ray revealed a pneumothorax on the right side, very likely a spontaneous pneumothorax of the type that can occur in young people.

Scenario 16

The following scenario illustrates the emergency care of a patient with a gastrointestinal complaint.

You and Sandy have decided to try a new outdoor experience this summer. Sandy's mother has agreed to keep the baby for a week while you two float the middle fork of the Tuna River. Because this is your first rafting experience, you've signed up with a rafting company managed by a friend of yours from a ski patrol in a neighboring state. You know that his guides are experienced and qualified.

The trip will take 5 days, part of which will be through the deep and narrow Tuna Canyon, where you'll have no access to civilization for 2 days. You have all the personal supplies recommended by the rafting company, plus your backpacking emergency care kit.

Twenty eager "river runners" climb into the rafts early the first morning about a day's run from the entrance to the canyon. The first night is spent on a large sandbar. The roar of the river keeps everyone but the guides from sleeping soundly.

The next morning, the guides prepare a ranch-style breakfast. You notice that Sandy leaves half of her breakfast untouched. When you ask why, she says that dinner the night before bothered her stomach and she isn't feeling very hungry, although she feels okay otherwise. She spent a long time at the latrine and mentions to you that she is constipated and her abdomen hurts when she tries to have a bowel movement. After breakfast, camp is packed, the rafts loaded, and the rafters shove off into the swift river.

By late afternoon, Sandy clearly is not feeling well. She has curled up in the bottom of the raft and is lying on her side with her hips flexed and her knees drawn up. She looks pale and, when questioned, says that she has a dull ache in her abdomen. When you ask her where it hurts she points to the area around her navel. She finished her menstrual period about 2 weeks earlier and thinks she may be having some ovulation pain. Bob, a trip leader who has had wilderness-EMT training, notices Sandy's discomfort and asks whether she's okay, but she shrugs him off and says she'll be fine.

When you reach the next camping place, Sandy crawls into her sleeping bag as soon as the tent is up. By now, she looks quite ill and you are growing increasingly worried about her.

You question her more carefully and learn that she started to have midabdominal discomfort during the previous night. She has no appetite and feels nauseated. She ate a small amount of breakfast but no lunch, although she has been able to drink water. She doesn't want any dinner.

During the day, the pain moved down into her right lower quadrant. She doesn't recall having any symptoms of head cold, sore throat, earache, cough, chest pain, or shortness of breath. Her bowel movements were normal until that morning. She has had no pain on urination and has no pain anywhere else in her body.

You take a thermometer from your emergency care kit and take an oral temperature. It is 100.4°F. Her pulse is strong, regular, and faster than normal and you count it at 100 beats/min. She is breathing at 16 breaths/min.

You warm your hands against your body, then palpate her bare abdomen, starting in the left lower quadrant. There is no tenderness until you move around to the right lower quadrant, where she winces when you apply slight pressure. You lay your ear on her bare abdomen. The bowel sounds seem normal; at least you don't hear the rushes you have heard in the past with patients who had gastroenteritis.

You ask her a few more questions, most of which you think you know the answers to already. She reaffirms that she has never had any serious illnesses, is taking no drugs except for an occasional Tylenol for headache, and was feeling fine before the trip started. She has had no surgery except a tonsillectomy.

Taking a flashlight and tongue blade out of the emergency care kit, you look at her throat. It is a normal red color with no white spots. Feeling under the sides of her jaw, you find no swelling or tenderness.

With deep concern, you seek out Bob and take him aside.

You: "Bob, I'm afraid Sandy has a significant problem. She's had abdominal pain since last night. It started off in the midabdomen and then moved into her right lower quadrant. She has no appetite, is nauseated, and has a temperature of 100.4°F. She was constipated this morning and her stomach hurt when she tried to move her bowels. She's also very tender in the right lower quadrant. Her bowel sounds are normal, and she has no symptoms of a respiratory or urinary infection. I'm not sure what's going on, but I don't think it's just the stomach flu, and I'm afraid it might be serious. Do you have a radio?"

Bob: "No, I'm afraid we don't. The nearest place to get help is where we leave the canyon about 10 miles downstream. We can't get there before noon tomorrow. It'll be dark in an hour so, unfortunately, we can't continue tonight."

You: "Looks like we'll have to do the best we can tonight, then get moving at first light. As I recall from my Outdoor Emergency Care classes, we shouldn't give her anything to eat or drink and should get her to a doctor as soon as possible. Until we can get out of here in the morning, we'd better keep an eye on her."

Bob: "You're right. I'll have a look at her, too."

Bob dons latex gloves and goes into the tent, where he spends a few minutes assessing Sandy. His findings are the same as yours.

Bob: "She has an acute abdomen. In the wilderness-EMT course I took, if you couldn't get a patient with an acute abdomen to a hospital right away, they recommended giving small sips of water and antibiotics. We have some cephalexin in the medical kit, and some oral Demerol for pain."

You: "That sounds reasonable to me."

Bob gets the medications from the medical kit and hands them to you, telling you to summon him if Sandy's condition worsens. You go into the tent and explain to Sandy what is going to happen, trying to keep the worry out of your voice. She swallows an antibiotic capsule and a Demerol pill with some water and manages to keep them down.

You can hear Bob talking to the other rafters, explaining the situation while the guides are fixing supper. You stay awake most of the night, listening to Sandy moan intermittently as she sleeps fitfully. She takes a sip of water every now and then and on one occasion vomits a cupful into a pan. You inspect the vomit with a flashlight; it is clear, yellow stomach contents without any blood. Toward morning, she seems more comfortable and falls into a deep sleep for an hour.

You awake with a start. It is still dark but you can hear someone moving around outside, clanking pots and pumping the stove. In a few minutes the others are starting to stir.

Leaving Sandy, you help with a quick breakfast, breaking camp, and loading the rafts, then get her out of the tent, into a drysuit, and onto a raft. She tells you the pain has diminished, and you reassess her abdomen, finding it generally tender and slightly distended. She swallows a few sips of water, then vomits it back up. It's getting light as the rafts shove off into the river.

The rest of the trip through the canyon seems to take forever. Sandy is able to keep two more antibiotic capsules down. Finally, you make shore on a sandy beach where a dirt road reaches the river. One of the guides runs off up the road to the nearest house, about 2 miles away. A half hour later, a large four-wheel-drive pickup arrives in a cloud of dust with a friendly rancher at the wheel.

When you arrive at the hospital 20 miles away, Sandy is taken immediately to surgery, where she is found to have an inflamed appendix with a walled-off abscess around an area of perforation. Ten days later, thanks to intravenous antibiotics, she can join you on a flight home.

Medical Emergencies
Scenario 17

The following scenario describes how to manage a serious medical emergency that may occur in the nonurban setting.

You are having a late lunch in the Midway Chalet when you notice a commotion a few tables away. A middle-aged man has knocked a soft drink cup off his tray and is slumped in his chair. A woman about the same age—probably his wife—rises from her chair and quickly moves around the table to the man. He is holding his hand over his chest, and his face is gray.

You get up and walk over to the pair. As you approach, you can see beads of sweat on the man's forehead and an anguished look on his face.

You: "Hello, sir, I'm Constance Vigil of the High Range Ski Patrol. Can I help you?"

Patient: "Please!"

Wife: "Something's wrong with my husband. He's never been like this before. Honey, what's wrong?"

Patient: "I have a terrible pain in my chest. I can't breathe."

You: "Where is the pain?"

The patient point to the midsternum and tells you that the pain is there. You grasp his wrist and assess his pulse. It is regular, weak, and faster than normal. His breathing rate is slightly above normal.

You: "What's your name?"

Patient: "Max Doud."

You: "Have you ever had anything like this before?"

Patient: "No."

You: "How long ago did it start?"

Patient: "Just a few minutes ago."

You: "What does the pain feel like?"

Patient: "Like someone is squeezing my chest."

You: "Does the pain go anywhere from your chest?"

Patient: "To my left elbow."

You: "Have you ever had any heart trouble or high blood pressure?"

Patient: "Not that I know of."

You: "Excuse me a minute. I'm going to make a quick call on the radio."

You call the Midway patrol shack, not far away, telling the patroller who answers that you have a patient with chest pain. You request a toboggan, oxygen, a BVM device, and suction, and ask him to call the doctors' patrol member on duty. You also ask that he call the summit and have a patroller bring down the AED as soon as possible. Before signing off, you request that he summon an ALS ambulance from town. You then turn back to the patient.

You: "How are you feeling now?"

Patient: "Pretty bad. The pain's no better."

You: "Would you feel better if you were to lie down?"

Patient: "No. This is okay."

If anything, the patient looks worse. His breathing is faster and his pulse is faster and weaker. At this point, the Midway patroller arrives with the portable oxygen, BVM device, and a V-Vac suction unit. You open the tank and pressurize the gauges.

You: "I'm going to put this oxygen mask on your face and give you some oxygen. This should make you feel better and less short of breath."

Patient: "Thanks, I need it."

You put a nonrebreathing mask on the patient's face and turn the flow rate up to 15 L/min. The patient looks more relaxed. Suddenly, his eyes roll back in his head and he starts gasping as he sags back into the chair. You have your hand on his radial pulse; all of a sudden, you cannot feel it.

Shaking his shoulder, you ask him if he is okay. There is no answer. His wife starts to wail. Quickly, you lift him from the chair and lay him supine on the floor. Pulling your pocket mask from your emergency care belt, you take the mask off his face and plug the oxygen tubing into the nipple on the pocket mask. He continues to gasp occasionally. You perform the head tilt–chin lift technique, place the pocket mask over his face, and deliver two rescue breaths. You quickly feel for the carotid pulse. It is absent.

While locating your hand position on the patient's chest, you turn to the Midway patroller.

You: "Joe, we have a full code. Call the base and have them send up a Thiokol ASAP."

You give the patient 15 chest compressions at a rate of 80/min, while rapidly counting "*one*-and-two-and...." You give two more rescue breaths, then two more cycles of chest compressions and rescue breaths.

By this time, Joe is back at the patient's side and takes over chest compressions after you give the last two rescue breaths. He gives five compressions this time. The two of you intersperse each set of five compressions with a rescue breath using the pocket mask. The patient's color, which had become a ghastly blue, is starting to pink up a little.

After a few minutes, Dr. Karen Fixx comes in the door, followed by the summit patroller carrying the AED. You continue CPR as the physician turns on the defibrillator. She attaches the two electrodes to the patient's chest. You stop CPR.

Doctor: "This is a semiautomated machine that gives you verbal and visual prompts to tell you what to do."

Machine: "Shock advised."

Doctor: "All stand clear!"

Everybody moves away from the patient. Dr. Fixx pushes the "Shock" button. The patient jumps as a shock is delivered. After a few seconds, the AED emits a shock advised warning.

Dr. Fixx pushes the "Shock" button again. The patient jumps as a shock is delivered. After another few seconds, the machine advises against delivering another shock.

You feel for the patient's carotid pulse. This time, you can feel a faint pulse that is soon steady and stronger. The patient is starting to breathe on his own. You attach the oxygen to the BVM device, and you and Joe start supporting the patient's breathing.

The sound of a diesel motor outside the chalet signals the arrival of the big Thiokol. The patient is quickly carried outside and loaded into its bed, head downhill. You ride with Dr. Fixx and Joe in back with the patient, taking all of the emergency equipment with you, in case more problems occur en route to the waiting ambulance. The patient's wife rides down in the cab with the driver.

The patient is fortunate that you were right there when he had a cardiac arrest, CPR was started immediately, and the defibrillator was available promptly. You have managed two other cardiac arrest patients in your patrol career, but resuscitation efforts were, unfortunately, unsuccessful. *This one,* you think to yourself with satisfaction, *looks like he's going to make it.*

Environmental Emergencies
Scenario 18

The following scenario describes how to manage a patient with a typical environmental emergency.

You've had a busy weekend day as hill chief. It's 5 p.m. and you're waiting for the Midway sweep chief to arrive from his station so the hill can be closed.

There's a commotion outside and the area manager enters, accompanied by a worried teenager. He introduces the young woman as Sophie Moore and tells you that her boyfriend skied out of bounds off the side of upper Big Elk run around 3 p.m. and hasn't come back. She was supposed to meet him at the cafeteria an hour ago. He also tells you that he thinks an off-area rescue is needed, and the sheriff has asked the patrol to run it.

Nodding in agreement, you begin to question Sophie. She tells you that her boyfriend, 17-year-old Hart Dogge, is an expert skier who prefers powder to groomed runs. He's in good health and good physical condition. They had lunch together and he ate a large meal. Hart has done some summer backpacking but has had no special training in winter camping or cold-weather survival. He was wearing blue jeans, a turtle-neck shirt, a pair of ski gloves, and an insulated ski jacket but no hat.

Sophie doesn't believe he was carrying any matches or other emergency gear. She was with him when he left the side of Upper Big Elk and followed him about 100 yards before deciding that she had better traverse back to the run. She tells you that she can show you where they left the run. She wanted him to come back with her, but he insisted on continuing and said he would meet her later at the lodge cafeteria.

Quickly, you round up two senior patrollers who have taken the National Ski Patrol's Advanced Mountain Travel and Rescue Course and brief them on the problem. You place the assistant hill chief in charge of selecting the backup party and someone to cover the radio at the base. You then send a patroller for some candy bars from the base lodge and retrieve the backpacks, emergency care kit, and the Heatpac from the off-area cache.

You don't have your mountaineering skis with you, but it sounds as if alpine gear will work because the topography is all downhill from upper Big Elk to the road. There's a fiberglass Akja toboggan at the summit warming hut, and if you can locate the young man, it can probably be brought down to transport him if needed.

Dusk is falling as nine patrollers and Sophie get on the lower chair and head for the top. It is 18°F, and the forecast calls for clear and cold weather. The plan is for three patrollers to stay at the summit with a radio and the Akja, two to ski all the way down Big Elk looking for tracks coming back into the ski area, and one to go back down with Sophie after she shows you where Hart went. The other three will follow Hart's tracks, and the sheriff's deputies will patrol the road to find him if he eventually skis out by himself. All the rescuers have radios.

Sophie points to where she and Hart skied under the boundary rope on the right-hand side of the run; only their two tracks are there to follow. After sending Sophie and her escort down the mountain, you and your two colleagues turn on headlamps and ski one after the other down through the dense timber, following the tracks. It is 6 p.m. In a few minutes, one set of tracks turns back and starts traversing back toward the run—obviously Sophie's tracks.

After about 30 minutes, it is pitch dark. You are down in a deep valley between two ridges and the ground is becoming more level. The tracks continue ahead of you. You note that Hart is definitely a good

powder and tree skier; there are no signs that he has fallen. After another 15 minutes, you are forced to walk on the level through the deep snow.

You periodically report your position to the summit by radio. The timber is becoming thicker; in some places you can barely get between the small lodgepole pine trees. Hart's tracks start turning to the left, going back uphill. You see some places where the snow is disturbed, where he probably fell. No doubt he was tiring and decided to try to climb back up to the run.

Following the tracks uphill is becoming harder and harder, and you're getting hungry. The three of you stop, take your climbing skins from the off-area packs, put them on your skis, and each have a candy bar before continuing.

Suddenly, you find two skis in the snow where Hart apparently took off his skis and started to walk directly uphill in the deep snow. You tell yourself it was a good thing that he didn't leave his poles behind as well. You suspect you'll find him soon, and you report your findings to the summit by radio. In a few minutes, you have to take your own skis off in order to follow his trail because it is so steep. You strap the skis to your packs and steady yourselves with your poles. It is 7 p.m.

Although you are all in excellent shape, the three of you are breathing heavily as you fight your way uphill through the deep snow. Finally, you reach the top of the ridge and find yourselves in a flat clearing. You put your skis on again and follow the foot trail in the snow. It's starting to wander from side to side, and you think that Hart must be exhausted by now.

You know where you are; you are in the clearing that drops off from the middle dogleg on Big Elk run, about one quarter mile below the dogleg. You think that Hart must have been very disappointed not to find the run when he reached the top of the ridge. He would have to climb the next ridge to reach it from here and probably doesn't have enough strength left. You report the situation to the summit by radio.

Up ahead, at the end of the tracks you see a dark object in the snow between two trees. The tracks lead to it. Excitedly, you hurry to the object. Your headlight beam catches a white face with tousled, dark hair. The boy is sitting in the snow, leaning against a log, shivering occasionally. You glance at your watch: it is 8 p.m.

You: "Hello, Hart, are you okay? I'm Ben Schussen from the High Range Ski Patrol."

Patient (weakly): "Hi, I'm pretty cold."

You: "Well, we're going to get you warmed up and give you a ride down to the road."

You assess the patient's pulse and find that it is somewhat weak, regular, and slower than normal. His respirations are also slower than normal.

You: "Let's take your temperature. Do you think you can keep this in your mouth for a few minutes?"

Patient: "Okay."

You take your hypothermia thermometer out of its case, shake the mercury down, and place the tip under Hart's tongue, asking him to keep his lips tight around the thermometer. You then pause and press the radio transmission key and call the summit patroller.

You: "We have a 10-23, and we need the toboggan. Bring it down to the middle dogleg on Big Elk run, but instead of going to the left, go straight down off area, headed for the road. You'll pick up our tracks in about 400 yards."

After the summit patroller confirms, you open the off-area pack and take out a waterproof, fleece-lined casualty bag, a long Therm-A-Rest pad, and the Heatpac. One of the other patrollers is digging a small trench that will keep Hart out of the wind, and the other is gathering wood for a fire. You inflate the pad and place it in the snow, placing the casualty bag on top of it. You look at the thermometer, which has a reading of 91°F. You note to yourself that the patient has a core or rectal temperature of 92°F, which is cold but not too cold.

You and another patroller gently help Hart into the casualty bag. His inner clothes are wet with sweat, but the bag is waterproof and windproof. You assemble the Heatpac, placing a cartridge into the chamber and turning the reversed D cell around so it will power the fan. You light the fuse; a cloud of smoke pours out for a moment and then the device settles down with a hum. You attach the Y-shaped split tubing and push it up under the patient's shirt, placing the combustion chamber in its insulated container on his upper thighs. Then you lace up the casualty bag.

By this time, the fire is blazing at one end of the trench. You carefully slide the patient on the pad into the other end of the trench and place a folded space blanket between the fire and the snow so that it reflects the fire's heat toward the patient. His breathing has speeded up and he is more alert.

You: "Do you feel any better now?"

Patient: "I'm starting to feel warmer."

You: "The toboggan will be here shortly."

In about 30 minutes you hear two patrollers thrashing the heavy toboggan through the dense timber. After they arrive, it takes only a few minutes to load the patient into the Akja, put out the fire, and start off downhill. As you approach the road, you see the lights of several cars ahead, one of them a sheriff's vehicle with its light-bar flashing red and blue. The patient and Akja are loaded into a large four-wheel-drive vehicle and taken up to the patrol room, about 2 miles away. Hart's parents and Sophie are waiting for him. By the time you arrive, he is awake, alert, talking coherently, and feeling a lot better. His oral temperature is 96°F. It is 9 p.m.

It takes you 30 minutes to debrief. The patient is sent home with his parents, somewhat subdued when he realizes he will lose his season pass for this episode. The parents are instructed to check in with the emergency department of a nearby hospital when they get home.

Emergency Care of Infants and Children
Scenario 19

The following scenario was adapted from a 1995 *Ski Patrol Magazine* article by Mark Frank, MD, and Gerard Glancy, MD. The article describes how to manage an unresponsive child.

You are a member of the patrol at Mount Shred, a major snowboarding center. While covering the hill's halfpipe area with Mary, another patroller, you watch as a girl who is about 6 years old enjoys a good run. Suddenly, the child loses control and flies off the side of the halfpipe into a nearby stand of trees. A boy about 12 years old, who you assume is the little girl's brother, races over from the other side of the halfpipe. You immediately radio the aid room and rush to the scene.

When you arrive, the girl is lying on the ground, and her body position suggests that she struck a tree and fell backwards. Her helmet is behind her on the snow. There is a bleeding laceration over her right eye and a bruise over her left jaw.

You and Mary take off your skis, put on latex gloves, and approach the child. By this time, the boy has reached the scene.

Boy: "That's my sister! Is she okay?"

Mary: "It looks like she took a bad spill. We'll tend to her. Are your parents nearby?"

Boy: "They're down at the lodge. I'll go get them."

Mary: "Tell them to meet us at the aid room at the base."

While Mary gives directions to the boy, you focus

on the little girl. Stabilizing her head with your hand, you shake her shoulder gently.

You: "Honey, are you all right? My name is Chris and I'm with the ski patrol. I'm here to help you."

The girl does not respond. You immediately start to assess the ABCs. Her airway is open and her breathing is strong but labored. Her carotid pulse is strong and fast.

After the child's brother left to find the parents, you ask Mary to stabilize the girl's head and neck and keep the airway open with the jaw-thrust maneuver. You take off your aid belt, open it, and begin the rapid body survey. The child's pupils are round and equal, and both respond to your penlight. You place a sterile compress over the oozing scalp laceration and secure it with a self-adhering roller bandage.

Moving downward, you note that there is blood in the girl's mouth, one tooth is pointing at an abnormal angle, and another is missing. You perform a finger sweep, which dislodges the loose tooth and produces the missing one. Carefully, you remove the two teeth, holding each by the crown, and place them in a small plastic bag to tape to the child's jacket so they won't get lost.

The child's breathing seems to be less labored. After measuring from the corner of her mouth to the angle of her jaw, you select the proper oropharyngeal airway from your belt and insert it into place. You then radio dispatch.

You: "Dispatch, we have an unresponsive child, approximately 6 years old, with a rapid pulse and a scalp laceration. We need a toboggan, the pediatric Stifnecks, a pediatric backboard, oxygen, suction, and some help. Please arrange for helicopter transport."

You recheck the patient's carotid pulse and find it's 180 beats/min. The girl is breathing at a rate of 24 breaths/min. You continue the rapid body survey. There are no obvious neck abnormalities. Unzipping the child's jacket and pushing her shirt and longjohn top up, you assess the child's chest and find that there are no obvious wounds and both sides are moving symmetrically as she breathes.

You then pull down the clothing on her upper body and slide her ski pants down to temporarily expose her abdomen. There are no obvious abnormalities. You assess the extremities and find no deformities or swelling and note that the child isn't wearing a medical alert bracelet or necklace. She doesn't respond to a painful pinch of each extremity and doesn't move spontaneously.

Two patrollers arrive with the toboggan and one of them begins to administer oxygen by nonrebreathing mask at 15 L/min. The other patroller carefully applies a suitable pediatric Stifneck collar.

Next, you log roll the child onto her side for a moment while you quickly assess her back. Finding no abnormalities, you roll her onto the pediatric long backboard. A folded blanket is placed under her torso to put her in the correct anatomic position. Your fellow patrollers strap the girl's trunk and lower extremities securely into place and immobilize her head to prepare her for transport off the mountain.

Before starting down, you conduct the ongoing assessment; she is still a U on the AVPU scale. Her respirations are 24 breaths/min and regular, and her pulse is 60 beats/min and regular. Her pulse is at the bottom of the normal pulse range for her age. You begin to worry about increasing intracranial pressure. Her capillary refill is normal.

The patient is taken carefully and as rapidly as possible to the base by toboggan. As you near the base lodge you see the girl's brother and parents waiting at the door to the aid room. The LifeFlight helicopter roars overhead as it prepares to land.

Two weeks later, the patrol receives a thank-you card and the good news that the child had just been released from the hospital after undergoing removal of a subdural hematoma.

Scenario 20

The following scenario was adapted from a 1995 *Ski Patrol Magazine* article by Mark Frank, MD, and Gerard Glancy, MD. This scenario describes how to manage a responsive adolescent.

A local school is sponsoring a downhill race for participants between age 8 and 14 years at your ski area, Ego Alley Resort, and you're providing course coverage. As one young racer skis down the course, he loses control in one of the turns and begins sliding across the run. Just before coming to a stop, he bounces off one of the poles supporting the barrier fence. Both of his skis fly off. As he lies there, he starts to scream and clutches his left thigh with both hands.

You ski toward him, noting that he makes no attempt to get up. By the time you arrive, his parents are already there. They're talking to him as you take off your skis.

Father: "Johnny, why didn't you see that patch of ice? It was obvious! Get up and finish the race!"

Johnny (crying): "My leg hurts."

Father: "It's probably only a charley horse. If you get up now, you may still be able to finish in the top 10!"

You: "Hi, my name is Ken and I'm with the ski patrol. Is there anything I can do to help?"

Father: "You can help Johnny get back on his skis to finish the race."

You: "I saw your son fall, and I was concerned he may have hurt himself. Is it okay if I check him over to see if he's all right?"

Father: "Well, okay, but that's a very expensive, ultra-thin racing suit, so be careful with it."

You: "How old is Johnny?"

Father: "Nine."

You: "Johnny, I'm going to check your thigh and see what's happened."

Johnny is still crying loudly and holding his left thigh. He nods his head affirmatively. You take off your jacket and put it around him, leaving his helmet on to keep his head warm.

His airway is obviously open and he's breathing well. You grasp his near wrist and assess the radial pulse. It's strong although it seems to be somewhat more rapid than normal. You put on a pair of gloves and continue the rapid body survey, placing emphasis on the site of injury. As you work, you try to engage Johnny in small talk regarding siblings, pets, hobbies, and school to help him relax.

Assessment of the left thigh discloses marked tenderness at its midportion. There's no obvious deformity, but you aren't sure about swelling. You compare it with the opposite thigh. You reach down and unbuckle his left ski boot, rebuckling it in a looser setting.

You: "Johnny, can you feel your toes?"

Johnny: "Yes."

You: "Do you have any trouble moving your leg or thigh?"

Johnny (sobbing): "I can't move it. It hurts too much."

You: "Can you wiggle your toes without them hurting?"

Johnny: "Yes."

You: "Did you hit your head or hurt your neck?"

Johnny: "No."

You: "Do you hurt anywhere else besides your thigh?"

Johnny: "No."

You (to Johnny's parents): "I'm concerned that

Johnny's hurt his leg bad enough that he shouldn't ski on it. I'll call for a toboggan and some equipment so we can get him down to the aid room."

Father: "If you think he hurt his leg, I want a doctor to come up here right away and examine it before you touch him!"

You: "I'm sorry, but we aren't able to do that at this ski area. The ski patrol is trained in the initial care of these injuries, and we'll be happy to assist your son. I recommend that we splint his leg and get him safely off the mountain to our aid room before he gets any colder. Splinting will also help the pain a lot. Meanwhile, I can radio for a physician to meet us at the aid room."

You radio the summit for a toboggan, pediatric femur traction splint, oxygen, and some help. Next, you radio the aid room and ask them to page the physician on call to meet you there in about 20 minutes.

While you wait, you perform the rapid body survey and find no other obvious injuries or painful areas. However, after comparing the left midthigh with the right, you believe that the left midthigh is now slightly swollen. There is no sign of any blood on the patient's left pant leg. You unbuckle his other ski boot.

The ongoing assessment shows no changes. The patient's mental status is normal, his respirations are normal at 16 breaths/min, and his pulse is strong and 100 beats/min. Speaking with a confident and comforting tone, you're as honest as possible as you tell the boy what's going to happen. You assure him that you'll inform him before you do anything. You also let him know that the pain in his thigh will increase momentarily when the traction splint is being put in place, but that he'll feel better once traction is applied.

The toboggan arrives and you start oxygen using a nonrebreathing mask at 15 L/min. Johnny tries to be brave but cries harder, holding his mother's hand as the traction splint is applied. Johnny is loaded into the toboggan, covered with a blanket and tarp, and transported to the aid room, accompanied by his parents.

Later, the physician on call tells you that Johnny fractured his left femur.

Advanced Assessment

Scenario 21

This scenario describes how to manage a patient with a serious medical problem.

As part of a family reunion, you are taking six cousins from the East on a 4-day backpacking trip into the high country northeast of Grandstone National Park. They have all hiked parts of the Appalachian Trail but before now have never been above 6,000' for very long.

appendix a

Your party's gear is packed and the seven of you take your four-wheel-drive wagon and your four-door sedan up to the Lady of the Lake trailhead. You take the lead and ask Andy, who used to be a ski patroller at Mount Scree in Vermont, to herd the stragglers from the rear. You set a steady, rhythmic pace and stop at regular intervals to admire the view and the many small meadows with their colorful patches of flowers. Everyone is somewhat short of breath from the altitude, but no one lags behind.

Camp that night is near the lower end of Aerie Lake, at an altitude of 9,500′. Several members of the group take their spinning gear out as soon as they spot the huge brown trout in the deep water at the bottom of a nearby small cliff, but it is shrimp-hatch time and they don't have any luck.

You prepare an impressive spread for supper: fresh pasta from Bernadelli's in town (complete with their famous homemade sauce), freeze-dried vegetables, garlic bread, and pistachio instant pudding. Everyone is in their sleeping bags by 8:30 p.m., with plans to fish for grayling in an inlet creek the next morning and then scramble up Wolverine Peak for a view of the entire mountain range.

You usually don't sleep well your first night at altitude, and this night is no exception. Several times you hear some stirring from the other tent, and once a flashlight beam plays briefly on the side of your tent. It sounds like someone is walking up the path to where you have established a latrine. You have dropped off into a deep sleep when you are suddenly awakened by a disturbance at the tent entrance.

"Ben, come out here, please. Something's wrong with Bill." It's Andy, and he looks worried. You pick up your pile jacket, strap on your camp sandals, and squirm out through the entrance. The sun is just coming up over the ridge to the east. You glance at your watch: it is 6 a.m.

Andy tells you that Bill got up several times during the night to go out and is now lying in his sleeping bag. He is complaining of being short of breath and weak.

You crawl into the tent. Cousin Bill, a 36-year-old computer programmer, is lying on his side. There is enough light for you to see his face, which is pale with beads of sweat on the forehead. He looks anxious.

You unzip the bag, reach in, and grasp his wrist. "Andy, get me your flashlight, please." Bill's pulse is regular, strong, and faster than normal. His breathing is faster than normal but not labored.

You: "Bill, what's wrong?"

Patient: "I'm not sure. I'm very weak and can't get my breath."

You: "When did it start?"

Patient: "I was okay when I went to bed…maybe a little tired from the walk in. I woke up at about midnight and had to use the latrine in a hurry. On the way back from the latrine I was more short of breath and my legs felt pretty weak, and for a few minutes I wasn't sure I would make it back to the tent. I felt better after I got back into my bag and fell asleep again. About 2 hours later, I had to get up and have another bowel movement. On the way back I was weak and short of breath again. I got back to sleep but I'm not feeling any better. I'm still weak and short of breath, and I'm starting to feel sick to my stomach."

You: "Do you have a headache or any dizziness?"

Patient: "No headache, but I feel dizzy."

You: "Do you mean you're lightheaded or do you actually have trouble with your balance? Is the tent going around in circles?"

Patient: "Lightheaded, I guess."

You: "What was the bowel movement like? Did you look at it? Was it diarrhea? Did you have any cramps?"

Patient: "It was soft but not diarrhea. I couldn't see much, it was too dark and my flashlight battery is weak. No cramps."

You: "Have you had a cold, sore throat, chills, fever, nausea, vomiting, or diarrhea during the last week or so?"

Patient: "No."

You: "Have you had any other changes in your bowel habits?"

Patient: "The bowel movements have been pretty dark the last few days."

You: "Have you had any indigestion, like heartburn or sour stomach?"

Patient: "Some sour stomach. I've used a lot of Rolaids the last two weeks."

At this point, you're puzzled. Bill's airway, breathing, and circulation seem to be basically all right but stressed, with a fast heart rate and breathing rate. You know that you should consider acute mountain sickness in anyone who isn't feeling well above 6,000′. Also, you know that there's a lot of stomach flu going around, but it does not sound like a typical case of that. You need to assess his neck and chest.

You don a pair of gloves. Pulling down the neck of Bill's T-shirt, you look at his neck. The veins are not distended. You don't feel any tender nodes under the jaw, and there are no tender areas or swelling. The trachea is in the midline.

Pulling the T-shirt up around the patient's neck, you look at his chest. Both sides are moving symmetrically as he breathes. You put your ear to both sides of the chest and don't hear any rattles, wheezes, or other noise. The breathing sounds are loud and equal on both sides. You move on to assess the patient's abdomen.

With the tips of your fingers, you palpate the abdomen, starting in the right upper quadrant. Each time you push in with your fingers, you ask, "Does this hurt?" When you reach the epigastric area, he winces. You can hear some loud gurgles. There are no other tender areas.

You have a feeling that you are forgetting something... Airway, Breathing, Circulation. That's it! Circulation includes bleeding.

You: "Andy, do me a favor. Run up to the latrine and tell me what Bill's bowel movement looks like. Seriously."

Andy is back in a few minutes.

Andy: "There's a lot of reddish-black B.M. in the latrine."

The pieces of the puzzle are coming together. Bill probably has an ulcer and is bleeding from it. You remember reading about bleeding ulcers in Outdoor Emergency Care.

You: "Bill, have you ever had an ulcer?"

Patient: "I had one 3 years ago, but it cleared up with Prilosec and antibiotics."

You: "Does this feel anything like that ulcer?"

Patient: "Maybe so."

You: "You mentioned a sour stomach. What happens when you eat?"

Patient: "It gets better but then comes back in an hour or so."

You: "Are you taking any regular medicine besides the Rolaids?"

Patient: "No."

You: "Have you had any other medical problems in the past? Any allergies?"

Patient: "No."

You: "Anything else we need to know about you?"

Patient: "I've always been healthy, but more tired lately. Probably because we've been awfully busy at work. I had a hard time getting time off to come on this trip."

You give Bill some reconstituted powdered milk, instant Cream of Wheat, and Mylanta from your aid pack. You give the car keys to another cousin, Mike, a marathon runner, who has agreed to return to the trailhead and call for a helicopter.

As it turns out, Bill has only one more bowel movement, his pulse slows, and his color returns to some extent before he is helicoptered out to a hospital early that afternoon. A duodenal ulcer is found on the endoscopic exam. It was not bleeding actively by then, so your emergency care may have helped. You resolve to leave Bernadelli's famous pasta sauce off of future menus.

Scenario 22

This scenario illustrates the assessment and care of a patient with multiple injuries.

It's a beautiful June day in the Granite Mountains. High Range Ski Area has been closed for 6 weeks, but you're still not ready to quit skiing. You, your wife, Sandy, and two other couples have just driven up the switchbacks of the Whitetail Highway to 10,000' where there is plenty of snow and an abundance of steep chutes to choose from. You and your friends brought several vehicles so that you can leave a half-dozen switchbacks below to ferry you back after you ski the Granite Creek Headwall.

You hoped to have the site to yourselves, but there are five other cars at the turnoff by the top of the headwall. It's only 7 a.m., so the snow is still in good condition. There's time to make a dozen runs before it turns to mush in the hot June sun.

Several other skiers are getting into their bindings as you brake to a stop. It takes a few minutes to limber up and click into your own bindings. The right-hand chute is narrow but in excellent condition as you jump-turn down the 50° section at the top and break out into the wider, easier terrain below. You're puffing a little when you reach the bottom. Sandy is right behind you, demonstrating the smooth, effortless technique you've always envied. The other four arrive a few minutes apart.

At the end of the third run, you're starting to feel it a little in your quads. You skid to a stop and look up the chute. Sandy is halfway down and in good form.

She joins you, breathing easily in the thin air. As you both look uphill, the next skier is coming down. You don't recognize him; he must be from one of the other cars parked at the turnoff.

As you watch, the skier suddenly loses his balance during a turn, falls forward, and starts to cartwheel. Both skis fly off. You think his poles must still be with him, but there is such a cloud of snow that you're not sure. You hear Sandy gasp as he hits a small rock out-crop and launches into the air, picking up speed as he hits the snow headfirst. From there he tumbles over and over, bounces off one side of the gully, and finally slides to a halt about 100 yards above you. You and Sandy kick your skis off and run toward him. As you run, you reach behind to make sure your aid belt is still there.

The skier, a man in his early 20s, is lying on his back and not moving. As you reach his side, you rap-idly take in the scene and reach for a pair of latex gloves. There is some blood on the snow near his head. His cap is gone, and his eyes are closed. You're not sure if he is breathing. His right thigh is twisted at an unusual angle.

After donning the gloves and encouraging Sandy to do the same, you steady his head with your hand, shake his shoulder, and call loudly: "Buddy, are you okay?" There is no answer. His face is pale with beads of sweat on his forehead.

You move around behind the patient and stabilize his head and neck while you thrust his jaw forward. As you bend your ear to his mouth and nose, you're relieved to hear the air moving in and out. Next, you feel for his carotid pulse under the neck of his pullover; it's strong and regular, but a little too fast. You can see his chest lifting; his breathing rate seems normal. Looking at his dark hair, you see blood trick-ling through it on the right temporoparietal area of the scalp and running down his cheek.

Sandy takes over the jaw-thrust maneuver and manual stabilization of the patient's head and neck while you reach into the aid belt and retrieve an oral airway, a flashlight, and a tongue blade. You check the airway for size by placing it against his cheek. You open the patient's mouth and use the tongue blade to push the tongue out of the way. He does not gag. There's no blood in his mouth, and his teeth look normal. You slip the oral airway in place.

Quickly, you assess the patient's eyes and pupils; both pupils are round and respond to the light of your flashlight, but the right one is slightly larger than the left. You evaluate the patient's responsiveness using the AVPU scale. He is not alert, and he does not respond to verbal stimulus. You pinch the skin of his inner arm through his jacket, and he stirs and moans. Next, you pinch the tip of his right index finger gently but firmly, then the tip of his left index finger. He withdraws the right hand but not the left. You repeat the pinch on the skin of both lower legs; he moves the right leg slightly but not the left. You determine that the patient scores a P on the AVPU scale but is moving only the left side of his body.

The patient has a serious head injury and may be starting to lateralize, but he may also be in early shock. You know that head injuries by themselves don't cause shock, so something else must be going on.

Turning back to the patient's head, you find a large laceration that's oozing blood. Gently feeling the scalp around the laceration, you can't feel any depression or irregularities.

By this point, one of the other two couples has arrived, and you ask the woman, Jenny, to hand you a sterile compress from the plastic bandage bag. You place the sterile compress over the laceration as Jenny's husband, Mike, who is a fellow patroller, removes his aid belt and dons a pair of latex gloves. Mike places direct pressure on the wound while you attend to the rest of the patient's head and face.

There is no blood in either ear and the sides of the jaw are symmetrical. Moving to the patient's neck, you run your fingers down the spinous processes of the seven cervical vertebrae but don't find any step-off deformities or lumps. On the front of the neck, the veins are flat, there are no open wounds, bruises, or swelling, and the trachea is in the midline.

You reassess the patient's breathing and pulse. The breathing rate has increased and is now at 28 breaths/min. The carotid pulse is 110 beats/min and seems weaker. Moving quickly to the patient's chest, you open his jacket and place a hand on each side of his chest. Both sides expand equally. Lifting his pullover, you run both hands down the ribs on each side while you inspect the skin. There are no wounds, bruises, or swelling of the upper chest, but when you reach the lower chest you find a large bruise over the lower right ribs. Moving down to the abdomen, you notice that he moans when you press on his right upper quadrant beneath the costal angle. You press the sides of the pelvis together and backward; they seem solid and he doesn't moan.

Proceeding downward to the lower extremities, you run your hands over both thighs. The midthigh of his right leg is swollen beneath his jeans, and he moans again when you press on the swollen area. The lower extremities are otherwise normal.

At this point, you see the other couple, Pete and Jane, approaching, accompanied by two young skiers—possibly the patient's friends. You reflect a moment. You have a skier who took a bad fall with lots of kinetic energy, bounced off some rocks, cartwheeled, and tumbled. He is responsive only to pain, has a large scalp laceration and maybe an early blown pupil on the right. His left side isn't moving as well as his right in response to pain. To you, this indicates a serious head injury that is getting worse.

In addition, he has a rising pulse and respiratory rate, evidence of injuries to the lower right chest and upper right abdomen, and a probable right femur fracture. Possible lung and liver injury, as well as a possible femoral fracture, can be the cause of early shock.

You turn to the patient's two friends and begin to question them.

You: "Hi, I'm Ben Schussen from the High Range Ski Patrol. Is this man a friend of yours?"

Friend: "Yes, he's Oliver de Place. He's a senior at the university. What happened to him?"

You: "He took a bad fall and tumbled all the way down the chute. He's unconscious, badly hurt, and may be going into shock. He has injuries to his head, chest, abdomen, a probable femur fracture, and a possible neck injury. Do you have a car parked down there at the turnout?"

Friend: "Yes."

You: "This is an emergency. I need you to get in your car and drive quickly to the restaurant at the entrance to the canyon, just before the switchbacks start up."

You reach into your aid belt and pull out a pen and a small notebook.

You: "Here's some paper so you can write this down. Call the county sheriff and tell him about your friend, where he is, that he fell about 1,000′ down the Granite Creek headwall, he's injured his head, chest, abdomen, femur, and possibly his neck, and that he's going into shock. We need the ALS ambulance from the town hospital with a doctor or paramedic, and some help from the sheriff's office right away. Tell them we need a backboard, traction splint, oxygen, BVM device, suction, a basket stretcher, and at least six people to carry him out to the road. We need a LifeFlight helicopter from the city to meet us in town. Do you have all that?"

Friend: "You bet. I'm writing it down. I'm on my way."

As he leaves, you finish the rapid body survey by assessing the patient's upper extremities and running your hand behind his back from the base of the neck to the tailbone. With Mike's help, you remove both boots and check the pulses in both feet. Both are easy to find and strong. Then you take a pair of paramedic shears from your aid belt and cut the patient's right pant leg open to the hip. There is a large swelling in the middle of the thigh but no blood or open wounds.

You, Mike, Pete, and Sandy then align the patient into the anatomic position, straightening his right lower extremity with axial traction. While maintaining the extremity traction and head/neck stabilization, the four of you carefully roll him a quarter turn onto his side while Jenny places several parkas on the snow under him.

You talk to the patient's other friend and are able to get some sketchy details about his medical history. He has no illnesses, doesn't take any medications, doesn't have allergies, and has always been healthy although somewhat impulsive and carefree. He's been skiing for two seasons, has never taken any lessons, and this is the first time he's skied the headwall. His favorite summer sport is motorcycle racing.

The patient is evacuated to town on a long backboard without incident, with a traction splint on his right lower extremity. He was immediately flown to City Hospital, where he spent the next 5 weeks, 2 weeks of which were on a ventilator in the Surgical Intensive Care Unit.

Luckily, the patient didn't fracture his neck. You heard that he required a craniotomy to remove a right epidural hematoma followed immediately by a laparotomy to sew up a laceration in his liver. His fractured femur was treated with an intramedullary nail a week later. Three months after he was released from the hospital, you found out that he was back on his motorcycle.

Rescue Techniques
Scenario 23

This scenario illustrates a typical extrication problem.

You and three friends have planned a day of rock climbing. At the last minute, Lucky decided not to go because of a bout of vomiting and diarrhea, so you, Tom, and Spike drive to the Rosebud Lake road and park at a turnout just past a bridge over Rosebud Creek. From there it is about one quarter mile to the base of the Central Spire, through a small wooded area and up a boulder field.

Instead of climbing in two teams of two as originally planned, you have to climb in one team of three. To save time, you decide to alternate leads and leave a fixed rope to protect the third man. He follows, self-belayed by two jumars while the first man belays the second man up the next pitch.

The climb is going well until the start of the second pitch, a difficult one to the right of a wall. The middle part involves a 40′ traverse to the right along a narrow ledge, an area of tricky climbing on some loose rock, and then some small faces alternating with small ledges leading back toward the wall. Tom leads and you follow.

You clean the chocks as you go and note that the rope you are trailing for Spike to climb now hangs straight down about 30′ to the left of the bad section. After you join Tom, you have a fleeting feeling that you probably should have left some of the protection in for Spike to take out.

You tie off Spike's fixed rope securely to the anchor, tell him that it is ready, then belay Tom up the next pitch. You notice some motion on Spike's rope, then it tightens and you know he has started up. Tom's pitch is easy and in 10 minutes you hear his "Off belay!"

Suddenly, you hear a cry from below. Looking over, you see Spike hanging free in his harness next to the wall. He yells something; you can hardly hear it over the noise of the creek in the valley, but it sounds like "Help!" You call to Tom that Spike's been hurt and to come back down. In a few minutes, Tom has rappelled back down to join you, and you both rappel down to Spike.

You: "What's wrong?"

Spike: "I hurt my shoulder."

Spike is holding his left arm away from his chest, supporting his forearm with his right hand. You and Tom pull him over to a small ledge, where he can stand. Tom threads a descending ring onto two slings and ties them around a nearby horn. As soon as the anchor is ready, you clip Spike into it.

You: "What happened?"

Spike: "I fell off that loose stuff over there and swung into the wall. I hit my shoulder. It hurts bad and I can't move it."

You: "Did you hurt anything else?"

Spike: "No."

You: "What about your head and neck? You sure took some fiberglass off your helmet."

Spike: "I bounced my head off the wall, but my head and neck feel okay."

You: "What about your back?"

Spike: "It feels okay."

You: "Were you knocked out at all?"

Spike: "No."

You: "Let me see you move your fingers."

Spike wiggles the fingers of his left hand, then squeezed your hand when you ask him to. When you scrape your fingernail over the skin on the back of his left hand, he tells you he can feel it. You assess the injured shoulder. Running your finger from the sternum to the point of the shoulder along the clavicle, you note that the surface of the clavicle is smooth, regular, and nontender. When you get to the shoulder, you note that the point of the shoulder is sharp and squared off.

Spike (groaning): "This is really sore. I gotta sit down."

You: "Okay, I'll steady you. Be careful you don't slip."

You pinch the skin over the left deltoid muscle and then the right.

You: "Can you feel this? Does it feel the same on both sides?"

Spike: "Yes."

You: "Can you move your shoulder at all?"

Spike: "No."

You: "Because it hurts or because it's weak?"

Spike: "Because it hurts."

You: "I think your shoulder may be dislocated. Let me check a few other things, then we'll get you splinted and out of here."

You quickly assess Spike's head, neck, and back, while asking if he hit his chest or pelvis. He says there is no pain anywhere else. His pupils are round, regular, equal, and respond to light. His mouth is normal, there is no obvious bleeding from the mouth or nose, and you see no obvious facial injuries. You do not remove the helmet, because he'll need it for evacuation. There is no tenderness or swelling of the neck, particularly over the spinous processes. There is no tenderness or obvious deformities of the back either, especially the spinous processes of the vertebrae, which you examine through his jacket.

You open your small backpack and take out a long length of 1″ nylon webbing, two triangular bandages, and a spare fleece jacket that you fold into a tight bundle and place between Spike's arm and his chest. You make a sling out of one triangular bandage and cradle his left arm in it, then fold the second bandage into a wide cravat and use it to secure his arm to his chest.

You: "Spike, you can't rappel with your bad shoulder. Since I'm bigger than Tom, what we're going to do is make a harness with this long sling so that you can sit on my back. Tom is going to belay the two of us while we rap off to the ground. Good thing we have a spare rope. If we tie two of the ropes together, they'll reach."

Spike: "Okay."

Meanwhile, Tom has retrieved and coiled the two ropes, and has taken the third one out of his pack and uncoiled it.

You: "Spike, stand up where you are. Tom is going to make the harness. I'll back up to you so Tom can strap you on my back."

Tom centers the sling at the middle of Spike's upper back, then runs an end around each side of the chest under the armpit and crosses the ends over Spike's chest. You back up to Spike and half-squat so he can straddle your back. Tom runs an end over each of your shoulders, then across your chest like an X, through Spike's legs, around his hips, and across your waist, where you tie the ends securely. The system feels solid.

Tom slips the end of one of the two 150′ ropes through the descending ring on the anchor, ties the two ropes together, and throws the coiled ends of the ropes out into space. They reach the ground easily. You tie the belay rope to your harness and Spike's harness, and Tom sets up a belay using a Munter hitch. You set up your rappel with a figure-eight descender clipped to your harness and slowly back to the edge while Tom keeps you tightly on belay. Leaning back, you brace your legs wide apart as you walk over the edge.

All goes well; Spike is solidly attached to your back and able to balance himself with his feet as you descend. You lean to the opposite side to keep his injured shoulder away from the rock. Fortunately, it's a sheer wall all the way to the ground, without any loose rock. You reach the ground without incident and

within a few minutes, Tom rappels down to join you.

It takes about 30 minutes to negotiate the boulder field. Spike walks slowly and carefully, and you and Tom support him as necessary. A few minutes later, you're in the car and headed for town.

Scenario 24

The following scenario illustrates how to extricate an injured skier from a difficult location.

It's March 1 at High Range Ski Area. Several storms in a row have dumped 3′ of powder on the mountain's 8′ base, and cold temperatures have kept it in good condition. Early Saturday morning, the parking lot is full of the powder hounds' 4 × 4 vehicles. The lines waiting for the lifts to start are as long as you've ever seen them.

You're looking for some good skiing yourself, especially on presweep, and you're not disappointed. You have first duty at the summit, but after that you plan to make at least one run down through the trees in Powder Park, the best ungroomed area on the mountain. First duty is quiet and you are standing outside the hut, ready to get into your bindings, when your replacement arrives. He's covered with snow, so you know where he's been.

About halfway through the park, you hear a shout and catch sight of a woman gesticulating wildly. Curious, you leave the untracked area and ski toward her across an area of powder-covered bumps. She is pointing to a clump of trees where a set of tracks leads toward a huge spruce whose lower branches are buried in the snow.

Skier: "Sir, my friend is down under that tree and can't get out! Can you help him?"

You nod your head and motion for her to follow you. As you approach the tree, you see that the tracks appear to ski right into the closest lower branches, which are bare of snow. The tracks disappear in a hole in the snow underneath the branches.

You pole up to the hole, part the branches, and look into the gloomy snow well that surrounds the trunk of the tree. A young man is upside down in the well, his skis tangled in the lower branches and his head buried in the snow. One ski pole is still strapped to his right wrist; the other is nowhere in sight.

You quickly get out of your skis, lower yourself into the hole, bend down, and start digging the snow away from his face. Out of the corner of your eye, you note that his right arm seems to be bent at an abnormal angle. You call out to the patient and ask if he is okay.

There is no answer. You quickly pull off your ski gloves and thrust his jaw forward, opening his airway, and place your ear close to his mouth and nose. You hear a faint gasp and a cough. He is breathing slowly. You quickly open your aid pack and put on a pair of latex gloves, then you open the patient's mouth and perform the finger sweep. There is no snow in his mouth. You palpate the carotid artery and find that his pulse is strong and regular with a rate that is slightly faster than normal.

You key your lapel mike and call Summit. When Summit replies you describe the situation.

You: "There's been an accident in Powder Park, just to the left of the opening of the lower chute. I need a toboggan, long backboard, KED, oxygen, suction, two snow shovels, an ax and saw, and at least six patrollers."

When you again ask the patient if he's okay, he responds with a moan. His eyes remain closed but he is now breathing well and his pulse is strong. You call to his friend, asking her to take your skis and make an upright X in the snow with them to guide the other patrollers. You keep his jaw thrust forward with one hand while you enlarge his breathing space some more with your other hand. Because the patient is moaning, he probably has a gag reflex and won't tolerate an oral airway. You shift yourself around so you can stabilize his head and neck better. It's quite a trick; this is the first time you've tried it on someone who is hanging upside down. While waiting, you introduce yourself to the patient's friend and explain what you are doing.

After what seems like hours but is really more like 10 minutes, the toboggan arrives, followed shortly by a crowd of fellow patrollers. They survey the scene and receive a briefing from you, and then one of them takes the shovel and starts to enlarge the entrance to the well, being careful not to dislodge any snow that is supporting the patient. The patient's skis are left on for the moment since they are wedged into the branches and supporting his legs. The oxygen backpack and portable hand-suction unit are brought up, and one of the patrollers crowds into the hole with you, ready to use them. Fortunately, the oxygen tubing is about 6' long. The patroller places a nonrebreathing mask on the patient's face and adjusts the flow to 15 L/min.

You: "I think the best course of action is to dig out this hole until enough of us can get in here to raise the patient and slide the backboard under him. We have to assume that he has both a neck and a head injury. I haven't had time to look closely, but I think

his right arm may be broken. Rick, take a look at the arm and then get ready to support and stabilize the shoulders and arms with Keith. Ted and Sue, you get ready to support and stabilize the hips. Jack, as soon as you have enough snow shoveled out of the way, support his legs and get his skis off. Rick, after you check the arm, get the ax and saw and clear away those lower branches. Careful that you don't jar him. Before anyone else comes down into the hole, get that backboard in here."

In just a few minutes, the hole is big enough so you can maneuver. You have the patient's head and neck stabilized manually, two patrollers are supporting the shoulders and arms, two the hips, and one the legs. Rick has assessed the right arm and reports that there is swelling and some crepitus at its midportion. The radial pulse at the right wrist is strong. The skis and pole are off. The backboard is down in the hole, and the patient's friend is ready to slide it in place under him.

You: "The idea is to lift and pivot his body clockwise like a log until he is horizontal, face up, and the backboard can be slid under him and its ends braced on the sides of the hole. I'll call the signals. We'll move him about 12" at a time, pivoting around his hips so that his legs rotate down and the rest of his body rotates up until he is horizontal. As you move him, bring his legs together and his arms to his sides. Keep the shoulders and hips at right angles to the spine, and keep the spine straight. Okay, everybody ready? Raise his upper body 12" on three. One, two, three."

The patient's upper body is raised 12" toward the horizontal and the legs lowered 12".

You: "Another 12", on three. One, two, three."

Slowly and smoothly, the patient is pivoted into the faceup, horizontal position, the backboard is slid under him, and he is lowered onto it. Ted takes an adjustable adult-size Stifneck collar out of the backboard stuffsack and applies it to the patient's neck.

By now, the patient's eyes are open and he is starting to stir and moan. Carefully, the six of you carry him on the board a few feet out into the open snow where there is room to work. You continue to manually stabilize the patient's head and neck.

Ted quickly conducts a rapid body survey and finds no injuries except the fracture of the right arm. He then takes two SAM splints from his aid packs, doubles them, shapes them into troughs, and applies them to the inside and outside of the patient's right arm, fixing them in place with 3″ Kling. The right arm's radial pulse is strong both before and after splinting.

After splinting the patient's arm, Ted aligns his extremities and straps him to the board with padding under his head, under the small of his back, and on both sides of his legs. Jack then secures the patient's splinted right upper extremity to his body using two cravats and a modified sling and swathe arrangement. Since the toboggan has to go down a steep chute to get out of the park, you decide to supplement the standard over-the-shoulder straps with groin straps.

Relieved of your duty at the head and neck, you take a flowsheet form out of your aid pack and start filling it out. You begin the ongoing assessment: the patient now has a strong, steady pulse of 90 beats/min; he is breathing well at 16 breaths/min; his pupils are round, regular, and equal; and, because he opens his eyes and looks at you when you call his name, he scores a V on the AVPU scale. Before being strapped down, he was moving all three uninjured extremities spontaneously and withdrawing them when you pinched them.

The toboggan has been brought alongside and the tarpaulin and sleeping bag opened. The patient is placed on the backboard into the toboggan, and the sleeping bag is closed. You strap him in securely because you have a steep toboggan run ahead; if he has to vomit you plan to tip the entire toboggan on its side and use the V-Vac suction unit. There was some discussion as to whether he should be transported head uphill or head downhill; because of his altered mental status, the original breathing problem, and the steepness of the route, you opt to position him with his head uphill.

In a few minutes, the patient is on his way to the base with Ted skiing beside him to monitor his airway, breathing, and oxygen, and watch for early signs of vomiting. There is one steep, narrow part of the chute where the toboggan will need to be belayed down, but fortunately the patroller who brought the toboggan remembered that in Powder Park you always bring along a lift evacuation sack with 150′ of goldline, a longhorn figure-eight descender, slings, and a locking carabiner.

Scenario 25

This scenario illustrates how to extricate two injured people from a difficult location.

It has been a pleasant spring day with a warming snowpack, rivulets at the base lodge, and mud in the parking lot. You and two other patrollers, Jan and Joe, are among the last to leave. You are putting your skis on the car when you see two skiers come out of the bar and climb into an old red sedan. Mud flies as they accelerate out of the parking lot, turn onto the road, and disappear down the mountain at a high speed.

As you enter the final curve before turning onto the main highway, you see a car in the ravine ahead; the taillights are still on and the bumper is resting against a large tree at the edge of the road. It looks like the red sedan. You pull over to the side of the road and turn on your emergency blinkers. The three of you jump out of the car with aid packs in hand and approach the accident site. The snow is heavy, wet, and about 2′ deep.

The front end of the two-door sedan is crumpled against the tree. There is a figure in each bucket seat: the driver, who is bent forward over the steering wheel, and the passenger, who has slid slightly forward on the seat and is lying on his left side with his head and chest on the seat, his left knee bent, his left hip flexed and internally rotated, and his abdomen and left lower extremity under the dashboard. Neither person is wearing a seatbelt, and neither one is moving. There is a star-shaped crack in the driver's side of the windshield. You don't smell any gasoline.

You try to open the driver's door and find it locked. Jan tries the other door. It isn't locked but is bent and won't open. You give Joe your keys and ask him to get the lug wrench out of the trunk of your car. The car is stable as it rests against the tree, and it appears safe to try to access the two individuals.

You open your aid pack and take out a pair of latex gloves and a roll of 2″ adhesive tape. Quickly, you tear off four long strips and lay them on the left rear window in the form of an eight-pointed star. Using the sharp end of the lug wrench, you give the window a hard blow at its lower rear corner. The tempered glass turns white as it fractures into many small pieces, most of which stay in place. With the blunt end of the lug wrench, you knock a large hole in the glass that allows you to reach in and flip the front door latch open with the end of the lug wrench. The door opens easily.

You reach in across the driver to turn off the ignition and notice that the top of the steering wheel is cracked and bent forward. There is a distinct odor of beer in the car. Neither patient has stirred, but you can see that the driver is breathing. There is a pool of blood on the dashboard in front of the steering wheel. You quickly pull on the pair of rubber gloves.

Jan squeezes into the rear seat. She moves to the right side behind the passenger, reaches forward, and opens the window of the passenger door. You follow her, then reach forward over the back of the driver's seat to manually stabilize the driver's head and neck. Blood is dripping down his face from a large cut on his forehead. The skin of his face is cool and moist. Jan helps you pull the driver back against the seat while you use the jaw-thrust maneuver to maintain his airway.

You ask the driver if he is okay. The driver stirs and moans, but his eyes remain closed. His respirations are rapid and shallow. You feel for his carotid pulse: it is regular, strong, and somewhat faster than normal.

Jan puts on a pair of rubber gloves, leans forward over the back of the seat, and loudly asks the passenger whether he is okay. The passenger moans and his eyes open. Meanwhile, a pair of headlights approach from the rear.

Jan: "I think he said 'No.'"

You: "Joe, stop that car. Have them call for an ambulance from the nearest phone. Tell them we have a car accident up here with two victims, both with head injuries and possible neck injuries."

The car slows to a stop and Joe recognizes two lift operators from the ski area. He delivers the message and they drive away.

Jan manually stabilizes the passenger's head and neck.

Jan: "The passenger is breathing well at a normal rate. He has a strong carotid pulse and responds to verbal stimuli. His skin is cold and clammy. I see no obvious bleeding."

You: "Joe, we need to keep these folks stabilized and maintain their airways. Please conduct rapid body surveys on them while we're waiting for the ambulance. Start with the driver because he has a big cut on his forehead, is bleeding, and has labored breathing. Don't forget your gloves."

After donning gloves, Joe leans in the door and assesses the driver's head, announcing his findings as he goes. At 24 breaths/min, the driver's breathing is rapid and appears to be adequate. The carotid pulse is still regular and strong, at 100 beats/min. Blood is dripping from a 2″ cut on his forehead. Aside from some bruising of the right upper and lower eyelids, Joe finds no other open or closed wounds. He takes a sterile compress from his aid pack, applies it to the wound, and anchors it by wrapping a 2″ self-adhering roller bandage around the patient's head.

Next, Joe assesses the neck, chest, and abdomen. The neck shows no open or closed wounds and no deformities. Joe opens the driver's jacket and pulls up his turtleneck shirt. There are no obvious open chest wounds, but there is a large ecchymosis in the center of the chest. Fortunately, both sides of the chest are moving equally as the patient breathes.

Joe then unfastens the driver's ski pants and assesses the abdomen as well as possible. There are no obvious open or closed wounds, he finds no distention, and the patient does not flinch when Joe presses on all four abdominal quadrants. Joe presses the iliac crests together and then backward. There is no crepitus and the driver does not flinch.

Joe palpates the driver's lower and upper extremities through the clothing and finds no obvious swellings or deformities. Both radial pulses are strong. The driver moves all four extremities in response to a painful stimulus. Joe slips a hand behind the driver's neck and back and runs it down as many of the spinous processes as he can. He notices no deformities or swelling and the driver does not flinch.

Moving around to the right of the car, Joe reaches through the window and, with some difficulty, assesses the passenger's ABCs. The patient's breathing is adequate at 16 breaths/min, and the carotid pulse is strong and regular at 90 beats/min.

There is no obvious bleeding and no abnormalities of the neck or chest. Because of the patient's position, the abdomen cannot be assessed. There is a large blue area of swelling on the passenger's forehead. The pupils are normal and both respond to light. The mouth and nose appear normal. There are no obvious abnormalities of the upper extremities or back.

Joe: "There is a dent in the dashboard near this guy's knee. His hip is flexed and internally rotated. I'll bet he dislocated his left hip."

You hear a siren in the distance and in a few minutes the headlights and flashing red lights of the ambulance appear around the bend ahead, followed by a highway patrol car. The ambulance pulls to a halt on the other side of the road. You recognize the two attendants as Skip and Cliff, an EMT-B and a paramedic you have worked with before.

You: "Hello, guys. We have two patients here. The driver is a V on the AVPU scale. His pulse is 100 and breathing is 24 and labored. He has a large laceration on his forehead and a steering wheel injury to his chest. The passenger is also a V on the AVPU. His pulse is 90, his breathing 16. He has a bruise on his forehead and a possible dislocated left hip. Neither one was wearing a seatbelt, and this car doesn't have airbags."

After a rapid survey of the scene, Skip and Cliff unload the extrication kit, trauma bag, oxygen apparatus, two long backboards, two KEDs, a portable oxygen tank, and a wheeled cot-stretcher from the ambulance. Cliff puts on a pair of rubber gloves and removes two rigid collars from the trauma bag. While you continue to maintain manual stabilization of the driver's head and neck, Cliff quickly repeats Joe's urgent survey, finding no additional abnormalities of the head, anterior neck, chest, abdomen, pelvis, and extremities.

The compress over the head laceration shows some blood at its center, but there is no active bleeding coming from beneath the compress. Cliff palpates the patient's back and posterior neck through the clothing, again finding no abnormalities. He then applies the rigid collar and brings over the oxygen tank, attaching a nonrebreathing mask to the patient's face with the oxygen flow turned to 15 L/min.

Meanwhile, Skip has sprung the lock of the passenger's door with a pry bar and has opened the door, providing good access to the patient. As Jan continues to stabilize the head and neck and Joe the trunk, Skip puts on rubber gloves and reassesses the passenger, including the abdomen and both upper and lower extremities. He finds nothing that Joe did not find in his rapid body survey and agrees with Joe's assessment of the probability of a dislocated left hip. Skip applies a rigid collar, and Cliff brings over a second oxygen apparatus and uses a nonrebreathing mask to start the patient on oxygen at 15 L/min.

Just then, you note an increase in the driver's breathing rate. You notify Cliff, who repeats the ABCs. The driver's breathing rate is now 30 breaths/min, and his carotid pulse is 120 beats/min. The patient must be extricated as soon as possible; there is no time to apply an extrication vest. Cliff calls to Skip, who, with Joe's help, brings the wheeled stretcher and a long backboard over to the car. Skip forces the left door as far forward as possible, springing its hinges.

While you continue to stabilize the driver's head and neck, Cliff supports the driver's chest and Skip frees his legs from the pedals. Skip then carefully moves into the back seat, and the three of you rotate the driver so that his back is facing the open doorway, his hips and knees are bent, and his feet are between the bucket seats. You carefully keep his head and neck aligned with his trunk during these maneuvers.

Joe moves the stretcher with the backboard on it so

that one end is at the door opening. He raises it to seat level and slides the end of the backboard under the driver's buttocks. The driver's chest and abdomen are carefully lowered onto the board and slid axially until his body is centered and his legs can be straightened and lowered onto the board. Oxygen is continued at 15 L/min.

Cliff reassesses the driver and finds that his pupils are normal and he continues to respond to verbal stimuli. His pulse has slowed somewhat, probably because he is now supine. His respirations are unchanged, and his blood pressure is 100/90 mm Hg. Despite the likelihood of compression injury to the anterior chest, both sides continue to move symmetrically, and his skin color is good. No open or closed abdominal wounds or tender areas are discovered. Responses to pain in his four extremities are normal and symmetrical, and he moves all four extremities spontaneously.

Meanwhile, Jan and the highway patrolman are applying a KED to the passenger. They slip the device between the seat and the patient's back and secure the patient's body to the device by the body side flaps, thoracic straps, and right groin strap. They leave the left groin strap unfastened because of the flexion and internal rotation of the patient's injured left hip. They pad the back of his head to maintain the head and neck in the neutral position and secure the head using the side flaps and foam straps across the forehead and the rigid collar.

By this time, you and Skip have moved the driver on the backboard over to the ambulance and placed him on the squad bench. Cliff helps Jan place the passenger on a long backboard by carrying the wheeled stretcher back over to the right-hand door, placing it in the snow, laying the second board on it, raising the stretcher to seat level, and putting the foot of the backboard carefully under the passenger's buttocks. Next they rotate the passenger, with the KED in place, to the side with his back facing the open door, slide him onto the lower end of the backboard, lay him flat, and then slide him headward until he's in the middle of the backboard. The dislocated left hip is manually stabilized in place during this maneuver.

Before the patient is strapped securely to the backboard, Skip performs an ongoing assessment on the passenger as well as can be done with the KED in place. Skip pays special attention to the lower abdomen and pelvis, which could not be thoroughly assessed in the patient's original cramped position.

The passenger's pulse and breathing rate are

unchanged and his blood pressure is 140/90 mm Hg. Cliff reassesses the patient's pupils, head, and neck and finds no changes. The abdomen shows no open or closed wounds, no distention, and no areas of tenderness. Aside from the obvious left hip injury, no other abnormalities are found in his four extremities. The ambulance's pulse oximeter shows that the blood oxygen saturation of both the driver and passenger are 98% with administration of oxygen at 15 L/min.

Skip will drive the ambulance, and Cliff will be in back with the two patients. Because Cliff will be very busy with two patients, they ask you to ride along to the hospital to help Cliff. You agree; Jan and Joe will meet you at the hospital. As the ambulance drives off, a tow truck from town arrives to remove the wrecked vehicle.

Snowsports and Mountain Biking Injuries
Scenario 26

Based on a scenario by Rob Bates, MD, in a 1995 issue of *Ski Patrol Magazine*, this scenario describes how to handle serious injuries sustained by a backcountry skier.

It is 2 p.m. on an overcast day in February. You have just returned to High Range Ski Area after 3 days in the backcountry, where you helped teach an advanced mountaineering course to fellow members of your nordic ski patrol. The course went well, and the skiing was good, with 1' to 2' of fresh snow. As you prepare to conduct a critique of the course, a backcountry skier bursts into patrol headquarters.

You: "Can I help you?"

Skier: "Yes, there's been an accident about 4 miles up the Ridge Crest Trail, in the big bowl. Six of us were skiing the bowl when my friend Mel triggered a big slide. It carried him about 200 yards and slammed him into a snag. We found him right away—he was only partly buried—but his leg is broken."

You: "When did the accident happen?"

Skier: "About an hour ago."

You: "Does he have any other injuries besides his leg?"

Skier: "I don't think so."

You: "Was he unconscious?"

Skier: "No."

You: "Did he having any trouble breathing?"

Skier: "No."

You: "Who is with him?"

Skier: "There were six of us altogether. Two of us skied out and the other three stayed with him. When we left, they were digging a pit for shelter and starting a fire."

Further questioning reveals that the patient, a 24-year-old student, is in good health and is an expert backcountry telemark skier. The party was well supplied with emergency rescue equipment, including avapoles (ski poles that can be joined together to form an avalanche probe pole), shovels, and avalanche transceivers. They had ample food, spare clothing, and a few emergency care supplies, but no emergency care training.

You tell the other nordic patrol members to assemble at the aid room and retrieve the rescue packs, a two-part Cascade toboggan, oxygen, and the backcountry emergency care kit for a possible ground evacuation. You then ask the nurse in charge of the aid room to arrange for a helicopter evacuation. The nearest helicopter is down for repairs, so one from the east side of the mountains is dispatched. The helicopter pilot reports that although borderline weather conditions are forecast for flying over the mountains, he'll give it a shot. You decide to proceed with ground evacuation, at least for backup.

Enough radios are on hand to give one to each of your patrollers, and the radios are compatible with a radio carried by the helicopter pilot. Fortunately, your topographic map includes the rescue area.

Within 30 minutes of the notification, the nordic patrol heads out, carrying the two toboggan halves and the other gear on pack frames and led by the patient's friend. Soon you are traveling up a relatively steep, forested valley that is broken up by avalanche chutes and snow-covered streams. You see evidence of recent slides higher up on the steeper slopes but not where the trail crosses. Each person is wearing an avalanche transceiver, packing a shovel, and either using avapoles or carrying collapsible probes.

You and the other patrollers cross each chute one at a time, 100' apart, with your waist belts and safety straps unbuckled, wrists out of the pole straps, parkas zipped, and hoods on. When you are halfway to the avalanche scene, the helicopter flies overhead. The pilot radios that he can't land at the scene but has located a clearing near a frozen lake about a mile away.

You arrive at the scene 2 hours after leaving the lodge. The patient is lying on several parkas, out of the wind in a snow pit with a fire at one side, accompanied by his friends. His leg is supported on clothing but not splinted. The area looks fairly secure from further avalanche danger.

You assess the patient's radial pulse and note that the patient's pulse is strong, regular, and faster than normal.

You: "Hi, I'm Rocky Montayne from the High Range Nordic Ski Patrol. We're here to get you fixed up and moved over to the helicopter landing site. How are you feeling?"

Patient: "Thanks for coming. I'm Mel Suerte. I'm having a lot of pain in my left hip and leg and can't feel my left foot."

The patient's voice is quiet and stressed. His respirations appear normal.

You: "Can you wiggle your toes?"

Patient: "No, not on the left."

You: "Do you hurt anywhere else? How about your head, neck, and back?"

Patient: "They feel okay."

You: "Were you knocked out?"

Patient: "No."

You put on a pair of rubber gloves and ask the patient whether he remembers what happened. He's able to remember the avalanche clearly and appears oriented times four (to person, place, time, and event). The other patrollers are assembling the supplies and connecting the two halves of the toboggan.

You assess the patient's left lower extremity. Both the thigh and leg are swollen and deformed. Palpating the extremity through the clothing, you note marked tenderness involving the mid- to lower thigh and midcalf.

You ask another patroller to manually stabilize the patient's thigh and leg, and you carefully remove the boot. The patient cannot feel or move his ankle and toes. You are unable to feel any pulses in the foot or ankle.

You ask a third patroller to use a seam ripper on the patient's left pant leg from the ankle to the hip to expose the extremity so it can be assessed for bleeding and evidence of open fracture. While this is being done, you start the rapid body survey.

You record a radial pulse of 110 beats/min and a breathing rate of 28 breaths/min. Assessing the head, you find no evidence of any wounds, swelling, or tenderness. The pupils are round, regular, and equal, and they respond to your penlight. There is no sign of bleeding from the patient's mouth or ears. As you

assess his neck, you note mild tenderness over the midcervical spinous processes. You ask two patrollers to manually stabilize the head and neck and apply a rigid collar.

By this time, the left lower extremity is exposed. There are no signs of blood or open wounds, although there is tight swelling and some deformity of the midthigh and midcalf.

Returning to the chest, you find equal expansion on both sides and no rib tenderness or obvious soft-tissue injuries. The abdomen is soft and nontender, and there is no pain when you press on the iliac crests. The femoral pulses are strong and equal. The right lower extremity and both upper extremities are unremarkable. There is no obvious tenderness or deformity of the thoracic and lumbosacral spine.

While the patient's left lower extremity is manually stabilized, two patrollers replace his boot and apply a Kendrick traction device, using minimal traction. Next, they apply an extrication vest and, with the aid of three other patrollers, use the bridge lift to raise the patient high enough so that the toboggan can be slid underneath him. The patient is then lowered onto a sleeping bag, which is wrapped around him, and strapped into the toboggan. You let the helicopter pilot know that the patient is packaged for transport and that you are leaving for the makeshift landing zone.

One patroller pulls the toboggan from the front and one controls it from behind while you and the others break trail. The route to the helicopter is mostly downhill and you make good time, detouring occasionally to avoid potential avalanche runout zones.

You arrive at the helicopter at 5 p.m., where you are greeted by a flight nurse and an EMT. The patient is transferred to a long backboard for the flight, and the extrication vest is left in place. The patient's vital signs show a blood pressure of 98/70 mm Hg, respirations of 28 breaths/min, and a pulse of 120 beats/min. He continues to be responsive but somewhat lethargic. The helicopter leaves as soon as the patient is loaded.

Later, you obtain a report from the hospital. The emergency physician found closed, displaced fractures of the left femur, tibia, and fibula, and a complete tear of the left popliteal artery. X-rays of the cervical spine were normal. At surgery, the artery was repaired and the fractures stabilized by open reduction and internal fixation. Despite initial concerns that amputation might be necessary, the surgeon was able to save the patient's left foot. All four ligaments of the right knee were torn, even though field assessment showed no tenderness, swelling, or deformity and the patient did not complain of discomfort. Knee reconstruction was deferred to a later date.

You realize that if the patient had not been cared for and transported effectively and rapidly, he might have lost his left leg and foot.

Scenario 27

This scenario describes how to handle a medical problem in the backcountry.

You are spending the weekend with a friend who lives in Alpine City, which is a gateway community about 2 miles from Grandstone National Park and is a base for snowmobilers and backcountry skiers. Your friend, a forest ranger and first responder, is a member of the local snowmobile rescue team.

The two of you are finishing your lunch when his radio interrupts with a transmission from the leader of a visiting backcountry ski group that is staying in a hut about 4 miles from town. A member of the group is sick and they are requesting she be transported back to town by snowmobile. Details are sketchy, but she is short of breath, dizzy, trembling, and having trouble walking. As far as they know, she has not been injured.

You and your friend quickly mount two snowmobiles and drive to the firehouse in the middle of town where the rescue toboggan is stored. When you arrive, you find two other members of the rescue group ahead of you. You quickly load your emergency care gear, oxygen, suction, a trauma kit, and a whole-body vacuum splint into the toboggan, hitch it to a snowmobile, and head for the scene.

Arriving at the hut, which is at an altitude of about 7,500', you find a 25-year-old woman lying on a cot. She is in respiratory distress, her face is pale, and her hands and feet are trembling intermittently.

You: "Hi, I'm Rocky Montayne from the High Range Nordic Ski Patrol and this is Tim Burr from the U.S. Forest Service. Can we help you?"

Patient: "Yes, thanks for coming. I'm Selma Schwin. I don't feel well at all."

You grasp the patient's wrist and note that the skin is cool and the pulse is strong with a normal rate. Her breathing rate is about twice the normal rate.

You: "What happened to you?"

Patient: "Well, I've been here 3 days. Day before yesterday, we skied up here from town and then telemarked the hills around the lake. Yesterday, I felt very tired, was short of breath, and had trouble with my balance. I slept about 17 hours yesterday and felt

better this morning, so we went skiing again. I felt dizzy and short of breath again, so we called for help."

You: "Have you ever skied at this altitude before?"

Patient: "Yes, I've skied in the Alps without any trouble. We were at Steamboat telemarking from the summit at 12,000' last month and I didn't have any trouble then."

You: "Have you had this type of shortness of breath before?"

Patient: "I've had trouble with hyperventilation before."

You: "Have you hurt yourself skiing recently?"

Patient: "No."

You: "Has anything happened recently that might upset you?"

Patient: "Well, I was riding my bike a week ago when I was hit by a car. The driver ran a red light, knocked me off the bike, and I fell on my side and left wrist. My side is black and blue, and my wrist still hurts."

You: "Did you go to the emergency department?"

Patient: "Yes, they x-rayed my wrist and said it wasn't fractured."

You: "Do you have any chest pain, headache, nausea, vomiting, or diarrhea? Have you had a cold or the flu recently?"

Patient: "No."

You: "Are you having your menstrual period right now?"

Patient: "Yes."

You ask Pat, one of the rescue team members, to start administering oxygen to the patient by nasal cannula at 4 L/min. You then proceed to ask her about allergies, medicines or drugs taken, any past illnesses or injuries, and anything else that might be significant. The answers are all negative.

You perform the rapid body survey as the patient continues to hyperventilate. Her scalp, pupils, nose, ears, and mouth are unremarkable. Her neck isn't stiff and there are no palpable lymph nodes. Opening her jacket, you inspect her chest. Both sides are moving equally. You hear no abnormal breath sounds with your unaided ear.

Moving to the abdomen, you find no tenderness or abnormal masses. You examine her lower extremities through her clothing. She winces as you palpate her left thigh and calf. You slide the fleece pant leg up and assess the calf directly. There is some purplish-yellow discoloration and the calf is definitely swollen and tender. You confirm this by comparing it with the opposite calf. The patient winces as you bend the foot upward at the ankle and says that this causes pain in the calf.

You pull her fleece trousers down low enough to expose her upper thighs. The lateral left thigh is tender with purplish-yellow discoloration. You then assess her upper extremities and back, finding no further abnormalities except for some tenderness in the wrist at the base of the left thumb. You mention that if her wrist doesn't improve, she should have it x-rayed again. You wonder how she could have skied this morning on her left leg.

You now try to fit things together. Acute mountain sickness doesn't fit exactly, because although it could occur at this altitude, she has had no trouble much higher than this in the past. She certainly has had enough happen to her recently to make her anxious, so this could be benign hyperventilation. However, she did have the bicycle accident a week ago and might have a blood clot in her left leg that could be spreading to her lungs. The most important priority is to transport her to the nearest medical center where she can be properly diagnosed and treated.

You bundle the patient into a sleeping bag, place her in the toboggan, and transport her to town, administering oxygen by nonrebreathing mask at 15 L/min. In town, she is transferred by ambulance to the nearest hospital, 100 miles away. The ambulance attendants check her blood oxygen saturation with the oxygen off and find it is 98%, which is normal; in fact, it is unusually good for an altitude of 7,500′.

You later hear that in the hospital emergency department, a chest x-ray is normal, a Doppler examination for blood clots in the left lower extremity is negative, and a lung scan for blood clots in the lungs is negative.

The patient appeared to have benign hyperventilation secondary to stress, anxiety, and the effects of altitude. You hear that 2 days later, she was telemarking again.

Triage

Scenario 28

The following scenario focuses on triage in action.

You are a professional ski patroller at Destination Resort, a large ski and snowboard area served by a gondola as well as multiple chairlifts. You are patrolling a high bowl above the gondola when you hear over the radio that there has been a derailment. Eight gondola cars have fallen to the ground.

You arrive at the first gondola car and see nine victims inside. You report quickly to patrol headquarters, point to a spot outside, and say, "All of you who can walk, move over here." Three of the nine are able to do so. Your survival scans reveal the following (the patients are not listed in the order in which you scanned them):

1. A middle-aged woman who is screaming hysterically. She has a large lump on her forehead and a deformed wrist. Her respirations and pulse are normal. She tells you that she hurt her head and wrist when the gondola fell.

2. A middle-aged man who is lying in the gondola wreckage, unresponsive, breathing normally, groaning, and spontaneously moving all four extremities. His pulse is palpable and strong.

3. An older man with an obvious crushed chest. He is not breathing and has no detectable pulse.

4. A young woman who is lying quietly. Her skin is pale, cold, and clammy, her respirations are rapid and shallow, and her pulse is fast and weak. She complains weakly of abdominal pain.

5. An obnoxious middle-aged man who is yelling, cursing, and threatening to sue the resort. He does not appear to be hurt.

6. A young man who is lying quietly on his side, complaining of pain in his back between the shoulder blades. His breathing appears normal, and his pulse is palpable and strong. He says he cannot move his legs.

7. An elderly woman who appears basically healthy and vigorous for her age. She is in respiratory distress and is complaining of chest pain. Her pulse is strong and fast, and her respirations are more than 30 breaths/min. A brief inspection of the pain site discloses a flail segment of the chest wall.

8. A middle-aged woman who seems calm and does not appear to be injured.

9. A teenage girl who is lying quietly. Her respirations are shallow, irregular, and more than 30 breaths/min, although they improve somewhat with the jaw-thrust maneuver. Her pulse is rapid and weak, and the skin of her wrist is cold and clammy. She does not respond to your voice.

How should these patients be classified, and what do you do? Write down your analysis of the scene before reading the analysis below.

Analysis

You assign patients 4 and 7 **red** priority because of impending shock and hypoxia, respectively, and because with simple care and rapid transport, they have a reasonable chance of survival. You assign patients 2 and 6 **yellow** priority because, although seriously injured, they appear to be stable enough to wait for transport. You classify patient 3 **black** priority and patients 1 and 8 **green** priority.

Because patient 8, who is calm, appears to be sensible, you ask her to try to quiet patient 1; if this is unsuccessful, patient 1 should be moved to **yellow** priority.

Patient 5, who would otherwise be assigned green priority because he appears uninjured, might be moved up to **red** priority for immediate transport to get him out of everyone's hair. However, a rapid, tactful request for his help might calm him down by giving him something to do.

You assign patient 9 **yellow** priority because, although her survival scan indicates that she is red priority, her chance of survival is less than patients 4 and 7, and she requires more care than they do. As soon as more help arrives you can move her up to red priority.

You perform basic salvage maneuvers on patients 4 and 9. For patient 4, these actions include a rapid search for external bleeding and elevating her legs 12″; for patient 9, you open the airway, elevate her legs 12″, and also conduct a rapid search for external bleeding. You recruit a green-priority patient to maintain patient 9's airway.

As soon as more help arrives, you assist patient 7's breathing, transport patients 4, 7, (and 9, if possible), and monitor patients 9, 2, and 6. After patients 9, 2, and 6 are transported, you transport patients 1, 8, 3, and 5.

Scenario 29

The following scenario illustrates how to manage a patient with multiple injuries and other problems.

You have summit duty on a calm morning 2 days after a severe storm covered High Range Ski Area with 2′ of heavy powder. The Drainage, a steep, heavily forested, ungroomed area to the north, has just been opened after the patrol skied it without finding any evidence of unstable snow.

You are ready to go off duty when the phone rings. It's the hill chief.

Chief: "Ben, there's been an avalanche in the Drainage at the narrow runout chute. We have a report of a buried snowboarder. Mike's on his way up on a snowmobile with a witness and Tami's coming with her avalanche dog. Get ready to take a hasty party down as soon as you get some patrollers off the Number 2 chair. Be careful."

You know exactly where the Drainage slid; it slid there once before, many years ago. Your radio sputters with an announcement from the hill chief, directing all available patrollers to report to the summit for an avalanche search.

You quickly take six transceivers out of the avalanche locker in the summit shack, then go to the shed where the avalanche gear is stored. Opening the shed, you pull out four shovels, some flagging, and the large bundle of probe poles, and carry them over to the side of the lift unloading ramp. Returning to the summit shack, you get the oxygen backpack from the closet. You see two patrollers on a chair, ready to unload, and wave them over.

The whine of the snowmobile announces Mike's arrival with the witness, a young man in his late 20s who is pale but calm. Leaving word with the lift operator, you distribute transceivers, probes, and shovels. Then, shouldering the oxygen backpack yourself, you follow the witness into the Drainage.

The heavy powder makes travel difficult, but in less than 10 minutes you arrive at the top of the chute. There is a 2′ fracture line above an icy base with a large pile of debris at the bottom. The witness points out where he last saw the victim, a young man in his early 20s named Harry Slab. You mark the point-last-seen with flagging, then carefully make your way down the icy avalanche bed to the upper margin of the debris pile.

You determine that because the area above the chute has been well skied by the patrol, it is stable. You and the other three patrollers spread out and slowly descend toward the toe of the avalanche, looking for clues, kicking at the snow, and probing at likely areas. After 10 minutes, you reach the toe without finding any sign of the victim.

A shout from the top announces Tami's arrival with Loki, a 4-year-old German shepherd. Tami takes off her skis, gives Loki the command to "check it out," and they start to descend the chute. Loki ranges from side to side, sniffing the snow. They reach the toe of the slide without finding anything, then start up again. The dog stops suddenly above a large tree at the north side of the slide and starts to dig and bark.

Everyone converges on the spot with shovels and probes. You take off the oxygen backpack, then start to dig carefully to the side of the dog and uncover the tip of a snowboard. The dog is called off, and two of you dig rapidly, uncovering what appears to be the patient's right thigh and hip. The patient's thigh is twisted and bent at an abnormal angle. Now that you know his body orientation, it is easy to locate his head. Even though the risk of another slide is probably small, you direct one patroller to act as an avalanche lookout.

There is a small air space around the patient's face, with some ice in its walls. The patient is not breathing. As soon as you've excavated enough space around the patient's head, you start rescue breathing using a pocket mask from your emergency care belt. After two rescue breaths, you assess the carotid pulse. It is faint, fast, and regular. You continue rescue breathing, adding oxygen from the tank at 15 L/min.

One of the rescuers, Bill, radios patrol headquarters to report the successful find. He is told that there is a toboggan on the way down from the summit. He asks patrol headquarters to request a helicopter, which should arrive about the time the toboggan reaches the base with the patient.

By this time, the patient's head, neck, and most of his trunk are exposed. You are stabilizing the patient's head and neck with both palms while you hold the pocket mask over his face with your fingers. Bill retrieves the hand-powered suction unit from the oxygen backpack, lays it at your side, and switches the oxygen tubing to the BVM device. You remove the pocket mask, and Bill deftly inserts an oropharyngeal airway, then fits the mask of the BVM device into place. You hold the BVM device while you continue to stabilize the patient's head and neck. Bill starts squeezing the ventilation bag at a rate of one breath every 5 seconds. With each ventilation, the patient's chest rises beneath his parka.

Meanwhile, the others have uncovered the patient's upper and lower extremities and removed the snowboard.

Mark begins the rapid body survey. The patient's neck appears normal; there are no open wounds or tracheal deviation. Upon assessing the chest, you find that the right side is flattened compared with the left, and the skin over this area crackles as you run your hand across it. You ask Mark whether there is paradoxical motion of the right side of the chest, and he replies that there is not and that there is good chest rise on each side with the ventilations. You remember that paradoxical motion occurs only when patients breathe

for themselves, not when they are being ventilated.

The patient's abdomen appears normal. The right thigh is angulated at its midpoint with the leg and foot rotated externally and with a definite bulge in the midthigh area compared with the left. You assess the patient's radial pulse and find it is weak with a rate of 120 beats/min, which means that his systolic blood pressure is at least 80 mm Hg.

Mark runs his hand down the patient's posterior neck and back. There are no obvious deformities, although the mechanism of injury suggests the strong possibility of neck or back injury. A blanket is carefully pushed under and around the patient. You ask Mark to call patrol headquarters and have someone bring down a backboard and a traction splint, if they're not already on the way.

A shout from the top of the chute announces the arrival of two more patrollers with the toboggan. Mark reaches the toboggan handler by radio, suggesting that the toboggan be belayed down to the incident site. Three additional patrollers arrive carrying a long backboard and a Sager splint.

The Sager splint is applied to the patient's right lower extremity and traction is initiated. The extremity straightens and rotates into the normal, anatomic position in the splint. You and Bill continue to ventilate the patient, stopping every few minutes to see if he has started to breathe on his own.

After the traction splint is in place, the long backboard is laid next to the patient and six of you raise the patient carefully out of the hole without altering his position. You and the others slide the board under him and carefully align him into the anatomic position on the board before applying a rigid collar.

By this time, the patient is starting to moan and stir. He is securely strapped to the board, then lifted into the toboggan and covered with a blanket and tarp. Opinions differ regarding whether his head should be uphill or downhill. You all conclude that his head should be uphill because his respiratory system is probably compromised more by his respiratory arrest and crushed chest than his circulatory system is by his probable hypovolemia and hypothermia.

The board is moved forward in the toboggan so that there is room for the oxygen tank and a patroller at the rear by the patient's head. You have the biggest hands; therefore, you are elected to man the BVM device. In the past, you have practiced using one hand to stabilize a patient's head and neck and keep the mask in place while squeezing the bag with the other hand, so you know you can do it. The first 200 yards of the route to the base is steep, so you fashion an "umbilical cord" with a short length of 1" webbing from your emergency care belt and tie yourself to the rear of the toboggan so you won't fall forward.

The toboggan is slowly belayed down the remaining 50 yards of the avalanche debris and arrives at the base 10 minutes after reaching the gentler slopes 150 yards beyond.

By this time, the patient is starting to breathe irregularly on his own, and you continue to support him with the BVM device. Once you reach the aid room, you take the patient's blood pressure, which is 90/40 mm Hg. His pulse is 105 beats/min. You hear the throbbing of the helicopter rotor becoming louder in the distance.

Hazardous Plants and Animals
Scenario 30

The following scenario describes how to manage a case of poisoning occurring in the outdoors.

You and your wife, Sandy, have decided to take the baby and spend the weekend in an isolated campground in the Granite Range, about 100 miles from town. You leave right after work on Friday. After turning off the main highway, you drive about 50 miles on a secondary road over a high pass.

The campground is situated where a raging cascade drops through a high mountain valley and empties into the main drainage. It is late June—too warm for good high mountain skiing and, anyway, you want to introduce your 12-month-old son to car camping. You pick a site at the back of the campground, not too close to the creek, next to an expensive, three-season dome tent pitched beside a four-wheel-drive vehicle.

It is almost dark when you finish supper and start on the dishes. The baby is in his playpen. There is a commotion at the next campsite, where two couples in their late 20s have just finished eating. One of the men is lying on the ground, groaning. The others seem to be standing around, watching him helplessly, so you decide to find out if they need assistance.

You: "Hi, I'm Ben Schussen. Is something wrong?"

Woman: "Yes, there's something wrong with my husband. He says he has a terrible stomachache and is nauseated. Look at the way he's drooling. I don't know what to do. Are you a doctor?"

You: "No, but I'm on the ski patrol at High Range Ski Area. When did this start?"

Woman: "Just after he finished supper, a few minutes ago."

You bend down to observe the patient more closely. He is doubled up and in obvious pain. His breathing is rapid. You check his radial pulse, which is rapid and strong. His face is pale, and beads of sweat cover his forehead. There is saliva all over the top of his shirt.

You: "Was he all right before supper?"

Woman: "Yes. We went on a hike and he seemed his normal self."

You ask Sandy to get the emergency care kit out of the truck and then ask the woman what her husband had for supper.

Woman: "We had some venison, fried potatoes, mixed vegetables, and cake for dessert."

You: "Has anyone else been feeling sick?"

Woman: "No."

You: "Did he eat anything that the rest of you didn't eat?"

Woman: "Come to think of it, he did. He found some yampa by the side of the creek on the way back and dug up some roots. I boiled them for him. Nobody else ate any."

You: "What's his name?"

Woman: "Don Eaton."

You take a pair of latex gloves from the kit, put them on, then pull up the patient's shirt and assess his abdomen. There is no distention.

You: "Don, what did this plant that you ate look like?"

Patient (gasping): "Like a typical yampa. You know, the little cream-colored flowers that look like Queen Anne's lace. But the root didn't taste quite right."

You: "How much did you eat?"

Patient: "Two, maybe three pieces."

You press each abdominal quadrant in turn, and ask the patient whether anything hurts. The patient indicates that the epigastric area is tender.

You: "Did you save any of the yampa?"

Patient: "Yes, there's some there under the tent flap."

You hurry over to the side of the tent and retrieve several roots from under the flap. One of them has a stem with several leaves still attached to it. It looks like a small water hemlock. Don must have mistaken it for yampa. On the way back you take a dishpan, canteen, and cup from the table.

You: "You better get rid of it—I think it's making you sick. Here, drink this cup of water and I'll help you throw it up."

You help the patient sit up and he is able to drink the water. You take a spoon off the table and gag him with the handle. He vomits a large amount of stomach contents into the dishpan.

You: "Don't throw that away, we need to save it."

You point to the four-wheel-drive vehicle parked next to the patient's tent and ask whose it is. The other man indicates that it is his.

You: "Mrs. Eaton, your husband is quite ill and should be taken to a hospital as soon as possible. I'll send my wife Sandy to the nearest phone to call an ambulance from Sylvan City. Then, we'll load him into the back of the vehicle and meet the ambulance on the pass."

You turn back to the patient. He has stopped moaning but doesn't seem as alert. His respirations seem slower and less deep. You turn to Sandy and speak to her quietly.

You: "Take the baby with you and head for the trading post up the road. Call Sylvan City, tell them who we are, and tell them that we have a man with probable water hemlock poisoning and we'll be bringing him in. We need an ambulance to meet us on the pass for a transfer. Tell them to send a doctor with it if they can, or at least a paramedic. I'll be back as soon as I can."

Sandy zips up the tent and heads for the truck with the baby. You turn to the other man.

You: "Help me load him into the back of this rig. We'll need a pad for him to lie on and the pan for him to throw up in. I have a bucket with a lid in the tent that we can save the vomit in. Put that plant in a bag and bring it along."

In a few minutes everything is ready. The patient, his wife, and you sit in the back seat with your emergency care kit. The driver seems somewhat hesitant and wants to take down the tent and pack up the camp before leaving, but after the patient has a grand mal seizure in the back of his vehicle, he becomes more convinced that the situation is urgent.

You reassess the patient. His airway is open, and his respirations are regular but shallow, about 16 breaths/min. His pulse is regular at 120 beats/min and definitely weaker than it was a short while ago. You

open your kit and take out a set of oropharyngeal airways and your pocket mask. You try to remember the signs and symptoms of water hemlock poisoning. You do know that it is probably the most toxic native American plant; even a single bite of water hemlock can be fatal.

It is 100 miles to the nearest hospital. With luck, you have only 50 miles to go before you meet the ambulance. You prepare yourself to start basic life support, which you are fairly certain the patient will need soon.

Water Emergencies

Scenario 31

The following scenario illustrates the type of complex emergency care problem that can occur with water-related sports.

You, your wife Sandy, and the baby are spending a weekend at a friend's vacation house on a large lake. The shore is ringed with cottages, most of which have boat docks and small sand beaches. By midmorning, many sailboats and small motorboats are out in the lake, and a few swimmers are braving the chilly waters. You have your canoe on top of your new four-wheel-drive vehicle and are planning to have lunch at a picturesque, uninhabited inlet across the lake.

A family reunion seems to be going on at the next cabin. A half dozen teenagers in swimwear are playing volleyball on the beach while their parents sit talking under beach umbrellas. They finish their game and race each other to the end of the pier where they dive into the water, then reappear shortly and stroke awkwardly toward a floating dock 50 yards farther out in the lake.

After they have pulled themselves onto the dock, they seem agitated and keep glancing shoreward, calling someone's name. The parents rise from their chairs and hurry to the shore edge. You can't make out the details of the exchange of shouts, but there is obviously something wrong.

You tell Sandy that something is wrong and you are going to check it out. Sandy scoops up the baby and follows you as you jog over to the group of parents.

You: "What's wrong?"

Parent: "George is missing. They all dove off the end of the pier and he didn't come up."

You: "My wife and I have taken some lifesaving training; we'll see what we can do. Have someone notify the sheriff and call an ambulance right away."

You kick off your sandals, peel off your T-shirt, and run to the end of the pier. About 20′ out, you see something red in the water. You carefully step down into the water and swim out to the object, using a strong breaststroke and keeping your eyes on that area. When you reach it, you see that it is a teenage boy wearing a pair of red shorts, floating face down in the water just below the surface, near a buried piling.

You: "Sandy, I've found him! Come in and give me a hand."

Sandy hands the baby to one of the women, drops her windbreaker, pulls a mouth shield out of her purse, and runs to the end of the pier. Meanwhile, you approach the teenager's head. Lowering your feet, you find that the water is about 4′ deep and you can easily stand on the bottom. You grasp both of his arms, straighten his elbows, and extend his arms over his head, sandwiching his head between his biceps. You then walk forward a few feet so that his body floats to the surface. You turn his body toward you as a unit until he is face up, with his head and neck cradled by your left elbow. At this point Sandy joins you, reaches the patient's side, and opens his airway with the jaw-thrust maneuver, asking loudly, "George, are you okay?"

There is no answer. She applies the mouth shield and immediately gives two rescue breaths of 2 seconds each. She listens carefully and watches the patient's chest, which rises with the rescue breaths. She feels the carotid pulse, and finds that it is fast and regular. She then starts rescue breathing, giving one breath every 5 seconds. The two of you start walking slowly and carefully toward the shore, continuing rescue breathing as you keep his face above water and his head and neck stabilized.

By the time you reach a depth of 2′, you're close to shore. You call several of the parents into the water to help you get the patient onto dry land. After explaining the principles of the direct ground lift-and-carry, you are able to change his head and neck stabilization to the standard manual type, shift his arms to the side of his body, and raise him out of the water using three parents plus the two of you. The lift produces no significant spine motion that you can detect. The five of you slowly and carefully carry the patient a few feet up on the beach and lower him supine onto the sand. Sandy assesses his breathing and carotid pulse. The pulse is still strong and regular, but he does not breathe spontaneously. She then resumes rescue breathing.

You hear an approaching siren, and in a minute the ambulance arrives and two EMTs join you, carrying a long backboard, oxygen tank, portable suction unit, and trauma kit. By now, the patient is taking an occasional gasping breath on his own. One of the EMTs starts to assist the patient's breathing, using a BVM device with oxygen at 15 L/min. The other EMT pulls out an eardrum temperature-measuring device. When you raise your eyebrows, he remembers that the ear canal is probably full of water and checks the rectal temperature instead; it is 98°F. The temperature is down 1.5° because of the cold lake water, but there is no serious hypothermia.

Sandy pinches one of the patient's fingertips and the tip of one of his toes to test his ability to move in response to pain. There is no response in the lower extremities. There is a slight amount of shoulder flexion in the upper extremities.

You think that the patient probably has a fractured neck with some spinal cord injury, as well as a submersion injury, and you are glad you were careful to stabilize his head and neck. Maybe you spared him a few nerve fibers that he can use later on.

After a few minutes of ventilation and oxygenation, the patient's breathing is deeper and regular. The four of you quickly log roll him onto his side and then back onto the backboard. His breathing continues to be assisted with the BVM device. Just after you finish strapping him securely to the board, he starts to retch. You quickly tip the board on its side while one of the EMTs clears his mouth with the portable electric suction unit. He vomits a large amount of lake water mixed with stomach contents onto the sand.

You help the EMTs carry the patient to the ambulance and load him onto the gurney. With lights flashing and siren screaming, the ambulance drives off, followed by a sedan carrying the boy's parents. By now, the other teens have returned to the shore, and you spend a few minutes warning them of the dangers of diving into shallow water.

Appendix B

Skill Guides

Contents

(CPI) = Critical Performance Indicator

VITAL SIGNS DETERMINATION

Objective: To demonstrate the ability to determine a set of baseline vital signs.

SKILL	YES	NO	NOTATIONS
• Initiates BSI precautions.			(CPI)
Level of Responsiveness (LOR)			
• Assesses the patient's LOR using the AVPU scale.			
• Determines the patient's pupil diameter and reaction to light.			
Pulse			
• Palpates the radial pulse and determines the rate.			(CPI)
• Describes the rhythm and strength.			
• Palpates the carotid pulse and determines the rate.			(CPI)
• Palpates the dorsalis pedis pulse, as necessary, and determines the rate.			
Respirations			
• Assesses the rise and fall of the chest wall for 30 seconds to determine the respiratory rate.			(CPI)
• Assesses respirations with respect to rhythm, effort, depth, and noise.			
Blood Pressure by Auscultation or Palpation			
• Applies the blood pressure cuff to the arm above the elbow, centering it over the brachial artery.			
• Inflates the cuff while auscultating the brachial pulse or palpating the radial pulse.			
• Continues to inflate the cuff to 20 mm Hg above the point at which the pulse is no longer heard or felt.			
• Slowly releases the pressure, noting when pulse is first heard or felt (systolic) and again when sound is absent (diastolic by auscultation only). Reports the values.			(CPI)

	YES	NO	
Did the trainee or OEC technician adequately demonstrate the performance criteria of this skill?			

COMMENTS

(CPI) = Critical Performance Indicator

USE OF OXYGEN AND AIRWAY ADJUNCTS—OROPHARYNGEAL AND NASOPHARYNGEAL AIRWAYS

Objective: To demonstrate the correct use of oropharyngeal and nasopharyngeal airways.

SKILL	YES	NO	NOTATIONS
• Initiates BSI precautions.			(CPI)
• Selects proper size oropharyngeal airway by measuring from the corner of the mouth to the angle of the jaw. OR • Selects proper size nasopharyngeal airway by measuring from the tip of the nose to the earlobe. Coats the airway with a water-soluble lubricant.			
• If using an oral airway, opens the mouth using an appropriate technique.			
• Inserts the airway using an appropriate technique.			(CPI)

Did the trainee or OEC technician adequately demonstrate the performance criteria of this skill?			

COMMENTS

(CPI) = Critical Performance Indicator

USE OF OXYGEN AND AIRWAY ADJUNCTS—SUCTIONING OF THE ORAL CAVITY

Objective: To demonstrate the correct use of suctioning equipment.

SKILL	YES	NO	NOTATIONS
• Initiates BSI precautions.			(CPI)
• Assembles, turns on, and tests device.			
• Opens the mouth using the crossed-finger technique.			
• Inserts rigid tip catheter without suction applied (measures length from corner of mouth to angle of jaw and inserts catheter no farther than distance measured).			
• Applies suction for no longer than 15 seconds while the rigid catheter is twisted or rotated during withdrawal.			(CPI)

	YES	NO	
Did the trainee or OEC technician adequately demonstrate the performance criteria of this skill?			

COMMENTS

(CPI) = Critical Performance Indicator

USE OF OXYGEN AND AIRWAY ADJUNCTS—ADMINISTRATION OF OXYGEN

Objective: To demonstrate the correct use of oxygen equipment.

SKILL	YES	NO	NOTATIONS
• Initiates BSI precautions.			(CPI)
• Assembles oxygen cylinder and regulator, and checks for leaks.			(CPI)
• Chooses a delivery device by patient need. —Selects nonrebreathing oxygen mask, connects to regulator, prefills the regulator, and initially adjusts oxygen flow to 12 to 15 L/min. —Selects nasal cannula, connects to regulator, and adjusts oxygen to 6 L/min maximum.			(CPI)
• Applies the appropriate oxygen delivery device to the patient and verifies that the patient receives oxygen. If using a nonrebreathing mask, readjusts the flow rate to keep the bag half-full on inhalation.			(CPI)
• When finished providing oxygen, closes the oxygen tank.			
• Bleeds regulator device to "0."			

Did the trainee or OEC technician adequately demonstrate the performance criteria of this skill?			

COMMENTS

appendix b

(CPI) = Critical Performance Indicator

USE OF OXYGEN AND AIRWAY ADJUNCTS— USE OF POCKET MASK FOR ARTIFICIAL VENTILATION

Objective: To demonstrate the correct use of oxygen equipment for artificial ventilation.

SKILL	YES	NO	NOTATIONS
• Initiates BSI precautions.			(CPI)
• Assembles mask components as necessary, using device specific one-way valve.			
• Sizes and inserts correctly sized oropharyngeal or nasopharyngeal airway using appropriate technique.			
• Connects oxygen to pocket mask.			
• Adjusts oxygen supply to 15 L/min.			
• Maintains open airway and mask seal.			
• Demonstrates adequate ventilation (rate and depth) on a manikin.			(CPI)

	YES	NO	
Did the trainee or OEC technician adequately demonstrate the performance criteria of this skill?			

COMMENTS

(CPI) = Critical Performance Indicator

USE OF OXYGEN AND AIRWAY ADJUNCTS—
USE OF BAG-VALVE-MASK FOR ARTIFICIAL VENTILATION

Objective: To demonstrate the correct use of oxygen equipment for artificial ventilation.

SKILL	YES	NO	NOTATIONS
• Initiates BSI precautions.			(CPI)
• Assembles bag-valve-mask components, including reservoir.			
• Sizes and inserts a correctly sized oropharyngeal or nasopharyngeal airway using appropriate technique.			
• Connects oxygen supply to bag-valve-mask.			
• Adjusts oxygen supply to 15 L/min.			
• Maintains open airway and mask seal.			
• Demonstrates adequate ventilation (rate and depth) on a manikin.			(CPI)

Did the trainee or OEC technician adequately demonstrate the performance criteria of this skill?			

COMMENTS

(CPI) = Critical Performance Indicator

PATIENT ASSESSMENT—UNRESPONSIVE PATIENT

Objective: To demonstrate the ability to determine the baseline condition of an unresponsive patient and to make an appropriate transport decision.

SKILL	YES	NO	NOTATIONS
Scene Size-Up			
• Initiates BSI precautions.			(CPI)
• Determines that the scene is safe.			
• Determines the nature of illness (NOI) and/or the mechanism of injury (MOI).			(CPI)
• Notes the number of patients and the responsiveness of each.			
• Evaluates the need to disentangle or extricate the patient(s). Considers c-spine immobilization.			
• Notes the need for personnel or equipment.			
Initial Assessment—Unresponsive Patient			
• Confirms general impression of the patient and/or level of responsiveness (LOR).			
• Assesses airway, breathing, and circulation (ABCs).			(CPI)
• Assists breathing or performs CPR, as necessary.			
• Checks for severe bleeding: intervention = control bleeding.			(CPI)
• Calls for transport, equipment, assistance, and/or EMS as needed.			
Rapid History and Physical Exam			
• Performs the rapid body survey.			(CPI)
• Provides interventions and maintains spinal immobilization as needed.			(CPI)
• Obtains baseline vital signs.			(CPI)
• Obtains SAMPLE history from witnesses.			
• Transports patient off the hill.			(CPI)
• Performs a detailed physical exam as necessary.			
• Performs ongoing assessment.			

	YES	NO	
Did the trainee or OEC technician adequately demonstrate the performance criteria of these skills?			

COMMENTS

(CPI) = Critical Performance Indicator

PATIENT ASSESSMENT—RESPONSIVE TRAUMA PATIENT

Objective: To demonstrate the ability to determine the baseline condition and specific injury or injuries in a responsive trauma patient.

SKILL	YES	NO	NOTATIONS
Scene Size-Up			
• Initiates BSI precautions.			(CPI)
• Determines that the scene is safe.			
• Determines the nature of illness (NOI) and/or the mechanism of injury (MOI).			(CPI)
• Notes the number of patients and the responsiveness of each.			
• Evaluates the need to disentangle or extricate the patient(s). Considers c-spine immobilization.			
• Notes the need for personnel or equipment.			
Initial Assessment—Responsive Patient			
• Offers to assist/obtains the patient's consent.			
• Confirms general impression of the patient and/or level of responsiveness (LOR).			
• Assesses airway, breathing, and circulation (ABCs).			(CPI)
• Assists breathing or performs CPR, as necessary.			
• Checks for severe bleeding: intervention = control bleeding.			(CPI)
• If the patient has abnormal ABCs or presents a poor general impression, the rescuer performs the rapid body survey, obtains baseline vital signs, obtains the SAMPLE history, and provides rapid transport.			
• Obtains the chief complaint.			
• Calls for transport, equipment, assistance, and/or EMS as needed.			(CPI)
Focused History and Physical Exam—Trauma Patient			
• Conducts a trauma-focused physical exam of the area of chief complaint; confirms chief complaint.			
• Obtains SAMPLE history.			
• Exposes and inspects only what is necessary to determine the appropriate emergency care.			
• Stabilizes and maintains the patient's body temperature.			
• Determines the appropriate baseline vital signs.			
• Provides care for the chief complaint: interventions.			
• Transports patient off the hill.			
• Performs a detailed physical exam as necessary.			
• Performs ongoing assessment.			
Did the trainee or OEC technician adequately demonstrate the performance criteria of these skills?			

COMMENTS

(CPI) = Critical Performance Indicator

PATIENT ASSESSMENT—RESPONSIVE MEDICAL PATIENT

Objective: To demonstrate the ability to determine the baseline condition and specific complaint of a responsive patient with a medical problem.

SKILL	YES	NO	NOTATIONS
Scene Size-Up			
• Initiates BSI precautions.			(CPI)
• Determines that the scene is safe.			(CPI)
• Determines the nature of illness (NOI) and/or the mechanism of injury (MOI).			
• Notes the number of patients and the responsiveness of each.			
• Evaluates the need to disentangle or extricate the patient(s). Considers c-spine immobilization.			
• Notes the need for personnel or equipment.			
Initial Assessment—Responsive Patient			
• Offers to assist/obtains the patient's consent.			
• Confirms general impression of the patient and/or level of responsiveness (LOR).			
• Assesses airway, breathing, and circulation (ABCs).			(CPI)
• Assists breathing, or performs CPR as necessary.			(CPI)
• Checks for severe bleeding: intervention = control bleeding.			(CPI)
• If the patient has abnormal ABCs or presents a poor general impression, the rescuer performs the rapid body survey, obtains baseline vital signs, obtains the SAMPLE history, and provides rapid transport.			
• Obtains the chief complaint.			(CPI)
• Calls for transport, equipment, assistance, and/or EMS as needed.			
Focused History and Physical Exam—Medical Patient			
• Obtains the SAMPLE history using OPQRST.			(CPI)
• Conducts a medical-focused physical exam of the area of chief complaint; confirms chief complaint.			(CPI)
• Stabilizes and maintains the patient's body temperature.			
• Determines the appropriate baseline vital signs.			
• Provides care for the chief complaint: interventions = as needed.			(CPI)
• Transports the patient off the hill.			
• Performs a detailed physical exam as necessary.			
• Performs ongoing assessment.			
Did the trainee or OEC technician adequately demonstrate the performance criteria of these skills?			

COMMENTS

(CPI) = Critical Performance Indicator

PATIENT ASSESSMENT—RAPID BODY SURVEY

Objective: To demonstrate the ability to perform a rapid body survey on a patient.

SKILL	YES	NO	NOTATIONS
• Initiates BSI precautions.			(CPI)
• Maintains c-spine immobilization, as necessary.			(CPI)
• Does not expose the patient unnecessarily.			
• Performs the head-to-toe, hands-on, clothes-on exam using the DCAP-BTLS mnemonic to assess the patient.			
• Examines the head (skull, facial bones, pupils, ears, nose, mouth).			
• Examines and palpates the neck (cervical spine, anterior neck, medical-alert tags).			
• Examines and palpates the chest (noting any abnormalities and deformities).			
• Examines and palpates the abdomen (all quadrants). and pelvis.			
• Examines and palpates each lower extremity (noting any abnormalities, and evaluating circulation, motion, and sensation [CMS]).			
• Examines and palpates each upper extremity (noting any abnormalities, evaluating CMS, and looking for medical-alert tags).			
• Examines and palpates the back and buttocks.			

Did the trainee or OEC technician adequately demonstrate the performance criteria of these skills?			

COMMENTS

(CPI) = Critical Performance Indicator

PATIENT ASSESSMENT—DETAILED PHYSICAL EXAM AND ONGOING ASSESSMENT

Objective: To demonstrate the ability to perform a detailed physical exam and ongoing assessment.

SKILL	YES	NO	NOTATIONS
• Initiates BSI precautions.			(CPI)
Detailed Physical Exam—Patient Is in a Warm Shelter			
• Performs a head-to-toe systematic exam.			
• Examines the head (skull, facial bones, pupils, ears, nose, mouth).			
• Examines and palpates the neck (cervical spine, anterior neck, medical-alert tags).			
• Examines and palpates the chest (noting any abnormalities and deformities).			
• Examines and palpates the abdomen (all quadrants) and pelvis.			
• Examines and palpates each lower extremity (noting any abnormalities, and evaluating circulation, motion, and sensation [CMS]).			
• Examines and palpates each upper extremity (noting any abnormalities, evaluating CMS, and looking for medical-alert tags).			
• Examines and palpates the back and buttocks.			
• Updates and records the level of responsiveness (LOR) and vital signs, including the pulse, respirations, and blood pressure.			
• Cares for all problems found.			
• Reevaluates transport decision.			
Ongoing Assessment			
• Repeats the initial assessment.			
• Updates and records the patient's vital signs.			
• Repeats the focused assessment.			
• Reevaluates interventions and adjusts as needed.			

Did the trainee or OEC technician adequately demonstrate the performance criteria of these skills?			

COMMENTS

(CPI) = Critical Performance Indicator

BLEEDING CONTROL/SHOCK MANAGEMENT

Objective: To demonstrate the ability to control severe bleeding and manage shock.

SKILL	YES	NO	NOTATIONS
Bleeding Control			
• Initiates BSI precautions.			(CPI)
• Recognizes the severity of the bleeding and gives it proper priority.			
• Exposes the wound site.			
• Applies direct pressure using a dressing.			(CPI)
• Elevates the wound site above the level of the heart.			
• Maintains direct pressure and elevation; applies additional dressing if needed.			
• Applies direct pressure to the appropriate arterial pressure point if bleeding has not been controlled.			
• Bandages the wound and immobilizes as necessary.			(CPI)
Shock Management			
• Determines if patient is showing signs and symptoms of shock.			
• Applies high-concentration oxygen.			
• Initiates steps to prevent heat loss from the patient.			
• Properly positions the patient.			
• Provides for rapid transport.			

Did the trainee or OEC technician adequately demonstrate the performance criteria of this skill?			

COMMENTS

(CPI) = Critical Performance Indicator

GENERAL MANAGEMENT OF FRACTURES

Objective: To demonstrate the care and splinting of fractures. This will include angulated or displaced fractures, long bone fractures, and fractures at or near a joint.

Note: *Any device chosen must be applied correctly and in accordance with its manufacturer's instructions. If the device chosen for the upper extremity is "soft" (eg, sling and swathe), all of the objectives must be met.*

SKILL	YES	NO	NOTATIONS
• Initiates BSI precautions.			(CPI)
• Assesses the limb, surrounding joints, and mechanism of injury (MOI) to determine the presence and location of fractures and/or dislocations.			
• Assesses circulation, motion, and sensation (CMS) of the limb.			(CPI)
• Manually stabilizes the fracture site and the limb. (Note: *Continuous manual stabilization must be maintained until a splint is applied and secured.*)			
• If there is no distal circulation, realigns the limb by straightening each joint individually and applies axial traction at the nearest distal joint or end of the limb until unusual resistance is met or circulation returns.			(CPI)
• Monitors the patient for indications of unusual resistance or excessive pain during alignment.			
• Aligns the limb to near-anatomically correct position.			
• Positions, applies, and secures splint without excessive movement of the limb, ensuring that all voids are filled.			
• Ensures that the fracture site, the joints above and below the injury, and the limb are immobilized.			(CPI)
• Reassess the CMS of the limb.			(CPI)

	YES	NO	
Did the trainee or OEC technician adequately demonstrate the performance criteria of this skill?			

COMMENTS

(CPI) = Critical Performance Indicator

MANAGEMENT OF AN OPEN FRACTURE

Objective: To demonstrate the control of bleeding associated with an open fracture and immobilization of the limb.

SKILL	YES	NO	NOTATIONS
• Initiates BSI precautions.			(CPI)
• Assesses the limb, joint, and mechanism of injury (MOI) to determine the presence and location of a fracture and/or dislocation.			
• Assesses the circulation, motion, and sensation (CMS) of the limb.			
• Controls any bleeding that is present. —Exposes the fracture site. —Uses direct and indirect pressure, as appropriate. —Uses the pressure point, if necessary.			(CPI)
• Dresses and bandages the wound.			(CPI)
• Prepares the immobilization device for use, taking into account any abnormal anatomic positioning of the limb.			
• Manually stabilizes the fracture site and the limb. (Note: *Continuous manual stabilization must be maintained until a mechanical device is applied and completely secured.*)			
• If there is no distal circulation, realigns the limb until unusual resistance is met or circulation returns.			(CPI)
• Aligns the limb to near-anatomically correct position.			
• Positions, applies, and secures the device without any excessive movement of the limb, ensuring that all voids are filled.			(CPI)
• Makes sure that the fracture site, the joints above and below the injury, and the limb are immobilized.			
• Reassesses the CMS of the limb.			

	YES	NO	
Did the trainee or OEC technician adequately demonstrate the performance criteria of this skill?			

COMMENTS

(CPI) = Critical Performance Indicator

TRACTION SPLINTING

Objective: To immobilize a fracture of the femur using a traction-splinting device.

SKILL	YES	NO	NOTATIONS
• Initiates BSI precautions.			(CPI)
• Assesses the limb using DCAP-BTLS, and notes the mechanism of injury to determine the presence and location of a fracture.			
• Manually stabilizes the fracture site and limb. (Note: *Continuous manual stabilization must be maintained until a splint is applied and secured.*)			
• Assesses the circulation, motion, and sensation (CMS) of the limb.			(CPI)
• Realigns the limb if needed. (Note: *Manual traction should be applied at the knee until the limb is straightened and the ankle hitch is applied.*)			(CPI)
• Applies an ankle hitch.			
• Prepares the immobilization device and materials to be used.			
• Positions the splint properly under the limb and against the ischial tuberosity or pelvic bone (depending on the splint type) without excessive movement or elevation of the limb.			(CPI)
• Applies the splint, including any necessary cradles, supports, etc.			
• Applies mechanical traction at the ankle.			
• Secures the limb properly in the splint.			
• Reassesses the CMS function of the limb.			

	YES	NO	NOTATIONS
Did the trainee or OEC technician adequately demonstrate the performance criteria of this skill?			

COMMENTS

(CPI) = Critical Performance Indicator

SKI BOOT REMOVAL

Objective: To demonstrate the removal of a typical ski boot without compromising an injured leg.

Note: *The decision to remove a ski boot from an injured leg is based on local protocols.*

SKILL	YES	NO	NOTATIONS
• Initiates BSI precautions.			(CPI)
• Stabilizes and manually immobilizes the lower leg and the ski boot.			(CPI)
• While maintaining manual immobilization, spreads boot shell as wide as possible, pulling tongue out or opening rear entry boot. Loosens all devices and provides instructions to assisting OEC technician.			
• With the boot shell held open and the leg immobilized, applies tension to the boot. Firmly and smoothly pulls and rotates boot off the foot.			
• Monitors patient for indications of excessive pain or resistance. Stops or modifies procedure as appropriate.			
• Assesses distal circulation, motion, and sensation (CMS), swelling, displacement, bruising, etc. in injured extremity.			(CPI)
• Prepares to splint the lower extremity.			

	YES	NO	
Did the trainee or OEC technician adequately demonstrate the performance criteria of this skill?			

COMMENTS

(CPI) = Critical Performance Indicator

SPINAL IMMOBILIZATION

Objective: To demonstrate spinal immobilization techniques using a long or short spinal immobilization device.

Note: *The use of a web strap system is the method of choice. Any device chosen must be applied correctly and in accordance with the manufacturer's instructions.*

SKILL	YES	NO	NOTATIONS
• Initiates BSI precautions.			(CPI)
• Uses manual stabilization techniques to firmly stabilize the head and neck. (Note: *Continuous manual stabilization must be maintained until the head is mechanically immobilized and secured.*)			(CPI)
• Assesses mechanism of injury and neurologic functions to determine nature and extent of injury. This assessment must include circulation, motion, and sensation (CMS) in the patient's extremities.			
• Applies a rigid collar (or equivalent) without excessive movement of the head/neck.			
• Transfers the patient as a unit onto spinal immobilization device without excessive movement, maintaining spinal integrity, and properly positions patient on spinal immobilization device.			
• Fills any voids present under the neck or along the spine as necessary.			
• Adequately secures the torso and pelvis to the spinal immobilization device. (Note: *The torso and extremities must be mechanically secured before the head and neck.*)			(CPI)
• Secures the patient's extremities to the immobilization device.			
• Secures the patient's head to the spinal immobilization device.			(CPI)
• Reassesses the CMS in the patient's extremities.			

	YES	NO	
Did the trainee or OEC technician adequately demonstrate the performance criteria of this skill?			

COMMENTS

(CPI) = Critical Performance Indicator

APPLICATION OF A STANDING BACKBOARD

Objective: To demonstrate the application of a backboard on a standing patient who may have a spinal injury.

SKILL	YES	NO	NOTATIONS
• Initiates BSI precautions.			(CPI)
• The first rescuer stands behind the patient and manually stabilizes the patient's head and neck in an anatomically neutral position.			(CPI)
• A second rescuer applies a rigid cervical collar.			
• The second rescuer then inserts the backboard from the side, under the first rescuer's arm and behind the patient.			
• Two rescuers stand facing the patient, one on either side. Each inserts one hand under the patient's armpit and grasps the handhold on the board near or slightly above the armpit.			
• Two rescuers grasp a handhold near the top of the board with their free hands.			
• A fourth rescuer stabilizes the foot of the board.			
• Lowers the board to the ground while manual stabilization of the head and neck is continually maintained.			(CPI)
• Centers the patient by axial sliding, and straps him or her to the board using standard techniques.			(CPI)

	YES	NO	
Did the trainee or OEC technician adequately demonstrate the performance criteria of this skill?			

COMMENTS

(CPI) = Critical Performance Indicator

HELMET REMOVAL

Objective: To demonstrate the correct removal of a helmet from a trauma patient who may have a head or neck injury or obstructed airway.

SKILL	YES	NO	NOTATIONS
• Initiates BSI precautions.			(CPI)
• The patient's head and neck is manually stabilized by placing a hand on each side of the helmet, fingers holding the patient's mandible. A second rescuer unbuckles the chin strap.			
• The second rescuer manually stabilizes the patient's head and neck at the occiput and chin.			(CPI)
• The first rescuer spreads the sides of the helmet and begins to ease it off the patient's head.			(CPI)
• The second rescuer slides his or her hand up the neck to the back of the head and prevents flexion of the neck.			
• The first rescuer resumes manual stabilization of the cervical spine.			
• The patient is immobilized as appropriate.			

	YES	NO	
Did the trainee or OEC technician adequately demonstrate the performance criteria of this skill?			

COMMENTS

(CPI) = Critical Performance Indicator

EXTRICATION FROM DIFFICULT POSITIONS (JAMS AND PRETZELS)

Objective: To safely move an injured patient, especially one with a suspected neck or back injury, into a supine, anatomically neutral position on the ground or onto a backboard.

SKILL	YES	NO	NOTATIONS
• Initiates BSI precautions.			(CPI)
• Performs scene size-up and initial patient assessment.			
• Calls for help (additional equipment, personnel, and EMS transport).			
• Provides necessary interventions (maintains airway, performs CPR, controls bleeding, etc.).			(CPI)
• Stabilizes the cervical spine.			(CPI)
• When additional personnel arrive, manually stabilizes the three reference points (head, shoulders, and hips).			
• Checks circulation, motion, and sensation (CMS) of all limbs.			
• Uses axial, smooth motions in small increments, and aligns one extremity at a time.			
• Aligns all body parts into position 1 (progressing from higher to lower numbered position) as early as possible unless pain or resistance occurs.			(CPI)
• Positions patient on a backboard, maintaining spinal integrity at all times.			
• Stabilizes the patient on a backboard and reassesses CMS.			(CPI)
• Reassesses patient status and interventions, and continues with care, evacuation, and transport.			

Did the trainee or OEC technician adequately demonstrate the performance criteria of this skill?			

COMMENTS

(CPI) = Critical Performance Indicator

LIFTING TECHNIQUES—LONG-AXIS DRAG

Objective: To demonstrate techniques to move a patient over snow or other smooth terrain.

SKILL	YES	NO	NOTATIONS
• Initiates BSI precautions.			(CPI)
• Maintains manual stabilization of the patient's head and neck throughout the maneuver. —Headward drag: supports or cradles the upper torso. —Footward drag: supports or cradles the ankles and lower torso.			(CPI)
• Moves in a crouched position, pulling the patient slowly and smoothly about 12″ at a time.			
• Repositions self and repeats the drag until reaching the desired location.			

Did the trainee or OEC technician adequately demonstrate the performance criteria of this skill?			

COMMENTS

(CPI) = Critical Performance Indicator

LIFTING TECHNIQUES—LOG ROLL

Objective:	To demonstrate manual lifting techniques to move patients onto other devices.

SKILL	YES	NO	NOTATIONS
• Initiates BSI precautions.			(CPI)
• Manually stabilizes the head and neck in an anatomically neutral position.			(CPI)
• Positions sufficient rescuers on the same side of the patient with rescuers' hands placed on the opposite side of the patient's body. Moves the patient as a unit, taking body mass into consideration.			
• Rolls the patient toward the rescuers on command from the leader (at the head) onto the uninjured side if possible, keeping the body in line. (The patient's arm may be alongside the body or elevated based on local protocol.)			(CPI)
• Places the spinal immobilization device beside the patient and underneath as far as possible without excessive movement.			
• Rolls the patient onto the device on command from the leader, keeping the body in line.			(CPI)

Did the trainee or OEC technician adequately demonstrate the performance criteria of this skill?			

COMMENTS

(CPI) = Critical Performance Indicator

LIFTING TECHNIQUES—MULTIPLE-PERSON DIRECT FROM THE GROUND

Objective: To demonstrate manual lifting techniques to move patients onto other devices.

SKILL	YES	NO	NOTATIONS
• Initiates BSI precautions.			(CPI)
• Manually stabilizes the head and neck in an anatomically neutral position.			

• Determines the number of lifters available:
  • 5 people—3 to lift, 1 at head, 1 to move the device.
  • 6 people—4 to lift, 1 at head, 1 to move the device.			

• Prepares and positions all of the equipment needed.			
• Explains the commands, procedures, and hand positions for the lift.			
• Executes the lift and slides the device into place, lifting the patient as a unit.			(CPI)

	YES	NO	
Did the trainee or OEC technician adequately demonstrate the performance criteria of this skill?			

COMMENTS

(CPI) = Critical Performance Indicator

LIFTING TECHNIQUES—BRIDGING

Objective: To demonstrate manual lifting techniques to move patients onto other devices.

SKILL	YES	NO	NOTATIONS
• Initiates BSI precautions.			(CPI)
• Manually stabilizes the head and neck in an anatomically neutral position.			

• Determines the number of lifters available:
  • 5 people—3 to lift, 1 at head, 1 to move the device.
  • 6 people—4 to lift, 1 at head, 1 to move the device.			

• Prepares and positions all of the equipment needed.			
• Positions the lifters and has them form a bridge over the patient, head-to-shoulder or shoulder-to-shoulder. (Note: *All lifters must use the same configuration whether it be head-to-shoulder or shoulder-to-shoulder.*)			
• Explains the commands, procedures, and hand positions for the lift.			
• Positions hands underneath the patient to lift at points of body mass (shoulders, hips).			
• Executes the lift and slides the device into place, lifting the patient as a unit.			(CPI)

Did the trainee or OEC technician adequately demonstrate the performance criteria of this skill?			

COMMENTS

(CPI) = Critical Performance Indicator

LIFTING TECHNIQUES—LIFT INTO A TOBOGGAN

Objective: To demonstrate loading and securing a patient into a toboggan.

SKILL	YES	NO	NOTATIONS
• Initiates BSI precautions.			(CPI)

• Assesses
   —position of the patient in the toboggan.
   —nature and extent of the injury.
   —patient responsiveness.
   —patient mobility (ability to assist).
   —number of people able to assist.
   —terrain (steep or flat).
   —conditions (icy/hard; poor footing; soft, deep powder).
   —type of toboggan (with or without basket stretcher), height of edges, and number of handles.			

• Positions the toboggan and all of the other equipment.			
• Ensures all lifters are in appropriate position.			
• Performs the lift smoothly without compromising the injury.			(CPI)
• Ensures that the patient clears the side of the sled.			(CPI)
• Positions any equipment (skis, snowboard, oxygen tank) properly and secures the patient with straps.			

	YES	NO	
Did the trainee or OEC technician adequately demonstrate the performance criteria of this skill?			

COMMENTS

Appendix C

Emergency Care Kits

Warren D. Bowman, MD, FACP

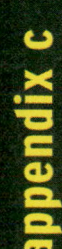

Emergency Care Kits

Although improvisation can serve emergency care providers well, quality patient care usually depends on having appropriate equipment. Rescuers must carry with them or have ready access to a wide variety of emergency care materials—everything from bandages and splints to oropharyngeal airways and extrication vests.

The amount and type of equipment carried in an emergency care kit depends on its intended use. For instance, a kit carried by a nordic patroller in a remote area will differ somewhat from one carried by an alpine patroller at a major resort with prompt access to a hospital. Materials carried by a paramedic or search and rescue team member will vary from those packed by a recreationalist on a 3-day backpacking trip.

The following lists are suggestions only and can be modified to suit individual needs. Prescription medications are marked with an asterisk (*), and controlled substances are marked with two asterisks (**) except where listed as part of a physician's kit. Controlled substances include narcotics, sleeping pills, tranquilizers, and other drugs that may potentially be abused. They can be prescribed only by a physician registered with the Drug Enforcement Administration (DEA) of the US Department of Justice. The physician is given a DEA number that must be included on every prescription written for a controlled substance.

In each list, the quantity of each item (dressing, bandages, pills, etc) is the *minimum* quantity recommended. The actual quantity depends on the number of people to be served by the kit and the time that may elapse before the kit can be replenished.

Note: All emergency care kits must be checked frequently so that the items can be replaced or restored after they have been used. Moreover, kits and equipment must be examined at least once a year so that deteriorated, expired, or outdated supplies and equipment can be replaced.

Ski Patrol Emergency Care Equipment

The emergency care supplies and equipment used in ski patrol operations are quite varied and can depend on the environment in which the patroller works. For instance, materials for alpine patrollers will differ to some extent from those for nordic patrollers, and equipment in avalanche-prone areas will differ from that stocked in slide-free areas.

Contents for an Alpine Patrol Belt or Vest

- Four triangular bandages, folded as cravats
- Two rolls of self-adhering roller bandage: one 2″, one 3″
- Six prepackaged bandage strips (eg, Curad, Band-Aids)
- Roll of 2″ adhesive tape, waterproof
- Nine assorted sterile compresses: three each of three sizes
- Pocket knife (eg, Swiss Army knife)
- Safety pins: two large, two medium
- Several resealable plastic bags (eg, Ziploc) of various sizes
- Paramedic shears or bandage scissors
- Several clean tongue blades in a plastic bag
- Two pairs of disposable rubber gloves in a plastic 35-mm film canister or plastic bag
- Pocket mask (preferable) or a disposable mouth shield (each should have a one-way valve with O_2 port)
- Small flashlight
- Lighter or matches in a waterproof container
- Notebook and "space pen" (or other writing implement capable of writing on wet paper)
- Flow sheet for vital signs
- Release-of-responsibility form

Additional Considerations

- Tube of instant glucose (eg, Glutose)
- Blood glucose test strips (eg, Chemstrip bG)
- SAM splint
- 50′ of $1/8$″ braided nylon cord
- Three oropharyngeal airways: one each for an adult, child, and infant

- Ankle hitch with 30" of ⅛" to ¼" braided nylon cord for pulling traction
- Seam ripper
- Plastic storage bags, several sizes
- Tools such as a screwdriver, pliers, small wrench, or "Leatherman" tool
- Cigarette lighter
- Map of the ski area
- Fire starter
- Avalanche transceiver (on each individual)
- Avalanche probe
- Avalanche shovel
- Biohazard bag for disposal of contaminated materials used on scene

Contents for a Nordic Patrol Emergency Care Kit

- Four or more cravats
- Three rolls of self-adhering roller bandage: one each of three sizes
- Roll of 2" adhesive tape, preferably waterproof
- Sterile, nonadhesive gauze compresses, assorted sizes
- Four trauma dressings: two large, two medium
- Prepackaged bandage strips (eg, Curad, Band-Aid)
- Povidone-iodine (eg, Betadine) swabs
- Petroleum jelly (eg, Vaseline) gauze
- 4' of plastic wrap (folded or rolled) or four large plastic storage bags
- 3" rubberized bandage (eg, Ace bandage)
- Two pairs of disposable rubber gloves
- SAM splint
- Three oropharyngeal airways: one each for an adult, child, and infant
- Pocket mask with a one-way valve and oxygen intake nipple
- Tube of instant glucose (eg, Glutose)
- Tweezers or splinter forceps
- Paramedic shears or bandage scissors
- Single-edge razor blade or a No. 15 scalpel blade in a sterile packet
- Four safety pins: two large, two medium

- Steel sewing needle
- Ankle hitch with 30" of ⅛" to ¼" braided nylon cord for pulling traction
- Seam ripper
- Spreader for ski pole splint or similar device for constructing a traction splint
- Hypothermia thermometer
- Flashlight or preferably headlamp
- Notebook and space pen
- Flow sheet for vital signs
- Lighter or matches in a waterproof container
- Fire starter

Optional

- Rewarming device for a hypothermic patient (HEATPAC, chemical heating pads, or hot air inhalation device)
- Pneumatic splints
- Kendrick Traction Device
- Urinal or pee bottle
- Blood glucose test strips
- Bottle of 10% povidone-iodine (eg, Betadine) solution
- Physiologic saline solution for irrigating*
- 30-mL syringe and 18-gauge needle or catheter for irrigating
- Twelve 25-mg diphenhydramine (Benadryl) capsules
- Twenty 325-mg aspirin or acetaminophen tablets
- Sleeping bag
- Survival equipment (eg, bivy bag, stove, signal flare, signal mirror)
- Lighter
- For avalanche-prone areas: shovel, collapsible probe, transceiver

Additional Considerations

- Twelve doses of pain medication, eg, tablets of acetaminophen with 30-mg of codeine** (Tylenol No. 3) or 100-mg tablets of propoxyphene with acetaminophen** (Darvocet-N 100)
- Injectable epinephrine* (eg, AnaKit, EpiPen) for anaphylactic reactions

appendix c

Contents for a Toboggan Pack

- Ensolite to pad bottom of toboggan
- Blankets or a sleeping bag
- Waterproof cover
- Quick splint
- Canvas stretcher
- Cravats and padding material

Additional Considerations
(items usually kept at the top of the hill)

- Long and short backboards
- Pneumatic splints
- Traction splints
- Extra sleeping bags
- Oxygen pack (described below)
- Trauma pack (described below)
- Medical pack (described below)
- Automated external defibrillator
- Extra toboggan packs
- Portable suction (manual or electric)

Oxygen pack: oxygen cylinder(s) with regulator(s), bag-valve-mask (BVM) devices (adult and pediatric sizes), suction apparatus, oxygen tubing, nonrebreathing masks (adult and pediatric sizes), and nasal cannulae (adult and pediatric sizes), oropharyngeal and nasopharyngeal airways

Trauma pack: cravats, self-adhering roller bandage, rubberized bandage (eg, Ace), waterproof adhesive tape (eg, 1″ and 2″), sterile compresses, petroleum jelly (eg, Vaseline) gauze, trauma dressings, SAM splints, a Sager or other traction splint, rigid collars (adult and pediatric sizes), oropharyngeal and nasopharyngeal airways, rubber gloves, an extrication vest, and biohazard (red) bags

Medical pack: injectable epinephrine (eg, AnaKit, EpiPen), oral glucose (eg, Glutose), blood glucose measuring equipment, asthma inhaler, oropharyngeal and nasopharyngeal airways, tongue blades, rubber gloves, stethoscope, a blood pressure cuff, pulse oximeter, biohazard (red) bags, and a sharps container

Patrol Aid Room Equipment

The following are the minimum number of items. Final selection should be based on local needs and consultation with area management and the patrol's medical advisor or consultant and OEC instructors.

Basic Equipment

- Cots or beds
- Bedpans and urinals
- Warming mechanism for cold patients (infrared lamps, electric blankets, hot water bottles, heating pads, etc)
- Portable screen or curtains for privacy
- Emergency care cabinet (see contents listed below)
- Oxygen equipment
- Suction equipment
- BVM devices
- Pocket masks with one-way valves and O_2 inlets
- Sink with running water, soap, towels
- Toilet
- Waste receptacles
- Containers for infectious waste and contaminated clothing
- Telephone and radio
- Pipe cutter (for shortening impaled objects)
- Large container for warm water for rewarming a frozen hand or foot

Contents of Emergency Care Cabinet

- Self-adhering roller bandages
- Prepackaged bandage strips
- Butterfly bandages or Steristrips
- Sterile dressings: assorted sizes, including nonadhering types
- Standard thermometer
- Low-reading thermometer
- Cravats
- Tweezers or splinter forceps

- Ring cutter
- Plastic bags for making a cold pack with snow
- Adhesive tape, assorted widths
- Single-edge razor blades
- 10% povidone-iodine (Betadine) solution or other skin preparation solution
- Tincture of benzoin
- Sewing kit
- Safety pins
- Paramedic shears
- Bandage scissors
- Disposable gowns
- Disposable face shields
- Disposable rubber gloves, including sterile pairs
- Disposable paper cups
- Rubbing alcohol
- Wash pan, large, metal or plastic
- Emesis basin
- Urinal
- Laboratory thermometer for measuring water temperature in frostbite rewarming
- Stethoscope
- Blood pressure cuff
- Oral and nasopharyngeal airways
- Flashlight
- Tongue blades
- Sanitary napkins
- Blood glucose measuring equipment: (eg, One Touch II blood glucose meter, Chemstrip bG)
- Pulse oximeter
- Sterile physiologic saline solution
- Incident and other report forms

Medical Kit for Ski Patrol Physician or Paramedic

The following are the minimum number of items. Final determination should be made by conferring with area management and the patrol medical advisor (or consultant) and members of the physician patrol, if any.

- Intravenous fluids, IV sets, IV needles
- Cardiac monitor/defibrillator (or automated external defibrillator)
- Endotracheal intubation kit with endotracheal tubes
- Drugs (see Physician/Paramedic and Search-and-Rescue Kits later in this appendix)
- Equipment for needle thoracotomy and cricothyroidotomy
- Flutter valve (eg, Heimlich)
- Chest tube set and insertion pack
- Small oto-ophthalmoscope set

Recreational Emergency Care Kit

The amount of equipment carried in a recreational emergency care kit depends on the length of the planned trip, the difficulty of obtaining medical help, the number of party members, and the type of transportation. The requirements of a 1-day, cross-country ski tour are obviously different than those of a 4-week, Alaskan expedition.

As mentioned previously, the following lists are suggestions only and can be modified to suit individual needs. In each instance, the number of each item recommended is the minimum number. To determine how much of each item to take, consider the number of people in the party and the total trip time, with emphasis on minimal weight and bulk, low cost, maximum chance of use, favorable weight/bulk/cost-to-benefit ratio, and opportunities for multiple uses.

Contents of a Basic Kit

A basic kit (▶ Table C-1) is suitable for a day trip or to be carried by each member of a party on a multiday trip. It can be stored in a small stuff sack.

Table C-1 Contents of a Basic Kit

Items	Comments
Two cravats	Use as a bandage or sling.
One or two rolls of 3″ or 4″ self-adhering roller bandage (eg, Kling or Kerlix)	Use as bandaging material. Roll of 2″ adhesive tape, preferably waterproof can be torn in half lengthwise to make 1″ tape. Small strips can be torn off to make butterfly bandages. Can also be used for blister prevention and treatment.
Six or more prepackaged bandage strips	Use for small wounds.
Four sterile gauze compresses, 3″ x 4″ or 4″ x 4″ (nonadhering—Telfa or equivalent)	Can be cut up and used with pieces of tape to make small bandages (if you don't want to carry regular prepackaged bandage strips).
Twenty 325-mg aspirin or 500-mg acetaminophen (eg, Tylenol) and/or 200-mg ibuprofen tablets (eg, Advil, Nuprin, Motrin)	For headache and other mild pain, take one or two every 3 hours as needed. Take ibuprofen with food. Ibuprofen is preferred if there is a risk of frostbite (two twice daily with food during hazardous conditions). Persons younger than 18 years should not take aspirin because it can cause Reye's syndrome in those with flu-like symptoms.
Sunscreen or sunblock	See Chapter 15.
Lip balm	Use a type that stays relatively soft in cold weather and has a proper SPF number (see Chapter 15).
Multiuse knife with scissors and tweezers (Swiss Army knife)	For various uses.
Safety pins	For various uses; include large sizes to improvise an upper extremity splint by pinning the patient's sleeve to the front of his or her jacket.
Plastic sandwich bags	For various uses; fill with snow to improvise a cold pack.
Personal medications, if any	Patients with diabetes should include pills or a tube of oral glucose as well as diabetes-control medicine (pills, insulin with injection equipment) and blood or urine glucose measuring equipment. Consider carrying two ampules of glucagon with injection equipment if insulin is being used.
Water purification equipment (purifying tablets, water filter)	One filter set or bottle of tablets for every two people.
Small flashlight or headlamp with spare batteries and bulbs	A headlamp may be preferred because its use frees both hands.
Pair of disposable rubber gloves	Keep in a 35-mm film canister or plastic bag.
Optional	
Sheet of moleskin	For blister prevention and treatment (some prefer this to 2″ tape).
Antacid (eg, Di-gel, Tums) or antacid/anti-gas preparation (eg, Mylanta)	A combination of an antacid and an antigas preparation may be preferred for the increased intestinal gas common at altitude.
Small, foil-packaged, disposable, moist towelettes	For hand washing if no water is available.
Barrier device (pocket mask, face shield)	For protection against the patient's saliva during rescue breathing or CPR.

Table C-1 Contents of a Basic Kit—continued

Items	Comments
Optional for a Multiday Trip	
Sleeping pills** of choice, if desired, with directions for use (Consult a physician.)	Try these out at home to be sure they are effective. Use with caution above 12,000′ (3,658 m) because they may interfere with acclimatization and cause altered mental status. Sleeping aids such as ear plugs and eye shields alone may be sufficient.
Pee bottle	Anyone who has had to get out of a warm sleeping bag to make a nocturnal pit stop knows what this is for. Women may wish to add a Sani-Fem funnel.

Contents of a Master Kit

A master kit (▶ **Table C-2**) is designed for multiday recreational tours. Each party should have one master kit, which can be carried in a nylon stuff-sack, with breakables in a separate, hard-sided container.

Table C-2 Contents of a Master Kit

Items	Comments
Additional cravats to provide at least six per party	At least six are needed to improvise a traction splint from ski poles or to strap a patient to an improvised long backboard.
Twelve additional sterile, nonadhering gauze compresses	
Four trauma pads: two medium, two large (eg, ABD pads or Surgipads)	
3″ rubberized bandage (eg, Ace)	
Four extra self-adhering roller bandages, two each of 2″ and 3″	
Six tongue blades	For various uses; improvise a finger splint or wrap several together with duct tape or adhesive tape to make an all-purpose hand and forearm splint.
30″ of ⅛″ to ¼″ braided nylon cord	For setting up a pulley for a traction splint.
Spreader for ski pole splint, such as an 8″ piece of ski pole with two holes in it	The ski pole tips go in the holes (see Figure D-1).
Seam ripper	Use instead of cutting expensive clothing.
Sewing needle (can be part of a sewing kit)	For various uses, including care of blisters and ingrown toenails.

appendix c

Table C-2 Contents of a Master Kit—continued

Items	Comments
Small bottle of antiseptic cleanser (10% povidone-iodine [eg, Betadine] solution or chlorhexidine gluconate [Hibiclens])	Dilute povidone-iodine 1:10 with clean water for care of high-risk wounds.
Thermometer	The rectal type is more versatile. For cold weather trips, a low-reading thermometer is recommended instead of, or in addition to, a standard clinical one.
Single-edge razor blade or packaged sterile No. 15 scalpel blade, splinter forceps	For incising and draining abscesses and removing splinters.
30-mL syringe, No. 18-gauge needle, and splash shield	For wound irrigation.
Turkey-baster syringe or 60-mL syringe and Foley catheter	For upper airway suction.
Two extra pairs of disposable rubber gloves (consider sterile ones)	For dressing open wounds or to avoid contact with moist body fluids.
Pocket mask with a one-way valve	To increase the effectiveness of rescue breathing and to help avoid contact with the patient's saliva.
Notebook and "space pen"	To record vital signs and other important data.
Oropharyngeal and nasopharygeal airways (at least two sizes such as large and small adult)	To manage the airway of an unresponsive patient.

Medications

5-g tube of ophthalmic ointment (eg, Polysporin*)	Can be used in the eyes or on the skin for eye infections or infected cuts. Apply 3 times daily.
Twenty-four 25-mg or 12 50-mg diphenhydramine hydrochloride (Benadryl) capsules	For itching, hives, and drug reactions, administer one 50-mg or two 25-mg capsules every 4 hours as needed. The 25-mg size is nonprescription medication.
Alternatives: Loratadine* (Claritin), Dexchlorpheniramine* (Polaramine), *Fexofenadine (Allegra).	Consult a physician for the appropriate doses.
Twelve 30-mg tablets of acetaminophen with 30-mg of codeine** (Tylenol No. 3)	For pain, administer one to two tablets every 3 hours as needed. Drugs containing codeine can also be used for diarrhea, with one tablet given every 3 hours, as needed.
Alternatives: 100-mg tablets of propoxyphene and acetaminophen** (Darvocet-N 100), or tramadol** (Ultram)	Consult a physician for the appropriate doses.

Table C-2   Contents of a Master Kit—continued

Items	Comments
Optional	
SAM splint	Use as a small, multipurpose fixation splint or as an improvised rigid collar. Can be improvised using sticks or tongue blades wrapped with duct tape or adhesive tape.
Kendrick traction device	Use as an alternative to the ski pole traction splint.
Twelve 2.5-mg tablets of diphen-oxylate with atropine sulfate** (eg, Lomotil)	For diarrhea, take one or two tablets every 3 hours as needed.
Alternative: 2-mg capsules of loperamide (Imodium A-D)	Administer two capsules with the first loose bowel movement, then one with each subsequent movement (no more than four in each 24-hour period). Loperamide is a nonprescription medication.
Six 25-mg prochlorperazine* (Compazine) rectal suppositories	For vomiting, one suppository is inserted every 12 hours as needed. Insert one suppository every 4 hours as needed.
Alternative: 25-mg promethazine* (Phenergan) suppositories	Prochlorperazine is preferred for persons at high altitude.
Optional for Those with Special Training and Licensing	
10- or 12-gauge over-needle catheter (eg, Angiocath) and sharps container	For relief of tension pneumothorax.
Foley catheter with lubricating jelly	For urinary retention.
Cricothyroidotomy set	For upper airway obstruction not relieved by simple techniques.
Additional Considerations	
Twelve 100-mg meperidine** (Demerol) tablets	For severe pain, half a tablet or one tablet is taken every 3 hours as needed.
Alternatives: Oxycodone† or hydrocodone† and acetaminophen capsules (Tylox, Percodan, Vicodin)	One tablet is taken every 3 hours as needed. (†These are strong narcotics.)
Injectable epinephrine* (AnaKit, EpiPen)	For anaphylactic reactions. (It is preferable to have a susceptible person carry his or her own kit as well.)
Cellular phone, Global Positioning System (GPS) unit	These devices can be helpful when it's necessary to call for help or in locating your precise position.
For extended trips into remote country, you may wish to add:	
Several packets of powdered sport drink (eg, Gatorade) or Oralyte (see Appendix D)	Use as an electrolyte-replacement solution.

appendix c

Table C-2 Contents of a Master Kit—continued

Items	Comments
20 cotrimoxazole DS* (Septra DS, Bactrim DS) tablets	This is a good, inexpensive, multipurpose single antibiotic. One tablet is taken twice daily for at least 7 days.
or	
Twenty 500-mg ciprofloxacin* (Cipro) tablets	Another good, albeit expensive, multipurpose single antibiotic. Take one tablet twice daily for at least 7 days. Children, teenagers younger than 18 years, and pregnant women should not take this medication.
or	
One medication from each of the following two groups of antibiotics:	Offers broader coverage than a single antibiotic, but is more complicated to use.
1. Twenty-one 250- to 500-mg amoxicillin* capsules, one three times daily, or 250- to 500-mg amoxicillin-clavulanate* (Augmentin) three times daily *Alternatives:* 250- to 500-mg cephalexin* (Keflex) four times daily; 250-mg Cefaclor* (Ceclor) three times daily; 250-mg cefuroxime* (Ceftin) twice daily; 400-mg erythromycin ethyl succinate* (EES 400) four times daily	1. For upper and lower respiratory tract infections, wound and skin infections, and high-risk wounds (those which are likely to become seriously infected). The medication should be taken for at least 7 days.
2. Fourteen 100-mg doxycycline* tablets, one twice daily *Alternatives:* 250-mg tetracycline* tablets, one four times daily	2. For urinary tract infections and dysentery. Tetracyclines should not be taken with milk or dairy products or close to meals. An exaggerated sunburn reaction may occur, especially in persons at high altitude or on snow. The drug should be discontinued at the first sign of unusual skin redness. Pregnant women, nursing mothers, and children younger than 8 years should not take tetracyclines.

Note: If no improvement is experienced with a drug in one group after 2 days, switch to a drug in the other group.

Table C-2 Contents of a Master Kit—continued

Items	Comments
Suggested for High Altitude	
Twelve or more 250-mg acetazo-lamide* (Diamox) tablets	See Appendix D.
Thirty 4-mg dexamethasone* (Decadron or Hexadrol) tablets	See Appendix D.
Six 10-mg and 20 long-acting (30-mg) nifedipine* (Procardia)	See Appendix D.
Suggested for Developing Countries	
Twenty 500-mg ciprofloxacin* (Cipro) tablets or cotrimoxazole* (Septra DS, Bactrim) tablets	For dysentery, one tablet is taken twice daily for 7 to 10 days. See Appendix D.
Pills for malaria prophylaxis if needed	Consult a physician. Immunocompromised persons (those with AIDS and other diseases that affect the immune system) and those with increased susceptibility to traveler's diarrhea (persons who have had stomach surgery or lack gastric acid) should consult a physician regarding medication for prophylaxis of traveler's diarrhea.
Optional for Women	
Seven clotrimazole (Mycelex 7) vaginal suppositories	For yeast vaginitis. Insert one at bedtime for 1 week. See Appendix D.
Alternative: One 150-mg fluconazole* (Diflucan) tablet	One dose
Fourteen 500-mg metronidazole* (Flagyl) tablets	For all other types of vaginitis, one tablet is taken twice daily for 1 week (see Appendix D). This drug should not be given if the person is pregnant or has been drinking alcohol. If one medication is ineffective, switch to the other.
Suggested for Snake Country (see Chapter 13)	
Optional	
Constriction band (eg, a wide rubber tourniquet type)	To delay absorption of snake venom.

Contents of a Wilderness Search and Rescue (SAR) Emergency Care Kit

Dressings, Bandages, and Wound Care

- Ten 4" x 4" nonadhesive gauze compresses
- Four trauma dressings: two medium, two large (eg, ABD pads or Surgipads)
- Four self-adhering roller bandages, two 2", two 3"
- Two packs of povidone-iodine (eg, Betadine) swabs or a bottle of 10% solution
- One 500-mL bottle and splash shield of physiologic saline* and sterile 30-mL syringe with a sterile 18-gauge needle for wound irrigation
- Sharps container
- Two packets of Vaseline gauze
- One roll each of ½", 1", and 2" adhesive tape, preferably waterproof
- 4' of plastic wrap, folded or rolled
- Twenty-four prepackaged bandage strips
- Steristrips, ⅛" and ¼"
- Two 3" rubberized bandages
- Two 2" rubberized bandages
- Twelve plastic storage bags: six small, six medium
- Four pairs of disposable rubber gloves, nonsterile
- Two pairs of disposable rubber gloves, sterile
- Two disposable face shields
- Biohazard bags

Splints and Backboards

- Rigid collars: two adjustable adult Stifnecks plus one or two Stifneck child sizes (you can improvise a child-size collar from a SAM splint)
- Sager splint or Kendrick traction device
- Pneumatic splint for lower extremity, long size
- Kendrick extrication device or Oregon Spine Splint II
- Eight cravats
- Two SAM splints
- One backboard (SKED, Ferno-Washington), preferably a lightweight one or one that can break in half if backpacking is required

Cardiorespiratory

- Six oropharyngeal airways, two each of three sizes (adult, child, and infant)
- Six nasopharyngeal airways, two each of three sizes (adult, child, and infant)
- Pocket mask with one-way valve and oxygen intake nipple
- Suction apparatus (V-Vac or portable, battery-operated unit)
- Three BVM devices: two adult and one child size

Drugs

Consider drugs suggested for the recreational emergency care master kit. Add an epinephrine injection kit* (AnaKit, EpiPen) for anaphylactic reactions, sublingual nitroglycerin tablets* (Nitrostat, 0.4 mg, or Nitro-spray) for angina pectoris, instant glucose (Glutose) for hypoglycemia, and activated charcoal for poisoning.

Other

- Lightweight stethoscope
- Blood pressure cuff
- Clinical thermometer
- Hypothermia thermometer
- Blood glucose test equipment
- Small pulse oximeter
- Paramedic shears
- Bandage scissors
- Triage tags for labeling
- Urinal or pee bottle
- Small flashlight
- Single-edge razor blade
- Seam ripper
- Steel sewing needle
- Lubricant jelly
- Safety pins
- Tweezers or splinter forceps
- Notebook and space pen
- Headlamp

Additional Items for Cold Weather

- Hypothermia rewarming equipment such as chemical heating pads, HEATPAC, a device for heating inspired air
- Container large enough to rewarm a frozen hand or foot
- Laboratory thermometer to measure water temperature
- Extra sleeping bag or casualty bag
- Tent

Optional, Depending on Manpower and Transport Capacity

- Oxygen backpack (two tanks, regulator, nonrebreathing masks, nasal cannulae, and tubing)

Wilderness SAR Physician/Paramedic Kit

- Stethoscope
- Blood pressure cuff
- Small otoscope/ophthalmoscope with tongue blades
- Cricothyroidotomy set
- Endotracheal intubation kit
- Spare batteries
- 14-gauge Intracath for needle thoracotomy
- Flutter valve (Heimlich or improvised from a finger of a rubber glove)
- Several spare 20- to 35-mL syringes
- Intravenous fluids: liter bags of lactated Ringer's solution and liter bags of normal saline solution
- IV administration sets
- 18- and 20-gauge Intracath needles
- Sharps container
- 1" adhesive tape
- ½" adhesive tape, preferably waterproof
- Alcohol swabs

- Parenteral drugs (include sterile syringes and needles for injection):
  - Meperidine
  - Morphine
  - Prochlorperazine or Promethazine
  - Furosemide
  - Epinephrine 1:1000
  - Naloxone
  - Aminophylline (requires a 50-mL syringe)
  - Diphenhydramine
  - Diazepam
  - 50% glucose (requires a 50-mL syringe)
  - Dexamethasone
  - Glucagon

Optional

- Chest tube set and insertion pack
- Water seal apparatus and bag of sterile water
- Nasogastric tubes
- Foley catheter (18-F) with collection bag, clamp, and lubricant
- Povidone-iodine swabs
- Monitor/defibrillator or automated external defibrillator
- Pulse oximeter
- AED
- ACLS drugs‡: (include IV bags, needles and tubing, additional sterile syringes and needles):
  - Aspirin
  - Atropine
  - Epinephrine 1:10,000
  - Verapamil
  - Procainamide
  - Digoxin
  - Lidocaine
  - Morphine
  - Adenosine
  - Nitroglycerin
  - Vasopressin

‡ Questionable whether carrying these ACLS drugs would improve survival at all in the wilderness context. Best scenario would be rapid defibrillation with an AED.

Appendix D

Principles of Wilderness Emergency Care

Warren D. Bowman, MD, FACP

Principles of Wilderness Emergency Care

The information in this appendix is included as a guide for wilderness travelers, including members of recreational parties, wilderness search and rescue (SAR) teams, mountain rescue groups, and nordic ski patrols. For these purposes, the term "wilderness" means any area where:

- there is no "9-1-1" to call,

- no sophisticated medical facilities exist and your only emergency care equipment is what you bring or can improvise,

- communications are primitive or nonexistent,

- you may be stranded by severe environmental conditions, or

- evacuation to medical care is usually prolonged or delayed.

For most people, the word "wilderness" evokes an image of thick woods or high, snow-covered mountains, but wilderness can also mean arctic ice, subarctic tundra, the desert, the seashore, a tropical savannah or rain forest, the ocean, the underwater world, caverns, and wild rivers.

Exposure to the wilderness can be brief or prolonged. In a sense, an alpine skier caught in a blizzard on a mountaintop is in wilderness, but only briefly unless he or she strays outside the ski area boundary. Nordic skiers or hikers on a day trip may be in wilderness for a time, as may cavers in a deep cavern, kayakers in a canyon, scuba divers in the water's depths, pilots downed in the desert, or mountaineers at significant heights. Small-boat sailors, inhabitants of isolated villages, and victims of urban disasters whose electricity is cut off and whose medical facilities and communications have been destroyed can all be said to be in the wilderness.

Wilderness is usually remote but, in some cases, areas of true wilderness are so close to inhabited areas that sophisticated rescue teams or helicopter crews with advanced life support capability can reach a patient within an hour or two of notification.

Successful wilderness existence requires a respect for the forces of nature and at least some wilderness survival training and equipment. Rescuers who operate in nonurban areas also need training in *wilderness emergency care*.

The basics of this care have been addressed throughout this textbook and should be quite familiar to you by now. In most cases, emergency care of injuries and illnesses in the wilderness follows the same principles as emergency care anywhere. Most differences are due to lack of equipment, need for improvisation, and the need to care for a patient over a longer period, during which the injury or illness may evolve or be modified by the environment.

The content in this appendix is mainly designed for your personal edification and protection. Some of this information goes *far beyond* what rescuers are legally authorized to do in most states unless they are physicians, physician's assistants, or nurse practitioners. This is particularly true of the sections on reducing dislocations and the use of prescription drugs.

Even though such procedures may be medically indicated, their inclusion does not imply that the National Ski Patrol endorses procedures or practices that go beyond the usual levels of emergency care described in the body of this text.

Wilderness emergency care differs from urban or even outdoor emergency care in the following ways:

- It is practiced in the wilderness environment, where extreme conditions of heat, cold, altitude, and weather are common and difficulties in obtaining food, water, and shelter are significant. Dangers such as snow avalanches, rockfalls, flash floods, forest fires, and lightning may be present. Hazardous microorganisms, insects, marine animals, land animals, and plants may endanger the health of wilderness travelers, and preexisting medical conditions may recur or flare up at awkward times.

- Definitive medical care may be many hours or days away because of distance, adverse environmental conditions, problems with infrastructure caused by natural or manmade disasters, lack of transportation, or difficulties in communication.

- Illnesses rarely seen elsewhere, such as acute mountain sickness, deep frostbite, and wild-animal mauling, may occur.

- It may be desirable to train able laypersons to carry out advanced procedures for common injuries and illnesses in which a delay in treatment of more than a few hours or days might have significant but otherwise preventable adverse effects. The emphasis is on simple procedures requiring a minimum of training and equipment but with the potential for saving life or limb.

- Rescuers need to learn extended care (basic nursing care) of an injured or ill person so they can provide for the patient's ordinary day-to-day requirements until medical assistance can be reached.

- Certain standard urban protocols such as those for cardiac arrest may be unrealistic or even hazardous to rescuers.

- Ordinary illnesses and injuries can occur in the wilderness as easily, and at times more easily, than at home, and can be even more inconvenient.

- The amount of first aid equipment that can be carried by the average wilderness recreational group, or even the best-equipped wilderness search and rescue group with helicopter support, is limited; improvisation *will* be necessary.

Wilderness emergency care can be rendered at several levels of complexity and sophistication. The simplest level is first aid or first responder care for informal recreational groups that carry limited emergency supplies and equipment and rely on improvisation. More sophisticated levels are wilderness first responder (WFR) and wilderness emergency medical technician (WEMT) care, which may be available in larger, more experienced groups, including guided parties with more elaborate emergency capabilities.

The next highest level is search and rescue (SAR) emergency care, in which rescuers trained at an advanced EMT or paramedic level may be available and rescue kits may include fairly complex and sophisticated supplies and equipment. The highest level is expeditionary emergency care and care given by medical workers in isolated villages. In these situations, personnel are highly trained, supplies are plentiful, medical equipment is usually sophisticated, and there is less emphasis on choosing equipment based on its portability.

Nineteenth century German statesman Otto von Bismarck once said that "politics is the art of the possible." The same can be said about the inherent nature of wilderness emergency care. Rescuers cannot carry the equivalent of a hospital emergency department on their backs. Instead, they must make do with carefully chosen but limited equipment and rely on thorough training, sharp assessment skills, ingenuity, and the ability to improvise. Patients who are seriously injured or ill may die despite the best care provided in a modern hospital. Thus, rescuers should have a realistic view of their limitations, yet resolve to keep skills honed and do their best at all times.

Because rescuers who are *prepared* for potential wilderness hazards can avoid many otherwise

inevitable difficulties, prevention is emphasized in previous sections of this textbook and in this appendix. You will enjoy your wilderness experiences more when you have the training and equipment to prevent most problems and deal successfully with those that are unpreventable. However, *do not overestimate your capabilities*. If a member of a wilderness party is significantly ill or injured, the group must abort the trip and transport the patient to medical care.

Each member of a wilderness party should start out in good basic health, in good physical condition, and be free of acute or chronic infectious disease. If health questions arise, the party leader should require a physician's certificate of physical ability sufficient for the anticipated level of physical stress. Many minor physical abnormalities and well-controlled medical conditions are stable enough to allow wilderness travel. Such conditions include mild hypertension, minor valvular heart disease, hay fever, asthma, diabetes, and similar ailments.

Other conditions rule out wilderness travel because they can flare up under the stress of high altitude or long hours on the trail and be difficult to treat in isolated circumstances. These conditions include active peptic ulcers; known kidney, bladder, or gallbladder stones; coronary artery disease; chronic obstructive pulmonary disease; metastatic cancer; clotting or bleeding disorders; and a history of severe, recurrent high-altitude illness.

Disabilities of the musculoskeletal system, such as active rheumatoid arthritis; recurrent, severe back pain; and severe knee and hip joint disease also preclude excursions into the wilderness. People with the mild form of sickle cell anemia known as sickle cell trait are susceptible to spleen infarctions during high-altitude travel and have even been known to die during strenuous exercise.

Consult a physician familiar with wilderness medical problems if you are unsure of whether you or a fellow group member is fit to join a particular trip.

Before setting out on an excursion into the wilderness, *all group members should be up-to-date on routine immunizations, especially tetanus*. The party leader should ask whether any party members have a significant health impairment and whether medication is taken for any specific conditions. People who take tranquilizers, antidepressants, anticholinergics, or beta-blockers on a regular basis may be more susceptible to wilderness stresses. For example, beta-blockers—commonly used to treat high blood pressure—can cause chronic fatigue, depression, and deconditioning marked by poor exercise tolerance and poor recovery from strenuous exercise.

Anyone who has had an anaphylactic reaction to food, drugs, or stings should carry an emergency kit containing epinephrine (adrenalin) and an antihistamine. At least one other party member should know how to use these kits. Any group member who wears prescription eyeglasses should carry a spare pair, and contact lens wearers should carry a pair of regular glasses as well. Contact lenses can actually freeze to the eyes under severe winter conditions.

Persons with diabetes should take adequate supplies of necessary medications and other equipment (insulin, syringes, needles, antidiabetic pills, glucagon, oral glucose preparations, and test kits to obtain glucose levels in blood or urine). In case of an emergency, patients with diabetes should pack extra supplies, some of which should be carried by another party member who may be required to administer the medication to the person with diabetes. On a trip that includes a person with diabetes who requires insulin, at least one other party member should know how to give insulin injections. Patients with diabetes should carry extra food for emergency snacks at all times.

If you want formal instruction in wilderness emergency care, a number of organizations teach Wilderness-EMT and Wilderness First Responder courses. In most cases, participants must already be trained at the Outdoor Emergency Care, EMT-Basic, or First Responder level. You can get a list of available courses from the Wilderness Medical Society or the National Association for Search and Rescue. Contact information for these organizations can be found at www.OECzone.com.

Patient Assessment in the Wilderness

Patient assessment in the wilderness is much the same as in the outdoors in general, except emergency care in the wilderness is even more reliant on skillful and thorough assessment. Extreme environmental conditions may delay detailed assessment until shelter has been reached. Clothing should be cut or torn only as a last resort. Rescuers should be thoroughly familiar with the assessment of both injured and ill patients, as described in Chapter 7.

Cardiac Arrest in the Wilderness

Guidelines for starting and stopping CPR, while reasonable and appropriate in a *traditional* environment, might not be relevant in the wilderness.

Studies have shown that patients with out-of-hospital cardiac arrest due to ventricular fibrillation have a dismal survival rate when treated with CPR alone, even when the collapse is witnessed. The best results—30% survival—have been obtained with bystander CPR, defibrillation within 4 minutes, and advanced cardiac life support within 8 minutes. Therefore, in a remote area where an automated external defibrillator is unavailable and advanced cardiac life support is many hours or days away, *CPR has little or no chance of success.* In addition, administering CPR under wilderness conditions may put group members in serious danger because of physical hazards and the risk of exhaustion.

Some reasonable conclusions can be drawn based on these facts, which elicit certain suggestions regarding CPR in remote areas. Since the following measures were legal only in a few states at the time of this writing, they are suggestions only.

First, in a wilderness setting you may wish to try a single precordial thump (a sudden, sharp blow with your fist placed over the patient's heart) if the arrest was witnessed, since this may restore the patient's normal heart rhythm. Second, because CPR may be ill-advised in a remote environment it should not be attempted at all if:

- the patient is in cardiac arrest caused by trauma
- the patient is a drowning victim who has been immersed for more than an hour
- the cardiac arrest was unwitnessed and the time of onset is unknown
- the patient is hypothermic with an incompressible chest
- the patient appears to be dead, based on rigor mortis (stiffening) or livor mortis (discoloration of the body parts next to the ground), lethal injuries, or a body core (rectal) temperature below 60°F (16°C)
- giving CPR would be hazardous to rescuers

Moreover, after 30 minutes of CPR with no signs of life, further CPR is probably useless and may reasonably be discontinued. Administering CPR to a patient who is being evacuated by backboard or toboggan is very difficult, if not impossible. Unless an ambulance or helicopter can be brought in rapidly, chances of survival are minimal. *Exceptions* to this include the following:

- The patient is hypothermic and has a *compressible* chest
- The patient has another condition *complicated* by significant hypothermia (core temperature < 90°F [32°C]) (such as avalanche burial and near-drowning in cold water)
- The patient is in cardiac and/or respiratory

arrest caused by lightning injury (see Chapter 15) or drug overdose (see Chapter 13)

In these instances, the prognosis is theoretically more favorable and you should give CPR aggressively.

Respiratory Arrest in the Wilderness

The outlook in a patient, especially a child, who has a pulse but is in respiratory arrest is more favorable than that of a patient in cardiac arrest. Rescuers should continue rescue breathing as long as they are able to do it without becoming exhausted or endangering themselves.

Extended Patient Care (Nursing Care) in the Wilderness

In addition to requiring specific care for injuries and illnesses, patients in the wilderness have certain basic requirements for survival, which, for the most part, their rescuers share. These include the following:

- Oxygen
- Shelter
- Normal body temperature
- Water
- Food
- Assistance with natural processes such as eating, drinking, urinating, and defecating
- Psychological support
- Basic faith and the will to live

Paying attention to these requirements will ensure that the patient is in the best possible physical condition during stabilization and transport to definitive medical care.

The initial care of an injured or ill person is no different in the wilderness than anywhere else. While one rescuer performs the initial assessment and gives immediate care as described in Chapter 7, other party members construct a shelter and prepare to stabilize the patient's body temperature.

In cold weather, place insulation beneath and around the patient, cover the patient's head and neck, and replace wet clothing with dry clothing. Also, lay the patient in a sleeping bag, start a fire or stove, and erect a tent or prepare a snow shelter.

In hot weather, rig a tarp or other shelter as protection against the sun, and in desert conditions prepare a cool surface for the patient to lie on, either by scraping away the upper 6″ of hot earth or by building a platform with backpacks or natural materials. Add or sub-

tract clothing as appropriate to protect the patient against the sun or to prevent a rise in body temperature.

The mechanisms for stabilizing body temperature are always impaired by injury or illness, so both hypothermia and hyperthermia can develop more easily in an injured or ill person than in a healthy individual. The rescue party must also look to its own safety, since party members are subject to the same environmental stresses as the patient.

After caring for urgent problems and stabilizing the patient's body temperature, proceed with the focused history and physical exam, treat less urgent problems, and then perform the detailed physical exam, as appropriate, so that nothing is missed. In cold weather, expose one small body area at a time for examination.

Normal daily requirements for food and fluid are discussed in Chapter 2. Daily fluid requirements may increase substantially at high altitude, in hot weather, or with vomiting, diarrhea, extensive burns, or profuse perspiring. Give fluids in the form of plain water, soup, bouillon, flavored fruit drinks, or electrolyte-containing sport drinks such as Gatorade or Exceed.

Limit the intake of caffeine-containing beverages such as tea, cocoa, and coffee because caffeine is a diuretic and may increase fluid loss through the kidneys, thereby contributing to dehydration. Alcohol should not be drunk for the same reason. When a patient is losing large amounts of fluid through vomiting, diarrhea, or extensive burns, measure or estimate the amount of fluid lost and try to replace the lost fluid volume-for-volume with bouillon, sport drinks, or other electrolyte-containing fluids.

The World Health Organization has recommended a standard electrolyte-replacement solution for diarrheal illness, designed for use in underdeveloped countries where such illnesses are endemic. This solution, called Oralyte, contains 90 milliequivalents (mEq) of sodium, 20 mEq of potassium, 80 mEq of chloride, 30 mEq of bicarbonate, and 111 millimoles of glucose per liter. It is prepared by mixing 3.5 g of table salt, 2.5 g of sodium bicarbonate (baking soda), 1.5 g of potassium chloride (available in many pharmacies), and 20 g of glucose in a liter of clean water just before use. The solution can be flavored to taste with small amounts of powdered lemonade or another flavoring agent.

Packets containing the right proportions of these compounds can be purchased in some parts of the world, or they can be made up beforehand and carried in emergency care kits. Oralyte is better than sport drinks for initial replacement of fluids lost by vomiting and diarrhea because it contains more electrolytes. After the patient improves, sport drinks can be used instead if desired.

In patients with diarrhea, fluid losses sometimes can be reduced by giving drugs that slow the motility of the bowel (see Stomach and Bowel Problems later in this appendix). Patients who are vomiting because of an illness that does not interfere greatly with stomach or bowel function, such as acute mountain sickness, headache, or mild gastroenteritis, may be able to eat and drink if vomiting can be controlled with an antivomiting suppository such as promethazine (Phenergan) or prochlorperazine (Compazine). Side effects of these drugs are similar; they include drowsiness, dizziness, blurred vision, rash, and low blood pressure. Muscle spasms, especially of the neck, occur occasionally, especially with prochlorperazine. These effects can be relieved by the antihistamine diphenhydramine (Benadryl), which is available without prescription (two 25-mg capsules taken immediately by mouth).

Do not give anything, including drugs, by mouth to patients who are vomiting because of a head or abdominal injury, who have altered responsiveness, or who may have surgery within 6 to 8 hours.

Some SAR groups include members who are trained and licensed to give intravenous (IV) fluids, which are very useful in these circumstances. An average daily IV fluid prescription for a patient unable to eat or drink is 2,500 mL of 5% glucose in 0.45% ("half-normal") physiologic saline solution with 20 mEq of potassium chloride added per liter. If the patient is also vomiting or having diarrhea, estimate the additional fluid losses and replace this lost fluid volume with equal amounts of the same solution, or with lactated Ringer's solution, in addition to the daily fluid prescription. In most cases, normal kidneys select what the body needs and excrete the remainder.

Collect and measure the volume of all urine excreted by the patient. If urine output is less than 500 mL (17 ounces) per 24 hours, the patient is probably dehydrated and needs more fluid. Urine is normally light yellow when hydration is adequate, but it may be orange in patients with severe injury or illness or even in healthy persons who have been exercising heavily. Liver disease with jaundice turns urine cola colored; vitamin tablets containing riboflavin (vitamin B_2) turn urine bright yellow.

Liquids are a more urgent requirement than food, because a healthy person can go without eating for many days without permanent damage. Patients who are nauseated and would vomit ordinary amounts of liquid may be able to tolerate frequent sips of small amounts. Those who are able to tolerate solid food should eat a light, bland diet. Water, oatmeal, Cream of Wheat, bland soup, broth, Jell-O, bread, hard candy, and sweet herb tea are usually well tolerated. The patient should be allowed to eat as desired and not be forced to eat.

Rescuers must also make provisions for the patient to urinate or defecate if necessary. A wide-mouth screw-top polyethylene bottle ("pee bottle") with a capacity of 1 pint to 1 quart (500 to 1,000 mL) can be used as a urinal. Search-and-rescue teams can carry lightweight commercially marketed plastic urinals.

Patients can defecate in the supine position if they are placed on carefully arranged clothing, on an Ensolite pad with a hole cut in it, or if positioned over a hole dug in the ground or snow. Always ask patients whether they need to urinate or defecate and allow them to do so before packaging them on a backboard.

Unconscious or severely injured patients may be unable to urinate. Members of SAR groups and expeditions should obtain the special training necessary to insert Foley catheters, which should be included in their emergency care kits. If no catheter is available, nothing can be done except to evacuate the patient with a pee bottle or urinal strategically placed to catch urine that may be voided spontaneously. It is important to prevent the patient's clothing from becoming wet with urine, especially in cold weather.

When caring for an injured or ill patient in the wilderness, adequate pain relief is necessary for humanitarian reasons and has some value in preventing shock. Serious wilderness travelers may wish to have their physicians prescribe pain medicines such as acetaminophen with codeine (Tylenol with codeine), meperidine (Demerol), propoxyphene with acetaminophen (Darvocet-N 100), or tramadol hydrochloride (Ultram), so that small amounts of these drugs can be carried for personal use. Try pain medications at home first on headaches and other painful conditions to ensure that they are effective in relieving pain and do not cause undesirable side effects.

Side effects of acetaminophen with codeine and meperidine are similar and can include lightheadedness, dizziness, sleepiness, shortness of breath, nausea, vomiting, and constipation. Meperidine can also cause sweating and respiratory depression. Propoxyphene can cause dizziness, sleepiness, nausea, and vomiting. Tramadol can cause dizziness, nausea, constipation, headache, and sleepiness.

As with all drugs in emergency care kits, the containers should be labeled with the name of the medicine, the date the prescription was filled, the person's name, the prescribing physician's name, and directions for use. Ask your druggist to add the expiration date of the lot as well.

Leaders of prolonged wilderness trips should consider requiring *each* trip member to carry such drugs since current state and federal regulations do not allow a rescuer to give these drugs to a patient unless the rescuer is appropriately licensed or under physician supervision. However, in general, the patient may *take* such drugs on his or her *own* responsibility and may be assisted if necessary. No one should take a drug to which he or she is known to be allergic.

For extended wilderness trips and expeditions, injectable pain medication is useful—especially for patients who cannot swallow pills—but must be administered by an individual who is trained and authorized to inject it. Several drug manufacturers market injectable codeine, meperidine, and morphine in convenient, prefilled, single-dose containers. These pain medications, however, should *not* be given to patients with head injuries or high altitude cerebral edema.

Rescuers must not rely on pain medication to the extent that they neglect traditional emergency care procedures for reducing pain, such as aligning and splinting fractures or applying cold packs to sprains.

Adhere to the usual habits of cleanliness and sanitation as closely as possible in the wilderness. Carry biodegradable soap and use it to wash your hands after urination or a bowel movement, before cooking and eating, and before dressing open wounds. Cover food to protect it from flies. Also be sure to carry and put on rubber gloves before handling vomitus, feces, and other secretions of a patient. If soap is unavailable, wash your hands in plain water or snow.

Defecate *downhill* and at least 200' from camp, water sources, or snow to be melted for water. Bury feces and burn used toilet paper. Do not camp closer than 100' from a water source such as a lake, stream, or spring.

Providing the patient with psychological support (see Chapter 16) is extremely important to reinforce faith and the will to live, and to encourage optimism, patience, and cooperation. Apprise the patient of emergency care procedures as you go along, but refrain from discussing troubling aspects of emergency care or evacuation within the patient's hearing range. Rescuers should remain calm, unhurried, and deliberate, and avoid the appearance of indecision, pessimism, fear, or panic. You can discuss the general situation with the patient, but remain positive. Warn the patient in advance if you are going to perform procedures that might be unpleasant or painful.

Encourage a patient with a minor injury or illness to *self-evacuate*, but make sure at least one other party member accompanies him or her. When evacuating a patient with a severe injury or illness, the party must decide whether to use their resources alone or send for help. This will depend on the weather; party size; training; available equipment; distance and type of terrain involved; the type of injury or illness and the patient's condition; and the availability of local SAR groups, helicopters, and other assistance. Generally speaking, unless the weather is excellent, the party is strong and well-equipped, the route is short and easy, and the patient is comfortable and stable, the best course of action is to make a comfortable camp and send for help. Send the two strongest party members, and encourage any other members who are demoralized or otherwise a liability to go as well. Send along a written note that includes each patient's name, gender, age, type of injury or illness, current condition, and the emergency care being given. Also describe the party's resources, the location in detail (map coordinates are preferred), the names, addresses, and telephone numbers of relatives to notify, and any other pertinent information.

If the party is so small that it will be necessary to leave a patient alone in order to reach help, leave an adequate supply of food, fuel, and water within the patient's reach and assure him or her that you will return with help.

If evacuation is possible, stabilize the patient before he or she is moved. "Stabilizing the patient" means that you control bleeding, clean and bandage all wounds, stabilize fractures, and help the patient take care of any urgent physical needs, such as urination and defecation. Pain should be controlled, by medication if appropriate. The patient's body temperature should be stable and the attendants should be fed, rested, and ready to go.

The Wilderness Medical Society in its most recent (2001) Practice Guidelines recommends that in any person with one or more of the following conditions, further travel be postponed and/or preparations for evacuation be made:

1. Sustained or progressive physiologic deterioration as indicated by orthostatic dizziness (dizziness upon standing up), syncope (fainting), tachycardia or bradycardia (an abnormally slow or fast heart rate), dyspnea (labored breathing), altered mental status, progressive weakness,

intractable vomiting and/or diarrhea, an inability to tolerate oral fluids, or the return of loss of responsiveness following a head injury. In other words, if patients are not improving, they must get out!

2. Debilitating pain

3. Inability to sustain travel at a reasonable pace due to a medical problem

4. Passage of blood by mouth or by rectum, if not from an obviously minor source

5. Signs and symptoms of serious high altitude illness

6. Infections that progress despite appropriate treatment

7. Chest pain that is not clearly musculoskeletal in origin

8. Development of a dysfunctional psychological status that impairs the safety of the person or the group

Travel may continue if it is toward definitive care in the case of items 3, 4, and 8, or when descending in the case of serious high-altitude illness (item 5).

Wilderness Injuries

Wilderness injury management follows the same basic principles as management of any injury, except for certain modifications to avoid infection, impaired circulation, or other complications that can arise during a lengthy evacuation.

In the case of a fracture or dislocation, check circulation, motion, and sensation (CMS) during assessment, before and after alignment and splinting, and at regular intervals thereafter.

It is particularly important to monitor circulation of an injured extremity to detect changes caused by swelling and tight splinting, because reduced circulation increases the risk of gangrene and, in cold weather, frostbite. Maintain the injured patient's temperature at a normal level.

Lacerations and Other Open Wounds

In the wilderness, improperly treated open wounds can partially immobilize a patient because of pain, stiffness, swelling, and infection, making self-evacuation difficult. Pay particular attention to high-risk wounds, defined as those more likely to become seriously infected, such as:

- Human or animal bites
- Open fractures or dislocations
- Wounds with exposed ligaments or tendons
- Large and/or ragged wounds
- Wounds containing considerable dirt and/or devitalized tissue

After bleeding is controlled, all open wounds should be cleaned to prevent infection (as outlined in Chapter 8). In addition, unless the patient is allergic to iodine, disinfect high-risk wounds by pouring a 1% solution of povidone-iodine (Betadine) directly onto the wound. The povidone-iodine solution can be prepared on the spot by adding nine parts of clean water to one part of the standard 10% stock solution. Then, cover the wound with a sterile dressing moistened with 1% povidone-iodine solution, stabilize it, and transport the patient to medical care. Antibiotics are recommended to prevent infection in high-risk wounds (see Antibiotics later in this appendix).

An impaled object should be cut to a manageable size, if possible. If you can remove it easily, consider doing so if the object will otherwise interfere with patient packaging and transport.

Small wounds can be closed with butterfly bandages or sterile tape (SteriStrips), but large wounds should be bandaged open, except in cold weather when they should be taped closed to prevent cold injury. A new type of skin adhesive, octylcyanoacrylate (Dermabond) is useful for closing small wounds in the wilderness that otherwise would require suturing. It is not generally available, but you may be able to obtain it through your local hospital with the help of your physician. If you plan to carry it in your aid kit, seek instructions for use from a physician.

If at all possible, avoid wrapping tape completely around an extremity, since the tape may cause a tourniquet-like effect if the extremity swells. Abrasions heal faster if they can be kept moist. They should be cleaned with mild soap and clean water and covered with Saran Wrap or a special dressing such as Opsite.

Dressings can be improvised from clean material such as pillowcases, sheets, towels, underclothing, shirts, and sanitary napkins. Clean toilet paper and paper tissues are absorbent and can be used if nothing better is available. You can improvise bandages from pack straps, belts, strips torn from clothing, cord, or nylon webbing. Kerchiefs and bandannas can be used as cravats and triangular bandages. Rolled T-shirts can also be used as cravats, and clean socks suffice as hand or foot bandages. You can make occlusive dressings by placing plastic sandwich or garbage bags over sterile compresses.

The immunization status of a patient with an open wound will determine whether tetanus prophylaxis should be considered as soon as medical help is reached.

Fractures

The most important emergency care for any fracture is stabilization by splinting. Because of the need to "pack light," few wilderness travelers are able to carry a large variety of premade splints, although air splints and malleable metal splints, such as the SAM splint, are lightweight and easy to carry, especially by large parties and SAR groups.

Splints must usually be improvised from natural materials, ski poles, ice axes, ice hammers, and parts of packs such as hip pads and shoulder straps. Below

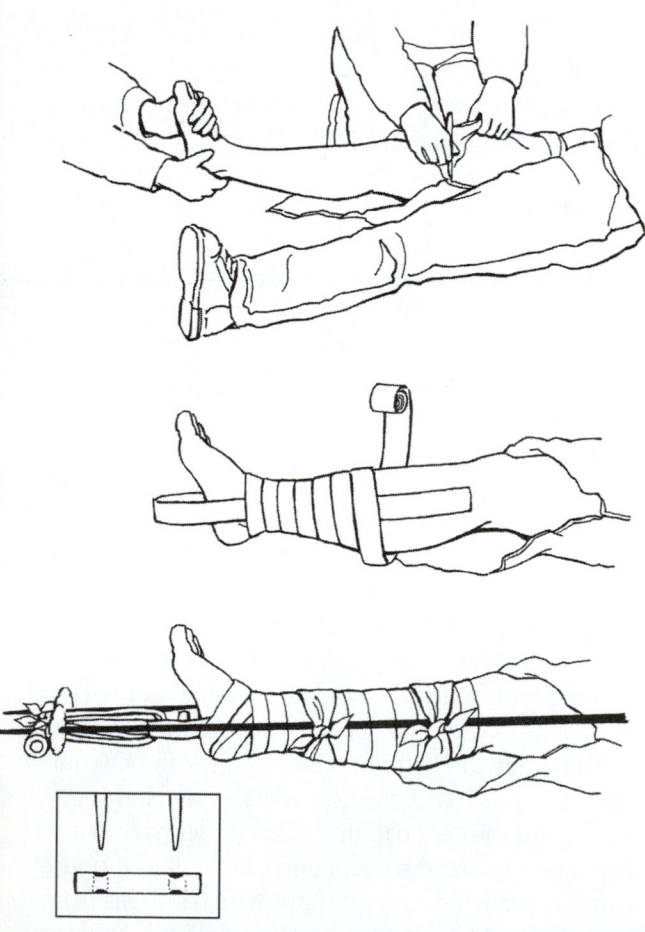

Figure D-1 Modified traction splinting for a fractured femur. (Detail box shows spreader made from a section of a ski pole, with two holes drilled in it.)

timberline, you can cut tree branches and small trees to use as splinting materials. Short fixation splints can be improvised from six or more small, straight branches laid side-by-side, cross-braced with two or more short branches, and wrapped with duct tape.

A sling can be improvised by pinning the shirt sleeve to the shirt with a large safety pin ("blanket pin"), or by pulling the tail of a T-shirt up over the forearm and pinning it to the shirt breast. You can make an all-purpose forearm and hand splint from two pairs of socks: ask the patient to hold one rolled sock in the palm of his or her hand and then pull two to three socks up over the hand and wrist like a mitten. Uninjured body parts can serve as splints, ie, a fractured upper arm can be splinted against the chest wall with a sling and swathe, and a fractured hip can be splinted by tying both lower extremities together.

In addition to receiving the care for a high-risk wound, a patient with an open fracture should take antibiotics (see Antibiotics later in this appendix).

The most significant modification of traditional splinting in the wilderness is that involving the emergency care of a fractured femur. The standard emergency care for a fracture of the middle half to three fifths of the femur is traction splinting, but traction applied to a boot for more than an hour can cause loss of the dorsalis pedis pulse, pain, and pressure damage to the ankle tissues. Even when a padded traction harness is used, traction applied to a bare foot or foot with a stocking can cause pain and injury if applied for more than a few hours.

Therefore, unless evacuation time will be short, avoid putting pressure on the ankle entirely by using the following method (◄ **Figure D-1**): remove the patient's boot and sock(s), roll up the pant leg or open it with a seam ripper, and apply a strip of 2"-wide adhesive tape from just below the knee down one side of the leg, under the sole of the foot, and then up the other side of the leg so that a stirrup is formed. Next, wrap the leg from toes to knee with an elastic bandage. Make sure that the bandage is firm but not too tight and that the color and temperature of the toes remain normal. Insert a piece of wood into the loop of the stirrup to serve as a spreader to keep pressure off the sides of the ankle. Then apply a traction type of splint (described in Chapter 24), which can be an improvised canoe paddle-, single ski-, or ski pole-traction splint or a commercial splint such as the Hare, Sager, or Kendrick traction device. The stirrup prevents you from replacing the sock on the foot, so keep the patient's foot warm by wrapping it with spare clothing. Unwrap the clothing at intervals to inspect the toes for color, warmth, sensation, and motion.

Dislocations

In line with accepted emergency care, standard teaching protocol in this text is to treat a dislocation by splinting it in the position found without attempting to straighten or align it unless circulation or nerve supply is impaired.

However, a dislocation is usually more painful than a fracture and causes considerable pressure on joint cartilage and other structures, resulting in additional injury.

When a dislocation is splinted in the position found, ligaments, tendons, and nerves are stretched more and circulation is more often impaired than when a fracture is splinted this way. Therefore, when medical help is more than a few hours away, there is considerable justification for attempting to align a dislocation to restore a normal anatomic position.

Alignment usually provides marked pain relief, eases evacuation, and may prevent future disability. This type of alignment is called *relocation* of the dislocation.

The process of relocation should be slow and steady, with no quick jerks. If one attempt is unsuccessful or causes severe pain, abandon further attempts at relocation and splint the dislocation in the most comfortable position.

Relocation works best if it can be done *immediately* after the dislocation, before muscles go into spasm, before the injured part stiffens, and while it is still numb. Otherwise, you should encourage the patient to take a dose of pain medication and delay the relocation until the medication has time to work—about 45 minutes to an hour.

For the following techniques, the author is indebted to Joseph Serra, MD, whose pioneering work in this area has greatly improved the management of wilderness injuries.

Shoulder Dislocations

In the wilderness, the shoulder is the most commonly dislocated joint, and the injury is usually an anterior dislocation. The mechanism is a force applied with the shoulder in abduction and external rotation, such as a high brace while kayaking, a slip while the arm is over the head with the hand wedged in a crack, or a fall on an externally rotated, outstretched hand. A dislocation can also result from a hard fall with a direct blow to the shoulder, but this is often complicated by a *fracture* of the upper end of the humerus. Therefore,

the following descriptions of techniques for relocating an anterior shoulder dislocation do *not* apply to a dislocation caused by a direct blow to the shoulder.

Before and after any attempt at alignment or relocation, check and document CMS—especially with regard to the axillary nerve. If, at any point during relocation, CMS deteriorates, stop and splint the dislocation in the position found.

Several methods are available for relocating an uncomplicated shoulder dislocation. In every case, follow the CMS check by carefully putting several of your fingers into the patient's axilla (armpit). You can usually palpate the head of the humerus, which feels like a ball, in the anterior part of the axilla. Then, move the extremity slightly. A grating sound or feeling means a fracture is also present.

If there is any possibility of a fracture, stop at this point and splint the shoulder as described in Chapter 24. Fortunately, fracture-dislocations of the shoulder are rare in young, healthy persons unless strong forces are involved and/or the dislocation is caused by a direct fall on the shoulder.

An excellent, safe method for relocating a dislocated shoulder is to have the patient lie prone on an elevated platform such as a large, flat rock or log that is high enough to allow the injured extremity to hang free. Tie a 10-lb weight to the patient's wrist (▼ **Figure D-2**). The gradual pull will usually relocate the shoulder within 1 to 1½ hours.

If an elevated platform is unavailable or the method is unsafe due to severe weather conditions, try the following technique (▶ **Figure D-3A**). Have the patient sit on the ground while you kneel next to him or her, facing the patient's injured side. An assistant should sit behind the patient opposite you and anchor the patient

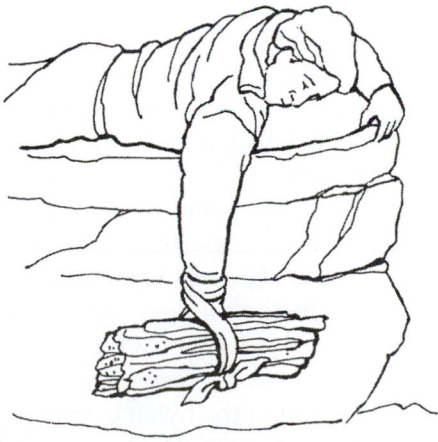

Figure D-2   Using gravity to relocate a dislocated shoulder.

Figure D-3   Using two rescuers to relocate a dislocated shoulder.

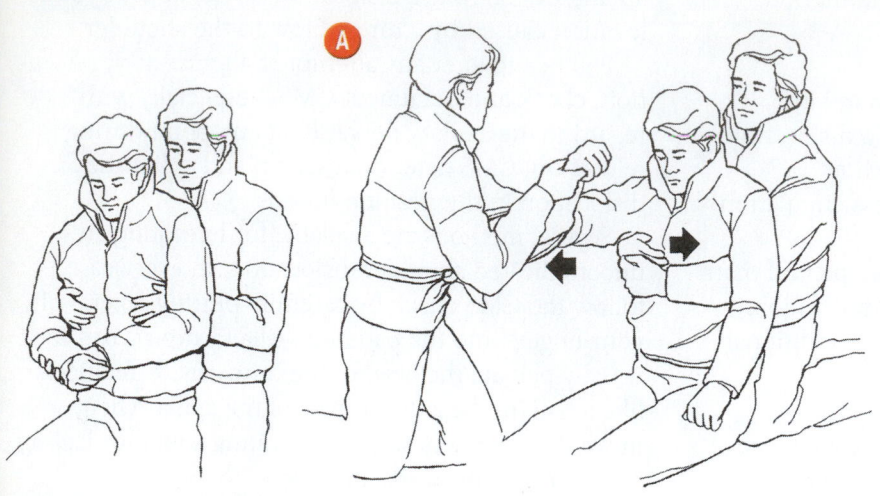

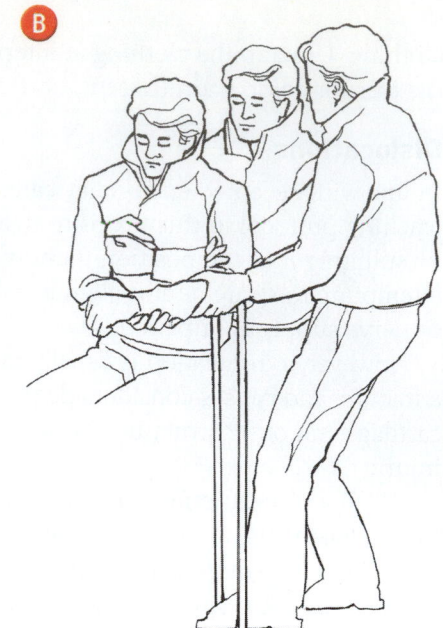

by wrapping both arms or a sling around the patient's chest. You then tie two cravats *securely* together with square knots to make a large loop, slip the loop over your head, and work it down around your waist. The loop should be large enough so that you can pull it out in front of your waist about 8″ to 12″.

Next, grasp the patient's injured upper extremity, flex the elbow to a right angle with the forearm pointing upward, slip the free end of the loop over the patient's hand, and work it down just distal to the bend of the elbow.

Then, keeping the patient's forearm bent with both hands, slowly lean backward while your assistant applies countertraction in the opposite direction. The shoulder should slip back into place, frequently with an audible pop. The patient often sighs with relief as the pain disappears.

A variation of this technique (▲ **Figure D-3B**) can be performed in a narrow space such as on a ledge, or in a canoe or other watercraft. Tie a loop using about 5′ of 1″ nylon webbing. The patient should be seated with the arm on the injured side hanging straight down and the elbow bent to a right angle so that the forearm is horizontal.

If possible, have an assistant kneel or sit behind the patient with his or her arms wrapped around the patient's chest below the armpits for stabilization. Stand next to the patient's injured side. Then slip the upper part of the nylon loop over the patient's forearm and work it back to just distal to the elbow. Place one foot in the lower part of the nylon loop and, while holding the patient's forearm firmly and keeping the

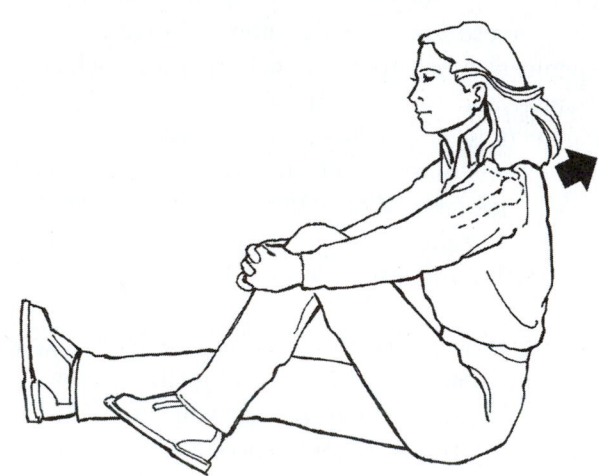

Figure D-4   Self-relocation of a dislocated shoulder.

patient's elbow bent, step down firmly on the loop, thus putting downward pressure on the humerus and allowing its head to slip back into the shoulder joint. It helps to slightly rotate the elbow externally while you are applying the downward pressure.

If you happen to dislocate your shoulder and no help is available, self-relocation is sometimes successful if done immediately. It is easier if the shoulder has been dislocated before. The method is as follows: Sit on the ground and bend the knee on the side of the dislocated shoulder (▲ **Figure D-4**). Grasp the knee with both hands, interlocking your fingers firmly. Shift your hands medially so that the extremity on the injured side is tight and the normal one lax, concentrating the force on

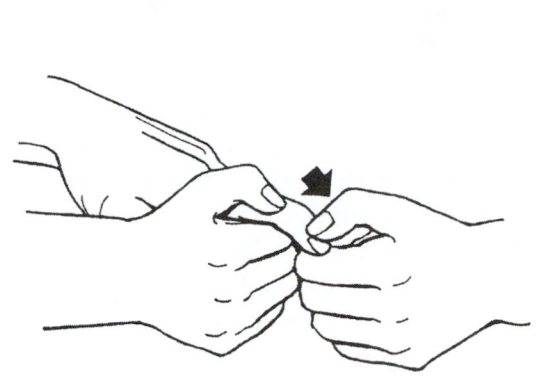

Figure D-5   Relocating a dislocated finger.

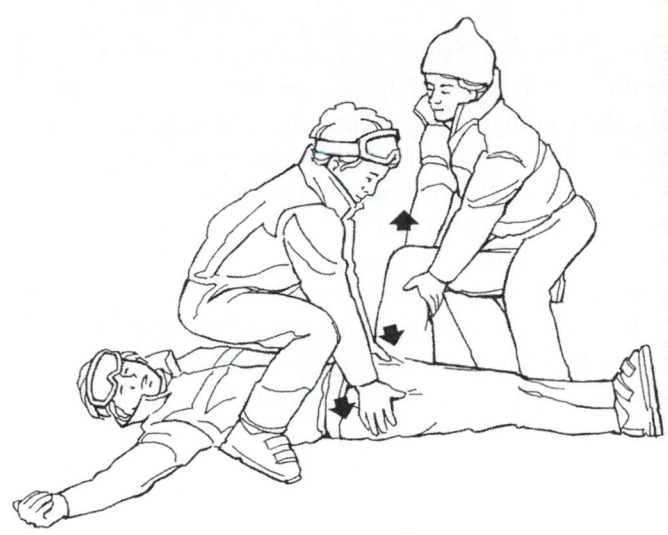

Figure D-6   Relocating a dislocated hip.

the injured side. Slowly lean back and straighten your hip and the shoulder will slip back into place.

After relocation, an injured upper extremity should be stabilized with a sling and swathe until medical help is obtained, or for at least 1 week.

Elbow Dislocations

When an elbow is dislocated, the forearm is usually forced backward on the upper arm, producing a marked deformity, in which the point of the elbow is much farther back than it should be and a large notch is visible above the olecranon process.

When seen from the front, the forearm on the involved side appears shorter than the opposite, normal forearm. If this characteristic is not evident, the patient probably has a fracture above the elbow rather than a dislocated elbow. When seen from the side, the dimension of the elbow from front to back is greater than normal and there is a bulge in front of the elbow. The circulation and nerve supply of the forearm and hand are frequently compromised. Crepitus should be absent; if present, a fracture is likely.

To relocate a dislocated elbow, pull steadily on the forearm with the elbow partly flexed while an assistant holds the upper arm tightly. The normal shape of the elbow should be restored and the notch above the olecranon process should disappear. Stabilize the relocated elbow as described in Chapter 25.

Finger Dislocations

To relocate a dislocated finger, firmly hold the part of the patient's finger proximal to the dislocation. With the other hand, partly flex the finger distal to the disloca-

tion, while pulling on it and pushing the base of the dislocated part back into position (◄ **Figure D-5**). Splint the relocated finger using an all-purpose forearm and hand splint (improvised as necessary). If the patient requires some mobility of the hand to self-evacuate, "buddy-tape" the injured finger to an adjacent, uninjured finger with a gauze pad placed between the two fingers.

Hip Dislocations

Attempting to relocate a dislocated hip in the field is justifiable because a prolonged hip dislocation interrupts the blood supply to the head of the femur, eventually causing its death and making a total hip replacement operation likely.

The most common type of hip dislocation is a posterior dislocation. The lower extremity is characteristically bent at the hip, rotated inward, and adducted. Attempts to move the hip are very painful.

The relocation technique (▲ **Figure D-6**) is as follows: have an assistant straddle the patient, facing the patient's feet, and place one hand on each side of the front of the pelvis to provide countertraction. Straddle the leg on the patient's injured side, holding it tightly between your legs, and gently bend the patient's knee to 90°. Bend your own knees slightly and grasp the back of the patient's leg tightly just below the knee with your interlocked hands. Next, exert steady traction in an upward direction by straightening your knees while the assistant leans hard on the patient's pelvis.

After relocation, put padding between the knees and ankles, tie the lower extremities together, and transport the patient on a long backboard, improvised if necessary.

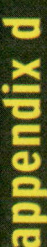

appendix d

Patella Dislocations

In the case of a patella dislocation, ask the patient to flex the hip so the thigh is at a right angle to the trunk, which relaxes the quadriceps muscle on the front of the thigh. Then gently straighten the knee while pushing the patella back toward its normal location at the front of the knee joint. The extremity should then be splinted in extension.

If the patient must self-evacuate, a "walking splint" can be fashioned with a short Ensolite or Therm-A-Rest pad wrapped around the extremity to keep the knee straight. The patient should use a cane improvised from a ski pole, ice ax, or stick.

Knee Dislocations

Because of the knee's strong ligamentous and muscular attachments, its dislocation requires great force. Most of the major ligaments of the knee must be torn for the joint to dislocate.

A dislocated knee is usually unstable, and the circulation and nerve supply are usually impaired. Amputation will likely result if the dislocation cannot be reduced within 6 to 8 hours. Therefore, there is considerable reason to attempt relocation in a wilderness setting.

Relocation consists of simple axial traction to realign the joint so that the leg and foot are in the most normal position possible and the pulses in the foot are the strongest.

Afterward, immobilize the extremity in a long-leg type of fixation splint, being sure to monitor and document CMS at 15-minute intervals. If any functions become compromised, remove the splint and realign the injury in the position that gives the strongest pulses in the foot.

Ankle Dislocations

An ankle dislocation is almost always a fracture-dislocation, so impairment of the circulation and nerve supply are a danger.

Wilderness emergency care consists of relocating the ankle with simple axial traction to return the foot to a normal position with strong pulses (▼ Figure D-7) and stabilizing the extremity with a fixation splint.

Monitor and document CMS functions at 15-minute intervals after relocation. If any functions become compromised, remove the splint and realign the injury in the position that gives the strongest pulses in the foot.

Sprains

The standard assessment and emergency care for an ankle sprain is addressed in Chapter 25. In wilderness conditions, a patient with an ankle sprain may have to self-evacuate. A sturdy hiking, mountaineering, or telemark boot alone may provide the necessary support, but an adhesive-tape boot (▼ Figure D-8) is usually needed to stabilize the sprain enough to allow locomotion. Remove the patient's boot and sock(s) and consider shaving the lower leg and foot before applying the tape.

Hold the patient's foot at a right angle to the leg and apply overlapping vertical and horizontal strips of tape that are 1″ wide and 20″ to 30″ long. Leave no skin showing between strips. Run vertical strips from the

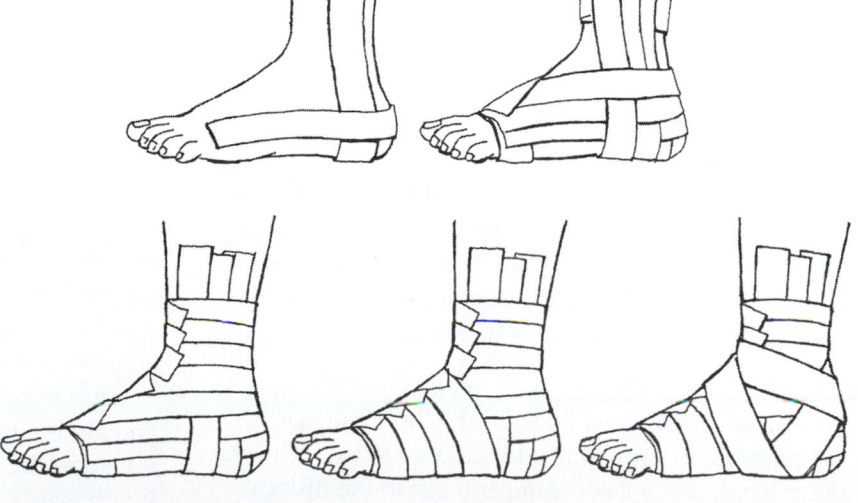

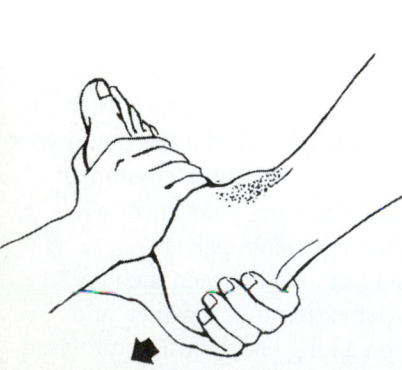

Figure D-7   Relocating a dislocated ankle.

Figure D-8   An adhesive-tape boot can support a sprained ankle.

lower leg on the *uninjured* side across the sole of the foot and up the opposite side of the ankle; run horizontal strips from the top of the foot around the back of the heel to the other side of the top of the foot.

Alternate application of these vertical and horizontal strips. Avoid ring-like strips extending all the way around the ankle or foot at the same level because, if swelling occurs, they may act as tourniquets.

Continue taping until most of the ankle, lower leg, and posterior two thirds of the foot are covered. Conclude with a figure-of-8 wrap around the ankle, heel, and arch to stabilize the arch and provide additional heel stabilization. Then replace the patient's sock and boot on the foot. Usually the patient will need one less sock on the injured foot because of the thickness of the tape.

Note: It is less painful to remove the tape if it is peeled off *from top to bottom.*

Injuries to the Head, Spine, Chest, Abdomen, and Pelvis; Multiple Injuries

Rockfall accidents, falls while climbing, and high-speed skiing and snowboarding accidents can cause multiple injuries similar to those seen in motor vehicle accidents. Serious head, neck, back, chest, abdominal, pelvic, and extremity injuries can occur singly or in various combinations, sorely taxing the emergency care skills of rescuers. The immediate care of these injuries is described in the assessment chapter and in the chapters on specific injuries. Give the patient oxygen, if available, and take steps to keep the airway open even though this may be difficult if there are facial injuries. In the unresponsive patient without a gag reflex, insert an oropharyngeal airway if available. Nasopharyngeal airways also can be used in appropriate circumstances.

It is useful to have the ability to give intravenous fluids, to intubate or perform a cricothyroidotomy when the upper airway cannot be opened by usual measures, and to insert a needle or tube into the chest for a tension pneumothorax. However, these techniques go beyond the skill levels appropriate to this textbook since they require special training, licensing, and equipment.

Open Abdominal Wound

A loop of bowel protruding through an open abdominal wound can be successfully replaced if discovered and treated *immediately.* Replace the loop as aseptically as possible (ie, avoid getting dirt and germs on it) and tape the wound shut. If much time has elapsed, however, the loop will swell and be impossible to replace. In this case, it should be covered with a clean—preferably sterile—cloth moistened with warm physiologic saline or clean water with $^1/_2$ teaspoon of table salt added per quart, preferably disinfected or brought to a boil and then cooled (see Figure 19-13).

Keep the dressing moist during evacuation, using repeated applications of one of the above solutions warmed to body temperature.

Spine Injury

According to standard emergency care protocols, a patient with a suspicious mechanism of injury must be immobilized on a long backboard (see Chapter 26), even if the patient has no signs or symptoms of spine or spinal cord injury.

Because of the difficulty of obtaining or improvising a backboard and transporting a boarded patient, many authorities feel that in wilderness conditions, a patient with a normal mental status and *no* signs or symptoms of spine or spinal cord injury need not be boarded on the basis of mechanism of injury alone. In this case, the patient *must* have:

- full range of spinal motion,
- normal motor and sensory function,
- no spine pain, tenderness, or deformity,
- no distracting painful injuries,
- no alcohol or sedative drug consumption.

In addition, enough time should have elapsed since the accident to allow any initial numbness to disappear. Since it is difficult to improvise a serviceable long backboard, safe evacuation of a patient with a neck or back injury is almost impossible if you have to rely solely upon the resources of a small, poorly equipped party. In almost every case, it is preferable to camp on the spot and send for help rather than try to evacuate a seriously injured patient who is partly immobilized with substandard equipment.

If the patient *must* be moved because of incoming bad weather or a hazardous location, a backboard can be improvised as described in Chapter 27. At times, a vest-type device can be improvised using the patient's packframe and adding groin straps.

Backcountry rescue groups usually use a whole-body vacuum splint or the combination of a vest-type device, such as the Kendrick Extrication Device or Oregon Spine Splint II, and a backboard such as the Ferno-Washington or SKED.

Shock

In the wilderness, shock is most often caused by one of the following conditions:

- Loss of whole blood from the circulation because of
  1. severe or uncontrolled external bleeding
  2. internal bleeding from a fractured femur, fractured pelvis, or multiple injuries
  3. internal bleeding from a bleeding ulcer or ruptured ectopic pregnancy
- Loss of the fluid part of the blood because of:
  1. severe vomiting or diarrhea
  2. extensive burns
- Heart attack with cardiogenic shock
- Spinal cord injury with neurogenic shock

There is no effective field emergency care for any of these conditions except for controlling bleeding and trying to replace fluids lost by vomiting or diarrhea. Any care to be given is designed to buy time until the patient can reach a hospital. When a patient has a condition commonly known to cause shock, anticipate shock and make arrangements to contact help or evacuate the patient as soon as possible, *before* shock actually develops.

In the hospital, a patient in shock is initially treated by replenishing the blood volume with whole blood, plasma, and intravenous fluids. Although it is rarely possible or practical to transfuse whole blood in the field, rescue groups can carry intravenous fluids as long as they have members who are trained and licensed to administer them. Such groups should use physician input to develop protocols for managing shock in patients.

Lactated Ringer's solution and physiologic saline are the best standard intravenous preparations to carry for treating shock.

In cold weather, intravenous preparations must be protected from freezing. Rescuers often accomplish this by carrying the bags of fluid inside clothing against the body. Portable intravenous fluid warmers are also available.

Minor Problems

Although certainly not threatening to life or limb, minor injuries can mar an otherwise rewarding wilderness excursion. Early recognition and management can keep minor problems from turning into bigger ones.

Blisters

Blisters are annoying injuries produced when a sock wrinkle or ill-fitting boot rubs repeatedly against the skin. Blisters are most common on the heels, toes, and soles of the feet.

The best treatment is prevention. Always wear at least two pairs of socks—preferably a thin inner pair made of a slick material such as polypropylene or silk next to the skin, plus one or two outer pairs of heavy wool—so that friction tends to occur between sock layers rather than between the sock and your skin. Cut your toenails before a trip and wear properly broken-in boots that are correctly fitted for length so that the toes will not jam against the tip of the boot during downhill travel.

If a sore spot develops, call for a halt, immediately remove the boot and socks, and look for a reddened area of skin. Overlay this area with protective material such as Spenco Adhesive Knit, a piece of moleskin, or four layers of 2"-wide adhesive tape. In the absence of these materials, duct tape has been used successfully. Replace the socks, making sure they are not creased or wrinkled, and lace the boot snugly enough to prevent the foot, and especially the heel, from moving around inside it.

If a blister has already developed (and you discover it before it has already broken), protect it by overlaying it with several layers of tape. Cut holes slightly larger than the blister in the bottom layers ▼ **Figure D-9**. Clean and dress a broken blister as you would any other open wound.

Occasionally, a blister is so painful or awkwardly located that it has to be drained. First, wash your hands with soap and water, then wash the skin with an antiseptic solution. Sterilize a needle over a flame, allow it to cool, and insert it under the skin about 1/4" from the edge of the blister. Push it up into the blister,

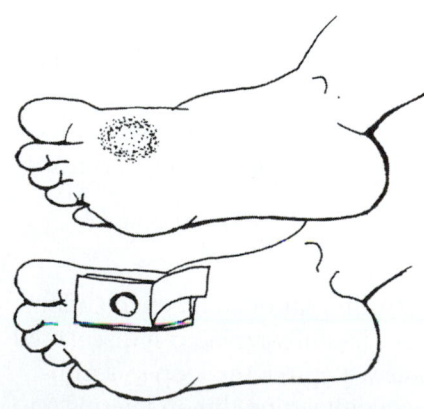

Figure D-9 Protecting a blister with tape.

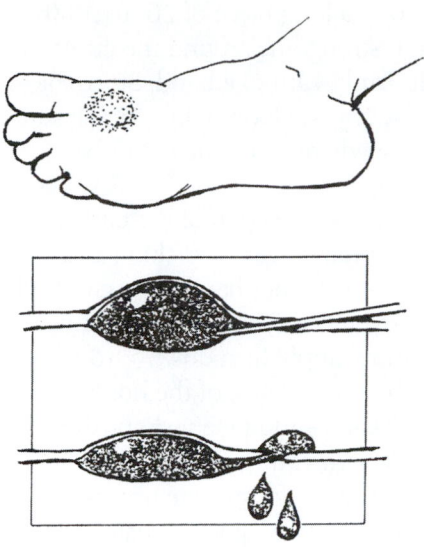

Figure D-10 Draining a blister.

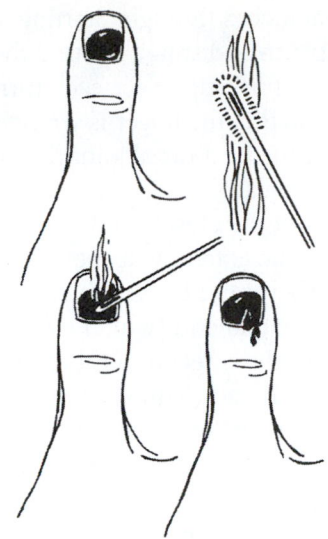

Figure D-11 Draining a subungual hematoma.

and withdraw it while pressing on the blister
(▲ **Figure D-10**). Bandage the drained blister.

Subungual Hematoma

Subungual hematoma, or bleeding under the nail, most often occurs when a hard object such as a hammer or rock strikes a fingertip or toetip with enough force to break blood vessels underneath the nail. Pressure from the bleeding causes severe, throbbing pain, and assessment reveals a large, tender, semilunar, reddish-purple hematoma under the nail. The pain can be relieved by draining the hematoma.

Wash the fingertip or toetip with soap and water, then heat a piece of thin, rigid wire (eg, a straightened paper clip or the blunt end of a needle from a sewing kit) on a stove or over a candle flame (a match flame is not hot enough) until it is red-hot. Next, press the red-hot end firmly into the nail at the center of the hematoma and allow it to burn through the nail
(▶ **Figure D-11**). Maintain close control so that the hot object does not penetrate too far.

A "pop" and sudden "give" means that the object is through the nail. When the object is withdrawn, it is usually followed by a gush of blood and the pain is relieved. Bandage the nail with a small commercial bandage strip.

Jewelry Removal

Immediately remove all jewelry from an injured upper extremity. If a ring is not quickly removed and the finger swells, the ring will act like a tourniquet, reducing circulation in the finger. Fortunately, the fol-

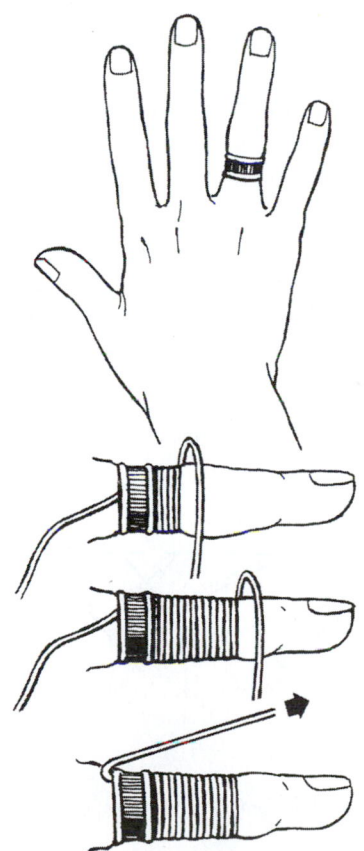

Figure D-12 Removing a ring from a swollen finger.

lowing technique is simple, almost always works, and spares a valuable ring (▲ **Figure D-12**).

You will need a small spool of strong thread or dental floss. First, soap the finger well. Work the loose end of the thread or floss under the ring in a proximal direction and pull several inches through. Starting just distal to the ring, wind the thread snugly around the finger, working toward the fingertip. Place each turn next to the previous one so that the finger is wrapped solidly from the ring over the next distal joint down to the midpoint of the next phalanx.

Note that the pressure of the closely laid thread reduces the swelling to some extent. Cut the thread at the spool end, leaving several inches of loose thread. Then, pull the proximal end (which you worked under the ring) in the direction of the fingertip. This will cause the thread to unwind off the finger, pulling the ring over the joint and off the finger in the process. If this doesn't work, and if the ring is starting to act as a tourniquet, you may be able to saw the ring off with the file from a Swiss Army knife or cut the ring with a pair of wire cutters.

Fishhook Removal

There are two techniques for removing a fishhook embedded in the skin. If the barb is already through the skin or just under the skin where it can easily be pushed through, cut it off with a wire cutter or side-cutter pliers and back the hook out of the hole (▼ Figure D-13).

The second method consists of disengaging the barb of the hook from the tissues so that it can be directly backed out of the hole (▼ Figure D-14). If the hook has more than one barb, cut off the barbs that are not

buried in the skin. Loop a long piece of 20- to 30-lb test line or other thin, strong line around the curve of the hook and grip it firmly with one hand. Since the hook will be pulled out by the loop of line, make sure that no one is standing where he or she might be struck by the hook.

Next, determine the exact location of the barb and the direction of penetration by gently rocking and rotating the hook with your other hand, trying to find the position of least resistance. Then, while holding the hook in this position, apply firm downward pressure with your thumb on the shank of the hook (directly over the barb) and simultaneously push up on the eye of the hook with your index finger. This disengages the barb of the hook from the tissues. While maintaining this pressure, quickly snatch the hook out by pulling on the line at a slightly upward angle with the first hand.

If the eye and shank parts of the hook have broken off, you may be able to remove the hook with the same technique but with a pair of pliers instead of a loop of line.

Finally, clean the wound with germicidal soap. Afterwards, the patient should consider getting tetanus prophylaxis, depending on immune status. If signs of infection develop, the patient should see a physician.

This technique is unsuitable when a hook is embedded in an area of the body where it is difficult to apply strong downward pressure on the shank,

Figure D-13   Removing a fishhook with a wire cutter.

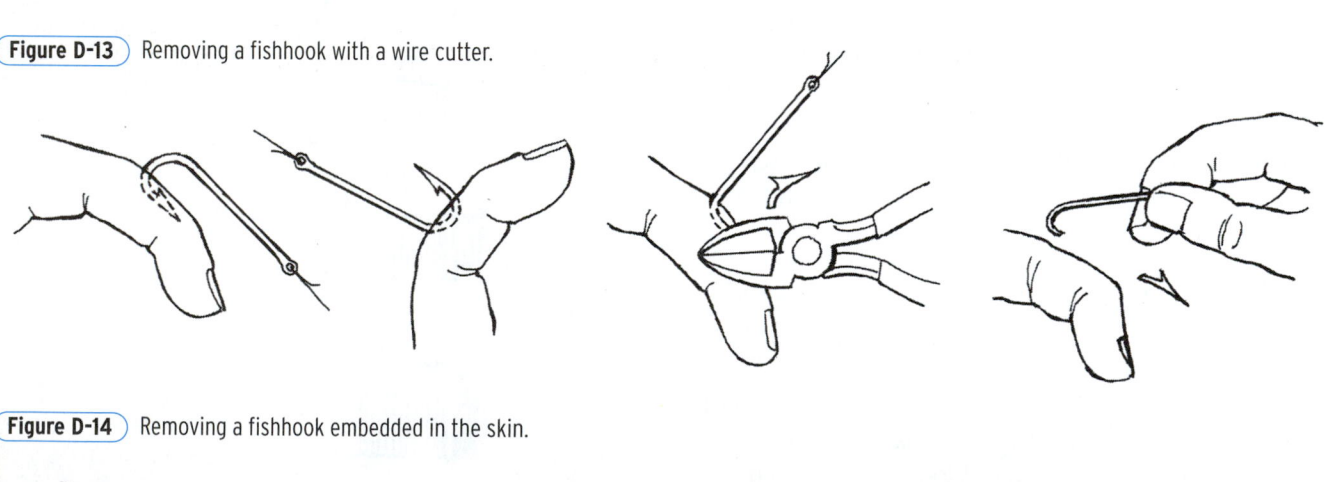

Figure D-14   Removing a fishhook embedded in the skin.

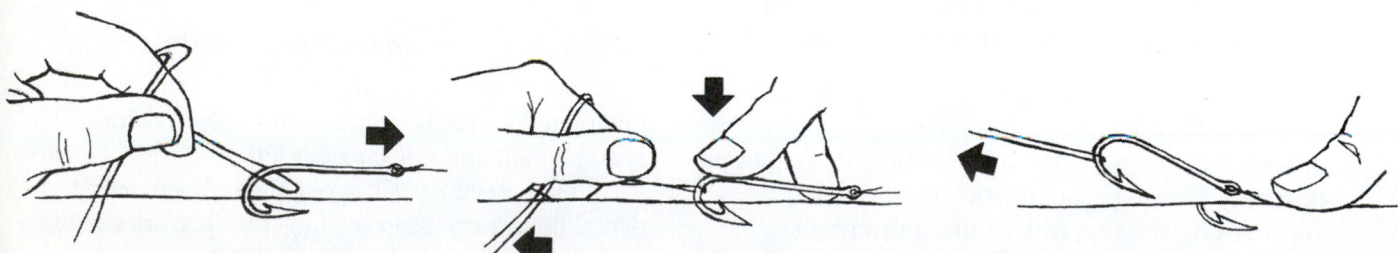

eg, the sides of the neck, earlobes, and around the eyes. A hook cannot be removed by this method when the barb has already come through the skin. If the hook is in an eyeball, cut off the line at the base of the hook, stabilize and bandage the eye, and take the patient to an emergency department ophthalmologist as soon as possible.

Skin Cracks

Small, painful skin cracks are annoyances that mainly affect the fingertips. Common in winter and in dry climates, skin cracks can be prevented to some extent by liberal use of hand cream and by avoiding frequent hand washings. Eating moderate amounts of fat plus a serving of Jell-O several times a week may help prevent skin cracks.

Before you go to bed, apply a dab of thick greasy ointment (such as Vaseline or Bag Balm) to the crack, cover it with a Band-Aid then secure this with several turns of breathable plastic tape around the finger.

In some cases, you can squeeze the crack shut and apply a small amount of Super Glue or Dermabond special skin adhesive to keep it sealed. Both types of glue are waterproof and protect the skin while the skin heals underneath, but they usually have to be reapplied at least once a day. Any residual glue will eventually fall off as the surface area of healing skin is shed normally.

Ingrown Toenail

Improper toenail-cutting techniques and ill-fitting footwear occasionally cause a nail to grow into the soft tissues of the side of the toe. The nail of the great toe is most commonly involved.

In serious cases, especially when the area around the nail edge becomes infected, a physician should be consulted. Minor cases can be treated by using a thin rigid object such as the blunt end of a needle to tease a small wad of cotton under the edge of the nail, thus elevating the nail edge out of the irritated toe tissues. Monitor the cotton and replace it if it works loose.

As the nail grows, its tip and edge will grow past the tissues rather than into them, and after a few weeks the cotton can be removed. Until then, avoid putting pressure on the nail by wearing thinner socks, wider boots, or possibly by removing a piece of the boot over the affected toe.

An ingrown toenail can be prevented by cutting the nail straight across rather than rounding it off, cutting off sharp nail corners, and by cutting nails long enough so that the corners extend past the soft tissues.

Leg Cramps

Because of demands placed on lower-extremity muscles by unaccustomed use, many wilderness travelers suffer from leg cramps. At times, excessive perspiration with a loss of salt may contribute. The cramps occur most often in the evening or night of the first few days of a trip. Treatment consists of massaging the muscle and stretching it in the direction opposite the cramp.

Nocturnal cramps can be prevented to some extent by taking a 325-mg tablet of quinine sulfate or two 25-mg tablets of diphenhydramine (Benadryl) nightly at bedtime. Quinine requires a prescription.

Side effects of quinine include blurred vision, ringing in the ears, dizziness, headache, nausea, and vomiting; side effects of diphenhydramine include sleepiness, dizziness, and abdominal pain.

Splinter Removal

Like most outdoor recreationists, wilderness travelers occasionally get a splinter, sliver, or thorn imbedded in their skin. The appropriate care is to first wash the involved area with soap and water, then use a sterile (flamed) sewing needle to free one end of the object so it can be grasped and pulled out with a small forceps. The tweezers from a Swiss Army knife may work but a better tool is a special splinter forceps (available at most pharmacies).

Use of Prescription Drugs

Federal and state laws prohibit laypersons from prescribing or dispensing prescription drugs. Moreover, transporting and even using the prescription drugs described in this appendix may be illegal under various state and/or federal statutes *unless* the drugs in the individual's possession have been prescribed for him or her by a physician and this fact is documented by labels that give the individual's name, the physician's name, and directions for use.

Nevertheless, since under certain conditions the proper drug may prevent or control serious illness or even save a life, wilderness travelers may wish to become familiar with the carefully selected drugs described in this appendix. These can be obtained by prescription from their physicians for inclusion in personal first aid kits. Prescription drugs *should not* be offered to others.

No one should take a drug to which he or she has a known allergy. Common allergic reactions to both prescription and nonprescription drugs include hives and a generalized skin rash. More serious reactions include fever, arthritis, and anaphylactic shock. If skin changes develop or a person starts to feel unwell while taking a drug, he or she should consider stopping that drug immediately.

The drugs and doses mentioned in the following sections are for *adults*. Those wishing to obtain drugs for children's use should consult a pediatrician. No pregnant woman should take any drug, including those mentioned in this appendix, without approval from an obstetrician.

Cold Injuries

The prevention and emergency care of cold injuries are discussed in Chapters 2 and 15. The current recommendation for emergency care of a patient with frostbite is to leave blisters unopened and protect them from damage. However, blister fluid contains prostaglandins and other substances that can injure tissues. For this reason, some authorities recommend removing pink (but not purple or bloody) blister fluid by sterile aspiration with a syringe and needle. In addition, if self-evacuation on foot is required, collapsing such blisters may make it easier.

There is evidence that nonsteroidal anti-inflammatory drugs such as ibuprofen (Advil, Nuprin, Motrin) may help prevent some of the tissue injury associated with frostbite. Ibuprofen can be purchased in 200-mg tablets without a prescription. If frostbite is suspected, immediately begin taking the ibuprofen in a dosage of two tablets twice daily with food. The major side effects of ibuprofen are epigastric distress, heartburn, nausea, and vomiting. Before using ibuprofen in the wilderness, try it at home to make sure you tolerate it.

High-Altitude Illness

The prevention and care of the illnesses of high altitude are discussed in Chapter 15.

For severe acute mountain sickness (AMS), high-altitude cerebral edema (HACE), and high-altitude pulmonary edema (HAPE), oxygen is very useful, if available. It is given by nasal cannula at 4 to 6 L/min or mask at a rate of 8 to 15 L/min, but even 1 L/min will help when supplies are limited. Because oxygen supplies are always finite, simultaneously begin preparations for descent. A portable hyperbaric chamber, the Gamow Bag, has been shown to be as effective as medical oxygen. It can be carried by large mountaineering groups and expeditions and is also useful at high-altitude resorts.

Physicians advocate a number of drugs for their use in preventing or treating high-altitude illness. Acetazolamide (Diamox), a carbonic anhydrase inhibitor, has definite value in preventing AMS, particularly in rescuers who do not have time to ascend slowly. The dose is 125 to 250 mg by mouth every 12 hours for 3 to 4 days. Start the medication 24 hours before ascent (or, for rescuers, as soon as possible), or at the first sign of discomfort, which usually begins at 10,000′ to 12,000′ (3,048 to 3,657 m). Side effects include tingling in the extremities and intolerance to carbonated beverages.

For mild AMS, take aspirin, acetaminophen, or tablets of acetaminophen with 30-mg of codeine (Tylenol No. 3) for headache, plus 125 to 250 mg of acetazolamide every 12 hours for 2 to 3 days to speed acclimatization. For nausea and vomiting, take 10 mg of prochlorperazine (Compazine) orally every 4 hours or 25 mg by rectal suppository every 12 hours as needed. Because prochlorperazine also stimulates breathing, it is preferred over other antinausea agents such as prometh-azine (Phenergan).

When treating severe AMS, acetazolamide can be used but is of less value. Nifedipine (Procardia, Adalat) is useful in preventing and treating HAPE, probably because of its ability to reduce pulmonary artery pressure. The treatment dose is one 10-mg capsule chewed and swallowed for fast effect, followed by 30 mg of a long-acting form (Procardia XL 30) every 12 to 24 hours.

For prevention in HAPE-prone individuals, give 30 mg of the long-acting preparation at bedtime on the third and second days before ascent, increasing to 30 mg every 12 hours on the day of the ascent. Mountaineers who intend to carry nifedipine in their first aid kits are advised to try it out at home beforehand to see if it causes significant side effects such as dizziness, headache, weakness, or low blood pressure.

Dexamethasone, taken in an initial oral or intramuscular dose of 6 mg followed by 4 mg every 6 hours, is helpful in reducing increased intracranial pressure in patients with HACE. It is also useful in preventing AMS in those who cannot take acetazolamide or in rescuers who ascend quickly to very high altitude. The prevention dose is 4 mg every 6 hours starting several hours before ascent and continuing for several days. Side effects of short-term use include epigastric discomfort, heartburn, nausea, vomiting, muscle weakness, and sodium retention with edema.

It cannot be emphasized too strongly that *no* drug or device should be relied upon alone to correct severe

AMS, HAPE, or HACE; the definitive treatment is *rapid descent*.

Antibiotics

Because infectious diseases can occur in the wilderness, it is wise for travelers who expect to be far from civilization for very long to carry antibiotics and have some idea of the indications for their use.

The principal antibiotic-requiring infections likely to be seen are upper and lower respiratory tract infections, dysentery, urinary tract infections, and wound and skin infections. Antibiotics are also used to prevent infection in high-risk wounds.

The principal bacteria to worry about are streptococci (including *S pneumoniae*—previously called *Pneumococcus*) and *Haemophilus influenzae*, which cause respiratory infections; *Campylobacter, Shigella, Salmonella,* and toxin-producing *Escherichia coli,* which cause dysentery and urinary infections; *Proteus,* which cause urinary infections; and staphylococci and streptococci, which cause skin infections.

Under ideal circumstances, the causative microorganism should be identified by culture in each illness and its sensitivity tested so that the correct antibiotic can be chosen. However, the wilderness traveler does not have this luxury and must rely on a small number of carefully selected antibiotics and some general rules of thumb to choose the best drug based on the signs and symptoms of a given illness, the organism(s) most likely responsible, and the known spectrum of activity of each drug. Fortunately, this empiric process is not difficult and is frequently successful.

Many different antibiotics are available and are quite safe when used according to directions by individuals who are not allergic to them. Except as noted later, antibiotics should be taken for 7 to 10 days.

The traveler who will be out a week or more and will be more than 2 or 3 days from the trailhead should carry antibiotics in his or her first aid kit. Experts disagree on how many antibiotics should be carried and which ones should be chosen. Choices are dictated to some extent by cost and by the diseases typically found in the geographic area to be visited. The following recommendations are based on the author's personal experience in North America. Those who will be traveling on other continents, and especially in developing countries, are advised to consult a physician knowledgeable in travel medicine. There are also a number of excellent travelers' medical guidebooks available.

If you wish to carry a single, inexpensive, multiple-purpose antibiotic, the best choice is probably cotrimoxazole (trimethoprim/sulfamethoxazole, or TMP/SMZ) in the double strength (DS) size, which has some activity against all the bacteria mentioned above except for *Campylobacter* and perhaps staphylococci. The dose is one DS tablet twice daily. The principal side effects are nausea, vomiting, loss of appetite, and an allergic skin rash.

Another good single, multiple-purpose, but more expensive antibiotic is ciprofloxacin (Cipro), a quinolone that has some activity against all the bacteria mentioned above. It has less activity against streptococci than does cotrimoxazole but more activity against *Salmonella, Shigella,* and toxin-producing *E coli*. Its dose is one 500-mg tablet twice daily. Side effects are uncommon but can include nausea, vomiting, diarrhea, abdominal pain, and headache. Children, teenagers younger than 18 years, pregnant women, and nursing mothers should not take ciprofloxacin because of the potential for adverse side effects.

A better alternative may be to carry two separate antibiotics: (a) a semisynthetic penicillin, a cephalosporin, or erythromycin; and (b) tetracycline or a tetracycline derivative such as doxycycline. Together, these two groups of drugs are likely to control most infections that may be contracted in the wilderness in temperate latitudes. Large expeditions, groups traveling to developing countries—especially in the tropics—or rescue groups may wish to include additional antibiotics, including parenteral (injectable) forms for patients who are vomiting or unable to swallow.

Amoxicillin, a semisynthetic penicillin, has good activity against bacteria that cause upper and lower respiratory tract infections, urinary tract infections, and wound and skin infections. Unlike cephalosporins, it is also active against *Salmonella* and *Shigella*. It is taken in a dose of 250 to 500 mg every 8 hours. It is probably best to chose a brand in which amoxicillin is combined with potassium clavulanate (Augmentin). Clavulanate is a beta-lactamase blocker that increases the action of amoxicillin against staphylococci, *Haemophilus, E coli, Proteus,* and other important pathogens. Unfortunately, the addition of clavulanate markedly increases the cost. Side effects include nausea, vomiting, diarrhea, vaginitis, allergic skin rash, and hives. The prevalence of penicillin allergy makes semisynthetic penicillins less useful than cephalosporins for guided groups and large parties.

Cephalosporins are active against all the important organisms except *Campylobacter, Salmonella, Shigella,* and toxin-producing *E coli*. They are effective in upper and lower respiratory infections, skin infections, and urinary tract infections. Cephalexin (Keflex), a moderately priced example, is given in a dose of 250 to 500 mg four times daily. Other, probably better but more expensive, choices are cefaclor (Ceclor) at a dosage of 250 mg three times daily, and cefuroxime (Ceftin) at a dosage of 250 to 500 mg twice daily. Side effects are uncommon but include nausea, vomiting, diarrhea, vaginitis, and occasionally an allergic skin rash.

Erythromycin is active against streptococci, some staphylococci, and some *Haemophilus* infections. It is also active against *Mycoplasma* (a common cause of bronchitis), amoebae, and *Campylobacter,* but not against other dysentery organisms. The dosage of the ethyl succinate form is 400 mg four times daily. Delayed-release forms (taken at a dosage of 500 mg twice daily) are also available. Side effects include occasional nausea, vomiting, diarrhea, and abdominal discomfort.

Doxycycline and other tetracyclines are active against rickettsial diseases (typhus, Rocky Mountain spotted fever), undulant fever, tularemia, plague, Lyme disease, *Mycoplasma* infections, *E coli* infections, amoebae, and to some extent streptococci and *Haemophilus* infections. They are also active against *Chlamydia* (a common cause of sexually transmitted diseases and some eye infections) and to a lesser extent against *Shigella*. The dose of doxycycline is 100 mg twice daily. Tetracycline is taken in a dosage of 250 mg four times daily, at least 1 hour before or 2 hours after eating. Avoid milk and milk products while taking tetracycline and its derivatives. Pregnant women, nursing mothers, and children younger than age 8 years should not take this drug because it stains developing teeth.

Because the effectiveness of tetracyclines deteriorates with age, supplies should be replaced yearly (fortunately, they are inexpensive). Patients taking a tetracycline, especially doxycycline, occasionally experience severe sun reactions, which can be prevented to some extent by wearing protective clothing and liberally applying a sunscreen with a high SPF value (see Chapter 15). Other side effects include abdominal discomfort, nausea, vomiting, diarrhea, black tongue, sore mouth, vaginitis, and anal discomfort.

To obtain drugs with the longest shelf life, tell the pharmacist that the drugs are to be used in a first aid kit. Request that the expiration date be typed on each label and try to protect drugs from temperature extremes.

For *empiric treatment* of severe colds, coughs, and sore throats, amoxicillin, amoxicillin/clavulanate, a cephalosporin, erythromycin, or—in the case of a single, multiple-purpose antibiotic—either cotrimoxazole or ciprofloxacin are useful. This is especially true if the patient is producing a yellow or green discharge from the chest or nose, or has white spots on the tonsils, an earache, high fever, or swollen and tender neck glands beneath the mandible. These antibiotics should also be taken for suspected pneumonia or pleurisy, skin and wound infections, abscesses, and to prevent infection in high-risk wounds, open fractures, and open wounds of the chest and abdomen (if the patient is able to swallow).

Suspected urinary or prostate infections may clear up with amoxicillin, amoxicillin/clavulanate, a tetracycline, a cephalosporin, cotrimoxazole or ciprofloxacin. These are also the most useful antibiotics for severe diarrhea, except doxycycline is favored over tetracycline and cephalosporin (see Stomach and Bowel Problems later in this appendix).

If there is no improvement after 48 hours of treatment with an antibiotic from one group, substitute a member of the other group. Except as noted later in this appendix, antibiotics that are producing the desired improvement should be taken for a minimum of 7 days.

Treat abscesses and wound infections with hot packs as well as antibiotics, and cover them with dressings moistened with 1% povidone-iodine solution (10% solution diluted 1:10 with clean water), unless the patient is allergic to iodine. A wound that becomes swollen, hot, red, tender, and painful is probably infected, especially if it drains pus. If the wound has been taped closed, remove the tape and allow the wound to drain. Apply hot, wet packs to the wound four times daily for 30 minutes to speed healing.

Make a hot pack by heating a cloth in clean water, wringing excess water from it, folding it, and placing it against the wound. Test the temperature of the hot pack against your own (cleaned) skin to make sure that it will not burn the patient.

Suspect an abscess in any patient with fever who has a hot, swollen, red, tender area in the skin or a muscle. Apply hot packs as described above to speed the formation of pus, which will collect in a shiny, yellow or reddish spot on the surface of the abscess. To allow pus to drain, clean this spot with an antiseptic (10% povidone-iodine solution), and nick it with a razor blade or sharp knife sterilized over a flame. Try to introduce a small, sterile gauze wick (cut from a sterile gauze pad with sterilized scissors) into the abscess cavity to help it drain and keep it from sealing off prematurely. Continue applying hot packs to promote continued drainage of the pus.

Treat small, infected cuts by applying an antibiotic ointment such as Polysporin three times daily. The ophthalmic form can be used both on the skin and in the eye for conjunctivitis, which is characterized by a red, sore eye that may discharge pus. Unless conjunctivitis clears rapidly, evacuate the patient.

Stomach and Bowel Problems

The type of food usually consumed in the wilderness (freeze-dried food, candy, nuts, lunch meat, dried fruit, cheese) frequently produces an unusual amount of intestinal gas and softer-than-normal stools. Some individuals may experience cramps, usually in the lower abdomen. Gas may accumulate in the left upper abdomen, causing pressure or sharp pains in the chest that may be mistaken for more serious illnesses. These symptoms usually disappear when the offending foods are removed from the diet.

Occasionally, patients with altitude sickness, headache, food poisoning, or gastroenteritis may vomit. Vomiting can usually be controlled with medicated rectal suppositories such as prochlorperazine (Compazine) in 25-mg doses inserted every 12 hours as necessary, or promethazine (Phenergan) in 25-mg doses inserted every 4 to 6 hours as necessary.

Mild diarrhea, often caused by food or gastroenteritis, can be controlled by taking nonprescription loperamide (Imodium) in 2-mg tablets, two with the first loose bowel movement, then one tablet with each subsequent bowel movement up to four in each 24-hour period. Side effects include abdominal pain, nausea, vomiting, constipation, sleepiness, fatigue, and dry mouth. An alternative is to take prescription diphenoxylate/atropine sulfate (Lomotil) in a dose of one 2.5-mg tablet every 4 hours as needed. Side effects include numbness of the extremities, sleepiness, dizziness, constipation, and inability to urinate. Bismuth subsalicylate (Pepto-Bismol) is also quite useful in treating mild to moderately severe diarrhea but is bulky to carry—especially the liquid form. It should not be taken by patients who are allergic to aspirin. The dosage is two tablespoonfuls or two tablets four times daily.

Patients with severe diarrhea and diarrhea accompanied by chills, fever, severe cramps, and blood or pus in the stool should *not* use these drugs, but should start taking an antibiotic and be evacuated, staying hydrated as well as possible. The antibiotics of choice in order of effectiveness are ciprofloxacin, cotrimoxa-

zole, amoxicillin or amoxicillin-clavulanate, and doxycycline. Bismuth subsalicylate should not be taken with doxycycline because it inactivates the antibiotic.

Giardiasis, caused by the protozoan *Giardia lamblia*, is a hazard for wilderness travelers in temperate as well as tropical climates. Symptoms include gastric distress, mild diarrhea, and foul-smelling flatus. The condition does not respond to any of the antibiotics previously mentioned but can be effectively treated with metronidazole (Flagyl), a drug mentioned later in the section on Special Problems of Women. Fortunately, the incubation period for giardiasis is long enough that, except for extended trips, the patient is usually back home before severe symptoms develop.

When patients with any kind of stomach or bowel disturbance are able to eat, they should be given a simple carbohydrate-containing light diet consisting of broth, bland soup, tea, Jell-O, pudding, and toast. They should avoid milk, spices, rich foods, and fruit juices at first. Dehydration should be corrected as described earlier.

Any patient with persistent or severe abdominal pain should be evacuated promptly (see the section on Acute Abdomen in Chapter 13).

Proper sanitation and attention to water and food supplies will often prevent much gastrointestinal misery. Always wash your hands after defecation and before eating. When washing dishes, rinse off soap thoroughly since it is a gastrointestinal irritant. Keep food covered in order to protect it from flies. Native food should be avoided in developing countries, unless it can be peeled or has been well cooked shortly after being prepared and is still hot. In developing countries, do not eat raw vegetables, unpeeled fruit, cooked food that has cooled, or food that has been exposed to flies. Avoid iced drinks because the ice may be contaminated. Drink only bottled, boiled, or disinfected water.

Respiratory Problems

People with head colds or sore throats should avoid wilderness trips because the stressful environment may bring on complications such as pneumonia or a sinus infection. Suspect pneumonia or pleurisy in a person who has a cough with fever or chest pain, especially if the cough is producing yellow or green sputum and the pain is located in the side of the chest underneath the armpit or beneath the scapula and is aggravated by deep breathing and coughing. Patients with suspected pneumonia or other severe respiratory infections should take amoxicillin, amoxicillin/clavulanate, a cephalosporin, erythromycin, cotrimoxazole, or ciprofloxacin and be evacuated promptly to medical care.

Urinary Problems

Symptoms of urinary tract infection include painful urination, frequent voiding of small amounts of urine, a feeling that the bladder has not been emptied, chills, fever, and backache in the costovertebral angle. The patient should drink plenty of fluids.

In mild cases, the patient should take cotrimoxazole, one DS tablet twice daily, ciprofloxacin at a dose of 500 mg twice daily, amoxicillin, or amoxicillin/clavulanate, one tablet three times daily, for at least 3 days. In moderate-to-severe cases with chills, fever, and prostration, the drug should be taken for 10 days. Cephalosporins, doxycycline, or tetracycline also have some effect.

If you have no antibiotics, 500 mg of vitamin C taken three times daily is of value.

Special Problems of Women

Wilderness travel without the customary amenities of civilization may pose special problems for women. Vaginal infections (vaginitis) that may occur can be divided into two general types for purposes of treatment.

Yeast infections, characterized by thick, whitish discharge and severe itching, usually respond promptly to clotrimazole vaginal suppositories (Mycelex 7, available without prescription), inserted once daily at bedtime for 7 days. Side effects are rare, but include local irritation and vomiting. An oral prescription drug, fluconazole (Diflucan), is also available, which is very effective when given in a *single* dose of 150 mg. Side effects include headache, nausea, abdominal pain, and diarrhea.

Other types of vaginitis commonly involve a thinner, yellowish discharge, sometimes with an objectionable odor. These infections are usually caused by either *Trichomonas vaginalis* or *Gardnerella vaginalis*. They both usually respond to one 500-mg tablet of metronidazole (Flagyl) taken twice daily for 7 days. While taking metronidazole, the patient should not drink alcohol because the combination produces symptoms similar to those associated with Antabuse (flushing, copious sweating, severe headache, vomiting, dyspnea, and heart irregularities). Pregnant woman should not take metronidazole, but can take clotrimazole suppositories, which have some activity against *Trichomonas*. Side effects of metronidazole include abdominal pain, nausea, vomiting, diarrhea, and a metallic taste in the mouth.

Women who customarily have menstrual cramps should carry a medication such as Midol that they have previously found to give relief. Otherwise, one or two 200-mg tablets of ibuprofen (nonprescription Advil, Nuprin) taken three to four times daily with food are usually effective. Prescription pain pills such as acetaminophen with codeine (Tylenol with codeine) and propoxyphene with acetaminophen (Darvocet-N 100) also can be used.

Glossary

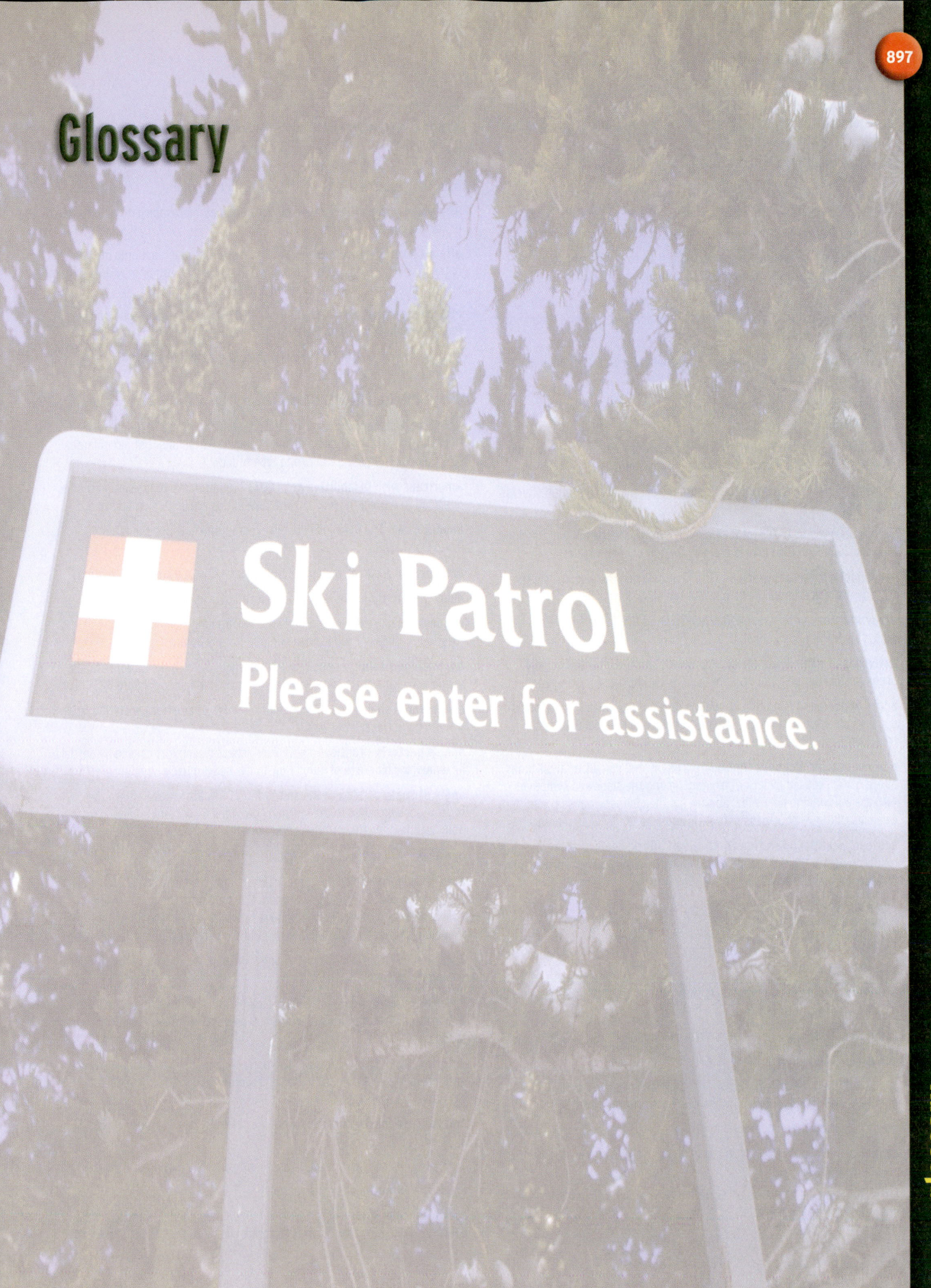

abandonment Failure to continue service or care of another that by law one is required to complete.

abdomen The body cavity that contains the major organs of digestion and excretion.

abduction Motion of a limb away from the midline.

abortion Delivery of the fetus and placenta before 20 weeks; miscarriage.

abrasion Loss or damage of the superficial layer of skin as a result of a body part rubbing or scraping across a rough or hard surface.

absence seizure Seizure that may be characterized by a brief lapse of attention in which the patient may stare and does not respond. Also known as petit mal seizure.

acceleration The process of increasing speed; the rate of change of velocity with respect to time.

acclimatization The process by which the body adjusts to a new environment.

acetabulum The depression on the lateral pelvis where its three component bones join, in which the femoral head fits snugly.

acidosis A pathologic condition resulting from the accumulation of acids in the body.

acromioclavicular (A/C) joint A simple joint where the bony projections of the scapula and the clavicle meet at the top of the shoulder.

acromioclavicular separations The joint between the clavicle and the acromion of the scapula at the point of the shoulder.

acromion The lateral extension of the spine of the scapula that forms the highest point of the shoulder.

activities of daily living (ADL) The basic activities a person usually accomplishes during a normal day, such as eating, dressing, and washing.

acute abdomen A condition of sudden onset of pain within the abdomen, usually indicating peritonitis; demands immediate medical or surgical treatment.

acute mountain sickness (AMS) A condition that can occur at altitudes above 6,500', caused by lack of oxygen. Among the signs and symptoms of AMS are a throbbing headache, apathy, lightheadedness, nausea, vomiting, weakness, fatigue, shortness of breath, and a generally ill appearance.

acute myocardial infarction (AMI) Heart attack; death of heart muscle following obstruction of blood flow to it. Acute in this context means "new" or "happening right now."

Adam's apple The firm prominence in the upper part of the larynx formed by the thyroid cartilage.

adaptive athlete An individual who is physically or mentally challenged and participates in a sport.

addiction A state of overwhelming obsession or physical need to continue the use of a drug or agent.

adduction Motion of a limb toward the midline.

adolescents Children between 12 and 18 years of age.

advanced life support (ALS) Advanced lifesaving procedures, some of which are now being provided by the OEC technician and the EMT-B.

aerobic capacity The body's ability to take, transport, and use oxygen.

agonal respirations Occasional, gasping breaths that occur after the heart has stopped.

air embolism The presence of air in the veins, which can lead to cardiac arrest if it enters the heart.

airway The upper airway tract or the passage above the larynx, which includes the nose, mouth, and throat. The lower airway includes the larynx, trachea, bronchi, and alveoli.

allergen A substance that causes an allergic reaction.

allergic reaction The body's exaggerated immune response to an internal or surface agent.

altered level of consciousnes A mental state in which patients may be unresponsive, combative, or confused, may thrash about, or may drift into and out of an alert state; also called altered mental status.

altered mental status A change in the way a person thinks and behaves that may signal disease in the central nervous system.

alveoli The air sacs of the lungs in which the exchange of oxygen and carbon dioxide takes place.

ambient temperature The temperature of the surrounding environment.

American Standard System A safety system for oxygen cylinders larger than size D, designed to prevent the accidental attachment of a regulator to a cylinder containing the wrong type of gas.

Americans with Disabilities Act (ADA) Comprehensive legislation that is designed to protect individuals with disabilities against discrimination.

amniotic sac The fluid-filled, baglike membrane in which the fetus develops.

amputation A complete separation from the body by cutting or tearing.

anaphylactic shock Severe shock caused by allergic reactions.

anaphylaxis An extreme, possibly life-threatening systemic allergic reaction that may include shock and respiratory failure.

anatomic position The position of reference in which the patient stands facing you, arms at the side, with the palms of the hands forward.

aneurysm A swelling or enlargement of a part of an artery, resulting from weakening of the arterial wall.

angina pectoris Transient (short-lived) chest discomfort caused by partial or temporary blockage of blood flow to the heart muscle.

angle of Louis A ridge on the sternum that lies at the level where the second rib is attached to the sternum; provides a constant and reliable bony landmark on the anterior chest wall.

anorexia Lack of appetite for food.

anoxic Diminished oxygen in the arterial blood despite normal ability of the blood to contain and carry oxygen. May be due to reduced oxygen supply, respiratory obstruction, reduced surface area in the lungs for exchange of gases, or inadequate respiratory movements.

anterior The front surface of the body; the side facing you in the standard anatomic position.

anterior cruciate ligament (ACL) Ligament in the knee that runs from the posterior femur to the anterior tibia, preventing forward dislocation of the tibia.

anterior superior iliac spines The bony prominences of the pelvis (ilium) at the front on each side of the lower abdomen just below the plane of the umbilicus.

anterograde (posttraumatic) amnesia Inability to remember events after an injury.

antidote A substance that is used to neutralize or counteract a poison.

anus The terminal end of the rectum.

aorta The main artery, which receives blood from the left ventricle and delivers it to all the other arteries that carry blood to the tissues of the body.

aortic valve The one-way valve that lies between the left ventricle and the aorta. It keeps blood from flowing back into the left ventricle after the left ventricle ejects its blood into the aorta. One of four heart valves.

apex (plural: apices) The tip or the topmost portion of a structure.

Apgar score A scoring system for assessing the status of a newborn that assigns a number value to each of five areas of assessment.

aphasia The inability to communicate verbally.

apnea Absence of breathing.

appendix A small tubular structure that is attached to the lower border of the cecum in the right lower quadrant of the abdomen.

arterial rupture Rupture of a cerebral artery that may contribute to interruption of cerebral blood flow.

arteriole The smallest branch of an artery leading to the vast network of capillaries.

artery A blood vessel, consisting of three layers of tissue and smooth muscle that carries blood away from the heart.

articular cartilage A pearly layer of specialized cartilage covering the articular surfaces (contact surfaces on the ends) of bones in synovial joints.

aspiration The introduction of vomit or other foreign material into the lungs.

assault Placing an individual in a position without consent in which the individual fears physical harm will occur.

assault and battery The illegal infliction of injury to a person by physical means, the act of which was initiated with a wrongful or evil intent.

asthma A disease of the lungs in which muscle spasm in the small air passageways and the production of large amounts of mucus result in airway obstruction.

asystole Complete absence of heart electrical activity.

ataxia Loss of muscle coordination leading to difficulty in maintaining balance and inability to walk.

atherosclerosis A disorder in which cholesterol and calcium build up inside the walls of blood vessels, eventually leading to partial or complete blockage of blood flow.

athetoid cerebral palsy A disorder in which a person makes constant, slow writhing movements.

atrium One of two (right and left) upper chambers of the heart. The right atrium receives blood from the vena cava and delivers it to the right ventricle. The left atrium receives blood from pulmonary veins and delivers it to the left ventricle.

attention deficit disorder (ADD) Neurologic syndrome that is usually hereditary. Symptoms include distractibility, short attention span, impulsiveness, hyperactivity, and restlessness that interfere with everyday function.

auscultation A method of listening to sounds within an organ with a stethoscope.

autism A developmental neurologic disorder that includes severe problems with communication and behavior.

automated external defibrillation (AED) A portable electrical device that is capable of analysis of heart rhythms by an on-board computer and making the medical decision to use or withhold the use of an electrical shock capable of stopping the uncontrolled fibrillation of the heart muscle. This device is designed to be used out of the hospital environment by lay persons with a minimum of training.

autonomic dysreflexia (AD) A condition in which the body below the spine injury level does not have ability to sense and react normally to certain stimuli.

autonomic (involuntary) nervous system The part of the nervous system that regulates functions that are not controlled by conscious will, such as digestion and sweating.

avalanche probe A long pole used to search for a body buried in the snow.

avalanche transceiver An electronic device that can emit a signal and also receive a signal from another transceiver. Worn by people in avalanche-prone terrain to assist rescue in the event of avalanche burial.

AVPU A mnemonic for assessing a patient's level of responsiveness by determining whether a patient is Awake and alert, responsive to Verbal stimulus or Pain, or Unresponsive; used principally in the initial assessment.

avulse To pull or tear away.

avulsion An injury in which soft tissue either is torn completely loose (amputation) or is hanging as a flap.

axon The long process of a neuron.

backboard A device that is used to immobilize a patient who is suspected of having a hip, pelvic, spinal, or lower-extremity injury. Also called a spineboard, trauma board, or long board.

bag-valve-mask (BVM) device A device with a face mask attached to a ventilation bag containing a reservoir and connected to oxygen; delivers more than 90% supplemental oxygen.

ball-and-socket joint Joint that allows rotation as well as bending.

barrier device A protective item, such as a pocket mask with a valve, that limits exposure to a patient's body fluids.

basal metabolism Heat produced by constant internal metabolic processes (50 kcal per square meter of body surface per hour in an average person).

basic life support (BLS) Noninvasive emergency lifesaving care that is used to treat airway obstruction, respiratory arrest, or cardiac arrest.

basket stretcher A rigid stretcher commonly used in technical and water rescues that surrounds and supports the patient yet allows water to drain through holes in the bottom. Also called a Stokes litter.

Battle's sign Bruising behind an ear over the mastoid process that may indicate skull fracture.

behavior How a person functions or acts in response to his or her environment.

behavioral crisis The point at which a person's reactions to events interfere with activities of daily living.

bending trauma An impact that tends to momentarily reverse the normal forward curve of the spine.

biceps The large muscle that covers the front of the humerus.

bilateral A body part that appears on both sides of the midline.

bile ducts Ducts that convey bile between the liver and the intestine.

bilirubin A yellow compound that is a byproduct of the normal breakdown of red blood cells. It is removed by the liver and excreted through the bile into the intestines.

birth canal The vagina and cervix.

blood pressure The pressure that the blood exerts against the walls of the arteries as it passes through them.

bloody show A plug of pink-tinged mucus that is discharged when the cervix begins to dilate.

blowout fracture Fracture of the orbit or of the bones that support the floor of the orbit.

blunt injury Injury to the head in which the brain has been injured but the skin is unbroken.

body In physics, any mass of matter that is distinct from other masses of matter.

body substance isolation (BSI) An infection control concept and practice that assumes that all body fluids are potentially infectious.

brachial artery The major vessel in the upper extremity that supplies blood to the arm.

bradycardia A heart rate of less than 60 beats/min in children or less than 80 beats/min in infants.

brain The controlling organ of the body and center of consciousness; functions include perception, control of reactions to the environment, emotional responses, and judgment.

brain stem The part of the central nervous system that controls virtually all functions that are necessary for life, including the cardiac and respiratory systems.

breath-holding syncope Loss of consciousness caused by a decreased breathing stimulus.

breath sounds An indication of air movement in the lungs, usually assessed with a stethoscope.

breech presentation Delivery in which the buttocks come out first.

bridge lift A lift performed by four or more rescuers. Each rescuer braces his or her head against the shoulder of an opposite rescuer, allowing lifting to occur with the arms instead of the back.

bronchi The tubular air passages of the lungs.

bronchioles The smallest of the bronchi.

burnout A condition of chronic fatigue and frustration that results from mounting stress over time.

burns An injury in which the soft tissue receives more energy than it can absorb without injury from thermal heat, frictional heat, toxic chemicals, electricity, or nuclear radiation.

calcaneus The heel bone.

camber The arch that is formed when a ski or snowboard is placed on a flat surface, with the middle of the board higher than the tip and tail.

capillary Any one of the small blood vessels that connect arteriole and venule and through whose walls various substances pass into and out of the interstitial tissues and then on to the cells.

capillary refill A test that evaluates distal circulatory system function by squeezing (blanching) blood from an area such as a nail bed and watching the speed of its return after releasing the pressure.

capillary vessels The fine end-divisions of the arterial system that allow contact between cells of the body tissues and the plasma and red blood cells.

carbon dioxide retention A condition characterized by a chronically high blood level of carbon dioxide in which the respiratory center no longer responds to high blood levels of carbon dioxide.

cardiac arrest A state in which the heart fails to generate an effective and detectable blood flow; pulses are not palpable in cardiac arrest, even if muscular and electrical activity continues in the heart.

cardiogenic shock A state in which not enough oxygen is delivered to the tissues of the body, caused by low output of blood from the heart. It can be a severe complication of a large acute myocardial infarction, as well as other conditions.

cardiovascular fitness Conditioning the heart and circulatory system to meet an active body's changing needs for blood.

carotid artery The major artery that supplies blood to the head and brain.

carpometacarpal joint The joint between the wrist and the metacarpal bones; the thumb joint.

casualty collection area A designated location where victims of a mass-casualty incident may be taken for triage and initial medical care prior to transport to a hospital.

catheter A hollow, cylindrical structure that drains or delivers fluids.

cecum The first part of the large intestine, into which the ileum opens.

central nervous system (CNS) The brain and spinal cord.

cerebellum One of the three major subdivisions of the brain, sometimes called the "little brain"; coordinates the various activities of the brain, particularly body movements.

cerebral edema Swelling of the brain.

cerebral embolism Obstruction of a cerebral artery caused by a clot that was formed elsewhere in the body and traveled to the brain.

cerebral palsy (CP) A disability resulting from brain injury before, during, or shortly after birth.

cerebrovascular accident (CVA) An interruption of blood flow to the brain that results in the loss of brain function.

cerebrum The largest part of the three subdivisions of the brain, sometimes called the "gray matter"; made up of several lobes that control movement, hearing, balance, speech, visual perception, emotions, and personality.

cervical spine The portion of the spinal column consisting of the first seven vertebrae that lie in the neck.

cervix The lower one-third, or neck, of the uterus.

chest compliance The ability of the chest to fully expand when air is drawn in on inhalation.

chief complaint The reason a patient called for help; also, the patient's response to general questions such as "What's wrong?" or "What happened?"

child abuse Any improper or excessive action that injures or otherwise harms a child or infant; includes neglect and physical, sexual, and emotional abuse.

chronic bronchitis Irritation of the major lung passageways, from either infectious disease or irritants such as smoke.

chronic obstructive pulmonary disease (COPD) A slow process of dilation and disruption of the airways and alveoli, caused by chronic bronchial obstruction.

circulation, motion, sensation (CMS) An abbreviation for what to check in an injured extremity.

circulatory system The complex arrangement of connected tubes, including the arteries, arterioles, capillaries, venules, and veins, that moves blood, oxygen, nutrients, carbon dioxide, and cellular waste throughout the body.

clavicle The collarbone; it is lateral to the sternum and medial to the scapula.

closed abdominal injury Any injury of the abdomen caused by a nonpenetrating instrument or force, in which the skin remains intact; also called blunt abdominal injury.

closed chest injury Injury to the chest in which the skin is not broken, usually due to blunt trauma.

closed fracture A fracture in which the overlying skin is not broken.

closed injury Injury in which damage occurs beneath the skin or mucous membrane but the surface remains intact.

coagulation Formation of clots to plug openings in injured blood vessels and stop blood flow.

coccyx The last four vertebrae of the spine; the tailbone.

cognitive disability Damage or deterioration in any portion of the brain that affects the ability to process information, coordinate and control the body, and/or move in space.

colic Acute, intermittent cramping abdominal pain.

command post A designated center where an incident commander establishes a location to oversee and coordinate the response activities.

common cold A viral infection usually associated with swollen nasal mucous membranes and the production of fluid from the sinuses and nose.

communicable disease Any disease that can be spread from person to person, or from animal to person.

compartment syndrome Swelling in a confined space that produces dangerous pressure; may cut off blood flow or damage sensitive tissue.

compensated shock The early stage of shock, in which the body can still compensate for blood loss.

complete airway obstruction Occurs when a foreign body completely obstructs the patient's airway. Patients cannot breathe, talk, or cough.

compression (blunt) trauma Trauma caused by an impact between a body part and a blunt object; impact may cause injury without penetrating soft tissues or internal organs and cavities.

concussion A temporary loss or alteration of part or all of the brain's abilities to function without actual physical damage to the brain.

conduction The transmission of heat, sound waves, nerve impulses, or electricity by contact.

congestive heart failure (CHF) A disorder in which the heart loses part of its ability to effectively pump blood, usually as a result of damage to the heart muscle and usually resulting in a backup of fluid into the lungs.

conjunctiva The delicate membrane that lines the eyelids and covers the exposed surface of the eye.

conjunctivitis Inflammation of the conjunctiva.

connecting nerves Nerves in the brain and spinal cord that connect the motor and sensory nerves.

consent Permission to render care.

contagious An infectious disease that is capable of being transmitted from one person to another.

contamination The presence of infective organisms or foreign bodies such as dirt, gravel, or metal.

continuous quality improvement (CQI) A system of internal and external reviews and audits of all aspects of the OEC program and the EMS system.

contusion A bruise without a break in the skin.

convection Transmission of heat by a moving gas or liquid.

core The central nervous system, heart, lungs, liver, and other important internal organs of the body.

core curriculum The essential curriculum content that must be covered in every OEC course.

core temperature The temperature of the central part of the body (eg, the heart, lungs, and vital organs).

cornea The transparent tissue layer in front of the pupil and iris of the eye.

coronary artery A blood vessel that carries blood and nutrients to the heart muscle.

costal arch A bridge of cartilage that connects the ends of the sixth through tenth ribs with the lower portion of the sternum.

costovertebral angle An angle that is formed by the junction of the spine and the tenth rib.

cot (wheeled ambulance stretcher) A specially designed stretcher that can be rolled along the ground. A collapsible undercarriage allows it to be loaded into the ambulance. Also called an ambulance cot, gurney, or pram.

cranial nerves Specialized nerves that arise directly from the brain, and provide specific function.

cranium The area of the head above the ears and eyes; the skull. The cranium contains the brain.

crepitus A grating or grinding sensation caused by fractured bone ends or joints rubbing together.

cricoid cartilage A firm ridge of cartilage that forms the lower part of the larynx.

cricoid pressure Pressure on the cricoid cartilage; applied to inhibit gastric distention and aspiration of vomitus in the unconscious patient.

cricothyroid membrane A thin sheet of fascia that connects the thyroid and cricoid cartilages that make up the larynx.

critical incident stress debriefing (CISD) A confidential group discussion of a severely stressful incident that usually occurs within 24 to 72 hours of the incident.

critical incident stress management (CISM) A process that confronts the responses to critical incidents and defuses them, directing the emergency services personnel toward physical and emotional equilibrium.

croup An infectious disease of the upper respiratory system that may cause partial airway obstruction and is characterized by a barking cough; usually seen in children.

crowning The appearance of the infant's head at the vaginal opening during labor.

crushing injury An injury caused by compression that involves both direct tissue injury and injury caused by circulation disturbance resulting from pressure on blood vessels.

cyanosis A bluish-gray skin color that is caused by reduced levels of oxygen in the blood.

DCAP-BTLS A mnemonic for assessment in which each area of the body is evaluated for Deformities, Contusions, Abrasions, Punctures/Penetrations, Burns, Tenderness, Lacerations, and Swelling.

deaf Partially or completely incapable of hearing.

deceleration The process of decreasing speed; eg, when a skier's body abruptly loses speed upon colliding with a tree.

decompensated shock The late stage of shock, when blood pressure is falling.

decompression sickness A painful condition seen in divers who ascend too quickly, in which gas, especially nitrogen, forms bubbles in blood vessels and other tissues; also called "the bends."

deep Farther inside the body and away from the skin.

deep frostbite A full- or partial-thickness freezing of a body part, most commonly the hands and feet.

defibrillation To shock a fibrillating (chaotically beating) heart with specialized electrical current in an attempt to restore a normal rhythmic beat.

dehydration A state in which fluid losses are greater than fluid intake into the body, leading to shock and death if untreated.

delirium tremens (DTs) A severe withdrawal syndrome seen in alcoholics who are deprived of ethyl alcohol; characterized by restlessness, fever, sweating, disorientation, agitation, and convulsions; can be fatal if untreated.

dependent lividity Blood settling to the lowest point of the body, causing discoloration of the skin.

depression A persistent mood of sadness, despair, and discouragement; depression may be a symptom of many different mental and physical disorders, or it may be a disorder on its own.

dermis The inner layer of the skin, containing hair follicles, sweat glands, nerve endings, and blood vessels.

detailed physical exam The part of the assessment process in which a detailed area-by-area exam is performed on patients whose problems cannot be readily identified or when more specific information is needed about problems identified in the focused history and physical exam.

diabetic coma Unconsciousness caused by dehydration, very high blood glucose levels, and acidosis in diabetes.

diabetic ketoacidosis (DKA) A form of acidosis in uncontrolled diabetes in which certain acids accumulate when insulin is not available.

diaphoretic Characterized by profuse sweating.

diaphragm A muscular dome that forms the undersurface of the thorax, separating the chest from the abdominal cavity. Contraction of the diaphragm (and the chest wall muscles) brings air into the lungs. Relaxation allows air to be expelled from the lungs.

diastole The relaxation, or period of relaxation, of the heart, especially of the ventricles.

diastolic blood pressure The lowest point of the blood pressure curve.

diastolic pressure The pressure that remains in the arteries during the relaxing phase of the heart's cycle (diastole) when the left ventricle is at rest.

diffusion A process in which molecules move from an area of higher concentration of molecules to an area of lower concentration.

digestion The processing of food that nourishes the individual cells of the body.

dilation Widening of a tubular structure such as a coronary artery.

diphtheria An infectious disease in which a membrane lining the pharynx is formed that can severely obstruct passage of air into the larynx.

direct ground lift A lifting technique that is used for patients who are found lying supine on the ground with no suspected spinal injury.

direction Route, course, path.

disability Any restriction in or lack of ability to perform an activity in the manner or within the range considered normal for a human being.

disarticulation An amputation that occurs at a joint.

disaster A widespread event that disrupts community resources and functions, in turn threatening public safety, citizens' lives, and property.

dislocation Disruption of a joint in which ligaments are damaged and the bone ends are no longer in normal contact.

displaced fracture A fracture in which bone fragments are separated from one another and not in anatomic alignment.

distal Nearer to the tips of the extremities.

distracted The action of pulling the spine along its length.

distraction trauma Trauma caused by stretching.

diving reflex Slowing of the heart rate caused by submersion in cold water.

dorsal The posterior surface of the body, including the back of the hand.

dorsalis pedis artery The artery on the anterior surface of the foot.

dorsiflexion Upward flexion of the foot.

Down syndrome A common genetic condition resulting in mental and physical anomalies.

drowning Death from suffocation by submersion in water.

duodenum The first part of the small intestine, which connects the stomach to the jejunum.

dysarthria The inability to pronounce speech clearly, often a result of blood flow to the right hemisphere of the brain.

dyslexia Condition characterized by a significant delay in one or more areas of learning.

dysphagia Difficulty in swallowing.

dyspnea Shortness of breath or difficulty breathing.

dystonic cerebral palsy A condition in which an individual's muscles are extremely rigid.

ecchymosis Discoloration of the skin associated with a closed wound; bruising.

eclampsia Convulsions (seizures) resulting from severe hypertension in the pregnant woman.

ectopic pregnancy A pregnancy that develops outside the uterus, typically in a fallopian tube.

edema The presence of abnormally large amounts of fluid between cells in body tissues, causing swelling of the affected area.

electrolytes Certain salts and other chemicals that are dissolved in body fluids and cells.

embolus A blood clot or other substance in the circulatory system that travels to a blood vessel where it causes blockage.

emergency medical services (EMS) A multidisciplinary system that represents the combined efforts of several professionals and agencies to provide prehospital emergency care to the sick and injured.

emergency medical technician (EMT) An EMS professional who is trained and licensed by the state to provide emergency medical care in the field.

emergency move A move in which the patient is dragged or pulled from a dangerous scene before initial assessment and care are provided.

emesis Vomiting.

emphysema A disease of the lungs in which there is extreme dilation and eventual destruction of pulmonary alveoli with poor exchange of oxygen and carbon dioxide; it is one form of chronic obstructive pulmonary disease (COPD).

EMT-Basic An EMT who has training in basic emergency care skills, including automated external defibrillation, use of a definitive airway adjunct, and assisting patients with certain prescribed medications.

EMT-Intermediate An EMT who has extensive training in advanced life support, including intubation, IV (intravenous) therapy, pharmacology, cardiac monitoring, and other advanced assessment and treatment skills.

EMT-Paramedic An EMT who has extensive training in advanced life support including intubation, IV skills, pharmacology, cardiac life support and advanced assessment and treatment skills. Additionally, EMT-Paramedics are required to complete a lengthy supervised internship.

endocrine system The complex message and control system that integrates many body functions, including the release of hormones.

energy The capacity for doing work.

envenomation The act of injecting venom.

epidermis The outer layer of skin, which is made up of cells that are sealed together to form a watertight protective covering for the body.

epiglottis A thin, leaf-shaped valve that allows air to pass into the trachea but prevents food or liquid from entering.

epiglottitis An infectious disease in which the epiglottis becomes inflamed and enlarged and may cause upper airway obstruction.

epilepsy Recurrent episodes of seizures caused by an abnormal focus of electrical activity within the brain that may cause impaired responsiveness, abnormal movements, or psychic, sensory, or autonomic disturbances.

epinephrine A substance produced by the body (commonly called adrenaline), and a drug produced by pharmaceutical companies that increases pulse rate and blood pressure; the drug of choice for an anaphylactic reaction.

epistaxis Nosebleed.

esophagus A collapsible tube that extends from the pharynx to the stomach; contractions of the muscle in the wall of the esophagus propel food and liquids through it to the stomach.

eustachian tube The internal auditory canal that connects the middle ear to the nasal cavity.

evaporation Conversion of a liquid into a vapor.

evisceration The displacement of organs outside of the body.

exhalation The part of the breathing process in which the diaphragm and the intercostal muscles relax, forcing air out of the lungs.

expressed consent A type of consent in which a patient gives express authorization for provision of care or transport.

extend To straighten.

external auditory canal The ear canal; leads to the tympanic membrane.

extremity lift A lifting technique that is used for patients who are supine or in a sitting position with no suspected extremity or spinal injuries.

extrication Removal of a patient from entrapment or a dangerous situation or position, such as from a rock slide, avalanche, wrecked vehicle, industrial accident, or building collapse.

extrication vest A vest-shaped device made of fabric strengthened with lightweight materials to form a lightweight and collapsible short backboard; designed to temporarily immobilize the trunk, head, and neck of a patient in a confined area such as an automobile seat or tree well when a long backboard cannot be used. Common types are the Kendrick extrication device (KED) and Oregon Spine splint.

eyes-forward position A head position in which the patient's eyes are looking straight ahead and the head and torso are in line.

fallopian tube Long, slender tube that extends from the uterus to the region of the ovary on the same side, and through which the ovum passes from ovary to uterus.

fascia A sheet or band of tough fibrous connective tissue; lies deep under the skin and forms an outer layer for the muscles.

febrile seizures Convulsions that result from sudden high fevers, particularly in children.

femoral artery The principal artery of the thigh that supplies blood to the lower extremities.

femoral head The proximal end of the femur, articulating with the acetabulum to form the hip joint.

femur The thigh bone; the longest and one of the strongest bones in the body.

fetus The developing, unborn infant inside the uterus.

fibula The lateral of the two bones of the lower leg.

first responder The first medically trained individual, such as a patroller, search and rescue personnel, police officer, or other rescuer, to arrive at the scene of an emergency to provide initial medical assistance.

flail chest A condition in which three or more ribs are fractured in two or more places, or in association with a fracture of the sternum, so that a segment of chest wall is effectively detached from the rest of the thoracic cage.

flex To bend.

flexible stretcher A stretcher that can become smaller for carrying and storage but when in use will wrap around the patient to provide support and stabilization.

floating ribs The eleventh and twelfth ribs, which do not attach to the sternum through the costal arch.

flutter valve A one-way valve that allows air to leave the chest cavity but not return. Formed by taping three sides of an occlusive dressing to the chest wall, leaving the fourth open as the valve.

focused history and physical exam The part of the assessment process, either trauma or medical, in which the patient's major complaints or any problems that are immediately evident are further and more specifically evaluated.

foramen magnum A large opening at the base of the skull through which the brain connects to the spinal cord.

force Any action that changes the state of rest or motion of a body to which that force is applied.

four-person log roll The recommended procedure for moving a patient with a suspected spinal injury from the ground to a long spine board.

Fowler's position The position in which the patient is sitting up or semisitting with the knees bent.

fracture A break in the continuity of a bone.

frostbite Damage to tissues as the result of exposure to cold; frozen body parts.

frostnip A mild cold injury caused by cold-induced superficial blood vessel constriction.

fulcrum point The hinge-like point about which a lever turns.

full-thickness (third-degree) burn A burn that affects all skin layers and may affect the subcutaneous layers, muscle, bone, and internal organs, leaving the area dry, leathery, and white, dark brown, or charred.

functional disorder A disorder in which there is no known identifiable physiologic reason for the abnormal functioning of an organ or organ system.

gag reflex A normal reflex mechanism that causes retching; activated by touching the soft palate or the back of the throat.

gallbladder A sac on the undersurface of the liver that collects bile from the liver and discharges it into the duodenum through the common bile duct.

gangrene Tissue death followed by bacterial invasion and putrification; usually caused by loss of blood supply.

gastric distention A condition in which air fills the stomach as a result of high volume and pressure during artificial ventilation.

general adaptation syndrome The body's three-stage response to stress. First, stress causes the body to trigger an alarm response, followed by a stage of reaction and resistance, and then recovery, or if the stress is prolonged, exhaustion.

generalized seizure Seizure characterized by severe twitching of all the body's muscles that may last several minutes or more; also known as a grand mal seizure.

genital system The male and female reproductive systems.

Glasgow Coma Scale A method of assessing a patient's level of consciousness by scoring the patient's response to eye opening, motor response, and verbal response.

glenoid fossa The part of the scapula that joins with the humeral head to form the glenohumeral joint.

globe The eyeball.

glucose One of the basic sugars; it is the primary fuel, along with oxygen, for cellular metabolism.

Golden Hour The time from injury to definitive care, during which treatment of shock or traumatic injuries should occur because survival potential is the best.

good air exchange A term used to distinguish the degree of distress in a patient with a partial airway obstruction. With good air exchange, the patient is still conscious and able to cough forcefully, although wheezing may be heard.

greater trochanter A bony prominence on the proximal lateral side of the thigh, just below the hip joint.

guarding Involuntary muscle contractions (spasm) of the abdominal wall, an effort to protect the inflamed abdomen.

hair follicles The small organs in the skin that produce hair.

hallucinogen An agent that produces false perceptions in any one of the five senses.

handicapped A term used to describe a person with an impairment that substantially limits one or more of life's activities.

head tilt–chin lift maneuver A combination of two movements to open the airway by tilting the forehead back and lifting the chin; used for non-trauma patients.

heart A hollow muscular organ that receives blood from the veins and propels it into the arteries.

heart rate (pulse) The wave of pressure that is created by the heart's contracting and forcing blood out the left ventricle and into the major arteries.

heartburn A type of indigestion characterized by a burning sensation in the epigastric area or beneath the sternum and often accompanied by increased saliva production. A new acronym that involves heartburn is GERD (gastroesophageal reflux disease). This indicates that the contents of the stomach regurgitate into the lower esophagus.

heat cramps Painful muscle spasms usually associated with vigorous activity in a hot environment.

heat exhaustion A form of heat injury in which the body loses significant amounts of fluid and electrolytes because of heavy sweating; also called heat prostration or heat collapse.

heatstroke A life-threatening condition of severe hyperthermia caused by exposure to excessive natural or artificial heat, marked by warm, dry skin; severely altered mental status; and often irreversible coma.

Heimlich maneuver A technique for relieving upper-airway obstruction due to a foreign body by giving quick, repetitive upper abdominal thrusts.

hematemesis Vomiting blood.

hematoma The collection of blood in a space, tissue, or organ due to a break in the wall of a blood vessel.

hematuria The presence of blood in the urine.

hemiparesis Weakness on one side of the body.

hemophilia A congenital condition in which the patient lacks one or more of the blood's normal clotting factors.

hemoptysis The spitting or coughing up of blood.

hemorrhage Profuse bleeding.

hemorrhagic stroke One of the two main types of stroke; occurs as a result of bleeding inside the brain.

hemothorax Collection of blood in the chest.

hernia The protrusion of a loop of an organ or tissue through an abnormal body opening.

high altitude cerebral edema (HACE) A serious complication of acute mountain sickness, characterized by swelling of the brain, ataxia, and altered mental status.

high altitude pulmonary edema (HAPE) A type of high-altitude illness characterized by the lungs filling with edema fluid.

hinge joint A joint that can bend and straighten but cannot rotate; these joints restrict motion to one plane.

histamine A substance released by the immune system in allergic reactions that is responsible for many of the symptoms of anaphylaxis.

hollow organs Structures through which materials pass, such as the stomach, small intestines, large intestines, ureters, and bladder.

hormone A chemical substance that regulates the activity of body organs and tissues; produced by a gland.

host The organism or individual that is attacked by the infecting agent.

humerus The supporting bone of the upper arm that joins with the scapula (glenoid) to form the shoulder joint and with the ulna and radius to form the elbow joint.

hyperbaric chamber A chamber, usually a small room, pressurized to more than atmospheric pressure.

hyperextension Extreme or abnormal extension.

hyperflexion Extreme or abnormal flexion.

hyperglycemia Abnormally high glucose level in the blood.

hypertension Blood pressure that is higher than the normal range.

hyperthermia A condition in which core temperature rises to 101°F (38.3°C) or more.

hyperventilation Rapid or deep breathing that lowers blood carbon dioxide levels below normal.

hyphema Bleeding into the anterior chamber of the eye, obscuring part or all of the iris.

hypnotic A sleep-inducing effect or agent.

hypoglycemia A condition characterized by low blood glucose levels.

hypotension Blood pressure that is lower than the normal range.

hypothermia A condition in which the internal body temperature falls below 95°F (35°C), usually as a result of prolonged exposure to cool or freezing temperatures.

hypovolemic shock A condition in which low blood volume, due to either massive internal or external bleeding or extensive loss of body water, results in inadequate perfusion.

hypoxia A dangerous condition in which the body tissues and cells do not have enough oxygen.

hypoxic drive A "backup system" to control respiration; senses drops in the oxygen level in the blood.

ileus Paralysis of the bowel, arising from any one of several causes; stops contractions that move material through the intestine.

iliac crest The rim, or wing, of the pelvic bone.

ilium One of three bones that fuse to form the pelvic ring.

impairment Any loss or abnormality of psychological, physiologic, or anatomic structure or function.

implied consent Type of consent in which a patient who is unable to give consent is given treatment under the legal assumption that he or she would want treatment.

incident commander The individual who has overall command of the scene in the field.

incontinent Loss of bowel and bladder control due to a generalized seizure.

infancy The first year of life.

infarcted cells Cells in the brain that die as a result of loss of blood flow to the brain.

infarction Death of a body tissue, usually caused by interruption of its blood supply.

infection The abnormal invasion of a host or host tissues by organisms such as bacteria, viruses, or parasites, with or without signs or symptoms of disease.

infectious disease A disease that is caused by infection.

inferior The part of the body, or any body part, nearer to the feet.

inferior vena cava One of the two largest veins in the body; carries blood from the lower extremities and the pelvic and abdominal organs into the heart.

informed consent Permission for treatment given by a competent patient after the potential risks, benefits, and alternatives to treatment have been explained.

ingestion Swallowing; taking a substance by mouth.

inguinal ligament The tough, fibrous ligament that stretches between the lateral edge of the pubic symphysis and the anterior superior iliac spine.

inhalation The active, muscular part of breathing that draws air into the airway and lungs.

initial assessment The part of the assessment process that helps you to identify any immediately or potentially life-threatening conditions so that you can initiate lifesaving care.

injury A specific damage or wound.

insulators Materials that resist transmission of electricity, heat, or sound.

insulin A hormone produced by the pancreas that enables sugar in the blood to enter the cells of the body; used in synthetic form to treat and control diabetes mellitus.

insulin shock Unconsciousness or altered mental status in a patient with diabetes caused by significant hypoglycemia; usually the result of excessive exercise and activity or failure to eat after a routine dose of insulin.

intentional tort A wrong inflicted by one person against another person (a victim) after thoughtful consideration and directed by a conscious, reasonable mind. The wrong or violation must cause a physical, mental, or emotional injury to the victim, and if these elements are all present, the law gives the victim a remedy, usually in money.

intercostal muscles The muscles between the ribs.

intervention An urgent measure that interrupts assessment in order to care for a condition that threatens life or limb and requires immediate care.

intervertebral disk The cushion that lies between two vertebrae.

inversion Reversal of a normal relationship. The turning or rotation of the foot about its long axis so that the sole points inward.

involuntary Not performed willingly; not subject to control.

involuntary activities The actions that we do not consciously control.

involuntary muscle A muscle whose contractions are not under conscious control.

iris The muscle and surrounding tissue behind the cornea that dilate and constrict the pupil, regulating the amount of light that enters the eye; pigment in this tissue gives the eye its color.

irreversible shock The final stage of shock, resulting in death.

ischemia A lack of oxygen that deprives tissues of necessary nutrients, resulting from partial or complete blockage of blood flow; potentially reversible since permanent injury has not yet occurred.

ischemic cells Cells in the brain that receive enough blood after a cerebrovascular accident to stay alive but not to function properly.

ischemic stroke One of the two main types of stroke; occurs when blood flow to a particular part of the brain is cut off by a blockage (eg, a clot) inside a blood vessel.

ischium One of three bones that fuse to form the pelvic ring.

jams and pretzels Techniques for aligning and extricating a patient found in an awkward position or confined location.

jaundice A yellow skin or sclera color that is caused by liver disease or dysfunction.

jaw-thrust maneuver Technique to open the airway by placing the fingers behind the angle of the jaw and bringing the jaw forward; used when a patient may have a cervical spine injury.

joint (articulation) The place where two bones come into contact.

joint capsule The fibrous sac with synovial lining that encloses a joint.

kidneys Two retroperitoneal organs that excrete the end products of metabolism as urine and regulate the body's salt and water content.

kinetic energy Energy associated with motion.

Kussmaul respirations Deep, rapid breathing; usually the result of an accumulation of certain acids when insulin is not available in the body.

labored breathing Breathing that requires visibly increased effort; characterized by grunting, stridor, and use of accessory muscles.

laceration A smooth or jagged open wound.

lacrimal glands The glands that produce fluids to keep the eye moist; also called tear glands.

large intestine The portion of the digestive tube that encircles the abdomen around the small bowel, consisting of the cecum, the colon, and the rectum.

glossary

laryngospasm A severe constriction of the larynx and vocal cords.

lateral Parts of the body that lie farther from the midline; also called outer structures.

Law of Conservation of Energy In physics, the law that holds that energy can be neither created nor destroyed but may be changed from any form to any other form.

layer A single thickness spread out or covering a surface.

learning disorders A lack of order or impairment with learning skills.

lens The transparent part of the eye through which images are focused on the retina.

leukotrienes Chemical substances that contribute to anaphylaxis; released by the immune system in allergic reactions.

ligament A band of fibrous tissue that connects bones to bones, and supports and strengthens a joint.

limb presentation A delivery in which the presenting part is a single arm, leg, or foot.

liver A large solid organ that lies in the right upper quadrant immediately below the diaphragm; it produces bile, stores sugar for immediate use by the body, and produces many substances that help regulate immune responses.

log roll A technique used to roll a patient 180° (usually from prone to supine) or to the side so that a backboard or blanket can be slipped underneath without bending or twisting the spine.

long-axis drag (axial slide) A technique of moving a patient by sliding him or her in the direction of the long axis of the patient's body.

lumbar spine The lower part of the back, formed by the lowest five nonfused vertebrae; also called the dorsal spine.

lumbar vertebrae Vertebrae of the lumbar spine.

lumen The inside diameter of an artery or other hollow structure.

magnitude Great size, strength, or extent.

mandible The bone of the lower jaw.

manic-depressive A mentally ill person with a cyclic affective psychosis in which there are alternating moods of depression and mania (madness, characterized by excessive excitement).

manubrium The upper quarter of the sternum.

mass-casualty incident (MCI) An emergency situation involving more than one patient, that can place such a great demand on equipment or personnel that the system is stretched to its limit or beyond.

mastoid process The prominent bony mass at the base of the skull about 1" posterior to the external opening of the ear.

maxilla The bone that forms the upper jaw on either side of the face and contains the upper teeth, the orbit of the eye, the nasal cavity, and the palate.

mechanism of injury (MOI) The way in which traumatic injuries occur; the forces that act on the body to cause damage.

medial Parts of the body that lie closer to the midline; also called inner structures.

medial collateral ligament Condensation or thickening of the medial joint capsule of the knee, that provides medial stability to the knee joint; most frequently injured knee ligament in snowsports.

medical control Physicians' instructions that are given directly by radio (online/direct) or indirectly by protocol/guidelines (off-line/indirect), as authorized by the medical director of the service program.

medical director The physician who develops the protocols for a management group or authorizes the OEC technician or EMT to perform emergency medical care in the field.

medical group supervisor The individual named to coordinate the activities of emergency medical personnel.

medicolegal A term relating to medical jurisprudence (law) or forensic medicine.

meninges Three distinct layers of tissue that surround and protect the brain and the spinal cord within the skull and the spinal canal.

mental disorder An illness with psychological or behavioral symptoms and/or impairment in functioning, caused by a social, psychological, genetic, physical, chemical, or biologic disturbance.

mental retardation (MR) A below average intellectual capacity from birth or childhood associated with difficulties in learning and socialization.

metabolism Chemical reactions that provide the body's energy; the process by which energy is made available for the uses of the organism.

midaxillary line An imaginary vertical line drawn through the middle of the axilla (armpit), parallel to the midline.

midclavicular line An imaginary vertical line drawn through the middle portion of the clavicle and parallel to the midline.

midline An imaginary vertical line drawn from the middle of the forehead through the nose and the umbilicus (navel) to the floor.

motion The action or process of change of position.

motor fitness The possession of strength, power, balance, agility, flexibility, and endurance.

motor nerves Nerves that carry information from the central nervous system to the muscles.

mucous membrane The lining of body cavities and passages that are in direct contact with the outside environment.

mucus A watery substance secreted by the mucous membranes that lubricates the body openings.

multigravida A woman who has had previous pregnancies.

multipara A woman who has had more than one live birth.

multiple sclerosis (MS) A neurologic condition that causes weakness or paralysis of the extremities, loss of stamina, and balance difficulties.

muscular dystrophy (MD) Progressive and irreversible muscle wasting.

musculoskeletal system The bones and voluntary muscles of the body.

myocardial contusion A bruise of the heart muscle.

myocardium Heart muscle.

nasal cannula An oxygen delivery device in which oxygen flows through two small, tubelike prongs that fit into the patient's nostrils.

nasopharyngeal (nasal or trumpet) airway Airway adjunct inserted into the nostril of a conscious patient who is not able to maintain a natural airway.

nasopharynx The part of the pharynx that lies above the level of the roof of the mouth, or soft palate.

National Ski Patrol (NSP) A federally chartered education association servicing the snowsports and outdoor recreation communities by providing exceptional education programs.

nature of illness (NOI) Effort to determine the general type of illness.

nausea An unpleasant sensation in the epigastrium that often leads to vomiting.

near drowning Survival, at least temporarily, after suffocation in water.

negligence Lacking in due care or concern.

negligence suit A court action that decides the issue of who should be responsible for damage caused to a person (plaintiff) by someone (defendant) who commits a careless or reckless act. This suit allows the court to determine not only who is at fault, but also the amount of money required to be paid to restore or compensate the plaintiff.

neonatal The first month after birth.

nervous system The system that controls virtually all activities of the body, both voluntary and involuntary.

neurogenic shock Circulatory failure caused by paralysis of the nerves that control the size of the blood vessels, leading to widespread dilation; seen in spinal cord injuries.

Newton's First Law of Motion A body at rest will tend to remain at rest and a body in motion will tend to remain in motion unless acted upon by an outside force.

nondisplaced fracture A simple crack in the bone that has not caused the bone to move from its normal anatomic position; also called a hairline fracture.

nonrebreathing mask A combination mask and reservoir bag system that is the preferred way to give oxygen in the prehospital setting; delivers up to 90% inspired oxygen.

nonrotational fall Occurs when a skier falls forward over the ski tips, which tends to bend the leg over the front edge of the boot.

nuchal cord An umbilical cord that is wrapped around the infant's neck.

occiput The most posterior portion of the skull.

occlusion Blockage, usually of a tubular structure such as a blood vessel.

occlusive dressing Dressing made of Vaseline gauze, aluminum foil, or plastic, that prevents air and liquids from entering or exiting a wound.

Occupational Safety and Health Administration (OSHA) The federal regulatory compliance agency that develops, publishes, and enforces guidelines concerning safety in the workplace.

OEC technician An individual who has training in basic emergency care skills, including using airway adjuncts, assisting patients with medications, splinting, providing emergency care for environmental illnesses and injuries, spinal injuries, and ski and other outdoor injuries, using special equipment, performing techniques used in difficult or prolonged transport, and in some cases, automated external defibrillation.

olecranon process The bony projection of the ulna at the elbow to which the triceps muscle tendon is attached.

ongoing assessment The part of the assessment process in which problems are reevaluated and responses to treatment are assessed.

open abdominal injury An injury of the abdomen caused by a penetrating or piercing instrument or force, in which the skin is lacerated or perforated and the cavity is opened to the atmosphere; also called penetrating injury.

open chest injury Injury to the chest in which the chest wall itself is penetrated by a fractured rib or some external object.

open fracture Any break in a bone in which the overlying skin has been violated.

open head injury Injury to the head in which a penetrating object has caused scalp lacerations, contusions, hematomas, and obvious skull deformities.

open injury An injury in which there is a break in the surface of the skin or the mucous membrane, exposing deeper tissue to potential contamination.

opioids Any drug or agent with actions similar to morphine.

OPQRST The six pain questions: Onset, Provoking factors, Quality, Radiation, Severity, Time.

optic nerve A cranial nerve that transmits visual information to the brain.

orbit The eye socket, made up of the maxilla and zygoma.

organic brain syndrome Temporary or permanent dysfunction of the brain, caused by a disturbance in the physical or physiologic functioning of brain tissue.

oropharyngeal (oral) airway Airway adjunct inserted into the mouth to keep the tongue from blocking the upper airway and to make suctioning the airway easier.

oropharynx A tubular structure that extends vertically from the back of the mouth to the esophagus and trachea.

ostomy bag An appliance that attaches by special adhesive to the abdominal wall of some people who have had abdominal surgery.

Outdoor Emergency Care (OEC) A comprehensive prehospital care education and training program for nonurban settings.

ovary A female gland that produces sex hormones and ova (eggs).

overland wheeled stretcher A stretcher on a wheel assemble used in outdoor conditions; the most commonly used device in outdoor rescue.

palmar The front region of the hand.

palpate Examine by touch.

pancreas A flat, solid organ that lies below and behind the liver and the stomach; it is a major source of digestive enzymes and produces the hormone insulin.

pancreatitis Inflammation of the pancreas.

paradoxical motion The motion of the portion of the chest wall that is detached in a flail chest; the motion—in during inhalation, out during exhalation—is exactly the opposite of normal chest wall motion during breathing.

parietal regions The areas between the temporal and occiput regions of the cranium.

partial airway obstruction Condition in which an obstruction leaves the patient able to exchange some air, but also causes some degree of respiratory distress.

partial pressure The percentage of total pressure accounted for by a specific gas, such as oxygen or carbon dioxide. For example, at sea level the partial pressure of oxygen is 160 mm Hg (21% of the total atmospheric pressure of 760 mm Hg).

partial-thickness (second-degree) burn A burn affecting the epidermis and some portion of the dermis but not the subcutaneous tissue, characterized by blisters and skin that is white to red, moist, and mottled.

patella The kneecap; a specialized bone that lies within the tendon of the quadriceps muscle.

pathogen A microorganism that is capable of causing disease in a susceptible host.

pedal edema Swelling of the feet and ankles caused by collection of fluid in the tissues; a possible sign of congestive heart failure (CHF).

pediatrics A specialized medical practice devoted to the care of the young.

pelvic cavity The cavity in the lowest part of the trunk. Continuous with the abdominal cavity, it contains the bladder, rectum, and female reproductive organs.

glossary

pelvis A cone-shaped bony ring made up of the right and left pelvic bones joined in front at the pubis and in back to the sacrum at the sacroiliac joints. Each pelvic bone is made up of three fused bones: the ilium, ischium, and pubic bones. The pelvis contains the pelvic cavity.

penetrating wound An injury resulting from a sharp, pointed object.

penetration trauma Trauma caused by a sharp object moving at a moderate to high speed that penetrates the skin, or by a moving body striking a narrow, pointed object.

perfusion The circulation of blood within an organ or tissue in adequate amounts to meet the cells' current needs.

pericardial tamponade Compression of the heart due to a buildup of blood or other fluid in the pericardial sac.

pericardium The fibrous sac that surrounds the heart.

perineum The area of skin between the vagina and the anus.

peripheral nervous system The part of the nervous system that consists of 31 pairs of spinal nerves and 12 pairs of cranial nerves. These peripheral nerves may be sensory nerves, motor nerves, or connecting nerves.

peristalsis The wave-like contraction of smooth muscle by which the ureters or other tubular organs propel their contents.

peritoneal cavity The abdominal cavity.

peritoneum The membrane lining the abdominal cavity (parietal peritoneum) and covering the abdominal organs (visceral peritoneum).

peritonitis Inflammation of the peritoneum.

phantom foot syndrome A mechanism responsible for anterior cruciate ligament injury when the tail of the ski acts as a lever pointing in a direction opposite to that of the foot. Occurs when the thigh rotates internally when the knee is hyperflexed, as when novices try to stop by sitting down.

pin-indexing system A system established for portable cylinders to ensure that a regulator is not connected to a cylinder containing the wrong type of gas.

pinna The external, visible part of the ear.

placenta Tissue attached to the uterine wall that nourishes the fetus through the umbilical cord.

placenta abruptio Premature separation of the placenta from the wall of the uterus.

placenta previa A condition in which the placenta develops over and covers the cervix.

plaintiff The party that institutes a suit in a court.

plantar The bottom of the foot.

plasma A sticky, yellow fluid that carries the blood cells and nutrients and transports cellular waste material to the organs of excretion.

platelets Tiny, disk-shaped elements that are much smaller than the cells; they are essential in the initial formation of a blood clot.

pleura The serous membrane covering the lungs and lining the thoracic cavity, completely enclosing a potential space known as the pleural space.

pleural effusion A collection of fluid between the lung and chest wall that may compress the lung.

pleural space The potential space between the parietal pleura and the visceral pleura. It is described as "potential" because under normal conditions, the lungs fill this space.

pleuritic chest pain Sharp, stabbing pain in the chest that is worsened by a deep breath or other chest wall movement; often caused by inflammation or irritation of the pleura.

pneumatic antishock garment (PASG) An inflatable device that covers the legs and abdomen; used to splint the lower extremities or pelvis, or to control bleeding in the lower extremities, pelvis, or abdominal cavity.

pneumonia An infectious disease of the lung that damages lung tissue.

pneumothorax A partial or complete accumulation of air in the pleural space.

point tenderness Tenderness that is sharply localized at the site of the injury, found by gently palpating along the bone with the tip of one finger.

poison A substance whose chemical action could damage structures or impair function when introduced into the body.

polydipsia Excessive thirst persisting for long periods of time despite reasonable fluid intake; often the result of excessive urination.

polyphagia Excessive eating; in diabetes, the inability to use glucose properly can cause a sense of hunger.

polyuria The passage of an unusually large volume of urine in a given period; in diabetes, this can result from wasting of glucose in the urine.

poor air exchange A term used to distinguish the degree of distress in a patient with a partial airway obstruction. With poor air exchange, the patient has a weak, ineffective cough, increased difficulty breathing, possible cyanosis, and may produce a high-pitched noise on inhalation (stridor).

portable stretcher A stretcher with a strong, rectangular tubular metal frame and fabric stretched across it.

position of function A hand position in which the wrist is slightly dorsi-flexed and all finger joints are moderately flexed.

posterior The back surface of the body; the side away from you in the standard anatomic position.

posterior tibial artery The artery just posterior to the medial malleolus; it supplies blood to the foot.

postictal state Period following a seizure that lasts between 5 and 30 minutes, characterized by labored respirations and some degree of altered mental status. Also called **postictal period**.

postpolio syndrome After-effects of poliomyelitis, a viral infection of the spinal cord which may cause either broadly distributed or local paralysis. Years after the initial paralysis, the person may exhibit fatigue, shortness of breath, and balance problems.

posttraumatic stress disorder (PTSD) A delayed stress reaction to a prior incident. This delayed reaction is the result of one or more unresolved issues concerning the incident that might have been alleviated with the use of critical incident stress management.

potential energy The position of a body in a gravity field with respect to its own parts or another body.

power grip A technique in which the litter or backboard is gripped by inserting each hand under the handle with the palm facing up and the thumb extended, fully supporting the underside of the handle on the curved palm with the fingers and thumb.

power lift A lifting technique in which the rescuer's back is held upright, with legs bent, and the patient is lifted when the rescuer straightens the legs to raise the upper body and arms.

pregnancy-induced hypertension A condition of late pregnancy that also involves headache, visual changes, and swelling of the hands and feet; also called preeclampsia.

preschool-age Children between 3 to 6 years of age.

presentation The position in which an infant is born; the part of the infant that appears first.

pressure point A point where a blood vessel lies near a bone; useful when direct pressure and elevation do not control bleeding.

priapism A continuous and painful erection of the penis caused by certain spinal injuries and some diseases.

primary triage The initial triage performed on the scene of a mass-casualty incident.

primigravida A woman who is experiencing her first pregnancy.

primipara A woman who has had one live birth.

prolapse of the umbilical cord A situation in which the umbilical cord comes out of the vagina before the infant.

prone position The position in which the body is lying face down.

prostate gland A small gland that surrounds the male urethra where it emerges from the urinary bladder; it secretes a fluid that is part of the ejaculatory fluid.

proximal Structures that are closer to the trunk.

psychogenic A symptom or illness that is caused by mental or emotional factors as opposed to physical ones.

psychogenic shock Shock caused by a sudden, temporary reduction in blood supply to the brain that causes fainting (syncope).

psychosis Any severe mental disorder characterized by deterioration of normal intellectual and social functioning and by partial or complete withdrawal from reality.

pubic symphysis A hard bony prominence that is found in the midline in the lowermost portion of the abdomen.

pubis One of three bones that fuse to form the pelvic ring.

public accommodation A legally recognized business, organization, group, or other legal entity that affords a service, trade, or work to the general public, or may be controlled by the federal government because of its connection with interstate commerce or trade.

pulmonary artery The major artery leading from the right ventricle of the heart to the lungs; it carries oxygen-poor blood.

pulmonary circulation The closed circuit of the circulatory system that includes the lungs. Blood is pumped from the right side of the heart through the lungs and back to the left side of the heart.

pulmonary contusion A bruise of the lung.

pulmonary edema A buildup of fluid in the lungs, usually as a result of congestive heart failure, also from high altitude.

pulmonary embolism A blood clot that breaks off from a large vein and travels to the blood vessels of the lung, causing obstruction of blood flow.

pulmonary veins The four veins that return oxygenated blood from the lungs to the left atrium of the heart.

pulse The wave of pressure created as the heart contracts and forces blood out the left ventricle and into the major arteries.

pulse oximetry An assessment method that measures oxygen saturation of hemoglobin in the capillary beds.

pupil The circular opening in the middle of the iris that admits light to the back of the eye.

putrefaction Decomposition of body tissues.

quadrants The way to describe the sections of the abdominal cavity. Imagine two lines intersecting at the umbilicus dividing the abdomen into four equal areas.

quality control Ensuring that the appropriate emergency care standards of training are met by OEC technicians on each call; this is the responsibility of the medical director.

rabid Describes an animal that is infected with rabies.

raccoon eyes Bruising under the eyes that may indicate skull fracture.

radial artery The major artery in the forearm; it is palpable at the wrist on the thumb side.

radiation A continuation of an area of pain or discomfort; gives the sensation that the pain is moving (radiating) away from the origin.

radius The bone on the thumb side of the forearm; most important in wrist function.

rales A crackling breath sound caused by the flow of air through liquid in the lungs; a sign of lower airway obstruction.

rapid body survey A quick, hands-on, clothes-on examination of the entire body during the initial assessment; designed to be performed on site before reaching shelter.

rapid history and physical exam A part of the assessment process for an unresponsive or a responsive trauma patient with a significant mechanism of injury with a goal of evacuating the patient to definitive care as quickly as possible.

Raynaud's syndrome A disease of the hands and feet, characterized by intermittent spasm of the small arteries of the fingers and toes caused by exposure to cold.

recovery position The preferred body position for an unconscious patient with no suspected spine injury. The patient lies on his or her side with the opposite knee flexed and the head cushioned on the hand. Also called the semiprone, rescue, stable side, or NATO position.

rectum The lowermost end of the colon.

red blood cells Cells that carry oxygen to the body's tissues; also called erythrocytes.

reduce To return a dislocated joint or fractured bone to its normal position; set.

referred pain Pain felt in an area of the body other than the area where the cause of pain is located.

refresher An annual continuing education program designed by the NSP and required for its members to review one third of the entire OEC curriculum.

rehabilitation area The area that provides protection and treatment to firefighters and other personnel working at an emergency. Here, workers are medically monitored and receive any needed care as they enter and leave the scene.

renal pelvis A cone-shaped collecting area that connects the ureter and the kidney.

respiration A general term for the process of exchanging oxygen and carbon dioxide between the atmosphere and the body cells. Frequently used as a synonym for breathing.

respiratory system All the structures of the body that contribute to the process of breathing, consisting of the upper and lower airways and their component parts.

responsiveness The way in which a patient responds to external stimuli, including verbal stimuli (sound), tactile stimuli (touch), and painful stimuli.

retina The light-sensitive area of the eye where images are projected; a layer of cells at the back of the eye that changes the light image into electrical impulses, which are carried by the optic nerve to the brain.

retinal detachment Separation of the retina from its attachments at the back of the eye.

retractions Movements in which the skin pulls in around the ribs during inspiration.

retrograde amnesia The inability to remember events leading up to a brain injury.

retroperitoneal Behind the abdominal cavity.

rewarm To raise the body temperature of a patient with hypothermia, or to raise the temperature of a part affected with frostbite.

rhonchi Coarse breath sounds heard in patients with chronic mucus in the airways.

rib One of 12 paired, curved bones that form and support the chest wall.

rigor mortis Stiffening of the body, is a definitive sign of death.

rotational fall A fall that causes the foot to turn outward, forcing the leg outward at the knee.

rotational trauma Trauma caused by a twisting force.

Rule of Nines A system that assigns percentages to sections of the body, allowing calculation of the amount of skin surface involved in the burn area.

sacrum One of three bones (sacrum and two pelvic bones) that make up the pelvic ring; consists of five fused sacral vertebrae.

safety officer The individual responsible for protecting mass-casualty incident response personnel and victims from unseen hazards or dangers.

salivary glands The glands that produce saliva to keep the mouth and pharynx moist.

SAMPLE history A key brief history of a patient's condition to determine Signs/Symptoms, Allergies, Medications, Pertinent past history, Last oral intake, and Events leading to the illness/injury.

scalp The thick skin covering the cranium, which usually bears hair.

scaphoid A proximal boat-shaped bone of the carpus (bones of the wrist joint) on the radial side.

scapula The shoulder blade.

scene size-up A quick assessment of the scene and the surroundings made to provide information about its safety and the mechanism of injury or nature of illness, before you enter and begin patient care.

schizophrenia A group of mental disorders characterized by disturbances of thinking, mood, and behavior. With schizophrenia, there is an altered concept of reality and in some cases delusions and hallucinations. Mood changes include inappropriate emotional responses and loss of empathy. Withdrawn, regressive, and bizarre behavior may be noted.

school-age Children between 6 and 12 years of age.

sciatic nerve The major nerve in the lower extremity; controls much of muscle function in the leg and sensation in the entire leg and foot.

sclera The tough, fibrous white portion of the eye that protects the more delicate inner structures.

scoop stretcher A stretcher that is designed to be split into two or four sections that can be fitted around a patient who is lying on the ground or other relatively flat surface; also called a split litter.

scuba A system that delivers air to the mouth and lungs at various atmospheric pressures, increasing with the depth of the dive; stands for **self-contained underwater breathing apparatus**.

sebaceous glands Glands in the dermis that produce an oily substance called sebum, which discharges along the shafts of the hairs.

secondary triage An in-depth reassessment of a patient's condition that allows for a change in triage category.

sector commander The individual delegated to oversee and coordinate activity in an incident command sector; works under the incident commander.

sedative A substance that decreases activity and excitement.

seizure Generalized, uncoordinated muscular activity associated with loss of responsiveness; a convulsion.

Sellick maneuver A technique that is used to prevent gastric distention in which pressure is applied on the cricoid cartilage.

semen Seminal fluid ejaculated from the penis and containing sperm.

seminal vesicles Storage sacs for sperm and seminal fluid, which empty into the urethra at the prostate.

sensitization Developing a sensitivity to a substance that initially caused no allergic reaction.

sensory nerves Nerves that transmit sensory input, such as touch, taste, heat, cold, and pain, from the body to the central nervous system.

septic shock Shock caused by severe bacterial infection.

shaken baby syndrome Bleeding within the head and damage to the cervical spine of an infant who has been intentionally and forcibly shaken; a form of child abuse.

shell The skin, muscles, and extremities of the body.

shock A condition that develops when the circulatory system is not able to deliver sufficient blood to body organs, resulting in organ failure and eventual death if untreated.

shock position The position that has the head and torso (trunk) supine and the lower extremities elevated 6" to 12". This helps to increase blood flow to the brain; also referred to as the *modified Trendelenburg's position*.

shoulder girdle The proximal portion of the upper extremity, made up of the clavicle, the scapula, and the humerus.

shoulder separation Usually caused by a direct blow or hard fall onto the shoulder that forces the acromion part of the scapula forward and tears the ligaments that attach it to the clavicle.

sign An objective finding that can be seen, heard, felt, smelled, or measured.

skeletal muscle Striated muscles that are attached to bones and usually cross at least one joint.

skeleton The framework that gives us our recognizable human form; also designed to allow motion of the body and protection of vital organs.

skier's thumb A sprain or fracture of the structures at the base of the thumb that occurs when the thumb is bent backward during a fall.

skier's toe Characterized by pain in the big toe caused by repeated dorsiflexion.

skin The outer covering of the body, made up of the outer epidermis and the inner dermis.

small intestine The portion of the digestive tube between the stomach and the cecum, consisting of the duodenum, jejunum, and ileum.

smooth muscle A muscle that is not under voluntary control, found in the respiratory, circulatory, digestive, urinary, and reproductive systems. Smooth muscles help carry out much of the body's automatic internal work. They are called "smooth" because they lack the striations found in skeletal muscle.

sniffing position An upright position in which the patient's head and chin are thrust slightly forward and the patient appears to be sniffing; most commonly seen in children.

snowblindness Sunburn of the conjunctiva of the eye.

snowboarder's ankle Fracture of the talus (the support structure for both the tibia and fibula).

solid organs Solid masses of tissue where much of the chemical work of the body takes place (eg, the liver, spleen, pancreas, and kidneys).

somatic (voluntary) nervous system The part of the nervous system that regulates our voluntary activities, such as walking, talking, and writing.

spastic cerebral palsy A condition in which there is constant, involuntarily contraction of an individual's muscles.

sphincters Circular muscles that encircle and, by contracting, constrict a duct, tube, or opening.

spina bifida (SB) A congenital malformation of the spinal column (usually the bony spine in the same area) in which segments of the spine fail to fuse, allowing the spinal cord to protrude.

spinal canal The tunnel in which the spinal cord lies; formed by the successive vertebral arches.

spinal column The bony column, composed of 33 vertebrae, that forms the main support for the body and protects the spinal cord.

spinal cord An extension of the brain, composed of virtually all the nerves carrying messages between the brain and the rest of the body. It lies inside of, and is protected by, the spinal canal.

spinal cord injury (SCI) Damage to the spinal cord resulting from trauma.

splint A flexible or rigid appliance used to protect and maintain the position of an injured extremity.

spontaneous pneumothorax Pneumothorax that occurs when a weak area on the lung ruptures in the absence of major injury, allowing air to leak into the pleural space.

spontaneous respirations Breathing in a patient that occurs with no assistance.

sprain A joint injury involving damage to supporting ligaments, and partial or complete temporary dislocation of bone ends.

stable A patient whose vital signs and mental status are normal and unchanging, and there is no significant MOI or NOI.

staging area manager The individual responsible for ensuring that resources are available, positioned, deployed, and properly allocated.

stair chair A lightweight folding device that is used to carry a conscious, seated patient up or down stairs.

standard of care What the specific area has chosen to use as its methods of providing the care to the ill and injured patients.

standard of training The tools to facilitate training OEC technicians to operate in a variety of situations, using an assortment of equipment.

START Simple Triage And Rapid Treatment system of initial (primary) triage.

status epilepticus The term used to describe a continuous seizure, or multiple seizures without a return to consciousness, for 30 minutes or more.

sternocleidomastoid muscles The muscles on either side of the neck that allow movement of the head.

sternum The breastbone.

stimulant An agent that produces an excited state.

stoma Opening in the neck that connects the trachea directly to the skin; also a port created on the abdominal wall to facilitate excrement.

stomach The saclike organ between the esophagus and the duodenum where food is mixed with gastric juice to form a semifluid substance that is passed on to the intestines for further digestion.

strain Stretching or tearing of a muscle; also called a muscle pull.

strangulation Complete obstruction of blood circulation in a given organ as a result of compression or entrapment, an emergency situation causing death of tissue.

striated muscle Muscle that has characteristic stripes, or striations, under the microscope; voluntary, or skeletal, muscle.

stridor A harsh, high-pitched inspiratory sound that is often heard in acute laryngeal (upper airway) obstruction; may sound like crowing and be audible without a stethoscope.

stroke A loss of brain function in certain brain cells that do not get enough oxygen. Usually caused by obstruction of the blood vessels in the brain that feed oxygen to those brain cells.

stroke and brain trauma A condition that results when part of the brain becomes anoxic from loss of blood supply.

styloid process A long, pointed process of a bone.

subcutaneous emphysema The presence of air in soft tissue; palpation produces a characteristic crackling sensation.

subcutaneous tissue Tissue, largely fat, that lies directly under the dermis and serves as an insulator of the body.

substance abuse The knowing misuse of any substance to produce some desired effect.

sucking chest wound An open or penetrating chest wall wound through which air passes during inspiration and expiration, creating a sucking sound.

sun protection factor (SPF) A number that refers to how much longer skin protected by a sunscreen can be exposed to the sun before becoming red (compared to unprotected skin).

sunburn A superficial or partial-thickness burn caused by ultraviolet light in the medium-wave range (UVB) with a wavelength of 290 to 320 nanometers.

superficial Closer to or on the skin.

superficial (first-degree) burn A burn affecting only the epidermis, characterized by skin that is red but not blistered or actually burned through.

superior The part of the body, or any body part, nearer to the head.

superior vena cava One of the two largest veins in the body; carries blood from the upper extremities, head, neck, and chest into the heart.

supine Lying face up.

supine hypotensive syndrome A drop in blood pressure caused when the heavy uterus of a supine, third-trimester pregnant patient obstructs the vena cava, lowering blood return to the heart.

glossary

supine position The position in which the body is lying face up.

sweat glands The glands within the dermis that secrete sweat.

symphysis The joint that is held together with fibrous tissue allowing slight, limited motion.

symptom A subjective finding that the patient feels but that can be identified only by the patient.

syncope Fainting.

systole The contraction, or period of contraction, of the heart, especially that of the ventricles.

systolic blood pressure The highest point of the blood pressure curve.

systolic pressure The increased pressure along an artery with each contraction (systole) of the ventricle.

tachycardia Rapid heart rhythm, more than 100 beats/min.

tachypnea Rapid respirations.

talus A bone of the foot that forms the distal portion of the ankle joint and supports the tibia and fibula.

technical rescue team A team of individuals trained for special or hazardous rescue situations.

temporal regions The lateral portions on each side of the cranium.

temporomandibular joint (TMJ) The joint formed where the mandible and cranium meet, just in front of the ear.

tendon A tough, ropelike cord of fibrous tissue that attaches a skeletal muscle to a bone.

tension pneumothorax An expanding collection of air outside the lung that places pressure on the heart and blood vessels.

terminal velocity A final speed of fall reached when the air resistance equals the pull of gravity.

testicle A male genital gland that contains specialized cells that produce hormones and sperm.

thoracic cage The chest or rib cage.

thoracic spine The 12 vertebrae that lie between the cervical vertebrae and the lumbar vertebrae. One pair of ribs is attached to each of the thoracic vertebrae.

thorax The chest cavity that contains the heart, lungs, esophagus, and great vessels (the aorta and the two venae cavae).

thrombosis Clotting of the cerebral arteries that may result in the interruption of cerebral blood flow and subsequent stroke.

thyroid cartilage A firm prominence of cartilage that forms the upper part of the larynx; the Adam's apple.

tibia The larger of the two lower leg bones responsible for supporting the major weight-bearing surface of the knee and the ankle; the shinbone.

tidal volume The amount of air that is exchanged with each breath.

toboggan A rescue sled found on most ski slopes. Construction and features vary to accommodate a variety of terrain and snow conditions. Comes with two or four handles. Rescuer steers the toboggan from within or outside the front handles. On steep or difficult terrain a second rescuer uses a tail rope or the second set of handles for better stability in the rear.

toddler The period following infancy until 3 years of age.

tolerance The need for increasing amounts of a drug to obtain the same effect.

tonic-clonic seizure A seizure that features rhythmic back-and-forth motion of an extremity and body stiffness.

tonsil tip A large, semirigid suction tip recommended for suctioning the pharynx; also called a Yankauer tip.

topographic anatomy The superficial landmarks of the body that serve as guides to the structures that lie beneath them.

torso The trunk without the head and limbs.

tourniquet The bleeding control method of last resort that occludes arterial flow; used only when all other methods have failed and the patient's life is in danger.

toxin A poison or harmful substance.

trachea The windpipe; the main trunk for air passing to and from the lungs.

traction The act of exerting a pulling force on a structure.

tragus The small, rounded, fleshy bulge that lies immediately anterior to the ear canal.

transient ischemic attack (TIA) A disorder of the brain in which brain cells temporarily stop working because of insufficient oxygen, causing stroke-like symptoms that resolve completely within 24 hours of onset.

transportation area The area in a mass-casualty incident where ambulances and crews are organized to transport patients from the treatment area to receiving hospitals.

transportation officer The individual in charge of the transportation sector in a mass-casualty incident, who assigns patients from the treatment area to waiting ambulances in the transportation area.

trauma The effect of a force applied to the body; often used interchangeably with injury; a physical or psychological wound or injury.

treatment area Location in a mass-casualty incident where patients are brought after being triaged and assigned a priority, where they are reassessed, treated, and monitored until transport to the hospital.

treatment officer The individual, usually a physician, who is in charge of and directs EMS personnel at the treatment area in a mass-casualty incident.

Trendelenburg's position The position in which the body is supine with the head lower than the feet.

triage The process of sorting patients based on the severity of injury and medical need, to establish treatment and transportation priorities.

triage area Designated area in a mass-casualty incident where the triage officer is located and patients are initially triaged before being taken to the treatment center.

triage officer The individual in charge of the incident command triage area, who directs the sorting of patients into triage categories in a mass-casualty incident.

triage tag A tag attached to a patient in a mass-casualty incident that indicates the person's triage category and specific injuries or vital signs. The triage tag is typically used once patients undergo secondary triage at a treatment area.

triceps The largest muscle that covers the back of the humerus.

tripod position An upright position where the patient leans forward onto outstretched arms and thrusts the head and chin slightly forward to keep the airway open.

turbinates Layers of bone within the nasal cavity.

tympanic membrane The eardrum, which lies between the external and middle ear.

type I diabetes The type of diabetic disease that usually starts in childhood and requires insulin for proper treatment and control.

type II diabetes The type of diabetic disease that usually starts in later life and often can be controlled through diet and oral medications.

ulna The bone on the small finger side of the forearm.

ulnar artery One of the major arteries of the forearm; it can be palpated at the wrist on the ulnar side (at the base of the fifth finger).

umbilical cord The conduit connecting mother to infant via the placenta; contains two arteries and one vein.

unified command Incident command process shared by the various agency area commanders (fire, rescue, EMS, law enforcement).

universal precautions Protective measures that have traditionally been developed by the Centers for Disease Control and Prevention (CDC) for use in dealing with objects, blood, body fluids, or other potential exposure risks of communicable disease.

unresponsive A patient who is less than alert, ie, less than A on the AVPU scale.

unstable A patient whose vital signs or mental status are abnormal or changing, or in whom there is a significant MOI or NOI.

ureter A small, hollow tube that carries urine from the kidneys to the bladder.

urethra The canal that conveys urine from the bladder to outside the body.

urinary bladder A sac behind the pubic symphysis made of smooth muscle that collects and stores urine.

urinary system The organs that control the discharge of certain waste materials filtered from the blood and excreted as urine.

urticaria Small spots of generalized itching and/or burning that appear as multiple raised areas on the skin; hives.

uterus The muscular organ where the fetus grows, also called the womb; responsible for contractions during labor.

vagina A muscular distensible tube that connects the uterus with the vulva (the external female genitalia); also called the birth canal.

vasa deferentia (vas deferens) The spermatic duct of the testicles.

veins Tubular vessels that carry blood from the tissues back to the heart.

velocity Speed. The magnitude of velocity is the body's speed, and the direction of velocity is the body's direction of motion.

ventilation Exchange of air between the lungs and the air of the environment, either spontaneously by the patient or with assistance from a rescuer.

ventral The anterior surface of the body.

ventricle One of two (right and left) lower chambers of the heart. The left ventricle receives blood from the left atrium (upper chamber) and delivers blood to the aorta. The right ventricle receives blood from the right atrium and pumps it into the pulmonary artery.

ventricular fibrillation Disorganized, ineffective twitching of the ventricles, resulting in no blood flow and a state of cardiac arrest.

ventricular tachycardia Rapid heart rhythm in which the electrical impulse begins in the ventricle (instead of the atrium), which may result in inadequate blood flow and eventually deteriorate into cardiac arrest.

vertebrae The 33 bones that make up the spinal column.

visual impairment Disability involving reduction or loss of vision, usually described in terms of acuity or range. Classifications include legal blindness, partial sightedness, or total blindness.

vital signs The key signs that are used to evaluate the patient's overall condition, including respirations, pulse, blood pressure, level of consciousness, and skin characteristics.

voluntary Spontaneous, arising from one's own free will

voluntary activity Actions that we consciously perform, in which sensory input determines the specific muscular activity.

voluntary muscle Muscle that is under direct voluntary control of the brain and can be contracted or relaxed at will; skeletal, or striated, muscle.

vomit The verb form refers to ejection of stomach contents through the mouth due to the contraction of the muscles of the stomach.

vomitus Vomited material.

weapons of mass destruction Biological, chemical, and nuclear warfare mediums used for mass destruction, more prevalent in wartime and more closely associated with the military.

wheal A raised, swollen, well-defined area on the skin resulting from an insect bite or allergic reaction.

wheeze A high-pitched, whistling breath sound, characteristically heard on expiration in patients with asthma or COPD.

wheezing A whistling breath sound caused by air traveling through narrowed air passages within the bronchioles; a sign of lower airway obstruction.

white blood cells Blood cells that play a role in the body's immune defense mechanisms against infection; also called leukocytes.

windburn Irritation of the skin caused by exposure to wind; resembles superficial sunburn.

Winter Emergency Care (WEC) The original name of the OEC course. Also used to identify the core curriculum that targets the winter environment.

xiphoid process The narrow, cartilaginous lower tip of the sternum.

zygomas The quadrangular bones of the cheek, articulating with the frontal bone, the maxillae, the zygomatic processes of the temporal bone, and the great wings of the sphenoid bone.

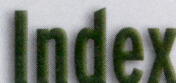

Index

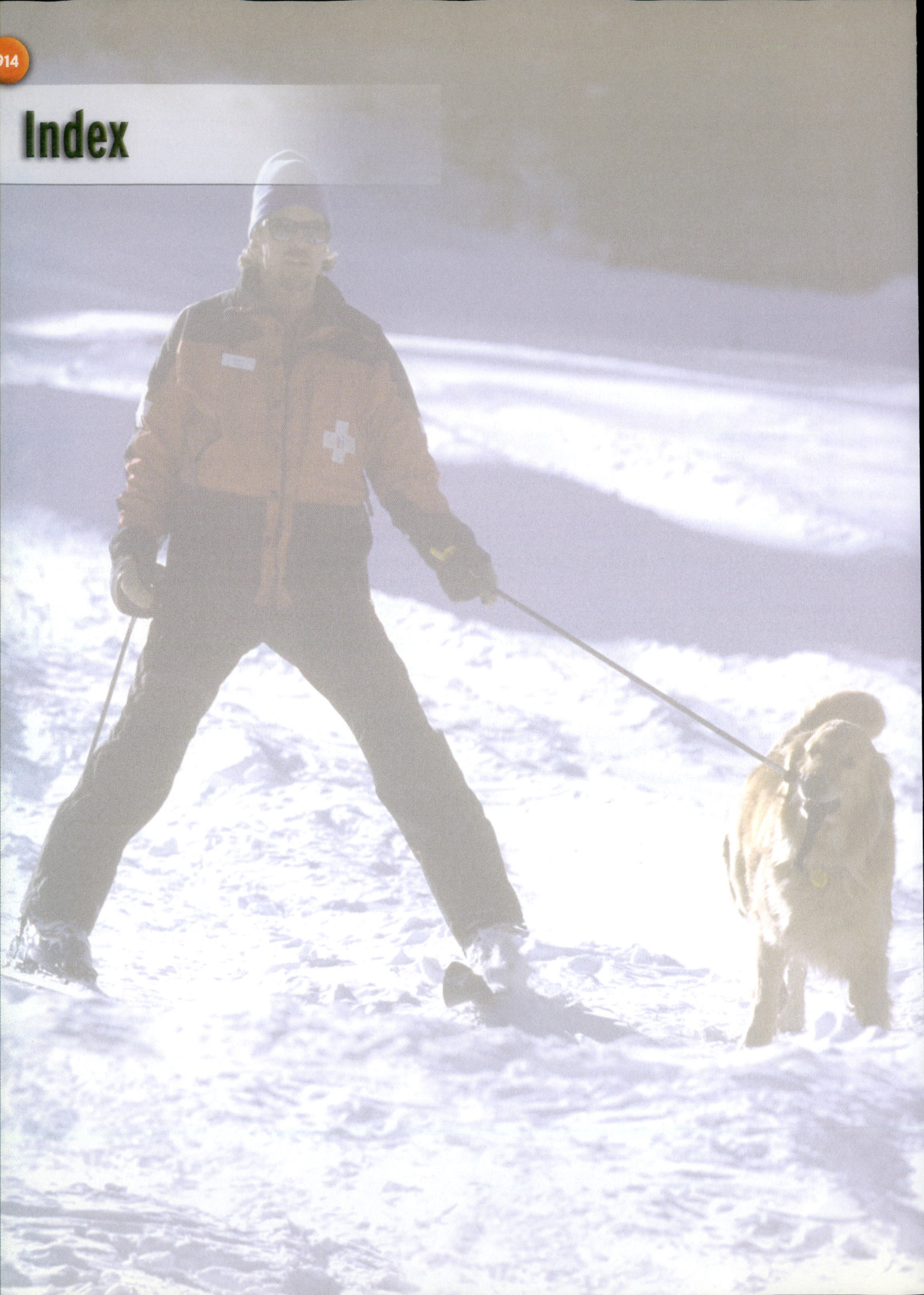

index

index

Additional Credits

Cover

Upper Left © 1993 Photodisc

Upper Right Annabel Spencer/Scott Markewitz Photography

Lower Left Mark Doolittle, International Mountain Bike Association

Lower Right © 1999 Eyewire

Section 1

Opener © 2001 Brian Robb

Chapter 1
1-1 Charles S. Shimanski, The American Alpine Club
1-2 Mark Doolittle, International Mountain Bike Association
1-4 David Johe, MD

Chapter 2
Opener Mark Doolittle, International Mountain Bike Association
2-2 Reproduced with permission from Pugh, L.G.C.E., *Journal of Physiology,* 1957, London, 135: 590-610
2-3 Reproduced with permission from Houston, C.S., *Going Higher,* Little Brown, 80, 1987
2-14 Courtesy of the US Dept. of Agriculture and the US Dept. of Health and Human Services
2-16 (lt.) Rick Heltebrake, Snow Summit Mountain Resort
2-18 © George Kochaniec/CORBIS/Sygma

Chapter 3
3-1 © Richard Shock/Stone
3-2 © Michael Heller/911 Pictures
3-7 © Matthew McVay, Tony Stone Worldwide

Chapter 5
5-8 © L.I. Inc./Custom Medical Stock Photo

Section 2

Opener © 1999 Eyewire

Chapter 6
6-37 © Eddie Sperling

Section 3

Opener © 1993 Photodisc

Chapter 7
7-11 John Dobson, MD

Section 4

Opener © 1993 Photodisc

Chapter 11
11-16 Adapted from *CPR for Family and Friends,* © 2000, American Heart Association

Chapter 13
13-13 © Andrea Randolph
13-23 © Brad Robertson, MD
13-25a © Charles Seaborn/Stone
13-25b © Doug Perrine/Innerspace Visions
13-25c © Kevin McDonnell/Photo

Chapter 14
14-11 Salomon North America
14-15 Dana Jordan, Cascade Toboggan

Chapter 15
Opener Bud Frantz, Class VI River Runners;
15-20 Charles S. Shimanski, The American Alpine Club

Chapter 16
Opener © Steve Cole/Photodisc

Chapter 17
Opener © Eyewire
17-10 Courtesy of David J. Burchfield, MD
17-11 From *Mayo Clinic Complete Book of Pregnancy and Baby's First Year.* © 1994 Mayo Foundation for Medical Education and Research, Rochester, MN. Reprinted with permission.
17-12 From *Mayo Clinic Complete Book of Pregnancy and Baby's First Year.* © 1994 Mayo Foundation for Medical Education and Research, Rochester, MN. Reprinted with permission.
17-13 From *Mayo Clinic Complete Book of Pregnancy and Baby's First Year.* © 1994 Mayo Foundation for Medical Education and Research, Rochester, MN. Reprinted with permission.

Section 5

Opener © 1999 Eyewire

Chapter 19
19-6 © English/Custom Medical Stock Photo

Chapter 21
Opener St. Anthony's Central Hospital, Trauma Services

Chapter 23
23-6 Courtesy of John Dobson, MD

Chapter 24
24-4A, 24-6, 24-9, 24-10, 24-11, 24-14, 24-16, 24-19 Courtesy of John Dobson, MD
24-33 Harley Schwarz

Chapter 25
25-1, 25-5, 25-8, 25-9, 25-12, 25-16, 25-17, 25-20, 25-21, 25-22, 25-25, 25-26, 25-32, 25-34, 25-38, 25-40, 25-41, 25-43, 25-44, 25-48, 25-49, 25-50, 25-54, 25-56, 25-58, 25-59 Courtesy of John Dobson, MD
25-53 © Science Photo Library/Photo Researchers

Section 6

Opener © 1993 Photodisc

Chapter 27
27-26, 27-27 Dana Jordan, Cascade Toboggan

Chapter 28
Opener Doug Stewart, Colorado Mountain College
28-1 Brad Odekirk, *Summit Daily News*

Chapter 29
Opener Doug Stewart, Colorado Mountain College
29-1 Brad Odekirk, *Summit Daily News*

Section 7

Opener © 1999 Eyewire

Chapter 30
Opener © Scott T. Baxter/Getty Images
30-28 Courtesy of Marianne Gausche-Hill, MD

Chapter 31
31-2 John Carr, Special Olympics Colorado
31-4 Seth Roberts, National Sports Center for the Disabled

Appendix A

Opener © 2001 Brian Robb

Appendix B

Opener Charles S. Shimanski, The American Alpine Club

Appendix C

Opener © 2001 Brian Robb

Appendix D

Opener Bud Frantz, Class VI River Runners

Glossary

Opener © 2001 Brian Robb

Index

Opener © 2001 Brian Robb

Unless otherwise indicated, photographs have been supplied by Brian Robb, London Schertzer, Ingrid Tistaert, the National Ski Patrol, the American Academy of Orthopaedic Surgeons, Maryland Institute of Emergency Medical Services System, PhotoDisc, and Jones and Bartlett Publishers. Illustrations are by Reata Bitter, Bitter-Sweet Studios; Rolin Graphics; Imagineering; and Graphic World.

additional credits